# THE
# 5-Minute Veterinary Consult Ferret and Rabbit

# THE
# 5-MINUTE
# VETERINARY
# CONSULT

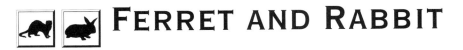

# FERRET AND RABBIT

*Barbara L. Oglesbee, DVM, DABVP*
*Westminster Veterinary Group*
*Westminster, California*
*Clinical Associate Professor,*
*College of Veterinary Medicine*
*Ohio State University*
*Columbus, Ohio*

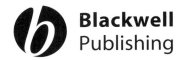
**Blackwell**
Publishing

© 2006 Blackwell Publishing
All rights reserved

Blackwell Publishing Professional
2121 State Avenue, Ames, Iowa 50014, USA

Orders:      1-800-862-6657
Office:      1-515-292-0140
Fax:         1-515-292-3348
Web site:    www.blackwellprofessional.com

Blackwell Publishing Ltd
9600 Garsington Road, Oxford OX4 2DQ, UK
Tel.: +44 (0)1865 776868

Blackwell Publishing Asia
550 Swanston Street, Carlton, Victoria 3053, Australia
Tel.: +61 (0) 3 8359 1011

First edition, 2006

**Library of Congress Cataloging-in-Publication Data**

Oglesbee, Barbara L.
  The 5-minute veterinary consult : ferret and rabbit / Barbara L. Oglesbee.
    p. cm.
  Includes bibliographic references and index.
  ISBN-13: 978-0-7817-9399-5 (alk. paper)
  ISBN-10: 0-7817-9399-8 (alk. paper)
  1. Ferret—Diseases—Handbooks, manuals, etc. 2. Rabbits—Diseases—Handbooks,
manuals, etc. 3. Veterinary Medicine Diseases—Handbooks, manuals, etc. I. Title.

  SPF997.5.F47O35 2007
  636.976'628—dc22

The last digit is the print number: 9 8 7 6 5 4 3 2

I dedicate this book with love to my children, Alexandra and Ian, the center of my world, for their patience and support, and for the sacrifice required to give Mom time to write.

# PREFACE

The popularity of rabbits and ferrets as companion animals has increased exponentially in recent years. With this increase, veterinarians in general small animal practice, emergency clinics, and even canine and feline specialty practice are often faced with the difficult challenge of evaluating these often unfamiliar species. Although excellent, in-depth textbooks exist, much of the current information available on these species is scattered in multiple journals, periodicals, conference proceedings, bulletins, veterinary magazines, and internet resources. For the busy practitioner to keep abreast of all of these resources is a daunting task, especially for those simultaneously striving to keep current in canine and feline medicine. *The 5-Minute Veterinary Consult: Ferret and Rabbit* is designed to bring this information together in a concise, readily accessible format.

*The 5-Minute Veterinary Consult: Ferret and Rabbit* is a quick reference with a unique format that provides consistency and breadth of coverage unparalleled by other texts. Like other editions in *The 5-Minute Veterinary Consult* series, the ferret and rabbit edition is divided into topics based on presenting problems and diseases. Each topic has an identical format, which makes it easy to find information. Detailed, up-to-date information on the diagnosis and treatment options for all disorders commonly encountered in these species are readily accessible. Individual topics are thoroughly covered within a few pages so that there is little need to cross-reference to other topics within the text.

To make this information quickly available, the book is divided by species into separate sections for ferrets and rabbits, with tabs to help quickly identify the section required. Within each species section, topics are organized alphabetically so that each can be readily located. A detailed contents and index are also provided to help the reader efficiently find the desired topic. The Appendixes contain a formulary of commonly used medications, reference ranges for laboratory values, and unique biological characteristics for each species. Also included is a full-color bookmark with anatomical drawings of the rabbit and ferret.

I am fortunate and pleased to have had the assistance of several outstanding experts in the field of companion exotic medicine to serve as a panel of reviewers for every topic presented in this work. Their input has significantly strengthened the text and greatly enhanced the depth and scope of coverage of each topic. Unlike canine and feline medicine, the amount of information available on the disorders of rabbits and ferrets that has been generated by controlled studies is limited. Much of our cumulative knowledge is based on the shared experience of practicing exotic animal veterinarians. Because of this, many topics in rabbit and ferret medicine are controversial. I have made every attempt to present information with as little bias as possible, and this was facilitated by having each topic reviewed. However, the reader is encouraged to utilize the list of Suggested Reading printed at the end of each topic for additional information and viewpoints.

All topics in this work have been updated within the past year of publication. My goal is to revise the text every three years, to be certain that the content is current. Additionally, I hope to expand the pool of experts, both for content review and for the list of contributors. The openness and camaraderie that exists within our emerging field of companion exotic animal medicine has been essential to its growth. I would welcome any input that you could give to make future editions more useful. Please send your comments to:

Dr. Barbara Oglesbee

# Acknowledgments

I would like to express my gratitude to the reviewers of this text. The expertise of all of the reviewers has significantly strengthened the text and greatly enhanced the depth and scope of coverage of each topic. Thanks goes especially to Dr. Michael Murray, Dr. Evelyn Ivey, and Dr. Tia Greenberg for their extensive effort and willingness to work within a limited time-frame.

Special acknowledgment and thanks to Dr. Branson Ritchie, who has collaborated with me on our larger goal, *The 5-Minute Veterinary Consult: Avian and Exotic*. This future work is in progress and will combine the current text with reptilian and avian species to create a single resource for companion exotic species.

I would like to acknowledge all exotic practioners who have contributed in one way or an-other to our cumulative knowledge base. Much of what we know of companion exotic animal medicine is based on the shared experience of these veterinarians, without which this text would not have been possible. I would like to especially acknowledge Drs. Katherine Quesenberry, James Carpenter, Susan Brown, Karen Rosenthal, and Avery Bennett, who have so effectively educated veterinarians worldwide in the area of small mammal medicine and surgery.

Lastly, I would like to gratefully acknowledge Drs. Larry P. Tilley and Francis W.K. Smith, Jr., whose insight and innovation pioneered *The 5-Minute Veterinary Consult* series.

# REVIEWERS

DAVE CHAPMAN, DVM
   All Creatures Care Cottage Veterinary
      Hospital
   Costa Mesa, California

TIA GREENBERG, DVM
   Westminster Veterinary Group
   Westminster, California

EVELYN IVEY, DVM, DABVP—AVIAN
   Glenolden Animal Hospital
   Glenolden, Pennsylvania

MATTHEW S. JOHNSTON, DVM,
DABVP—AVIAN
   Assistant Professor of Zoological
      Medicine
   Colorado State University
   Fort Collins, Colorado

MICHAEL MURRAY, DVM
   Avian and Exotic Clinic of the Monterey
      Peninsula
   Monterey, California

KAREN ROSENTHAL, DVM, MS,
DABVP—AVIAN
   Director of Special Species Medicine
   Associate Professor of Special Species
      Medicine
   Abaxis Chair of Special Species
      Medicine
   Matthew J. Ryan Veterinary Hospital at
      the University of Pennsylvania
   Philadelphia, Pennsylvania

# CONTENTS

| TOPIC |
|---|

**FERRET**

| | |
|---|---|
| Adrenal Disease (Hyperadrenocorticism) | 2 |
| Alopecia | 5 |
| Anorexia | 7 |
| Ascites | 9 |
| Ataxia | 11 |
| Campylobacteriosis | 13 |
| Canine Distemper Virus | 15 |
| Cardiomyopathy, Dilated | 17 |
| Cardiomyopathy, Hypertrophic | 19 |
| Clostridial Enterotoxicosis | 21 |
| Coccidiosis | 23 |
| Congestive Heart Failure | 24 |
| Cough | 27 |
| Cryptosporidiosis | 29 |
| Dermatophytosis | 30 |
| Diabetes Mellitus | 32 |
| Diarrhea | 35 |
| Dyschezia and Hematochezia | 38 |
| Dysphagia | 40 |
| Dyspnea and Tachypnea | 42 |
| Dystocia and Fetal Death | 44 |
| Dysuria and Pollakiuria | 45 |
| Ear Mites | 47 |
| Eosinophilic Gastroenteritis | 48 |
| Epizootic Catarrhal Enteritis | 50 |
| Fleas and Flea Infestation | 53 |
| Gastritis | 55 |
| Gastroduodenal Ulcers | 58 |
| Gastrointestinal and Esophageal Foreign Bodies | 61 |
| Giardiasis | 64 |
| Gingivitis and Periodontal Disease | 65 |
| Heartworm Disease | 66 |
| Helicobacter Mustelae | 68 |
| Hepatomegaly | 71 |
| Hydronephrosis | 73 |
| Hyperestrogenism | 74 |
| Hypersplenism | 77 |

| TOPIC | |
|---|---|
| Hypoglycemia | 79 |
| Inflammatory Bowel Disease | 81 |
| Influenza Virus | 83 |
| Insulinoma | 85 |
| Lower Urinary Tract Infection | 88 |
| Lymphadenopathy (Lymphadenomegaly) | 90 |
| Lymphoplasmacytic Enteritis and Gastroenteritis | 92 |
| Lymphosarcoma | 94 |
| Mast Cell Tumor | 97 |
| Megaesophagus | 98 |
| Melena | 100 |
| Multiple Myeloma | 102 |
| Nasal Discharge (Sneezing, Gagging) | 104 |
| Neoplasia, Digestive System | 106 |
| Neoplasia, Integumentary | 107 |
| Neoplasia, Musculoskeletal and Nervous System | 108 |
| Obesity | 109 |
| Otitis Externa and Media | 111 |
| Paresis and Paralysis | 113 |
| Parvovirus Infection (Aleutian Disease Virus [ADV]) | 115 |
| Petechia/Ecchymosis/Bruising | 117 |
| Pleural Effusion | 119 |
| Pneumonia, Aspiration | 121 |
| Pneumonia, Bacterial | 123 |
| Pneumonia, Mycotic | 125 |
| Pododermatitis and Nail Bed Disorders | 127 |
| Polyuria and Polydipsia | 129 |
| Pregnancy Toxemia | 131 |
| Proliferative Bowel Disease | 132 |
| Prostatitis and Prostatic Abscesses | 134 |
| Prostatomegaly | 136 |
| Pruritus | 138 |
| Ptyalism | 140 |
| Pyometra and Stump Pyometra | 142 |
| Rabies | 145 |
| Rectal and Anal Prolapse | 147 |
| Regurgitation | 148 |
| Renal Failure | 150 |
| Renomegaly | 153 |
| Salmonellosis | 155 |
| Sarcoptic Mange | 157 |
| Splenomegaly | 159 |
| Urinary Tract Obstruction | 161 |
| Urogenital Cystic Disease (Paraurethral Cysts) | 164 |
| Urolithiasis | 167 |
| Vaginal Discharge | 170 |
| Vomiting | 172 |
| Weight Loss and Cachexia | 174 |

| TOPIC | |
|---|---|

**RABBIT**

| | |
|---|---|
| Abscessation | 178 |
| Alopecia | 182 |
| Anorexia and Pseudoanorexia | 184 |
| Anterior Uveitis | 187 |
| Anticoagulant Rodenticide Poisoning | 190 |
| Arthritis—Osteoarthritis | 192 |
| Arthritis—Septic | 194 |
| Ataxia | 196 |
| Cataracts | 199 |
| Cheek Teeth (Molar and Premolar) Malocclusion and Elongation | 201 |
| Cheyletiellosis (Fur Mites) | 205 |
| Clostridial Enteritis/Enterotoxicosis | 207 |
| Coccidiosis | 210 |
| Congestive Heart Failure | 212 |
| Conjunctivitis | 215 |
| Constipation (Lack of Fecal Production) | 219 |
| Dermatophytosis | 223 |
| Diarrhea, Acute | 225 |
| Diarrhea, Chronic | 228 |
| Dyspnea and Tachypnea | 231 |
| Dysuria and Pollakiuria | 234 |
| Ear Mites | 236 |
| Encephalitozoonosis | 238 |
| Encephalitis and Meningoencephalitis | 241 |
| Encephalitis Secondary to Parasitic Migration | 244 |
| Epiphora | 245 |
| Epistaxis | 248 |
| Exophthalmos and Orbital Diseases | 250 |
| Facial Nerve Paresis/Paralysis | 254 |
| Fleas and Flea Infestaton | 257 |
| Gastric Dilation | 259 |
| Gastrointestinal Foreign Bodies | 262 |
| Gastrointestinal Hypomotility and Gastrointestinal Stasis | 266 |
| Head Tilt (Vestibular Disease) | 270 |
| Heat Stroke and Heat Stress | 273 |
| Hematuria | 275 |
| Hypercalciuria and Urolithiasis | 277 |
| Incisor Malocclusion and Overgrowth | 280 |
| Incontinence, Urinary | 284 |
| Lameness | 286 |
| Lead Toxicity | 288 |
| Lower Urinary Tract Infection | 290 |
| Mastitis, Cystic and Septic | 293 |
| Melena | 295 |
| Myxomatosis | 297 |
| Nasal Discharge and Sneezing | 298 |

| TOPIC | |
| --- | --- |
| Neck and Back Pain | 301 |
| Nephrolithiasis and Ureterlithiasis | 303 |
| Obesity | 306 |
| Otitis Externa and Media | 308 |
| Otitis Media and Interna | 311 |
| Paresis and Paralysis | 314 |
| Pasteurellosis | 317 |
| Pinworms (Oxyurids) | 320 |
| Pneumonia | 321 |
| Poisoning (Intoxication) | 324 |
| Polyuria and Polydipsia | 326 |
| Pruritus | 328 |
| Ptyalism (Slobbers) | 330 |
| Pyoderma | 333 |
| Pyometra and Nonneoplastic Endometrial Disorders | 336 |
| Rabies | 339 |
| Red Eye | 341 |
| Renal Failure | 344 |
| Rhinitis and Sinusitis | 347 |
| Seizures | 350 |
| Shope Papilloma Virus | 353 |
| Spondylosis Deformans | 354 |
| Stertor and Stridor | 356 |
| Thymoma/Thymic Lymphoma | 359 |
| Tooth Root Abscesses (Apical Abscesses) | 360 |
| Toxoplasmosis | 364 |
| Treponematosis (Rabbit Syphilis) | 366 |
| Trichobezoars | 367 |
| Ulcerative Pododermatitis (Sore Hocks) | 371 |
| Urinary Tract Obstruction | 374 |
| Uterine Adenocarcinoma | 377 |
| Vaginal Discharge | 379 |
| Vertebral Fracture or Luxation | 381 |
| Weight Loss and Cachexia | 384 |
| | |
| Appendix I Common Dosages for Ferrets | 388 |
| Appendix II Normal Values for Ferrets | 392 |
| Appendix III Common Dosages for Rabbits | 394 |
| Appendix IV Normal Values for Rabbits | 397 |
| Appendix V Toxic Plants and Their Clinical Signs—Antidotes and Treatment | 399 |
| | |
| Index | 403 |

# FERRET

# ADRENAL DISEASE (HYPERADRENOCORTICISM)

 **BASICS**

## DEFINITION
- Spontaneous hyperadrenocorticism is a disorder resulting in excessive production of estrogens, androgens, and estrogen-related compounds by the adrenal cortex.
- Cortisol concentrations are not significantly elevated.
- Clinical signs are due to the deleterious effects of the elevated circulating estrogen and androgen concentrations on multiple organ systems. Clinical signs caused by the space occupying effects of the tumor may also be seen.

## PATHOPHYSIOLOGY
- Ferret adrenal disease is caused by excessive secretion of sex steroids from adrenocortical hyperplasia, adrenal adenomas, or carcinoma.
- Unilateral disease is somewhat more common than bilateral adrenal disease.
- Hyperadrenocorticism resulting from pituitary corticotroph tumors or hyperplasia oversecreting ACTH has not been documented in the ferret.
- Iatrogenic hyperadrenocorticism resulting from excessive exogenous administration of glucocorticoids has not been reported in ferrets.

## SYSTEMS AFFECTED
- Ferret adrenal disease is a multisystemic disorder.
- Signs referable to the skin or reproductive tract predominate.
- Bone marrow suppression may also occur.
- The degree to which each system is involved varies; in some patients signs referable to one system may predominate; others have several systems involved to a comparable degree.

## GENETICS
Unknown; however, a genetic predisposition is suspected since many of the ferrets in North America come from similar breeding stock

## INCIDENCE/PREVALENCE
Considered one of the most common disorders in ferrets. Over 95% of ferrets with bilaterally symmetric progressive alopecia have ferret adrenal disease.

## GEOGRAPHIC DISTRIBUTION
Ferret adrenal disease is seen more commonly in ferrets in North America as compared to those in Europe. This may be due to genetics, early neutering practices, or differing husbandry practices.

## SIGNALMENT

### Breed Predilections
N/A

### Predominant Sex
Seen primarily in neutered animals—equal incidence in male and female animals. Females may be presented for evaluation more frequently than males because of the prominent appearance of vulvar swelling.

### Mean Age and Range
Generally a disorder of middle-aged animals, 3–4 years old. The reported age range is 1–7 years.

## SIGNS

### General Comments
- Severity may vary greatly, depending on the duration and magnitude of sex steroid excess.
- In some cases, the space-occupying and catabolic effects of the neoplastic process contribute.

### Historical and Physical Examination Findings
- Alopecia is the most common clinical sign. Hair loss often begins in late winter or early spring; hair initially may regrow later in the year, followed by progressive alopecia the following spring. Bilaterally symmetric alopecia begins in the tail region and progresses cranially. In severe cases, the ferret will become completely bald. In most cases, the skin has a normal appearance.
- About 30% of affected ferrets are pruritic; secondary pyoderma is sometimes seen.
- Swollen vulva in spayed females is extremely common.
- Stranguria due to urogenital cysts or prostatic hyperplasia in males—common, often life-threatening consequence; large urogenital cysts can be palpable; occasionally occurs in females as well
- Sexual aggression or return of sexual behavior in neutered animals
- Thinning of the skin, muscle atrophy, and pot-bellied appearance in chronic disease
- Occasionally, mammary gland hypertrophy
- Rarely, anemia, polydipsia, and polyuria
- Occasionally, affected adrenal gland is palpably enlarged.
- Splenomegaly is a common, usually incidental finding.

## CAUSES
Functional adrenal hyperplasia, adenoma, or adenocarcinomas most common

## RISK FACTORS
Evidence suggests that adrenal disease may be related to neutering at an early age. The gonads and adrenals arise embryonically from the urogenital ridge; some gonadal cells are likely present in the adrenals. Stimulation of these cells by pituitary gonadotropin may cause hypertrophy of these steroid-secreting cells.

 **DIAGNOSIS**

## DIFFERENTIAL DIAGNOSIS
- For alopecia and pruritus: seasonal alopecia, pyoderma, flea-allergy dermatitis, dermatophytes, mast cell tumor, cutaneous lymphoma
- For swollen vulva in spayed females: ovarian remnant, intact female
- For stranguria: cystitis, urolithiasis

## CBC/BIOCHEMISTRY/URINALYSIS
- Usually normal
- Rarely, in chronic cases, hemogram may show nonregenerative anemia, leukopenia, or thrombocytopenia due to estrogen excess.
- Leukocytosis is seen in ferrets with abscessed urogenital cysts or stump pyometra.
- Hypoglycemia may be present—usually due to concurrent insulinoma since many ferrets in this age range will also have pancreatic tumors
- Urinalysis may reveal decreased specific gravity in polyuric animals (rare)

## OTHER LABORATORY TESTS
- Elevations in plasma estradiol, androstenedione, and 17-hydroxyprogesterone combined are most diagnostic (available through the Clinical Endocrinology Laboratory, Department of Comparative Medicine, University of Tennessee). Plasma concentration of these steroids often decline precipitously following surgical removal of the affected gland and resolution of clinical signs.
- Elevation in serum estrogens alone in males is diagnostic; however, in females estrogens may be elevated due to either adrenal disease or an ovarian remnant.
- Elevations in serum cortisol are rarely seen.
- Unlike the diagnosis in dogs, ACTH response test and low-dose dexamethasone suppression tests are not diagnostic and are not pertinent to the diagnosis. Likewise, urinary cortisol:creatinine ratio is not useful in the diagnosis of adrenal disease in ferrets.

## IMAGING
- Radiographs occasionally demonstrate enlarged adrenal glands.
- In ferrets with prostatomegaly or urogenital cysts, single or multiple soft tissue density structures may be visible around the urinary bladder.
- Ultrasonography can be very useful for demonstrating adrenal gland enlargement, depending on the experience of the ultrasonographer. Ideally, the affected gland should be identified prior to surgery.
- Examine the spleen, pancreas, mesenteric lymph nodes, and liver for concurrent disease, especially in older ferrets.

## DIAGNOSTIC PROCEDURES
- Exploratory laparotomy—may be the only option for definitive diagnosis (see surgical considerations below).
- Human chorionic gonadotropin (hCG) challenge test in spayed females with swollen vulva. 100 IU of hCG IM once, administer at least 7–10 days following onset of vulvar swelling. If swelling subsides 3–4 days postinjection, an ovarian remnant is

# ADRENAL DISEASE (HYPERADRENOCORTICISM)

likely. Some ovarian remnants do not respond to a single injection of hCG, requiring a second injection 7–10 days later. If the vulva remains swollen after repeat injection, adrenal disease is most likely the cause.

## PATHOLOGIC FINDINGS
• Gross examination reveals enlargement of the adrenal gland, irregular surface or discoloration of the affected gland, cysts, or differences in texture within the affected gland.
• Occasionally, bilateral tumors are found.
• Invasion into the liver, kidney, vena cava, or other abdominal organs in some patients with adrenal adenocarcinoma
• Metastasis rarely occurs.
• In females, stump pyometra may be seen.
• Microscopically—adrenocortical hyperplasia, adrenocortical adenoma or carcinoma, or leiomyosarcoma

## TREATMENT

### APPROPRIATE HEALTH CARE
• Ferret adrenal disease may be treated with adrenalectomy or managed medically. The decision as to which form of treatment is appropriate is multifactorial; which gland is affected (left vs. right), surgeon's experience and expertise, severity of clinical signs, age of the animal, concurrent diseases, and financial issues should be considered.
• Surgical removal of the affected adrenal gland(s) is often curative. This procedure may require special surgical expertise, especially if the right adrenal gland is diseased. (See surgical considerations, below.)
• Medical treatment (see medications, below) may cause a sufficient reduction in clinical signs. Depending on the circumstances, medical treatment may be preferred. However, medical treatment is not curative, must be administered lifelong, and has no effect on adrenal tumor size or potential metastasis.
• If clinical signs are limited to cosmetic appearance (alopecia), some owners may elect not to treat at all. Owners should be advised that metastasis, although rare, does occur, the space occupying and catabolic effects of neoplasia may become significant, and males may develop prostatic disease that can cause life-threatening urethral obstruction.
• Hospitalization is usually required for patients with urethral obstruction due to prostate disease, for severely depressed patients, and during the postsurgical recovery period for those undergoing adrenalectomy.

### NURSING CARE
N/A

### DIET
Normal diet is returned 2–6 hours post-surgery.

## CLIENT EDUCATION
• If surgical treatment is opted, the affected adrenal gland can usually be identified and removed during exploratory laparotomy, even if the affected gland could not be identified by preoperative imaging techniques.
• If the right or both adrenal glands are affected, surgical treatment is more difficult and referral may be required, depending on the surgeon's experience.
• If medical treatment is opted owners should be advised that medical treatment is life-long, that metastasis, although rare, may occur, the space occupying and catabolic effects of neoplasia may become significant, and males may develop prostatic disease that can cause life-threatening urethral obstruction.

## SURGICAL CONSIDERATIONS
• Adrenalectomy is often curative for unilateral adrenocortical hyperplasia, adenomas, and adenocarcinomas.
• Both adrenals should be observed and palpated. Normal glands are light pink with homogenous color and density, 2–3 mm in width, and 6–8 mm in length. Indications for removal include gross enlargement of the adrenal gland, irregular surface or discoloration, cysts, or differences in texture within the affected gland.
• Several techniques for adrenalectomy have been advocated, and problems may be associated with each surgical option, depending on the surgeon's expertise. Refer to suggested reading list for a more detailed description of surgical procedures.
• Left adrenalectomy is generally a relatively uncomplicated procedure.
• Right adrenalectomy requires special surgical expertise. Proximity of the right adrenal to the vena cava and the potential for vena cava invasion by malignant tumors make complete excision a high-risk procedure. Referral to a surgeon or clinician with experience is recommended when possible.
• Many practitioners advocate debulking, rather than complete removal of the right adrenal, as this procedure carries less risk of life-threatening complications. If this method is chosen, signs of clinical disease will return, necessitating repeat surgery or medical therapy alone.
• If both adrenals are affected, removal of the left adrenal gland and a subtotal adrenalectomy of the right gland are often recommended. Eventually, however, the ferret is likely to become symptomatic, requiring complete removal of the remaining gland or medical management.
• Removal of both adrenals may cause iatrogenic adrenal insufficiency (Addison's disease), requiring close monitoring and medical management.
• Always explore the entire abdominal cavity during surgery since concurrent liver disease, gastrointestinal tract disease, insulinoma, lymphoma, or other neoplastic diseases are extremely common. Biopsy the liver and any enlarged lymph nodes to check for metastases.

## MEDICATIONS

### DRUG(S) OF CHOICE
Medical treatment of adrenal disease:
• Successful treatment of adrenal disease has been anecdotally reported using leuprolide acetate, a GNRH analog. This is a potent inhibitor of gonadotropin secretion and acts to suppress LH and FSH and to downregulate their receptor sites. It is available as a 1- or 4-month depot injection and has been anecdotally reported to alleviate the dermal and reproductive organ signs of adrenal disease in ferrets. Reported dosages: Lupron 30-day depot, 100–250 µg/kg IM q4w until signs resolve, then q4–8w prn, lifelong. Larger ferrets often require the higher end of the dose range. This drug has no effect on adrenal tumor growth or metastasis. Side effects include dyspnea, lethargy, and local injection site irritation. Anecdotal reports suggest that Lupron is more successful in alleviating clinical signs in patients with hyperplasia or adenomas; adenocarcinomas may be less likely to respond.
• Flutamide (10 mg/kg PO q12–24h) inhibits androgen uptake and binding in target tissues, and is used in the treatment of androgen-responsive prostatic tumors in humans. It has been used to reduce the size of prostatic tissue and treat alopecia in ferrets with adrenal disease. This drug has no effect on adrenal tumor growth or metastasis. Side effects may include gynomastia and hepatic injury; monitor liver enzyme concentrations during therapy. Therapy is expensive and may be cost prohibitive for some clients.
• Melatonin (0.5–1.0 mg/animal q24h prn, administered 7–9 hours after sunrise) has been used to control breeding activity in ferrets and mink, and has been anecdotally used in ferrets with adrenal disease to successfully alleviate clinical signs of alopecia, aggressive behavior, vulvar swelling and prostatomegaly. Alleviation of clinical signs may be more likely in patients with adrenal hyperplasia or adenoma; adenocarcinomas are less likely to respond. Melatonin has no demonstrated effect on adrenal tumor growth or metastasis. Also available in an implant form approved by the FDA for use in mink.
If surgical treatment is opted:
• In ferrets with concurrent insulinoma or if a combination of left and subtotal right adrenalectomy is performed, administer post-operative prednisone 0.25–0.5 mg/kg PO q12h for 1 week, then gradually tapering the dose over 1–2 weeks.

## ADRENAL DISEASE (HYPERADRENOCORTICISM)

• If subtotal or total bilateral adrenalectomy is performed, long-term post-operative treatment with glucocorticoids is often necessary. The dosage is titrated to the individual patient and tapered to the lowest dosage interval necessary to prevent clinical signs of hypoadrenocorticism. Many ferrets have accessory adrenal tissue, and some may be weaned from exogenous steroids completely if carefully monitored. However, some ferrets do become critically ill due to hypoadrenocorticism even with prednisone supplementation, and treatment with mineralocorticoid may also be required. Treatment is initiated based on clinical signs and electrolyte status (signs typically occur within days to week postoperatively). Dosages have been extrapolated from feline dose; Florinef (fludrocortisone acetate) 0.05–0.1 mg/kg PO q24h or divided q12h or Deoxy-corticosterone pivalate (DOCP) 2 mg/kg IM q21d. Carefully monitor electrolyte status.

### CONTRAINDICATIONS
N/A

### ALTERNATIVE DRUGS
• Anastrozole (0.1 mg/kg PO q24h until signs resolved, then on a week on/week off basis prn) is an aromatase inhibitor used to inhibit the production of estrogens.
• Bicalutamide (5 mg/kg PO q24h until signs resolved, then on a week on/week off basis prn) inhibits testosterone at receptor sites.
• Mitotane (o,p'-DDD) may be palliative in rare cases for ferrets with adrenal hyperplasia, not effective in the treatment of adenomas or adenocarcinomas, rarely effective; side effects can be severe.
• Ketoconazole is not effective in the treatment of ferret adrenal disease.

### PRECAUTIONS
• The use of mitotane may cause iatrogenic hypoadrenocorticism and hypoglycemia if an undetected insulinoma is present. Use with extreme caution if at all.
• Pregnant women should avoid handling Anastrozole or Bicalutamide

 FOLLOW-UP

### PATIENT MONITORING
• Response to therapy is evident by remission of clinical signs, particularly hair regrowth, regression of vulvar swelling, and reduction in the size of urogenital cysts or prostatic tissue. Urogenital signs usually resolve within days of surgery.
• Monitor serum glucose concentrations following surgery, since many ferrets have concurrent insulinomas and develop postoperative hypoglycemia.
• Following unilateral adrenalectomy or subtotal adrenalectomy, monitor for return of clinical signs, since tumor recurrence is common. Clinical signs typically develop 1 year or more postoperatively.
• In ferrets with bilateral adrenalectomy, monitor for the development of Addison's disease (lethargy, weakness, anorexia, periodic evaluation of serum electrolytes).

### PREVENTION/AVOIDANCE
There is some evidence suggesting that neutering after 6 months of age may decrease the incidence of disease.

### POSSIBLE COMPLICATIONS
• Recurrence of tumor or development of tumor in the remaining gland in patients with unilateral or subtotal bilateral adrenalectomy
• Metastasis in patients with carcinomas
• Invasion of right adrenal tumors into the vena cava or liver
• Cachexia due to the catabolic effects of neoplasia
• Development of postoperative hypoglycemia in patients with concurrent undiagnosed insulinoma
• Addison's disease or death in ferrets with bilateral adrenalectomy

### EXPECTED COURSE/PROGNOSIS
• Following surgical removal of the affected gland(s), a reduction in vulvar swelling is seen within 2 days to 2 weeks, and the haircoat returns to normal within 2–4 months. A reduction in size of paraurethral cysts may occur as soon as 1–2 days postoperatively.
• Response to medical therapy may vary with tumor type; anecdotal reports suggest a range of days to months for alleviation of signs. Insufficient data exist to predict the outcome of long-term therapy.
• Prognosis is variable and depends on tumor type, age of animal, presence of concurrent disease, and mode of treatment.
• Ferrets with adrenal hyperplasia or adenomas often live 2 or more years, even with no treatment. Dermal and/or urogenital signs will worsen without treatment.
• Carcinomas rarely metastasize. If metastasis occurs, the prognosis is fair to poor.

 MISCELLANEOUS

### ASSOCIATED CONDITIONS
Insulinomas, lymphoma, and/or nonspecific splenomegaly are often concurrently found in ferrets with adrenal disease.

### AGE-RELATED FACTORS
Older animals are more likely to have concurrent heart disease, renal disease, or other neoplasia.

### ZOONOTIC POTENTIAL
N/A

### PREGNANCY
N/A

### SYNONYMS
Hyperadrenocorticism

### SEE ALSO
• Hyperestrogenism
• Insulinoma
• Lower urinary tract obstruction
• Prostatomegaly
• Pyometra
• Urogenital cystic disease

### ABBREVIATIONS
• ACTH = adrenocorticotropic hormone
• GNRH = gonadotropin-releasing hormone
• hCG = human chorionic gonadotropin

*Suggested Reading*
Antinoff N. Urinary disorders in ferrets. Semin Avian Exotic Pet Med 1998;7(2):89–92.
Beeber NL. Abdominal surgery in ferrets. Vet Clin North Am Exot Anim Pract 2000;3(3):647–662.
Fox JG, Marini RP. Diseases of the endocrine system. In: Fox JG, ed. Biology and Diseases of the Ferret. 2nd Ed. Baltimore: Williams & Wilkins, 1998.
Ludwig L, Aiken S. Soft tissue surgery. In: Quesenberry KE, Carpenter JW, eds. Ferrets, Rabbits and Rodents: Clinical Medicine and Surgery. St. Louis: WB Saunders, 2004:121–134.
Paul-Murphy J, Ramer J. Melatonin use in ferret adrenal gland disease. Proc North Am Vet Conf 2000;897.
Pollock CGT. Urogenital diseases. In: Quesenberry KE, Carpenter JW, eds. Ferrets, Rabbits and Rodents: Clinical Medicine and Surgery. St. Louis: WB Saunders, 2004:79–90.
Quesenberry KE, Rosenthal KL. Endocrine disease. In: Hillyer EV, Quesenberry KE, eds. Ferrets, Rabbits and Rodents: Clinical Medicine and Surgery. Philadelphia: WB Saunders, 1997.
Rosenthal KL, Peterson ME: Evaluation of plasma androgen and estrogen in ferrets with hyperadrenocorticism. J Am Vet Med Assoc 1996;209:1097–1102.
Rosenthal KL, Peterson ME, Quesenberry KE, et al. Hyperadrenocorticism associated with adrenocortical tumors or nodular hyperplasia of the adrenal gland in ferrets: 50 cases (1987–1991). J Am Vet Med Assoc 1993;203:271–275.
Weiss CA, Scott MV: Clinical aspects and surgical treatment of hyperadrenocorticism in the domestic ferret: 94 cases (1994–1996). J Am Anim Hosp Assoc 1997;33:487–493.
Wheeler J, Bennet RA. Ferret abdominal surgical procedures. Part I. Adrenal gland and pancreatic beta-cell tumors. Compend Contin Educ Pract Vet 1999;21(9):815–822.

# BASICS

## DEFINITION
- Extremely common disorder in ferrets
- Characterized by a complete or partial lack of hair in areas where it is normally present
- May be associated with a multifactorial cause
- May be the primary problem or only a secondary phenomenon

## PATHOPHYSIOLOGY
- Multifactorial causes
- All of the disorders represent a disruption in the growth of the hair follicle from endocrine abnormalities, infection, or trauma.

## SYSTEMS AFFECTED
- Skin/exocrine
- Endocrine/metabolic

## SIGNALMENT
- No specific age or sex predilection
- Ferret adrenal disease, the most common cause of alopecia, is seen primarily in middle-aged (3–7 years old) neutered animals—equal incidence in male and female animals

## SIGNS
- The pattern and degree of hair loss are important for establishing a differential diagnosis.
- Large diffuse areas of alopecia—indicate a follicular dysplasia or metabolic component
- Multifocal patches of alopecia—most frequently associated with folliculitis from bacterial, mycotic, or parasitic infection
- May be acute in onset or slowly progressive

## CAUSES
- Endocrine—ferret adrenal disease, seasonal alopecia in intact animals; ferret adrenal disease is the most common cause of alopecia in pet ferrets
- Infectious—bacterial pyoderma, dermatophytosis; most often a secondary problem
- Parasitic—ear mites, fleas, sarcoptic mange
- Neoplastic—cutaneous lymphoma, mast cell tumor
- Immunologic—contact dermatitis has been anecdotally reported in ferrets. Cutaneous lesions resembling urticaria or histologic lesions characteristic of allergic reactions in other species have also been anecdotally reported; however, there are no confirmed cases of atopy, food allergy, or other allergic dermatitis in ferrets.
- Nutrition—particularly fat or protein deficiencies; may be seen in ferret fed a vegetable-based diet

## RISK FACTORS
N/A

# DIAGNOSIS

## DIFFERENTIAL DIAGNOSIS
### Differentiating Causes
Pattern and degree—important features for formulating a differential diagnosis

### Symmetrical
- Ferret adrenal disease—over 95% of neutered ferrets with bilaterally symmetric alopecia have adrenal disease. Hair loss often begins in late winter or early spring; hair initially may regrow later in the year, followed by progressive alopecia the following spring. Alopecia begins in the tail region and progresses cranially. In severe cases, the ferret will become completely bald. In most cases, the skin has a normal appearance, although skin thickening may appear. Some ferrets are pruritic and secondary pyoderma is occasionally seen. Other signs related to adrenal disease, such as a swollen vulva in spayed females, may be seen.
- Seasonal flank alopecia—in intact animals (or females with ovarian remnant), bilaterally symmetric alopecia begins at the tail base and progresses throughout the breeding season (March–August for females, December–July for males). Alopecia is not as extensive as in ferrets with adrenal disease.
- Hyperestrogenism (females)—symmetrical alopecia of the flanks and perineal and inguinal regions with enlarged vulva and mammary glands

### Multifocal to Focal
- Ear mites—partial to complete alopecia caudal to the ears; waxy brown aural discharge; excoriations around pinna
- Fleas—patchy alopecia at tail base and in cervical and dorsal thoracic region; excoriations; secondary pyoderma
- Sarcoptic mange—two forms reported—generalized with diffuse alopecia and intense pruritus and local form affecting the feet with secondary pododermatitis
- Bacterial folliculitis—multifocal area of circular alopecia to coalescing large areas of hair loss; epidermal collarettes
- Dermatophytosis—partial to complete alopecia with scaling; with or without erythema; not always ringlike; may begin as small papules
- Neoplasia—cutaneous lymphoma, cutaneous epitheliotropic lymphoma (mycoses fungoides)–diffuse, generalized truncal alopecia with scaling and erythema, later nodule and plaque formation; mast cell tumor—focal alopecia with pruritus, scaling, and often covered with black crusts

## CBC/BIOCHEMISTRY/URINALYSIS
- Inflammatory leukocytosis with neutrophilia may be seen with pyoderma.
- Lymphocytosis may be seen with cutaneous lymphoma.
- Nonregenerative anemia, leukopenia, or thrombocytopenia with estrogen excess

## OTHER LABORATORY TESTS
Ferret adrenal disease—elevations of serum estradiol, androstenedione, and 17-hydroxyprogesterone combined are most diagnostic (available through the University of Tennessee Clinical Endocrinology Laboratory, Department of Comparative Medicine).

## IMAGING
Ultrasonography—evaluate adrenal glands for evidence of ferret adrenal disease; generally requires an ultrasonographer experienced in evaluating ferret adrenal glands

## DIAGNOSTIC PROCEDURES
- Response to therapy as a trial
- Fungal culture
- Skin scraping
- Cytology
- Skin biopsy

# TREATMENT
- Treatment must be specific to the underlying cause to be successful.
- Ferret adrenal disease—may be treated with adrenalectomy or managed medically. The decision as to which form of treatment is appropriate is multifactorial; which gland is affected (left vs. right), surgeon's experience, severity of clinical signs, age of the animal, concurrent diseases, and financial issues should be considered.
- Hyperestrogenism—OHE or surgical removal of ovarian remnant
- Mast cell tumor—surgical excision

# MEDICATIONS

## DRUG(S) OF CHOICE
- Varies with specific cause
- Ear mites—ivermectin 1% (Ivomec, Merck AgVet) diluted 1:10 in propylene glycol—instill 0.4 mg/kg divided into each ear topically and repeat in 2 weeks; do not use topical and parenteral ivermectin concurrently. Thiabendazole product (Tresaderm, Merck AgVet) at cat dosages has also been used topically; however, treatment failures are common due to owner compliance and the small size of the ear canal. Selamectin (Revolution, Pfizer) topical application of the cat dosage has been anecdotally reported to be effective.
- Fleas—fipronil (Frontline, Rhone Merieux) 1/5–1/2 of cat pipette applied topically q60d. Imidacloprid (Advantage, Bayer) 1 cat dose divided onto 2–3 spots

## ALOPECIA

topically q30d. Selamectin (Revolution, Pfizer) topical application of the cat dosage has been anecdotally reported to be effective; 5% carbaryl powders applied topically q7d × 3–6 treatments. Topical pyrethrin products that are safe for use in puppies and kittens may be applied topically q7d.
• Sarcoptic mange—ivermectin 0.2–0.4 mg/kg SC q14d for 3 to 4 doses. Selamectin (Revolution, Pfizer) topical application of the cat dosage has been anecdotally reported to be effective.
• Bacterial folliculitis—shampoos and antibiotic therapy, preferably based on culture and susceptibility testing; good initial choices include amoxicillin/clavulanate (12.5 mg/kg PO q12h), cephalexin 15–25 mg/kg PO q12h, or trimethoprim/sulfa 15–30 mg/kg PO q12h
• Dermatophytosis—lime sulfur dip q7d has been used successfully; may be antipruritic; has antiparasitic, antibacterial, and antifungal properties; disadvantages are bad odor and staining; miconazole cream for focal lesions
• Demodicosis—rarely occurs; the use of amitraz (Mitaban, Upjohn) applied topically to affected area 3–6 times q14d has been reported
• Neoplasia—various chemotherapy protocols

### CONTRAINDICATIONS
Do not administer topical and systemic ivermectin simultaneously.

### PRECAUTIONS
*Ivermectin*
Anecdotally associated with birth defects when used in pregnant jills

*Topical Antiparasitic Agents*
• Fipronil, imidacloprid, and selamectin—off-label use; no reports of toxicity; however, use is not widespread and safety has not been evaluated; use with caution
• Flea shampoos, sprays, or powders—use cautiously and sparingly to minimize ingestion during grooming.
• Antibacterial shampoos—use cautiously as may cause excessive dryness and pruritus.

### POSSIBLE INTERACTIONS
None

### ALTERNATIVE DRUGS
Ferret adrenal disease—leuprolide acetate, an LHRH agonist, is a potent inhibitor of gonadotropin secretion and acts to suppress LH and FSH and to downregulate their receptor sites. The use of this compound has been anecdotally reported to treat adrenal-associated alopecia in ferrets. It is available as a 1- or 4-month depot injection. Reported dosages: Lupron 30-day depot, 100–250 µg/kg IM q4w until signs resolve, then q4–8w prn, lifelong. This drug has no effect on adrenal tumor growth or metastasis.

 **FOLLOW-UP**

### PATIENT MONITORING
Varies with cause

### POSSIBLE COMPLICATIONS
N/A

 **MISCELLANEOUS**

### ASSOCIATED CONDITIONS
Other types of neoplasia, especially insulinoma and lymphoma, are often found in ferrets with adrenal disease.

### AGE-RELATED FACTORS
N/A

### ZOONOTIC POTENTIAL
Dermatophytosis can cause skin lesions in people.

### PREGNANCY
Avoid griseofulvin and ivermectin in pregnant animals.

### SYNONYMS
None

### SEE ALSO
• Dermatophytosis
• Ear mites
• Adrenal disease
• Fleas

• Hyperestrogenism
• Lymphosarcoma
• Mast cell tumors

### ABBREVIATIONS
LHRH = luteinizing hormone–releasing hormone
OHE = ovariohysterectomy

*Suggested Reading*
Clyde VL. Practical treatment and control of common ectoparasites in exotic pets. Vet Med 1996;91(7):632–637.
Fox JG, Marini RP. Diseases of the endocrine system. In: Fox JG, ed. Biology and Diseases of the Ferret. 2nd Ed. Baltimore: Williams & Wilkins, 1998.
Kelleher SA. Skin diseases of the ferret. Vet Clin North Am Exotic Anim Pract 2001;4(2):565–572.
Orcutt C. Dermatologic diseases. In: Quesenberry KE, Carpenter JW, eds. Ferrets, Rabbits and Rodents: Clinical Medicine and Surgery. St. Louis: WB Saunders, 2004:79–90.
Patterson MM, Kirchain SM. Comparison of three treatments for control of ear mites in ferrets. Lab Anim Sci 1999;49(6):655–657.
Rosenthal KL. Endocrine disorders of ferrets: insulinoma and adrenal gland disease. 21st Annu Waltham/OSU Symp Treat Small Anim Dis: Exotics1997;35–38.
Rosenthal KL. Ferret and rabbit endocrine disease diagnosis. In: Fudge AM, ed. Laboratory Medicine, Avian and Exotic Pets. Philadelphia: WB Saunders, 2000.
Scott D. Dermatoses of pet rodents, rabbits and ferrets. In: Scott D, Miller W, Ariffen C, eds. Small Animal Dermatology. 5th Ed. Philadelphia: WB Saunders, 1995.

*Portions Adapted From*
Rhodes KH. Alopecia. In: Tilley LP, Smith FWK, Jr., eds. The 5-Minute Veterinary Consult: Canine and Feline, 3rd Ed. Baltimore: Lippincott Williams & Wilkins, 2004.

# BASICS

## DEFINITION
• The lack or loss of appetite for food; appetite is psychologic and depends on memory and associations, compared with hunger, which is physiologically aroused by the body's need for food; the existence of appetite in animals is assumed.
• The term pseudoanorexia is used to describe animals that have a desire for food but are unable to eat because they cannot prehend, chew, or swallow food.

## PATHOPHYSIOLOGY
• Anorexia is most often associated with systemic disease but can be caused by many different mechanisms.
• The control of appetite is a complex interaction between the CNS and the periphery.
• Appetite regulation is more appropriately viewed as neuropharmacologic interactions mediated via neurotransmitters rather than as anatomic centers in the hypothalamus.
• The regulation of food intake also depends on the peripheral control of appetite.
• The gastric distension theory suggests that gastric distension promotes satiety, which is probably hormonally mediated.
• Beyond the stomach, satiety can be induced by placing food in the small intestine.
• Inflammatory, infectious, metabolic, or neoplastic diseases can cause inappetence, probably as a result of the release of a variety of chemical mediators.

## SYSTEMS AFFECTED
All body systems are affected; breakdown of the intestinal mucosal barrier is particularly important in sick patients.

## SIGNALMENT
Depends on the underlying cause

## SIGNS
• Refusal to eat is a common complaint presented by ferret owners, because a poor appetite is strongly associated with illness.
• Reluctance to eat may be the only abnormality identified after an evaluation of the patient history and physical examination; this is typical in ferrets with many types of gastrointestinal tract diseases or psychologic causes of anorexia.
• Patients with disorders causing dysfunction or pain of the face, neck, oropharynx, and esophagus may display an interest in food but be unable to complete prehension and swallowing (pseudoanorexia).
• Pseudoanorectic patients commonly display weight loss, halitosis, excessive drooling, difficulty in prehension and mastication of food, dysphagia, and odynophagia (painful eating).

• Odynophagia is exhibited as repeated efforts at swallowing and vocalization when eating.
• Most underlying causes of pseudoanorexia can be identified by a thorough examination of the face, neck, oropharynx, and esophagus for traumatic lesions, masses, foreign bodies, dental disease, ulceration, and neuromuscular dysfunction.
• Clinical signs in true anorexia vary and are related to the underlying cause.

## CAUSES

### Anorexia
• Almost any systemic disease process
• Gastrointestinal disease is one of the most common causes—especially gastrointestinal foreign body, gastric ulceration, ECE, or infiltrative bowel diseases.
• Endocrine disease—especially insulinoma
• Metabolic disease—especially hepatic or renal disease
• Neoplasia involving any site—especially lymphoma
• Cardiac failure
• Pain
• Infectious disease
• Respiratory disease
• Neurologic disease
• Psychologic—unpalatable diets, alterations in routine or environment, stress
• Toxicosis and drugs
• Musculoskeletal disorders
• Acid-base disorders
• Miscellaneous—motion sickness, high environmental temperature, etc.

### Pseudoanorexia
• Any disease process that interferes with the swallowing reflex
• Diseases causing painful prehension and mastication, stomatitis, glossitis, gingivitis (e.g., physical agents, caustics, bacterial infections, viral infections, foreign bodies, uremia), oral or glossal neoplasia (especially squamous cell carcinoma), neurologic disorders (rabies, tetanus, CNS lesions), musculoskeletal disorders (mandible fracture or subluxation), dental disease, salivary gland disorders, and retrobulbar abscess
• Diseases causing oropharyngeal dysphagia (much less common in ferrets), glossal disorders (neurologic, neoplastic), pharyngitis, pharyngeal neoplasia, retropharyngeal disorders (lymphadenopathy, abscess, hematoma, sialocele), neuromuscular disorders (CNS lesions, botulism)
• Diseases of the esophagus—esophagitis, neoplasia, and neuromuscular disorders (unusual in ferrets)

## RISK FACTORS
N/A

# DIAGNOSIS

## DIFFERENTIAL DIAGNOSIS
• Gastrointestinal disease is the most common cause of anorexia in ferrets, followed by systemic disease.
• Obtain a minimum database (CBC, biochemistry, radiographs) to help eliminate the possibility of underlying medical disorders.
• Questioning about the patient's interest in food and its ability to prehend, masticate, and swallow food, along with a thorough examination of the animal's oropharynx, face, and neck, will help identify pseudoanorexia; if the owners are poor historians, the patient should be observed while eating.
• A thorough history regarding the animal's environment and diet, other animals and people in the household, and any recent changes involving any of these helps identify psychologic anorexia.
• Any abnormalities detected in the physical examination or historical evidence of illness mandates a diagnostic workup for the identified problem.

## CBC/BIOCHEMISTRY/URINALYSIS
Abnormalities vary with different underlying diseases and causes of pseudoanorexia and anorexia.

## OTHER LABORATORY TESTS
Special tests may be necessary to rule out specific diseases suggested by the history, physical examination, or minimum database (see other topics on specific diseases).

## IMAGING
• If underlying disease is suspected but no abnormalities are revealed by the physical examination or minimum database, perform abdominal radiography and abdominal ultrasonography to identify hidden conditions such as gastrointestinal tract disease, hepatic disease, or neoplasia. Consider thoracic radiography to rule out cardiac or pulmonary disease.
• The need for further diagnostic imaging varies with the underlying condition suspected (see other topics on specific diseases).

## DIAGNOSTIC PROCEDURES
Vary with underlying condition suspected (see other topics regarding specific diseases)

## ANOREXIA

### TREATMENT
- Treat underlying cause.
- Symptomatic therapy includes attention to fluid and electrolyte derangements, reduction in environmental stressors, and modification of the diet to improve palatability.
- Most ferrets will accept high-calorie diets such as Eukanuba Maximum Calorie diet (Iams Co., Dayton, OH), Feline a/d (Hills Products, Topeka, KS), or Clinicare Feline liquid diet (Abbott Laboratories, North Chicago, IL); may also add dietary supplement such as Nutri-Cal (EVSCO Pharmaceuticals, Buena, NJ) to increase caloric content to these foods.
- Warming the food to body temperature or offering via syringe may increase acceptance. Administer these supplements several times a day.
- Resting energy requirement for ferrets is 70 kcal/kg bw per day (sick ferrets have higher requirements). Clinicare Feline contains 1 kcal/mL; Eukanuba Maximum Calorie diet contains 2 kcal/mL.
- Techniques for providing enteral nutrition include force-feeding or placement of nasogastric, esophagostomy, gastrostomy, or jejunostomy tubes.
- Parenteral nutrition may be provided via infusion through a polyurethane jugular catheter using a syringe pump.

### MEDICATIONS
#### DRUG(S) OF CHOICE
- Depends on the underlying cause
- Gastrointestinal antisecretory agents are helpful to treat, and possibly prevent, gastritis in anorectic ferrets. Ferrets continually secrete a baseline level of gastric hydrochloric acid and, as such, anorexia itself may predispose to gastric ulceration. Those successfully used in ferrets include omeprazole (0.7 mg/kg PO q24h), famotidine (0.25–0.5 mg/kg PO, IV, SC q12–24h), and cimetidine (5–10 mg/kg PO, SC, IM q8h).
- Analgesics may promote appetite in painful conditions; Carprofen 1 mg/kg PO q12–14h

- Metoclopramide (0.2–0.4 mg/kg SC, PO IM) or cisapride (0.5 mg/kg PO q8h–12h; available from various compounding pharmacies) may be useful if anorexia is associated with delayed gastric emptying or ileus.

#### CONTRAINDICATIONS
Avoid antiemetics or promotility agents if gastrointestinal obstruction is present or suspected.

#### PRECAUTIONS
Use non-steroidal anti-inflammatory agents with caution in ferrets with gastrointestinal or renal disease.

#### POSSIBLE INTERACTIONS
N/A

#### ALTERNATIVE DRUGS
N/A

### FOLLOW-UP
#### PATIENT MONITORING
Body weight and hydration to determine if management is effective

#### POSSIBLE COMPLICATIONS
- Dehydration, malnutrition, and cachexia are most likely; these exacerbate the underlying disease.
- Ferrets secrete a baseline level of gastric hydrochloric acid and may develop gastric ulcerations when anorectic.
- Hepatic lipidosis is a possible complication of anorexia, especially in obese ferrets.
- Breakdown of the intestinal mucosal barrier is a concern in debilitated patients.

### MISCELLANEOUS
#### ASSOCIATED CONDITIONS
Hypoglycemia may occur in anorectic ferrets with insulinoma, kits, and cachectic patients and in some medical conditions (e.g., advanced liver disease).

#### AGE-RELATED FACTORS
Nutritional support and/or glucose-containing fluids may be necessary to treat or prevent hypoglycemia in anorectic kits, ferrets with insulinoma or emaciated ferrets.

#### ZOONOTIC POTENTIAL
N/A

#### PREGNANCY
N/A

#### SYNONYMS
Inappetence

#### SEE ALSO
- Epizootic Catarrhal Enteritis
- Eosinophilic gastroenteritis
- Gastroduodenal ulcers
- Gastrointestinal and esophageal foreign bodies
- Insulinoma
- Lymphoplasmacytic enteritis and gastroenteritis
- Lymphosarcoma

#### ABBREVIATIONS
CNS = central nervous system
ECE = epizootic catarrhal enteritis
IBD = infiltrative bowel disease

*Suggested Reading*

Finkler MR. Ferret colitis. In: Kirk RW, Bonagura JD, eds. Kirk's Current Veterinary Therapy XI: Small Animal Practice. Philadelphia: WB Saunders, 1992.

Fox JG. Diseases of the gastrointestinal system. In: Fox JG, ed. Biology and Diseases of the Ferret. 2nd Ed. Baltimore: Williams & Wilkins, 1998.

Hoefer HL, Bell JA. Gastrointestinal Diseases. In: Quesenberry KE, Carpenter JW, eds. Ferrets, Rabbits and Rodents: Clinical Medicine and Surgery. St. Louis: WB Saunders, 2004:25–40.

Jenkins JR. Rabbit and ferret liver and gastrointestinal testing. In: Fudge AM, ed. Laboratory Medicine, Avian and Exotic Pets. Philadelphia: W.B. Saunders, 2000.

Jenkins C, Bassett JR. Helicobacter infection. Compend Contin Edu Pract Vet 1997;19(3):267–279.

Marini RP, Fox JG, Taylor NS, et al. Ranitidine bismuth citrate and clarithromycin, alone or in combination, for eradication of Helicobacter mustelae infection in ferrets. Am J Vet Res 1999;60(10):1280–1286.

Williams BH, Kiupel M, West KH, et al. Coronavirus-associated epizootic catarrhal enteritis in ferrets. J Am Vet Med Assoc 2000;217:526–530.

*Portions Adapted From*

Walker MC. Anorexia. In: Tilley LP, Smith FWK, Jr., eds. The 5-Minute Veterinary Consult: Canine and Feline, 3rd Ed. Baltimore: Lippincott Williams & Wilkins, 2000.

# BASICS

## DEFINITION
The escape of fluid, either transudate or exudate, into the abdominal cavity between the parietal and visceral peritoneum

## PATHOPHYSIOLOGY
Ascites can be caused by the following:
• CHF and associated interference in venous return
• Depletion of plasma proteins associated with inappropriate loss of protein from renal or gastrointestinal disease—protein-losing nephropathy or enteropathy, respectively
• Obstruction of the vena cava or portal vein, or lymphatic drainage due to neoplastic occlusion
• Overt neoplastic effusion
• Peritonitis—infective or inflammatory
• Electrolyte imbalance, especially hypernatremia
• Liver cirrhosis

## SYSTEMS AFFECTED
• Cardiovascular
• Gastrointestinal
• Renal/urologic
• Hemic/lymph/immune

## SIGNALMENT
No age or sex predisposition

## SIGNS
• Episodic weakness, rear limb paresis or ataxia
• Lethargy
• Abdominal distension
• Abdominal discomfort when palpated
• Dyspnea from abdominal distension or associated pleural effusion
• Anorexia
• Weight gain

## CAUSES
• CHF
• Hypoproteinemia
• Renal disease
• Cirrhosis of liver
• Ruptured bladder
• Peritonitis
• Abdominal neoplasia
• Abdominal hemorrhage

## RISK FACTORS
N/A

# DIAGNOSIS

## DIFFERENTIAL DIAGNOSIS

### Differentiating Abdominal Distension Without Effusion
• Organomegaly—splenomegaly (most common), renomegaly (renal cysts), and hepatomegaly
• Obesity—extremely common
• Abdominal neoplasia
• Pregnancy
• Gastric dilatation (rare)

### Differentiating Diseases
• Transudate—right-sided CHF, hypoproteinemia, cirrhosis of liver, renal disease, and ruptured bladder
• Exudate—peritonitis, abdominal neoplasia, and hemorrhage

## CBC/BIOCHEMISTRY/URINALYSIS
• Neutrophilic leukocytosis occurs in patients with systemic infection.
• Albumin is low in patients with impaired liver synthesis, gastrointestinal loss, or renal loss.

### Liver Enzymes
• Low to normal in patients with impaired liver synthesis
• High in patients with liver inflammation and chronic passive congestion

### BUN and Creatinine
• High in patients with renal failure
• BUN low in patients with impaired liver synthesis

### Glucose
Low in patients with concurrent insulinoma or impaired liver synthesis

## OTHER LABORATORY TESTS
• To detect hypoproteinemia—protein electrophoresis

## IMAGING
• Thoracic and abdominal radiography to evaluate cardiac size and rule out organomegaly
• Ultrasonography of the heart, liver, spleen, pancreas, kidney, bladder, and abdomen can often determine cause.

## DIAGNOSTIC PROCEDURES
• Abdominocentesis—remove approximately 1–3 mL of abdominal fluid via aseptic technique; a portion of the sample for bacterial culture and antibiotic sensitivity
• Allows characterization of the fluid type and determination of potential underlying cause (following parameters extrapolated from canine and feline data)

### Transudate
• Clear and colorless
• Protein <2.5 g/dL
• Specific gravity <1.018
• Cells <1000/mm³—neutrophils and mesothelial cells

### Modified Transudate
• Red or pink; may be slightly cloudy
• Protein 2.5–5.0 g/dL
• Specific gravity >1.018
• Cells <5000 /mm³—neutrophils, mesothelial cells, erythrocytes, and lymphocytes

### Exudate (Nonseptic)
• Pink or white; cloudy
• Protein 2.5–5.0 g/dL
• Specific gravity >1.018
• Cells 5,000–50,000/mm³—neutrophils, mesothelial cells, macrophages, erythrocytes, and lymphocytes

### Exudate (Septic)
• Red, white, or yellow; cloudy
• Protein >4.0 g/dL
• Specific gravity >1.018
• Cells 5,000–100,000/mm³—neutrophils, mesothelial cells, macrophages, erythrocytes, lymphocytes, and bacteria

### Hemorrhage
• Red; spun supernatant clear and sediment red
• Protein >5.5 g/dL
• Specific gravity 1.007–1.027
• Cells consistent with peripheral blood
• Does not clot

### Urine
• Clear to pale yellow
• Protein >2.5 g/dL
• Specific gravity 1.000–1.040
• Cells 5,000–50,000/mm³—neutrophils, erythrocytes, lymphocytes, and macrophages

## ASCITES

### TREATMENT
• Can design treatment on an outpatient basis, with follow-up or inpatient care, depending on physical condition and underlying cause
• If patients are markedly uncomfortable when lying down or become more dyspneic with stress, consider removing enough ascites to reverse these signs.
• Dietary salt restriction may help control transudate fluid accumulation due to CHF, cirrhosis, or hypoproteinemia, but this may be difficult to achieve in ferrets.
• For exudate ascites control, address the underlying cause; corrective surgery may be indicated, followed by specific therapeutic management (e.g., tumor removed, abdominal bleeding controlled, blood transfusion administered).

### MEDICATIONS
**DRUG(S) OF CHOICE**
• Patients with liver insufficiency or CHF—diuretics such as furosemide (1–4 mg/kg PO, SC, IV, IM q8h–12h); sodium restriction possibly helpful, but difficult to achieve in ferrets
• Patients with hypoproteinemia and associated ascitic fluid accumulation—can treat as above with the addition of hetastarch (6% hetastarch in 0.9% NaCl); administer an IV bolus (10–20 mL/kg) slowly over 2–3 hours, then as a constant rate infusion of 1–2 mL/kg/hr for 24 hours; hetastarch increases plasma oncotic pressure and pulls fluid into the intravascular space.
• Systemic antibiotic therapy is dictated by bacterial identification and sensitivity testing in patients with septic exudate ascites.

**CONTRAINDICATIONS**
N/A

**PRECAUTIONS**
N/A

**POSSIBLE INTERACTIONS**
N/A

**ALTERNATIVE DRUGS**
N/A

### FOLLOW-UP
**PATIENT MONITORING**
• Varies with the underlying cause
• Check sodium, potassium, BUN, creatinine, and weight fluctuations periodically if the patient is maintained on a diuretic.

**POSSIBLE COMPLICATIONS**
Aggressive diuretic administration may cause hypokalemia

### MISCELLANEOUS
**ASSOCIATED CONDITIONS**
N/A

**AGE-RELATED FACTORS**
N/A

**ZOONOTIC POTENTIAL**
N/A

**PREGNANCY**
N/A

**SYNONYMS**
Abdominal effusion

**SEE ALSO**
• CHF
• Lymphosarcoma
• Neoplasia, digestive system

**ABBREVIATIONS**
• BUN = blood urea nitrogen
• CHF = congestive heart failure

*Suggested Reading*
Fox JG. Diseases of the gastrointestinal system. In: Fox JG, ed. Biology and Diseases of the Ferret. 2nd Ed. Baltimore: Williams & Wilkins, 1998.
Hoefer HL, Bell JA. Gastrointestinal diseases. In: Quesenberry KE, Carpenter JW, eds. Ferrets, Rabbits and Rodents: Clinical Medicine and Surgery. St. Louis: WB Saunders, 2004:25–40.
Jenkins JR. Rabbit and ferret liver and gastrointestinal testing. In: Fudge AM, ed. Laboratory Medicine, Avian and Exotic Pets. Philadelphia: W.B. Saunders, 2000.
Rosenthal K. Management of cardiac disease in ferrets. Waltham/OSU Symp Treatment Sm Anim Dis 1997;Sept.

*Portions Adapted From*
Thornhill JA. Ascites. In: Tilley LP, Smith FWK, Jr., eds. The 5-Minute Veterinary Consult: Canine and Feline, 3rd Ed. Baltimore: Lippincott Williams & Wilkins, 2003.

# BASICS

## DEFINITION
• A sign of sensory dysfunction that produces incoordination of the limbs, head, and/or trunk
• Three clinical types—sensory (proprioceptive), vestibular, and cerebellar; all produce changes in limb coordination, but vestibular and cerebellar ataxia also produce changes in head and neck movement.

## PATHOPHYSIOLOGY

### Sensory
• Proprioceptive pathways in the spinal cord relay limb and trunk position to the brain.
• When the spinal cord is slowly compressed, proprioceptive deficits are usually the first signs observed, because these pathways are located more superficially in the white matter and their larger-sized axons are more susceptible to compression than are other tracts.
• Generally accompanied by weakness owing to early concomitant upper motor neuron involvement

### Cerebellar
• The cerebellum regulates, coordinates, and smooths motor activity.
• Proprioception is normal, because the ascending proprioceptive pathways to the cortex are intact; weakness does not occur, because the upper motor neurons are intact.
• Inadequacy in the performance of motor activity; strength preservation; no proprioceptive deficits

### Vestibular—Unusual in Ferrets
• Diseases that affect the vestibular receptors, the nerve in the inner ear, or the nuclei in the brainstem cause various degrees of disequilibrium with ensuing vestibular ataxia.
• Affected animal leans, tips, falls, or even rolls toward the side of the lesion; may be accompanied by head tilt

## SYSTEMS AFFECTED
Nervous—spinal cord (and brainstem); cerebellum; vestibular system

## SIGNALMENT
Any age or sex

## SIGNS
• Important to define the type of ataxia to localize the problem

• Only hindlimbs affected—likely weakness due to systemic or metabolic disease (most common cause of ataxia in ferrets) or a spinal cord disorder
• Only one limb involved—consider a lameness problem.
• All or both ipsilateral limbs affected—cerebellar
• Head tilt—vestibular (rare)

## CAUSES

### Metabolic
Most Common Cause of Rear Limb Ataxia
• Hypoglycemia from insulinomas—extremely common cause
• Electrolyte disturbances—especially with gastrointestinal foreign bodies, severe hepatic disease, or sepsis
• Anemia—seen with hyperestrogenism, leukemia, and CRF

### Neurologic
Spinal Cord—Most Common Neurologic Cause
• Neoplastic—primary bone tumors (especially chondroma, chondrosarcoma); multiple myeloma and metastatic tumors that infiltrate the vertebral body (especially lymphoma)
• Traumatic—intervertebral disc herniation; fracture or luxation
• Vascular—hematomyelia due to the effects of hyperestrogenism (rare)
• Infectious—discospondylitis (rare); myelitis (not reported in ferrets but should be considered)

### Cerebellar
• Neoplastic—any tumor of the CNS (primary or secondary) localized to the cerebellum
• Infectious—CDV; rabies (rear limb ataxia may be the only clinical sign in ferrets with rabies) and any other CNS infection affecting the cerebellum
• Inflammatory, idiopathic, immune-mediated—ADV-induced encephalomyelitis
• Toxic—metronidazole

### Vestibular
• Infectious—CDV; otitis media or interna (rare)
• Neoplastic
• Traumatic
• Inflammatory, immune-mediated—ADV-induced meningoencephalomyelitis
• Toxic—metronidazole

### Miscellaneous
• Respiratory compromise
• Cardiac compromise
• Drugs—acepromazine; antihistamines; antiepileptics

## RISK FACTORS
N/A

# DIAGNOSIS

## DIFFERENTIAL DIAGNOSIS
• Differentiate the types of ataxia.
• Differentiate from other disease processes that can affect gait—musculoskeletal; metabolic; cardiovascular; respiratory.
• Musculoskeletal disorders—typically produce lameness and a reluctance to move
• Systemic illness and endocrine, cardiovascular, and metabolic disorders—can cause ataxia, especially of the pelvic limbs; usually other signs present such as weight loss, inappetence, ptyalism, hair loss, murmurs, arrhythmias, or collapse with exercise; suspect a non-neurologic cause and obtain minimum data from hemogram, biochemistry analysis, and urinalysis.
• Head tilt or nystagmus—likely vestibular
• Intention tremors of the head or hypermetria—likely cerebellar; sometimes metabolic disease
• Only limbs affected—likely spinal cord dysfunction. If all four limbs affected: lesion is in the cervical area or is multifocal to diffuse. Only pelvic limbs affected: may be metabolic disease or spinal cord dysfunction; spinal lesion is anywhere below the second thoracic vertebra

## CBC/BIOCHEMISTRY/URINALYSIS
Normal unless metabolic cause (e.g., hypoglycemia, electrolyte imbalance, and anemia)

## OTHER LABORATORY TESTS
• Hypoglycemia—simultaneous fasting glucose and insulin determination—may be supportive of a diagnosis of insulinoma if the insulin assay used has been validated for use in ferrets. Do not fast the ferret for longer than 4–6 hours. Monitor blood glucose concentrations every 30–60 minutes and discontinue testing when glucose concentration falls below 60 mg/dL.
• Anemia—differentiates as nonregenerative or regenerative on the basis of the reticulocyte count or bone marrow aspirate.
• Electrolyte imbalance—correct the problem; see if ataxia resolves.
• Serum electrophoresis—hypergammaglobulinemia (gammaglobulins >20% of total protein) seen in ferrets with ADV
• IFA—to rule out CDV; can be performed on peripheral blood, buffy coat smears, or conjunctival or mucous membrane scrapings.

## IMAGING
• Spinal radiographs—if spinal cord dysfunction suspected
• Bullae radiographs—if peripheral vestibular disease suspected (rare in ferrets); CT or MRI scans superior but more expensive

## ATAXIA

• Thoracic radiographs—identify neoplasia, cardiopulmonary disease
• CT or MRI—if cerebellar disease suspected; evaluate potential brain disease
• Abdominal ultrasonography—if neoplasia, hepatic, renal, adrenal, or pancreatic dysfunction suspected
• Echocardiography—if cardiac disease suspected

### DIAGNOSTIC PROCEDURES
• CSF—may confirm nervous system causes
• Myelography—may establish evidence of spinal cord compression. Use 22-g spinal needle; infuse iohexol (0.25–0.50 mL/kg)
• Location for CSF tap or myelography—atlanto-occipital region or L5–L6 region

### TREATMENT
• Usually outpatient, depending on the severity and acuteness of clinical signs
• Exercise—restrict if spinal cord disease suspected
• Client should monitor gait for increasing dysfunction or weakness; if paresis worsens or paralysis develops, other testing is warranted.

### MEDICATIONS

### DRUG(S) OF CHOICE
Not recommended until the source or cause of the problem is identified

### CONTRAINDICATIONS
N/A

### PRECAUTIONS
N/A

### POSSIBLE INTERACTIONS
N/A

### ALTERNATIVE DRUGS
N/A

### FOLLOW-UP

### PATIENT MONITORING
Periodic neurologic examinations to assess condition

### POSSIBLE COMPLICATIONS
• Depend on the underlying cause
• Spinal cord or neuromuscular disease—progression to weakness and possibly paralysis
• Hypoglycemia—seizures, stupor, coma

### MISCELLANEOUS

### ASSOCIATED CONDITIONS
N/A

### AGE-RELATED FACTORS
N/A

### ZOONOTIC POTENTIAL
Rabies—rare cause of ataxia in ferrets, but when present has extreme zoonotic potential. Rabies cases must be strictly quarantined and confined to prevent exposure to humans and other animals. Local and state regulations must be adhered to carefully and completely.

### PREGNANCY
N/A

### SYNONYMS
N/A

### SEE ALSO
• Parvovirus (ADV)
• Gastrointestinal foreign body
• Insulinoma
• Paresis and paralysis
• See specific diseases

### ABBREVIATIONS
• ADV = Aleutian disease virus (parvovirus)
• CDV = canine distemper virus
• CSF = cerebrospinal fluid
• CT = computed tomography
• IFA = immunofluorescent antibody test
• MRI = magnetic resonance imaging
• PNS = peripheral nervous system

*Suggested Reading*

Antinoff N. Musculoskeletal and neurologic diseases. In: Quesenberry KE, Carpenter JW, eds. Ferrets, Rabbits and Rodents: Clinical Medicine and Surgery. St. Louis: WB Saunders, 2004:115–120.

Caplan ER, Peterson ME, Mulles HS, et al. Diagnosis and treatment of insulin-secreting pancreatic islet cell tumors in ferrets: 57 cases (1986–1994). J Am Vet Med Assoc 1996;209:1741–1745.

Hoefer HL. Cardiac disease in ferrets. Proc North Am Vet Conf 1995; 577–578.

Une Y, Wakimoto Y, Kakano Y, et al. Spontaneous Aleutian disease in a ferret. J Vet Med Sci 2000;62(5):553–555.

*Portions Adapted From*

Shell LG. Ataxia. In: Tilley LP, Smith FWK, Jr., eds. The 5-Minute Veterinary Consult: Canine and Feline, 3rd Ed. Baltimore: Lippincott Williams & Wilkins, 2003.

BASICS

## OVERVIEW
• *Campylobacter jejuni*—fastidious, microaerophilic, Gram-negative curved bacteria; often isolated from the gastrointestinal tract of healthy ferrets and other mammals; usually not a primary cause of gastrointestinal disease in ferrets
• Disease seen in immunosuppressed animals; may be copathogen with other enteric pathogens (bacterial, viral, or protozoal). Ferrets with inflammatory bowel disease or intestinal lymphoma may become symptomatic.
• Infection—fecal–oral route from contamination of food, water, fresh meat (poultry, beef), and the environment
• Invasion of gastrointestinal mucosa—hematochezia; leukocytes in feces; ulceration; edema; congestion of intestine; bacteremia; occasionally septicemia and abortion; bacteria shed in feces for weeks to months
• Healthy adult ferrets often asymptomatic carriers—shedding of organism in feces carries health risk to owners and other household pets (cats, dogs)

## SIGNALMENT
Clinical disease more common in young or immunosuppressed animals

## SIGNS
• Diarrhea—ranges from mucous-like and watery to bloody or bile streaked; common; may be chronic
• Tenesmus common
• Fever (mild or absent), anorexia, and intermittent vomiting may accompany diarrhea.
• Young animals (up to 6 months of age)—clinical signs most severe; attributable to enterocolitis/diarrhea
• Adults—usually asymptomatic carriers

## CAUSES AND RISK FACTORS
• *C. jejuni*
• Kennels with poor sanitation and hygiene and fecal buildup in the environment
• Young animals—debilitated, immunosuppressed, or parasitized (e.g., *Giardia*, Coccidia, *Desulfovibrio* spp.)
• Nosocomial infection may develop in hospitalized patients.
• Adults—concurrent gastrointestinal disease (e.g., ECE, clostridia, *Salmonella*, *Giardia*, cryptosporidia, IBD, lymphoma)

 DIAGNOSIS

## DIFFERENTIAL DIAGNOSIS
• Signalment, history, physical examination, and fecal examination (direct smear and bacterial culture) enable diagnosis in most cases.
• Distinguish from other causes of acute enterocolitis.
• Bacterial enterocolitis—*Salmonella*, *Clostridium* spp.
• Parasitic enterocolitis—*Giardia*, *Isospora*, cryptosporidia
• Viral enterocolitis—ECE
• Dietary indiscretion or intolerance
• Inflammatory or infiltrative bowel disease

## CBC/BIOCHEMISTRY/URINALYSIS
• CBC—usually normal
• Biochemistry abnormalities—effects of diarrhea and dehydration (e.g., azotemia, electrolyte disturbances)

## OTHER LABORATORY TESTS
N/A

## IMAGING
N/A

## DIAGNOSTIC PROCEDURES
• Fecal leukocytes—in gastrointestinal tract and stool
• Fecal culture—microaerophilic at about 42°C for 48 hours on special *Campylobacter* blood agar plates

### Direct Examination of Feces
• Gram stain—make a smear of watery stool on a glass slide; heat fix; use Gram stain; leave counterstain (safranin) on for longer than usual.
• Wet mount—drop a small amount of stool (if not watery, mix with a small amount of saline or broth) on a glass slide; add a cover slip; view on phase or dark-field objective; note large numbers of curved, highly motile bacteria (characteristic darting motility).

 TREATMENT
• Mild enterocolitis—outpatient
• Severe enterocolitis—inpatient, especially immature patients; isolate
• Mild dehydration—oral fluid therapy with an enteric fluid replacement solution
• Severe dehydration—intravenous fluid therapy with balanced polyionic isotonic solution (e.g., lactated Ringer's)

 MEDICATIONS

## DRUG(S) OF CHOICE
• Treat any identified copathogens with the appropriate medication.
• Antibiotics—recommended for signs of systemic illness (e.g., fever or dehydration, diarrhea) and in immune-suppressed patients
• Erythromycin—10 mg/kg PO q6h for 5 days
• Chloramphenicol—25–50 mg/kg PO q12h for 5 days
• Neomycin—10–20 mg/kg PO q6h for 5 days; may be effective
• Metronidazole—15–20 mg/kg PO q12h for 5 days; may be effective
• Penicillins and ampicillin—potentially ineffective

## CONTRAINDICATIONS/POSSIBLE INTERACTIONS
Antidiarrheal drugs that reduce intestinal motility are contraindicated.

 FOLLOW-UP

## PATIENT MONITORING
Repeat fecal culture after completion of treatment.

## PREVENTION/AVOIDANCE
• Good hygiene (hand washing)
• Routinely clean and disinfect runs, food, and water bowls

## POSSIBLE COMPLICATIONS
Bacteremia, septicemia, and abortion

## EXPECTED COURSE AND PROGNOSIS
• Adults—usually self-limiting
• Juveniles with severe or persistent enterocolitis—treat with antibiotics

## CAMPYLOBACTERIOSIS

 MISCELLANEOUS

**ASSOCIATED CONDITIONS**
Concurrent infection with other pathogenic bacteria, enteric parasites, or viruses

**AGE-RELATED FACTORS**
Young animals at greatest risk

**ZOONOTIC POTENTIAL**
High potential to infect humans

**PREGNANCY**
Experimental infection with *Campylobacter* has been reported to cause abortion in pregnant jills.

**ABBREVIATIONS**
• ECE = epizootic catarrhal enteritis
• IBD = infiltrative bowel disease

*Suggested Reading*

Fox JG. Bacterial and mycoplasmal diseases. In: Fox JG, ed. Biology and Diseases of the Ferret. 2nd Ed. Baltimore: Williams & Wilkins, 1998:321–354.

Fox JG. Enteric bacterial infections. In: Greene CE, ed. Infectious Diseases of the Dog and Cat. Philadelphia: WB Saunders, 1998:226–229.

Hoefer HL, Bell JA. Gastrointestinal diseases. In: Quesenberry KE, Carpenter JW, eds. Ferrets, Rabbits and Rodents: Clinical Medicine and Surgery. St. Louis: WB Saunders, 2004:25–40.

*Portions Adapted From*

Legendre AM. Campybacteriosis. In: Tilley LP, Smith FWK, Jr., eds. The 5-Minute Veterinary Consult: Canine and Feline, 3rd Ed. Baltimore: Lippincott Williams & Wilkins, 2003.

# CANINE DISTEMPER VIRUS

## BASICS

### DEFINITION
- An acute contagious disease with respiratory, cutaneous, gastrointestinal, and CNS manifestations
- Caused by CDV, a Morbillivirus in the Paramyxoviridae family
- Distemper is uniformly fatal in ferrets.

### PATHOPHYSIOLOGY
- Natural route of infection—airborne and droplet exposure through contact with affected animals or fomites
- From the nasal cavity, pharynx, and lungs, macrophages carry the virus to local lymph nodes, where virus replication occurs; spreads via viremia to the surface epithelium of respiratory, gastrointestinal, and urogenital tracts and to the CNS
- Viremia occurs within 2 days of exposure, and virus can be detected in nasal exudates within 5–13 days postexposure.
- Incubation period is 7–10 days.
- In unvaccinated ferrets—death occurs from 12–35 days postexposure, depending on the strain of virus.

### SYSTEMS AFFECTED
- Multisystemic—all lymphatic tissues; surface epithelium in the respiratory, alimentary, and urogenital tracts; endocrine and exocrine glands
- Nervous—skin; gray and white matter in the CNS

### GENETICS
N/A

### INCIDENCE/PREVALENCE
- Ferrets—sporadic outbreaks in unvaccinated colonies and animal shelters
- Wildlife (raccoons, skunks, foxes)—fairly common

### GEOGRAPHIC DISTRIBUTION
Worldwide

### SIGNALMENT

#### Species
- Most species of the order Carnivora—Canidae, Hyaenidae, Mustelidae, Procyonidae, Viverridae
- Felidae families—recent; large cats in California zoos and in Tanzania

#### Breed Predilection
N/A

#### Mean Age and Range
Young animals are more susceptible than are adults.

#### Predominant Sex
N/A

### SIGNS
- Catarrhal phase occurs 7–10 days postexposure—fever, serous nasal and ocular discharge, sneezing, depression, and anorexia
- 10–15 days following exposure, a characteristic, erythematous, pruritic rash appears on the chin and lips and spreads caudally to the inguinal area.
- Mucopurulent nasocular discharge occurs with secondary bacterial infections; crusts appear on the eyes, nose, and chin.
- Hardening of the footpads (hyperkeratosis) and nose is common.
- Coughing is common, since the primary site of virus replication is the lungs; secondary bacterial pneumonia is common in ferrets not treated with antibiotics.
- Vomiting, diarrhea, and melena occurs in some ferrets.
- CNS—CNS signs are seen in many infected ferrets; signs often (but not always) occur following systemic disease; depends on the virus strain; either acute gray matter disease (seizures and myoclonus with depression) or subacute white matter disease (incoordination ataxia, paresis, paralysis, and muscle tremors); meningeal signs of hyperesthesia and cervical rigidity may be seen in both.

### CAUSES
- CDV, a Morbillivirus within the Paramyxoviridae family; same virus that infects dogs; closely related to measles virus, rinderpest virus of cattle, and phocine (seal) and dolphin distemper viruses
- Secondary bacterial infections frequently involve the respiratory and gastrointestinal systems.

### RISK FACTORS
Contact of nonimmunized animals with CDV-infected animals (ferrets, dogs, or wild carnivores)

## DIAGNOSIS
A presumptive diagnosis of CDV may be made in any unvaccinated ferret with fever and characteristic respiratory and cutaneous signs.

### DIFFERENTIAL DIAGNOSIS
- Influenza virus—CDV can be difficult to differentiate from influenza virus during the early, catarrhal phase. Influenza is self-limiting, whereas CDV will progress and dermatologic signs will follow.
- Enteric signs—differentiate from *Helicobacter*, ECE, gastrointestinal foreign body, and inflammatory bowel disease. Respiratory or dermatologic signs seen with CDV do not occur with these diseases.
- CNS signs—rabies

### CBC/BIOCHEMISTRY/URINALYSIS
Lymphopenia during early infection

### OTHER LABORATORY TESTS
An immunofluorescent antibody (IFA) test can be performed on peripheral blood, buffy coat smears, or conjunctival or mucous membrane scrapings. False negatives may occur. Vaccination will not affect the results.

### IMAGING
Radiographs—determine the extent of pneumonia; lung lobe consolidation is common.

### DIAGNOSTIC PROCEDURES
Postmortem diagnosis—histopathology, immunofluorescence and/or immunocytochemistry, virus isolation, and/or PCR; preferred tissues from lungs, stomach, urinary bladder, lymphs, and brain

### PATHOLOGIC FINDINGS

#### Gross
- Mucopurulent discharges—from eyes and nose, bronchopneumonia, catarrhal enteritis, and skin pustules; probably caused by secondary bacterial infections; commonly seen
- Generalized dermatitis
- Footpads and nose—hyperkeratosis
- Lungs—patchy consolidation as a result of interstitial pneumonia

#### Histologic
- Intracytoplasmic eosinophilic inclusion bodies—frequently found in epithelium of the bronchi, liver, and urinary bladder; also seen in reticulum cells and leukocytes in lymphatic tissues
- Inclusion bodies in the CNS—glial cells and neurons; frequently intranuclear; can also be found in cytoplasm
- Staining by fluorescent antibody or immunoperoxidase may detect viral antigen where inclusion bodies are not seen.

## TREATMENT

### APPROPRIATE HEALTH CARE
Inpatients and in isolation to prevent infection of other ferrets and dogs

### NURSING CARE
- Symptomatic supportive care may prolong the life of the animal by days to weeks; however, CDV is uniformly fatal in ferrets.
- Intravenous fluids—with anorexia and diarrhea

### ACTIVITY
Limited

## CANINE DISTEMPER VIRUS

### DIET
Depends on the extent of gastrointestinal involvement; offer meat baby foods if anorectic.

### CLIENT EDUCATION
Inform client that mortality rate is 100%.

### SURGICAL CONSIDERATIONS
N/A

## MEDICATIONS

### DRUG(S) OF CHOICE
• Antiviral drugs—none known to be effective
• Antibiotics—to reduce secondary bacterial infection, because CDV is highly immunosuppressive

### CONTRAINDICATIONS
Corticosteroids—do not use, because they augment the immunosuppression and may enhance viral dissemination.

### PRECAUTIONS
N/A

### POSSIBLE INTERACTIONS
N/A

### ALTERNATIVE DRUGS
N/A

## FOLLOW-UP

### PATIENT MONITORING
• Monitor for signs of pneumonia or dehydration from diarrhea in the acute phase of the disease.
• Monitor for development of rash or hyperkeratosis.
• Monitor for CNS signs.

### PREVENTION/AVOIDANCE
• Avoid infection of kits by isolation to prevent infection from wildlife (e.g., raccoons, foxes, skunks) or from CDV-infected dogs or ferrets.
• Recovered dogs are not carriers.

### Vaccines
• MLV-CD—prevents infection and disease. Only chick embryo–adapted vaccines should be used in ferrets. Vaccines available include PureVax (Merial, Athens, GA), and Fervac-D (United Vaccines Inc., Madison, WI). Canine or ferret tissue culture–adapted vaccines can induce disease and should never be used.
• Begin vaccination at 6–8 weeks of age, and vaccinate every 3–4 weeks until the ferret is 14 weeks old, followed by annual boosters.
• Killed vaccines do not offer reliable, consistent protection.

### Maternal Antibody
Most kits lose protection from maternal antibody at 6–12 weeks of age.

### POSSIBLE COMPLICATIONS
Hypersensitivity reactions to CDV vaccination are common and may be fatal; premedication with diphenhydramine (0.5–2.0 mg/kg PO, IM, IVq8–12h) may prevent reaction; monitor closely following vaccination for collapse, vomiting, hemorrhagic diarrhea, or shock.

### EXPECTED COURSE AND PROGNOSIS
• Death—12–35 days after infection; mortality rate approximately 100%
• Euthanasia—owner may elect once definitive diagnosis is made.

## MISCELLANEOUS

### ASSOCIATED CONDITIONS
Secondary bacterial rhinitis and pneumonia

### AGE-RELATED FACTORS
Unvaccinated ferrets of any age are extremely susceptible to infection followed by death due to CDV.

### ZOONOTIC POTENTIAL
Possible that humans may become subclinically infected with CDV; immunization against measles virus also protects against CDV infection.

### PREGNANCY
In utero infection of fetuses—occurs in dogs, but has not been documented in ferrets

### SYNONYMS
• Paramyxovirus
• Hard pad disease

### ABBREVIATIONS
• CDV = canine distemper virus
• CNS = central nervous system
• ECE = epizootic catarrhal enteritis
• PCR = polymerase chain reaction
• MLV = modified live virus

*Suggested Reading*

Antinoff N. Musculoskeletal and neurologic diseases. In: Quesenberry KE, Carpenter JW, eds. Ferrets, Rabbits and Rodents: Clinical Medicine and Surgery. St. Louis: WB Saunders, 2004:115–120.

Benson KG, Paul-Murphy J, Ramer JC. Evaluating and stabilizing the critical ferret: basic diagnostic and therapeutic techniques. Compend Contin Edu Pract Vet 2000;22:490–497.

Fox JG, Pearson RC, Gorham JR: Viral diseases. In: Fox JG, ed. Biology and Diseases of the Ferret. 2nd Ed. Baltimore: Williams & Wilkins, 1998.

Hoover JP, Baldwin CA, Rupprecht CE. Serologic response of domestic ferrets (Mustela putorius furo) to canine distemper and rabies virus vaccines. J Am Vet Med Assoc 1989;194(2):234–238.

Williams BH. Ferret microbiology and virology. In: Fudge AM, ed. Laboratory Medicine, Avian and Exotic Pets. Philadelphia: WB Saunders, 2000:334–342.

Williams BH. Therapeutics in ferrets. Vet Clin North Am Exotic Anim Pract 2000;3(1):131–153.

*Portions Adapted From*

Appel MJG. Canine Distemper. In: Tilley LP, Smith FWK, Jr., eds. The 5-Minute Veterinary Consult: Canine and Feline, 3rd Ed. Baltimore: Lippincott Williams & Wilkins, 2003.

# BASICS

## DEFINITION
Dilated cardiomyopathy is a disease of the ventricular muscle characterized by systolic myocardial failure and an enlarged, volume-overloaded heart that leads to signs of congestive heart failure (CHF) or low cardiac output.

## PATHOPHYSIOLOGY
• Myocardial failure leads to reduced cardiac output and CHF.

## SYSTEMS AFFECTED
• Cardiovascular
• Respiratory—pulmonary edema
• Renal/urologic—prerenal azotemia
• All organ systems are affected by reductions in cardiac output

## INCIDENCE/PREVALENCE
Exact incidence/prevalence has not been documented; however, cardiac disease is common in ferrets, and dilated cardiomyopathy is the most commonly diagnosed heart disease in ferrets.

## SIGNALMENT
Middle-aged to older ferrets; 4 years average age; no sex predilection

## SIGNS

### Historical Findings
*Signs Related to Low Cardiac Output*
• Weakness—usually manifested as rear limb weakness, ataxia, or paresis
• Anorexia
• Depression
• Some ferrets are asymptomatic.
*Signs Related to CHF*
• Dyspnea
• Tachypnea
• Abdominal distension in animals with ascites, hepatomegaly, or splenomegaly (splenomegaly often an incidental finding)

### Physical Examination Findings
• Cardiac auscultation—the heart is located more caudally in the thoracic cavity, extending from the caudal border of the seventh to eighth rib; may hear soft systolic heart murmur, gallop rhythm, or other arrhythmia
• Breath sounds are muffled if there is pleural effusion; crackles if there is pulmonary edema
• Prolonged capillary refill time or cyanosis possible
• Posterior paresis
• Pulse deficits possible with atrial fibrillation, ventricular premature contractions, and paroxysmal ventricular tachycardia.
• Jugular pulses possible from tricuspid regurgitation, arrhythmias, or right-sided CHF
• Hepatomegaly with or without ascites

• Splenomegaly (may be related to congestion, or an incidental finding in older ferrets)
• Hypothermia

## CAUSES AND RISK FACTORS
The underlying etiology of idiopathic dilated cardiomyopathy remains unknown. Taurine deficiency is not believed to be a cause.

# DIAGNOSIS

## DIFFERENTIAL DIAGNOSIS
• Rear limb weakness—consider metabolic disease including hypoglycemia (especially insulinoma); anemia (hyperestrogenism, blood loss from gastrointestinal tract, leukemia, CRF); gastrointestinal foreign body; neurologic disease including CNS or spinal cord disease; CDV or rabies
• Pleural effusion—mediastinal lymphoma, other neoplasia, abscess, chylothorax
• Cough—infection (influenza virus, CDV, bacterial tracheitis, bronchitis, pneumonia); neoplasia; heartworm disease
• Dyspnea—neoplasm (mediastinal lymphoma), primary pulmonary disease, pleural effusion, trauma resulting in diaphragmatic hernia, pulmonary hemorrhage, pneumothorax, airway obstruction due to foreign body
• Myocardial failure secondary to long-standing congenital or acquired left ventricular volume overload diseases

## CBC/BIOCHEMISTRY/URINALYSIS
Routine hematologic tests and urinalysis are usually normal unless altered by severe heart failure (e.g., prerenal azotemia, high ALT, hyponatremia), therapy for heart failure (e.g., hypokalemia, hypochloremia), or concurrent disease

## OTHER LABORATORY TESTS
Heartworm serologic testing—ELISA (Snap heartworm antigen test, Idexx Laboratories)

## IMAGING

### Radiographic Findings
• Radiography often shows pleural effusion or pulmonary edema.
• The cardiac silhouette typically is enlarged in a globoid manner.
• Hepatomegaly, splenomegaly, or ascites may be seen.
• Important tool for ruling out mediastinal lymphoma in dyspneic ferrets

### Echocardiographic Findings
• Echocardiography is the diagnostic modality of choice.
• Characteristic findings include thin ventricular walls, enlarged left ventricular end-systolic and end-diastolic dimensions, left atrial enlargement, and low fractional shortening.

## DIAGNOSTIC TESTS

### Electrocardiography
• Often is normal and may not be helpful in the diagnosis
• Ferrets resist attachment of alligator clips; use padded clips, soft clips, or isoflurane anesthesia to perform ECG; active ferrets may be distracted and will remain still when fed Nutri-Cal while the ECG is being performed
• Pronounced respiratory sinus arrhythmias are common in normal ferrets and should not be overinterpreted.
• The ECG of normal ferrets differs from the feline ECG in that R waves are taller, and a short QT interval and/or elevated ST segment are commonly seen.
• Both ventricular and supraventricular arrhythmias can be seen.
• First- or second-degree heart block are common findings both in normal ferrets and ferrets with DCM.
• May show left atrial or ventricular enlargement patterns

### Pleural Effusion Analysis
Pleural effusion typically is a modified transudate. Analysis of the pleural effusion is important to rule out other causes of pleural effusion such as pyothorax, lymphosarcoma, or chylothorax.

## PATHOLOGIC FINDINGS
• Heart:body ratio is increased.
• Ventricle walls are thin and the lumen is enlarged.
• Valve anatomy is normal.
• Histopathology shows myocardial degeneration, necrosis, and myocardial fibrosis.

# TREATMENT

## APPROPRIATE HEALTH CARE
• Severely dyspneic, weak, or anorectic ferrets in congestive heart failure should be treated as inpatients.
• Mildly affected animals can be treated as outpatients.

## NURSING CARE
• Thoracocentesis is both therapeutic and diagnostic. If there is significant pleural effusion, drain each hemithorax with a 20-gauge butterfly catheter after the ferret is stable enough to be handled. When performing thoracocentesis be aware that the heart is located much more caudally within the thorax in the ferret as compared to dogs and cats. Sedation (midazolam 0.3–1.0 mg/kg IM, SC, or ketamine 10–20 mg/kg IM plus diazepam 1–2 mg/kg IM) or anesthesia with isoflurane by mask may be necessary.
• Supplemental oxygen therapy is beneficial for ferrets in congestive heart failure.

## CARDIOMYOPATHY, DILATED

• Minimize handling of critically dyspneic animals. Stress can kill!
• If hypothermic, external heat (incubator or heating pad) is recommended.

### ACTIVITY
Restrict if possible.

### DIET
Most anorectic ferrets will accept high-calorie dietary supplements such as Clinicare Feline liquid diet (Abbott Laboratories, North Chicago, IL), canned chicken human baby foods, and Eukanuba Maximum Calorie diet (Iams Co., Dayton, OH). A low-sodium diet is not palatable to ferrets.

### CLIENT EDUCATION
Emphasize potential signs associated with progression of disease and adverse side effects of medication.

### SURGICAL CONSIDERATIONS
N/A

## MEDICATIONS

### DRUG(S) OF CHOICE
• Furosemide is recommended at the lowest effective dose to eliminate pulmonary edema and pleural effusion. If the ferret is in fulminant cardiac failure, administer furosemide at 2–4 mg/kg q8–12h IM or IV. Initially, furosemide should be administered parenterally. Long-term therapy should be continued at a dose of 1–2 mg/kg q8–q12h PO. The pediatric elixir is generally well accepted.
• Nitroglycerin (2% ointment) 1/16–1/8 inch applied topically to hairless areas can be used in conjunction with diuretics in the acute management of congestive heart failure to further reduce preload. Nitroglycerin will lower the dose of furosemide and is particularly useful in patients with hypothermia or dehydration.
• Enalapril is recommended for long-term maintenance to reduce afterload and preload. Begin with a dose of 0.25–0.5 mg/kg PO q48h and increase to q24h dosing if well tolerated (see precautions). Enalapril can be compounded into a suspension by a compounding pharmacy for ease of administration.
• Digoxin is recommended to strengthen contractility at a dose of 0.005–0.01 mg/kg PO q12–24h. If serum digoxin concentrations remain low, this dose may be increased to q12h dosing. Be certain to monitor serum digoxin concentrations and clinical signs of toxicity at this dose.
• In the case of atrial fibrillation, slowing of the ventricular rate response may be achieved with chronic administration of digoxin combined with propanolol (0.2–1.0 mg/kg q8–12h).
• Therapeutic goal is obtaining a ventricular rate between 180 and 250 bpm at rest.

### CONTRAINDICATIONS
Digoxin should be avoided in severe uncontrolled paroxysmal ventricular tachycardia.

### PRECAUTIONS
• Ferrets are very sensitive to the hypotensive effects of ACE inhibitors and may become weak and lethargic. The dosage should be reduced if this side effect is observed or hypotension is documented.
• Beta blockers and calcium channel blockers are negative inotropes and may have an acute adverse effect on myocardial function, although recent human studies have suggested that chronic administration of beta blockers may be of benefit in DCM.
• The combination of diuretics and ACE inhibitors may result in azotemia, especially in patients with severe heart failure or preexisting renal dysfunction.
• Overzealous diuretic therapy may cause dehydration and hypokalemia.
• Digoxin dose should be reduced if renal insufficiency is documented or suspected.

### POSSIBLE INTERACTIONS
Renal dysfunction and hypokalemia predispose to digitalis intoxication

### ALTERNATIVE DRUGS
• Other vasodilators, including hydralazine, may be used instead of or in addition to an ACE inhibitor. Dosages have been anecdotally extrapolated from feline dosages; however, their use is not widespread, and efficacy and safety are unknown (beware of hypotension).
• Other beta blockers, such as atenolol, carvedilol, or metoprolol, can be used instead of propranolol to help control ventricular response rate in atrial fibrillation. Dosages have been anecdotally extrapolated from feline dosages; however, their use is not widespread, and efficacy and safety are unknown.

## FOLLOW-UP

### PATIENT MONITORING
• Repeat thoracic radiographs in 1 week to determine efficacy of therapy.
• Periodically monitor electrolyte and renal parameters.
• Digoxin concentrations should be measured 2 weeks after initiating therapy. Therapeutic range (as extrapolated from dogs and cats) is between 1 and 2 ng/dL 8–12 hours postpill.
• Monitor blood pressure in ferrets treated with Enalapril.

### PREVENTION/AVOIDANCE
N/A

### POSSIBLE COMPLICATIONS
• Sudden death due to arrhythmias
• Iatrogenic problems associated with medical management (see above)

### EXPECTED COURSE AND PROGNOSIS
• Always fatal
• Patients can usually experience a good quality of life for 6–24 months following diagnosis.

## MISCELLANEOUS

### ASSOCIATED CONDITIONS
Ferrets with heart disease often have concurrent insulinoma, adrenal disease, or neoplasia.

### AGE-RELATED FACTORS
Prevalence increases with age.

### ZOONOTIC POTENTIAL
N/A

### PREGNANCY
N/A

### SYNONYMS
Congestive cardiomyopathy

### SEE ALSO
• Dyspnea and tachypnea
• Heartworm disease
• Lymphosarcoma

### ABBREVIATIONS
• ACE = angiotensin-converting enzyme
• ALT = alanine aminotransferase
• CDV = canine distemper virus
• CNS = central nervous system
• CRF = chronic renal failure
• DCM = dilated cardiomyopathy
• ELISA = enzyme-linked immunosorbent assay
• FS% = percent fractional shortening

### Suggested Reading
Rosenthal KL. Respiratory diseases. In Quesenberry KE, Carpenter JW, eds. Ferrets, Rabbits and Rodents: Clinical Medicine and Surgery. St. Louis: WB Saunders, 2004:72–78.
Petrie JP, Morrisey JK. Cardiovascular and other diseases. In: Quesenberry KE, Carpenter JW, eds. Ferrets, Rabbits and Rodents: Clinical Medicine and Surgery. St. Louis: WB Saunders, 2004:58–71.

### Portions Adapted From
DeFrancesco TC. Cardiomyopathy, Dilated—Cats. Miller MW. Cardiomyopathy, Dilated—Dogs. In: Tilley LP, Smith FWK, Jr., eds. The 5-Minute Veterinary Consult: Canine and Feline, 3rd Ed. Baltimore: Lippincott Williams & Wilkins, 2003.

# CARDIOMYOPATHY, HYPERTROPHIC

## BASICS

### OVERVIEW
• Hypertrophic cardiomyopathy is a rare disease in ferrets characterized by concentric hypertrophy (increased wall thickness) of the ventricular free wall or the intraventricular septum of the nondilated left ventricle.
• The disease occurs independently of other cardiac disorders that may cause concentric hypertrophy (e.g., aortic stenosis) or systemic disorders. Hypertrophy secondary to hypertension or hyperthyroidism has not been reported in ferrets.
• Increased LV wall thickness leads to impaired ventricular filling (due to lack of compliance).
• High left ventricular filling pressure develops, causing left atrial enlargement.
• Mitral insufficiency may develop secondary to structural and/or functional changes of the mitral valve.
• Pulmonary venous hypertension causes pulmonary edema. Some ferrets develop biventricular failure (i.e., pulmonary edema, pleural effusion, and rarely ascites).

### SIGNALMENT
• The incidence of HCM in ferrets is very low, such that accurate accounts of signalment are lacking.
• HCM appears to be more common in young ferrets as compared to DCM, which is seen more often in ferrets > 4 years old.

### SIGNS

#### Historical Findings
• Asymptomatic (frequently)
• Sudden death (especially during anesthesia)
*Signs Related to Low Cardiac Output*
• Weakness—usually manifested as rear limb weakness, ataxia, or paresis
• Anorexia
• Depression
*Signs Related to Congestive Heart Failure*
• Dyspnea
• Tachypnea

#### Physical Examination Findings
• May be normal
• Tachycardia
• Arrhythmia
• Systolic murmur in some animals
• Muffled heart sounds, lack of chest compliance, and dyspnea characterized by rapid shallow respirations may be associated with pleural effusion.
• Dyspnea and louder than normal lung sounds and crackles if pulmonary edema is present
• Arrhythmia in some animals

### CAUSES AND RISK FACTORS
The cause of hypertrophic cardiomyopathy is unknown. Genetic abnormalities in genes coding for myocardial contractile proteins have been documented in humans and in cats but not in ferrets.

## DIAGNOSIS

### DIFFERENTIAL DIAGNOSIS
• Rear limb weakness—consider metabolic disease including hypoglycemia (especially insulinoma); anemia (hyperestrogenism, blood loss from gastrointestinal tract, leukemia, CRF); gastrointestinal foreign body; neurologic disease including CNS or spinal cord disease; CDV or rabies
• Pleural effusion—mediastinal lymphoma, other neoplasia, abscess, chylothorax
• Cough—infection (influenza virus, CDV, bacterial tracheitis, bronchitis, pneumonia); neoplasia; heartworm disease
• Dyspnea—neoplasm (mediastinal lymphoma), primary pulmonary disease, pleural effusion, trauma resulting in diaphragmatic hernia, pulmonary hemorrhage, pneumothorax, airway obstruction due to foreign body
• Ascites, abdominal distension—consider hypoproteinemia, severe liver disease, ruptured bladder, peritonitis, abdominal neoplasia, and abdominal hemorrhage.
• Infiltrative cardiac disorders
• Other causes of CHF

### CBC/BIOCHEMISTRY/URINALYSIS
• Results usually normal
• Prerenal azotemia in some animals

### OTHER LABORATORY TESTS
Heartworm serologic testing—ELISA (Snap heartworm antigen test, Idexx Laboratories)

### IMAGING

#### Radiography
• May be normal
• Generalized cardiomegaly and LA or LV enlargement may be seen
• Pulmonary edema or pleural effusion or both in some animals
• The different forms of cardiomyopathy cannot be differentiated by radiography

#### Echocardiography
• Marked thickening of the left ventricular free walls and interventricular septum
• Normal or reduced left ventricular lumen
• Left atrial enlargement
• Normal or high fractional shortening
• Mitral regurgitation
• Hypovolemia may cause the heart wall to appear thickened, mimicking HCM.

### OTHER DIAGNOSTIC PROCEDURES

#### Electrocardiography
• May be normal
• Sinus tachycardia (HR >280) is common.
• Atrial premature complexes and ventricular premature complexes occasionally

### PATHOLOGIC FINDINGS
• Abnormal heart:body weight ratio
• Nondilated left ventricle with hypertrophy of intraventricular septum or left ventricular free wall
• Left atrial enlargement
• Myocardial scarring

## TREATMENT
• Outpatient management unless in congestive heart failure
• Oxygen if dyspneic
• Minimize handling of critically dyspneic animals. Stress can kill!
• Thoracocentesis is both therapeutic and diagnostic. If there is significant pleural effusion, drain each hemithorax with a 20-gauge butterfly catheter after the ferret is stable enough to be handled. When performing thoracocentesis be aware that the heart is located much more caudally within the thorax in the ferret as compared to dogs and cats. Sedation (midazolam 0.3–1.0 mg/kg IM, SC, or ketamine 10–20 mg/kg IM plus diazepam 1–2 mg/kg IM) or anesthesia with isoflurane by mask may be necessary.
• Warm environment if hypothermic

## MEDICATIONS

### DRUG(S) OF CHOICE

#### Beta Blockers
• Dosage—propranolol (0.2–1.0 mg/kg q8–12h) or atenolol (3.125–6.25 mg/ferret PO q24h)
• Beneficial effects may include slowing of sinus rate and correcting atrial and ventricular arrhythmias.
• Role in asymptomatic patients unresolved

#### Diltiazem
• Dosage—3.75–7.5 mg/ferret PO q12h
• Beneficial effects may include slower sinus rate, resolution of supraventricular arrhythmias, improved diastolic relaxation, and peripheral vasodilation, but this has not been documented in ferrets.
• Role in asymptomatic patients unresolved

### Furosemide
• Indicated to treat pulmonary edema, pleural effusion, and ascites
• Dosage—for acutely dyspneic animals: 2–4 mg/kg q8–12h IM or IV. Initially, furosemide should be administered parenterally.
• Once pulmonary edema resolves, taper the dosage to the lowest that controls edema (usually1–2 mg/kg q12h PO) for long-term therapy). The pediatric elixir is generally well accepted.
• Not indicated in asymptomatic patients

### Nitroglycerin 2% Ointment
• Venodilation lowers atrial filling pressures, thereby reducing pulmonary edema and pleural effusion.
• May be used in the acute stabilization of ferrets with severe pulmonary edema or pleural effusion
• Dosage—1/16–1/8 inch applied topically to non-haired areas can be used in conjunction with diuretics in the acute management of congestive heart failure.
• When used intermittently, it may be useful for long-term management.

### CONTRAINDICATIONS/POSSIBLE INTERACTIONS
• Positive inotropic drugs should be avoided.
• The use of a calcium channel blocker in combination with a beta blocker should be avoided because clinically significant bradyarrhythmias can develop in other small animals and are likely to also occur in ferrets.
• The use of potent arteriolar dilators should be avoided in patients with dynamic LV outflow tract obstruction. However, the use of milder vasodilators such as ACE inhibitors in patients with congestive heart failure is generally well tolerated.

• Overzealous diuretic therapy may cause dehydration and hypokalemia.

### PRECAUTIONS
• Atenolol, enalapril, propanolol, and diltiazem may all cause lethargy, anorexia and hypotension.

### ALTERNATIVE DRUGS

#### Enalapril
• Dosage—0.25–0.5 mg/kg PO q48h and increase to q24h dosing if well tolerated
• Ferrets are very sensitive to the hypotensive effects of ACE inhibitors and may become weak and lethargic. The dosage should be reduced if this side effect is observed or hypotension is documented.
• The combination of diuretics and ACE inhibitors may result in azotemia, especially in patients with severe heart failure or pre-existing renal dysfunction

## FOLLOW-UP
• Reevaluation depends on the severity of the clinical signs. Reevaluation with radiography and echocardiography may be useful to characterize disease progression and make appropriate medication adjustments.
• Observe closely for signs of dyspnea, lethargy, weakness, anorexia, and posterior paralysis.
• If treating with enalapril, monitor renal function and blood pressure.
• Due to the rarity of this condition in ferrets, information regarding prognosis is lacking. In ferrets with severe congestive heart failure or other complications, prognosis is generally guarded.

## MISCELLANEOUS

### ABBREVIATIONS
• ACE = angiotensin-converting enzyme
• CDV = canine distemper virus
• CHF = congestive heart failure
• CNS = central nervous system
• CRF = chronic renal failure
• DCM = dilated cardiomyopathy
• ELISA = enzyme-linked immunosorbent assay
• HCM = hypertrophic cardiomyopathy
• LV = left ventricle
• LA = left atrium

### Suggested Reading
Fox JG. Other systemic diseases. In: Fox JG, ed. Biology and Diseases of the Ferret. 2nd Ed. Baltimore: Williams & Wilkins, 1998:307–320.

Hoefer HL. Cardiac disease in ferrets. Proc North Am Vet Conf 1995;577–578.

Rosenthal K. Management of cardiac disease in ferrets. Waltham/OSU Symp Treatment Sm Anim Dis 1997; Sept.

Rosenthal KL. Respiratory diseases. In: Quesenberry KE, Carpenter JW, eds. Ferrets, Rabbits and Rodents: Clinical Medicine and Surgery. St. Louis: WB Saunders, 2004:72–78.

Petrie JP, Morrisey JK. Cardiovascular and other diseases. In: Quesenberry KE, Carpenter JW, eds. Ferrets, Rabbits and Rodents: Clinical Medicine and Surgery. St. Louis: WB Saunders, 2004:58–71.

### Portions Adapted From
Smith FWK, Jr., Keene, BW. Cardiomyopathy, Hypertropic—Cats. Kienle, RD. Cardiomyopathy, Hypertropic—Dogs. In: Tilley LP, Smith FWK, Jr., eds. The 5-Minute Veterinary Consult: Canine and Feline, 3rd Ed. Baltimore: Lippincott Williams & Wilkins, 2003.

# CLOSTRIDIAL ENTEROTOXICOSIS

 BASICS

## OVERVIEW

• Clostridial enterotoxicosis is a relatively uncommon disease in ferrets. Two clinical syndromes may be seen with clostridial enterotoxicosis. One is a syndrome characterized by diarrhea due to enterotoxin production by certain strains of enteric *Clostridium perfringens* (CP). The second, more serious syndrome is characterized by acute gastrointestinal bloating due to gas production by CP organisms.
• CP is a common enteric inhabitant generally found in the vegetative form living in a symbiotic relationship with the host.
• Certain strains of CP appear to be genetically capable of producing enterotoxin that binds to the enteric mucosa, alters cell permeability, and results in cell damage and/or subsequent cell death. Depending on the strain of organism and host defenses, CP may cause mild disease with anorexia and diarrhea or life-threatening disease with severe abdominal distention, gastrointestinal bloating, and, in some cases, peracute death.
• Enterotoxin production is associated with enteric sporulation of CP.
• A number of intrinsic host-related factors appear to influence enterotoxin production and pathogenicity of CP.

## SIGNALMENT

• A relatively uncommon disease in ferrets; often a copathogen
• No age or sex predilections

## SIGNS

### General Comments

Clinical syndromes are associated with either diarrhea or serious, life-threatening disease associated with severe gastrointestinal bloating.

### Historical Findings

• Most common—large or small bowel diarrhea, often green in color with mucous, small amounts of fresh blood, small scant stools, and tenesmus with an increased frequency of stools; other signs include anorexia, abdominal discomfort, or generalized unthriftiness.
• Occasionally, acute severe bloating of the stomach and/or small intestines with gas occurs ("bloat syndrome"). The severity of signs depends on the degree of gastric/intestinal distension, which may vary from moderate to severe. Signs include acute depression, ptyalism, anorexia, weakness, collapse, or acute death. Owners may note progressive abdominal distension.
• May be a history of prolonged antibiotic use

• Severe acute "bloat syndrome" has been associated with overeating of meat or household garbage.
• May be a nosocomial (hospital-acquired) disease with signs precipitated during or shortly following hospitalization or boarding.

### Physical Examination Findings

*Mild to Moderate Diarrhea*
• Abdominal discomfort and gas or fluid-filled intestines may be detected on palpation.
• May be evidence of blood or mucous in the feces

*Bloat Syndrome*
• Abdominal distension
• Tympanic cranial abdomen
• Tachycardia
• Tachypnea
• Signs of hypovolemic shock (e.g., pale mucous membranes, decreased capillary refill time, weak pulses)

## CAUSES AND RISK FACTORS

• Not known if enterotoxigenic CP is a true acquired infection or an opportunistic pathogen
• Only certain strains of CP can produce enterotoxin, and certain animals are affected clinically.
• Disease may be associated with small intestinal bacterial overgrowth.
• Clostridia overgrowth may occur secondary to prolonged antibiotic use.
• Stress factors to the gastrointestinal tract, dietary change, concurrent disease, or hospitalization may initiate disease.
• Bloat syndrome has been reported following overeating of meat or unsanitary feeding conditions, but has also been seen following hospitalization and/or surgical procedures.
• Overgrowth of CP may occur secondary to gastrointestinal foreign bodies or other concurrent gastrointestinal disease.

 DIAGNOSIS

Patients with chronic intermittent clinical signs—always evaluate during the onset of episodes.

## DIFFERENTIAL DIAGNOSIS

• More common causes of diarrhea in ferrets include ECE and infiltrative gastrointestinal tract diseases (lymphoma, inflammatory bowel disease).
• Consider all causes of diarrhea, including systemic or metabolic disease, as well as specific intestinal disorders.

• For bloat syndrome, consider gastrointestinal foreign bodies, aerophagia, or gastrointestinal outflow obstruction.

## CBC/BIOCHEMISTRY/URINALYSIS

• With mild/moderate diarrhea—usually normal
• With bloat syndrome, expect hemogram abnormalities consistent with acute inflammation and hemoconcentration/shock; electrolyte abnormalities and acid-base alterations may be seen.

## OTHER LABORATORY TESTS

Fecal direct examination, fecal flotation, zinc sulfate centrifugation to rule out gastrointestinal parasites in patients with diarrhea

### Microbiology

Anaerobic fecal cultures may demonstrate high concentrations of CP organisms but occasionally are negative due to the fastidious nature of the organism.

### Fecal Cytology

• Large numbers of CP spores in the feces in a patient with evidence of clinical disease.
• Cytology—make a thin fecal smear on a microscope slide, air-dry or heat fix, and stain with Diff-Quick or Wright's stain or use malachite green, a specific spore stain.
• CP spores have a "safety-pin" appearance—an oval structure with a dense body at one end of the spore wall; bacteria with terminal spores may also be seen.
• Examine for spores shortly after onset of clinical signs.

## IMAGING

• Radiographs may be normal in ferrets with mild to moderate disease; occasionally, excessive amount of gas is visible in the large and/or small bowel.
• With bloat syndrome, moderate to severe gastric, small and/or large bowel gas distension

## DIAGNOSTIC PROCEDURES

• Exploratory laparotomy may be needed to evaluate the extent of gastric pathology and to rule out gastrointestinal foreign bodies, neoplasia, and intestinal inflammatory diseases.
• Abdominocentesis and cytology may help determine if perforation has occurred in ferrets with gastric bloat.

## PATHOLOGIC FINDINGS

With bloat syndrome, grossly dilated, thin-walled stomach and intestines; diffuse necrosis of mucosa on histologic examination

# TREATMENT

## APPROPRIATE HEALTH CARE

### Diarrhea:
• Most patients with mild to moderate diarrhea can be treated as outpatients.
• Hospitalize when diarrhea is severe, resulting in dehydration and electrolyte imbalance; administer supportive fluids on the basis of hydration status.

### Bloat Syndrome:
• Bloat syndrome requires inpatient management.
• Patients require immediate medical therapy with special attention to establishing improved cardiovascular function and gastric decompression.
• Shock/fluid therapy should accompany gastric decompression; give isotonic fluids at the rate of 90 mL/kg within the first 30–60 minutes, the general treatment of choice for hypovolemic (shock) patients.
• Supportive fluids on the basis of hydration status are recommended for animals not in shock.
• First try gastric decompression by orogastric intubation with an appropriately sized rubber catheter; light sedation with narcotics may facilitate this process.
• Decompression by other techniques such as trocarization and in-dwelling catheters may be necessary if orogastric intubation is not successful; these techniques have not been described in ferrets.
• Orogastric intubation may need to be repeated to maintain gastric decompression.

# MEDICATIONS

## DRUG(S) OF CHOICE

### Antibiotics
• Most patients respond well to appropriate antibiotic therapy (e.g., amoxicillin 20 mg/kg PO, SC q12h, clindamycin 5.5–10 mg/kg PO q12h, or metronidazole 15–20 mg/kg PO q12h).
• Patients with chronic disease may require prolonged antibiotic therapy.

• For pain relief with mild to moderate gastrointestinal distention—butorphanol (0.05–0.5 mg/kg IM, SC q8–12h) or buprenorphine (0.01–0.05 mg/kg SC, IM, IV q12h)
• For patients with life-threatening gastric bloat—corticosteroids such as dexamethasone sodium phosphate (4–8 mg/kg slow IV) or prednisolone sodium succinate (22 mg/kg slow IV) used to stabilize membranes, aid in cardiovascular support, and potentially help with treatment and prevention of reperfusion injury

## CONTRAINDICATIONS
N/A

## PRECAUTIONS
Rapid administration of prednisolone sodium succinate may cause vomiting.

## POSSIBLE INTERACTIONS
N/A

## ALTERNATIVE DRUGS
N/A

# FOLLOW-UP

## PATIENT MONITORING
• Monitor patients closely for recurrence of dilation or cardiorespiratory decompensation.
• Response to therapy supports the diagnosis; repeat diagnostics are rarely necessary.

## PREVENTION/AVOIDANCE
Infection is associated with environmental contamination; disinfection is difficult.

## POSSIBLE COMPLICATIONS
• Gastrointestinal necrosis or rupture may occur after treatment.
• Gastric dilation may recur.

## EXPECTED COURSE AND PROGNOSIS
• Most animals with mild to moderate diarrhea respond well to therapy; chronic patients may require long-term therapy; failure to respond suggests concurrent disease; further diagnostic evaluation is indicated.
• The prognosis is fair to grave following gastrointestinal bloat, depending on the degree of distension and time elapsed to treatment.

# MISCELLANEOUS

## ASSOCIATED CONDITIONS
Frequently other enteric disease

## AGE-RELATED FACTORS
N/A

## ZOONOTIC POTENTIAL
Unknown

## PREGNANCY
N/A

## SYNONYMS
Bloat syndrome

## SEE ALSO
• ECE
• Gastrointestinal foreign body
• Inflammatory bowel disease

## ABBREVIATION
ECE = epizootic catarrhal enteritis

### Suggested Reading

Finkler MR. Ferret colitis. In: Kirk RW, Bonagura JD, eds. Kirk's Current Veterinary Therapy XI: Small Animal Practice. Philadelphia: WB Saunders, 1992.

Fox JG. Diseases of the gastrointestinal system. In: Fox JG, ed. Biology and Diseases of the Ferret. 2nd Ed. Baltimore: Williams & Wilkins, 1998.

Harrenstein L. Critical care of ferrets, rabbits and rodents. Semin Avian Exotic Pet Med 1994;3(4):217–228.

Harrison SG, Borland ED. Deaths in ferrets (Mustela putorius) due to Clostridium botulinum type C. Vet Rec 1973 93(22)576-7.

Hoefer HL, Bell JA. Gastrointestinal diseases. In: Quesenberry KE, Carpenter JW, eds. Ferrets, Rabbits and Rodents: Clinical Medicine and Surgery. St. Louis: WB Saunders, 2004:25–40.

Jenkins JR. Rabbit and ferret liver and gastrointestinal testing. In: Fudge AM, ed. Laboratory Medicine, Avian and Exotic Pets. Philadelphia: WB Saunders, 2000.

Rosenthal K. Update on ECE disease in ferrets. Proc North Am Vet Conf 2000;1017–1018.

### Portions Adapted From

Twedt DC. Clostridial Enterotoxicosis. In: Tilley LP, Smith FWK, Jr., eds. The 5-Minute Veterinary Consult: Canine and Feline, 3rd Ed. Baltimore: Lippincott Williams & Wilkins, 2003.

# COCCIDIOSIS

 ## BASICS

### OVERVIEW
• An enteric infection associated with *Isospora* spp. in pet ferrets; *Eimeria* spp. has been reported to cause disease in laboratory and free-ranging ferrets.
• Strictly host-specific (i.e., no cross-transmission)
• Usually asymptomatic infection; may cause moderate to severe clinical disease in young ferrets
• Asexual multiplication that occurs in intestinal epithelial cells causes cellular damage and disease
• Following asexual multiplication, sexual reproduction results in shedding of oocysts in the feces
• Oocysts become infective 1–4 days after shedding in the feces.
• May be copathogen with *Desulfovibrio* sp. (proliferative bowel disease)
• Occasionally, hepatic infection in young ferrets

### SIGNALMENT
Young ferrets, usually 6–16 weeks of age

### SIGNS
• Often asymptomatic
• Rectal prolapse
• Watery-to-mucoid, sometimes blood-tinged, diarrhea
• Tenesmus
• Weakness, lethargy, dehydration, and weight loss with severe infection or hepatic infection
• Thickened, ropy intestines and enlarged mesenteric lymph nodes may be palpable.
• With hepatic involvement, may see jaundice

### CAUSES AND RISK FACTORS
• Infected ferrets contaminating environment with oocysts of *Isospora* spp. or *Eimeria* spp.
• Stress
• Enteric infection with *Desulfovibrio* sp. or other copathogens

 ## DIAGNOSIS

### DIFFERENTIAL DIAGNOSIS
• Consider all causes of diarrhea, including systemic or metabolic disease, as well as specific intestinal disorders.
• Blood and mucous in stool is also seen with *Desulfovibrio* spp., clostridia, *Campylobacter*, and *Salmonella*. These organisms all can cause disease alone or be copathogens with Coccidia.
• Wasting, thickened gastrointestinal tract and palpable mesenteric lymph nodes—consider ECE, *Desulfovibrio* sp., clostridia, *Campylobacter*, and lymphoma.

### CBC/BIOCHEMISTRY/URINALYSIS
• Usually normal; may be hemoconcentrated if dehydrated
• Increased liver enzymes, bile acids with hepatic involvement

### OTHER LABORATORY TESTS
N/A

### IMAGING
N/A

### DIAGNOSTIC PROCEDURES
• Fecal examination for oocysts using routine fecal floatation
• Oocysts range in size from 10–45 μm.

 ## TREATMENT
• Usually treated as an outpatient
• Inpatient if debilitated
• Fluid therapy if dehydrated

 ## MEDICATIONS

### DRUG(S) OF CHOICE
Sulfadimethoxine—50 mg/kg PO on the first day, then 25 mg/kg q24h for 9 days

### CONTRAINDICATIONS/POSSIBLE INTERACTIONS
N/A

 ## FOLLOW-UP
Fecal examination for oocysts 1–2 weeks following treatment

 ## MISCELLANEOUS

### AGE-RELATED FACTORS
Disease in young patients 6–16 weeks old

### SEE ALSO
• Epizootic Catarrhal Enteritis
• Dyschezia and hematochezia
• Proliferative bowel disease

### ABBREVIATION
ECE = epizootic catarrhal enteritis

### Suggested Reading
Bowman DD, ed. Georgi's Parasitology for Veterinarians. 6th Ed. Philadelphia: WB Saunders, 1994:95–97.
Fox JG. Diseases of the gastrointestinal system. In: Fox JG, ed. Biology and Diseases of the Ferret. 2nd Ed. Baltimore: Williams & Wilkins, 1998:273–290.
Fox JG. Parasitic diseases. In: Fox JG, ed. Biology and Diseases of the Ferret. 2nd Ed. Baltimore: Williams & Wilkins, 1998:375–392.
Hoefer HL, Bell JA. Gastrointestinal diseases. In: Quesenberry KE, Carpenter JW, eds. Ferrets, Rabbits and Rodents: Clinical Medicine and Surgery. St. Louis: WB Saunders, 2004:25–40.

# BASICS

## DEFINITION
• Left-sided congestive heart failure (L-CHF)—failure of the left side of the heart to advance blood at a sufficient rate to meet the metabolic needs of the patient or to prevent blood from pooling within the pulmonary venous circulation
• Right-sided congestive heart failure (R-CHF)—failure of the right side of the heart to advance blood at a sufficient rate to meet the metabolic needs of the patient or to prevent blood from pooling within the systemic venous circulation

## PATHOPHYSIOLOGY
• The most common cause of CHF in the ferret is DCM.
• L-CHF—low cardiac output causes lethargy, exercise intolerance, syncope, and prerenal azotemia. High hydrostatic pressure causes leakage of fluid from pulmonary venous circulation into pulmonary interstitium and alveoli. When fluid leakage exceeds ability of lymphatics to drain the affected areas, pulmonary edema develops.
• R-CHF—high hydrostatic pressure leads to leakage of fluid from venous circulation into the pleural and peritoneal space and interstitium of peripheral tissue. When fluid leakage exceeds ability of lymphatics to drain the affected areas, pleural effusion, ascites, and peripheral edema develop

## SYSTEMS AFFECTED
All organ systems can be affected by either poor delivery of blood or by the effects of passive congestion from backup of venous blood.

## INCIDENCE/PREVALENCE
Very common syndrome in clinical practice

## SIGNALMENT
Varies with cause

## SIGNS

### General Comments
Signs vary with underlying cause.

### Historical Findings
• Weakness, lethargy, exercise intolerance; manifested as rear limb paresis or paralysis in ferrets
• Anorexia
• Coughing and dyspnea
• Abdominal distension

### Physical Examination Findings
*L-CHF*
• Tachypnea
• Inspiratory and expiratory dyspnea when animal has pulmonary edema
• Pulmonary crackles and wheezes
• Prolonged capillary refill time

• Possible murmur or gallop
• Weak femoral pulses
*R-CHF*
• Rapid, shallow respiration if animal has pleural effusion
• Jugular venous distention or jugular pulse in some animals
• Hepatomegaly
• Splenomegaly (may be due to congestion or incidental finding in older ferrets)
• Ascites
• Possible murmur or gallop
• Muffled heart sounds if animal has pleural or pericardial effusion
• Weak femoral pulses
• Peripheral edema (very rare)

## CAUSES

### Pump (Muscle) Failure of Left or Right Ventricle
Idiopathic DCM is the most common cause of CHF in the ferret.

### Pressure Overload to Left Heart
Causes reported in other mammals, such as systemic hypertension, subaortic stenosis, or left ventricular tumors, have not yet been reported in ferrets. However, these causes should be considered because there is no reason that these diseases should not occur in ferrets, and they may be under-reported.

### Pressure Overload to Right Heart
• Heartworm disease is the most common cause of R-CHF in the ferret.
• Causes reported in other mammals, such as chronic obstructive pulmonary disease, pulmonary thromboembolism, pulmonic stenosis, right ventricular tumors, or primary pulmonary hypertension have not yet been reported in ferrets. However, these causes should be considered because there is no reason that these diseases should not occur in ferrets, and they may be under-reported.

### Volume Overload of the Left Heart
• Mitral valve endocardiosis
• Aortic insufficiency
• Ventricular septal defect anecdotally reported; other congenital defects have not been reported, but should be considered.

### Impediment to Filling of Left Heart
• Hypertrophic cardiomyopathy
• Pericardial effusion with tamponade
• Restrictive pericarditis
• Left atrial masses (e.g., tumors and thrombus), pulmonary thromboembolism, and mitral stenosis have not yet been reported in ferrets. However, these causes should be considered because there is no reason that these diseases should not occur in ferrets, and they may be under-reported.

### Impediment to Right Ventricular Filling
• Pericardial effusion
• Restrictive pericarditis

• Right atrial or caval masses and tricuspid stenosis have not yet been reported in ferrets. However, these causes should be considered because there is no reason that these diseases should not occur in ferrets, and they may be under-reported.

### Rhythm Disturbances
• Bradycardia (AV block)
• Tachycardia (e.g., atrial fibrillation, atrial tachycardia, and ventricular tachycardia)

## RISK FACTORS
• No heartworm prophylaxis
• Risk factors for other diseases have not been evaluated.

# DIAGNOSIS

## DIFFERENTIAL DIAGNOSIS
• Rear limb weakness—consider metabolic disease including hypoglycemia (especially insulinoma); anemia (hyperestrogenism, blood loss from gastrointestinal tract, leukemia, CRF); gastrointestinal foreign body; neurologic disease including CNS or spinal cord disease; CDV or rabies
• Pleural effusion—mediastinal lymphoma, other neoplasia, abscess, chylothorax
• Cough—infection (influenza virus, CDV, bacterial tracheitis, bronchitis, pneumonia), neoplasia, heartworm disease
• Dyspnea—neoplasm (mediastinal lymphoma), primary pulmonary disease, pleural effusion, trauma resulting in diaphragmatic hernia, pulmonary hemorrhage, pneumothorax, airway obstruction due to foreign body
• Ascites, abdominal distension—consider hypoproteinemia, severe liver disease, ruptured bladder, peritonitis, abdominal neoplasia, and abdominal hemorrhage.

## CBC/BIOCHEMISTRY/URINALYSIS
• CBC usually normal; may be stress leukogram
• Mild to moderately high alanine transaminase, aspartate transaminase, and serum alkaline phosphatase with R-CHF
• Prerenal azotemia in some animals

## OTHER LABORATORY TESTS
Heartworm serologic testing—ELISA (Snap heartworm antigen test, Idexx Laboratories)

## IMAGING

### Radiographic Findings
• Generalized cardiomegaly
• Pulmonary edema (L-CHF), pleural effusion or both are extremely common findings.
• Hepatomegaly, splenomegaly, or ascites may be seen (R-CHF).
• The different forms of cardiomyopathy cannot be differentiated by radiography.
• Important tool for ruling out mediastinal lymphoma in dyspneic ferrets

# CONGESTIVE HEART FAILURE

### Echocardiography
• Echocardiography is the diagnostic modality of choice to differentiate forms of cardiomyopathy, cardiac masses, heartworm disease, and pericardial effusion.
• Findings vary markedly with cause.

## DIAGNOSTIC PROCEDURES

### Electrocardiographic Findings
• Often is normal and, if so, not helpful in the diagnosis
• Ferrets resist attachment of alligator clips; use padded clips, soft clips, or isoflurane anesthesia to perform ECG; active ferrets may be distracted and will remain still when fed Nutri-Cal while the ECG is performed.
• Pronounced respiratory sinus arrhythmias are common in normal ferrets and should not be overinterpreted.
• The ECG of normal ferrets differs from the feline ECG in that R waves are taller, and a short QT interval and/or elevated ST segment are commonly seen.
• Both ventricular and supraventricular arrhythmias can be seen.
• First- or second-degree heart block are common findings both in normal ferrets and in ferrets with CHF.
• May show atrial or ventricular enlargement patterns
• Sinus tachycardia (HR > 280) is common.

### Abdominocentesis
Analysis of ascitic fluid in patients with R-CHF generally reveals modified transudate.

### Pleural Effusion Analysis
Pleural effusion typically is a modified transudate with total protein < 4.0 g/dL and nucleated cell counts < 2500/mL (these values have been extrapolated from other mammalian species to be used as a guideline). Analysis of the pleural effusion is important to rule out other causes of pleural effusion such as pyothorax, lymphosarcoma, or chylothorax.

## PATHOLOGIC FINDINGS
Cardiac findings vary with disease.

## TREATMENT

### APPROPRIATE HEALTH CARE
• Severely dyspneic, weak, or anorectic ferrets in congestive heart failure should be treated as inpatients.
• Mildly affected animals can be treated as outpatients.

### NURSING CARE
• Supplemental oxygen therapy for dyspneic animals
• Minimize handling of critically dyspneic animals. Stress can kill!

• Thoracocentesis is both therapeutic and diagnostic. If there is significant pleural effusion, drain each hemithorax with a 20-gauge butterfly catheter after the ferret is stable enough to be handled. When performing thoracocentesis be aware that the heart is located much more caudally within the thorax in the ferret as compared to dogs and cats. Sedation (midazolam 0.3–1.0 mg/kg IM, SC, or ketamine 10–20 mg/kg IM plus diazepam 1–2 mg/kg IM) or anesthesia with isoflurane by mask may be necessary.
• If hypothermic, external heat (incubator or heating pad) is recommended.

## ACTIVITY
Restrict activity.

## CLIENT EDUCATION
With few exceptions (e.g., heartworm disease), CHF is not curable.

## SURGICAL CONSIDERATIONS
N/A

## MEDICATIONS

### DRUG(S) OF CHOICE

#### Diuretics
• Furosemide is recommended at the lowest effective dose to eliminate pulmonary edema and pleural effusion. If the ferret is in fulminant cardiac failure, administer furosemide at 2–4 mg/kg q8–12h IM or IV. Initially, furosemide should be administered parenterally. Long-term therapy should be continued at a dose of 1–2 mg/kg q12h PO. The pediatric elixir is generally well accepted.
• Predisposes the patient to dehydration, prerenal azotemia, and electrolyte disturbances

#### Venodilators
• Nitroglycerin (2% ointment) 1/16–1/8 inch applied topically can be used in conjunction with diuretics in the acute management of CHF to further reduce preload. Nitroglycerin will lower the dose of furosemide and is particularly useful in patients with hypothermia or dehydration.
• May be useful in animals with chronic L-CHF when used intermittently

#### Digoxin
• Digoxin is used in animals with dilated cardiomyopathy at a dose of 0.005–0.01 mg/kg PO.
• Digoxin also indicated to treat supraventricular arrhythmias (e.g., sinus tachycardia, atrial fibrillation, and atrial or junctional tachycardia) in patients with CHF

### ACE Inhibitors
Enalapril is recommended for long-term maintenance to reduce afterload and preload. Begin with a dose of 0.25–0.5 mg/kg PO q48h and increase to q24h dosing if well tolerated (see precautions). Enalapril can be compounded into a suspension by a compounding pharmacy for ease of administration.

### Beta Blockers
• Dosage—propranolol (0.2–1.0 mg/kg q8–12h) or atenolol (3.125–6.25 mg/ferret PO q24h)
• Most useful in patients with hypertrophic cardiomyopathy
• Beneficial effects may include slowing of sinus rate and correcting atrial and ventricular arrhythmias.
• Role in asymptomatic patients unresolved

### Calcium Channel Blockers
*Diltiazem*
• Used to treat hypertropic cardiomyopathy
• Dosage—3.75–7.5 mg/ferret PO q12h
• Beneficial effects may include slower sinus rate, resolution of supraventricular arrhythmias, improved diastolic relaxation, and peripheral vasodilation, but they have not been documented in ferrets.

## CONTRAINDICATIONS
Positive inotropic drugs should be avoided in patients with HCM.

## PRECAUTIONS
• Ferrets are very sensitive to the hypotensive effects of ACE inhibitors and may become weak and lethargic. The dosage should be reduced if this side effect is observed or hypotension is documented.
• Atenolol, enalapril, propanolol and diltiazem may all cause lethargy, anorexia and hypotension.
• ACE inhibitors and digoxin must be used cautiously in patients with renal disease.
• Overzealous diuretic therapy may cause dehydration and hypokalemia.

## POSSIBLE INTERACTIONS
• The use of a calcium channel blocker in combination with a beta blocker should be avoided because clinically significant bradyarrhythmias can develop in other small animals and are likely to also occur in ferrets.
• Combination of high-dose diuretics and ACE inhibitors may alter renal perfusion and cause azotemia.

## ALTERNATIVE DRUGS
• Other vasodilators, including hydralazine, may be used instead of or in addition to an ACE inhibitor. Dosages have been anecdotally extrapolated from feline dosages; however, their use is not widespread, and efficacy and safety are unknown (beware of hypotension).

• Other beta blockers, such as atenolol, carvedilol, or metoprolol, can be used instead of propranolol to help control ventricular response rate in atrial fibrillation. Dosages have been anecdotally extrapolated from feline dosages; however, their use is not widespread, and efficacy and safety are unknown.

• Patients unresponsive to furosemide, vasodilators, and digoxin (if indicated) may benefit from combination diuretic therapy by adding spironolactone. Dosages have been anecdotally extrapolated from feline dosages; however, their use is not widespread, and efficacy and safety are unknown.

• Potassium supplementation if animal has hypokalemia; use potassium supplements cautiously in animals receiving ACE inhibitors or spironolactone.

## FOLLOW-UP

### PATIENT MONITORING
• Monitor renal status, electrolytes, hydration, respiratory rate and effort, heart rate, body weight, and abdominal girth.
• If azotemia develops, reduce the dosage of diuretic. If azotemia persists and the animal is also on an ACE inhibitor, reduce or discontinue the ACE inhibitor. Use digoxin with caution if azotemia develops.
• Monitor ECG if arrhythmias are suspected.
• Check digoxin concentration periodically. Therapeutic range (as extrapolated from dogs and cats) is between 1 and 2 ng/dL 8–12 hours postpill.

### PREVENTION/AVOIDANCE
• Minimize stress and exercise in patients with heart disease.

• Prescribing an ACE inhibitor early in the course of heart disease in patients with mitral valve disease and DCM may slow the progression of heart disease and delay onset of CHF. Consider this in asymptomatic animals if they have DCM or if they have mitral valve disease and radiographic or echocardiographic evidence of left heart enlargement.

### POSSIBLE COMPLICATIONS
• Sudden death due to arrhythmias
• Iatrogenic problems associated with medical management (see above)

### EXPECTED COURSE AND PROGNOSIS
Prognosis varies with underlying cause.

## MISCELLANEOUS

### ASSOCIATED CONDITIONS
N/A

### AGE-RELATED FACTORS
• DCM seen in young animals
• Degenerative heart conditions and HCM generally seen in middle-aged to old animals

### ZOONOTIC POTENTIAL
N/A

### PREGNANCY
N/A

### SYNONYMS
N/A

### SEE ALSO
• Cardiomyopathy, dilated
• Cardiomyopathy, hypertrophic
• Heartworm disease

### ABBREVIATIONS
• ACE = angiotensin-converting enzyme
• AV = atrioventricular block
• CBC = complete blood count
• CDV = canine distemper virus
• CHF = congestive heart failure
• CRF = chronic renal failure
• DCM = dilated cardiomyopathy
• ELISA = enzyme-linked immunosorbent assay
• HCM = hypertrophic cardiomyopathy

*Suggested Reading*

Fox JG. Other systemic diseases. In: Fox JG, ed. Biology and Diseases of the Ferret. 2nd Ed. Baltimore: Williams & Wilkins, 1998:307–320.

Hoefer HL. Cardiac disease in ferrets. Proc North Am Vet Conf 1995;577–578.

Keene BW, Bonagura JD. Therapy of heart failure. In: Bonagura JD, ed. Current Veterinary Therapy XII. Philadelphia: WB Saunders, 1995.

Rosenthal K. Management of cardiac disease in ferrets. Waltham/OSU Symp Treatment Sm Anim Dis 1997; Sept.

Rosenthal KL. Respiratory diseases. In: Quesenberry KE, Carpenter JW, eds. Ferrets, Rabbits and Rodents: Clinical Medicine and Surgery. St. Louis: WB Saunders, 2004:72–78.

Petrie JP, Morrisey JK. Cardiovascular and other diseases. In: Quesenberry KE, Carpenter JW, eds. Ferrets, Rabbits and Rodents: Clinical Medicine and Surgery. St. Louis: WB Saunders, 2004:58–71.

*Portions Adapted From*

Smith FWK, Jr., Tilley LP. Congestive Heart Failure, Left Sided and Congestive Heart Failure, Right Sided. In: Tilley LP, Smith FWK, Jr., eds. The 5-Minute Veterinary Consult: Canine and Feline, 3rd Ed. Baltimore: Lippincott Williams & Wilkins, 2004.

# COUGH

## BASICS

### DEFINITION
A sudden forceful expiration of air through the glottis, usually accompanied by an audible sound, which is preceded by an exaggerated inspiratory effort

### PATHOPHYSIOLOGY
• One of the most powerful reflexes in the body
• Induced by stimulation of either afferent fibers of the pharyngeal distribution of the glossopharyngeal nerves or sensory endings of the vagus nerves located in the larynx, trachea, and larger bronchi
• Begins with an inspiratory phase followed in sequence by an inspiratory pause, glottis closure, increased intrathoracic pressure, and glottis opening
• Serves as an early warning system for the pharynx and respiratory system and as a protective mechanism

### SYSTEMS AFFECTED
• Respiratory
• Musculoskeletal—because of the role played in the reflex by inspiratory and expiratory muscles of respiration
• Cardiovascular

### SIGNALMENT
No age or sex predilection

### SIGNS
N/A

### CAUSES
#### Upper Respiratory Tract Diseases
• Nasopharyngeal—rhinitis or sinusitis (influenza virus, bacterial, CDV); nasopharyngeal foreign body or tumor
• Laryngeal—inflammation, foreign body, injuries, tumors
• Tracheal—inflammation (inhalation of irritating substances and heat), infections (viral and bacterial), foreign body, tumor

#### Lower Respiratory Tract Diseases
• Bronchial—inflammation, infection (influenza, CDV, bacterial), foreign body
• Pulmonary/vascular—pulmonary edema, heartworm disease, tumor (especially lymphoma), infection, aspiration pneumonia

#### Other Diseases
• Pleural—tumor (mediastinal lymphoma), infection (bacterial and fungal), inflammation
• Esophageal—inflammation, foreign body, tumor

### RISK FACTORS
• Esophageal, gastroesophageal, and upper gastrointestinal disorders—predispose the patient to aspiration pneumonia
• Environmental factors—exposure to viral and bacterial diseases; exposure of ferrets to mosquitoes without effective heartworm prophylaxis

## DIAGNOSIS

### DIFFERENTIAL DIAGNOSIS
#### Similar Signs
Sneezing and coughing—expiratory events that may occur together in certain conditions (e.g., rhinitis, sinusitis, and regurgitation); may confuse both the owner and the history; forceful expiration of a sneeze: mouth usually closed; cough: mouth usually open

#### Causes
• Patterns and characteristics—may suggest underlying cause
• Nocturnal—may be associated with early stages of left-sided CHF
• Precipitated by exercise or excitement—frequently the result of inflammation or irritation involving the larynx, trachea, and bronchi
• Harsh and prolonged—suggests involvement of the major airways
• Productive—suggests fluid or mucous in the expectorated material
• Dry—indicates lack of mucous or fluid production

### CBC/BIOCHEMISTRY/URINALYSIS
• CBC—may suggest possible causes (e.g., neutrophilia with infection)
• Mild to moderate elevations in ALT—suggest liver congestion secondary to pulmonary disease or right heart failure

### OTHER LABORATORY TESTS
• Filaria serologic test—evaluate for heartworm disease; false negatives common as ferrets are rarely microfilaremic
• Serologic tests that identify adult *Dirofilaria immitis* antigen are of some use; however, false-negative results are common—ELISA (Snap heartworm antigen test, Idexx Laboratories)

### IMAGING
• Radiographs—particularly useful for evaluating patients with nasal, sinus, tracheal, cardiac, and lower respiratory tract disorders
• Thoracic ultrasound—useful for patients with primary cardiac disease and pleural effusion

### DIAGNOSTIC PROCEDURES
• Thoracocentesis—with pleural effusion
• CT scan—better evaluates nasal and sinus disorders
• Transtracheal wash with cytologic examination and culture—evaluates lower respiratory tract disorders

## TREATMENT
• Outpatient—unless CHF is diagnosed or marked alteration in pulmonary function or hemoptysis noted
• Exercise restriction—best enforced until a cause is established and corrected, especially when activity aggravates the condition
• Inform client that a wide variety of conditions can be responsible for the cough, and a fairly extensive workup may be required to define and treat the underlying cause.
• Surgical intervention—may be indicated for tumors involving the respiratory system

## MEDICATIONS

### DRUG(S) OF CHOICE
• Symptomatic treatment without other abnormalities—broad-spectrum antibiotics; bronchodilator-expectorant; appropriate follow-up evaluations
• Collect airway specimens for bacterial culture and sensitivity testing before administering antibiotics.
• Broad-spectrum antibiotics—for suspected infection when results of bacterial culture and sensitivity testing are pending (e.g., trimethoprim/sulfonamide at 15–30 mg/kg PO, SC q12h; enrofloxacin at 10–20 mg/kg PO, SC, IM q24h; or cephalexin 15–25 mg/kg PO q8–12h
• Bronchodilator (e.g., theophylline 4.25 mg/kg q8–12h) with or without the use of expectorants—may be beneficial for a variety of diseases affecting the trachea and lower respiratory airways
• Cough suppressants are rarely indicated in ferrets; avoid in patients with coughs secondary to bacterial respiratory infection and CHF.
• Therapeutic thoracocentesis—perform for any patient with a marked pleural effusion.

### CONTRAINDICATIONS
• Corticosteroids—do not use in animals with infectious causes of cough.
• Cough suppressants—do not use in any patient in which either a respiratory infection or clinically important heart disease is suspected.

## PRECAUTIONS
• Cough suppressants—indiscriminate use may obscure the warning signs of serious cardiac and pulmonary disorders and predispose the patient to serious complications or even death.
• Bronchodilator therapy—intravenous use of aminophylline may cause tachyarrhythmias.
• Diuretics—do not use in patients with primary airway disease; drying of secretions decreases clearance of mucous and exudate.

## POSSIBLE INTERACTIONS
Theophylline bronchodilators—clearance may be inhibited by other drugs (e.g., enrofloxacin and chloramphenicol); signs of toxicity may develop with the addition of such drugs.

## ALTERNATIVE DRUGS
N/A

 FOLLOW-UP

## PATIENT MONITORING
Follow-up thoracic radiographs—in 10–14 days with bronchopulmonary disease; in 3–4 weeks to monitor potential tumors

## POSSIBLE COMPLICATIONS
• Complete control does not guarantee resolution of the inciting cause.
• Serious respiratory dysfunction and even death may be caused by underlying disease.

 MISCELLANEOUS

## ASSOCIATED CONDITIONS
• Heavy breathing
• Dyspnea

## AGE-RELATED FACTORS
N/A

## ZOONOTIC POTENTIAL
N/A

## PREGNANCY
N/A

## SEE ALSO
• Canine distemper virus
• Congestive heart failure
• Influenza virus
• Nasal discharge (sneezing, gagging)
• Pneumonia, bacterial

## ABBREVIATIONS
• ALT = alanine aminotransferase
• CBC = complete blood count
• CDV = canine distemper virus
• CHF = congestive heart failure
• ELISA = enzyme-linked immunosorbent assay

*Suggested Reading*
Ettinger SJ. Coughing. In: Ettinger SJ, ed. Textbook of Veterinary Internal Medicine. 5th Ed. Philadelphia: WB Saunders, 2000:162–166.
Kendrick RE. Ferret respiratory diseases. Vet Clin North Am Exotic Anim Pract 2000;3(2):453–464.
Rosenthal KL. Respiratory diseases. In: Quesenberry KE, Carpenter JW, eds. Ferrets, Rabbits and Rodents: Clinical Medicine and Surgery. St. Louis, WB Saunders, 2004:72–78.
Petrie JP, Morrisey JK. Cardiovascular and other diseases. In: Quesenberry KE, Carpenter JW, eds. Ferrets, Rabbits and Rodents: Clinical Medicine and Surgery. St. Louis: WB Saunders, 2004:58–71.

*Portions Adapted From*
Harpster NK. Cough. In: Tilley LP, Smith FWK, Jr., eds. The 5-Minute Veterinary Consult: Canine and Feline, 3rd Ed. Baltimore: Lippincott Williams & Wilkins, 2003.

# CRYPTOSPORIDIOSIS

## BASICS

### OVERVIEW
• *Cryptosporidium* spp.—Coccidian protozoan; causes gastrointestinal disease in ferrets, dogs, cats, humans, calves, and rodents; ubiquitous in nature; worldwide distribution; enteric life cycle
• Infection and clinical disease may occur in immunosuppressed ferrets or as a copathogen with other primary gastrointestinal pathogens
• Infection—when sporulated oocysts are ingested, sporozoites are released and penetrate intestinal epithelial cells; after asexual reproduction, merozoites are released to infect other cells.
• Immunocompetent animals—asymptomatic
• Immunocompromised animals—intestinal disease

### SIGNALMENT
No sex or breed predilection

### SIGNS
• Most infections subclinical
• Yellow/beige diarrhea, anorexia, depression

### CAUSES AND RISK FACTORS
• Ingestion of contaminated water or feces; feeding raw meat
• Immunosuppression, corticosteroid therapy
• May be copathogen or secondary to ECE

## DIAGNOSIS

### DIFFERENTIAL DIAGNOSIS
• Dietary indiscretion or intolerance
• Parasites—giardiasis, coccidiosis
• Infectious agents—ECE, Aleutian disease virus, *Salmonella*, *Campylobacter*, *Clostridium*
• Organ disease—renal, hepatic
• Neoplasia—intestinal lymphoma, insulinoma
• Infiltrative diseases—inflammatory bowel disease

### CBC/BIOCHEMISTRY/URINALYSIS
Usually normal, unless an underlying immunosuppressive disease

### OTHER LABORATORY TESTS
N/A

### IMAGING
N/A

### DIAGNOSTIC PROCEDURES
• Fecal antigen detection test (ProSpecT Cryptosporidium Microtiter Assay; Color-Vue Cryptosporidium)—available; not extensively evaluated using ferret feces
• Sugar and zinc sulfate flotation—to concentrate fecal oocysts (oocysts are 3–6 μm so routine salt flotation often fails); oocysts best visualized after staining with modified acid-fast stain
• Submitting feces to a laboratory—mix one part 100% formalin with nine parts feces to inactivate oocysts and decrease health risk to laboratory personnel.
• Intestinal biopsy—cytologic and histopathologic identification of intracellular organisms; diagnostic but impractical; can produce false-negative results

### PATHOLOGIC FINDINGS
• Gross lesions—not well described in ferrets; possibly enlarged mesenteric lymph nodes; hyperemic intestinal mucosa; fix specimens in Bouin or formalin solution within hours of death because autolysis causes rapid loss of the intestinal surface containing the organisms.
• Microscopic lesions—parasites may be found on the tips of the brush border of intestinal villi; eosinophilic infiltration

## TREATMENT
• Disease is usually self-limiting. Treat underlying disease or copathogens. Most recover within 2–3 weeks.
• Mild diarrhea—oral glucose–electrolyte solution (Entrolyte, SmithKline)
• Severe diarrhea with dehydration—parental fluids

## MEDICATIONS

### DRUG(S) OF CHOICE
No reported efficacious treatment in ferrets

### CONTRAINDICATIONS/POSSIBLE INTERACTIONS
N/A

## FOLLOW-UP
• Monitor oocyst shedding in the feces 2–3 weeks in immunocompetent animals; longer shedding possible in immunocompromised ferrets
• Prognosis excellent if cause of immunosuppression can be overcome; most animals recover within 2–3 weeks.

## MISCELLANEOUS

### ZOONOTIC POTENTIAL
Warn clients of potential zoonotic transmission from organisms in feces and that immunocompromised people (HIV infection, chemotherapy, systemic corticosteroids) are at great risk.

### ABBREVIATIONS
ECE = epizootic catarrhal enteritis

### Suggested Reading
Fox JG. Diseases of the gastrointestinal system. In: Fox JG, ed. Biology and Diseases of the Ferret. 2nd Ed. Baltimore: Williams & Wilkins, 1998:273–290.
Fox JG. Parasitic diseases. In: Fox JG, ed. Biology and Diseases of the Ferret. 2nd Ed. Baltimore: Williams & Wilkins, 1998:375–392.
Bell JA. Gastrointestinal diseases. In: Quesenberry KE, Carpenter JW, eds. Ferrets, Rabbits and Rodents: Clinical Medicine and Surgery. St. Louis: WB Saunders, 2004:25–40.

### Portions Adapted From
Barr SC. Cryptosporidiosis. In: Tilley LP, Smith FWK, Jr., eds. The 5-Minute Veterinary Consult: Canine and Feline, 3rd Ed. Baltimore: Lippincott Williams & Wilkins, 2003.

# BASICS

## OVERVIEW
• A cutaneous fungal infection affecting the cornified regions of hair, nails, and occasionally the superficial layers of the skin
• Isolated organisms include *Microsporum canis* and *Trichophyton mentagrophytes*.
• Exposure to or contact with a dermatophyte does not necessarily result in an infection.
• Dermatophytes—grow in the keratinized layers of hair, nail, and skin; do not thrive in living tissue or persist in the presence of severe inflammation

## SIGNALMENT
• Uncommon disease of ferrets
• No age or sex predilection

## SIGNS

### Historical Findings
• Lesions may begin as alopecia, papules, or a poor hair coat.
• A history of previously confirmed infection or exposure to an infected animal or environment is a useful but not a consistent finding.

### Physical Examination Findings
• Often begins as papules and areas of alopecia
• Classic circular alopecia may be seen.
• Scales, crust, erythema—variable, usually in more advanced cases
• Thickening of the skin; hyperkeratosis seen in chronic disease
• Lesions may occur anywhere on the body.

## CAUSES AND RISK FACTORS
• Exposure to affected animals, including other ferrets and cats
• Poor management practices
• As in other species, immunocompromising diseases or immunosuppressive medications may predispose to infection, but this has not been demonstrated in ferrets.

# DIAGNOSIS

## DIFFERENTIAL DIAGNOSIS

### Differentiating Causes
• Ferret adrenal disease—rule out ferret adrenal disease, since this is the most common cause of alopecia and may occur in conjunction with dermatophytosis. Adrenal disease causes bilaterally symmetric alopecia. Hair loss often begins in late winter or early spring; hair initially may regrow later in the year, followed by progressive alopecia the following spring. Alopecia begins in the tail region and progresses cranially. In severe cases, the ferret will become completely bald. In most cases, the skin has a normal appearance, although some ferrets are pruritic and secondary pyoderma is occasionally seen. Other signs related to adrenal disease, such as a swollen vulva in spayed females, may be seen.
• Seasonal flank alopecia—in intact animals (or females with ovarian remnant), bilaterally symmetric alopecia begins at the tail base and progresses throughout the breeding season (March–August for females, December–July for males)
• CDV—characteristic rash usually follows a catarrhal phase characterized by nasoocular discharge, depression, and anorexia. A pruritic, erythematous rash appears on the chin and lips and spreads caudally to the inguinal area; pododermatitis is characterized by hyperkeratinization of the foot pads, erythema, and swelling. CDV is uniformly fatal, and signs other than dermatitis alone will be seen.
• Neoplasia—can be nodular, inflamed, swollen, or ulcerative, depending on tumor type. Mast cell tumors most common; appear as raised alopecic nodules; may become ulcerated or covered with a thick black crust; may be single or multiple, usually pruritic and found on neck and trunk
• Ear mites—partial to complete alopecia caudal to the ears; waxy brown aural discharge; excoriations around pinna; may be pruritic; differentiate by otic examination and skin scrape.
• Fleas—patchy alopecia at tail base and in cervical and dorsal thoracic region; pruritic; excoriations; secondary pyoderma sometimes seen
• Bacterial dermatitis—usually secondary infection—localized or multifocal areas of alopecia depending on primary cause; lesions may appear ulcerated; pruritus sometimes seen
• Sarcoptic mange—two forms reported—local form affecting the feet with intense pruritus and secondary pododermatitis, and generalized form with diffuse or focal alopecia and pruritus
• Demodicosis—extremely rare; has been reported in association with corticosteroid use; mites will be present on skin scrape.
• Hypersensitivity/contact irritant—uncommon cause; dermatitis localized to area of contact with irritant

## CBC/BIOCHEMISTRY/URINALYSIS
Not useful for diagnosis

## OTHER LABORATORY TESTS
To rule out ferret adrenal disease—elevations of serum estradiol, androstenedione, and 17-hydroxyprogesterone combined are most diagnostic (available through the University of Tennessee Clinical Endocrinology Laboratory, Department of Comparative Medicine).

## IMAGING
Ultrasonography—evaluate adrenal glands for evidence of ferret adrenal disease.

## DIAGNOSTIC PROCEDURES

### Fungal Culture
• Best means of confirming diagnosis
• Hairs that exhibit a positive apple-green fluorescence under Wood's lamp examination are considered ideal candidates for culture.
• Pluck hairs from the periphery of an alopecic area; do not use a random pattern.
• Test media—change to red when they become alkaline; dermatophytes typically produce this color during the early growing phase of their culture; saprophytes, which also produce this color, do so in the late growing phase; thus, it is important to examine the media daily.
• Positive culture—indicates existence of a dermatophyte; however, it may have been there only transiently, as may occur when the culture is obtained from the feet, which are likely to come into contact with a geophilic dermatophyte.

### Wood's Lamp Examination
Not a very useful screening tool; many pathogenic dermatophytes do not fluoresce; false fluorescence is common; lamp should warm up for a minimum of 5 minutes and then be exposed to suspicious lesions for up to 5 minutes; a true positive reaction associated with *M. canis* consists of apple-green florescence of the hair shaft; keratin associated with epidermal scales and sebum will often produce a false-positive fluorescence.

# TREATMENT

## APPROPRIATE HEALTH CARE
• May resolve spontaneously with no treatment
• Consider quarantine owing to the infective and zoonotic nature of the disease.
• Environmental treatment, including fomites, is important, especially in recurrent cases; diluted bleach (1:10) is a practical and relatively effective means of providing environmental decontamination; concentrated bleach and formalin (1%) are more effective at killing spores, but their use is not as practical in many situations; chlorhexidine was ineffective in pilot studies.

# MEDICATIONS

## DRUG(S) OF CHOICE
• Topical therapy and clipping—lime sulfur dip q7d has been used successfully; lime sulfur is odiferous and can stain; miconazole shampoo may also be effective for generalized lesions; miconazole creams or lotions may be used on focal lesions.

# DERMATOPHYTOSIS

• Griseofulvin—for treatment of refractory cases or severely affected animals; 25 mg/kg PO q12h for 4–6 weeks; administer with a high-fat meal; gastrointestinal upset is a possible common side effect; alleviate by reducing the dose or dividing the dose for more frequent administration.

## CONTRAINDICATIONS
N/A

## PRECAUTIONS
*Griseofulvin*
• Bone marrow suppression (anemia, pancytopenia, and neutropenia) reported in dogs and cats as an idiosyncratic reaction or with prolonged therapy; not yet reported in ferrets but may occur; weekly or biweekly CBC is recommended.
• Neurologic side effects reported in dogs and cats—monitor for this possibility in ferrets.
• Do not use during the first two trimesters of pregnancy; it is teratogenic.

## POSSIBLE INTERACTIONS
N/A

## ALTERNATIVE DRUGS
Ketaconazole—efficacy and safety in ferrets is unknown; hepatopathy reported in dogs and cats can be quite severe.

 FOLLOW-UP

## PATIENT MONITORING
Repeat fungal cultures toward the end of the treatment regimen and continue treatment until at least one culture result is negative.

## PREVENTION/AVOIDANCE
• Initiate a quarantine period and obtain dermatophyte cultures of all animals entering the household to prevent reinfection from other animals.
• Avoid infective soil, if a geophilic dermatophyte is involved.

## POSSIBLE COMPLICATIONS
False-negative dermatophyte cultures

## EXPECTED COURSE AND PROGNOSIS
• Many animals will "self-clear" a dermatophyte infection over a period of a few months.
• Treatment for the disease hastens clinical cure and helps reduce environmental contamination.

 MISCELLANEOUS

## ASSOCIATED CONDITIONS
N/A

## AGE-RELATED FACTORS
N/A

## ZOONOTIC POTENTIAL
Dermatophytosis is zoonotic.

## PREGNANCY
• Griseofulvin is teratogenic.
• Ketoconazole can affect steroidal hormone synthesis, especially testosterone.

## SYNONYMS
Ringworm

## ABBREVIATIONS
• CBC = complete blood count
• CDV = canine distemper virus

*Suggested Reading*

Kelleher SA. Skin diseases of the ferret. Vet Clin North Am Exotic Anim Pract 2001;4(2):565–572.

Fox JG. Mycotic diseases. In: Fox JG, ed. Biology and Diseases of the Ferret. 2nd Ed. Baltimore: Williams & Wilkins, 1998:393–403.

Orcutt C. Dermatologic diseases. In: Quesenberry KE, Carpenter JW, eds. Ferrets, Rabbits and Rodents: Clinical Medicine and Surgery. St. Louis: WB Saunders, 2004:79–90.

Williams BH. Ferret microbiology and virology. In: Fudge AM, ed. Laboratory Medicine, Avian and Exotic Pets. Philadelphia: WB Saunders, 2000:334–342.

*Portions Adapted From*

Gram WD. Dermatophytosis. In: Tilley LP, Smith FWK, Jr., eds. The 5-Minute Veterinary Consult: Canine and Feline, 3rd Ed. Baltimore: Lippincott Williams & Wilkins, 2003.

## BASICS

### OVERVIEW
• Disorder of carbohydrate, fat, and protein metabolism caused by an absolute or relative insulin deficiency
• Hyperglycemia may be caused by an insulin deficiency (similar to Type I diabetes), inhibition of insulin release from pancreatic beta cells, and peripheral resistance to insulin.
• Hyperglycemia may also be caused by excessive production and release of glucagon by a pancreatic glucagonoma.
• Mechanisms have not been well described in ferrets.
• Insulin deficiency impairs the ability of tissues (especially muscle, adipose tissue, and liver) to use carbohydrates, fats, and proteins.
• Impaired glucose use and ongoing gluconeogenesis cause hyperglycemia.
• Glucosuria develops, causing osmotic diuresis, polyuria, and compensatory weight loss; mobilization of free fatty acids to the liver causes both hepatic lipidosis and ketogenesis.

### SIGNALMENT
• Spontaneous diabetes appears to be very rare in ferrets.
• Diabetes is usually iatrogenic, secondary to pancreatectomy to treat insulinoma.
• No breed, sex, or age predilections have been described.

### SIGNS
• Early signs—polyuria and polydipsia (PU/PD), polyphagia, weight loss, and muscle wasting
• Later signs—anorexia, lethargy, depression, and vomiting
• Hepatomegaly and splenomegaly

### CAUSES AND RISK FACTORS
• Most common cause of hyperglycemia in ferrets is postoperative hyperglycemia following debulking of pancreatic beta cell tumors. Hyperglycemia is believed to be due to suppression of remaining islet cells by residual insulin from the removed tumors and will usually resolve spontaneously.
• Anecdotal reports of glucagonoma or combination of pancreatic insulinoma/glucagonoma exist; the relative incidence of these tumors is unknown.
• Spontaneous diabetes is uncommon in ferrets; causes and risk factors are unknown.

## DIAGNOSIS

### GENERAL COMMENTS
The diagnosis of diabetes is based on consistent elevation of plasma glucose concentration, combined with glucosuria, PU/PD, and weight loss. Identifying the cause of diabetes can be difficult. It has been suggested that some ferrets may have pancreatic glucagonoma alone or in combination with insulinoma. Documentation of glucagonoma is difficult since testing of serum glucagon concentration or immunohistochemical staining of biopsy samples are not readily available.

### DIFFERENTIAL DIAGNOSIS
• Renal glucosuria—usually does not cause PU/PD, weight loss, or hyperglycemia
• Stress hyperglycemia—no PU/PD or weight loss; blood glucose concentration normal if sample taken when animal is not stressed

### CBC/BIOCHEMISTRY/URINALYSIS
• Results of hemogram usually normal
• Glucose—>100 mg/dL is abnormal; persistent elevation of >300 mg/dL may warrant treatment; ferrets with diabetes have reported glucose >500 mg/dL.
• High SAP, ALT, and AST activities, and hypercholesterolemia and lipemia may be seen
• Increased BUN and creatinine possible if secondary nephritis
• Hypernatremia, hypokalemia, and hypophosphatemia may indicate severe decompensation.
• Glucosuria is a consistent finding.
• Ketonuria in late-stage disease not well documented in ferrets
• Urinary specific gravity may be low.
• Evidence of secondary bacterial cystitis possibly seen on the urinalysis

### OTHER LABORATORY TESTS
• Plasma insulin—diagnostic value of this test is questionable in ferrets; little is known about regulation of insulin release in ferrets. Low plasma insulin concentration with simultaneous hyperglycemia may suggest insulin deficiency. Be certain that the insulin assay used has been validated for use in ferrets.

• Plasma glucagons—to document glucagonoma. Testing is not readily available and assay must be validated for use in ferrets for results to be interpretable.

### IMAGING
Radiography and ultrasonography—useful to evaluate for concurrent or underlying disease (e.g., hepatic disease, adrenal disease, pancreatitis)

### DIAGNOSTIC PROCEDURES
N/A

### PATHOLOGIC FINDINGS
• Not well documented in ferrets
• Gross changes usually inapparent with spontaneous diabetes
• Histopathologic findings should be normal in cases of peripheral resistance to insulin or inhibition of insulin release. Vacuolar degeneration of the islets of Langerhans or low numbers of islet cells is possible with insulin deficiency.
• Immunohistochemical staining is necessary to demonstrate low numbers of beta cells or glucagonoma; however, this diagnostic tool is not readily available.
• Secondary nephritis may be seen.

## TREATMENT

### APPROPRIATE HEALTH CARE
• Hyperglycemia seen following pancreatectomy to treat insulinoma—usually resolves spontaneously without treatment. If hyperglycemia persists and the patient exhibits persistent clinical signs of diabetes (PU/PD, glucosuria, lethargy, increased appetite, and weight loss), treatment with insulin is generally indicated. Treatment with insulin is also indicated in ferrets that become ketoacidotic. Home regulation of postpancreatectomy hyperglycemia can be extremely difficult. Treatment of insulinoma by partial pancreatectomy is not usually curative, since some tumor is left behind, and eventually excessive amounts of insulin will again be released. Increased production of insulin, combined with exogenous insulin administration, may result in sudden, sometimes unexpected hypoglycemic episodes. Careful monitoring and client communication is necessary (see below).

# DIABETES MELLITUS

• If the animal is bright, alert, and well hydrated, intensive care and intravenous fluid administration are not required; start SC administration of insulin, beginning with NPH insulin 0.1 U/ferret SC q12h or Ultralente insulin 0.1 U/ferret SC q24. Dosages are empirical; careful monitorings required. Offer food at time of insulin injection and 4–6 hours later, and supply constant access to water; monitor closely for signs of illness (e.g., anorexia, lethargy, vomiting). Monitoring urine glucose may be helpful in alerting owners to impending hypoglycemic episodes (see follow up, below).

• Treatment of "sick" diabetic or ketoacidotic ferrets with inpatient intensive care; often a life-threatening emergency; goals are to correct the depletion of water and electrolytes, reverse ketonemia and acidosis, and increase the rate of glucose use by insulin-dependent tissues. Fluids—necessary to ensure adequate cardiac output and tissue perfusion and to maintain vascular volume; also reduce blood glucose concentration. IV administration of 0.9% saline is the initial fluid of choice; supplement with potassium when indicated.

• Volume determined by dehydration deficit plus maintenance requirements; replace over 24–48 h.

## DIET
• For hospitalized patients—offer high-quality ferret, feline w/d (Hills Products, Topeka, KS) or feline growth foods once the patient is stabilized. If this food is refused, try feeding chicken baby foods or critical care diets.

• Avoid soft, semimoist foods because they cause severe postprandial hyperglycemia.

• Diet at home—feed when each insulin injection is given and 4–6 hours following injection so that total food allotment is divided into four feedings.

## CLIENT EDUCATION
• Most ferrets with transient diabetes following partial pancreatectomy will either recover spontaneously or will require insulin treatment for short periods of time.

• Spontaneous diabetes can be a serious medical condition requiring lifelong insulin administration.

• Tight regulation of diabetes is difficult, and some ferrets do not improve with treatment.

• Discuss daily feeding and medication schedule and home monitoring of urine glucose. Many ferrets, especially those that are hyperglycemic following pancreatectomy, become suddenly and unexpectedly hypoglycemic. Warn owners that regulation is difficult. Discuss signs of hypoglycemia, home treatment, and when to call or visit a veterinarian.

• Clients are encouraged to keep a chart of pertinent information about the pet, such as urine dipstick results, daily insulin dose, and weekly body weight.

## SURGICAL CONSIDERATIONS
N/A

## MEDICATIONS

### DRUG(S) OF CHOICE
• Regular crystalline insulin—rapid bioavailability and short duration of action in cats and dogs; can be given by any parenteral route; used for patients with anorexia, vomiting, or ketoacidosis; can mix with other insulins

• NPH insulin—intermediate duration; bioavailability and duration is unknown in ferrets, but clinical experience suggests that these parameters are similar to those for cats; given SC q12h; initial dosage: 0.1 U per ferret; adjust the dosage according to individual response.

• Ultralente insulin—not widely used in ferrets; long-acting insulin; given SC, usually 0.1 U/ferret q24h; dosage extrapolated from feline regimens

• Species of origin of the insulin may affect pharmacokinetics; beef, pork, beef/pork, and human recombinant insulin are options; animal-origin insulins are being phased out; keep the pet on the same type and species of insulin if possible; when changing from an animal-origin to human recombinant insulin, lower the dosage and reregulate the animal.

### CONTRAINDICATIONS
N/A

### PRECAUTIONS
• Glucocorticoids, megestrol acetate, and progesterone cause insulin resistance.

• Hyperosmotic agents (e.g., mannitol and radiographic contrast agents) if the patient is already hyperosmolar from hyperglycemia

### POSSIBLE INTERACTIONS
Many drugs (e.g., NSAIDs, sulfonamides, miconazole, chloramphenicol, monoamine oxidase inhibitors, and beta blockers) potentiate the effect of hypoglycemic agents given orally; consult the product insert.

### ALTERNATIVE DRUGS
Therapy with oral administration of hypoglycemic agents is not commonly used in ferrets, since peripheral resistance to insulin (similar to Type II diabetes) has not been documented. Anecdotal reports suggest limited or unpredictable response to therapy.

## FOLLOW-UP

### PATIENT MONITORING
• Glucose curve—best method of monitoring. The owner feeds the pet, injects the insulin, and then brings the patient to the hospital for serial blood glucose testing every 1–2 hours, beginning about an hour after the injection. Animals receiving insulin q12h are followed for 12 hours, and those on insulin q24h are followed for 24 hours; the goal is to maintain blood glucose between 100 and 300 mg/100 mL for at least 20–22 h/day; however, tight regulation in ferrets may not be possible. Some ferrets respond little or not at all to insulin therapy.

• Urinary glucose monitoring—urine is tested for glucose and ketones before the meal and insulin injection; to use this as a regulatory method, the pet must be allowed to have trace to 1/4% glucosuria to avoid hypoglycemia. Insulin dosage is adjusted based on the amount of glycosuria present, the degree of PU/PD, appetite, and body weight. If no glucose is detected in the urine, discontinue insulin injections. Monitor serum glucose concentration to direct or withdraw future insulin therapy.

### PREVENTION/AVOIDANCE
N/A

### POSSIBLE COMPLICATIONS
• Seizure or coma with insulin overdose

• Continued production of insulin from remaining insulinoma postpancreatectomy, with resultant hypoglycemic episodes, seizure, coma, or death

• Progression of clinical signs associated with hyperglycemia despite insulin therapy

### EXPECTED COURSE AND PROGNOSIS
• Ferrets with hyperglycemia following partial pancreatectomy usually become euglycemic within 1–2 weeks after surgery. Insulin therapy, if required, is usually only temporarily indicated.

• Ferrets with spontaneous diabetes or those that continue to be hyperglycemic 2 weeks after pancreatectomy respond unpredictably to insulin and have a guarded to poor prognosis.

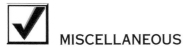

## MISCELLANEOUS

### ASSOCIATED CONDITIONS
- Insulinoma or glucagonoma
- Urinary tract infection and hepatic lipidosis may be sequelae to diabetes
- Ferret adrenal disease is seen concurrently in many ferrets with insulinomas

### SEE ALSO
- Insulinoma
- Polyuria and Polydipsia

### ABBREVIATIONS
- ALT = alanine aminotransferase
- AST = aspartate aminotransferase
- BUN = blood urea nitrogen
- NSAID = nonsteroidal antiinflammatory drug

*Suggested Reading*

Andrews GA, Myers NC, Chard-Bergstrom C. Immunohistochemistry of pancreatic islet cell tumors in the ferret (Mustela putorius furo). Vet Pathol 1997;34(5):387–393.

Fox JG, Marini RP. Diseases of the endocrine system. In: Fox JG, ed. Biology and Diseases of the Ferret. 2nd Ed. Baltimore: Williams & Wilkins, 1998

Hillyer EV. Ferret endocrinology. In: Kirk RW, Bonagura JD, eds) Kirk's Current Veterinary Therapy XI: Small Animal Practice. Philadelphia: WB Saunders, 1992.

Quesenberry KE, Rosenthal KL. Endocrine diseases. In: Quesenberry KE, Carpenter JW, eds. Ferrets, Rabbits and Rodents: Clinical Medicine and Surgery. St. Louis: WB Saunders, 2004:79–90.

Rosenthal KL. Ferret and rabbit endocrine disease diagnosis. In: Fudge AM, ed. Laboratory Medicine, Avian and Exotic Pets. Philadelphia: WB Saunders, 2000.

Weiss CA, Williams BH, Scott MV. Insulinoma in the ferret: clinical findings and treatment comparison of 66 cases. J Am Anim Hosp Assoc 1998;34:471–475.

*Portions Adapted From*

Wallace MS. Diabetes Mellitus, Uncomplicated In: Tilley LP, Smith FWK, Jr., eds. The 5-Minute Veterinary Consult: Canine and Feline, 2nd Ed. Baltimore: Lippincott Williams & Wilkins, 2000.

# DIARRHEA

## BASICS

### DEFINITION
Abnormal frequency, liquidity, and volume of feces

### PATHOPHYSIOLOGY
• Caused by imbalance in the absorptive, secretory, and motility actions of the intestines
• Diarrhea can result from a combination of factors.
• May or may not be associated with inflammation of the intestinal tract (enteritis)
• Foodstuffs and products of digestion exert osmotic forces. Ingestion of osmotically active foodstuffs that are poorly digestible, dietary malassimilation, malabsorption, or osmotically active medications (e.g., lactulose) can increase intestinal lumen osmotic force, which holds and draws fluid into the gut lumen, producing osmotic diarrhea. Fiber content contributes to the osmotic force exerted by a diet. Ferrets should not be fed a high-fiber or high-carbohydrate diet. The clinical signs of osmotic diarrhea often abate or resolve with fasting.
• Many of the infectious causes of diarrhea are related to increased secretion. Normally, the intestinal epithelium secretes fluid and electrolytes to aid in the digestion, absorption, and propulsion of foodstuffs. In disease states this secretion can overwhelm the absorptive activity and produce a secretory diarrhea.
• Inflammatory and infectious diarrhea—often produced by changes in secretion, motility, and absorptive ability; inflammation can also cause changes in intestinal wall permeability, causing loss of fluid and electrolytes and decreased absorptive ability.

### SYSTEMS AFFECTED
• Gastrointestinal
• Endocrine/metabolic—fluid, electrolyte, and acid-base imbalances

### SIGNALMENT
No specific age or gender predilection

### SIGNS

#### General Comments
• Patients can be placed into categories according to the severity of their illness. The extent of diagnostic workup and treatment are determined by the category.
• Mild illness—patients are alert, are active, and have no other clinical signs.
• Moderate illness—patients remain alert and active, but have other clinical signs such as anorexia, vomiting, or weight loss.
• Severe illness—patients are depressed, dehydrated, or listless and may also show signs listed under moderate illness.

#### Historical Findings
• Chewing habits—ferrets commonly ingest rubber toys, foam rubber, or cloth.
• History of diet change or ingestion of garbage or spoiled food
• History of recent exposure to other ferrets
• History of stress or other causes of immunosuppression

#### Small Bowel
• Larger volume of feces than normal
• Weight loss and polyphagia with malabsorption and maldigestion
• Melena
• Voluminous stools or "bird seed" consistency to feces may be seen with malabsorptive disorders.
• With many infectious diseases, especially ECE (aka "green slime disease"), feces are often mucoid and green.
• Diarrhea can be profuse and recurrent with severe weight loss.

#### Large Bowel
• Dark, liquid feces; fresh blood; green mucous or mucoid feces
• Frequency of defecation increased and volume often decreased
• Hematochezia, tenesmus, and/or mucous
• Dyschezia in ferrets with rectal or distal colonic disease
• Rectal prolapse, either intermittent or continuous, may be present.
• Weight loss and polyphagia

#### Physical Examination Findings
• Dehydration
• Emaciation
• Fecal staining of the perineum
• Poor haircoat—seen with chronic disease (infiltrative intestinal disease, hepatic disease, metabolic disorders)
• Abdominal distention may be due to thickened or fluid-filled intestinal loops, masses, ascites, or organomegaly (especially splenomegaly).
• Mesenteric lymph nodes are often palpably enlarged.

### CAUSES
• Bacterial infection–*Helicobacter mustelae* (most common bacterial infection), *Campylobacter* sp., *Clostridium* sp, and *Salmonella* sp. can be copathogens or primary pathogens in ferrets debilitated or stressed; *Mycobacterium avium-intracellulare* (rare)
• Viral infection—ECE (very common cause of diarrhea), rotavirus (rare)
• Infiltrative—lymphoplasmacytic gastroenteritis (very common cause), eosinophilic gastroenteritis (common), proliferative bowel disease common in young ferrets (*Desulfovibrio* sp.)
• Parasitic causes—Coccidia, *Giardia* (both are unusual and may be primary pathogens or secondary to ECE), *Cryptosporidium* spp. (rare)
• Neoplasia—lymphoma (common cause of diarrhea), adenocarcinoma

• Obstruction—foreign body, (common cause) neoplasia, intussusception
• Metabolic disorders—common; liver disease, renal disease
• Dietary—very common; diet changes, eating spoiled food, dietary intolerance
• Drugs and toxins—vaccine reaction (hemorrhagic diarrhea with CDV vaccination), plant toxins
• Maldigestion—hepatobiliary disease and pancreatitis (both are rare)

### RISK FACTORS
• Exposure to other ferrets
• Dietary changes or inappropriate diet
• Unsupervised chewing
• Feeding raw meat products
• Vaccine reaction

## DIAGNOSIS

### DIFFERENTIAL DIAGNOSIS

#### Differentiating Causes
• Melena and anorexia most common with *H. mustelae* or gastrointestinal foreign body
• Thickened intestinal loops and palpably enlarged mesenteric lymph nodes common with lymphoplasmacytic enteritis, eosinophilic enterocolitis, ECE, or lymphoma
• Bile-stained (green) mucous-covered diarrhea seen most commonly with ECE
• Granular, "bird seed"-like feces seen with maldigestive/malabsorptive disorders and ECE
• Tenesmus, dyschezia, and rectal prolapse in young ferrets with Coccidia or proliferative bowel disease
• A large amount of fresh blood in the feces is more common with salmonellosis.

### CBC/BIOCHEMISTRY
• Increased hematocrit and serum protein concentration seen with dehydration
• Anemia may be seen with chronic gastrointestinal bleeding
• TWBC elevation with neutrophilia may be seen with bacterial enteritis.
• TWBC elevation with lymphocytosis or normal TWBC with relative lymphocytosis can be suggestive of lymphoma
• Eosinophilia (as high as 35%) in ferrets with eosinophilic enterocolitis
• Hypoalbuminemia may be seen with protein loss from the intestinal tract, especially with proliferative bowel disease.
• Serum biochemistry abnormalities may suggest renal or hepatic disease; ALT elevations usually seen with ECE

### OTHER LABORATORY TESTS
• Fecal direct examination, fecal flotation, and zinc sulfate centrifugation may demonstrate gastrointestinal parasites.

• Fecal cytology—may reveal red blood cells or fecal leukocytes, which are associated with inflammatory bowel disease or invasive bacterial strains
• Fecal culture should be performed if abnormal bacteria are observed on the fecal Gram's stain or if *Salmonella* is suspected.

### IMAGING

#### Radiographic Findings
• Survey abdominal radiography may indicate intestinal obstruction, organomegaly, mass, foreign body, or ascites.
• Contrast radiography may indicate mucosal irregularities, mass, severe ileus, foreign body, stricture, or, rarely, thickening of the intestinal wall.
• Abdominal ultrasonography may demonstrate intestinal wall thickening, gastrointestinal mass, foreign body, ileus, or mesenteric lymphadenopathy. Hyperechogenicity may be seen with hepatic lipidosis or fibrosis; hypoechoic nodules are suggestive of hepatic necrosis, abscess, or neoplasia.

### OTHER DIAGNOSTIC PROCEDURES

#### Surgical Considerations
Exploratory laparotomy and surgical biopsy should be pursued if there is evidence of obstruction or intestinal mass and/or for definitive diagnosis of gastrointestinal inflammatory or infiltrative diseases or *H. mustelae*.

## TREATMENT
• Treatment must be specific to the underlying cause to be successful.
• Patients with mild disease usually respond to outpatient treatment.
• Patients with moderate to severe disease usually require hospitalization and 24-hour care for parenteral medication and fluid therapy.

### NURSING CARE

#### Fluid Therapy
• Essential in treatment of patients with diarrhea; route and type of fluids will depend on severity of disease.
• Subcutaneous and/or oral fluids may be sufficient in patients with mild disease.
• An IV route is most effective in patients that are severely dehydrated. Initially, a balanced fluid (e.g., lactated Ringer's solution) may be used.
• Correct electrolyte and acid-base disturbances in patients with moderate to severe disease
• Patients with hypoproteinemia may benefit from treatment with hetastarch (6% hetastarch in 0.9% NaCl); administer an IV bolus (10–20 mL/kg) slowly over 2–3 hours, then at a constant rate infusion of 1m/kg/h for 24 hours; hetastarch increases

plasma oncotic pressure and pulls fluid into the intravascular space.

### DIET
• Feed high-calorie diets, such as Eukanuba Maximum Calorie diet (Iams Co., Dayton, OH), Feline a/d (Hills Products, Topeka, KS), or Clinicare Feline liquid diet (Abbott Laboratories, North Chicago, IL) to emaciated animals in critical condition; may also add dietary supplement such as Nutri-Cal (EVSCO Pharmaceuticals, Buena, NJ) to increase caloric content of these foods
• Easily digestible, high-protein diets such as chicken baby food are often helpful in ferrets recovering from ECE or inflammatory bowel disease.
• Resting energy requirement for ferrets is approximately 70 kcal/kg body weight per day (sick ferrets have higher requirements). Clinicare Feline contains 1 kcal/mL; Eukanuba Maximum Calorie diet contains 2 kcal/mL.

### SURGICAL CONSIDERATIONS
• Exploratory laparotomy to remove foreign bodies or tumors

## MEDICATIONS

### DRUG(S) OF CHOICE

#### Antibiotic Therapy
• Indicated in patients with bacterial inflammatory lesions in the gastrointestinal tract; also indicated in patients with disruption of the intestinal mucosa evidenced by blood in the feces. Selection should be based on results of culture and susceptibility testing when possible.
• Some choices for empirical use while waiting for culture results include trimethoprim sulfa (15–30 mg/kg PO, SC q12h), amoxicillin (10–20 mg/kg PO, SC q12h), or enrofloxacin (10–20 mg/kg PO, SC IM q24h)
• Proliferative bowel disease—chloramphenicol (50 mg/kg, IM, SC, PO q12h)
• Giardiasis, anaerobic bacterial infections—metronidazole (15–20 mg/kg PO q12h)
• *H. mustelae*—amoxicillin (10 mg/kg PO q12h) plus metronidazole (20 mg/kg PO q12h) and bismuth subsalicylate (17 mg/kg PO q12h) for 2 weeks; or clarithromycin (12.5 mg/kg PO q8h) plus ranitidine bismuth citrate (this is not Zantac, ranitidine HCl) at 24 mg/kg PO q8h for 2 weeks

#### Gastrointestinal Antisecretory Agents
Are helpful to treat and possibly prevent gastritis in anorectic ferrets. Ferrets continually secrete a baseline level of gastric hydrochloric acid and, as such, anorexia itself may predispose to gastric ulceration. Those successfully used in ferrets include omeprazole (0.7 mg/kg PO q24h), famotidine (0.25–0.5 mg/kg PO, IV, SC q24h), and cimetidine (5–10 mg/kg PO, SC, IM q8h)

#### Corticosteroids
Often helpful in treatment of inflammatory bowel diseases (treat underlying disease whenever possible)—prednisone (1.25–2.5 mg/kg PO q24h); when signs resolve, gradually taper the corticosteroid dose to 0.5–1.25 PO mg/kg every other day.

#### Anticholinergics
Loperamide (0.2 mg/kg PO q12h) may be helpful in the symptomatic treatment of acute diarrhea (see contraindications/precautions).

### CONTRAINDICATIONS
• Anticholinergics in patients with suspected intestinal obstruction, glaucoma, intestinal ileus, liver disease, enterotoxin-producing bacteria and invasive bacterial enteritis
• Anticholinergics exacerbate most types of chronic diarrhea and should not be used for empirical treatment.

### PRECAUTIONS
• Loperamide may cause hyperactivity in ferrets.
• It is important to determine the cause of diarrhea. A general shotgun antibiotic approach may be ineffective or detrimental.
• Some ferrets will become anorectic when administered high doses of amoxicillin.

### POSSIBLE INTERACTIONS
N/A

### ALTERNATE DRUGS
See specific diseases for a more complete discussion of treatment.

## FOLLOW-UP

### PATIENT MONITORING
• Fecal volume and character, appetite, attitude, and body weight
• In patients with ECE, stool may not return to a normal consistency for several weeks. Occasionally, diarrhea will recur months after initial resolution of clinical signs.
• If diarrhea does not resolve, consider reevaluation of the diagnosis.

### POSSIBLE COMPLICATIONS
• Septicemia due to bacterial invasion of enteric mucosa
• Dehydration due to fluid loss

# DIARRHEA

## MISCELLANEOUS

### ASSOCIATED CONDITIONS
- Septicemia
- Rectal prolapse

### AGE-RELATED FACTORS
- Kits 4–6 weeks of age more susceptible to rotavirus
- Symptomatic *H. mustelae* more common in ferrets >3 years of age
- Older ferrets demonstrate more severe clinical signs with ECE.
- Proliferative bowel disease and Coccidia seen more commonly in ferrets <1 year of age

### ZOONOTIC POTENTIAL
- Cryptosporidiosis
- *Giardia*

### PREGNANCY
N/A

### SEE ALSO
- ECE Epizootic Catarrhal Enteritis
- Eosinophilic gastroenteritis
- Giardiasis

- *Helicobacter mustelae*
- Lymphophasmacytic enteritis and gastroenteritis
- Lymphosarcoma
- Proliferative bowel disease

### ABBREVIATIONS
- ALT = alanine aminotransferase
- CNS = central nervous system
- ECE = epizootic catarrhal enteritis
- TWBC = total white blood cell count

*Suggested Reading*

Finkler MR. Ferret colitis. In: Kirk RW, Bonagura JD, eds. Kirk's Current Veterinary Therapy XI: Small Animal Practice. Philadelphia: WB Saunders, 1992.

Fox JG. Diseases of the gastrointestinal system. In: Fox JG, ed. Biology and Diseases of the Ferret. 2nd Ed. Baltimore: Williams & Wilkins, 1998.

Fox JG: Parasitic diseases. In: Fox JG, ed. Biology and Diseases of the Ferret. 2nd Ed. Baltimore: Williams & Wilkins, 1998:375–392.

Fox JG, Marini RP. Helicobacter mustelae infection in ferrets: pathogenesis, epizootiology, diagnosis and treatment. Semin Avin Exotic Pet Med 2001;10(1):36–44.

Hoefer HL, Bell JA. Gastrointestinal diseases. In: Quesenberry KE, Carpenter JW, eds. In: Hillyer EV, Quesenberry KE, eds. Ferrets, Rabbits and Rodents: Clinical Medicine and Surgery. St Louis: WB Saunders, 2004:25–40.

Jenkins JR. Rabbit and ferret liver and gastrointestinal testing. In: Fudge AM, ed. Laboratory Medicine, Avian and Exotic Pets. Philadelphia: WB Saunders, 2000.

Williams BH, Kiupel M, West KH, et al. Coronavirus-associated epizootic catarrhal enteritis in ferrets. J Am Vet Med Assoc 2000;217:526–530.

*Portions Adapted From*

Duval DS. Diarrhea, acute. In: Tilley LP, Smith FWK, Jr., eds. The 5-Minute Veterinary Consult: Canine and Feline, 2nd Ed. Baltimore: Lippincott Williams & Wilkins, 2000.

## BASICS

### DEFINITION
• Dyschezia—painful or difficult defecation
• Hematochezia—bright red blood in the feces

### PATHOPHYSIOLOGY
• Result from various causes of inflammation or irritation of the rectum or anus
• Hematochezia may also occur with diseases of the colon.

### SYSTEMS AFFECTED
Gastrointestinal

### SIGNALMENT
• Coccidiosis and Proliferative Bowel Disease (PBD) are seen primarily in ferrets <6 months of age.
• No sex or age predilection in ferrets with other types of inflammatory bowel disease

### SIGNS

#### Historical Findings
• Crying out during defecation
• Tenesmus common
• Mucoid, bloody diarrhea in patients with colonic disease
• Severe weight loss, ataxia, weakness, muscle tremors, abdominal discomfort, or generalized unthriftiness in ferrets with severe PBD
• Anorexia, weight loss, muscle wasting, vomiting, ptyalism, and/or pawing at the mouth seen with other types of inflammatory bowel disease and ECE

#### Physical Examination Findings
• Inflammatory bowel diseases—cachexia; thickened, ropy intestines, enlarged mesenteric lymph nodes, and splenomegaly often palpable
• PBD—distal colon may be palpably thickened, mesenteric lymph nodes may be enlarged; fecal and urine staining of perineum; partial to complete rectal prolapse

### CAUSES

#### Colonic Disease
• Coccidiosis—most common cause in young ferrets
• Inflammation—IBD (lymphoplasmacytic gastroenteritis, eosinophilic gastroenteritis [EGE])
• Epizootic Catarrhal Enteritis (ECE)
• Neoplasia—lymphoma most common, adenocarcinoma
• Proliferative Bowel Disease (PBD [Desulfovibrio spp.])—unusual disease seen in young ferrets

#### Rectal/Anal Disease (Rare)
• Rectal or anal foreign body
• Trauma—bite wounds, etc.
• Neoplasia—adenocarcinoma, lymphoma

• Anal sacculitis or abscess—not usually a differential diagnosis since most ferrets purchased from pet shops have had the anal sacs removed by the breeding facility at a very young age

#### Extraintestinal Disease
• Prostatic disease—prostatic cysts, abscesses, or hyperplasia; seen in middle-aged ferrets with adrenal disease
• Fractured pelvis or hind limb
• Intrapelvic neoplasia

### RISK FACTORS
Stress, poor hygiene, concurrent disease

## DIAGNOSIS

### DIFFERENTIAL DIAGNOSIS
Dysuria, stranguria, or hematuria—abnormal findings on urinalysis, such as pyuria, crystalluria, bacteriuria with UTI or urolithiasis; hair loss and palpable caudal abdominal mass with urogenital cystic disease or prostatic hyperplasia

### CBC/BIOCHEMISTRY/URINALYSIS
• Usually normal
• May reflect underlying cause (e.g., inflammatory leukogram with infectious disease, eosinophilia with EGE, increased ALT with ECE)
• Hypoproteinemia with chronic diarrhea
• Dehydration—elevated PCV, TP, and azotemia; reflecting fluid loss from the gastrointestinal tract

### OTHER LABORATORY TESTS
Fecal direct examination, fecal flotation, and zinc sulfate centrifugation may demonstrate gastrointestinal parasites.

#### Microbiology
• Aerobic and anaerobic fecal cultures rule out clostridia or Salmonella
• Cultures for Desulfovibrio spp. are not useful, since they are intracellular organisms not usually shed in the feces.
• Fecal cytology may demonstrate clostridia or other organisms, increased white blood cell or red blood cell numbers

### IMAGING
• Pelvic radiographs may reveal urogenital cysts or prostatic disease, foreign body, or fracture.
• Ultrasonography may demonstrate prostatic disease or caudal abdominal masses.

### DIAGNOSTIC PROCEDURES
Definitive diagnosis of IBD or PBD requires biopsy and histopathology, usually obtained via exploratory laparotomy.

## TREATMENT
• Most patients with mild to moderate diarrhea can be treated as outpatients.
• Hospitalize when diarrhea is severe, resulting in dehydration and electrolyte imbalance; administer supportive fluids on the basis of hydration status.
• Rehydration is essential to treatment success in severely ill ferrets. Initially, a balanced fluid (e.g., lactated Ringer's solution) may be used.
• Supplementation with 5% dextrose is beneficial in anorectic, hypoglycemic patients.
• Patients with hypoproteinemia may benefit from treatment with hetastarch (6% hetastarch in 0.9% NaCl); administer an IV bolus (10–20 mL/kg) slowly over 2–3 hours; then as a constant rate infusion of 1 mL/kg/h for 24 hours; hetastarch increases plasma oncotic pressure and pulls fluid into the intravascular space.
• Proper, strict isolation procedures are essential in patients with suspected infectious diseases.

### DIET
Anorectic ferrets may refuse kibble but are often willing to eat canned cat foods, meat baby foods, or high-calorie liquid or paste dietary supplements.

## MEDICATIONS

### DRUG(S) OF CHOICE
• Depends on the underlying cause; see discussion under specific diseases.
• For Coccidia—sulfadimethoxine 50 mg/kg PO on the first day, then 25 mg/kg q24h or 9 days
• For PBD—chloramphenicol 50 mg/kg IM, SC, PO q12h × 14 days; elimination of signs supports the diagnosis.
• Antibiotics are indicated in most patients with hematochezia due to disruption of the intestinal mucosa. Selection should be based on results of culture and susceptibility testing when possible. Some choices for empirical use while waiting for culture results include trimethoprim sulfa (15–30 mg/kg q12h), amoxicillin (10–20 mg/kg PO, SC q12h), or enrofloxacin (10–20 mg/kg PO, SC, IM q24h).

### CONTRAINDICATIONS
N/A

# DYSCHEZIA AND HEMATOCHEZIA

**PRECAUTIONS**
N/A

**POSSIBLE INTERACTIONS**
N/A

**ALTERNATIVE DRUGS**
N/A

 **FOLLOW-UP**

**PATIENT MONITORING**
Monitor patients for recurrence of diarrhea or concurrent diseases such as gastrointestinal ulceration or enteric copathogens.

**POSSIBLE COMPLICATIONS**
• Rectal prolapse
• Dehydration, malnutrition, hypoproteinemia, anemia, and diseases secondary to therapy or resulting from the above mentioned problems
• May see fecal incontinence with rectal disease

 **MISCELLANEOUS**

**ASSOCIATED CONDITIONS**
N/A

**AGE-RELATED FACTORS**
• Coccidia and PBD more common in young ferrets

• Infiltrative (inflammatory, neoplastic) diseases more common in older ferrets

**ZOONOTIC POTENTIAL**
N/A

**PREGNANCY**
N/A

**SYNONYMS**
N/A

**SEE ALSO**
• Diarrhea
• Lymphoplasmacytic gastroenteritis
• PBD
• Rectal and anal prolapse

**ABBREVIATION**
• ECE = epizootic catarrhal enteritis
• IBD = inflammatory bowel disease
• PBD = proliferative bowel disease
• PCV = packed cell volume
• TP = total protein
• UTI = urinary tract infection

*Suggested Reading*

Fox JG. Diseases of the gastrointestinal system. In: Fox JG, ed. Biology and Diseases of the Ferret. 2nd Ed. Baltimore: Williams & Wilkins, 1998:273–290.

Fox JG. Parasitic diseases. In: Fox JG, ed. Biology and Diseases of the Ferret. 2nd Ed. Baltimore: Williams & Wilkins, 1998:375–392.

Fox JG, Murphy JC, Otto G, et al. Proliferative colitis in ferrets: epithelial dysplasia and translocation. Vet Pathol 1989;26(6):55–517.

Hoefer HL, Bell JA. Gastrointestinal diseases. In: Quesenberry KE, Carpenter JW, eds. Ferrets, Rabbits and Rodents: Clinical Medicine and Surgery. St. Louis: WB Saunders, 2004:25–40.

Jenkins JR. Rabbit and ferret liver and gastrointestinal testing. In: Fudge AM, ed. Laboratory Medicine, Avian and Exotic Pets. Philadelphia: WB Saunders, 2000.

Williams BH, Kiupel M, West KH, et al. Coronavirus-associated epizootic catarrhal enteritis in ferrets. J Am Vet Med Assoc 2000;217:526–530.

*Portions Adapted From*

Moore LE, Burrows CF. Dyschezia and Hematochezia. In: Tilley LP, Smith FWK, Jr., eds. The 5-Minute Veterinary Consult: Canine and Feline, 3rd Ed. Baltimore: Lippincott Williams & Wilkins, 2004.

# BASICS

## OVERVIEW
• Dysphagia may be defined as difficulty swallowing, resulting from the inability to prehend, form, and move a bolus of food through the oropharynx into the esophagus.
• Swallowing difficulties can be caused by mechanical obstruction of the oral cavity or pharynx, neuromuscular dysfunction resulting in weak or uncoordinated swallowing movements, or pain associated with prehension, mastication, or swallowing.

## SYSTEMS AFFECTED
• Neuromuscular
• Nervous
• Gastrointestinal
• Respiratory

## SIGNALMENT
No breed, sex, or age predilections have been described

## SIGNS
### Historical Findings
• Drooling, gagging, weight loss, ravenous appetite, repeated attempts at swallowing, swallowing with the head in an abnormal position, coughing (due to aspiration), regurgitation, painful swallowing, and occasionally anorexia are all possible.
• Ascertain onset and progression.
• Foreign bodies cause acute dysphagia; oropharyngeal disease may cause chronic or intermittent signs.

### Physical Examination Findings
• A thorough oral examination, with the patient sedated or anesthetized, if necessary, is most important.
• Observe for asymmetry, foreign body, inflammation, tumor, edema, abscessed teeth, and loose teeth.
• Observe the patient eating; this may localize the abnormal phase of swallowing.
• Perform a complete neurologic examination, with emphasis on the cranial nerves.

### Causes
• Pain because of dental disease (e.g., tooth fractures and abscess), mandibular trauma, stomatitis, glossitis, and pharyngeal inflammation may also disrupt normal prehension, bolus formation, and swallowing.
• Anatomic or mechanical lesions—consider pharyngeal inflammation (e.g., abscess, inflammation), pharyngeal or retropharyngeal foreign body, retropharyngeal lymphadenomegaly, neoplasia, temporomandibular joint disorders (e.g., luxation, fracture), mandibular fracture, and pharyngeal trauma.

• Neuromuscular disorders—megaesophagus has rarely been reported in the ferret. Cranial nerve deficits that impair prehension, bolus formation, and masticatory muscle myositis have not been reported in ferrets but should be considered.
• Rabies may cause dysphagia by affecting both the brainstem and peripheral nerves.
• Other CNS disorders, especially those involving the brainstem, should be considered if an anatomic, mechanical lesion or pain is not found.

# DIAGNOSIS

## DIFFERENTIAL DIAGNOSIS
• Must be differentiated from vomiting and regurgitation from esophageal disease
• Exaggerated or repeated efforts to swallow—characteristic of dysphagia; most useful means of distinguishing it from vomiting or regurgitation
• Vomiting is associated with abdominal contractions; dysphagia is not.

## CBC/BIOCHEMISTRY/URINALYSIS
• Inflammatory conditions may cause leukocytosis.
• High serum creatine phosphokinase activity may indicate a muscular disorder.

## OTHER LABORATORY TESTS
N/A

## IMAGING
• Obtain survey radiographs of the skull and neck; give particular attention to the mandibles and temporomandibular joint, teeth, and pharyngeal and retropharyngeal areas.
• Ultrasonography of the pharynx may be useful in patients with mass lesions and for obtaining ultrasound-guided biopsy specimens.
• Fluoroscopy, with or without positive contrast, is useful in evaluating pharyngeal movement in other mammals with suspected pharyngeal dysphagia and may have similar value in ferrets.
• CT and/or MRI may be useful to identify suspected intracranial mass

## DIAGNOSTIC PROCEDURES
• Excisional or incisional biopsies of a mass lesion
• Pharyngoscopy
• Electromyography of the pharyngeal musculature has been used in other small animals to confirm the presence of a neuromuscular disorder; usefulness in ferrets is unknown.

# TREATMENT
• Determine the underlying cause to develop a treatment plan and accurate prognosis.
• Direct primary treatment at the underlying cause.
• Nutritional support is important for all dysphagic patients.
• Patients with oral disease may be able to swallow a gruel or liquid diet; take care to avoid aspiration when feeding orally.
• Surgical excision of a mass lesion and foreign body may be curative or temporarily improve the signs of dysphagia.

# MEDICATIONS

## DRUG(S) OF CHOICE
Dysphagia is not immediately life-threatening; direct drug therapy at the underlying cause.

## CONTRAINDICATIONS
N/A

## PRECAUTIONS
• Use barium sulfate with caution in patients with evidence of aspiration.
• Use corticosteroids with caution or not at all in patients with evidence of, or at risk for, aspiration.

## POSSIBLE INTERACTIONS
N/A

## ALTERNATIVE DRUGS
N/A

# FOLLOW-UP

## PATIENT MONITORING
• Daily for signs of aspiration pneumonia (e.g., depression, fever, mucopurulent nasal discharge, coughing, and dyspnea)
• Body condition and hydration status daily; if oral nutrition does not meet requirements gastrostomy tube feeding may be necessary.

## POSSIBLE COMPLICATIONS
• Aspiration pneumonia is a common complication with swallowing disorders.
• Feeding multiple small meals with the patient in an upright position and maintaining this position for 10–15 minutes after feeding may help prevent aspiration of food.

# DYSPHAGIA

## MISCELLANEOUS

### ASSOCIATED CONDITIONS
Aspiration pneumonia

### AGE-RELATED FACTORS
• Young ferrets are more likely to ingest foreign objects and suffer facial trauma.
• Older ferrets are more likely to have oral pain from dental disease.

### ZOONOTIC POTENTIAL
• Consider rabies in any patient with dysphagia, especially if the animal's rabies vaccination status is unknown or questionable or it has been exposed to a potentially rabid animal.
• If a dysphagic animal dies of rapidly progressive neurologic disease, submit the head to a qualified laboratory designated by the local or state health department for rabies examination.

### PREGNANCY
N/A

### SYNONYMS
N/A

### SEE ALSO
• Pneumonia, aspiration
• Vomiting
• Weight loss and cachexia

### ABBREVIATIONS
• CNS = central nervous system
• CT = computed tomography
• MRI = magnetic resonance imaging

*Suggested Reading*

Blanco MC, Fox JG, Rosenthal K, et al. Megaesophagus in nine ferrets. J Am Vet Med Assoc 1994;205:444–447.

Hoefer HL, Bell JA. Gastrointestinal diseases. In: Quesenberry KE, Carpenter JW, eds. Ferrets, Rabbits and Rodents: Clinical Medicine and Surgery. St. Louis: WB Saunders, 2004:25–40.

Willard MD. Dysphagia and swallowing disorders. In: Kirk's Current Veterinary Therapy XI. Philadelphia: Saunders, 1992:572–577.

Williams BH, Weiss CA. Neoplasia. In: Quesenberry KE, Carpenter JW, eds. Ferrets, Rabbits and Rodents: Clinical Medicine and Surgery. St. Louis: WB Saunders, 2004:91–106.

*Portions Adapted From*

Longshore RC. Dysphagia. In: Tilley LP, Smith FWK, Jr., eds. The 5-Minute Veterinary Consult: Canine and Feline, 3rd Ed. Baltimore: Lippincott Williams & Wilkins, 2003.

# DYSPNEA AND TACHYPNEA

 **BASICS**

## DEFINITION
Dyspnea is the distressful feeling associated with difficult or labored breathing, tachypnea is rapid breathing (not necessarily labored), and hyperpnea is deep breathing. In animals, the term dyspnea often is applied to labored breathing that appears to be uncomfortable.

## PATHOPHYSIOLOGY
• Nonrespiratory causes of dyspnea may include abnormalities in pulmonary vascular tone (CNS disease, shock), pulmonary circulation, (CHF), oxygenation (anemia), or ventilation (obesity, ascites, abdominal organomegaly, musculoskeletal disease).
• Primary respiratory diseases may be divided into upper and lower respiratory tract problems; the latter can be subdivided into obstructive and restrictive causes.

## SYSTEMS AFFECTED
• Respiratory
• Cardiovascular
• Nervous (secondary to hypoxia)

## SIGNALMENT
Any

## SIGNS

### Historical Findings
• Orthopnea (recumbent dyspnea), restlessness, and poor sleeping may occur in ferrets with pleural space disease (mediastinal mass, effusions, abscesses, diaphragmatic hernias) or CHF.
• Exercise intolerance may occur with lower respiratory tract disease or CHF.
• Sneezing or naso-ocular discharge may be seen with upper respiratory infections.
• Coughing is rare in ferrets but may occur with dyspnea in ferrets with tracheal or LRT disease

### Physical Examination Findings
• Upper airway obstruction—stridor, stertor
• Pulmonary edema—fine inspiratory crackles
• Pneumonia—harsh inspiratory and expiratory bronchovesicular sounds
• Pleural effusion or diaphragmatic hernia—dull percussion and absent lung sounds ventrally, harsh lung sounds dorsally
• Mediastinal mass—noncompressible thorax
• Pyrexia (CDV, influenza, bacterial infections)
• Weight loss and poor hair coat in ferrets with chronic respiratory disease

## CAUSES

### Nonrespiratory Causes
• Cardiac disease (most common)—CHF, heartworm disease, severe arrhythmias, cardiogenic shock

• Neuromuscular disease—severe CNS disease (trauma, inflammation, neoplasia), rib fractures, spinal disease (trauma, disc extrusion), megaesophagus
• Mediastinal mass (lymphoma most common)
• Metabolic disease—acidosis, uremia
• Hematologic—anemia (estrogen toxicity, blood loss)
• Other—anxiety, pain, obesity, ascites, organomegaly, fever, heat stroke

### Respiratory Causes
*URT*
• Nasal obstruction—rhinitis/sinusitis (viral, bacterial, mycotic), granuloma, foreign body, neoplasia
• Laryngotracheal obstruction—foreign body, neoplasia
• Traumatic airway rupture
• Extraluminal tracheal compression—hilar lymphadenopathy (lymphoma)
*LRT*
• Obstructive—pulmonary edema (cardiogenic and noncardiac); pneumonia—viral (CDV, influenza), bacterial, and neoplasia (primary, metastatic) most common; mycotic, pulmonary contusion (trauma), consolidated lung lobe; pneumonitis (allergic, parasitic not documented in ferrets); intrathoracic tracheal disease (foreign body, neoplasia)
• Restrictive—pleural effusion caused by cardiac or pericardial disease; mediastinal masses (lymphoma); diaphragmatic hernias; hemothorax; pneumothorax; chylothorax

## RISK FACTORS
• Exposure to other ferrets
• Trauma, bite wounds
• CDV in poorly vaccinated animals
• Poor ventilation
• Immunosuppression

 **DIAGNOSIS**

## DIFFERENTIATING CAUSES
• Severe hypoglycemic episodes resulting in collapse in ferrets with insulinoma may be mistaken for dyspnea.
• Gagging and retching associated with nausea or vomiting may be mistaken for dyspnea.
• Tachypnea without dyspnea may be a physiologic response to fear, physical exertion, anxiety, fever, pain, or acidosis.
• Infectious causes (pneumonia, sinusitis/rhinitis) usually present with signs of systemic disease (emaciation, anorexia, depression).
• Primary cardiac disease often presents with a constellation of other signs (e.g., heart murmur, arrythmias, ascites).
• URT dyspnea is often more pronounced on inspiration.

• LRT dyspnea is more often associated with expiratory effort.
• Tracheal mass or foreign body may cause both inspiratory and expiratory dyspnea.
• Pleural space disease often presents as exaggerated thoracic excursions that generate only minimal airflow at the mouth or nose.

## CBC/BIOCHEMISTRY/URINALYSIS
• Hemogram—inflammatory leukocytosis (pneumonia, sinusitis), anemia with chronic disease
• Biochemistry panel—increased liver enzyme activity or bile acids (liver disease), increased CK (muscle wasting, heart disease)

## OTHER LABORATORY TESTS
• Cytologic examination, bacterial and mycotic culture—on samples from tracheal wash, deep nasal swabs, pleural fluid, or fine needle aspirates of masses
• Serologic tests that identify adult *Dirofilaria immitis* antigen are of some use; however, false-negative results are common—ELISA (Snap heartworm antigen test, Idexx Laboratories)
• Fluorescent antibody test for CDV—on blood or mucous membrane scrapings

## IMAGING

### Radiography
• Skull—may demonstrate nasal obstruction, sinusitis, bony destruction from neoplasia, or mycotic infections
• Thoracic—may reveal pulmonary diseases (small airway disease, pulmonary edema, and pneumonia), pleural space disease (effusions, mediastinal mass), pneumothorax, and hernias
• Cardiac shadow—cardiomegaly with heart disease
• Abdominal—organomegaly, ascites

### Ultrasonography
• Echocardiography to evaluate pericardial effusion, cardiomyopathy, heartworm disease, congenital defects, and valvular disease
• Thoracic ultrasound may be beneficial in some animals with mediastinal mass lesions, but the beam is often greatly attenuated by any air in surrounding lung lobes.
• Abdominal ultrasound may be used to evaluate masses or organomegaly.

## OTHER DIAGNOSTIC PROCEDURES
• Tracheal wash—cytology and culture
• Thoracocentesis—fluid analysis and culture

 **TREATMENT**
• Airway—if URT is obstructed, intubation (if possible) or tracheostomy may be required.

• Breathing—supply $O_2$ enrichment ($O_2$ cage or induction chamber) in a quiet environment. Ventilate only if animal has bradypnea or pulmonary arrest or is hypoventilating from exhaustion. If the hypoventilation is from pleural space disease, artificial ventilation and $O_2$ supplementation do little until chest is evacuated.
• Chest tap—may be both diagnostic and therapeutic in animals with pleural space disease. In acutely dyspneic animals, perform tap prior to radiography. A negative tap for air or fluid suggests solid pleural space (mass, abscess, or hernia) or primary pulmonary or cardiac disease.
• Surgery may be necessary to remove foreign bodies; obtain samples for biopsy or to debulk tumors, abscesses, or granulomas.

# MEDICATIONS

### DRUG(S) OF CHOICE
• Oxygen is the single most useful drug in the treatment of acute severe dyspnea.
• See primary disorder for definitive therapy.

### CONTRAINDICATIONS
• In animals with CHF and blunt chest trauma, iatrogenic fluid overload and pulmonary edema are potential problems. IV administration of crystalloids should be used judiciously.
• Respiratory rate and effort should be monitored carefully and frequently in these patients.

### PRECAUTIONS
Corticosteroids should be used with caution in patients with suspected infectious diseases.

### POSSIBLE INTERACTIONS
N/A

### ALTERNATE DRUGS
N/A

# FOLLOW-UP

### PATIENT MONITORING
• Repeat any abnormal tests.
• Radiographs—monitor response to therapy in animals with pulmonary disease. Pulmonary edema should be visibly improved within 12 hours of therapy, if effective therapy is used. Monitor the recurrence of pleural effusion, based on how quickly effusion accumulates.
• Cardiac ultrasound—3–12 weeks, depending on the condition

### POSSIBLE COMPLICATIONS
• Depends on the underlying disease
• Relapse, progression of disease, and death are common.

# MISCELLANEOUS

### ASSOCIATED CONDITIONS
• Lymphoma
• Splenomegaly

### ZOONOTIC POTENTIAL
Influenza virus

### PREGNANCY
N/A

### SYNONYMS
N/A

### SEE ALSO
See causes.

### ABBREVIATIONS
• CDV = canine distemper virus
• CHF = congestive heart failure
• CK = creatinine kinase
• CNS = central nervous system
• ELISA = enzyme-linked immunosorbent assay
• LRT = lower respiratory tract
• URT = upper respiratory tract

### Suggested Reading
Fox JG. Bacterial and mycoplasmal diseases. In: Fox JG, ed. Biology and Diseases of the Ferret. 2nd Ed. Baltimore: Williams & Wilkins, 1998:321–354.
Hoefer HL. Thoracic disease rule-outs in the ferret. Proc North Am Vet Conf 2001; 867–868.
Kendrick RE. Ferret respiratory diseases. Vet Clin North Am Exotic Anim Pract 2000;3(2):453–464.
Rosenthal K. Management of cardiac disease in ferrets. Waltham/OSU Symp Treatment Sm Anim Dis 1997;Sept.
Petrie JP, Morrisey JK. Cardiovascular and other diseases. In: Quesenberry KE, Carpenter JW, eds. Ferrets, Rabbits and Rodents: Clinical Medicine and Surgery. St. Louis: WB Saunders, 2004:58–71.
Rosenthal KL. Respiratory diseases. In: Quesenberry KE, Carpenter JW, eds. Ferrets, Rabbits and Rodents: Clinical Medicine and Surgery. St. Louis: WB Saunders, 2004:72–78.
Sasai H, Kato T, Sasaki S, et al. Echocardiographic diagnosis of dirofilariasis in a ferret. J Sm Anim Pract 2000;41(4):172–174.
Williams BH. Ferret microbiology and virology. In: Fudge AM, ed. Laboratory Medicine Avian and Exotic Pets. Philadelphia: WB Saunders, 2000:335–342.

### Portions Adapted From
Mason RA. Dyspnea, Tachypnea and Panting. In: Tilley LP, Smith FWK, Jr., eds. The 5-Minute Veterinary Consult: Canine and Feline, 3rd Ed. Baltimore: Lippincott Williams & Wilkins, 2003.

## DYSTOCIA AND FETAL DEATH

## BASICS

### OVERVIEW
- Dystocia is most commonly due to fetal malpositioning, fetal oversize, or fetal deformity.
- Litters must consist of at least three fetuses to induce parturition. Parturition should occur on day 41 of gestation for primiparous jills and day 41 or 42 for multiparous jills. If parturition does not occur after day 43, fetal death is likely.
- Parturition occurs quickly in normal jills with normal kits, with little signs of labor. Average length of labor is 2–3 hours, with an average of five kits born per hour.
- Nest building and mammary gland development occurs in the last week of pregnancy.

### SIGNALMENT
Intact females of breeding age (>4 months of age)

### SIGNS

#### Historical Findings
- Mating occurred 41–42 days prior to presentation.
- Mammary gland development within the last week

#### Signs
- Small litter size—no signs of parturition evident; less than four fetuses detected on abdominal palpation
- Dystocia—restlessness, crying out, irritability; labor lasting >4 hours

### CAUSES AND RISK FACTORS

#### Fetal
- Small litter size (<4 kits, normal litter size 8–10 kits) provides insufficient hormonal stimulus to induce parturition, resulting in fetal death.
- Oversize—results in dystocia: fetus weighing >14–20 g (normal size 8–10 g); fetal head deformity; anasarcous fetus
- Malposition in birth canal—dystocia

#### Maternal
- Small litter size—inadequate nutrition (ration containing <35% protein and 18% fat), breeding only once during estrus
- Abnormal pelvic canal from previous pelvic fracture
- Abnormality of the vaginal vault— stricture; hyperplasia; intraluminal or extraluminal mass
- Insufficient cervical dilation, poor uterine contractions, and ineffective abdominal press are rarely causes of dystocia in ferrets, but may occur in animals with underlying disease.

## DIAGNOSIS

### DIFFERENTIAL DIAGNOSIS
- Small litter size; insufficient to induce parturition—less than four fetuses evident on abdominal palpation, radiography, or ultrasound
- Pseudopregnancy—if fertilization fails, pseudopregnancy occurs following mating and lasts 40–42 days. Differentiate from pregnancy with small litter size by abdominal palpation, radiography, or ultrasound.

### CBC/BIOCHEMISTRY/URINALYSIS
- Depend on duration of condition—may be normal; may note hypoglycemia, dehydration, and hypocalcemia
- Perform analyses although results might not be available until after resolution of the condition.

### OTHER LABORATORY TESTS
N/A

### IMAGING
- Radiography (abdomen and pelvic area)— paramount; determines state of pregnancy, pelvic structure, number and malposition of fetuses, fetal oversize, and fetal death
- Ultrasonography—recommended for monitoring fetal viability

### DIAGNOSTIC PROCEDURES
N/A

## TREATMENT

### APPROPRIATE HEALTH CARE
- Small litter size—induce parturition at day 41–43 of gestation. Fetuses retained >43 days usually will not be viable.
- Dystocia—usually requires surgical delivery
- Inpatient—until delivery of all offspring and mother has stabilized
- Fluid replacement—balanced electrolyte solutions; for clinical dehydration
- Severely depressed jill—fluid and electrolyte balance must be restored before induction of anesthesia.

### SURGICAL DELIVERY
Indicated cesarean section—fetal malposition; fetal oversize; fetal stress; in utero fetal death; pelvic or vaginal obstruction; in jills with small litters if parturition does not occur within 8 hours of induction

## MEDICATIONS

### DRUG(S) OF CHOICE
To induce parturition in jills with small litters—prostaglandin F2a (Lutalyse) (0.5 mg/ferret IM) will generally result in delivery of kits within 3 hours. If unsuccessful, administer oxytocin 0.2–3.0 IU/kg SC, IM. If kits are not delivered within 8 hours, perform a cesarean section.

### CONTRAINDICATIONS
Oxytocin—contraindicated with obstructive dystocia of fetal or maternal cause and longstanding in utero fetal death

### PRECAUTIONS
N/A

### POSSIBLE INTERACTIONS
N/A

### ALTERNATIVE DRUGS
N/A

## FOLLOW-UP

### PATIENT MONITORING
Ultrasonography—to ensure that all fetuses are delivered

### POSSIBLE COMPLICATIONS
- Increased risk in future pregnancies
- Neonatal loss if treatment is not begun promptly

## MISCELLANEOUS

### ASSOCIATED CONDITIONS
N/A

### AGE-RELATED FACTORS
Young, primiparous jills are more likely to have small litters resulting in retained fetuses.

### ZOONOTIC POTENTIAL
N/A

### PREGNANCY
N/A

### SEE ALSO
N/A

*Suggested Reading*

Bell JA. Periparturient and neonatal diseases. In: Quesenberry KE, Carpenter JW, eds. Ferrets, Rabbits and Rodents: Clinical Medicine and Surgery. St. Louis: WB Saunders, 2004:50–57.

Fox JG, Pearson RC, Bell JA. Diseases of the genitourinary system. In: Fox JG, ed. Biology and Diseases of the Ferret. 2nd Ed. Baltimore: Williams & Wilkins, 1998:247–272.

Harrenstein L. Critical care of ferrets, rabbits and rodents. Semin Avian Exotic Pet Med 3(4):217–228, 1994.

Pollock CG. Urogenital diseases. In: Quesenberry KE, Carpenter JW, eds. Ferrets, Rabbits and Rodents: Clinical Medicine and Surgery. St. Louis: WB Saunders, 2004:41–49.

# BASICS

## DEFINITION
• Dysuria—difficult or painful urination
• Pollakiuria—voiding small quantities of urine with increased frequency

## PATHOPHYSIOLOGY
The urinary bladder and urethra normally serve as a reservoir for storage and periodic release of urine. Inflammatory and noninflammatory disorders of the lower urinary tract may decrease bladder compliance and storage capacity by damaging structural components of the bladder wall or by stimulating sensory nerve endings located in the bladder or urethra. Sensations of bladder fullness, urgency, and pain stimulate premature micturition and reduce functional bladder capacity. Dysuria and pollakiuria are caused by lesions of the urinary bladder and/or urethra and provide unequivocal evidence of lower urinary tract disease; these clinical signs do not exclude concurrent involvement of the upper urinary tract or disorders of other body systems.

## SYSTEMS AFFECTED
Renal/urologic—bladder, urethra, and prostate gland

## SIGNALMENT
N/A

## SIGNS

### Historical Findings
• Frequent trips to the litterbox
• Loss of housebreaking
• Tenesmus
• Feeding dog food or poor-quality cat foods in ferrets with urolithiasis
• Alopecia, increased sexual aggression, or vulvar swelling seen in ferrets with adrenal disease–associated urogenital cystic disease
• Anorexia, weight loss, and weakness in ferrets with chronic disease or urethral blockage

### Physical Examination Findings
• May be normal
• Caudal abdominal mass associated with the bladder (prostatic tissue or periurethral cysts)
• Turgid, painful bladder on abdominal palpation with obstruction or cystitis
• Thickened bladder wall on abdominal palpation or cystitis

## CAUSES

### Prostate Gland and Periurethral Tissues
• Urogenital cystic disease—associated with adrenal disease (periurethral cysts, prostatic cysts or hyperplasia, periprostatic cysts); most common cause of stranguria; can also occur in female ferrets
• Neoplasia—rare

### Urinary Bladder
• Urinary tract infection—bacterial; can be primary or secondary to urogenital cystic disease
• Urolithiasis
• Neoplasia (unusual)
• Trauma
• Iatrogenic—for example, catheterization, palpation, reverse flushing, overdistension of the bladder during contrast radiography, and surgery

### Urethra
• Extraluminal compression by urogenital cysts—most common
• Urethral plugs—in ferrets with abscessed urogenital cysts—thick, tenacious exudate from cysts enters urine in the bladder and may plug urethra
• Urinary tract infection
• Urethrolithiasis
• Neoplasia—local invasion by malignant neoplasms of adjacent structures
• Trauma
• Iatrogenic—see previous section

## RISK FACTORS
• Urogenital cysts are associated with ferret adrenal disease and the resultant excessive production of androgens. Males are at a higher risk of urinary tract obstruction secondary to urogenital cystic disease.
• Feeding dog foods or poor-quality cat foods, especially those that contain plant-based proteins, will predispose to development of urolithiasis.
• Diseases, diagnostic procedures, or treatments that (1) alter normal host urinary tract defenses and predispose to infection, (2) predispose to formation of uroliths, or (3) damage the urothelium or other tissues of the lower urinary tract
• Mural or extramural diseases that compress the bladder or urethral lumen

# DIAGNOSIS

## DIFFERENTIAL DIAGNOSIS

### Differentiate From Other Abnormal Patterns of Micturition
• Rule out polyuria—increased frequency and volume of urine
• Rule out urethral obstruction—stranguria, anuria, overdistended urinary bladder, signs of postrenal uremia

### Differentiate Causes of Dysuria and Pollakiuria
• Rule out urinary tract infection—hematuria; malodorous or cloudy urine; small, painful, thickened bladder
• Rule out prostatic or urogenital cystic diseases—alopecia, swollen vulva, increased sexual aggression, palpable caudal abdominal mass, depression, weakness, malodorous or cloudy urine

• Rule out urolithiasis—may see hematuria; palpable uroliths in urethra or bladder
• Rule out neoplasia—may see hematuria; palpable masses in urethra or bladder
• Rule out neurogenic disorders—rare finding; flaccid bladder wall; residual urine in bladder lumen after micturition; other neurologic deficits to hind legs, tail, perineum, and anal sphincter
• Rule out iatrogenic disorders—history of catheterization, reverse flushing, contrast radiography, or surgery

## CBC/BIOCHEMISTRY/URINALYSIS
• Results often normal. Lower urinary tract disease complicated by urethral obstruction may be associated with azotemia, hyperphosphatemia, acidosis, and hyperkalemia. Patients with concurrent pyelonephritis may have impaired urine-concentrating capacity, leukocytosis, and azotemia. Dehydrated patients may have elevated total plasma protein.
• Hemogram may rarely show nonregenerative anemia, leukopenia, or thrombocytopenia due to estrogen excess in ferrets with adrenal disease.
• Hypoglycemia may be present—usually due to concurrent insulinoma
• Disorders of the urinary bladder are best evaluated with a urine specimen collected by cystocentesis. Urethral disorders are best evaluated with a voided urine sample or by comparison of results of analysis of voided and cystocentesis samples. (Caution: Cystocentesis may induce hematuria.)
• Pyuria (normal value 0–5 WBC/hpf), hematuria (normal value 0–10 RBC/hpf), and proteinuria (normal value 0–33 mg/dL) may indicate abscessed urogenital cysts or urinary tract inflammation, but these are nonspecific findings that may result from infectious and noninfectious causes of lower urinary tract disease.
• Identification of bacteria in urine sediment suggests that urinary tract infection or abscessed urogenital cysts are causing or complicating lower urinary tract disease. Consider contamination of urine during collection and storage when interpreting urinalysis results.
• Identification of neoplastic cells in urine sediment indicates urinary tract neoplasia. Use caution in establishing a diagnosis of neoplasia based on urine sediment examination.
• Crystalluria occurs in some normal patients, patients with urolithiasis, or patients with lower urinary tract disease unassociated with uroliths.

## OTHER LABORATORY TESTS
• Quantitative urine culture—the most definitive means of identifying and characterizing bacterial urinary tract infections; negative urine culture results suggest a noninfectious cause.

## DYSURIA AND POLLAKIURIA

• Cytologic evaluation of urine sediment or urethral or vaginal discharges may help in evaluating patients with localized urinary tract disease.

• Elevations of serum estradiol, androstenedione, and 17-hydroxyprogesterone combined are most diagnostic for adrenal disease (available through the University of Tennessee Clinical Endocrinology Laboratory, Department of Comparative Medicine).

### IMAGING
Survey abdominal radiography, contrast urethrocystography and cystography, urinary tract ultrasonography, and excretory urography are important means of identifying and localizing causes of dysuria and pollakiuria.

### DIAGNOSTIC PROCEDURES
N/A

## TREATMENT

• Patients with nonobstructive lower urinary tract diseases are typically managed as outpatients; diagnostic evaluation may require brief hospitalization.

• Dysuria and pollakiuria associated with systemic signs of illness (e.g., pyrexia, depression, anorexia, vomiting, and dehydration) or laboratory findings of azotemia or leukocytosis warrant more aggressive diagnostic evaluation and initiation of supportive and symptomatic treatment.

• Treatment depends on the underlying cause and specific sites involved. See specific chapters describing diseases listed in section on causes.

• Clinical signs of dysuria and pollakiuria often resolve rapidly following specific treatment of the underlying cause(s).

## MEDICATIONS

### DRUG(S) OF CHOICE
• Depend on the underlying cause

• If bacterial cystitis is demonstrated, begin treatment with a broad-spectrum antibiotic. Some choices for empirical use while waiting for culture results include trimethoprim sulfa (15–30 PO, SC mg/kg q12h), amoxi-

cillin (10–20 mg/kg PO, SC q12h), or enrofloxacin (10–20 mg/kg PO, SC IM q24h). Modify antibacterial treatment based on results of urine culture and susceptibility testing.

### CONTRAINDICATIONS
Potentially nephrotoxic drugs (e.g., gentamicin) in patients who are febrile, dehydrated, or azotemic or who are suspected of having pyelonephritis, septicemia, or preexisting renal disease

### PRECAUTIONS
N/A

### POSSIBLE INTERACTIONS
N/A

### ALTERNATIVE DRUGS
N/A

## FOLLOW-UP

### PATIENT MONITORING
• Response to treatment by clinical signs, serial physical examinations, laboratory testing, and radiographic and ultrasonic evaluations appropriate for each specific cause

• Refer to specific chapters describing diseases listed in section on causes.

### POSSIBLE COMPLICATIONS
Refer to specific chapters describing diseases listed in section on causes.

## MISCELLANEOUS

### ASSOCIATED CONDITIONS
• Ferret adrenal disease

• Insulinomas are commonly seen in ferrets with adrenal disease.

• Ferrets on poor-quality diets are more prone to dental diseases.

### AGE-RELATED FACTORS
N/A

### ZOONOTIC POTENTIAL
N/A

### PREGNANCY
N/A

### SYNONYMS
N/A

### SEE ALSO
• Adrenal disease
• Lower urinary tract infection
• Urogenital cystic disease (periurethral cysts)
• Urinary tract obstruction
• Urolithiasis

### ABBREVIATIONS
• RBC = red blood cell
• WBC = white blood cell

*Suggested Reading*

Antinoff N. Urinary disorders in ferrets. Semin Avian Exotic Pet Med 1998;7(2):89–92.

Fox JG, Pearson RC, Bell JA. Diseases of the genitourinary system. In: Fox JG, ed. Biology and Diseases of the Ferret. 2nd Ed. Baltimore: Williams & Wilkins, 1998.

Hoefer HL. Rabbit and ferret renal disease diagnosis. In: Fudge AM, ed. Laboratory Medicine, Avian and Exotic Pets. Philadelphia: WB Saunders, 2000.

Li X, Fox JG, Erdman SE, et al. Cystic urogenital anomalies in ferrets (Mustela putorius furo). Vet Pathol 1996;33:150–158.

Marini RP, Esteves MI, Fox JG. A technique for catheterization of the urinary bladder in the ferret. Lab Anim 1994;28:155–157.

Palmore WP, Bartos KD. Food intake and struvite crystalluria in ferrets. Vet Res Commun 1987;11:519–526.

Pollock CG. Urogenital diseases. In: Quesenberry KE, Carpenter JW, eds. Ferrets, Rabbits and Rodents: Clinical Medicine and Surgery. St. Louis: WB Saunders, 2004:41–49.

Wheeler J, Bennett RA. Ferret abdominal surgical procedures. Part II. Gastrointestinal foreign bodies, splenomegaly, liver biopsy, cystotomy and ovariohysterectomy. Compend Contin Edu Pract Vet 1999;21(11):1049–1057.

*Portions Adapted From*

Kruger JM, Osborne CA. Dysuria and Pollakiuria. In: Tilley LP, Smith FWK, Jr., eds. The 5-Minute Veterinary Consult: Canine and Feline, 3rd Ed. Baltimore: Lippincott Williams & Wilkins, 2003.

# EAR MITES

## BASICS

### OVERVIEW
- *Otodectes cynotis* mite infestation is common in ferrets. Many ferrets are asymptomatic, but intense irritation of the external ear can also be seen.
- Sequelae to infestation are rare in ferrets; however, secondary bacterial or mycotic infections or otitis interna/media have been anecdotally reported. These sequelae are usually a consequence of overzealous cleaning of the ear canal.

### SIGNALMENT
No breed or sex predilection

### SIGNS
- Thick, red-brown or black crusts in the outer ear—may or may not be associated with mite infestation; this type of exudate is usually a normal finding in ferrets.
- Pruritus primarily located around the ears, head, and neck; occasionally generalized
- Alopecia and excoriations around the pinnae may occur, owing to the intense pruritus.
- Signs of otitis interna/media such as head tilt and vestibular signs have been anecdotally reported in ferrets with ear mites.

### CAUSES AND RISK FACTORS
*Otodectes cynotis*

## DIAGNOSIS

### DIFFERENTIAL DIAGNOSIS

#### Exudate in the Ear Canal
- Normal finding—most ferrets normally have a black to brown, crumbly exudate in the ear canal.
- Bacterial or mycotic otitis externa—rare in ferrets; may occur secondary to mite infestation; differentiate by microscopic examination of exudates.

#### Pruritus/Alopecia
- Fleas—patchy alopecia usually appears in other areas in addition to the head, especially tail region; finding flea dirt will help to differentiate.
- Sarcoptic mange—intense pruritus; can be generalized or localized to feet
- Contact dermatitis—usually ventral distribution
- Ferret adrenal disease—usually bilaterally symmetric alopecia, with or without pruritus, beginning at tail region and extending dorsally; however, it is possible to see unusual distributions of alopecia (such as the head alone) in ferrets with adrenal disease.

### CBC/BIOCHEMISTRY/URINALYSIS
Normal

### OTHER LABORATORY TESTS
N/A

### IMAGING
N/A

### DIAGNOSTIC PROCEDURES
- Ear swabs placed in mineral oil—usually a very effective means of identification
- Skin scrapings—identify mites, if signs are generalized; extremely rare in ferrets

## TREATMENT
- Contagious; important to treat all in-contact animals
- Thoroughly clean and treat the environment.
- Cleaning of the ear canal may not enhance treatment in the ferret. Overzealous cleaning of the ear canal may cause irritation, secondary bacterial or mycotic infections, or rupture of the tympanum.

## MEDICATIONS

### DRUG(S) OF CHOICE
- Ivermectin 1% (Ivomec, Merck Agvet)—use parenterally or topically; parenteral: 0.2–0.4 mg/kg SC q14d for 3–4 doses; topical treatment with ivermectin has been shown to be more effective in the treatment of ear mites. Topical: diluted 1:10 in propylene glycol—instill 0.4 mg/kg divided into each ear topically and repeat in 2 weeks; it is not necessary to clean the ears thoroughly to remove debris prior to topical administration of ivermectin since debris may aid in retention of medication in the canal. Do not use topical and parenteral ivermectin concurrently.
- Thiabendazole product (Tresaderm, Merck AgVet) at feline dosages has also been used as a topical; however, treatment failures are common due to owner compliance and the small size of the ear canal.

### CONTRAINDICATIONS
- Avoid overzealous cleaning of the ear canal.
- Ivermectin—do not use pregnant jills
- Do not use topical and parenteral ivermectin concurrently.

### PRECAUTIONS
All products discussed above are off-label use. Safety and efficacy has not been evaluated in ferrets. Use with caution, especially in young or debilitated animals.

### ALTERNATIVE DRUGS
Selamectin (Revolution) is effective in treating ear mites in dogs and cats and has been anecdotally used in ferrets at feline doses; however, safety, efficacy, and dosing has not been evaluated.

## FOLLOW-UP
- An ear swab and physical examination should be done 1 month after therapy commences.
- For most patients, prognosis is good.
- Infestation is more likely to recur or fail to respond to treatment with parenteral ivermectin or topical thiabendazole.

## MISCELLANEOUS

### ZOONOTIC POTENTIAL
The mites will also bite humans (rare).

### SEE ALSO
- Adrenal disease
- Dermatophytosis
- Fleas and Flea Infestation
- Pruritus

*Suggested Reading*

Fox JG. Parasitic diseases. In: Fox JG, ed. Biology and Diseases of the Ferret. 2nd Ed. Baltimore: Williams & Wilkins, 1998:375–392.

Kelleher SA. Skin diseases of the ferret. Vet Clin North Am Exotic Anim Pract 2001;4(2):565–572.

Orcutt C. Dermatologic diseases. In: Quesenberry KE, Carpenter JW, eds. Ferrets, Rabbits and Rodents: Clinical Medicine and Surgery. St. Louis: WB Saunders, 2004:79–90.

Patterson MM, Kirchain SM. Comparison of three treatments for control of ear mites in ferrets. Lab Anim Sci 1999;49(6): 655–7.

*Portions Adapted From*

Kuhl KA. Ear mites. In: Tilley LP, Smith FWK, Jr., eds. The 5-Minute Veterinary Consult: Canine and Feline, 2nd Ed. Baltimore: Lippincott Williams & Wilkins, 2000.

# EOSINOPHILIC GASTROENTERITIS

## BASICS

### DEFINITION
An inflammatory disease of the stomach and intestine, characterized by a transmucosal infiltration of eosinophils with resultant inflammation and thickening of the affected areas. Eosinophilic granulomas are often found in the mesenteric lymph nodes, and a peripheral eosinophilia is usually present.

### PATHOPHYSIOLOGY
• The underlying cause of the tissue and circulating eosinophilia is unknown. Although a parasitic or allergic cause has been suspected, parasites are usually not found, and allergies have not been well documented in ferrets.
• Eosinophils contain granules with substances that directly damage the surrounding tissues.

### SYSTEMS AFFECTED
Gastrointestinal—usually affects the small intestine; large intestine, stomach, and mesenteric nodes commonly affected and, occasionally, liver

### GENETICS
N/A

### INCIDENCE/PREVALENCE
• True incidence is unknown, but it is a relatively common cause of gastrointestinal tract disease in ferrets.
• Less common in ferrets than lymphoplasmacytic gastroenteritis

### GEOGRAPHIC DISTRIBUTION
N/A

### SIGNALMENT
*Mean Age and Range*
Young to middle-age; range—6 months to 4 years

*Predominant Sex*
None reported

### SIGNS
*Historical Findings*
Diarrhea with or without mucous or blood, anorexia, weight loss, and vomiting are the most common client complaints.

*Physical Examination Findings*
• Dehydration and emaciation
• Thickened intestinal loops and enlarged mesenteric lymph nodes may be palpated.
• Splenomegaly usually present—most often due to nonspecific, age-related change; rarely eosinophilic infiltration may occur.
• Hepatomegaly may be noted in few cases where infiltrates occur in the liver, or due to other, concurrent hepatic disease.

### CAUSES
• The cause is unknown. Theories include immune mediated, parasitic, or idiopathic.

• Idiopathic eosinophilic gastroenteritis; hypereosinophilic syndrome has been suggested, since some affected ferrets have a peripheral eosinophilia and, occasionally, eosinophilic infiltration into liver, spleen, lymph nodes, and skin.
• Immune-mediated—food allergy suspected; often associated with other forms of inflammatory bowel disease. Some ferrets respond very well to conversion to a novel protein source diet or respond to antiinflammatory or immunosuppressive doses of corticosteroids, suggesting a hypersensitivity reaction.
• Parasitic—parasites not usually found

### RISK FACTORS
N/A

## DIAGNOSIS

### DIFFERENTIAL DIAGNOSIS
• Common causes of weight loss, anorexia, diarrhea, and vomiting include gastrointestinal foreign body, lymphosarcoma, gastric ulcers, viral or bacterial enteritis, and other types of inflammatory bowel disease.
• Intestinal biopsy differentiates the other causes of inflammatory bowel disease from eosinophilic gastroenteritis.

### CBC/BIOCHEMISTRY/URINALYSIS
• Hemogram often reveals a peripheral eosinophilia (up to 35% eosinophils); however, this is not seen in every ferret with eosinophilic gastroenteritis.
• Panhypoproteinemia or hypoalbuminemia may be present due to protein-losing enteropathy.

### OTHER LABORATORY TESTS
Multiple fecal flotations and direct smears are needed to rule in or out intestinal parasitism; however, gastrointestinal parasites are rare in ferrets.

### IMAGING
• Plain abdominal radiographs provide little information.
• Barium contrast radiography may occasionally demonstrate thick intestinal walls and mucosal irregularities but does not provide any information about etiology or the nature of the thickening.
• Ultrasonography—to rule out other diseases; can be used to examine the liver, spleen, and mesenteric lymph nodes

### DIAGNOSTIC PROCEDURES
Definitive diagnosis requires biopsy and histopathology, usually obtained via exploratory laparotomy.

### PATHOLOGIC FINDINGS
• Stomach and intestinal tract may appear grossly normal, may appear diffusely thickened, or contain patchy, multifocal areas of thickening.

• Ulcerations and erosions may also be seen.
• Eosinophilic infiltrates can be patchy in the intestine; multiple biopsies may be necessary to obtain a diagnostic sample.
• Mesenteric lymph nodes are often grossly enlarged.
• Histopathology—affected areas of the gastrointestinal tract reveal a diffuse infiltrate of eosinophils into the lamina propria, submucosa, and occasionally the serosa; villous atrophy may be apparent; other inflammatory cell populations may be found along with eosinophils; focal eosinophilic granulomas may be seen in affected lymph nodes.

## TREATMENT

### APPROPRIATE HEALTH CARE
• Most can be treated on an outpatient basis.
• Patients that are dehydrated or emaciated or have other concurrent illnesses may require hospitalization until they are stabilized.

### NURSING CARE
If the patient is dehydrated or must be NPO because of vomiting, any balanced fluid such as lactated Ringer's solution is adequate (for a patient without other concurrent disease); otherwise, select fluids on the basis of secondary diseases.

### ACTIVITY
No need to restrict unless severely debilitated

### DIET
• Highly digestible diets with novel protein sources may be useful for eliciting remission, although an allergic cause has not been documented and little information is available regarding the efficacy of these diets. If attempted, choose feline diets since ferrets have high nutritional protein and fat requirements. Foods that have been anecdotally reported to elicit remission include feline lamb and rice diets, diets consisting exclusively of one type of meat (lamb, duck, turkey), or a "natural prey diet" consisting of whole rodents. If remission is elicited, continue diet for at least 8–13 weeks; this diet may need to be fed lifelong.
• Anorexic ferrets may refuse dry foods but are often willing to eat canned cat foods or pureed meats.

### CLIENT EDUCATION
• This can be a very frustrating disease to treat. Novel protein source trial diets are only occasionally effective, and client compliance is essential. Often clients have more than one ferret or give their ferrets treats and have difficulty feeding one exclusive type of food.
• In many cases, trial diets are ineffective. Some ferrets may never respond or may respond initially to medical therapy and diet

# EOSINOPHILIC GASTROENTERITIS

manipulation but become refractory to treatment with time.
• Explain the potential for long-term therapy.

## SURGICAL CONSIDERATIONS
N/A

## MEDICATIONS

### DRUG(S) OF CHOICE
• Corticosteroids—mainstay of treatment; prednisone (1.25–2.5 mg/kg PO q24h) for at least 1–2 weeks
• Gradually taper corticosteroids to 0.25–1 mg/kg qod; some ferrets will relapse when dosage is lowered and may require long-term therapy with higher doses of prednisone.
• Many ferrets fail to respond to prednisone therapy or initially respond but become refractory to treatment with time.

### CONTRAINDICATIONS
N/A

### PRECAUTIONS
In ferrets with concurrent infectious diseases, use corticosteroids with caution.

### POSSIBLE INTERACTIONS
N/A

### ALTERNATIVE DRUGS
• Other immunosuppressive drugs such as azathioprine (0.9 mg/kg PO q24–72h); has not been used extensively in ferrets; efficacy and safety have not been evaluated.
• Empirical use of antiparasitic agents has been advocated, although no parasitic causes have been documented and intestinal parasites are rare in ferrets. In general, these drugs are very safe to use, and a trial is unlikely to cause harm. Those used anecdotally include ivermectin (0.4 mg/kg SC once; repeat in 2 weeks) and metronidazole (15–20 mg/kg PO q12h × 2 weeks)

## FOLLOW-UP

### PATIENT MONITORING
• Initially frequent for some more severely affected patients; monitor severity of diarrhea and peripheral eosinophil counts.
• Patients with less severe disease—may be checked 2–5 weeks after the initial evaluation; monthly to bimonthly thereafter

### PREVENTION/AVOIDANCE
If a food intolerance or allergy is suspected or documented, avoid that particular item and adhere strictly to dietary changes.

### POSSIBLE COMPLICATIONS
• Weight loss, debilitation, and death in refractory cases
• Adverse effects of prednisone therapy (rare)

### EXPECTED COURSE AND PROGNOSIS
The prognosis is good to fair in those animals that respond clinically to corticosteroid and/or dietary therapy; poor to grave if clinical response is not observed

## MISCELLANEOUS

### ASSOCIATED CONDITIONS
Many affected ferrets also have splenomegaly (nonspecific in aged ferrets).

### AGE-RELATED FACTORS
N/A

### ZOONOTIC POTENTIAL
N/A

### PREGNANCY
N/A

### SYNONYMS
N/A

### SEE ALSO
• Anorexia
• Diarrhea
• Gastroenteritis, lymphoplasmacytic

### ABBREVIATIONS
NPO = nothing by mouth

*Suggested Reading*

Fox JG. Diseases of the gastrointestinal system. In: Fox JG, ed. Biology and Diseases of the Ferret. 2nd Ed. Baltimore: Williams & Wilkins, 1998.
Fox JG. Parasitic diseases. In: Fox JG, ed. Biology and Diseases of the Ferret. 2nd Ed. Baltimore: Williams & Wilkins, 1998:375–392.
Fox JG, Marini RP. Helicobacter mustelae infection in ferrets: pathogenesis, epizootiology, diagnosis and treatment. Semin Avin Exotic Pet Med 2001;10(1):36–44.
Hoefer HL, Bell JA. Gastrointestinal diseases. In: Quesenberry KE, Carpenter JW, eds. Ferrets, Rabbits and Rodents: Clinical Medicine and Surgery. St. Louis: WB Saunders, 2004:25–40.
Jenkins JR. Rabbit and ferret liver and gastrointestinal testing. In: Fudge Am, ed. Laboratory Medicine, Avian and Exotic Pets. Philadelphia: WB Saunders, 2000.
Palley LS, Fox JG. Eosinophilic gastroenteritis in the ferret. In: Kirk RW, Bonagura JD, eds. Kirk's Current Veterinary Therapy XI: Small Animal Practice. Philadelphia: WB Saunders, 1992.

# EPIZOOTIC CATARRHAL ENTERITIS

 **BASICS**

## DEFINITION
• An enteric disease characterized initially by anorexia, vomiting, and lethargy, followed by profuse green, mucous-covered diarrhea. Due to the characteristic diarrhea, pet owners refer to this disease as "green slime disease."
• Following the hypersecretory phase, chronic, intermittent, malabsorptive diarrhea is commonly seen.
• Typically high morbidity and low mortality rates are seen
• Clinical signs are usually seen within 48–72 hours following exposure to clinically affected ferrets or asymptomatic carriers.

## PATHOPHYSIOLOGY
• Initial lesions of epizootic catarrhal enteritis (ECE) are believed to be caused by an enteric coronavirus, although secondary bacterial and/or parasitic infections may contribute.
• Coronavirus infection causes lymphocytic infiltration, villous atrophy and blunting of intestinal villi, and vacuolar degeneration and necrosis of apical (villous tip) epithelium.
• Initial intestinal lesions cause hypersecretory, mucoid diarrhea and vomiting
• Following the hypersecretory phase, some ferrets recover with no further clinical signs; other ferrets develop chronic or intermittent disease due to villous atrophy and/or secondary/simultaneous infections.
• Hepatic degeneration and necrosis is often seen in ferrets with ECE; the mechanism for this has not been described.

## SYSTEMS AFFECTED
• Gastrointestinal—small intestinal villi and adjacent mucosal epithelium
• Hepatobiliary—hepatic degeneration and necrosis common
• Hemic/lymphatic/immune—mesenteric lymphoid hyperplasia
• Musculoskeletal—muscle wasting due to intestinal malabsorption
• Endocrine/metabolic—fluid, electrolyte, and acid-base imbalances

## INCIDENCE/PREVALENCE
• An extremely common cause of diarrhea in ferrets
• Seen most commonly in breeding facilities, animal shelters, pet stores, or wherever kits are reared
• Morbidity rates can reach 100% in these facilities or multiferret homes.

## GEOGRAPHIC DISTRIBUTION
Seen most commonly in North America

## SIGNALMENT
### Mean Age and Range
• Older ferrets more severely affected
• Young kits, 6–16 weeks of age, usually have mild to moderate disease or are asymptomatic carriers

### Predominant Sex
N/A

## SIGNS
### Historical Findings
• Exposure to other ferrets, either symptomatic or asymptomatic carriers (usually kits), is key to the diagnosis. Contact may be either direct or through fomites
• Within 48–72 hours of exposure, sudden onset of anorexia, lethargy, and often, repeated episodes of vomiting
• Diarrhea usually (but not always) seen—profuse, bright green colored, large mucous component; lasts several days and may recur
• Sudden profound weight loss common, especially in older animals with diarrhea
• In breeding facilities, pet stores, or multiferret households, all animals show varying degrees of clinical signs within a short period of time; younger animals are often less seriously affected
• Following the acute phase, chronic or intermittent diarrhea (often lasting months) is seen due to villous atrophy and subsequent malabsorption. Diarrhea is often granular ("bird seed" or "millet seed") in appearance and pale brown to green in color; mucous or fresh blood is sometimes seen.
• Some ferrets will appear to completely recover, then relapse weeks to months later.
• Lethargy, chronic wasting, and inappetence may be seen for weeks to months.

### Physical Examination Findings
• Dehydration, weight loss, and abdominal discomfort are consistent features.
• Thickened, ropy intestinal loops may be palpated.
• Occasionally enlarged mesenteric lymph nodes are palpable.
• Splenomegaly is a common, nonspecific finding.

## RISK FACTORS
• Ferrets from kennels, animal shelters, pet shops, or elsewhere where ferrets have congregated are at greatest risk.
• Older ferrets are at higher risk of severe infection, especially with concurrent insulinoma or gastrointestinal, cardiac, or adrenal disease.
• Copathogens such as parasites, viruses, and certain bacterial species (e.g., *Helicobacter mustelae*, *Campylobacter* spp., *Clostridium* spp. and *Cryptosporidium* spp.) hypothesized to exacerbate illness
• Crowding and poor sanitation increases the risk of infection, especially in kennels or animal shelters.

 **DIAGNOSIS**

## DIFFERENTIAL DIAGNOSIS
• Gastrointestinal foreign bodies—frequently cause similar signs, especially in young ferrets; often may differentiate by history
• *H. mustelae*—disease induced by *H. mustelae* often occurs secondary to ECE; likely related to stress and anorexia or general debility
• *Clostridium* spp, *Campylobacter* spp., *Salmonella* sp., or other enteric bacterial infections—should be considered as differential diagnoses. Enteritis caused by bacteria alone is uncommon. Generally, these agents are copathogens or secondary invaders.
• Gastrointestinal parasites—*Giardia*, Coccidia, *Cryptosporidium* spp. (may be primary pathogens or secondary to ECE)
• Lymphoma—may cause identical clinical signs; differentiate by characteristic ECE history and on plasma biochemistry—ALT often extremely elevated with ECE; elevated in lymphoma if hepatic involvement
• Metabolic disorders—liver disease, renal disease, pancreatic disease
• Dietary—diet changes, eating spoiled food, dietary intolerance
• Infiltrative—proliferative bowel disease (*Desulfovibrio* sp.), lymphoplasmacytic gastroenteritis, eosinophilic gastroenteritis
• Intussusception
• Toxin ingestion

## CBC/BIOCHEMISTRY/URINALYSIS
• Leukocytosis in ferrets with concurrent bacterial infections
• Increased PCV due to dehydration
• Increased ALT (often >700 U/L) and ALP commonly seen due to liver necrosis or mobilization of fat stores to liver
• Hypoproteinemia may be severe in patients with chronic disease
• Serum chemistry profiles help assess electrolyte disturbances, presence of azotemia associated with dehydration, hypoproteinemia, and hypoglycemia.

## OTHER LABORATORY TESTS
N/A

## IMAGING
• If done as part of the diagnostic workup, abdominal radiographs may reveal a generalized small intestinal ileus.
• Useful to rule in or out other causes of diarrhea

## DIAGNOSTIC PROCEDURES
• Definitive diagnosis requires biopsy and histopathology, usually obtained via exploratory laparotomy.
• Lymph node biopsy is indicated on enlarged mesenteric nodes.
• Fecal direct examination, fecal flotation, and zinc sulfate centrifugation many demonstrate gastrointestinal parasites (often co-pathogens).

# EPIZOOTIC CATARRHAL ENTERITIS

• Fecal cytology—may reveal RBC or fecal leukocytes, which can be associated with inflammatory bowel disease or invasive bacterial strains.
• Fecal culture should be performed if abnormal bacteria are observed on the fecal Gram's stain or if *Salmonella* is suspected (may be co-pathogens).
• Immunofluorescent staining of frozen sections of the small intestine—from fatal cases; may reveal viral antigen in cells lining the villus epithelium
• Electron microscopy—interpretation requires expertise.

## PATHOLOGIC FINDINGS

• Gross changes include hyperemia of the small intestine with green, mucoid diarrhea in the lumen in the acute phase. With chronic disease, there is a thinning of the intestinal wall with loss of villi.
• Mesenteric lymph nodes are often enlarged.
• Multifocal hepatic degeneration and necrosis are common.
• Histopathology reveals intestinal lymphocytic or lymphoplasmacytic inflammation and necrosis of apical epithelium, often with severe villus atrophy.

# TREATMENT

## APPROPRIATE HEALTH CARE

• Symptomatic and supportive
• Intensity depends on the severity of signs on examination.
• Prompt, intensive inpatient care favors treatment success.
• Proper, strict isolation procedures are essential.

## NURSING CARE

• Hospitalize patients that are dehydrated, anorectic, or severely debilitated.
• Rehydration is essential to treatment success in severely ill ferrets. Initially, a balanced fluid (e.g., lactated Ringer's solution) may be used.
• Correct electrolyte and acid-base disturbances in patients with moderate to severe disease.
• Patients with severe or chronic disease often develop hypokalemia. Supplementation methods and dosages are extrapolated from those used for canine or feline patients.
• Supplementation with 5% dextrose is beneficial in anorectic, hypoglycemic patients.
• Patients with hypoproteinemia may benefit from treatment with hetastarch (6% hetastarch in 0.9% NaCl); administer an IV bolus (10–20 mL/kg) slowly over 2–3 hours, then at a constant rate infusion of 1 mL/kg/hr for 24 hours; hetastarch increases plasma oncotic pressure and pulls fluid into the intravascular space.

## ACTIVITY

Restrict until symptoms abate.

## DIET

• Many affected ferrets will refuse kibble; however, most ferrets will accept high-calorie diets such as Eukanuba Maximum Calorie diet (Iams Co., Dayton, OH), Feline a/d (Hills Products, Topeka, KS), or Clinicare Feline liquid diet (Abbott Laboratories, North Chicago, IL); may also add dietary supplement such as Nutri-Cal (EVSCO Pharmaceuticals Buena, NJ) to increase caloric content to these foods.
• Warming the food to body temperature, or offering via syringe may increase acceptance.
• Administer these foods several times a day.
• Reported resting energy requirement for ferrets is 70 kcal/kg body weight per day (sick ferrets have higher requirements). Clinicare Feline contains 1 kcal/mL; Eukanuba Maximum Calorie diet contains 2 kcal/mL.
• Ferrets exhibiting malabsorptive diarrhea (characterized by grainy feces, weight loss) often respond well to a diet consisting of meat-based human baby foods and high-calorie dietary supplements until diarrhea resolves.

## CLIENT EDUCATION

• Inform owners about the need for thorough disinfection, especially if other ferrets are on the premises.
• Warn owners that malabsorptive diarrhea may persist for weeks to months, requiring long-term treatment.
• Warn owners that relapses are common following resolution of diarrhea.

## SURGICAL CONSIDERATIONS

N/A

# MEDICATIONS

## DRUG(S) OF CHOICE

• Treat secondary/concurrent infections (especially *H. mustelae*).
• Antibiotic therapy—indicated in patients with hypersecretory diarrhea or when secondary infections are identified. For empirical treatment, use broad-spectrum antibiotics such as trimethoprim sulfa (15–30 mg/kg PO, SC q12h), amoxicillin (10–20 mg/kg PO, SC q12h), or enrofloxacin (10–20 mg/kg PO, SC, IM q24h)
• Gastrointestinal antisecretory agents are helpful to treat, and possibly prevent, gastritis in anorectic ferrets. Ferrets continually secrete a baseline level of gastric hydrochloric acid and, as such, anorexia itself may predispose to gastric ulceration. Those successfully used in ferrets include omeprazole (0.7 mg/kg PO q24h), famotidine (0.25–0.5 mg/kg PO, IV q24h), and cimetidine (5–10 mg/kg PO, SC, IM q8h).

• Loperamide (0.2 mg/kg PO q12h) may be helpful in the symptomatic treatment of acute diarrhea (see precautions).
• For chronic, malabsorptive disease—administration of prednisone (0.25–1.0 mg/kg PO qod) may be helpful until signs abate.

## CONTRAINDICATIONS

N/A

## PRECAUTIONS

• Be certain that all secondary/concurrent bacterial or parasitic infections have been successfully treated prior to administering corticosteroid therapy.
• Loperamide may cause hyperactivity in ferrets; avoid in patients with suspected intestinal obstruction, glaucoma, intestinal ileus, liver disease, enterotoxin-producing bacteria, and invasive bacterial enteritis; do not use in patients with chronic diarrhea.

## POSSIBLE INTERACTIONS

N/A

## ALTERNATIVE DRUGS

N/A

# FOLLOW-UP

## PATIENT MONITORING

N/A

## PREVENTION/AVOIDANCE

No vaccine is currently available.

## POSSIBLE COMPLICATIONS

• Septicemia/endotoxemia
• Dehydration, death
• Intussusception

## EXPECTED COURSE AND PROGNOSIS

• Prognosis is guarded in severely affected ferrets.
• Prognosis is good for ferrets that receive prompt initial treatment and survive the initial crisis of illness.
• Many ferrets will develop chronic malabsorptive disease.
• Recurrence of signs of malabsorption or green diarrhea common in many ferrets for weeks to months following initial resolution of signs.

# MISCELLANEOUS

## ASSOCIATED CONDITIONS

• *H. mustelae*
• Lymphoplasmacytic enteritis
• Giardiasis
• Cryptosporidiosis

## AGE-RELATED FACTORS

• Older ferrets suffer a higher rate of severe illness.
• Young kits often have mild disease or are asymptomatic.

**ZOONOTIC POTENTIAL**
N/A

**PREGNANCY**
N/A

**SYNONYMS**
- Green slime disease
- Infectious hepatitis and enteritis of ferrets
- Ferret coronavirus

**SEE ALSO**
- Anorexia
- Diarrhea
- Gastroduodenal ulcers
- Lymphoplasmacytic enteritis and gastroenteritis
- Vomiting

**ABBREVIATIONS**
- ALP = alkaline phosphatase
- ALT = alanine aminotransferase
- PCV = packed cell volume
- RBC = red blood cell

*Suggested Reading*
Fox JG. Diseases of the gastrointestinal system. In: Fox JG, ed. Biology and Diseases of the Ferret. 2nd Ed. Baltimore: Williams & Wilkins, 1998:273–290.
Fox JG, Marini RP. Helicobacter mustelae infection in ferrets: pathogenesis, epizootiology, diagnosis and treatment. Semin Avin Exotic Pet Med 2001;10(1):36–44.
Hoefer HL, Bell JA. Gastrointestinal diseases. In: Quesenberry KE, Carpenter JW, eds. Ferrets, Rabbits and Rodents: Clinical Medicine and Surgery. St. Louis: WB Saunders, 2004:25–40.
Jenkins JR. Rabbit and ferret liver and gastrointestinal testing. In: Fudge AM, ed. Laboratory Medicine, Avian and Exotic Pets. Philadelphia: WB Saunders, 2000.
Rosenthal K. Update on ECE disease in ferrets. Proc North Amer Vet Conf 2000; 1017–1018.
Williams BH, Kiupel M, West KH, et al. Coronavirus-associated epizootic catarrhal enteritis in ferrets. J Am Vet Med Assoc 2000;217:526–530.

# FLEAS AND FLEA INFESTATION

## BASICS

### OVERVIEW
- Flea infestation—large number of fleas and flea dirt
- Heavy infestations may cause anemia, especially in young ferrets.
- Fleabite hypersensitivity has not been documented in ferrets; however, some ferrets appear to be significantly more pruritic than others, suggesting that a hypersensitivity reaction may exist in these animals.

### SIGNALMENT
- Incidence varies with climatic conditions and flea population.
- No age or sex predilection
- Clinical signs vary with individual animals.
- Young animals more likely to develop anemia

### SIGNS

*Historical Findings*
- History of flea infestation in other pets, including dogs and cats
- Some animals asymptomatic
- Biting, chewing, scratching, or excessive licking
- Signs of fleas and flea dirt

*Physical Examination Findings*
- Depends on the severity of the reaction and the degree of exposure to fleas (i.e., seasonal vs. year-round)
- Finding fleas and flea dirt
- Papules, alopecia, excoriations, and scaling, often in the tail region, but may appear anywhere
- Secondary bacterial infections sometimes seen
- Pale mucous membranes; tachycardia in anemic animals

### CAUSES AND RISK FACTORS
Exposure to other flea-infested animals within the household; keeping animals outdoors

## DIAGNOSIS

### DIFFERENTIAL DIAGNOSIS
- Ferret adrenal disease—rule out ferret adrenal disease, since this is the most common cause of alopecia and may occur in conjunction with fleas. Ferrets with adrenal disease may be extremely pruritic; secondary pyoderma may be present. Alopecia generally is symmetric, is gradual in onset, begins at the tail base, and progresses cranially. Other signs, such as vulvar swelling in females, are often seen. May be concurrent with flea infestation.

- *Otodectes* (ear mites)—usually not pruritic; lesions typically localized to areas surrounding ears; black/brown waxy exudate present
- Sarcoptic mange—unusual mite; sometimes may differentiate based on skin scraping, but mites not always present; therapeutic trial with ivermectin may differentiate; however, concurrent flea and *Sarcoptes* infestation may occur.
- Contact dermatitis—usually ventral distribution of lesions; acute onset

### CBC/BIOCHEMISTRY/URINALYSIS
Usually normal; hypereosinophilia inconsistently detected and not well documented

### OTHER LABORATORY TESTS
- Skin scrapings—negative
- Flea combings—fleas or flea dirt usually found in affected ferrets
- Cytology of ear exudates—no mites seen
- Serum estradiol, androstenedione, and 17-hydroxyprogesterone concentrations (available through the University of Tennessee Clinical Endocrinology Laboratory, Department of Comparative Medicine) to rule out ferret adrenal disease

### IMAGING
Abdominal ultrasound to rule out adrenal disease

### DIAGNOSTIC PROCEDURES
- Diagnosis usually based on historical information and distribution of lesions
- Fleas or flea dirt is supportive but occasionally may be difficult to find.
- The most accurate test may be response to appropriate treatment.

### PATHOLOGIC FINDINGS
- Superficial dermatitis occasionally seen
- Histopathologic lesions not well described

## TREATMENT

### CLIENT EDUCATION
Inform owners that controlling exposure to fleas is currently the only means of therapy.

## MEDICATIONS

### DRUG(S) OF CHOICE
- Corticosteroids—antiinflammatory dosages for symptomatic relief while the fleas are being controlled: prednisone 0.25–1.0 mg/kg q24h PO divided
- Antihistamines—use is anecdotal, generally not as effective as steroids: hydroxyzine (Atarax, Roerig) 2 mg/kg PO q8h; diphenhydramine (Benadryl, Parke-Davis) 0.5–2.0 mg/kg PO, IM, IV q8–12h; chlorpheniramine (Chlor-Trimeton, Squibb) 1–2 mg/kg PO q8–12h

- Fipronil (Frontline, Rhone Merieux)—monthly spot treatment for cats and dogs and spray treatment for dogs; activity against fleas and ticks; resistant to removal with water; dose 1/5–1/2 of cat pipette applied topically q60d; anecdotal dosage, safety, and efficacy not evaluated in ferrets
- Imidacloprid (Advantage, Bayer)—monthly spot treatment for cats and dogs; one cat dose divided into two to three spots topically q30d; anecdotal dosage, safety, and efficacy not evaluated in ferrets
- Selamectin (Revolution, Pfizer) topical application of the cat dosage has been anecdotally successful; safety and efficacy not evaluated in ferrets
- Systemic treatments—limited benefit because they require a fleabite to be effective; may help animals with flea infestation; Lufenuron (Program, Novartis) for cats, has been used anecdotally in ferrets at 30–45 mg/kg PO q30d; permethrin, available as a spot treatment, should not be used in ferrets
- Sprays and powders—usually contain pyrethrins and pyrethroids (synthetic pyrethrins) or carbaryl with an insect growth regulator or synergist; products labeled for use in kittens and puppies are anecdotally considered safe and generally effective; advantages are low toxicity and repellent activity; disadvantages are frequent applications and expense.
- Indoor treatment—fogs and premises sprays; usually contain organophosphates, pyrethrins, and/or insect growth regulators; apply according to manufacturer's directions; treat all areas of the house; can be applied by the owner; advantages are weak chemicals and generally inexpensive; disadvantage is labor intensity; premises sprays concentrate the chemicals in areas that most need treatment; safety of product usage in a ferret's environment is unknown.
- Professional exterminators—advantages are less labor-intensive; relatively few applications; sometimes guaranteed; disadvantages are strength of chemicals and cost; specific recommendations and guidelines must be followed; safety of product usage in a ferret's environment is unknown.
- Inert substances—boric acid, diatomaceous earth, and silica aerogel; treat every 6–12 months; follow manufacturer's recommendations; very safe and effective if applied properly
- Outdoor treatment—concentrated in shaded areas; sprays usually contain pyrethroids or organophosphates and an insect growth regulator; powders are usually organophosphates; products containing nematodes (*Steinerma carpocapsae*) are very safe and chemical-free.
- Antibiotics—may be necessary to treat secondary pyoderma, if severe

## CONTRAINDICATIONS
- Do not use flea collars on ferrets.
- Do not use organophosphate-containing products on ferrets.
- Do not use straight permethrin sprays or spot-ons on ferrets.

## PRECAUTIONS
- All flea-control products discussed above are off-label use. Safety and efficacy has not been evaluated in ferrets. Use with caution, especially in young or debilitated animals
- Prevent ferrets or their cagemates from licking topical spot-on products before they are dry.
- Pyrethrin/pyrethroid-type flea products—adverse reactions include depression, hypersalivation, muscle tremors, vomiting, ataxia, dyspnea, and anorexia.
- Toxicity—if any signs are noted, the animal should be bathed thoroughly to remove any remaining chemicals and treated appropriately.
- Rodents and fish are very sensitive to pyrethrins.

## POSSIBLE INTERACTIONS
With the exception of Lufenuron used concurrently with fipronil or imidacloprid, do not use more than one flea treatment at a time.

## ALTERNATIVE DRUGS
N/A

 **FOLLOW-UP**

## PATIENT MONITORING
- Pruritus and alopecia—should decrease with effective flea control; if signs persist evaluate for other causes or concurrent disease (e.g., ferret adrenal gland disease).

- Fleas and flea dirt—should decrease with effective flea control; however, absence is not always a reliable indicator of successful treatment in very sensitive animals.

## PREVENTION/AVOIDANCE
- See medications
- Year-round warm climates—may require year-round flea control
- Seasonally warm climates—usually begin flea control in May or June

## POSSIBLE COMPLICATIONS
- Secondary bacterial infections
- Adverse reaction to flea-control products

## EXPECTED COURSE AND PROGNOSIS
Prognosis is good, if strict flea control is instituted.

 **MISCELLANEOUS**

## ASSOCIATED CONDITIONS
N/A

## AGE-RELATED FACTORS
Use caution with flea-control products in young animals.

## ZOONOTIC POTENTIAL
In areas of moderate to severe flea infestation, people can be bitten by fleas; usually papular lesions are located on the wrists and ankles.

## PREGNANCY
Carefully follow the label directions of each individual product to estimate its safety; however, bear in mind that these products have not been used extensively in pregnant ferrets, and safety is unknown.

## SYNONYMS
N/A

## SEE ALSO
- Adrenal disease
- Dermatophytosis
- Ear mites
- Sarcoptic mange

## ABBREVIATIONS
N/A

*Suggested Reading*

Clyde VL. Practical treatment and control of common ectoparasites in exotic pets. Vet Med 1996;91(7):632–637.

Fisher MA, Jacobs DE, Hutchinson MJ, et al. Efficacy of imidacloprid on ferrets experimentally infested with the cat flea, Ctenocephalides felis. Compend Contin Edu Pract Vet 2001 23(4):8–10.

Fox JG. Parasitic diseases. In: Fox JG, ed. Biology and Diseases of the Ferret. 2nd Ed. Baltimore: Williams & Wilkins, 1998:375–392.

Kelleher SA. Skin diseases of the ferret. Vet Clin North Am Exotic Anim Pract 2001;4(2):565–572.

Orcutt C. Dermatologic diseases. In: Quesenberry KE, Carpenter JW, eds. Ferrets, Rabbits and Rodents: Clinical Medicine and Surgery. St. Louis: WB Saunders, 2004:79–90

*Portions Adapted From*

Kuhl KA, Greek JS. Fleas and Flea Control. In: Tilley LP, Smith FWK, Jr., eds. The 5-Minute Veterinary Consult: Canine and Feline, 2nd Ed. Baltimore: Lippincott Williams & Wilkins, 2002.

# BASICS

## DEFINITION
• Inflammation of the gastric mucosa
• Presence of gastric erosions and ulcers depends on the inciting cause and duration.

## PATHOPHYSIOLOGY
• Irritation of the gastric mucosa by chemical irritants, drugs, or infectious agents, resulting in an inflammatory response in the mucosal surface that may extend to involve submucosal layers
• Ferrets secrete a baseline level of gastric hydrochloric acid and may develop gastric ulcerations when anorectic.
• Immune-mediated disease may also produce chronic inflammation.

## SYSTEMS AFFECTED
• Gastrointestinal—esophagitis may result from chronic vomiting or gastroesophageal reflux.
• Respiratory—aspiration pneumonia is infrequently seen secondary to vomiting; it is more likely if concurrent esophageal disease exists or patient is debilitated.

## INCIDENCE/PREVALENCE
Relatively common, especially when due to *Helicobacter mustelae* or gastric foreign bodies

## SIGNALMENT
• Gastritis due to *Helicobacter* or gastric foreign bodies is seen most commonly in ferrets 3 months to 3 years of age.
• Gastric foreign bodies are more common in young (<2 years old) ferrets

## SIGNS

### Historical Findings
• Vomiting is a relatively uncommon sign of gastrointestinal tract disease in ferrets as compared to dogs or cats. When present, vomitus may be bile stained and may contain undigested food, flecks of blood, or digested blood ("coffee grounds").
• Weight loss and muscle wasting due to chronic anorexia is the most common sign of gastritis in ferrets.
• Ptyalism, pawing at the mouth, bruxism
• Diarrhea, sometimes with blood or mucous
• May see melena with ulceration
• Abdominal pain
• Lethargy, poor hair coat

### Physical Examination Findings
• Often normal
• May be thin with persistent anorexia
• May have pale mucous membranes with anemia from chronic blood loss
• Abdominal palpation may elicit cranial abdominal pain, splenomegaly, and/or enlarged mesenteric lymph nodes.

## CAUSES
• Infectious—*H. mustelae*, viral (ECE, distemper, ADV)
• Dietary indiscretion—foreign objects, trichobezoar, chemical irritants, spoiled foods
• Inflammatory—eosinophilic gastroenteritis, lymphoplasmacytic gastroenteritis
• Metabolic/endocrine disease—chronic liver disease, uremia
• Toxins—cleaning agents, heavy metals
• Drugs—NSAIDs, possibly glucocorticoids
• Miscellaneous—anorexia, stress

## RISK FACTORS
• Environmental—unsupervised/free-roaming pets are more likely to ingest inappropriate foods or materials, intentionally or unintentionally.
• Anorexia due to starvation, gastrointestinal or metabolic disease may cause gastric ulcers
• Potentially poor sanitary conditions and overcrowding may facilitate the spread of infection.
• Medications—NSAIDs, glucocorticoids

# DIAGNOSIS

## DIFFERENTIAL DIAGNOSIS
• For ptyalism, pawing at the mouth—insulinoma or other causes of hypoglycemia; any condition causing nausea (gastrointestinal lymphoma, hepatic or renal disease, lower intestinal tract disease)
• All the causes listed above are included in the differential diagnosis of gastritis; sometimes no identifiable cause is found for observed gastric inflammation.
• Idiopathic gastritis—diagnosis of exclusion; often characterized by a predominantly lymphoplasmacytic infiltrate (superficial or diffuse)

## CBC/BIOCHEMISTRY/URINALYSIS
• Hemogram usually unremarkable unless systemic disease present
• Hemoconcentration if severe dehydration
• Regenerative anemia with ulceration
• May see eosinophilia with eosinophilic gastroenteritis
• May see leukocytosis with neutrophilia and lymphocytosis with *Helicobacter*-induced disease
• Azotemia with low urine specific gravity in uremic gastritis
• Increased serum hepatic enzyme activities, or hypoalbuminemia with ECE or chronic hepatic disease

## OTHER LABORATORY TESTS
Fecal flotation—to screen for gastrointestinal parasitism

## IMAGING
• Survey abdominal radiographs—usually normal, but may reveal radiodense foreign objects, a thickened gastric wall, or gastric outlet obstruction with persistent gastric distension
• Contrast radiography—may detect foreign objects, outlet obstruction, delayed gastric emptying, or gastric wall defects
• Ultrasonography—may be used to evaluate stomach and intestinal wall thickness and gastric foreign objects; can be used to examine the liver, spleen, and mesenteric lymph nodes; may detect gastric wall thickening

## DIAGNOSTIC PROCEDURES
• Laparotomy for gastric biopsy and histopathology may be required for definitive diagnosis; if laparotomy is performed, so should biopsy, even if gastric mucosa appears normal.
• Many patients may be unsuitable candidates for surgery (severely debilitated, concurrent disease, or owner financial constraints). Alternatively, a presumptive diagnosis of *Helicobacter*-induced disease may be made based on identification of suggestive clinical signs, exclusion of other diagnoses, and a favorable response to empirical treatment.
• Foreign objects can occasionally be identified and retrieved via endoscopy. However, the small size of the patient and subsequent limitations on instrument size often limit the use of endoscopy.

## PATHOLOGIC FINDINGS
• *Helicobacter* gastritis—gastric mucosal ulceration and granular-appearing mucosa due to inflammatory reaction. Lesions appear most commonly in the pyloric antrum. On histopathologic examination, gastric spiral organisms seen on silver-stained sections; lymphoplasmacytic gastritis and lymphoid follicle hyperplasia
• Idiopathic gastritis—inflammatory infiltrates vary; most often lymphocytes and plasma cells; can see, eosinophils, and/or histiocytes
• Eosinophilic gastroenteritis—diffuse infiltrate of eosinophils into the lamina propria, submucosa, and, occasionally, the serosa; focal eosinophilic granulomas may be seen in affected lymph nodes.
• The distribution of lesions may be patchy, so take several biopsy specimens.

# TREATMENT

## APPROPRIATE HEALTH CARE
• Most patients are stable at presentation unless vomiting is severe enough to cause dehydration.
• Can typically manage as outpatient, pending diagnostic testing or undergoing clinical trials of special diets or medications
• If patient is dehydrated or vomiting becomes severe, hospitalize and institute appropriate IV fluid therapy.

## GASTRITIS

### NURSING CARE
N/A

### ACTIVITY
N/A

### DIET
• Ferrets rarely have intractable vomiting such that holding NPO for long periods is necessary. If holding NPO, monitor ferrets carefully for hypoglycemia. A fast >4 hours can be dangerous. Insulinomas are extremely common in middle-aged ferrets and may be the cause of signs of gastritis or may occur simultaneously with other causes of gastritis.
• Can use novel protein source if dietary allergy is suspected. Feed diets for a minimum of 3 weeks to assess adequacy of response.

### ANOREXIA
• Most ferrets will accept high-calorie diets such as Eukanuba Maximum Calorie diet (Iams Co., Dayton, OH), Feline a/d (Hills Products, Topeka, KS), or Clinicare Feline liquid diet (Abbott Laboratories, North Chicago, IL); may also add dietary supplement such as Nutri-Cal (EVSCO Pharmaceuticals, Buena, NJ) to increase caloric content to these foods.
• Warming the food to body temperature or offering via syringe may increase acceptance.
• Administer these foods several times a day.
• Reported resting energy requirement for ferrets is 70 kcal/kg body weight per day. Clinicare Feline contains 1 kcal/mL; Eukanuba Maximum Calorie diet contains 2 kcal/mL.

### CLIENT EDUCATION
• Gastritis has numerous causes.
• Diagnostic workup—may be extensive; usually requires a biopsy for a definitive diagnosis

### SURGICAL CONSIDERATIONS
• Gastrotomy for removal of foreign objects
• Surgical management if a mass is causing a gastric outflow obstruction
• Exploratory laparotomy may be required for definitive diagnosis.

 MEDICATIONS

### DRUG(S) OF CHOICE
• If *Helicobacter* infection is confirmed or suspected, institute appropriate therapy: amoxicillin (10 mg/kg PO q12h) plus metronidazole (20 mg/kg PO q12h) and bismuth subsalicylate (17–20 mg/kg PO q12h or 1 mL/kg of regular strength preparation [262 mg/15 mL] PO q12h)
• Gastrointestinal antisecretory agents are helpful to treat, and possibly prevent, gastritis in anorectic ferrets. Ferrets continually secrete a baseline level of gastric hydrochloric acid and, as such, anorexia itself may predispose to gastric ulceration. Those successfully used in ferrets include omeprazole (0.7 mg/kg PO q24h), famotidine (0.25–0.5 mg/kg PO, IV q12–24h), and cimetidine (5–10 mg/kg PO, SC, IM q8h).
• Sucralfate suspension (25 mg/kg PO q8h) protects ulcerated tissue (cytoprotection) by binding to ulcer sites.
• Administer antibiotic(s) with activity against enteric Gram-negatives and anaerobes parenterally if a suspected break in the gastrointestinal mucosal barrier or aspiration pneumonia
• Glucocorticoids (prednisone 1.25–2.5 mg/kg PO q24h; gradually taper to 0.25–1 mg/kg qod) may decrease inflammation in patients with chronic gastritis secondary to suspected immune-mediated mechanisms (eosinophilic or lymphoplasmacytic gastroenteritis).
• Antiemetics should be reserved for patients with refractory vomiting that have not responded to treatment of the underlying disease. Options include chlorpromazine (0.2–0.4 mg/kg SC, IM q8–12h) and metoclopramide.
• Metoclopramide (0.2–1.0 mg/kg PO, SC, IM q6–8h) or cisapride (0.5 mg/kg PO q8–12h) to increase gastric emptying and normalize intestinal motility when gastric emptying is delayed or duodenogastric reflux is present

### CONTRAINDICATIONS
• Do not use prokinetics (metoclopramide or cisapride) if gastric outlet obstruction is present.
• Alpha-adrenergic blockers such as chlorpromazine should not be used in dehydrated patients, since they can cause hypotension.

### PRECAUTIONS
N/A

### POSSIBLE INTERACTIONS
N/A

### ALTERNATIVE DRUGS
N/A

 FOLLOW-UP

### PATIENT MONITORING
• Resolution of clinical signs indicates a positive response.
• Monitor blood glucose concentration in animals held NPO for hypoglycemia, do not fast for >4 hours
• Repeat biopsy if signs decrease but do not resolve.

### PREVENTION/AVOIDANCE
• Avoid medications (e.g., NSAIDs) and foods that cause gastric irritation in the patient.
• Use antisecretory agents in anorectic ferrets
• Prevent unsupervised roaming and potential for dietary indiscretion.
• Avoid overcrowding and unsanitary conditions.

### POSSIBLE COMPLICATIONS
• Gastric erosions and ulcers with progressive mucosal damage, hemorrhage, and anemia from ulcers; perforation
• Aspiration pneumonia

### EXPECTED COURSE AND PROGNOSIS
Varies with underlying cause

 MISCELLANEOUS

### ASSOCIATED CONDITIONS
• Gastrointestinal foreign bodies
• Insulinoma, adrenal disease, lymphoma, and cardiac disease are common in middle-aged to older ferrets and may predispose to the development of gastric ulceration.

### AGE-RELATED FACTORS
Young animals are more likely to ingest foreign objects and have *Helicobacter*-induced gastritis.

### ZOONOTIC POTENTIAL
N/A

### PREGNANCY
N/A

### SYNONYMS
N/A

### SEE ALSO
• Eosinophilic gastroenteritis
• Gastroduodenal ulcer
• *Helicobacter mustelae*
• Lymphoplasmacytic gastroenteritis
• Vomiting

### ABBREVIATIONS
• ADV = Aleutian disease virus
• ECE = epizootic catarrhal enteritis
• NPO = nothing by mouth
• NSAIDs = nonsteroidal antiinflammatory drugs

*Suggested Reading*

Fox JG. Diseases of the gastrointestinal system. In: Fox JG, ed. Biology and Diseases of the Ferret. 2nd Ed. Baltimore: Williams & Wilkins, 1998.

Fox JG, Marini RP. Helicobacter mustelae infection in ferrets: pathogenesis, epizootiology, diagnosis and treatment. Semin Avin Exotic Pet Med 2001;10(1):36–44.

Hoefer HL, Bell JA. Gastrointestinal diseases. In: Quesenberry KE, Carpenter JW, eds. Ferrets, Rabbits and Rodents: Clinical Medicine and Surgery. St. Louis: WB Saunders, 2004:25–40.

Jenkins C, Bassett JR. Helicobacter infection. Compend Contin Edu Pract Vet 1997;19(3):267–279.

Jenkins JR. Rabbit and ferret liver and gastrointestinal testing. In: Fudge AM, ed. Laboratory Medicine, Avian and Exotic Pets. Philadelphia: WB Saunders, 2000.

Marini RP, Fox JG, Taylor NS, et al. Ranitidine bismuth citrate and clarithromycin, alone or in combination, for eradication of Helicobacter mustelae infection in ferrets. Am J Vet Res 1999;60(10):1280–1286.

Williams BH, Kiupel M, West KH, et al. Coronavirus-associated epizootic catarrhal enteritis in ferrets. J Am Vet Med Assoc 2000;217:526–530.

*Portions Adapted From*

Hart JR, Jr. Gastritis, Chronic. In: Tilley LP, Smith FWK, Jr., eds. The 5-Minute Veterinary Consult: Canine and Feline, 3rd Ed. Baltimore: Lippincott Williams & Wilkins, 2003.

# BASICS

## DEFINITION
Erosive lesions that extend through the mucosa and into the muscularis mucosa

## PATHOPHYSIOLOGY
• Gastroduodenal ulcers result from single or multiple factors altering, damaging, or overwhelming the normal defense and repair mechanisms of the gastric mucosal barrier.
• Factors that cause mucosal barrier damage and predispose to gastroduodenal ulcer formation include inhibiting the epithelial cell's ability to repair, decreasing the mucosal blood supply, and/or increasing gastric acid secretion.
• The risk of gastroduodenal ulcer formation increases with the number of insults to the gastric mucosal barrier.
• The most common cause of gastric ulceration is *Helicobacter mustelae*–induced disease.
• Ferrets secrete a baseline level of gastric hydrochloric acid and may develop gastric ulcerations when anorectic.

## SYSTEMS AFFECTED
• Gastrointestinal—gastric fundus and antrum are the most common sites of ulceration.
• Cardiovascular/hemic—acute hemorrhage may result in anemia with subsequent tachycardia, systolic heart murmur, and/or hypotension.
• Respiratory—tachypnea may be present with anemia; aspiration pneumonia possible secondary to vomiting.

## GENETICS
N/A

## INCIDENCE/PREVALENCE
• True incidence unknown; probably more common than clinically recognized
• *Helicobacter*-induced gastric ulceration is one of the most common causes of anorexia, melena, and vomiting in young ferrets.

## GEOGRAPHIC DISTRIBUTION
N/A

## SIGNALMENT

### Species/Breed Predilections
N/A

### Mean Age and Range
Most common in ferrets 3 months to 3 years of age

### Predominant Sex
N/A

## SIGNS

### General Comments
Some animals may be asymptomatic with significant gastroduodenal ulcer disease.

## SIGNS

### Historical Findings
Anorexia, ptyalism, bruxism, diarrhea, melena, vomiting, abdominal pain, weight loss, and weakness are the most common clinical signs. Many affected ferrets will paw at the mouth when nauseated.

### Physical Examination Findings
• May have signs of dehydration from fluid and electrolyte loss due to vomiting or diarrhea
• Pallor of the mucous membranes with chronic blood loss
• Weight loss—indicates chronic disease
• Poor haircoat or alopecia
• Fecal staining of the perineum
• Mesenteric lymph nodes are often palpably enlarged
• Splenomegaly is a common, usually nonspecific finding.
• Can be normal in patients with early or mild disease

## CAUSES
• *H. mustelae* is the most common cause of gastrointestinal ulcer disease in ferrets.
• Gastric foreign bodies
• Anorexia from any cause may cause gastric ulcers.
• Gastric neoplasia
• Metabolic disease—hepatic disease, renal failure
• Drugs—NSAIDs
• Gastritis—lymphocytic/plasmacytic gastroenteritis, eosinophilic gastroenteritis
• Stress/major medical illness—shock, severe illness, hypotension, trauma, major surgery, burns, heat stroke, sepsis
• Lead poisoning
• Neurologic disease—head trauma, intervertebral disk disease

## RISK FACTORS
• Stress, concurrent illness (e.g., ECE, other intestinal pathogens, insulinoma, lymphoma)
• Administration of ulcerogenic drugs (NSAIDs)
• Concurrent administration of NSAIDS and glucocorticoids
• Hypovolemic or septic shock

# DIAGNOSIS

## DIFFERENTIAL DIAGNOSIS
• For melena—esophageal disease (neoplasia, esophagitis, foreign body)—differentiate by contrast radiography and/or endoscopy; coagulopathies (DIC, anticoagulant rodenticide poisoning); nasal or oropharyngeal disease (neoplasia, fungal infection)—blood may be swallowed, and hematemesis and melena can occur; may differentiate on clinical signs and physical examination findings; Pepto-Bismol may cause black, tarry stools.

• For ptyalism, pawing at the mouth—insulinoma or other causes of hypoglycemia; any condition causing nausea (gastrointestinal lymphoma, hepatic or renal disease, lower intestinal tract disease)
• In young ferrets, gastrointestinal foreign bodies (in older ferrets trichobezoars) can cause identical clinical signs and may contribute to gastric ulceration.
• Similar clinical signs may be seen with gastrointestinal neoplasia, ECE, bacterial enteritis or inflammatory bowel disease.

## CBC/BIOCHEMISTRY/URINALYSIS
• Regenerative anemia seen with chronic blood loss and may be severe
• Panhypoproteinemia—may be present due to alimentary hemorrhage
• Leukocytosis with neutrophilia and lymphocytosis can be seen with *Helicobacter* infection; may see mature neutrophilia, left-shift neutrophilia with sepsis, and gastroduodenal ulcer perforation
• May see elevated BUN, creatinine, and isosthenuria—if ulcers are due to renal disease
• May see elevated liver enzymes, hyperbilirubinemia, and/or hypoalbuminemia—if ulcers are due to liver disease

## OTHER LABORATORY TESTS
• Fecal flotation—to screen for gastrointestinal parasitism
• For *Helicobacter*—culture usually requires gastric biopsy and specialized isolation techniques and media; success rates are low.

## IMAGING
• Radiography—usually normal with ulceration alone; helpful to rule out underlying disease (e.g., gastric foreign body) or other causes of gastrointestinal tract disease
• Gastrointestinal contrast studies rarely demonstrate mucosal irregularities or filling defects.
• Abdominal ultrasonography usually will not detect a gastroduodenal ulcer; it may identify a gastric or duodenal mass, gastric or duodenal wall thickening, and/or abdominal lymphadenopathy.

## DIAGNOSTIC PROCEDURES
• Gastric biopsy via laparotomy to diagnose *Helicobacter*-induced disease. Evidence of characteristic histologic lesions combined with documentation of the organism is needed to support *Helicobacter* infection as the cause of clinical disease. Exploratory laparotomy is also useful to evaluate the extent of gastric pathology and to rule out gastrointestinal foreign bodies, neoplasia, and intestinal inflammatory diseases.
• Many patients may be unsuitable candidates for surgery (severely debilitated, concurrent disease, or owner financial constraints). Alternatively, a presumptive diagnosis of *Helicobacter*-induced disease may be made based on identification of suggestive

# GASTRODUODENAL ULCERS

clinical signs, exclusion of other diagnoses, and a favorable response to empirical treatment.
• Endoscopy—may be used to identify ulcers or remove small foreign bodies; however, small patient size usually makes this procedure impractical.

## PATHOLOGIC FINDINGS
• Stomach—gastric mucosal ulceration and granular-appearing mucosa due to inflammatory reaction. Lesions appear most commonly in the pyloric antrum. On histopathologic examination, lymphocytic plasmacytic gastritis and lymphoid follicle hyperplasia are commonly seen, especially with *Helicobacter* infection.
• May identify *Helicobacter* spp. in gastric biopsy specimens (silver stains help identify *Helicobacter*)

# TREATMENT

## APPROPRIATE HEALTH CARE
• Treat any underlying causes.
• Can treat on an outpatient basis if the cause is identified and removed, vomiting is not excessive, and gastroduodenal bleeding is minimal
• Ferrets that are anorectic, vomiting, or dehydrated require hospitalization; treat as inpatients—those with severe gastroduodenal bleeding and/or ulcer perforation
• May need emergency management of hemorrhage or septic peritonitis

## NURSING CARE
• IV fluids to maintain hydration
• May need transfusions (whole blood or packed red blood cells) or oxygen-carrying hemoglobin solution infusions (Oxyglobin) in patients with severe gastroduodenal hemorrhage

## ACTIVITY
Restricted

## DIET
• If patient refuses normal diet, most will accept high-calorie diets such as Eukanuba Maximum Calorie diet (Iams Co., Dayton, OH), Feline a/d (Hills Products, Topeka, KS), or Clinicare Feline liquid diet (Abbott Laboratories, North Chicago, IL); may also add dietary supplement such as Nutri-Cal (EVSCO Pharmaceuticals, Buena, NJ) to increase caloric content to these foods.
• Warming the food to body temperature or offering via syringe may increase acceptance.
• Administer these supplements several times a day.
• Reported resting energy requirement for ferrets is 70 kcal/kg body weight per day. Clinicare Feline contains 1 kcal/mL; Eukanuba Maximum Calorie diet contains 2 kcal/mL.

## CLIENT EDUCATION
Explain the difficulty of establishing a diagnosis without invasive techniques such as gastric biopsy.

## SURGICAL CONSIDERATIONS
Surgical treatment is indicated if hemorrhage is uncontrolled and severe, gastroduodenal ulcer perforates, and/or potentially resectable tumor is identified.

# MEDICATIONS

## DRUG(S) OF CHOICE
• If *Helicobacter* infection is confirmed or suspected, institute appropriate therapy: amoxicillin (10 mg/kg PO q12h) plus metronidazole (20 mg/kg PO q12h) and bismuth subsalicylate (17–20 mg/kg PO q12h or 1 mL/kg of regular strength preparation [262 mg/15 mL] PO q12h) or clarithromycin (12.5 mg/kg PO q8h) plus ranitidine bismuth citrate (this is not Zantac, ranitidine HCl) at 24 mg/kg PO q8h for 2 weeks.
• Gastrointestinal antisecretory agents are helpful to treat, and possibly prevent, gastritis in anorectic ferrets. Ferrets continually secrete a baseline level of gastric hydrochloric acid and, as such, anorexia itself may predispose to gastric ulceration. Those successfully used in ferrets include omeprazole (0.7 mg/kg PO q24h), famotidine (0.25–0.5 mg/kg PO, IV q12–24h), ranitidine HCl (3.5 mg/kg PO q12h) and cimetidine (5–10 mg/kg PO, SC, IM q8h).
• Sucralfate suspension (25 mg/kg PO q8h) protects ulcerated tissue (cytoprotection) by binding to ulcer sites.
• Administer antibiotic(s) with activity against enteric Gram-negative bacteria and anaerobes parenterally if a suspected break in the gastrointestinal mucosal barrier or aspiration pneumonia

## CONTRAINDICATIONS
N/A

## PRECAUTIONS
N/A

## POSSIBLE INTERACTIONS
• Cimetidine may interfere with metabolism of other drugs.
• H$_2$-blockers prevent uptake of omeprazole by oxyntic cells.
• Sucralfate may alter absorption of other drugs.

## ALTERNATIVE DRUGS
N/A

# FOLLOW-UP

## PATIENT MONITORING
• Assess improvement in clinical signs.
• Can check PCV, TP, and BUN until they return to normal
• If vomiting persists or recurs after cessation of combination therapy, a biopsy may be needed to determine whether the infection has been eradicated.

## PREVENTION/AVOIDANCE
Avoid gastric irritants (e.g., NSAIDs) and stress.
Administer antisecretory agents to anorectic ferrets

## POSSIBLE COMPLICATIONS
• Gastroduodenal ulcer perforation and possible sepsis
• Severe blood loss requiring transfusion
• Aspiration pneumonia
• Death—sepsis, hemorrhage

## EXPECTED COURSE AND PROGNOSIS
• Varies with underlying cause
• Patients with malignant gastric neoplasia, renal failure, liver failure, sepsis, and gastric perforation—poor
• Gastroduodenal ulcers secondary to *Helicobacter* infection, inflammatory bowel disease, or NSAID administration—may be good to excellent, depending on severity

# MISCELLANEOUS

## ASSOCIATED CONDITIONS
N/A

## AGE-RELATED FACTORS
Neoplasia more common in older animals

## ZOONOTIC POTENTIAL
Further investigation needed to determine/evaluate a possible zoonotic potential for *Helicobacter* spp.

## PREGNANCY
Avoid metronidazole in pregnant animals.

## SYNONYMS
N/A

## ASSOCIATED CONDITIONS
• Gastrointestinal foreign bodies
• Insulinoma, adrenal disease, lymphoma, and cardiac disease are common in middle-aged to older ferrets and may predispose to the development of gastric ulceration.

## SEE ALSO
• Gastrointestinal and esophageal foreign bodies
• *Helicobacter mustelae*
• Inflammatory bowel disease
• Melena
• Vomiting

**ABBREVIATIONS**
- BUN = blood urea nitrogen
- DIC = disseminated intravascular coagulation
- ECE = epizootic catarrhal enteritis
- NSAIDs = nonsteroidal antiinflammatory drugs
- PCV = packed cell volume
- TP = total protein

*Suggested Reading*

Fox JG. Bacterial and mycoplasmal diseases. In: Fox JG, ed. Biology and Diseases of the Ferret. 2nd Ed. Baltimore: Williams & Wilkins, 1998.

Fox JG, Marini RP. Helicobacter mustelae infection in ferrets: pathogenesis, epizootiology, diagnosis and treatment. Semin Avin Exotic Pet Med 2001;10(1):36–44.

Hoefer HL, Bell JA. Gastrointestinal diseases. In: Quesenberry KE, Carpenter JW, eds. Ferrets, Rabbits and Rodents: Clinical Medicine and Surgery. St. Louis: WB Saunders, 2004:25–40.

Jenkins C, Bassett JR. Helicobacter infection. Compend Contin Edu Pract Vet 1997;19(3):267–279.

Marini RP, Fox JG, Taylor NS, et al. Ranitidine bismuth citrate and clarithromycin, alone or in combination, for eradication of Helicobacter mustelae infection in ferrets. Am J Vet Res 1999;60(10):1280–1286.

Wheeler J, Bennett RA. Ferret abdominal surgical procedures. Part II. Gastrointestinal foreign bodies, splenomegaly, liver biopsy, cystotomy and ovariohysterectomy. Compend Contin Edu Pract Vet 1999;21(11):1049–1057.

Williams BH. Ferret microbiology and virology. In: Fudge AM, ed. Laboratory Medicine, Avian and Exotic Pets. Philadelphia: WB Saunders, 2000.

*Portions Adapted From*

Mott J. Gastroduodenal Ulcer Disease. In: Tilley LP, Smith FWK, Jr., eds. The 5-Minute Veterinary Consult: Canine and Feline, 2nd Ed. Baltimore: Lippincott Williams & Wilkins, 2000.

# GASTROINTESTINAL AND ESOPHAGEAL FOREIGN BODIES

## BASICS

### DEFINITIION
A nonfood item located in the esophagus, stomach, or intestine

### PATHOPHYSIOLOGY
• Ferrets are extremely fond of chewing, especially on plastic, rubber toys, cloth, or vegetables. Therefore, gastrointestinal foreign bodies are a common occurrence. Trichobezoars acquired through grooming may also form gastrointestinal foreign bodies.
• Some small or easily deformed foreign bodies will pass through the gastrointestinal tract with the ingesta and will subsequently be eliminated from the body in the feces. Larger, nondeformable material may cause a partial or complete outflow obstruction, most commonly of the stomach or intestines.
• Ingestion of toxic foreign bodies, such as heavy metals, may cause a functional ileus, thereby contributing to foreign body retention.
• Retained objects of insufficient size to cause an outflow obstruction may cause a mechanical irritation to the mucosa.

### SYSTEMS AFFECTED
• Gastrointestinal—if an obstruction has occurred, the patient may become dehydrated from fluid loss via vomiting or regurgitation. If a perforation has occurred, mediastinitis or peritonitis may develop.
• Musculoskeletal—loss of muscle mass may occur due to inappetence.
• Multisystemic—heavy metal toxicosis can cause multisystemic changes.

### INCIDENCE/PREVALENCE
Exact incidence not reported; however gastrointestinal foreign bodies are one of the most common causes of clinical disease in pet ferrets.

### SIGNALMENT
• Younger ferrets (<2 years) are more likely to ingest toys or other objects.
• Trichobezoars are more commonly seen in older ferrets.

### Predominant Sex
N/A

### SIGNS

#### Historical Findings
*Esophagus*
• Esophageal foreign bodies are rare in ferrets.
• Regurgitation, ptyalism, anorexia, and persistent attempts at swallowing may be seen.
*Gastric*
• Inappetence, anorexia, weight loss, chronic wasting, and lethargy are the most common signs, especially with chronic partial obstruction.
• Signs of nausea such as ptyalism, bruxism, and pawing at the mouth are also common.
• Vomiting may also occur, but is seen less frequently than signs listed above.
• Pronounced weakness and reluctance to move are commonly seen in acute obstructions.
• Hematemesis and/or melena may be present if the foreign body has caused a gastric erosion or ulcer.
*Intestinal*
• Anorexia, lethargy, diarrhea, and bruxism are the most common signs.
• Diarrhea and vomiting may also occur.
• Melena may be present if the foreign body has caused intestinal erosion or ulcer.
• Depression and signs of pain such as reluctance to move occur in acute obstructions.

#### Physical Examination Findings
• May have signs of dehydration from fluid and electrolyte loss due to vomiting or diarrhea
• Pallor of the mucous membranes with chronic blood loss
• Pain may be elicited on abdominal palpation.
• Intestinal foreign bodies are occasionally palpable; gastric foreign bodies often are not.
• Gas- or fluid-filled stomach or intestines sometimes are palpable.
• Linear foreign bodies (although rare) may cause bunching of the intestines.
• Emaciation is seen in chronic cases.

### CAUSES
• Most retained foreign bodies are simply too large to pass through the intestinal tract.
• Gastrointestinal lymphoma, gastritis, or metabolic disease resulting in severe ileus may cause retention of a foreign object that would normally pass.
• Ferrets are particularly fond of chewing or swallowing rubber toys and foam rubber.

### RISK FACTORS
• Unsupervised access to toys or other objects to chew
• Underlying gastrointestinal tract disease

## DIAGNOSIS

### DIFFERENTIAL DIAGNOSIS
• Any disease that may cause ptyalism, bruxism, regurgitation, vomiting, anorexia, or weight loss should be considered in the differential diagnosis. The most common causes of these signs include gastrointestinal foreign bodies, *Helicobacter mustelae* gastritis, ECE, lymphoma, and inflammatory bowel diseases.

• *H. mustelae*-induced gastritis may cause similar clinical signs. *Helicobacter*-induced disease may be a primary pathogen and mimic gastrointestinal foreign bodies or may occur as a consequence of gastrointestinal foreign bodies (mechanical irritation of the gastric mucosa caused by the foreign body or stress).
• Differential diagnoses for ptyalism, pawing at the mouth—insulinoma or other causes of hypoglycemia; any condition causing nausea (gastrointestinal lymphoma, *Helicobacter*, ECE, hepatic or renal disease, lower intestinal tract disease)
• Melena and anorexia most common with *H. mustelae* or gastrointestinal foreign body
• Abdominal palpation may be helpful when differentiating causes of anorexia, weight loss, and gastrointestinal signs—thickened intestinal loops and palpably enlarged mesenteric lymph nodes are more common with eosinophilic enterocolitis, lymphoplasmacytic enteritis, ECE, or lymphoma and less likely with gastrointestinal foreign bodies.
• In patients with diarrhea, the character of diarrhea may be helpful in differentiating causes—bile-stained (green) mucous-covered diarrhea is seen most commonly with ECE; granular, "bird seed"-like feces is seen with maldigestive/malabsorptive disorders; tenesmus, dyschezia, and rectal prolapse is associated with colonic disease.

### CBC/BIOCHEMISTRY/URINALYSIS
• These tests are often normal.
• Inflammatory leukogram may be seen with foreign body–induced gastritis.
• PCV and TS elevation in dehydrated patients
• Anemia from gastric bleeding is rare.
• If the intestinal tract has been perforated, an inflammatory leukogram may be seen.

### OTHER LABORATORY TESTS
N/A

### IMAGING

#### Radiography
• Radiographs are valuable to delineate the type and location of some radiopaque foreign bodies, especially metallic substances. If gas is visualized in the mediastinum or pleural space, perforation of the esophagus should be considered. Gas distension of the stomach is sometimes observed with gastric foreign bodies. This gas occasionally may provide enough contrast to make the ingested object also visible.
• A sudden change in the diameter of intestinal loops is highly suggestive of foreign bodies. A mechanical ileus or displacement of bowel loops can sometimes (but not always) be seen. In many cases, however, radiographs can appear normal, especially in patients with a soft or foam rubber toy foreign body.

# GASTROINTESTINAL AND ESOPHAGEAL FOREIGN BODIES

• Localized free gas in the peritoneal cavity is seen with peritonitis resulting from gastrointestinal perforation.
• Plication of the intestines as observed with a linear foreign body is extremely rare in ferrets.

### Positive Contrast Radiography
A positive contrast study may reveal a delay in intestinal transit time and will sometimes document the presence of radiolucent objects. Barium is the contrast agent of choice to delineate a foreign body or ulceration. It is, however, contraindicated in ferrets with suspected perforation or intractable vomiting/regurgitation. In these instances, iohexol should be used.

### Ultrasonography
Abdominal ultrasound can be useful in documenting a gastric or intestinal foreign body.

## OTHER DIAGNOSTIC PROCEDURES
Upper gastrointestinal endoscopy may be used to diagnose esophageal and gastric foreign bodies. However, the small size of the patient and subsequent limitations on instrument size often limit the use of endoscopy. Endoscopy, when feasible, is superior to radiography in evaluating inflammation, punctures, lacerations, erosions, and ulcers.

## PATHOLOGIC FINDINGS
N/A

## TREATMENT

## APPROPRIATE HEALTH CARE
• Always treat as an inpatient. In the unusual instance in which the foreign object is successfully removed via endoscopy, the patient can go home the same day.
• Esophageal foreign bodies are considered an emergency since the incidence of complications increases with the length of time the foreign body is present.
• Gastric foreign bodies are considered an urgency rather than an emergency, unless the patient has evidence of gastric erosion or signs of toxicosis.
• Intestinal foreign bodies are usually an emergency since the incidence of complications increases with the length of time the foreign body is present.

## NURSING CARE
• Patients are usually anorectic or dehydrated. Fluid therapy using a balanced electrolyte solution should be administered prior to and during surgery.
• A warm, quiet environment should be provided for recovery.

## ACTIVITY
The patient may resume normal activity after the foreign body is removed.

## DIET
• If the ferret has been eating, the diet does not require modification. Most ferrets will resume eating soft food within 12–24 hours postsurgery.
• If the ferret refuses a normal diet, offer a high-calorie diet such as Eukanuba Maximum Calorie diet (Iams Co., Dayton, OH), Feline a/d (Hills Products, Topeka, KS), or Clinicare Feline liquid diet (Abbott Laboratories, North Chicago, IL); may also add a dietary supplement such as Nutri-Cal (EVSCO Pharmaceuticals, Buena, NJ) to increase caloric content to these foods
• Resting energy for ferrets is approximately 70 kcal/kg body weight per day (sick ferrets have higher requirements). Clinicare Feline contains 1 kcal/mL; Eukanuba Maximum Calorie diet contains 2 kcal/mL.

## CLIENT EDUCATION
• Discuss possible complications prior to treatment, especially if surgery is required.
• Remove objects commonly ingested from the environment, especially rubber toys.

## SURGICAL CONSIDERATIONS
• Esophageal foreign bodies are rare and may be removed via endoscopy.
• Gastric and intestinal foreign bodies are usually removed by surgery. This allows for assessment of the intestinal tract, liver, and spleen, along with biopsy specimen collection when indicated.
• Carefully observe the adrenals and pancreas, since concurrent disease is often present especially in the middle-aged to older animals.
• Objects in the stomach may occasionally be removed by flexible endoscopy. Endoscopy is less traumatic than surgery; however, object retrieval may be impaired due to the small size of the patient and subsequent limitations on instrument size.

## MEDICATIONS

## DRUG(S) OF CHOICE
• If gastric ulceration is evident, treatment for *H. mustelae* is indicated: amoxicillin (10 mg/kg PO q12h) plus metronidazole (20 mg/kg PO q12h) and bismuth subsalicylate (17 mg/kg PO q12h for at least 2 weeks); or clarithromycin (12.5 mg/kg PO q8h) plus ranitidine bismuth citrate (this is not Zantac, ranitidine HCl) at 24 mg/kg PO q8h) for 2 weeks
• Gastrointestinal antisecretory agents are helpful to treat, and possibly prevent, gastritis in anorectic ferrets. Ferrets continually secrete a baseline level of gastric hydrochloric acid and, as such, anorexia itself may predispose to gastric ulceration. Those successfully used in ferrets include omeprazole

(0.7 mg/kg PO q24h), famotidine (0.25–0.5 mg/kg PO, SC, IV q24h), ranitidine HCl (3.5 mg/kg PO q12h) and cimetidine (5–10 mg/kg PO, SC, IM q8h).
• Postoperative analgesics may promote appetite.

## CONTRAINDICATIONS
N/A

## PRECAUTIONS
N/A

## POSSIBLE INTERACTIONS
N/A

## ALTERNATIVE DRUGS
N/A

## FOLLOW-UP

## PATIENT MONITORING
• After the foreign body has been removed, assess the mucosa for damage. Mucosal ulceration may occur due to infection with *H. mustelae* or mucosal injury. Usually, the degree of mucosal injury is proportional to the length of time the object is within the gastrointestinal tract and the texture of the object.
• Monitor the patient for at least 2 months after the foreign body removal for evidence of stricture formation at the site of the foreign body.

## PREVENTION/AVOIDANCE
• The ferret should be closely supervised during times of access to potential foreign bodies.
• Avoid giving rubber toys to young ferrets.
• To prevent trichobezoars, administer a cat laxative regularly, especially during periods of heavy shedding.

## POSSIBLE COMPLICATIONS
Other than the possibility of stricture formation at the site of removal, complications following removal of gastric foreign bodies are rare.

## EXPECTED COURSE AND PROGNOSIS
• The prognosis following timely removal of an intestinal foreign body is usually good to excellent.
• Patients can usually be released within 36–48 hours.

## MISCELLANEOUS

## ASSOCIATED CONDITIONS
• Gastritis due to *H. mustelae*
• Gastrointestinal lymphoma
• Inflammatory bowel diseases (eosinophillic or lymphoplasmacytic)
• Insulinoma

# GASTROINTESTINAL AND ESOPHAGEAL FOREIGN BODIES

## AGE-RELATED FACTORS
• There is a higher incidence of foreign bodies in younger ferrets.
• Older ferrets are more likely to have concurrent diseases such as insulinoma or adrenal disease.
• Lymphoma may be seen in any age ferret.

## ZOONOTIC POTENTIAL
N/A

## PREGNANCY
N/A

## SYNONYMS
N/A

## SEE ALSO
• Anorexia
• Gastritis
• *Helicobacter mustelae*
• Insulinoma

• Lymphosarcoma
• Lymphoplasmacytic gastroenteritis

## ABBREVIATIONS
• ALT = alanine aminotransferase
• ECE = epizootic catarrhal enteritis
• PCV = packed cell volume
• TS = total solids

### Suggested Reading
Fox JG. Diseases of the gastrointestinal system. In: Fox JG, ed. Biology and Diseases of the Ferret. 2nd Ed. Baltimore: Williams & Wilkins, 1998:273–290.
Hoefer HL, Bell JA. Gastrointestinal diseases. In: Quesenberry KE, Carpenter JW, eds. Ferrets, Rabbits and Rodents: Clinical Medicine and Surgery. St. Louis: WB Saunders, 2004:25–40.

Marini RP, Fox JG, Taylor NS, et al. Ranitidine bismuth citrate and clarithromycin, alone or in combination, for eradication of *Helicobacter mustelae* infection in ferrets. Am J Vet Res 1999;60(10): 1280–6.
Wheeler J, Bennett RA. Ferret abdominal surgical procedures. Part II. Gastrointestinal foreign bodies, splenomegaly, liver biopsy, cystotomy and ovariohysterectomy. Compend Contin Edu Pract Vet 1999;21(11):1049–1057.

### Portions Adapted From
Jones BD. Esophageal and Gastrointestinal Foreign Bodies. In: Tilley LP, Smith FWK, Jr., eds. The 5-Minute Veterinary Consult: Canine and Feline, 1st Ed. Baltimore: Lippincott Williams & Wilkins, 1997.

# BASICS

## OVERVIEW
• Enteric infection with the protozoan parasite *Giardia* spp.
• Usually a copathogen with other enteric infectious agents; primary infection is rare.
• Water-borne transmission of cysts; dogs or cats in household may serve as reservoir.
• Motile (flagellated) organisms attach to surface of enterocytes in small intestine, especially duodenum through jejunum.
• Malabsorption syndrome with soft voluminous or grainy, "bird seed" appearing stools
• Importance as a reservoir for human infections not known

## SIGNALMENT
• Uncommon cause of gastrointestinal disease
• No breed, sex, or age predilections have been described.

## SIGNS
• May be asymptomatic
• Intermittent diarrhea, or may be acute with copathogens
• Soft, mucoid grainy "millet seed" or "bird seed" appearing feces
• Weight loss, poor hair coat
• Persistence may lead to chronic debilitation.

## CAUSES AND RISK FACTORS
• *Giardia* transmitted by oral ingestion of cysts, usually from water supplies. Ferrets are usually housed indoors and do not have access to most water sources; dogs or cats may serve as a reservoir within a household.
• Infection is often innocuous until a high parasite load develops.
• Debilitated ferrets, especially those with enteric disease (e.g., ECE, *Helicobacter*, gastrointestinal lymphoma), are more likely to shed *Giardia*. Treatment of both primary disease and giardiasis is usually necessary for resolution of clinical signs.

# DIAGNOSIS

## DIFFERENTIAL DIAGNOSIS
Other causes of maldigestion and malabsorption (e.g., ECE, gastrointestinal lymphoma, inflammatory bowel disease) are much more common.

## CBC/BIOCHEMISTRY/URINALYSIS
Usually normal; peripheral eosinophilia not documented, but may be suggestive

## OTHER LABORATORY TESTS
N/A

## IMAGING
N/A

## DIAGNOSTIC PROCEDURES
• Motile organisms, tear-drop–shaped, 10–18 × 7–15 μm; "falling leaf" appearance with two nuclei and flagella. Sometimes visible in fresh fecal wet mount with saline. Specimen should be <10 minutes old. Addition of iodine may enhance appearance.
• Cysts—seen as crescent shapes with zinc sulfate fecal flotation; 8–13 × 7–10 μm
• Fecal ELISA not superior to zinc sulfate flotation; usefulness in ferrets unknown
• Organisms are shed intermittently—lack of visualization does not rule out infection. Collect samples over several days to increase probability of identification.

# TREATMENT
Treat as outpatients unless debilitated or dehydrated.

# MEDICATIONS

## DRUG(S) OF CHOICE
• Metronidazole 15–20 mg/kg q12h for 2 weeks
• Treat all identified copathogens.

## CONTRAINDICATIONS/POSSIBLE INTERACTIONS
Metronidazole bitter taste; anorexia; vomiting; neurotoxic if overdosed

# FOLLOW-UP
Serial fecal examinations to confirm efficacy of treatment

# MISCELLANEOUS

## ZOONOTIC POTENTIAL
• *Giardia* is the most common intestinal parasite in humans residing in North America.
• *Giardia* spp. may not be highly host-specific; no conclusive evidence indicates that cysts shed by ferrets are infective for humans.

## ABBREVIATIONS
• ECE = epizootic catarrhal enteritis
• ELISA = enzyme-linked immunosorbent assay

*Suggested Reading*

Fox JG. Diseases of the gastrointestinal system. In: Fox JG, ed. Biology and Diseases of the Ferret. 2nd Ed. Baltimore: Williams & Wilkins, 1998.

Fox JG. Parasitic diseases. In: Fox JG, ed. Biology and Diseases of the Ferret. 2nd Ed. Baltimore: Williams & Wilkins, 1998:375–392.

Hoefer HL, Bell JA. Gastrointestinal diseases. In: Quesenberry KE, Carpenter JW, eds. Ferrets, Rabbits and Rodents: Clinical Medicine and Surgery. St. Louis: WB Saunders, 2004:25–40.

Jenkins JR. Rabbit and ferret liver and gastrointestinal testing. In: Fudge AM, ed. Laboratory Medicine, Avian and Exotic Pets. Philadelphia: WB Saunders, 2000.

*Portions Adapted From*

Jarvinen JA. Giardiasis. In: Tilley LP, Smith FWK, Jr., eds. The 5-Minute Veterinary Consult: Canine and Feline, 3rd Ed. Baltimore: Lippincott Williams & Wilkins, 2003.

# GINGIVITIS AND PERIODONTAL DISEASE

 BASICS

### OVERVIEW
• Gingivitis—a reversible inflammatory response of the marginal gumline; the earliest phase of periodontal disease
• Periodontal disease—inflammation of some or all of the tooth's support structures (gingiva, cementum, periodontal ligament, and alveolar bone)
• Caused by bacteria located in the gingival crevice; initially a pellicle forms on the enamel surface of a clean tooth; the pellicle is composed of proteins and glycoproteins deposited from saliva and gingival crevicular fluid; the pellicle attracts bacteria that soon adhere, forming plaque; the plaque thickens, eventually becomes mineralized, and transforms into calculus, which is rough and irritating to the gingival.
• Calculus formation is a common finding in ferrets, which occasionally leads to gingivitis; periodontal disease with bone loss and abscess formation is rare in ferrets.
• The severity of gingivitis is likely determined by the host's immunocompetency and local oral factors.

### SIGNALMENT
• Middle-aged to older ferrets
• Calculus formation is a common finding; gingivitis is occasionally seen; severe periodontal disease is rare.

### SIGNS
• Usually detected during routine wellness examinations
• Variable degrees of plaque and calculus formation
• Halitosis
• Erythremic or edematous gingiva
• Gingival surfaces may bleed easily on contact.
• Pustular discharge and bone loss uncommon finding
• Fractured canine teeth are a common finding in ferrets; pain is uncommon unless dental pulp is exposed.

### CAUSES AND RISK FACTORS
• Plaque accumulation
• Soft diet promotes gingivitis through accumulation of plaque.
• Chewing habits
• Lack of oral health care
• Metabolic diseases such as uremia may predispose.
• Specific bacterial pathogens and the role of aerobic vs. anaerobic bacteria and bacterial endotoxin formation have not been described in ferrets.

 DIAGNOSIS

### DIFFERENTIAL DIAGNOSIS
• Oral neoplasia
• Stomatitis

### CBC/BIOCHEMISTRY/URINALYSIS
May help identify risk factors

### OTHER LABORATORY TESTS
N/A

### IMAGING
• No radiographic changes are usually evident, since periodontal disease is not usually severe in ferrets.
• Radiographs are indicated if abscess or uncommon periodontal disease is suspected.

### DIAGNOSTIC PROCEDURES
• Anesthetized oral examination allows a more thorough visual examination of all dental surfaces; use of a periodontal probe may help distinguish between gingivitis and periodontitis (normal sulcal depths not described in ferrets; 1 mm in cats).
• The use of plaque-disclosing agents helps identify plaque and bacterial accumulations on enamel surfaces.
• Biopsy and histopathology to rule out oral neoplasia

 TREATMENT

• Modify behavior to avoid chewing hard objects and eliminate repetitive trauma, if possible.
• Regular dental prophylaxis can be performed before lesions develop.
• Hard food leaves less substrate on the teeth than soft food; chewing also helps to clean teeth mechanically.
• Professional periodontal therapy may reverse gingivitis.
• Dental cleaning—complete oral examination; supragingival removal of plaque and calculus; subgingival scaling; polishing; subgingival irrigation; extractions are rarely necessary.
• A gentle technique is necessary when cleaning; ferret teeth are more fragile than canine or feline teeth.

 MEDICATIONS

### DRUG(S) OF CHOICE
• Lactoperoxidase- and chlorhexidine-containing dentifrices are effective in retarding plaque but are difficult to use in ferrets.
• Topically applied chlorhexidine, 0.4% stannous fluoride gel, also reduces the inciting plaque formation.
• Antibiotics are generally not necessary in patients with mild gingivitis; for severe disease—clindamycin (5.5–10 mg/kg PO q12h) or clavulanic acid/amoxicillin (12.5 mg/kg PO q12h)

### POSSIBLE INTERACTIONS
N/A

### ALTERNATIVE DRUGS
N/A

 FOLLOW-UP

### PATIENT MONITORING
Regular oral reexaminations are necessary to determine the proper interval between periodontal therapies and assess the effectiveness of oral home care; these steps can cure gingivitis and help to avoid the progression to periodontitis.

### POSSIBLE COMPLICATIONS
Uncontrolled periodontitis invariably leads to tooth loss.

 MISCELLANEOUS

### ASSOCIATED CONDITIONS
N/A

### AGE-RELATED FACTORS
N/A

### ZOONOTIC POTENTIAL
None

*Suggested Reading*

Fox JG. Diseases of the gastrointestinal system. In: Fox JG, ed. Biology and Diseases of the Ferret. 2nd Ed. Baltimore: Williams & Wilkins, 1998:273–290.
Wiggs RB, Lobprise HB. Veterinary dentistry: principles and practice. Philadelphia: Lippincott-Raven, 1997.

*Portions Adapted From*

Klein T. Gingivitis. In: Tilley LP, Smith FWK, Jr., eds. The 5-Minute Veterinary Consult: Canine and Feline, 2nd Ed. Baltimore: Lippincott Williams & Wilkins, 2000.

# BASICS

## OVERVIEW
• Disease caused by infection with *Dirofilaria immitis*
• Worms may lodge in the right ventricle, cranial vena cava, or main pulmonary artery.
• Usually very low worm burden (range 1–21 adult worms, 1–2 more common); microfilaremia is less common (50–60% of infected ferrets).
• Severe cardiac disease may be seen in ferrets with very low worm burdens (one to two adults).
• High right ventricular afterload causes myocardial hypertrophy and, in some animals, CHF.
• Pulmonary hypertension and embolization occur, especially following adulticide therapy.

## SIGNALMENT
• May be seen in any age ferret
• Common disease in tropical and semi-tropical zones, especially along the Atlantic and Gulf coasts
• All unprotected ferrets are at risk in endemic regions.

## SIGNS

### General Comments
Clinical signs may vary from absent to mild–moderate signs (lethargy, anorexia) to signs of fulminant heart failure. Most ferrets, however, present with severe signs of CHF. Signs of CHF occur with very low adult worm burdens due to the small size of the ferret heart.

### Historical Findings
• Animals may be asymptomatic.
• Sudden death
• Coughing
• Weakness—usually manifested as rear limb weakness, ataxia, or paresis
• Anorexia
• Depression
• Cachexia
• Dyspnea, tachypnea
• Abdominal distension (ascites, hepatomegaly or splenomegaly) with right-sided CHF)
• Melena (rare)

### Physical Examination Findings
• Labored breathing, rales, or crackles—ferrets with severe pulmonary hypertension or pleural effusion
• Systolic murmur in some animals
• Muffled heart sounds, lack of chest compliance, and dyspnea characterized by rapid shallow respirations may be associated with pleural effusion.
• Tachycardia, ascites, and hepatomegaly indicate CHF.
• Occasionally, no abnormalities are found.

## CAUSES AND RISK FACTORS
• Infection with *D. immitis*
• Residence in endemic regions
• Lack of prophylaxis

# DIAGNOSIS

## DIFFERENTIAL DIAGNOSIS
• Other causes of CHF (e.g., dilated cardiomyopathy)
• Mediastinal lymphoma

## CBC/BIOCHEMISTRY/URINALYSIS
• Usually normal
• Mild to moderate anemia sometimes seen
• Eosinophilia and basophilia—not usually seen in ferrets with heartworm disease

## OTHER LABORATORY TESTS
• Modified Knott's test—limited usefulness; microfilaria are present in only approximately 50% of affected ferrets.
• Low worm burdens (fewer than five worms) and single-sex infections commonly result in false-negative results; negative result does not rule out heartworm disease.
• Serologic tests that identify adult *D. immitis* antigen are of some use; however, false-negative results are common—ELISA (Snap heartworm antigen test, Idexx Laboratories) appears to be most useful.
• Tests that detect circulating antibodies to immature and adult heartworm antigen—sensitivity and specificity for use in ferrets is unknown.

## IMAGING

### Radiographic Findings
• Pleural effusion is a very common finding.
• Cardiomegaly, right atrial enlargement, and enlarged vena cava are common; main pulmonary artery segment enlargement, and lobar arterial enlargement and tortuosity vary; but are usually absent.
• Parenchymal lung infiltrates of variable severity—surround lobar arteries; may extend into most or all of one or multiple lung lobes when thromboembolism occurs
• Diffuse, symmetrical, alveolar, and interstitial infiltrates occasionally occur.

### Echocardiographic Findings
• May be extremely helpful in the diagnosis when performed by an experienced practitioner
• Parallel, linear echodensities produced by heartworms may be detected in the right ventricle, right atrium, and pulmonary arteries.
• Sometimes unremarkable; may reflect right ventricular dilation and wall hypertrophy

## DIAGNOSTIC PROCEDURES

### Electrocardiographic Findings
• Usually normal

• Heart rhythm disturbances—occasionally seen (atrial fibrillation most common) in severe infection

## PATHOLOGIC FINDINGS
• Large right heart
• Pulmonary arterial myointimal proliferation
• Pulmonary thromboembolism
• Hepatomegaly and congestion in animals with right-sided CHF

# TREATMENT

## APPROPRIATE HEALTH CARE

### General Comments
• Treatment options include adulticide therapy followed by long-term treatment with prednisone and ivermectin (symptomatic animals), or treatment with prednisone and ivermectin alone (asymptomatic animals).
• Treatment with adulticide therapy carries the risk of complications from worm emboli and toxicity of the adulticide drug itself.
• Treatment with long-term ivermectin and prednisone allows a slower kill of adult heartworms and perhaps less risk of worm emboli. However, animals in fulminant heart failure may not survive long enough for this therapy to be effective.
• Sufficient evidence comparing the safety and efficacy of these treatment options does not exist; however, the prognosis with either option is fair to poor, especially in animals with fulminant signs of CHF. In general, the author prefers to administer adulticide therapy to animals with signs of CHF, whereas asymptomatic ferrets may not need adulticide therapy.

## NURSING CARE
• Symptomatic ferrets are often in fulminant heart failure and should be hospitalized and stabilized.
• Thoracocentesis is indicated in ferrets with pleural effusion. When performing thoracocentesis be aware that the heart is located much more caudally within the thorax in the ferret as compared to dogs and cats. Sedation (midazolam 0.3–1.0 mg/kg IM, SC) or ketamine (10–20 mg/kg IM plus diazepam 1–2 mg/kg IM) or anesthesia with isoflurane by mask may be necessary.
• It may be necessary to repeat thoracocentesis frequently to relieve dyspnea over a several month period.

## ACTIVITY
Severe restriction of activity required for at least 4–6 weeks after adulticide administration

# HEARTWORM DISEASE

## CLIENT EDUCATION

Reinfection can occur unless appropriate prophylaxis administered

## MEDICATIONS

### DRUG(S) OF CHOICE

Symptomatic ferrets—stabilize animals with right-sided CHF before adulticide treatment:

• Supplemental oxygen; thoracocentesis if indicated

• If the ferret is in fulminant cardiac failure, administer furosemide at 2–4 mg/kg q8–12h IM or IV. Initially, furosemide should be administered parenterally. Long-term therapy should be continued at a dose of 1–2 mg/kg PO q12h.

• Enalapril may be needed for long-term maintenance in ferrets with CHF to reduce afterload and preload. Begin with a dose of 0.25–0.5 mg/kg PO q48h and increase to q24h dosing if well tolerated.

• Prednisone is administered at a dose of 1 mg/kg PO q24h or divided q12h.

• Theophylline (4.25 mg/kg PO q8–12h) may be useful in severely dyspneic ferrets .

### Adulticide Treatment:

• Melarsomine dihydrochloride (Immiticid —protocols have been extrapolated from canine treatment as follows: Severely affected animals receive one injection 2.5 mg/kg IM), followed by two injections 24 hours apart 1 month later. Mild to moderately affected animals may receive two injections 24 hours apart, followed by one injection 1 month later. Administer deep IM injection using an insulin syringe; sedation is recommended to prevent movement and minimize local muscle necrosis.

• Begin administration of microfilaricide (ivermectin, 0.05 mg/kg PO q30d) concurrently with adulticide treatment. Treatment with ivermectin is continued monthly, year-round.

• Concurrent treatment with prednisone is essential to protect against pulmonary emboli. Begin administration of prednisone 1 mg/kg PO q24h or divided q12h concurrently with adulticide treatment. Treatment with prednisone is continued for at least 4 months.

### Alternative Treatment—Ivermectin and Prednisone Treatment Protocol

• For asymptomatic ferrets only; ferrets with signs of CHF should be given adulticide treatment. Monitor carefully for signs of CHF.

• Treat with ivermectin and prednisone as outlined above. Ivermectin will produce a gradual kill of adult worms; prednisone is used to treat thromboembolism.

## CONTRAINDICATIONS

Adulticide treatment with inpatients with renal failure or hepatic failure

## PRECAUTIONS

• Melarsomine dihydrochloride may cause local muscle necrosis; sudden death 12 hours postinjection has been anecdotally reported.

• Standard adulticide therapy in ferrets with severe infection is associated with high mortality due to subsequent pulmonary thromboembolism; may occur up to 3 months following adulticide therapy; concurrent prednisone therapy will significantly reduce this risk.

## POSSIBLE INTERACTIONS

None

## ALTERNATIVE DRUGS

Thiacetarsemide (Caparsolate), combined with heparin and aspirin therapy, has been used successfully; however, this treatment protocol is likely more toxic than treatment with melarsomine and has not been shown to have a greater survival rate.

## FOLLOW-UP

### PATIENT MONITORING

• Perform an antigen test 3–4 weeks after microfilaricide administration.

• Repeat thoracic radiographs periodically to determine efficacy of therapy.

### PREVENTION/AVOIDANCE

Heartworm prophylaxis should be provided for all ferrets at risk:

• Ivermectin—0.05 mg/kg PO q30d; dilute injectable formula in propylene glycol to a concentration of 0.5 mg/mL and dispense in a light protected bottle.

• Ivermectin (Heartgard Feline)—0.055 mg/ferret PO q30d; feline pill may be used; however, chewable tablets that have been broken in half must be discarded, as they will loose effectiveness once broken.

### POSSIBLE COMPLICATIONS

• Sudden death

• Postadulticide pulmonary thromboembolic complications—may occur up to 3–4 months after treatment

• Thrombocytopenia, disseminated intravascular coagulation

• Melarsomine adverse effects—sudden death within 12–24 hours of injection; pulmonary thromboembolism; injection site reaction (myositis); lethargy or depression; causes elevations of hepatic enzymes in dogs and possibly in ferrets

### EXPECTED COURSE AND PROGNOSIS

• Fair to guarded prognosis for animals with asymptomatic infection

• Postadulticide pulmonary complications likely in patients with moderate to severe infection

## MISCELLANEOUS

### ASSOCIATED CONDITIONS
N/A

### AGE-RELATED FACTORS
N/A

### ZOONOTIC POTENTIAL
N/A

### PREGNANCY
Adulticide treatment should be delayed if possible.

### SYNONYMS
N/A

### SEE ALSO
• Congestive heart failure
• Pleural effusion

### ABBREVIATIONS
• CHF = congestive heart failure
• ELISA = enzyme-linked immunosorbent assay

### Suggested Reading

Fox JG. Other systemic diseases. In: Fox JG, ed. Biology and Diseases of the Ferret. 2nd Ed. Baltimore: Williams & Wilkins, 1998:307–320.

Hoefer HL. Cardiac disease in ferrets. Proc North Am Vet Conf 1995;577–578.

Petrie JP, Morrisey JK. Cardiovascular and other diseases. In: Quesenberry KE, Carpenter JW, eds. Ferrets, Rabbits and Rodents: Clinical Medicine and Surgery. St Louis: WB Saunders, 2004:58–71.

Rosenthal K. Management of cardiac disease in ferrets. Waltham/OSU Symp Treatment Sm Anim Dis 1997;Sept.

Rosenthal KL. Respiratory diseases. In: Hillyer EV, Quesenberry KE, eds. Ferrets, Rabbits and Rodents: Clinical Medicine and Surgery. Philadelphia: WB Saunders, 1997:77–84.

Sasai H, Kato T, Sasaki S, et al. Echocardiographic diagnosis of dirofilariasis in a ferret. J Sm Anim Pract 2000;41(4):172–174.

Supakorndej P, Lewis RE, McCall JW, et al. Radiographic and angiographic evaluations of ferrets experimentally infected with Dirofilaria immitis. Vet Radiol Ultrasound 1995;36:23–25.

### Portions Adapted From

Calvert CA, Rawlings CA. Heartworm Disease—Dogs. In: Tilley LP, Smith FWK, Jr., eds. The 5-Minute Veterinary Consult: Canine and Feline, 3rd Ed. Baltimore: Lippincott Williams & Wilkins, 2003.

# BASICS

## DEFINITION

*Helicobacter mustelae* are microaerophilic, Gram-negative, urease-positive, spiral bacteria. *H. mustelae* infection in ferrets is associated with gastritis and peptic ulcerative disease.

## PATHOPHYSIOLOGY

• Nearly 100% of ferrets are colonized with *Helicobacter* by weaning. However, only a small percentage of these ferrets will develop clinically significant *Helicobacter*-associated disease. Disease is seen most commonly in ferrets that have been stressed or have other concurrent disease.
• The discovery of the association of *H. pylori* with gastritis, peptic ulcers, and gastric neoplasia has fundamentally changed the understanding of gastric disease in humans.
• Investigation of the relationship of gastric disease to *Helicobacter*-like organisms has resulted in the discovery of *H. mustelae* in ferrets as a cause of gastritis and peptic ulcers.
• Gastric colonization by *H. mustelae* can cause hypergastrinemia-induced peptic ulcer disease in ferrets; colonization usually results in diffuse antral gastritis, focal glandular atrophy, and superficial gastritis in the remainder of the stomach. Mucosal damage is the result of direct toxic effects of the bacteria and severe lymphoplasmacytic inflammatory reaction.
• *H. mustelae* has also been associated with gastric adenocarcinomas in ferrets.

## SYSTEMS AFFECTED

• Gastrointestinal
• Hemic/lymphatic/immune—mesenteric lymphoid hyperplasia
• Musculoskeletal—muscle wasting with severe disease
• Endocrine/metabolic—fluid, electrolyte, and acid-base imbalances

## GENETICS

N/A

## INCIDENCE/PREVALENCE

• *H. mustelae* is highly prevalent in ferrets—nearly 100% of ferrets are colonized by weaning. *H. mustelae* can be isolated from the feces of ferrets shortly after weaning, but shedding ceases by 20 weeks of age. Although *Helicobacter* can be found in a large percentage of ferrets, not all will become ill.
• Ferrets that are stressed are more likely to develop clinically significant disease.
• *Helicobacter*-induced disease is one of the most common causes of anorexia, melena, and vomiting in young ferrets.

## GEOGRAPHIC DISTRIBUTION

Seen more commonly in North America as compared to Europe. This may be due to variations in the pathogenicity of *Helicobacter* strains.

## SIGNALMENT

### Species/Breed Predilections
N/A

### Mean Age and Range
*Helicobacter*-induced disease is seen most commonly in ferrets 3 months to 3 years of age.

### Predominant Sex
N/A

## SIGNS

### Historical Findings
Anorexia, ptyalism, bruxism, diarrhea, melena, vomiting, abdominal pain, weight loss, and weakness are the most common clinical signs. Many affected ferrets will paw at the mouth when nauseated.

### Physical Examination Findings
• May be normal in patients with early or mild disease
• Pallor of the mucous membranes due to chronic blood loss is a common finding.
• May have signs of dehydration from fluid and electrolyte loss due to vomiting or diarrhea
• Weight loss—indicates chronic disease
• Poor haircoat or alopecia
• Fecal staining of the perineum
• Mesenteric lymph nodes are often palpably enlarged.
• Splenomegaly is commonly detected—usually a nonspecific finding

## CAUSES
*H. mustelae*

## RISK FACTORS
Stress, concurrent illness (e.g., ECE, other intestinal pathogens, insulinoma, lymphoma or other neoplasia)

# DIAGNOSIS

## GENERAL COMMENTS

• High *H. mustelae* spp. prevalence rates exist in ferrets; a combination of organism identification and demonstration of characteristic histologic lesions, or identification of organism and exclusion of other diagnoses are necessary to support a causal relationship between *Helicobacter* infection and clinical disease.
• A presumptive diagnosis may be made on identification of suggestive clinical signs, exclusion of other diagnoses, and a favorable response to empirical treatment.

## DIFFERENTIAL DIAGNOSIS

• In young ferrets gastrointestinal foreign bodies will cause identical clinical signs and may contribute to gastric ulceration; in middle-aged to older ferrets, trichobezoars are common GI foreign bodies.
• Gastric ulceration may result from stress or anorexia.
• Gastric ulcers may also be seen secondary to renal disease or the use of nonsteroidal antiinflammatory agents.
• Similar clinical signs may be seen with gastrointestinal neoplasia, ECE, *Salmonella* sp., or inflammatory bowel disease.

## CBC/BIOCHEMISTRY/URINALYSIS

• Regenerative anemia seen with chronic blood loss and may be severe
• May reflect fluid and electrolyte abnormalities secondary to vomiting and/or diarrhea
• Leukocytosis with neutrophilia and lymphocytosis is common.

## OTHER LABORATORY TESTS

• Culture—usually requires gastric biopsy and specialized isolation techniques and media; success rates are low.
• Serologic tests—assays developed for testing humans for antibody to *H. pylori* will cross-react with *H. mustelae*. The test is performed on whole blood. The usefulness of this test is questionable. A positive result does not necessarily indicate that *Helicobacter* is the cause of clinical disease, since nearly 100% of ferrets have been exposed to *H. mustelae* and will therefore have antibodies.

## IMAGING

• Radiography and ultrasonography—usually normal
• Gastrointestinal contrast studies rarely demonstrate mucosal irregularities or filling defects.

## DIAGNOSTIC PROCEDURES

• To establish a causal relationship between infection with *Helicobacter* and clinical signs, a gastric biopsy is needed. Exploratory laparotomy is often useful to evaluate the extent of gastric pathology and to rule out GI foreign bodies, neoplasia, and intestinal inflammatory diseases, but is not indicated in every case. Biopsy is performed via laparotomy. Evidence of characteristic histologic lesions combined with documentation of the organism is needed to support *Helicobacter* infection as the cause of clinical disease.
• Alternatively, a presumptive diagnosis may be made based on identification of suggestive clinical signs, exclusion of other diagnoses, and a favorable response to empirical treatment. Many patients may be unsuitable candidates for surgery (severely debilitated, concurrent disease, or owner financial constraints).

# HELICOBACTER MUSTELAE

• Urease test (also known as CLO test or *Campylobacter*-like organism test) of gastric biopsy specimens—identifies *Helicobacter*-like organisms; commercial tests are available for in-house use that typically yields results within minutes. The utility of this test is questionable, since most ferrets will be infected with *Helicobacter* and have positive test results. The mere presence of *Helicobacter* does not establish a casual relationship between organism and clinical signs.
• Examination of impression smears may reveal lymphoplasmacytic inflammatory reaction.

## PATHOLOGIC FINDINGS
Stomach—gastric mucosal ulceration and granular-appearing mucosa due to inflammatory reaction. Lesions appear most commonly in the pyloric antrum. On histopathologic examination, gastric spiral organisms seen on silver-stained sections; lymphoplasmacytic gastritis and lymphoid follicle hyperplasia

## TREATMENT

### APPROPRIATE HEALTH CARE
• Ferrets that are anorectic, vomiting, or dehydrated require hospitalization.
• Ferrets that will still eat and are not vomiting may be treated on an outpatient basis.
• There is no indication at present for treating asymptomatic animals with *Helicobacter* infection.

### NURSING CARE
• Fluid therapy using a balanced electrolyte solution should be administered to anorectic or dehydrated patients.
• A warm, quiet environment should be provided for recovery.

### ACTIVITY
N/A

### DIET
• If the normal diet is refused, offer a high-calorie diet such as Eukanuba Maximum Calorie diet (Iams Co., Dayton, OH), Feline a/d (Hills Products, Topeka, KS), or Clinicare Feline liquid diet (Abbott Laboratories, North Chicago, IL); may also add dietary supplement such as Nutri-Cal (EVSCO Pharmaceuticals, Buena, NJ) to increase caloric content to these foods
• Warming the food to body temperature or offering via syringe may increase acceptance.
• Administer these supplements several times a day.
• Reported basal energy requirement for ferrets is 70 kcal/kg body weight per day (sick ferrets have higher requirements). Clinicare Feline contains 1 kcal/mL; Eukanuba Maximum Calorie diet contains 2 kcal/mL.

## CLIENT EDUCATION
Explain the difficulty of establishing a definitive diagnosis without invasive techniques such as gastric biopsy.

## SURGICAL CONSIDERATIONS
N/A

## MEDICATIONS

### DRUG(S) OF CHOICE
• When possible, identify and treat all underlying diseases.
• Specific treatment for *Helicobacter*—the combination of amoxicillin (10–20 mg/kg PO q12h) plus metronidazole (20 mg/kg PO q12h) and bismuth subsalicylate (17 mg/kg PO q12h or 1 mL/kg of regular strength preparation [262 mg/15 mL] PO q12h) is an inexpensive treatment regimen that is usually effective. Treat for at least 2 (often 3–4) weeks.
• The combination of clarithromycin (12.5 mg/kg PO q8h) and ranitidine bismuth citrate (this is not Zantac, ranitidine HCl) at 24 mg/kg PO q8h for 2 weeks has also been effective in eradication of *Helicobacter* sp. Ranitidine bismuth citrate may not be commercially available. Anecdotal reports of substituting Ranitidine HCl (Zantac, GlaxoWellcome) at 3.5 mg/kg PO q12h exist. However efficacy is uncertain, since the additional bismuth citrate may be an important factor in eradicating infection.
• Other antisecretory agents successfully used in ferrets include omeprazole (0.7 mg/kg PO q24h), famotidine (0.25–0.5 mg/kg PO, IV q24h), and cimetidine (5–10 mg/kg PO, SC, IM q8h).
• Sucralfate suspension (25 mg/kg PO q8h) protects ulcerated tissue (cytoprotection) by binding to ulcer sites.

### CONTRAINDICATIONS
Avoid nonsteroidal antiinflammatory medications in ferrets with gastric ulcers.

### PRECAUTIONS
N/A

### POSSIBLE INTERACTIONS
• Cimetidine may interfere with metabolism of other drugs.
• Sucralfate may alter absorption of other drugs.

## FOLLOW-UP

### PATIENT MONITORING
• No noninvasive tests are currently available to confirm eradication of gastric *Helicobacter* spp.
• If clinical signs persist or recur after cessation of combination therapy, pursue other diseases as the cause.

## PREVENTION/AVOIDANCE
• Identify and treat any underlying disease.
• Gastrointestinal antisecretory agents are helpful to treat, and possibly prevent, gastritis in anorectic ferrets. Ferrets continually secrete a baseline level of gastric hydrochloric acid and, as such, anorexia itself may predispose to gastric ulceration.
• Avoid overcrowding and unsanitary conditions.

## POSSIBLE COMPLICATIONS
• Hemorrhage and anemia from ulcers
• Perforation
• Recurrence

## EXPECTED PROGNOSIS
• Most infections are eradicated by using the treatment regimen described above.
• Some ferrets with chronic infections are severely debilitated and will not respond to treatment.
• Recurrence is common, especially under stressful conditions. Repeat therapy may be necessary.

## MISCELLANEOUS

### ASSOCIATED CONDITIONS
• Gastrointestinal foreign bodies
• ECE

### AGE-RELATED FACTORS
Gastric *Helicobacter* organisms appear to be acquired at a young age.

### ZOONOTIC POTENTIAL
The high prevalence of *Helicobacter* spp. in ferrets raises the possibility that household pets may serve as a reservoir for the transmission of *Helicobacter* spp. to people; however, no cases have been documented.

### PREGNANCY
Avoid metronidazole in pregnant animals.

### SYNONYMS
Gastric spiral bacterial

### SEE ALSO
• Gastrointestinal foreign bodies
• Lymphoplasmacytic gastroenteritis
• Melena
• Vomiting

### ABBREVIATION
ECE = epizootic catarrhal enteritis
GI = gastrointestinal

### Suggested Reading
Fox JG. Bacterial and mycoplasmal diseases. In: Fox JG, ed. Biology and Diseases of the Ferret. 2nd Ed. Baltimore: Williams & Wilkins, 1998.
Fox JG, Marini RP. Helicobacter mustelae infection in ferrets: pathogenesis, epizootiology, diagnosis and treatment. Semin Avin Exotic Pet Med 2001;10(1):36–44.

Hoefer HL, Bell, JA. Gastrointestinal diseases. In: Quesenberry KE, Carpenter JW, eds. Ferrets, Rabbits and Rodents: Clinical Medicine and Surgery. St. Louis: WB Saunders, 2004:25–40

Jenkins C, Bassett JR. Helicobacter infection. Compend Contin Edu Pract Vet 1997;19(3):267–279.

Marini RP, Fox JG, Taylor NS, et al. Ranitidine bismuth citrate and clarithromycin, alone or in combination, for eradication of Helicobacter mustelae infection in ferrets. Am J Vet Res 1999;60(10): 1280–1286.

Wheeler J, Bennett RA. Ferret abdominal surgical procedures. Part II. Gastrointestinal foreign bodies, splenomegaly, liver biopsy, cystotomy and ovariohysterectomy. Compend Contin Edu Pract Vet 1999;21(11):1049–1057.

Williams BH. Ferret microbiology and virology. In: Fudge AM, ed. Laboratory Medicine, Avian and Exotic Pets. Philadelphia: WB Saunders, 2000.

*Portions Adapted From*

Simpson KW. Helicobacter Infection. In: Tilley LP, Smith FWK, Jr., eds. The 5-Minute Veterinary Consult: Canine and Feline, 2nd Ed. Baltimore: Lippincott Williams & Wilkins, 2000.

# HEPATOMEGALY

 BASICS

## DEFINITION
Large liver, detected on physical examination, abdominal radiography, ultrasonography, or direct visualization; liver normally 4.3% of body weight

## PATHOPHYSIOLOGY
Normal size—determined by sinusoidal capacitance; parenchymal or sinusoidal accumulation of cells, substrates, or storage products

### Diffuse or Generalized
• Inflammatory—immune-mediated or infectious hepatitis; classified according to cell type
• Congestion—impaired venous drainage
• Infiltration—cellular (usually neoplastic) invasion or accumulation of abnormal substances (glycogen, fat)
• Extramedullary hematopoiesis

### Nodular, Focal, or Asymmetric
• Neoplasia
• Hemorrhage
• Infection or inflammation

## SYSTEMS AFFECTED
• Gastrointestinal—gastric compression or displacement with severe condition
• Pulmonary—compromised ventilatory space

## SIGNALMENT
Middle-aged to older animals more commonly affected

## SIGNS

### Historical Findings
• Abdominal distention or palpable mass
• Icterus is rare in ferrets with liver disease.
• Depend on underlying cause

### Physical Examination Findings
• Liver palpable beyond costal margin (normal or small liver not readily palpable)
• May remain undetected in markedly obese patients

## CAUSES

### Neoplasia—Most Common Cause
• Primary hepatic—lymphoma; bile duct cystadenoma; hepatoma; hepatocellular carcinoma; bilary carcinoma
• Hemangioma or hemangiosarcoma
• Various metastatic tumors—especially islet cell carcinoma

### Inflammation
• Infectious hepatitis—inflammation secondary to chronic inflammatory bowel disease (e.g., eosinophilic gastroenteritis, lymphoplasmacytic gastroenteritis), ADV, ECE
• Acute hepatic necrosis—toxins, drugs, ischemia

### Venous Outflow Occlusion
High central venous pressure—right-sided congestive heart failure, cardiomyopathy, neoplasia, pericardial disease, heartworm disease, pulmonary hypertension, severe arrhythmia

### Infiltration
• Neoplasia
• Metabolic abnormalities—glycogen, lipid (hepatic lipidosis)

### Biliary Obstruction
• Pancreatic islet cell neoplasia; other neoplasms arising near or involving the bile duct
• Abscess
• Proximal duodenitis, duodenal foreign body

### Other
• Hepatic abscesses
• Extramedullary hematopoiesis
• Regenerative anemias
• Drugs—phenobarbital

## RISK FACTORS
• Neoplasia
• Chronic gastrointestinal tract disease
• Cardiac disease
• Heartworm disease
• Obesity complicated by anorexia—hepatic lipidosis

 DIAGNOSIS

## DIFFERENTIAL DIAGNOSIS

### Similar Signs
Distinguished from gastric, splenic, adrenal, or other cranial abdominal masses or effusions via radiographic and ultrasonographic imaging

### Causes
• History or physical examination findings—cardiac disorders (e.g., heart murmur, jugular distention, muffled heart sounds); significant anemia (pallor with or without jaundice)
• Parenchymal liver disease—may see lethargy, rear limb paresis, anorexia, weight loss, diarrhea, vomiting, hepatic encephalopathy, polydipsia and polyuria, ascites, and jaundice (rare)
• Ultrasonography—mass lesions, pancreatic disease

## CBC/BIOCHEMISTRY/URINALYSIS

### CBC
• May identify anemia and cause
• Leukogram—to identify underlying conditions (leukocytosis with neutrophilia with bacterial disease; may see lymphocytosis in young ferrets or lymphopenia in older ferrets with lymphoma; peripheral eosinophilia with eosinophilic gastroenteritis)
• Panhypoproteinemia or hypoalbuminemia is seen with protein-losing enteropathy.

### Biochemistry
• Moderate to high ALT and ALP with inflammatory disorders, primary hepatic neoplasia, hepatic lipidosis, or vacuolar hepatopathy
• Mild to moderately high liver enzymes with metastatic neoplasia, venous outflow obstruction, or infiltrative disorders
• Bilirubin is infrequently elevated in ferrets with liver disease.
• Hypergammaglobulinemia with ADV

## OTHER LABORATORY TESTS
• Serologic testing—to detect antibodies to ADV
• Heartworm testing—in endemic area

## IMAGING

### Abdominal Radiography
• Hepatomegaly—extension of a rounded liver margin caudal to the costal arch; caudal-dorsal displacement of stomach
• May suggest cause

### Thoracic Radiography
• Right and left lateral views—screen for metastasis and underlying disorders
• Cardiac, pulmonary, pericardial disorders

### Abdominal Ultrasonography
• Liver size and contour
• Abdominal effusions—distribution and echogenic patterns
• Diffuse enlargement with normal echogenicity—congestion, cellular infiltration, inflammation, extramedullary hematopoiesis
• Diffuse enlargement with hyperechoic parenchyma (minor nodularity)—lipidosis, glycogen accumulation, inflammation, diffuse early fibrosis
• Identify concurrent abdominal disease—liver, kidneys, intestines, lymph nodes
• Cannot differentiate benign from malignant disease

### Thoracic Ultrasonography
• Mediastinum—masses or lymphadenopathy
• Cardiac—functional abnormalities, masses

## OTHER DIAGNOSTIC PROCEDURES
• Fine-needle aspiration—23- or 25-gauge 2.5- to 3.75-cm (1- to 1.5-inch) needle; aspirated with ultrasound guidance
• Cytology—may reveal infectious agents, neoplasia, inflammation, or extramedullary hematopoiesis
• Hepatic biopsy—if findings suggest primary hepatic disease and imaging rules out other obvious diagnoses; via ultrasound-guided needle, laparoscopy, or laparotomy
• Microbial culture—aerobic and anaerobic bacterial

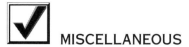
• Coagulation profile—before liver biopsy (limited information on normal ferrets available)
• Abdominal effusion paracentesis—cytology, protein content, cultures

## TREATMENT

### APPROPRIATE HEALTH CARE

• General supportive goals—eliminate inciting cause; optimize conditions for hepatic regeneration; prevent complications; reverse derangements associated with hepatic failure.
• Important derangements—dehydration and hypovolemia; hepatic encephalopathy; hypoglycemia; acid-base and electrolyte abnormalities; coagulopathies; gastrointestinal ulcerations; sepsis; endotoxemia

### NURSING CARE

• Hospitalize patients that are anorectic, dehydrated, or in heart or liver failure.
• Rehydration is essential to treatment success in severely ill ferrets.
• Fluids are usually supplemented with potassium chloride, 5% dextrose if anorectic or concurrent insulinoma.
• Heart failure or ascites—avoid sodium-rich fluids.

### ACTIVITY

Restricted; cage rest while undergoing primary therapy

### DIET

• If normal diet is refused, most ferrets will accept high-calorie dietary supplements such as Nutri-Cal (EVSCO Pharmaceuticals, Buena, NJ), or Clinicare Feline liquid diet (Abbott Laboratories, North Chicago, IL). Canned chicken human baby foods and Eukanuba Maximum Calorie diet (Iams Co., Dayton, OH) are usually accepted by anorectic ferrets.
• Warming the food to body temperature or offering via syringe may increase acceptance.
• Administer these supplements several times a day.
• Resting energy requirement is 70 kcal/kg body weight per day. Clinicare Feline con-

tains 1 kcal/mL; Eukanuba Maximum Calorie diet contains 2 kcal/mL.
• Restrict sodium—with cardiac failure or liver disease that causes ascites

### CLIENT EDUCATION

• Inform client that treatment depends on underlying cause.
• Warn client that many causes are life-threatening, although others are less serious and may be amenable to treatment.
• Inform client that a thorough workup is essential for attaining a definitive diagnosis.

### SURGICAL CONSIDERATIONS

Indicated for resection of primary or focal hepatic mass lesions (neoplasia, abscess)

## MEDICATIONS

### DRUG(S) OF CHOICE

• Cardiac causes—diuretics (e.g., furosemide) and an ACE inhibitor (enalapril) often warranted
• Infectious (e.g., bacterial) diseases—appropriate antimicrobial agents

### CONTRAINDICATIONS

Avoid hepatotoxic medications.

### POSSIBLE INTERACTIONS

N/A

### ALTERNATIVE DRUGS

N/A

## FOLLOW-UP

### PATIENT MONITORING

• Physical assessment and hepatic imaging—reassess liver size.
• CBC, biochemistry—assess progression of hepatic dysfunction.
• Thoracic radiographs, electrocardiography, and echocardiography—assess previous abnormalities.

### POSSIBLE COMPLICATIONS

Many causes are life-threatening.

✓ MISCELLANEOUS

### ASSOCIATED CONDITIONS

N/A

### AGE-RELATED FACTORS

N/A

### ZOONOTIC POTENTIAL

N/A

### PREGNANCY

N/A

### ABBREVIATIONS

• ACE = angiotensin-converting enzyme
• ADV = Aleutian disease virus
• ALP = alkaline phosphatase
• ALT = alanine aminotransferase
• CBC = complete blood count
• ECE = epizootic catarrhal enteritis

*Suggested Reading*

Hoefer HL, Bell, JA. Gastrointestinal diseases. In: Quesenberry KE, Carpenter JW, eds. Ferrets, Rabbits and Rodents: Clinical Medicine and Surgery. St. Louis: WB Saunders, 2004:25–40.

Jenkins JR. Rabbit and ferret liver and gastrointestinal testing. In: Fudge AM, ed. Laboratory Medicine, Avian and Exotic Pets. Philadelphia: WB Saunders, 2000.

Wheeler J, Bennett RA. Ferret abdominal surgical procedures. Part II. Gastrointestinal foreign bodies, splenomegaly, liver biopsy, cystotomy and ovariohysterectomy. Compend Contin Edu Pract Vet 1999;21(11):1049–1057.

Williams BH, Weiss CA. Neoplasia. In: Quesenberry KE, Carpenter JW, eds. Ferrets, Rabbits and Rodents: Clinical Medicine and surgery. St. Louis: WB Saunders, 2004:91–106.

Li X, Fox JG. Neoplastic diseases. In: Fox JG, ed. Biology and Diseases of the Ferret. 2nd Ed. Baltimore: Williams and Wilkins 1998:405–448.

*Portions Adapted From*

Richter KP, Center SA. Hepatomegaly. In: Tilley LP, Smith FWK, Jr., eds. The 5-Minute Veterinary Consult: Canine and Feline, 3rd Ed. Baltimore: Lippincott Williams & Wilkins, 2003.

# HYDRONEPHROSIS

## BASICS

### OVERVIEW
Causes progressive distension of the renal pelvis and diverticula, with atrophy of the renal parenchyma secondary to obstruction in most patients. The disease is usually unilateral and occurs secondary to complete or partial obstruction of the kidney or ureter by uroliths, neoplasia, retroperitoneal disease, and accidental ligation of the ureter during ovariohysterectomy.

### SIGNALMENT
Can be seen in either gender, although may be more common in young females due to inadvertent ligation of the ureter during ovariohysterectomy

### SIGNS
*Historical Findings*
• None in some animals
• Progressive abdominal distention
• May be referable to the cause of the obstruction

*Physical Examination Findings*
• Renomegaly
• Renal, abdominal, or lumbar pain
• Abdominal mass—bladder or periprostatic tissue

### CAUSES AND RISK FACTORS
Any cause of ureteral obstruction including uroliths; neoplasia; prostatic disease; retroperitoneal abscess, cysts, hematoma, or other mass; inadvertent ureteral ligation during ovariohysterectomy

## DIAGNOSIS

### DIFFERENTIAL DIAGNOSIS
• Other causes of renomegaly—especially renal cysts or neoplasia, which are much more common; abscess or granuloma also possible
• Pyelonephritis without obstruction

### CBC/BIOCHEMISTRY/URINALYSIS
• Normal in some patients
• Loss of urine-concentrating ability, hematuria, or pyuria in patients with underlying renal disease, neoplasia, or abscesses

### OTHER LABORATORY TESTS
Examination of fluid obtained during ultrasound-guided fine needle aspirate reveals urine.

### IMAGING
• Abdominal radiographs demonstrate renomegaly. Underlying problems such as urogenital cysts, prostatomegaly, uroliths, or abdominal masses may be detected.
• Ultrasonography reveals dilation of the renal pelvis and diverticula, with thinning of the renal parenchyma; dilation of the ureter may be detected in some animals.

### DIAGNOSTIC PROCEDURES
N/A

## TREATMENT

• Nephrectomy if the contralateral kidney is functioning normally. If the renal function is abnormal, kidney removal may not be necessary unless painful, infected, or neoplastic.
• Specific treatment depends on the cause and whether there is concurrent renal failure or other disease process (e.g., neoplasia, abscess). If obstruction is removable and sufficient renal function remains, removal of the affected kidney is not necessary.
• Emergency surgery rarely required; treat metabolic and electrolyte abnormalities prior to surgery.

## MEDICATIONS

### DRUG(S) OF CHOICE
N/A

## FOLLOW-UP

### PATIENT MONITORING
BUN, creatinine, and electrolytes

### EXPECTED COURSE AND PROGNOSIS
Depends on the cause, duration of obstruction, and presence or absence of concurrent infection. In cats and dogs, irreversible damage to the kidney usually begins 15–45 days after obstruction. If the obstruction is relieved within 1 week, renal damage is reversible; some function may be regained with relief of obstruction present for as long as 4 weeks. Insufficient data regarding return to function exist to make this assessment in ferrets.

## MISCELLANEOUS

### ABBREVIATION
BUN = blood urea nitrogen

*Suggested Reading*
Christie BA, Bjorling DE. Kidneys. In: Slatter D, ed. Textbook of small animal surgery. 2nd Ed. Philadelphia: Saunders, 1993:1428–1442.
Fox JG, Pearson RC, Bell JA. Diseases of the genitourinary system. In: Fox JG, ed. Biology and Diseases of the Ferret. 2nd Ed. Baltimore: Williams & Wilkins, 1998.
Pollock CGY. Urogenital diseases. In: Quesenberry KE, Carpenter JW eds. Ferrets, Rabbits and Rodents: Clinical Medicine and Surgery. St. Louis: WB Saunders, 2004:41–49.
Hoefer HL. Rabbit and ferret renal disease diagnosis. In: Fudge AM, ed. Laboratory Medicine, Avian and Exotic Pets. Philadelphia: WB Saunders, 2000.

*Portions Adapted From*
Berkovitch MG. Hydronephrosis. In: Tilley LP, Smith FWK, Jr., eds. The 5-Minute Veterinary Consult: Canine and Feline, 3rd Ed. Baltimore: Lippincott Williams & Wilkins, 2003.

# BASICS

## DEFINITION
High absolute or relative concentrations of feminizing sex hormones such as estradiol, estriol, and estrone. Severe aplastic anemia and blood loss due to abnormal clotting from estrogen-induced bone marrow suppression is the most common and severe effect of hyperestrogenism.

## PATHOPHYSIOLOGY
• Estrogens are produced by the ovary, testes, and adrenal cortex, and by peripheral conversion of precursor hormones.
• Severe hyperestrogenism is seen in intact females. Ferrets are seasonally polyestrous (breeding season March–August) and induced ovulators. Ovulation, followed by a pregnancy or pseudopregnancy lasting 41–43 days, is induced by stimulation of the cervix by mating or artificial means. Approximately half of unbred females will remain in estrus. Serum estrogen concentration will remain elevated for the remainder of the breeding season (6 months or more) in females that are not bred.
• Estrogen causes severe bone marrow suppression of erythroid, myeloid, and megakaryocytic cell lines. Females are at risk of developing life-threatening anemia and blood loss due to thrombocytopenia if allowed to remain in estrus for more than 1 month. Death usually occurs after 2 months of estrus.
• Hyperestrogenism is also occasionally seen in neutered ferrets of either gender with ferret adrenal disease. Adrenal cortical hyperplasia or neoplasia causes increased production of sex steroids and is one of the most common diseases of ferrets. The bone marrow suppressive effects of hyperestrogenism in ferrets with adrenal disease is usually mild.
• Other organs affected include the skin and urogenital tract.

## SYSTEMS AFFECTED
• Hemic/lymphatic/immune—aplastic anemia
• Urogenital—feminization, swollen vulva, pyometra, urogenital cysts
• Skin/exocrine—alopecia
• Neuromuscular—weakness, ataxia, or paresis from anemia; paresis or paralysis due to subdural hematoma formation (rare)

## GENETICS
N/A

## INCIDENCE/PREVALENCE
• Hyperestrogenism due prolonged estrus is less common in the United States, because most ferrets are neutered before arriving at pet stores at approximately 5–6 weeks of age.

• Up to 50% of unbred jills will develop bone marrow toxicity.
• Hyperestrogenism is a less common manifestation of ferret adrenal disease.

## SIGNALMENT
• Sexually mature females (>8–12 months of age)
• Endogenous hyperestrogenism is most common in young, intact female ferrets. It is occasionally seen in neutered female or male ferrets due to estrogen-secreting adrenocortical tumors.

## SIGNS

### Historical Findings
• Prolonged estrus
• Bilaterally symmetric alopecia, usually beginning at the tail base and progressing cranially.
• Hematuria
• Melena
• Anorexia, depression, and lethargy
• Rear limb weakness, ataxia, paresis, or paralysis

### Physical Examination Findings
• Pale mucous membranes are manifestations of anemia and bone marrow suppression.
• Petechiation, ecchymosis, or other signs of hemorrhage
• Systolic murmur associated with anemia
• Large, turgid vulva
• Serous or purulent vaginal discharge
• Bilateral, symmetrical alopecia beginning at the tail base
• Periurethral cyst or abscess
• Cutaneous hyperpigmentation
• Fever and depression due to pneumonia, septicemia, or pyometra may be caused by neutropenia associated with bone marrow suppression.
• Splenomegaly
• Gynecomastia (rare)
• Galactorrhea (rare)

## CAUSES AND RISK FACTORS
• Failure to breed intact females
• Ovarian remnant in neutered females
• Ferret adrenal disease—estrogen-secreting adrenal tumors. Evidence suggests that adrenal disease may be related to neutering at an early age.

# DIAGNOSIS

## DIFFERENTIAL DIAGNOSIS
• Rule out adrenal disease (usually seen in ferrets >2 years of age; signs not as severe and slower in onset)
• Rule out ovarian remnant in neutered animals (seen in ferrets <2 years of age) by performing hCG challenge test (see below)

• For anemia—blood loss (trauma, gastric ulceration, fleas), rodenticide toxicity, severe hepatic disease, neoplasia, anemia of chronic disease, renal failure
• For alopecia—adrenal disease, seasonal alopecia, ectoparasites, mast cell tumor, and dermatophytosis

## CBC/BIOCHEMISTRY/URINALYSIS
• Nonregenerative anemia (clinical signs usually apparent when PCV falls to <20%), thrombocytopenia (hemorrhage occurs when platelet counts fall below 20,000/μL), and leukocytosis initially, followed by leukopenia
• Use caution when interpreting the PCV from ferrets in which blood was collected under isoflurane anesthesia. Artifactual lowering of the PCV, sometimes as much as 40% below the actual PCV, may occur in ferrets under isoflurane anesthesia.
• Normal PCV (46–61%), erythrocyte count ($17.0 \times 10^6$ cells/μL), and reticulocyte count (10%) are higher in ferrets than other mammals.
• Hematuria

## OTHER LABORATORY TESTS
• High serum estrogen (estradiol) concentration to help confirm a suspected diagnosis
• Examination of vaginal cytology may reveal numerous cornified cells or purulent exudate in ferrets with pyometra.

## IMAGING
Radiography and ultrasonography to detect enlarged adrenals in ferrets with adrenal disease

## DIAGNOSTIC PROCEDURES
• Examination of bone marrow aspirate reveals hypoplasia of the myeloid, erythroid, and megakaryocytic lines.
• In spayed females with swollen vulva—hCG challenge test: 100 IU of hCG IM once at least 2 weeks following onset of vulvar swelling; if swelling subsides 3–4 days postinjection, an ovarian remnant is likely. Some ovarian remnants do not respond to a single injection of hCG, requiring a second injection 2 weeks later. If the vulva remains swollen, adrenal disease is most likely the cause.

## PATHOLOGIC FINDINGS
• Gross examination—swollen vulva, pale mucous membranes, petechia and ecchymosis, tan–pink bone marrow, hemorrhage in gastrointestinal tract, uterus or urinary bladder, hydrometra or pyometra, pneumonia, subdural hemorrhage in brain or spinal cord; enlargement of the adrenal gland(s) seen with adrenal disease
• Histopathologic examination—hypocellular bone marrow, hemosiderosis in liver, spleen and lymph nodes, suppurative pneumonia or metritis may be seen.

# HYPERESTROGENISM

## TREATMENT

### APPROPRIATE HEALTH CARE
Hospitalization is required in ferrets exhibiting clinical signs related to anemia or hemorrhage. Asymptomatic ferrets in estrus < 1 month may be treated on an outpatient basis.

### NURSING CARE
• Indications for whole blood transfusion are the same as those for dogs or cats. In general, most ferrets will benefit from a transfusion when the PCV falls below 15%, depending on clinical signs. Identifiable blood groups have not been demonstrated in ferrets, and transfusion reactions are unlikely. However, administration of dexamethasone sodium phosphate 4–6 mg/kg IV once prior to transfusion has been recommended as a precaution. Healthy, large males with a normal PCV are the most appropriate blood donors. Up to 0.6% of donor's body weight can be safely collected (usually, 6–12 mL, depending on the size of the ferret and volume required). Collect blood from anesthetized donor ferret via the anterior vena cava or jugular vein into a syringe with 1 mL acid citrate dextrose anticoagulant per 6 mL of blood. (Volume of blood to be transfused is estimated in the same manner as for cats.) Ideally, blood should be filtered during administration to the recipient. Administer blood slowly with a 21- to 22-gauge catheter into a large vein such as the jugular, or via an interosseous catheter if a vein is not accessible. Follow transfusion with IV administration of 0.9% NaCl to meet maintenance and dehydration needs.
• Supportive care, such as fluid therapy, warmth, and adequate nutrition, is required for recovery.

### ACTIVITY
Limited if anemic

### DIET
If normal diet is refused, most ferrets will accept high-calorie diets such as Eukanuba Maximum Calorie diet (Iams Co., Dayton, OH), Feline a/d (Hills Products, Topeka, KS), or Clinicare Feline liquid diet (Abbott Laboratories, North Chicago, IL); may also add dietary supplement such as Nutri-Cal (EVSCO Pharmaceuticals, Buena, NJ) to increase caloric content to these foods. Warming the food to body temperature or offering via syringe may increase acceptance.

### CLIENT EDUCATION
• Seek medical attention for any ferret remaining in estrus for more than 2 weeks.
• Ferrets with complications such as thrombocytopenia, pyometra, and pneumonia are poor surgical risks and often do not respond well to medical treatment.
• Nonbreeding females should be neutered.

### SURGICAL CONSIDERATIONS
• Ovariohysterectomy is the treatment of choice. This is usually a relatively safe procedure in ferrets with PCVs >30. Ferrets with PCVs <30 will usually require a blood transfusion prior to surgery. Ferrets that are extremely anemic, thrombocytopenic, and with secondary infections such as pneumonia or pyometra are poor surgical risks and should be stabilized if possible prior to surgery (transfusion as needed and medical treatment with hCG—see below).
• Perform celiotomy in ferrets with ovarian remnant. Ovarian tissue may be small and is located at the caudolateral pole of the kidney. These ferrets are usually not severely anemic presurgery, but a blood transfusion may be required if intraoperative hemorrhage is extensive.
• Ferret adrenal disease may be treated with adrenalectomy or managed medically. The decision as to which form of treatment is appropriate is multifactorial; which gland is affected (left vs. right), surgeon's experience and expertise, severity of clinical signs, age of the animal, concurrent diseases, and financial issues should be considered.

## MEDICATIONS

### DRUG(S) OF CHOICE
• hCG—administer 100 IU per ferret IM to stimulate ovulation and to end estrus. Signs of estrus (particularly vulvar swelling) should diminish within 3–4 days. If signs are still apparent 1 week posttreatment, repeat the injection. Treatment is only effective after day 10 of estrus.
• Administer antibiotics to treat secondary infections.
• Other supportive care measures include administration of iron dextran (10 mg/kg IM once), anabolic and corticosteroids have also been used.
• A purified polymerized Hb product (Oxyglobin, Biopure Corp., Cambridge, MA) has been used successfully in ferrets for which fresh, whole ferret blood was not available for transfusion. Anecdotal reports suggest that slow administration of 11–15 mL/kg over a 4-hour period can be used without adverse effects.

### CONTRAINDICATIONS
Do not use myelosuppressive chemotherapeutic agents in patients with bone marrow suppression.

### PRECAUTIONS
N/A

### ALTERNATIVE DRUGS
• GnRH—20 μg per ferret IM or SC may also be used to stimulate ovulation. Injection may be repeated q 1–2 weeks as needed. Treatment is only effective after day 10 of estrus.
• Anabolic steroids such as stanozolol (0.5 mg/kg PO, SQ q12h) have been advocated for use in anemic ferrets; safety and efficacy have not been evaluated.

## FOLLOW-UP

### PATIENT MONITORING
Monitor response to treatment by remission of clinical signs—reduction in vulvar swelling is good initial indicator of response to treatment. Repeat CBC 1–2 weeks posttreatment to monitor bone marrow response.

### PREVENTION/AVOIDANCE
• Perform ovariohysterectomy on all females not used for breeding.
• Do not allow intact females to remain in heat for longer than 2 weeks—induce ovulation by breeding or administration of hCG.

### POSSIBLE COMPLICATIONS
• Death due to blood loss and anemia during or following surgery. This is particularly a risk in severely anemic and thrombocytopenic patients that do not respond immediately to treatment with hCG.
• Death due to bronchopneumonia or septicemia
• Hemolysis following transfusion
• Permanent suppression of bone marrow (rare)

### EXPECTED COURSE/PROGNOSIS
• Estrus will be terminated within 1 week postadministration of hCG in 95% of ferrets.
• Signs of estrus will usually resolve within 1 week of surgery for removal of ovarian remnant, ovariohysterectomy, or adrenalectomy.
• Ferrets with a PCV >25% usually carry a good prognosis and respond to treatment with hCG. Perform ovariohysterectomy following termination of estrus to prevent future episodes
• Ferrets with a PCV of 15–25% or below carry a fair to guarded prognosis, depending on the severity of clinical signs and other factors such as age and concurrent diseases. Intensive medical treatment and, in some cases, multiple transfusions are required prior to or following ovariohysterectomy.

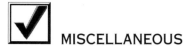

## MISCELLANEOUS

### ASSOCIATED CONDITIONS
- Pyometra
- Paraurethral cysts
- Insulinoma or lymphoma are commonly seen in ferrets with adrenal disease.
- Splenomegaly is a common, nonspecific finding.

### AGE-RELATED FACTORS
Females <2 years of age are most likely to develop hyperestrogenism due to ovarian remnant or prolonged estrus. Females >2 years of age are more likely to develop a milder degree of hyperestrogenism due to adrenal disease

### ZOONOTIC POTENTIAL
N/A

### PREGNANCY
N/A

### SYNONYMS
N/A

### SEE ALSO
- Adrenal disease
- Pyometra and Stump Pyometra

### ABBREVIATIONS
- CBC = complete blood count
- GnRH = gonadotropin-releasing hormone
- Hb = hemoglobin
- hCG = human chorionic gonadotropin
- PCV = packed cell volume

*Suggested Reading*

Bell JA. Periparturient and neonatal diseases. In: Quesenberry KE, Carpenter JW, eds. Ferrets, Rabbits and Rodents: Clinical Medicine and Surgery. St. Louis: WB Saunders, 2004:50–57.

Benson KG, Paul-Murphy J, Ramer JC. Evaluating and stabilizing the critical ferret: basic diagnostic and therapeutic techniques. Compend Contin Edu Pract Vet 2000;22:490–497.

Fox JG, Pearson RC, Bell JA. Diseases of the genitourinary system. In: Fox JG, ed. Biology and Diseases of the Ferret. 2nd Ed. Baltimore: Williams & Wilkins, 1998.

Hillyer EV. Ferret endocrinology. In: Kirk RW, ed. Current Veterinary Therapy XI. Philadelphia: WB Saunders, 1992.

Ludwig L, Aiken S. Soft tissue surgery. In: Quesenberry KE, Carpenter JW, eds. Ferrets, Rabbits and Rodents: Clinical Medicine and Surgery. St. Louis: WB Saunders, 2004:121–134.

Marini RP, Jackson LR, Esteves MI, et al. The effect of isoflurane on hematologic variables in ferrets. Am J Vet Res 1994;55:1497.

Orcutt CJ. Fluids and critical care in small mammals. Proc of North Amer Vet Conf 2001;886.

Pollock CG. Urogenital diseases. In: Quesenberry KE, Carpenter JW, eds. Ferrets, Rabbits and Rodents: Clinical Medicine and Surgery. St. Louis: WB Saunders, 2004:41–49.

Ryland LM. Remission of estrus associated anemia following hysterectomy and multiple blood transfusions in a ferret. J Am Vet Med Assoc 1982;181:820–822.

Wheeler J, Bennett RA. Ferret abdominal surgical procedures. Part II. Gastrointestinal foreign bodies, splenomegaly, liver biopsy, cystotomy and ovariohysterectomy. Compend Contin Edu Pract Vet 1999;21(11):1049–1057.

Williams BH. Therapeutics in ferrets. Vet Clin North Am Exotic Anim Pract 2000;3(1):131–153.

*Portions Adapted From*

Kern MR. Hyperestrogenism. In: Tilley LP, Smith FWK, Jr., eds. The 5-Minute Veterinary Consult: Canine and Feline, 2nd Ed. Baltimore: Lippincott Williams & Wilkins, 2000.

# HYPERSPLENISM

## BASICS

### OVERVIEW
Hypersplenism is a syndrome in which red or white blood cells are removed at an abnormally high rate by the spleen, resulting in one or more cytopenias. Hypersplenism is a rare cause of splenomegaly in ferrets.

### SIGNALMENT
No breed, sex, or age predilections have been described.

### SIGNS
• Signs are referable to anemia, leukopenia, and thrombocytopenia—weakness, anorexia, depression, lethargy, petechia, pale mucous membranes, tachycardia
• Abdominal distension; splenomegaly usually palpable

### CAUSES AND RISK FACTORS
Unknown

## DIAGNOSIS

### GENERAL COMMENTS
Diagnosis is based on the presence of one or more cytopenias, ruling out other causes of splenomegaly, and resolution of cytopenia with splenectomy.

### DIFFERENTIAL DIAGNOSIS
• Other causes of splenomegaly—neoplasia (lymphoma, hemangiosarcoma), extramedullary hematopoiesis, congestion, lymphoid hyperplasia from chronic antigenic stimulation, and age-related changes are all much more common causes of splenomegaly.
• Other cranial organomegaly or masses
• Other causes of cytopenias—hyperestrogenism, lymphoma, chronic disease, heavy metal toxicosis, blood loss; all are much more common

### CBC/BIOCHEMISTRY/URINALYSIS
• Anemia, leukopenia, and/or thrombocytopenia with splenomegaly suggest hypersplenism
• Use caution when interpreting the PCV from ferrets in which blood was collected under isoflurane anesthesia. Artifactual lowering of the PCV, sometimes as much as 40% below the actual PCV may occur in ferrets under isoflurane anesthesia.
• CBC useful in ruling out other causes of splenomegaly—leukocytosis indicates infectious or inflammatory conditions; lymphocytosis may suggest lymphoma; regenerative anemia may indicate blood loss; eosinophilia suggests hypereosinophilic syndrome.

### OTHER LABORATORY TESTS
N/A

### IMAGING
#### Abdominal Radiography
• Confirms or detects splenomegaly
• May be useful to rule out other causes of splenomegaly—gastrointestinal tract disease, adrenal disease, insulinoma, neoplasia

#### Abdominal Ultrasonography
• Diffuse enlargement with normal parenchyma—may be noted with hypersplenism, congestion, or cellular infiltration
• Useful to rule out other causes of splenomegaly—nodular abnormalities seen with neoplasia, hematoma
• Can identify concurrent abdominal diseases affecting liver, kidneys, intestines, and lymph nodes

### DIAGNOSTIC PROCEDURES
#### Fine Needle Aspiration—To Rule out Other Causes of Splenomegaly
Procedure—place patient in right lateral or dorsal recumbency; use a 23- or 25-gauge (1- to 1.5-inch) needle and 5-mL syringe; diffuse: may aspirate without ultrasonography; nodular: requires ultrasound guidance; anesthesia or tranquilization may be required.

#### Bone Marrow Aspiration
• Indicated with cytopenias before splenectomy (spleen may be the main source of circulating blood cells)
• Marrow may be normal or hypercellular with hypersplenism.

## TREATMENT

### APPROPRIATE HEALTH CARE
• Blood transfusion may be indicated in severely anemic animals.
• Indications for whole blood transfusion are the same as those for dogs or cats. In general, most anemic ferrets will benefit from a transfusion when the PCV falls below 15%, depending on clinical signs. Identifiable blood groups have not been demonstrated in ferrets, and transfusion reactions are unlikely. However, administration of dexamethasone sodium phosphate 4–6 mg/kg IV once prior to transfusion has been recommended as a precaution. Healthy, large males with a normal PCV are the most appropriate blood donors. Up to 0.6% of donor's body weight can be safely collected (usually 6–12 mL, depending on the size of the ferret and volume required). Collect blood from anesthetized donor ferret via the anterior vena cava or jugular vein into a syringe with 1 mL acid citrate dextrose anticoagulant per 6 mL of blood. (Volume of blood to be transfused is estimated in the same manner as for cats.) Ideally, blood should be filtered during administration to the recipient. Administer blood slowly with a 21- to 22-gauge catheter into a large vein such as the jugular or via an intraosseous catheter if a vein is not accessible. Follow transfusion with IV administration of 0.9% NaCl to meet maintenance and dehydration needs.
• Supportive care, such as fluid therapy, warmth, and adequate nutrition, is required for recovery.

### SURGICAL CONSIDERATIONS
#### Splenectomy
• Indicated for hypersplenism—removal of spleen results in resolution of cytopenias. Procedure is similar to that performed in dogs or cats. Do not remove spleen unless hypersplenism or neoplasia is diagnosed.
• Exploratory laparotomy—permits direct evaluation of all abdominal organs for diagnosis and treatment of other underlying causes of splenomegaly

## MEDICATIONS

### DRUG(S) OF CHOICE
• Administer antibiotics to treat secondary infections if indicated.
• Other supportive care measures for anemic patients include administration of iron dextran (10 mg/kg IM once), anabolic or corticosteroids
• A purified polymerized Hb product (Oxyglobin, Biopure Corp., Cambridge, MA) has been used successfully in ferrets for which fresh, whole ferret blood was not available for transfusion. Slow administration of 11–15 mL/kg over a 4-hour period has been used without adverse effects.

### CONTRAINDICATIONS
N/A

### PRECAUTIONS
N/A

### POSSIBLE INTERACTIONS
N/A

### ALTERNATIVE DRUGS
N/A

## FOLLOW-UP

### PATIENT MONITORING
Monitor CBC, including thrombocyte count, postoperatively. Resolution of cytopenia indicates successful treatment.

### POSSIBLE COMPLICATIONS
Postoperative sepsis—uncommon complication after surgery

## MISCELLANEOUS

### ASSOCIATED CONDITIONS
N/A

**AGE-RELATED FACTORS**
N/A

**ZOONOTIC POTENTIAL**
N/A

**PREGNANCY**
N/A

**SEE ALSO**
- Hyperestrogenism
- Lymphosarcoma
- Splenomegaly

**ABBREVIATIONS**
- CBC = complete blood count
- Hb = hemoglobin
- PCV = packed cell volume

*Suggested Reading*

Hillyer EV. Working up the ferret with a large spleen. Proc North Am Vet Conf 1994; 819–821.

Ludwig L, Aiken S. Soft tissue surgery. In: Quesenberry KE, Carpenter JW, eds. Ferrets, Rabbits and Rodents: Clinical Medicine and Surgery. St. Louis: WB Saunders, 2004:121–134.

Petrie JP, Morrisey JK. Cardiovascular and other diseases. In: Quesenberry KE, Carpenter JW, eds. Ferrets, Rabbits and Rodents: Clinical Medicine and Surgery. St. Louis: WB Saunders, 2004:58–71.

Wheeler J, Bennett RA. Ferret abdominal surgical procedures. Part II. Gastrointestinal foreign bodies, splenomegaly, liver biopsy, cystotomy and ovariohysterectomy. Compend Contin Edu Pract Vet 1999;21(11):1049–1057.

# HYPOGLYCEMIA

## BASICS

### DEFINITION
Abnormally low blood glucose concentration

### PATHOPHYSIOLOGY

*Mechanisms Responsible for Hypoglycemia*
- Excess insulin or insulinlike factors (e.g., insulinoma and iatrogenic insulin overdose); insulinoma most common cause in ferrets
- Reduction of hormones needed to maintain normal serum glucose (e.g., iatrogenic hypoadrenocorticism)
- Reduced hepatic gluconeogenesis (e.g., hepatic disease, sepsis)
- Overuse (sepsis, neoplasia)
- Reduced intake or underproduction (e.g., kits, severe malnutrition or starvation)

### SYSTEMS AFFECTED
- Nervous
- Musculoskeletal

### SIGNALMENT
Variable, depending on the underlying cause

### SIGNS
- Most animals have episodic signs
- Weakness
- Nausea—ptyalism, pawing at the mouth
- Ataxia
- Lethargy and depression
- Muscle fasciculation
- Posterior paresis
- Abnormal mentation (star-gazing)
- Exercise intolerance
- Abnormal behavior
- Stupor
- Collapse
- Seizures (rare)
- Some animals appear normal aside from findings associated with underlying disease.

### CAUSES

*Endocrine*
- Insulinoma—most frequent cause of hypoglycemia; one of the most common diseases seen in pet ferrets
- Iatrogenic insulin overdose
- Iatrogenic hypoadrenocorticism

*Hepatic Disease*
- Severe hepatitis (e.g., toxic and inflammatory)
- Cirrhosis

*Overuse*
- Neoplasia
- Sepsis

*Reduced Intake/Underproduction*
- Young kits
- Severe malnutrition or starvation

### RISK FACTORS
- Low energy intake predisposes hypoglycemia in patients with conditions causing overuse and underproduction.
- Fasting, excitement, exercise, and eating may increase the risk of hypoglycemic episodes in patients with insulinoma.

## DIAGNOSIS

### DIFFERENTIAL DIAGNOSIS
- Patients with hyperinsulinism—signs of hypoglycemia or a normal physical examination
- Patients with cirrhosis and severe hepatitis—usually have other signs of their disease (e.g., gastrointestinal signs, icterus, and ascites or edema).
- Patients with sepsis—critical; usually in shock; pyrexia or hypothermia revealed by examination; may have gastrointestinal signs
- Patients with iatrogenic hypoadrenocorticism—waxing, waning, nonspecific signs (e.g., vomiting, diarrhea, melena, and weakness); addisonian patients that present in a crisis usually display hypovolemia and hyperkalemia rather than hypoglycemia (e.g., shock, bradycardia, and dehydration).

### LABORATORY FINDINGS

*Drugs That May Alter Laboratory Results*
N/A

*Disorders That May Alter Laboratory Results*
- Lipemia, hemolysis, and icterus may interfere with spectrophotometric assays.
- Delayed serum separation artificially lowers glucose concentration; must separate serum after collection to prevent cellular glucose use
- Refrigerate or freeze serum sample not analyzed within 12 hours.
- Blood glucose reagent strips require whole blood.
- Measure glucose concentration in whole blood immediately following collection.

### CBC/BIOCHEMISTRY/URINALYSIS
- Hypoglycemia <70 mg/dL in most patients with insulinoma (normal value 90–100 mg/dL)
- Normoglycemia is seen in some patients, due to counterregulatory hormone production (epinephrine, glucocorticoids, glucagon, etc.). If insulinoma is suspected but the patient is normoglycemic, perform a carefully monitored fast for no longer than 4 hours. Serum glucose concentrations of <60 mg/dL are highly suggestive.
- Patients with cirrhosis, severe hepatitis, and hepatic neoplasia may have anemia associated with chronic disease, high liver enzyme activities, hyperbilirubinemia, hypoalbuminemia, and low urinary specific gravity.

### OTHER LABORATORY TESTS
- Simultaneous fasting glucose/insulin determination—may be helpful (but usually not necessary) when insulinoma is suspected; high plasma insulin in the face of hypoglycemia suggests insulinoma.
- Fasting and postprandial serum bile acids—indicated when functional hepatic disease is suspected; however, normal values in ferrets have not been reported.
- Bacterial culture of blood—indicated when sepsis is suspected

### IMAGING
- Abdominal radiography and ultrasonography—useful in patients with neoplastic processes (may see organomegaly or masses) as well as cirrhosis (microhepatica, hyperechogenicity) and severe hepatitis (hepatomegaly); pancreatic insulinomas are rarely detectable radiographically, but may be seen on ultrasonic examination if sufficiently large.
- Thoracic radiography—to detect metastasis if neoplasia is suspected

### DIAGNOSTIC PROCEDURES
Ultrasound-guided or surgical biopsy—useful to evaluate for cirrhosis, hepatitis, and neoplasia

## TREATMENT
- Treat as inpatients animals with clinical hypoglycemia; treat underlying disease.
- If able to eat (i.e., responsive, no vomiting), feeding should be part of initial treatment.
- If unable to eat, start continuous fluid therapy with 2.5% dextrose; if clinical signs persist, use a 5% dextrose solution.
- Surgery may be indicated if insulinoma is the cause of hypoglycemia.

## MEDICATIONS

### DRUG(S) OF CHOICE

*Emergency/Acute Treatment*
- In hospital—administer 50% dextrose, 0.25–2.0 mL IV slow bolus (1–3 minutes) to effect. Do not continue to administer once clinical signs begin to abate, or dextrose will cause a release of insulin and rebound hypoglycemia.
- At home—do not attempt to have the owner administer medication orally during a seizure; hypoglycemic seizures usually abate within 1–2 minutes; if a seizure is prolonged, recommend transportation to hospital; if a short seizure has ended or other signs of a hypoglycemic crisis exist, recommend rubbing corn syrup, honey, or 50% dextrose on the buccal mucosa using a cotton swab, followed by 2 mL/kg of the

same solution orally once the patient can swallow; then, seek immediate attention.
• Initiate frequent feeding (4–6 small meals a day) of a diet consisting of high-quality animal protein and low in simple sugars or, if unable to eat, continuous fluid therapy with 2.5% dextrose

### Long-Term Treatment
• See insulinoma for treatment of insulinoma.
• Young kits with hypoglycemia—increase the frequency of feeding (nursing or hand feeding).
• Other causes of hypoglycemia require treating the underlying disease and do not usually need long-term treatment.

### CONTRAINDICATIONS
• Insulin

### PRECAUTIONS
• 50% dextrose causes tissue necrosis and sloughing if given extravascularly; never administer dextrose in concentrations over 5% without confirmed vascular access.
• Administering a dextrose bolus without following with frequent feedings or continuous IV fluids with dextrose can predispose to subsequent hypoglycemic episodes.
• Barbiturates and diazepam in patients with hypoglycemic seizures—they do not treat the cause of the seizure and they may worsen hepatoencephalopathy.

### POSSIBLE INTERACTIONS
N/A

### ALTERNATIVE DRUGS
N/A

 **FOLLOW-UP**

### PATIENT MONITORING
• At home—for return or progression of clinical signs of hypoglycemia; assess serum glucose if signs recur.

• Single, intermittent serum glucose determinations may not truly reflect the glycemic status of the patient because of normal production of counterregulatory hormones.
• Other monitoring is based on the underlying disease.

### POSSIBLE COMPLICATIONS
Recurrent, progressive episodes of hypoglycemia

 **MISCELLANEOUS**

### ASSOCIATED CONDITIONS
Prolonged hypoglycemia can cause transient (hours to days) to permanent blindness from laminar necrosis of the occipital cerebral cortex.

### AGE-RELATED FACTORS
Neonatal animals have poor glycogen storage capacity and a reduced ability to perform gluconeogenesis; thus, short periods of fasting can cause hypoglycemia.

### ZOONOTIC POTENTIAL
N/A

### PREGNANCY
• Hypoglycemia can lead to weakness and dystocia.
• Pregnancy coupled with fasting causes hypoglycemia in rare instances.

### SYNONYMS
N/A

### SEE ALSO
• Insulinoma
• See specific causes

### ABBREVIATIONS
N/A

*Suggested Reading*

Caplan ER, Peterson ME, Mulles HS, et al. Diagnosis and treatment of insulin-secreting pancreatic islet cell tumors in ferrets: 57 cases (1986–1994). J Am Vet Med Assoc 1996;209:1741–1745.

Fox JG, Marini RP. Diseases of the endocrine system. In: Fox JG, ed. Biology and Diseases of the Ferret. 2nd Ed. Baltimore: Williams & Wilkins, 1998.

Marini RP, Ryden EB, Rosenblad WD, et al. Functional islet cell tumor in six ferrets. J Am Vet Med Assoc 1993;202:430–433.

Quesenberry KE, Rosenthal KL. Endocrine diseases. In: Quesenberry KE, Carpenter JW, eds. Ferrets, Rabbits and Rodents: Clinical Medicine and Surgery. St. Louis: WB Saunders, 2004:79–90.

Rosenthal KL. Endocrine disorders of ferrets: insulinoma and adrenal gland disease. 21st Annu Waltham/OSU Symp Treat Small Anim Dis Exotics 1997;35–38.

Rosenthal KL. Ferret and rabbit endocrine disease diagnosis. In: Fudge AM, ed. Laboratory Medicine, Avian and Exotic Pets. Philadelphia: WB Saunders, 2000.

Weiss CA, Williams BH, Scott MV. Insulinoma in the ferret: clinical findings and treatment comparison of 66 cases. J Am Anim Hosp Assoc 1998;34:471–475.

*Portions Adapted From*

Crystal MA. Glucose, Hypoglycemia. In: Tilley LP, Smith FWK, Jr., eds. The 5-Minute Veterinary Consult: Canine and Feline, 2nd Ed. Baltimore: Lippincott Williams & Wilkins, 2002.

# INFLAMMATORY BOWEL DISEASE

## BASICS

### OVERVIEW
- A group of gastrointestinal diseases characterized by inflammatory cellular infiltrates in the lamina propria of the small or large intestine, with associated clinical signs
- An abnormal mucosal immune response to certain causative factors that results in the recruitment of inflammatory cells to the intestine and resultant cellular damage
- Inflammatory response is usually lymphocytic, lymphoplasmacytic, or eosinophilic.
- Lymphocytic infiltration into the lamina propria of the intestines is a common inflammatory response to many infectious agents or environmental stimuli.
- Plasmacytic infiltration indicates chronicity or a more severe inflammatory reaction.
- The cause of tissue eosinophilia is unknown; although a parasitic or allergic cause has been suspected, parasites are usually not found, and allergies have not been well documented in ferrets.
- The exact mechanisms, antigens, and patient factors involved in initiation and progression remain unknown.

### SIGNALMENT
No sex or age predilection

### SIGNS
- Anorexia
- Weight loss, muscle wasting
- Diarrhea, sometimes with blood or mucous
- Melena
- Vomiting
- Ptyalism, pawing at the mouth
- Physical examination—cachexia; thickened, ropy intestines, enlarged mesenteric lymph nodes, and splenomegaly often palpable

### CAUSES AND RISK FACTORS
- Pathogenesis is most likely multifactorial.
- Lymphocytic or lymphoplasmacytic infiltrates may be associated with *Helicobacter mustelae*, ECE, ADV, *Giardia*, *Salmonella*, *Campylobacter*, cryptosporidiosis, or other infectious agents.
- Meat proteins, food additives, artificial coloring, preservatives, and milk proteins may play a role.

## DIAGNOSIS

### DIFFERENTIAL DIAGNOSIS
- Intestinal lymphosarcoma resembles inflammatory bowel disease in both clinical presentation and physical examination findings.
- Gastrointestinal foreign body
- Infectious diseases (e.g., *H. mustelae*, ECE, giardiasis, salmonellosis, *Campylobacter enteritis*, cryptosporidiosis, mycobacteriosis)

### CBC/BIOCHEMISTRY/URINALYSIS
- Lymphocytic or lymphocytic/plasmacytic—results often normal; these tests help rule in or out some other differential diagnoses.
- Eosinophilic—hemogram may reveal a peripheral eosinophilia (up to 35% eosinophils).
- Panhypoproteinemia or hypoalbuminemia may be present due to protein-losing enteropathy.

### OTHER LABORATORY TESTS
- Fecal direct examination, fecal flotation, and zinc sulfate centrifugation may demonstrate gastrointestinal parasites.
- Fecal cytology—may reveal RBC or fecal leukocytes, which are associated with inflammatory bowel disease or invasive bacterial strains.
- Fecal culture should be performed if abnormal bacteria are observed on the fecal Gram's stain, or if *Salmonella* is suspected.

### IMAGING
- Plain abdominal radiographs provide little information.
- Barium contrast radiography may demonstrate thick intestinal walls and mucosal irregularities but does not provide any information about etiology or the nature of the thickening.
- Ultrasonography—may be used to measure stomach and intestinal wall thickness and to rule out other diseases; can be used to examine the liver, spleen, and mesenteric lymph nodes

### DIAGNOSTIC PROCEDURES
Definitive diagnosis requires biopsy and histopathology, usually obtained via exploratory laparotomy.

### PATHOLOGIC FINDINGS
Infiltration of intestines with inflammatory cells

## TREATMENT

### APPROPRIATE HEALTH CARE
Outpatient, unless the patient is debilitated from dehydration, hypoproteinemia, or cachexia

### NURSING CARE
If the patient is dehydrated or must be NPO because of vomiting, any balanced fluid such as lactated Ringer's solution is adequate (for a patient without other concurrent disease); otherwise, select fluids on the basis of secondary diseases.

### ACTIVITY
No need to restrict unless severely debilitated

### DIET
- Highly digestible diets with novel protein sources may be useful for eliciting remission, although an allergic cause has not be documented and little information is available regarding the efficacy of these diets. If attempted, choose feline diets since ferrets have high nutritional protein and fat requirements. Foods that have been anecdotally reported to elicit remission include feline lamb and rice diets, diets consisting exclusively of one type of meat (lamb, duck, turkey), or a "natural prey diet" consisting of whole rodents. If remission is elicited, continue diet for at least 8–13 weeks; this diet may need to be fed lifelong.
- Anorexic ferrets may refuse dry foods but are often willing to eat canned cat foods or pureed meats.

### CLIENT EDUCATION
- Emphasize to the client that inflammatory bowel disease is not necessarily cured as much as controlled.
- Relapses are common; the client must be prepared to be patient during the various food and medication trials that are often necessary to get the disease under control.
- A severely debilitated patient may need hospitalization and parenteral nutrition.

## MEDICATIONS

### DRUG(S) OF CHOICE
- Treat the underlying cause (e.g., *Helicobacter*, *Salmonella*, *Giardia*, etc) if found; if gastric lesions are present empirical treatment for *Helicobacter* is indicated.
- Prednisone (1.25–2.5 mg/kg PO q24h); when signs resolve, gradually taper the corticosteroid dose to 0.5–1.25 mg/kg every other day.
- Azathioprine (Imuran, GlaxoSmithKline) 0.9 mg/kg PO q24–72 hours has been anecdotally used to treat lymphoplasmacytic gastroenteritis with some success.
- Metronidazole (15–20mg/kg PO q12h)—has antibacterial and antiprotozoal properties; some evidence that it also has immune-modulating effects
- See specific diseases for more detailed discussion of treatment.

### CONTRAINDICATIONS
If secondary problems are present, avoid therapeutic agents that might be contraindicated for those conditions.

### PRECAUTIONS
See discussion under specific diseases.

### POSSIBLE INTERACTIONS
See discussion under specific diseases.

### ALTERNATIVE DRUGS
See discussion under specific diseases.

**FOLLOW-UP**

**PATIENT MONITORING**
• Periodic reevaluation may be necessary until the patient's condition stabilizes.
• No other follow-up may be required except yearly physical examinations and assessment during relapse.

**PREVENTION/AVOIDANCE**
N/A

**POSSIBLE COMPLICATIONS**
Dehydration, malnutrition, adverse drug reactions, hypoproteinemia, anemia, and diseases secondary to therapy or resulting from the above mentioned problems

**EXPECTED COURSE AND PROGNOSIS**
• Varies with specific type of inflammatory bowel disease
• See discussion under specific diseases.

 **MISCELLANEOUS**

**ASSOCIATED CONDITIONS**
See discussion under specific diseases.

**AGE-RELATED FACTORS**
N/A

**ZOONOTIC POTENTIAL**
N/A

**PREGNANCY**
N/A

**SYNONYMS**
N/A

**SEE ALSO**
• Anorexia
• Diarrhea
• Eosinophilic gastroenteritis
• Lymphoplasmacytic gastroenteritis

**ABBREVIATIONS**
• ADV = Aleutian disease virus
• ECE = epizootic catarrhal enteritis
• IBD = inflammatory bowel disease
• NPO = nothing by mouth
• RBC = red blood cell

*Suggested Reading*

Finkler MR. Ferret colitis. In: Kirk RW, Bonagura JD, eds. Kirk's Current Veterinary Therapy XI: Small Animal Practice. Philadelphia: WB Saunders, 1992.

Fox JG. Diseases of the gastrointestinal system. In: Fox JG, ed. Biology and Diseases of the Ferret. 2nd Ed. Baltimore: Williams & Wilkins, 1998.

Bell JA. Gastrointestinal diseases. In: Quesenberry KE, Carpenter JW, eds. Ferrets, Rabbits and Rodents: Clinical Medicine and Surgery. St Louis: WB Saunders, 2004:25–40.

Jenkins JR. Rabbit and ferret liver and gastrointestinal testing. In: Fudge AM, ed. Laboratory Medicine, Avian and Exotic Pets. Philadelphia: WB Saunders, 2000.

Palley LS, Fox JG. Eosinophilic gastroenteritis in the ferret. In: Kirk RW, Bonagura JD, eds. Kirk's Current Veterinary Therapy XI: Small Animal Practice. Philadelphia: WB Saunders, 1992.

*Portions Adapted From*

Diehl KJ. Inflammatory Bowel Disease. In: Tilley LP, Smith FWK, Jr., eds. The 5-Minute Veterinary Consult: Canine and Feline, 3rd Ed. Baltimore: Lippincott Williams & Wilkins, 2003.

# INFLUENZA VIRUS

 BASICS

## DEFINITION

A common, self-limiting viral respiratory disease of ferrets characterized by sneezing, rhinitis, fever, conjunctivitis, and occasionally pneumonia

## PATHOPHYSIOLOGY

Human influenza types A and B (class Orthomyxoviridae) are both pathogenic in ferrets. Transmission occurs from human to ferret or ferret to human. Virus replication occurs in the nasal mucosa, causing rhinitis and conjunctivitis within 48 hours following exposure. Occasionally, infection spreads to the lungs, causing pneumonia.

## SYSTEMS AFFECTED

• Respiratory—rhinitis; interstitial pneumonia
• Ophthalmic—acute serous conjunctivitis without keratitis or corneal ulcers
• Gastrointestinal—anorexia, occasionally vomiting

## GENETICS

None

## INCIDENCE/PREVALENCE

Common, especially in multiferret households or facilities or during influenza epizootics in humans

## GEOGRAPHIC DISTRIBUTION

Worldwide

## SIGNALMENT

No age or sex predilection

## SIGNS

### Historical Findings

• Sudden onset
• Anorexia
• Serous nasal or ocular discharge
• Sneezing
• Dyspnea or coughing if pneumonia occurs
• Lethargy
• Occasionally otitis
• Occasionally vomiting

### Physical Examination Findings

• Generally alert and in good condition
• Fever
• Conjunctivitis
• Serous naso-ocular discharge, becoming purulent with secondary bacterial infections

## CAUSES

• Human influenza types A and B, belonging to the class Orthomyxoviridae
• Secondary bacterial infections frequently occur

## RISK FACTORS

• Exposure to affected humans or ferrets
• Multiferret facilities

 DIAGNOSIS

## DIFFERENTIAL DIAGNOSIS

### General Comments

Diagnosis is usually presumptive, based on history of exposure to affected humans or other ferrets and presence of suggestive clinical signs.

### Differentiating Similar Causes

• CDV—the presence of other clinical signs will help to differentiate CDV from influenza virus infection. In ferrets with CDV, facial dermatitis (rash, crusts) and hyperkeratotic foot pads are seen following the onset of nasal discharge. These signs are followed by severe respiratory signs, neurologic signs, and death. Fluorescent antibody testing on conjunctival smears, mucous membrane scrapings, or blood smears can be used to diagnose CDV.
• Nasal foreign bodies—usually unilateral with purulent, mucopurulent, and blood-tinged discharge
• Dental-related disease—abscess, oronasal fistula—rare in ferrets; differentiate based on oral examination.
• Fungal infections—cryptococcosis, blastomycosis—also rare; chronic infection, whereas influenza is self-limiting
• Nasal tumors—usually associated with serosanguinous or blood-tinged discharges; may cause unilateral discharge initially, then progress to bilateral discharge as the disease extends through the nasal septum

## CBC/BIOCHEMISTRY/URINALYSIS

No characteristic or consistent findings; leukopenia in early infection; leukocytosis in ferrets with secondary bacterial infections

## OTHER LABORATORY TESTS

• Serologic testing not readily available and rarely necessary. A rising titer indicates active infection; however, clinical signs generally resolve prior to receiving test results.
• Fluorescent antibody test to rule out CDV—on conjunctival or mucous membrane scrapings or peripheral blood smears

## IMAGING

• Skull radiographs—to differentiate influenza from nasal tumors, fungal rhinitis, or dental disease
• Radiographs of the lungs—for evidence of pneumonia

## DIAGNOSTIC PROCEDURES

Cell cultures to isolate the virus—oral pharynx; lung tissue; secretions from the nose and conjunctiva may be used if obtaining a definitive diagnosis is necessary.

## PATHOLOGIC FINDINGS

• Gross—reddened, swollen mucosa in the upper respiratory tract; serous to mucoid nasal or discharge
• Histopathologic—vacuolar degeneration of epithelial cells, progressing to epithelial necrosis, with sloughing of epithelial cells and infiltration of inflammatory cells (chiefly neutrophils in the early phase, then mononuclear cells) followed by epithelial cell regeneration and hyperplasia

 TREATMENT

## APPROPRIATE HEALTH CARE

Outpatient, unless severe pneumonia occurs

## NURSING CARE

• Clean eyes and nose as indicated.
• Provide palatable foods (see diet, below).
• Fluid therapy using a balanced electrolyte solution should be administered to anorectic or dehydrated patients. Subcutaneous route is sufficient in most patients, unless severe secondary bacterial pneumonia is present.
• Oxygen—with severe pneumonia

## ACTIVITY

Patients should be restricted from contact with humans and other ferrets to prevent transmission of the disease.

## DIET

• No restrictions
• Special diets—may be needed to entice anorectic ferrets to resume eating. Canned chicken human baby foods, Eukanuba Maximum Calorie diet (Iams Co., Dayton, OH), or Clinicare Feline liquid diet (Abbott Laboratories, North Chicago, IL) are examples of foods accepted by anorectic ferrets. Warming the food or offering via syringe may increase acceptance.

## CLIENT EDUCATION

Discuss the potential for zoonosis.

## SURGICAL CONSIDERATIONS

None

 MEDICATIONS

## DRUG(S) OF CHOICE

• Broad-spectrum antibiotics—indicated for secondary bacterial infections (e.g., trimethoprim/sulfonamide 15–30 mg/kg PO, SC q12h); enrofloxacin (10–20 mg/kg PO, SC, IM q24h); or cephalexin (15–25 mg/kg PO q8–12h).
• Antihistamines such as chlorpheniramine (1.0–2.0 mg/kg PO q8–12h) or diphenhydramine (0.5–2.0 mg/kg PO, IM, IV q8–12h) may help to alleviate nasal discharge.

• Antiviral medications amantadine (Symmetrel, Endo Labs; 6 mg/kg PO q12h) has been used anecdotally to shorten clinical course of disease.
• Antibiotic eye ointments—to reduce secondary bacterial infections of the conjunctiva

### CONTRAINDICATIONS
None

### PRECAUTIONS
• Antiviral medications are off-label use; efficacy and safety are unknown.

### POSSIBLE INTERACTIONS
None

### ALTERNATIVE DRUGS
None

## FOLLOW-UP

### PATIENT MONITORING
• Monitor for development of dyspnea associated with pneumonia.
• Monitor for the development of secondary bacterial rhinitis, conjunctivitis or sinusitis.
• No specific laboratory tests needed for monitoring

### PREVENTION/AVOIDANCE
Avoid exposure to humans or ferrets exhibiting clinical signs of influenza.

### POSSIBLE COMPLICATIONS
• Interstitial pneumonia—most serious complication
• Secondary bacterial infections of the lungs or upper airways

### EXPECTED COURSE AND PROGNOSIS
• Clinical disease—usually appears within 48 hours after exposure
• Recovery is usually rapid, occurring within 7 days of the onset of clinical signs.
• Prognosis excellent, unless severe secondary bacterial infections develop

## MISCELLANEOUS

### ASSOCIATED CONDITIONS
N/A

### AGE-RELATED FACTORS
N/A

### ZOONOTIC POTENTIAL
High

### PREGNANCY
N/A

### SYNONYMS
N/A

### SEE ALSO
• Canine distemper virus
• Coughing
• Nasal discharge (sneezing, gagging)

### ABBREVIATION
CDV = canine distemper virus

*Suggested Readings*
Fox JG, Pearson RC, Gorham JR. Viral diseases. In: Fox JG, ed. Biology and Diseases of the Ferret. 2nd Ed. Baltimore: Williams & Wilkins, 1998.
Kendrick RE. Ferret respiratory diseases. Vet Clin North Am Exotic Anim Pract 2000;3(2):453–464.
Rosenthal KL. Respiratory diseases. In: Quesenberry KE, Carpenter JW, eds. Ferrets, Rabbits and Rodents: Clinical Medicine and Surgery. St. Louis: WB Saunders, 2004:72–78.
Williams BH. Ferret microbiology and virology. In: Fudge AM, ed. Laboratory Medicine, Avian and Exotic Pets. Philadelphia: WB Saunders, 2000:334–342.

# INSULINOMA

## BASICS

### DEFINITION
Pancreatic islet beta-cell neoplasm that secretes an excess quantity of insulin

### PATHOPHYSIOLOGY
Excessive insulin secretion leads to excessive glucose uptake and use by insulin-sensitive tissues and reduced hepatic production of glucose; this causes hypoglycemia and its associated clinical signs.

### SYSTEMS AFFECTED
• Nervous—star-gazing, ataxia, seizures, disorientation, abnormal behavior, collapse, and posterior paresis
• Musculoskeletal—weakness and muscle fasciculations
• Gastrointestinal—nausea, vomiting

### SIGNALMENT
• Insulinoma is one of the most common diseases seen in pet ferrets.
• Usually seen in ferrets over 2 years old; mean 5 years of age
• No sex predilection reported

### SIGNS

#### General Comments
• Signs are typically episodic
• The rate of decline of serum glucose concentration affects the type and severity of clinical signs.
• Signs may or may not be related to fasting, excitement, exercise, and eating.
• Ferrets usually demonstrate more than one clinical sign, and the signs progress with time.

#### Historical Findings
• Abnormal mentation, star-gazing, nausea (characterized by ptylism and pawing at the mouth), weakness, depression, ataxia, tremors, and stupor most common; also, seizures (generalized and focal), posterior paresis, vomiting, collapse, muscle fasciculations, abnormal behavior, polyuria and polydipsia, and exercise intolerance
• Many of the hypoglycemic episodes may go unwitnessed, giving owners the impression of an acute onset.

#### Physical Examination Findings
• Often within normal limits unless examined during a hypoglycemic episode, then clinical signs as noted above
• Pancreatic tumors are usually not palpable.
• Emaciation and muscle wasting seen in ferrets with chronic disease
• Splenomegaly often incidental finding on abdominal palpation
• Signs of concurrent ferret adrenal disease (especially alopecia) are commonly seen.

### CAUSES
Insulin-producing adenoma or carcinoma of the pancreas

### RISK FACTORS
Fasting, excitement, exercise, and eating may increase the risk of hypoglycemic episodes.

## DIAGNOSIS

### DIFFERENTIAL DIAGNOSIS
• For hypoglycemia—fasting, starvation, gastrointestinal disease, sepsis
• Seizures and collapse—must consider cardiovascular (e.g., syncope), metabolic (e.g., anemia most common; hepatoencephalopathy, hypocalcemia, and iatrogenic hypoadrenocorticism are rare causes), and neurologic (e.g., epilepsy, neoplasia, toxin, and inflammatory disease) causes
• Posterior paresis and weakness—consider cardiovascular (e.g., arrhythmias, heart failure, and pericardial effusion), metabolic (e.g., anemia, hypokalemia, hypocalcemia, and), neurologic and neuromuscular (e.g., spinal cord disease), and toxic (e.g., botulism, chronic organophosphate exposure, and lead poisoning) causes
• Muscle fasciculations—consider metabolic (e.g., electrolyte imbalances) and toxic (e.g., tetanus and strychnine poisoning) causes

### CBC/BIOCHEMISTRY/URINALYSIS
• Hypoglycemia <70 mg/dL in most patients with insulinoma (normal value 90–100 mg/dL)
• Normoglycemia is seen in some patients, due to counterregulatory hormone production (epinephrine, glucocorticoids, glucagon, etc.). If insulinoma is suspected but the patient is normoglycemic, perform a carefully monitored fast for no longer than 4 hours. Serum glucose concentrations of <60 mg/dL are highly suggestive.
• Be certain to perform serum glucose concentration testing immediately following venipuncture, since storage of serum not separated from red cells will cause a falsely lowered value.
• The practice of feeding flavored nutritional supplements or peanut butter to aid in restraint or venipuncture should be strictly avoided prior to or during collection of blood for serum glucose concentration, as this will cause a falsely elevated value.

### OTHER LABORATORY TESTS
• Simultaneous fasting glucose and insulin determination—results are not consistently reliable, insulin assay not readily available. If measuring insulin is elected, it should be measured along with serum glucose; a single insulin measurement alone is not meaningful. After initiating fast, collect blood samples hourly or bihourly for serum glucose

determination and serum storage; when the serum glucose drops below 60 mg/dL (usually within 2–4 hours), submit that sample for serum insulin determination. Be certain that the insulin assay used has been validated for use in ferrets. Interpretation: high insulin in the face of hypoglycemia, insulinoma likely; normal insulin in the face of hypoglycemia, insulinoma possible; low insulin with hypoglycemia, insulinoma less likely
• Determination of serum insulin concentration is not usually necessary. In most cases, the finding of hypoglycemia with suggestive clinical signs justifies a presumptive diagnosis.

### IMAGING
Abdominal radiography is often normal, except for splenomegaly (usually incidental finding). Pancreatic nodules or metastatic nodules in regional lymph nodes, spleen, or liver can sometimes be seen on abdominal ultrasonography. Concurrent adrenal tumor(s) are commonly found.

### DIAGNOSTIC PROCEDURES
N/A

### PATHOLOGIC FINDINGS
• Multiple nodules of variable size within the pancreas are usually seen.
• Most insulinomas can be identified grossly at surgery; often gentle palpation is required for detection. Occasionally no tumor can be identified grossly, but multiple small tumors are present within the pancreas; a biopsy is necessary to identify these.
• Metastasis is relatively uncommon; when it occurs areas include the regional lymph nodes, spleen, liver, and local adipose tissue.
• Micrometastasis within the pancreas is common.
• Histopathologically tumors appear as either carcinoma or adenoma, but both behave malignantly.

## TREATMENT

### APPROPRIATE HEALTH CARE
• Hospitalize for workup, surgery, and (if clinically hypoglycemic) treatment.
• Treat as outpatient if the owner declines surgery and the patient is not clinically hypoglycemic.

### NURSING CARE
• Mild signs of hypoglycemia may respond to oral dextrose or glucose.
• Administer 50% dextrose, 0.5–2.0 mL IV slow bolus (1–3 minutes) to effect control of seizures/severe hypoglycemic signs. Do not continue to administer once clinical signs begin to abate, or dextrose will cause a release of insulin and rebound hypoglycemia.

• Fluid therapy with 2.5% dextrose and 0.45% saline (increase to 5% dextrose in water if needed to control clinical signs) should follow dextrose bolus; alternatively, if the patient can eat, frequent feedings of an appropriate diet (see diet) may replace dextrose-containing fluids in some patients.

### ACTIVITY
Restricted

### DIET
• The first and most important aspect of management (with or without surgery)
• Feed 4–6 small meals a day.
• Should consist of high-quality animal proteins and be low in simple sugars; avoid semimoist food.

### CLIENT EDUCATION
• Owner should be aware of signs of hypoglycemia. Mild signs may be alleviated by administering honey or syrups orally (taking care to avoided being bitten), followed by a small, high-protein meal. If collapse or seizures occur, they should be instructed to seek immediate medical attention.
• Insulinomas are progressive, even with surgical treatment, since complete excision of all nodules is rarely possible.

### SURGICAL CONSIDERATIONS
• Surgery confirms the diagnosis, often improves survival time, can provide temporary (and occasionally, long-term) remission, and often improves response to medical treatment.
• In most cases multiple nodules are present. Nodules appear as white to pink raised areas on the surface of the pancreas; however, nodules may be buried within the parenchyma—careful palpation is required for detection. Debulk large nodules or perform a partial pancreatectomy if multiple small nodules are present. In most cases small, nonpalpable nodules remain, and clinical signs will eventually return.
• Occasionally, nodules are too small to detect by gross examination. If no nodules are detected, biopsy the pancreas and submit for histopathologic examination.
• Biopsy the spleen, liver, and regional lymph node to look for metastasis.
• Always explore the entire abdominal cavity—concurrent adrenal disease is extremely common.
• Administer 2.5% dextrose in 0.45% saline or 5% dextrose in water pre-, inter- and postoperatively. Withhold food for up to 6–12 hours postoperatively (monitor blood glucose concentrations), and then offer a bland diet. Continue fluid therapy SC or IV until the ferret is eating normally and released.
• Measure serum glucose concentration after surgery and every 6–12 hours until concentration reaches 60–80 mg/dL.

• If serum glucose concentration does not increase postoperatively, begin medical treatment.

## MEDICATIONS

### DRUG(S) OF CHOICE

*Emergency/Acute Therapy*
See nursing care above.

*Long-Term Therapy*
• Surgical therapy is preferred in otherwise healthy ferrets under 6 years of age. Medical therapy is often a better option in older ferrets, in those with concurrent disease, or if owners have financial constraints prohibiting surgery. Many ferrets will have similar survival times and symptom-free intervals with medical therapy alone.
• Medical therapy is indicated when clinical signs return in patients who had previous surgical therapy.
• Glucocorticoids (prednisone at an initial dosage of 0.5–1.0 mg/kg PO q12h; increased to 2 mg/kg PO q12h if needed)—initiate medical treatment if dietary modification alone is insufficient to prevent hypoglycemic episodes. Serum glucose concentration will usually stay in the range of 60–90 mg/dL and signs will abate initially with prednisone and diet modification. With time and progression of the tumor, more insulin will be released and clinical signs will recur. Gradually increase the dose of prednisone as signs of hypoglycemia recur.
• Diazoxide (Proglycem, Baker Norton Pharmaceuticals)—added after dietary modification and prednisone treatment are no longer effective. Reduce prednisone dose back to 1–1.25 mg/kg PO q12 and begin diazoxide at a dose of 5–20 mg/kg PO per day, divided q8–12h. Gradually increase diazoxide to 30 mg/kg PO per day (divided into 2–3 doses) if needed.

### CONTRAINDICATIONS
Insulin

### PRECAUTIONS
• Dextrose bolus—suitable for acute hypoglycemic crisis if followed by continuous dextrose-containing fluids or appropriate feeding; may precipitate further hypoglycemic crises if given alone
• Diazoxide—can cause gastrointestinal irritation; causes bone marrow suppression, cataract formation, aplastic anemia, tachycardia, and thrombocytopenia in humans
• Prednisone and diazoxide each may cause fluid retention and increase preload in ferrets with congestive heart failure.

### POSSIBLE INTERACTIONS
N/A

### ALTERNATIVE DRUGS
Octreotide, a synthetic somatostatin analogue, has been anecdotally used in some ferrets with mixed efficacy.

## FOLLOW-UP

### PATIENT MONITORING
• Postoperative in-hospital serum glucose determinations—monitor every 6–12 hours for the first 2–3 days or until euglycemic. Most ferrets will be euglycemic within 1–2 days after surgery. If hypoglycemia persists, treatment with prednisone is necessary.
• Some ferrets will develop transient hyperglycemia after debulking the pancreas. At home, the urine may be monitored for glucose two to three times daily for the next week. In most cases, hyperglycemia is transient (resolving in 1–2 weeks) and does not require treatment.
• Monitor fasting serum glucose concentration 2 weeks postsurgery or at initiation of medical therapy, then every 1–3 months thereafter.
• Following medical treatment—monitor at home for return or progression of clinical signs of hypoglycemia and adjust medication on the basis of clinical signs and serum glucose levels.

### PREVENTION/AVOIDANCE
For early detection of insulinoma, annual to semiannual measurement of blood glucose concentration is recommended in ferrets over 2–3 years of age.

### POSSIBLE COMPLICATIONS
• Rarely, iatrogenic pancreatitis occurs due to handling of the pancreas during surgery. Clinical signs include nausea, anorexia, and vomiting. Withhold food and continue fluid therapy with 5% dextrose until euglycemic and appetite returns.
• Postoperative hyperglycemia occasionally occurs and usually resolves without treatment. Rarely, hyperglycemia will persist, resulting in clinical signs of diabetes mellitus (in one case, postoperative diabetes was seen in a ferret with a mixed insulinoma/ glucagonoma). See diabetes mellitus in ferrets for treatment.

### EXPECTED COURSE AND PROGNOSIS
• With surgical treatment, relatively few ferrets will remain euglycemic long-term. Most ferrets will require medical treatment or second surgical debulking within 6 months. In one study the median euglycemic interval was 240 days, with an average survival time of 483 days. If clinical signs return, debulking pancreatic tumors a second time usually

# INSULINOMA

will result in another disease-free interval but generally does not increase survival time as compared to medical treatment.

• With medical treatment alone, clinical signs will be controlled for periods of 6 months to 2 years, depending on the number and type of tumor.

 **MISCELLANEOUS**

## ASSOCIATED CONDITIONS

Ferret adrenal disease and splenomegaly are commonly found in ferrets with insulinomas.

## AGE-RELATED FACTORS

Older ferrets may not benefit from surgery, since mean survival times are relatively equivalent with medical therapy alone in older animals.

## ZOONOTIC POTENTIAL

N/A

## PREGNANCY

N/A

## SYNONYMS

• Insulin-secreting tumor
• Beta-cell tumor

• Hyperinsulinism
• Islet cell tumor
• Islet cell adenocarcinoma
• Insulin-producing pancreatic tumor

## SEE ALSO

Hypoglycemia

## ABBREVIATION

N/A

*Suggested Reading*

Caplan ER, Peterson ME, Mulles HS, et al. Diagnosis and treatment of insulin-secreting pancreatic islet cell tumors in ferrets: 57 cases (1986–1994). J Am Vet Med Assoc 1996;209:1741–1745.

Fox JG, Marini RP. Diseases of the endocrine system. In: Fox JG, ed. Biology and Diseases of the Ferret. 2nd Ed. Baltimore: Williams & Wilkins, 1998.

Ludwig L, Aiken S. Soft tissue surgery. In: Quesenberry KE, Carpenter JW, eds. Ferrets, Rabbits and Rodents: Clinical Medicine and Surgery. St. Louis: WB Saunders, 2004:121–134.

Marini RP, Ryden EB, Rosenblad WD, et al. Functional islet cell tumor in six ferrets. J Am Vet Med Assoc 1993;202:430–433.

Quensenberry KE, Rosenthal KL. Endocrine diseases. In: Quesenberry KE, Carpenter JW, eds. Ferrets, Rabbits and Rodents: Clinical Medicine and Surgery. St. Louis: WB Saunders, 2004:79–90.

Rosenthal KL. Endocrine disorders of ferrets: insulinoma and adrenal gland disease. 21st Annu Waltham/OSU Symp Treat Small Anim Dis Exotics 1997;35–38.

Rosenthal KL. Ferret and rabbit endocrine disease diagnosis. In: Fudge AM, ed. Laboratory Medicine, Avian and Exotic Pets. Philadelphia: WB Saunders, 2000.

Weiss CA, Williams BH, Scott MV. Insulinoma in the ferret: clinical findings and treatment comparison of 66 cases. J Am Anim Hosp Assoc 1998;34:471–475.

Wheeler J, Bennet RA. Ferret abdominal surgical procedures. Part I. Adrenal gland and pancreatic beta-cell tumors. Compend Contin Educ Pract Vet 1999;21(9):815–822.

*Portions Adapted From*

Crystal MA. Insulinoma. In: Tilley LP, Smith FWK, Jr., eds. The 5-Minute Veterinary Consult: Canine and Feline, 2nd Ed. Baltimore: Lippincott Williams & Wilkins, 2002.

# LOWER URINARY TRACT INFECTION

 BASICS

## OVERVIEW
• Result of microbial colonization of the urinary bladder and/or proximal portion of the urethra
• Microbes, usually aerobic bacteria, ascend the urinary tract under conditions that permit them to persist in the urine or adhere to the epithelium and subsequently multiply. Urinary tract colonization requires at least transient impairment of the mechanisms that normally defend against infection. Inflammation of infected tissues results in the clinical signs and laboratory test abnormalities exhibited by patients.

## SYSTEMS AFFECTED
Renal/urologic—lower urinary tract

## INCIDENCE/PREVALENCE
Uncommon in ferrets as compared to cats and dogs

## SIGNALMENT
• More common in female ferrets than in males
• All ages are affected, but occurrence increases with age because of a greater frequency of other urinary lesions (e.g., uroliths, prostate or urogenital cystic disease, and tumors) that predispose to secondary urinary tract infection.

## SIGNS
### Historical Findings
• None in some patients
• Pollakiuria—frequent voiding of small volumes
• Dysuria
• Urinating in places that are not customary
• Hematuria and cloudy or malodorous urine in some patients
• Signs of adrenal disease, especially alopecia in many patients

### Physical Examination Findings
• No abnormalities in some animals
• Acute infection—bladder or urethra may seem tender on palpation.
• Palpation of the bladder may stimulate urination, even in normal ferrets.
• Chronic infection—wall of the bladder or urethra may be palpably thickened or abnormally firm.
• Urogenital cysts palpable in some ferrets with ferret adrenal disease

## CAUSES AND RISK FACTORS
• Most common—*Escherichia*, *Staphylococcus*, and *Proteus* spp.
• Conditions that cause urine stasis or incomplete emptying of the bladder such as urogenital cystic disease or urolithiasis predispose to lower urinary tract infection.

 DIAGNOSIS

## DIFFERENTIAL DIAGNOSIS
• Lower urinary tract infection may mimic other causes of pollakiuria, dysuria, hematuria, and/or outflow obstruction, the most common of which are urogenital cystic disease (paraurethral cysts) and urolithiasis.
• Ferrets with urogenital cysts usually have other signs of adrenal disease, especially bilaterally symmetric alopecia.
• Differentiate from other causes by urinalysis, urine culture, radiography, and ultrasonography.

## CBC/BIOCHEMISTRY/URINALYSIS
• Results of CBC and serum biochemistry normal
• Pyuria (normal value 0–1 WBC/hpf) is most commonly associated with urinary tract infection, but noninfectious urinary lesions can also cause pyuria. Hematuria (normal value 0–3 RBC/hpf) and proteinuria (normal value 0–33 mg/dL) indicate urinary tract inflammation, but these are nonspecific findings that may result from infectious and noninfectious causes of lower urinary tract disease.
• Some urogenital or periprostatic cysts may become secondarily infected, forming abscesses that drain into the urinary bladder or urethra. Thick, purulent exudate from these abscesses may mix with urine in the bladder, resulting in significant pyuria and bacteriuria. In some cases, this exudate can be thick enough to cause urethral blockage.
• Identification of bacteria in urine sediment suggests that urinary tract infection is causing or complicating lower urinary tract disease or may be seen in ferrets with abscessed urogenital cysts. If small numbers of bacteria are seen, consider contamination of urine during collection and storage when interpreting urinalysis results.

## OTHER LABORATORY TESTS
### Urine Culture and Sensitivity Testing
• Urine culture is necessary for definitive diagnosis.
• Correct interpretation of urine culture results requires obtaining the specimen in a manner that minimizes contamination, handling and storing the specimen so that numbers of viable bacteria do not change in vitro, and using a quantitative culture method. Keep the specimen in a sealed sterile container; if the culture is not started right away, the urine can be refrigerated up to 8 hours without an important change in the results.
• Cystocentesis is the preferred technique for obtaining urine for culture. Cystocentesis often must be performed under isoflurane anesthesia.

## IMAGING
Survey and contrast radiographic studies as well as ultrasound of the bladder or urethra may detect an underlying urinary tract lesion (i.e., urogenital cystic disease or urolithiasis).

## DIAGNOSTIC PROCEDURES
N/A

## PATHOLOGIC FINDINGS
N/A

 TREATMENT

## APPROPRIATE HEALTH CARE
Treat as outpatient unless another urinary abnormality (e.g., obstruction) requires inpatient treatment.

## CLIENT EDUCATION
Prognosis for cure of simple urinary tract infection is excellent; prognosis for complicated urinary tract infection depends on the underlying abnormality. Compliance with recommendations for treatment and follow-up evaluations is crucial for optimum results.

## SURGICAL CONSIDERATIONS
Except when a concomitant disorder requires surgical intervention, management does not involve surgery.

 MEDICATIONS

## DRUG(S) OF CHOICE
• Base choice of drug on results of sensitivity test.
• Antibiotics that concentrate in the urine are most appropriate. Initial choices include trimethoprim-sulfadiazine (15–30 mg/kg PO, SC q12h), cephalexin (15–30 mg/kg PO q8–12h), amoxicillin/clavulanate (12.5 mg/kg PO q12h) or enrofloxacin (10–20 mg/kg PO, SC, IM q24h).
• For acute, uncomplicated infection, treat with antimicrobial drugs for at least 2 weeks. Appropriate duration of treatment for complicated lower urinary tract infection depends on the underlying problem.

## PRECAUTIONS
• Because of potential nephrotoxicity with long-term administration, use aminoglycosides only when there are no alternatives.

# LOWER URINARY TRACT INFECTION

## FOLLOW-UP

### PATIENT MONITORING

• When antibacterial drug efficacy is in doubt, culture the urine 2–3 days after starting treatment. If the drug is effective, the culture will be negative.
• Continue treating at least 1 week after resolution of hematuria, pyuria, and proteinuria. Failure of urinalysis findings to return to normal while an episode of urinary tract infection is being treated with an effective antibiotic (i.e., as indicated by negative urine culture) generally indicates some other urinary tract abnormality (e.g., urogenital cysts, urolith, tumor). Rapid recrudescence of signs when treatment is stopped generally indicates either a concurrent urinary tract abnormality or that the infection extends into some deep-seated site (e.g., prostatic or renal parenchyma).
• Successful cure of an episode of urinary tract infection is best demonstrated by performing a urine culture 7–10 days after completing antimicrobial therapy.

### PREVENTION/AVOIDANCE

• Treat underlying adrenal disease in ferrets with urogenital cystic disease.
• Feed high-quality ferret or cat foods to avoid urolithiasis.

### POSSIBLE COMPLICATIONS

Failure to detect or treat effectively may lead to pyelonephritis.

### EXPECTED COURSE AND PROGNOSIS

• If not treated, expect infection to persist indefinitely. Associated health risks include development of extension of infection to other portions of the urinary tract (e.g., the kidneys) or beyond (e.g., septicemia and bacterial endocarditis).
• Generally, the prognosis for animals with uncomplicated lower urinary tract infection is good to excellent. The prognosis for animals with complicated infection is determined by the prognosis for the other urinary abnormality.

## MISCELLANEOUS

### ASSOCIATED CONDITIONS
• Struvite urolithiasis
• Diabetes mellitus
• Ferret adrenal disease

### AGE-RELATED FACTORS
Complicated infection is more common in middle-aged to old than in young animals.

### SYNONYMS
• Bacterial cystitis
• Urethrocystitis
• Urethritis

### SEE ALSO
• Adrenal disease
• Diabetes mellitus
• Dysuria and pollakiuria
• Urogenital cystic disease
• Urolithiasis

### ABBREVIATIONS
• CBC = complete blood count
• RBC = red blood cell
• WBC = white blood cell

*Suggested Reading*

Antinoff N. Urinary disorders in ferrets. Semin Avian Exotic Pet Med 1998;7(2):89–92.

Fox JG, Pearson RC, Bell JA. Diseases of the genitourinary system. In: Fox JG, ed. Biology and Diseases of the Ferret. 2nd Ed. Baltimore: Williams & Wilkins, 1998.

Hoefer HL. Rabbit and ferret renal disease diagnosis. In: Fudge AM, ed. Laboratory Medicine, Avian and Exotic Pets. Philadelphia: WB Saunders, 2000.

Li X, Fox JG, Erdman SE, et al. Cystic urogenital anomalies in ferrets (Mustela putorius furo). Vet Pathol 1996;33:150–158.

Pollock CG. Urogenital diseases. In: Quesenberry KE, Carpenter JW, eds. Ferrets, Rabbits and Rodents: Clinical Medicine and Surgery. St. Louis: WB Saunders, 2004:41–49.

Wheeler J, Bennett RA. Ferret abdominal surgical procedures. Part II. Gastrointestinal foreign bodies, splenomegaly, liver biopsy, cystotomy and ovariohysterectomy. Compend Contin Edu Pract Vet 1999;21(11):1049–1057.

*Portions Adapted From*

Lees GE. Lower Urinary Tract Infection. In: Tilley LP, Smith FWK, Jr., eds. The 5-Minute Veterinary Consult: Canine and Feline, 3rd Ed. Baltimore: Lippincott Williams & Wilkins, 2003.

# LYMPHADENOPATHY (LYMPHADENOMEGALY)

## BASICS

### DEFINITION
Abnormally large lymph nodes, generalized or localized to a single node or group of regional nodes

### PATHOPHYSIOLOGY
• Can result from hyperplasia of lymphoid elements, inflammatory infiltration, or neoplastic proliferation within the lymph node
• Because of their filtration function, lymph nodes often act as sentinels of disease in the tissues they drain; inflammation of any tissue is often accompanied by enlargement of the draining nodes, which most likely results from reactive lymphoid hyperplasia but may also be caused by extension of the inflammatory process into the nodes (lymphadenitis).
• Reactive hyperplasia involves proliferation of lymphocytes and plasma cells in response to antigenic stimulation.
• Lymphadenitis—implies active migration of neutrophils, activated macrophages, or eosinophils into the lymph node
• Neoplastic proliferation may be either primary (malignant lymphoma) or metastatic. Malignant lymphoma is the most common cause of lymphadenomegaly in ferrets.

### SYSTEMS AFFECTED
Hemic/lymph/immune

### SIGNALMENT
No breed, sex, or age predilection

### SIGNS
• Peripheral lymphadenomegaly or mild enlargement of mediastinal or mesenteric nodes typically do not directly cause clinical signs.
• Severe—may cause mechanical obstruction and interference with the function of adjacent organs, signs of which depend on the affected lymph node and may include dysphagia, regurgitation, respiratory distress, dyschezia, and limb swelling
• May be systemically ill from the underlying disease process

### CAUSES

#### Neoplasia
• Lymphoma—most common cause of lymphadenomegaly
• Metastatic neoplasia

#### Lymphoid Hyperplasia
• Localized or systemic infection caused by infectious agents of all categories (i.e., bacteria, viruses, and protozoa) when infection does not directly involve the node—most common cause of mesenteric lymphadenomegaly
• ADV infection—generalized hyperplasia
• Antigenic stimulation by factors other than infectious agents (e.g., inflammatory bowel disease)

#### Lymphadenitis
• Bacteria—capable of causing purulent lymphadenitis, which may progress to abscessation; a few (e.g., *Mycobacterium* spp.) induce granulomatous lymphadenitis (unusual in ferrets).
• Fungi—systemic infections from blastomycosis, cryptococcosis, and histoplasmosis (unusual)
• Eosinophilic—may be associated with allergic inflammation of the organ being drained by the affected lymph node; may be encountered in a patient with gastrointestinal eosinophilic disease or in a lymph node draining a mast cell tumor

### RISK FACTORS
• Malignant lymphoma—possibly close association with other ferrets with lymphoma
• Lymphadenomegaly caused by metastatic neoplasms—varies with the type of primary neoplasm
• Impaired immune function predisposes to infection and, therefore, to lymphadenitis.

## DIAGNOSIS

### DIFFERENTIAL DIAGNOSIS
• For peripheral lymphadenomegaly—subcutaneous fat can surround the peripheral lymph nodes and have a firm consistency, mimicking lymphadenomegaly. This is extremely common in obese ferrets. Fine needle aspiration is often nondiagnostic, since the node is hidden deep within the fat deposits; a lymph node biopsy is usually necessary to differentiate lymphoma from normal node surrounded by fat deposits.
• For mesenteric lymphadenomegaly—reactive nodes due to chronic gastrointestinal inflammatory or infiltrative disease such as *Helicobacter mustelae* gastritis, lymphoplasmacytic gastroenteritis, eosinophilic gastroenteritis, or ECE. Hyperplastic lymph nodes can resemble lymphosarcoma on both gross and histologic examination and may be difficult to distinguish. If the mesenteric lymph nodes are the only area of lymphocyte proliferation observed, hyperplasia is more likely than neoplasia.
• Palpable lymph nodes in normal ferrets—mandibular, prescapular, axillary, superficial inguinal, and popliteal nodes
• Severe lymph node enlargement—most likely to develop in patients with lymphoma
• Lesser degrees of enlargement—attributable to reactive hyperplasia, lymphadenitis, or neoplasia
• Extent of enlargement in patients with metastatic disease varies widely.
• Multiple lymph nodes affected throughout the body—likely the result of lymphoma or systemic infection that causes either lymphadenitis or lymphoid hyperplasia

• Abscessation and metastatic neoplasms usually affect a single lymph node.

### CBC/BIOCHEMISTRY/URINALYSIS
• Cytopenias—seen with lymphoma, anemia of chronic disease, stress, splenic disease, or neoplastic infiltration of the bone marrow; also seen with viral disease
• Lymphocytosis—may suggest lymphoid neoplasia; atypical lymphocytes in the blood help establish a diagnosis of lymphoid neoplasia.
• Eosinophilia—may occur in animals with lymphadenopathy owing to eosinophilic gastroenteritis; relation to parasitic disease has not been established.
• Neutrophilia, with or without a left shift—may develop in patients with lymphoid hyperplasia or neoplasia
• Hyperglobulinemia—may develop in patients with ADV, chronic inflammatory disease, or lymphoid neoplasia

### OTHER LABORATORY TESTS
N/A

### IMAGING
• Radiography and ultrasonography—involvement of lymph nodes within the body cavity
• Lesions associated with lymph node enlargement may be detected in other organs (e.g., pneumonia, gastroenteritis, or primary tumor in animals with lymphadenomegaly caused by metastatic neoplasia).

### DIAGNOSTIC PROCEDURES

#### Cytologic Examination
• Aspirates from affected lymph nodes may help determine the major category of lymphadenomegaly (i.e., hyperplasia, inflammation, or neoplasia). Successful fine needle aspiration of peripheral nodes is more difficult to perform in ferrets—the nodes are frequently surrounded by firm fat deposits.
• It is often difficult to distinguish severe lymphoid hyperplasia from malignant lymphoma based on fine needle aspirate alone; thus, a biopsy is usually necessary for diagnosis.
• Lymphoid hyperplasia and lymphoma may be difficult to distinguish on gross or histologic examination. If the peripheral or mesenteric lymph nodes are the only area of lymphocyte proliferation observed and the ferret is otherwise asymptomatic, sampling of more than one node and submitting to a pathology lab familiar with ferrets may be needed for an accurate diagnosis.
• Rarely, aspirates from lymph nodes affected by lymphadenitis contain high proportions of neutrophils, macrophages, and/or eosinophils, depending on the cause of the inflammation; specific infectious agents, such as bacteria and systemic fungi, may be evident.

# LYMPHADENOPATHY (LYMPHADENOMEGALY)

• Aspirates from lymph nodes containing metastatic neoplasia contain populations of cells that are not seen in normal nodes; the appearance of such cells varies widely, depending on the type of neoplasm.

## Other

• Since a diagnosis often cannot be made by cytologic examination, excisional biopsy is preferable to needle biopsy.
• The cytologic diagnosis of lymphoma should be confirmed by histopathologic examination of an excised lymph node, and sampling of more than one node may be needed for accurate diagnosis.

## TREATMENT

• Because of the many disease processes and specific agents that can cause lymphadenomegaly, treatment depends on establishing the underlying cause.
• In animals with lymphoma, treatment includes combination chemotherapy or corticosteroids alone.

## MEDICATIONS

### DRUG(S) OF CHOICE

Appropriate medications vary with the cause of lymph node enlargement.

### CONTRAINDICATIONS

N/A

### PRECAUTIONS

N/A

### POSSIBLE INTERACTIONS

N/A

### ALTERNATIVE DRUGS

N/A

## FOLLOW-UP

### PATIENT MONITORING

Lymph node size to assess efficacy of treatment

### POSSIBLE COMPLICATIONS

N/A

## MISCELLANEOUS

### ASSOCIATED CONDITIONS

• Lymph node hyperplasia is often a component or manifestation of systemic disease.
• Lymphoma may involve other organs (e.g., liver, spleen, intestines, kidneys, and skin) with a variety of clinical consequences.
• Many middle-aged to older ferrets with lymphoma have concurrent insulinoma or ferret adrenal disease.

### AGE-RELATED FACTORS

None

### ZOONOTIC POTENTIAL

Caution should be exercised when performing fine needle aspiration in animals that may have systemic fungal disease.

### PREGNANCY

N/A

### SEE ALSO

• Epizootic catarrhal enteritis
• *Helicobacter mustelae*
• Inflammatory bowel disease
• Lymphosarcoma

### ABBREVIATIONS

• ADV = Aleutian disease virus
• ECE = epizootic catarrhal enteritis

*Suggested Reading*

Fox JG. Diseases of the gastrointestinal system. In: Fox JG, ed. Biology and Diseases of the Ferret. 2nd Ed. Baltimore: Williams & Wilkins, 1998:273–290.

Fox JG, Marini RP. Helicobacter mustelae infection in ferrets: pathogenesis, epizootiology, diagnosis and treatment. Semin Avin Exotic Pet Med 2001;10(1):36–44.

Williams BH, Weiss CA. Neoplasia. In: Quesenberry KE, Carpenter JW, eds. Ferrets, Rabbits and Rodents: Clinical Medicine and Surgery. St. Louis: WB Saunders, 2004:91–106.

Li X, Fox JG. Neoplastic diseases. In: Fox JG, ed. Biology and Diseases of the Ferret. 2nd Ed. Baltimore: Williams & Wilkins, 1998:405–448.

*Portions Adapted From*

Rassnick, KH. Lymphadenomegaly. In: Tilley LP, Smith FWK, Jr., eds. The 5-Minute Veterinary Consult: Canine and Feline, 3rd Ed. Baltimore: Lippincott Williams & Wilkins, 2003.

# LYMPHOPLASMACYTIC ENTERITIS AND GASTROENTERITIS

## BASICS

### OVERVIEW
• A form of inflammatory bowel disease characterized by lymphocyte and/or plasma cell infiltration into the lamina propria of the stomach, intestine, or both
• Lymphocytic infiltration into the lamina propria of the intestines is a common inflammatory response to many infectious agents or environmental stimuli. Lymphocytic infiltration into the lamina propria of the stomach is abnormal and usually indicates significant disease.
• Plasmacytic infiltration indicates chronicity or a more severe inflammatory reaction.
• An abnormal immune response to infectious agents or environmental stimuli may be responsible for initiating gastrointestinal inflammation. Continued exposure to antigen, coupled with self-perpetuating inflammation, may result in disease.
• The exact mechanisms, antigens, and patient factors involved in initiation and progression remain unknown.

### SIGNALMENT
No sex or age predilection

### SIGNS
• Anorexia
• Weight loss, muscle wasting
• Diarrhea, sometimes with blood or mucous
• Melena
• Vomiting
• Ptyalism, pawing at the mouth
• Physical examination—cachexia; thickened, ropy intestines, enlarged mesenteric lymph nodes, and splenomegaly often palpable

### CAUSES AND RISK FACTORS
• Pathogenesis is most likely multifactorial.
• Gastric lesions are often associated with *Helicobacter mustelae*.
• Intestinal lesions may be associated with epizootic catarrhal enteritis (ECE), *Giardia*, *Salmonella*, *Campylobacter*, cryptosporidiosis, ADV, or other infectious agents.
• Meat proteins, food additives, artificial coloring, preservatives, and milk proteins may play a role.

## DIAGNOSIS

### DIFFERENTIAL DIAGNOSIS
• Intestinal lymphosarcoma
• Infectious diseases (e.g., *H. mustelae*, ECE, ADV, giardiasis, salmonellosis, *Campylobacter enteritis*, cryptosporidiosis, mycobacteriosis)
• Gastrointestinal foreign body

• Other infiltrative inflammatory bowel conditions (e.g., eosinophilic gastroenteritis)

### CBC/BIOCHEMISTRY/URINALYSIS
• May be normal
• Nonregenerative anemia and mild leukocytosis without a left shift sometimes seen
• Hypoproteinemia from protein-losing enteropathy

### OTHER LABORATORY TESTS
• Fecal direct examination, fecal flotation, and zinc sulfate centrifugation many demonstrate gastrointestinal parasites.
• Fecal cytology—may reveal RBC or fecal leukocytes, which can be associated with inflammatory bowel disease or invasive bacterial strains
• Fecal culture should be performed if abnormal bacteria are observed on the fecal Gram's stain, or if *Salmonella* is suspected.

### IMAGING
• Survey abdominal radiographs—usually normal
• Barium contrast studies—rarely reveal mucosal abnormalities or thickened bowel loops; generally not helpful in establishing a definitive diagnosis; can be normal even in individuals with severe disease

### DIAGNOSTIC PROCEDURES
• Definitive diagnosis requires biopsy and histopathology, usually obtained via exploratory laparotomy.
• Intestinal fluid can also be submitted for quantitative culture if bacterial overgrowth is suspected.
• Lymph node biopsy is indicated on enlarged mesenteric nodes.

### PATHOLOGIC FINDINGS
• Grossly, stomach and intestinal appearance can range from normal to edematous, thickened, and ulcerated.
• The hallmark histopathologic finding is an infiltrate of lymphocytes and, in some cases, plasma cells in the lamina propria.
• The distribution may be patchy, so take several biopsy specimens.

## TREATMENT

### APPROPRIATE HEALTH CARE
Outpatient, unless the patient is debilitated from dehydration, hypoproteinemia, or cachexia
• Patients that are dehydrated or emaciated and those with protein-losing enteropathies or other concurrent illnesses may require hospitalization until they are stabilized.

### NURSING CARE
If the patient is dehydrated or must be NPO because of vomiting, any balanced fluid such as lactated Ringer's solution is adequate (for a patient without other concur-

rent disease); otherwise, select fluids on the basis of secondary diseases.

### ACTIVITY
No need to restrict unless severely debilitated

### DIET
• Highly digestible diets with novel protein sources may be useful for eliciting remission, although an allergic cause has not be documented and little information is available regarding the efficacy of these diets. If attempted, choose feline diets since ferrets have high nutritional protein and fat requirements. Foods that have been anecdotally reported to elicit remission include feline lamb and rice diets, diets consisting exclusively of one type of meat (lamb, duck, turkey), or a "natural prey diet" consisting of whole rodents. If remission is elicited, continue diet for at least 8–13 weeks; this diet may need to be fed lifelong.
• Anorectic ferrets may refuse dry foods but are often willing to eat canned cat foods or pureed meats.

### CLIENT EDUCATION
Explain the difficulty in finding an underlying cause and therefore successful treatment. There is a potential for long-term therapy.

### SURGICAL CONSIDERATIONS
N/A

## MEDICATIONS

### DRUG(S) OF CHOICE
• Treat the underlying cause (eg., *Helicobacter*, *Salmonella*, *Giardia*, etc.) if found.
• If gastric lesions are present, empirical treatment for *Helicobacter* is indicated. The combination of amoxicillin (10 mg/kg PO q12h) plus metronidazole (20 mg/kg PO q12h) and bismuth subsalicylate (17 mg/kg PO q12h or 1 mL/kg of regular strength preparation [262 mg/15 mL] PO q12h) is an inexpensive treatment regimen that is usually effective. Treat for at least 2 weeks and up to 3–4 weeks. Alternatively, clarithromycin (12.5 mg/kg PO q8h or divided q12h) and ranitidine bismuth citrate (this is not Zantac, ranitidine HCl) at 24 mg/kg PO q8h for 2 weeks have also been effective.
• Prednisone (1.25–2.5 mg/kg PO q24h); when signs resolve, gradually taper the corticosteroid dose to 0.5–1.25 mg/kg every other day.
• Metronidazole (15–20mg/kg PO q12h × 2 weeks)—has antibacterial and antiprotozoal properties; some evidence that it also has immune-modulating effects

### CONTRAINDICATIONS
N/A

# LYMPHOPLASMACYTIC ENTERITIS AND GASTROENTERITIS

## PRECAUTIONS
• In ferrets with concurrent infectious diseases, use corticosteroids with caution.
• Metronidazole—can cause reversible neurotoxicity at high dosages; discontinuing the drug usually reverses the neurologic signs. Ferrets generally object to the taste.

## POSSIBLE INTERACTIONS
N/A

## ALTERNATIVE DRUGS
Other immunosuppressive drugs such as Azathioprine (Imuran, GalaxoSmithKline) 0.9mg/kg PO q24–72 hours has been anecdotally used to treat lymphoplasmacytic gastroenteritis with some success. Has not been used extensively in ferrets; efficacy and safety has not been evaluated.

## FOLLOW-UP

### PATIENT MONITORING
• For resolution of clinical signs
• Severely affected patients require frequent monitoring; adjust medications during these visits.
• Check patients with less severe disease 2–3 weeks after their initial evaluation and then monthly to bimonthly until immunosuppressive therapy is discontinued.

### PREVENTION/AVOIDANCE
If a food intolerance or allergy is suspected or documented, avoid that particular item and adhere strictly to dietary changes.

### POSSIBLE COMPLICATIONS
• Weight loss, debilitation, and death in refractory cases
• Adverse effects of prednisone therapy

## EXPECTED COURSE AND PROGNOSIS
• Variable, depending on the underlying cause
• Ferrets with mild inflammation—good to excellent prognosis for full recovery
• Patients with severe infiltrates, particularly if other portions of the gastrointestinal tract are involved or if an underlying cause cannot be found—more guarded prognosis
• Often the initial response to therapy sets the tone for a given individual's ability to recover.

## MISCELLANEOUS

### ASSOCIATED CONDITIONS
Many affected ferrets also have splenomegaly (nonspecific in aged ferrets).

### AGE-RELATED FACTORS
N/A

### ZOONOTIC POTENTIAL
*Giardia* and cryptosporidiosis have zoonotic potential.

### PREGNANCY
• Corticosteroids have been associated with increased incidence of congenital defects, abortion, and fetal death.
• Metronidazole is mutagenic in laboratory animals; avoid.

### SYNONYMS
N/A

## SEE ALSO
• Eosinophilic, gastroenteritis
• Epizootic catarrhal enteritis
• Gastrointestinal foreign bodies
• *H. mustelae*
• Parvovirus Infection (Aleutian disease virus)

## ABBREVIATIONS
• ADV = Aleutian disease virus
• ECE = epizootic catarrhal enteritis
• NPO = nothing by mouth
• RBC = red blood cell

*Suggested Reading*

Bell JA. Gastrointestinal diseases. In: Quesenberry KE, Carpenter JW, eds. Ferrets, Rabbits and Rodents: Clinical Medicine and Surgery. St. Louis: WB Saunders, 2004:25–40.

Finkler MR. Ferret colitis. In: Kirk RW, Bonagura JD, eds. Kirk's Current Veterinary Therapy XI: Small Animal Practice. Philadelphia: WB Saunders, 1992.

Fox JG. Diseases of the gastrointestinal system. In: Fox JG, ed. Biology and Diseases of the Ferret. 2nd Ed. Baltimore: Williams & Wilkins, 1998.

Fox JG. Parasitic diseases. In: Fox JG, ed. Biology and Diseases of the Ferret. 2nd Ed. Baltimore: Williams & Wilkins, 1998:375–392.

Jenkins JR. Rabbit and ferret liver and gastrointestinal testing. In: Fudge AM, ed. Laboratory Medicine, Avian and Exotic Pets. Philadelphia: WB Saunders, 2000.

Marini RP, Fox JG, Taylor NS, et al. Ranitidine bismuth citrate and clarithromycin, alone or in combination, for eradication of *Helicobacter mustelae* infection in ferrets. Am J Vet Res 1999:60(10):1280–6.

# BASICS

## DEFINITION
Proliferation of neoplastic lymphocytes in solid tissues, primarily in lymph nodes, bone marrow, and visceral organs

## PATHOPHYSIOLOGY
• Lymphocytic or lymphoblastic lymphoma is seen most commonly in ferrets.
• Less often, a polymorphic lymphoma resembling lymphoma associated with a viral etiology in other species is seen. A retroviral etiology has been proposed but not conclusively demonstrated in ferret lymphosarcoma. Clusters of disease seen in cohabiting ferrets are suggestive of a viral etiology.
• Gastric lymphosarcoma has been associated with chronic *Helicobacter mustelae* gastritis; a causative effect has not been established.
• T lymphocyte lymphosarcoma can be seen in epitheliotropic (cutaneous), periorbital, or mediastinal lymphoma.

## SYSTEMS AFFECTED
• Hemic/lymphatic/immune—generalized, often peripheral, lymphadenomegaly with or without splenic, hepatic, and/or bone marrow involvement and circulating malignant lymphocytes
• Gastrointestinal—infiltration of stomach, intestines, and associated lymph nodes
• Respiratory—proliferation of neoplastic lymphocytes in mediastinal lymph nodes, thymus, or, less commonly, the lungs
• Miscellaneous (extranodal)—proliferation of or invasion by neoplastic lymphocytes in the bone marrow and ocular, cutaneous, mucocutaneous, neural, renal, cardiac, and other tissues

## GENETICS
No documentation of genetic basis

## INCIDENCE/PREVALENCE
Although the exact incidence is not well documented, it is one of the most common diseases seen in pet ferrets; third most common neoplasm (following insulinoma and adrenal neoplasia).

## GEOGRAPHIC DISTRIBUTION
N/A

## SIGNALMENT

### Mean Age and Range
• Most common in ferrets 2–5 years of age
• Ferrets 1 year of age or younger often have only mediastinal involvement.
• Young ferrets (<2 years of age) tend to have a high-grade, rapidly progressing lymphoblastic lymphoma—visceral involvement, especially of the mediastinal nodes, thymus, spleen, and liver is most common.
• Middle-aged ferrets (4–7 years) commonly have multicentric lymphoma.

• Older ferrets may have either high- or low-grade lymphocytic lymphoma—lymphadenomegaly is the predominant early sign, with organ or bone marrow involvement usually occurring later in the course of disease.

### Predominant Sex
None

## SIGNS

### General Comments
Depend on anatomic form and stage of disease

### Historical Findings
• All forms of malignant lymphoma—nonspecific, anorexia, lethargy, weight loss—occurrence of clinical signs may be cyclical.
• Middle-aged ferrets may be asymptomatic (sometimes for years) or have nonspecific signs that wax and wane.
• Multicentric—possibly no signs in early stages; generalized, painless lymphadenomegaly most common; may note distended abdomen secondary to hepatomegaly, splenomegaly, or ascites; anorexia, weight loss, and depression with progression of disease
• Gastrointestinal—anorexia, weight loss, lethargy, vomiting, diarrhea, abdominal discomfort, melena, tenesmus with mesenteric lymphadenomegaly
• Mediastinal—seen most often in younger ferrets—anorexia; weight loss; drooling; labored breathing; regurgitation; exercise intolerance secondary to mass(es) and/or effusion; coughing; difficulty swallowing
• Cutaneous—solitary or multiple masses; cutaneous epitheliotropic lymphoma (mycosis fungoides) may be pruritic with dermal thickening and crusting or ulcerated.
• Solitary form—depends on location; splenic form: abdominal distention, discomfort; periorbital lymphosarcoma: facial deformity, protrusion of the globe; spinal cord lymphosarcoma: quickly progressing posterior paresis may be seen; kidney: signs of renal failure

### Physical Examination Findings
• Multicentric—generalized, painless, irregular, movable, large lymph node(s) with or without hepatosplenomegaly
• Gastrointestinal—marked weight loss, possibly palpable abdominal mass or thickened gut loops
• Mediastinal—noncompressible cranial thorax; dyspnea—often induced by physical examination; tachypnea; muffled heart sounds secondary to pleural effusion
• Extranodal—splenic: splenomegaly due to extramedullary hematopoiesis (EMH) or splenic lymphoma; cutaneous: raised plaques, thickened, crusted dermis; neural: dementia, seizures, and paralysis; renal:

renomegaly and renal failure; cardiac: arrhythmias

## CAUSES
No cause proven—a viral etiology has been proposed.

## RISK FACTORS
Possible exposure to other ferrets with lymphosarcoma within the household possible risk factor

# DIAGNOSIS

## DIFFERENTIAL DIAGNOSIS
• For peripheral lymphadenomegaly—subcutaneous fat can surround the peripheral lymph nodes and have a firm consistency mimicking lymphadenomegaly. This is very common in obese ferrets. Fine needle aspiration is often nondiagnostic, since the node is hidden deep within the fat deposits; a lymph node biopsy is usually necessary to differentiate lymphoma from normal node surrounded by fat deposits.
• For mesenteric lymphadenomegaly—reactive nodes due to chronic gastrointestinal inflammatory or infiltrative disease such as *H. mustelae* gastritis, lymphoplasmacytic gastroenteritis, eosinophilic gastroenteritis, or ECE. Hyperplastic lymph nodes can resemble lymphosarcoma on both gross and histologic examination and may be difficult to distinguish. If the mesenteric lymph nodes are the only area of lymphocyte proliferation observed, hyperplasia is more likely than neoplasia.
• For mediastinal form—congestive heart failure, chylothorax, hemothorax
• Alimentary form—foreign body ingestion, intestinal ulceration, ECE, inflammatory bowel disease, intussusception, other gastrointestinal tumor
• Cutaneous form—mast cell tumor, other cutaneous neoplasm, chronic inflammatory disease

## CBC/BIOCHEMISTRY/URINALYSIS
• Anemia (PCV <45%) is common and may be severe in ferrets with leukemia.
• Both lymphocytosis and lymphopenia are commonly reported in ferrets with lymphoma.
• Lymphocytosis is a common finding, especially in young ferrets—lymphocyte counts of >3,500 cells/mm$^3$ or relative lymphocyte counts of >60% are suggestive of lymphoma; lymphoblastic leukemia (atypic lymphocytes with normal or low total lymphocyte numbers) is more common in young ferrets.
• Lymphopenia is often seen in older ferrets.
• Neutropenia and thrombocytopenia occasionally seen
• High ALT or ALP activity common
• Urinalysis usually normal

# LYMPHOSARCOMA

### OTHER LABORATORY TESTS
N/A

### IMAGING
• Thoracic radiography—may reveal sternal or tracheobronchial lymphadenomegaly, widened mediastinum, and pleural effusion
• Abdominal radiography—may reveal sublumbar or mesenteric lymphadenomegaly, intestinal mass, abdominal effusions, or hepatomegaly; splenomegaly is common due to EMH or splenic lymphoma.
• Ultrasonography—often necessary to detect lymphadenomegaly (or nodules in visceral organs)

### DIAGNOSTIC PROCEDURES
• Examine bone marrow aspirate when non-regenerative anemia, other cytopenia, or abnormal circulating lymphocytes are observed, and to assess prognosis associated with chemotherapy. Anecdotal reports suggest that if >50% of bone marrow sample contains malignant lymphocytes, patient is poor candidate for chemotherapy.
• Lymph node biopsy—may be diagnostic when peripheral lymphadenomegaly is present. The popliteal lymph nodes are most readily accessible. Hyperplastic lymph nodes can resemble lymphosarcoma on both gross and histologic examination and may be difficult to distinguish. If the peripheral lymph nodes are the only area of lymphocyte proliferation observed and the ferret is otherwise asymptomatic, sampling of more than one node and submitting to a pathology lab familiar with ferrets may be needed for an accurate diagnosis.
• FNA of mediastinal or mesenteric lymph nodes may be performed using ultrasound guidance. However, it is often difficult to differentiate hyperplasia from lymphoma based on an aspirate alone; exploratory laparotomy may be necessary for definitive diagnosis.

### PATHOLOGIC FINDINGS
• Cut section—homogenous, white masses, sometimes with areas of necrosis
• Monomorphic or polymorphic population of discrete round neoplastic cells that efface and replace parenchyma of lymph nodes and visceral organs or bone marrow

# TREATMENT

### GENERAL COMMENTS
• Many ferrets with lymphoma are asymptomatic, and the diagnosis is often incidental. It can be difficult to predict whether treatment is warranted in these cases. Many ferrets will remain asymptomatic for years with no treatment at all. In others, signs of disease may be cyclic and may wane with or without treatment, making evaluation of treatment success difficult.
• Treatment is indicated in young ferrets with aggressive lymphosarcoma or in middle-aged to older ferrets with clinical signs attributable to lymphoma.
• Older, debilitated ferrets are more likely to develop deleterious side effects to chemotherapy.

### APPROPRIATE HEALTH CARE
• Inpatient—intravenous chemotherapy and for debilitated, anorectic, or dehydrated patients
• Outpatient—after remission, some protocols allow owner to administer drugs orally at home; instruct owner to wear latex gloves when administering these drugs.

### NURSING CARE
• Fluid therapy—for animals with advanced disease and dehydrated patients
• Thoracocentesis or abdominocentesis—recommended with marked pleural or abdominal effusion

### ACTIVITY
Restrict in patients with low WBC or platelet count.

### DIET
N/A

### CLIENT EDUCATION
• Warn client that chemotherapy is rarely curative and relapse often occurs.
• Inform client that the side effects of chemotherapy drugs depend on the type used but are usually associated with the gastrointestinal tract and bone marrow.
• Note that the quality of life is good while the patient is receiving chemotherapy and while it is in remission; add that some protocols are associated with serious morbidity, whereas others have little morbidity.

### SURGICAL CONSIDERATIONS
• To relieve intestinal obstructions and remove solitary masses
• To obtain specimens for histopathologic examination

# MEDICATIONS

### DRUG(S) OF CHOICE
• Combination chemotherapy—many protocols exist with similar remission and survival times. Most are based on feline protocols. Ideally an oncologist should be consulted for recommendations. One protocol that has been used successfully by many practitioners, published in Quesenberry KE, Carpenter JW, eds. *Ferrets, Rabbits and Rodents: Clinical Medicine and Surgery* (see suggested reading), is a combination of prednisone, vincristine, and cyclophosphamide. Asparaginase can be added to this protocol if the patient has peripheral lymphadenopathy.
• Single-agent therapy (doxorubicin) or treatment with doxorubicin and prednisone has also been used as the sole protocol or as a rescue therapy.
• Corticosteroids alone—(prednisone 1 mg/kg PO q12h) is often effective in the short term (1–2 months). Do not begin treatment with prednisone alone if the owner is willing to undertake combination therapy; the response to combination therapy will be significantly diminished.
• Administer IV chemotherapeutic agents using an indwelling catheter under isoflurane anesthesia; alternatively, use a vascular access port or Broviac catheter placed in the jugular vein.
• Retinoids (isotretinoin 2 mg/kg PO q24h) have been used as a palliative treatment in ferrets with cutaneous epitheliotropic lymphoma with some success.

### CONTRAINDICATIONS
N/A

### PRECAUTIONS
• Use extreme caution when handling chemotherapeutic agents.
• Doxorubicin—use cautiously or not at all with poor cardiac contractility or arrhythmias; use cautiously in patients with > 50% of bone marrow replaced by cancer cells.
• L-asparaginase or doxorubicin—pretreat with diphenhydramine (0.5–2.0 mg/kg IM) 20 minutes before administration.

### POSSIBLE INTERACTIONS
All chemotherapy drugs must be given according to published protocols, because many have overlapping side effects.

### ALTERNATIVE DRUGS
Many alternative treatment protocols exist; consultation with an oncologist is recommended.

# FOLLOW-UP

### PATIENT MONITORING
• Signs of toxicity in ferrets receiving chemotherapy for lymphoma include anorexia, lethargy, weakness, vomiting, and hair loss.
• CBC and platelet count—24 hours prior to administration of cytotoxic agents; if severe leukopenia or neutropenia (WBC <1,500 cells/mm³; PCV <30%) is noted, discontinue therapy.
• Physical examination and cytologic or histologic evaluation on all nonresponsive lymph nodes

### PREVENTION/AVOIDANCE
N/A

### POSSIBLE COMPLICATIONS
• Leukopenia and neutropenia
• Vomiting and diarrhea
• Anorexia

- Cardiotoxicity—owing to doxorubicin
- Alopecia
- Sepsis
- Tissue sloughing—with extravasated dose

### EXPECTED COURSE AND PROGNOSIS

- Ferrets with mediastinal, splenic, cutaneous lymphoma or those with peripheral node involvement alone tend to respond well to chemotherapy. Many ferrets will live up to 2–3 years.
- Ferrets with polymorphic lymphoma respond poorly to chemotherapy, often present moribund, and do not survive long.
- Primary CNS, diffuse gastrointestinal, and multiorgan involvement—associated with poor response to treatment

 **MISCELLANEOUS**

### ASSOCIATED CONDITIONS

Insulinoma and adrenal disease are commonly found in ferrets with lymphoma.

### AGE-RELATED FACTORS

See above.

### ZOONOTIC POTENTIAL

None

### PREGNANCY

Treatment of pregnant ferrets is contraindicated.

### SYNONYMS

- Lymphoma
- Malignant lymphoma

### ABBREVIATIONS

- ALP = alkaline phosphatase
- ALT = alanine aminotransferase
- CBC = complete blood count
- CNS = central nervous system
- ECE = epizootic catarrhal enteritis
- EMH = extramedullary hematopoiesis
- PCV = packed cell volume
- WBC = white blood cell

*Suggested Reading*

Hutson CA, Kopit M, Walder E. Combination doxorubicin and orthovoltage radiation therapy, singe agent doxorubicin and high dose vincristine for salvage therapy of ferret lymphosarcoma. J Am Anim Hosp Assoc 1992:192:28:365–368.

Rassnick KM, Gould WJ, Flander JA. Use of a vascular access system for administration of chemotherapeutic agents to a ferret with lymphoma. J Am Vet Med Assoc 1995;206:500–504.

Rosenbaum MR, Affolter VK, Usborne AL, et al. Cutaneous epitheliotropic lymphoma in a ferret. J Am Vet Med Assoc 1995;209:1441–1444.

Williams BH, Weiss CA. Neoplasia. In: Quesenberry KE, Carpenter JW, eds. Ferrets, Rabbits and Rodents: Clinical Medicine and Surgery. St. Louis: WB Saunders, 2004:91–106.

Li X, Fox JG. Neoplastic diseases. In: Fox JG, ed. Biology and Diseases of the Ferret. 2nd Ed. Baltimore: Williams & Wilkins, 1998:405–448.

*Portions Adapted From*

Vonderharr MA. Lymphosarcoma—Dogs. In: Tilley LP, Smith FWK, Jr., eds. The 5-Minute Veterinary Consult: Canine and Feline, 2nd Ed. Baltimore: Lippincott Williams & Wilkins, 2000.

# MAST CELL TUMOR

## BASICS

### OVERVIEW
• Neoplasia arising from mast cells
• Histamine and other vasoactive substances released from mast cell tumors—may cause erythema and edema
• Mast cell tumors in ferrets are usually benign and do not metastasize.

### SIGNALMENT
• The most common skin tumor in ferrets
• Mean age reported as 4 years

### SIGNS

#### Historical Findings
• Patient may have had skin tumor for days to months at the time of examination.
• The tumor may have appeared to fluctuate in size or appearance; may have appeared to disappear completely only to recur
• Some tumors are extremely pruritic.
• Anorexia and vomiting, as seen in dogs with splenic or gastrointestinal tumors, have not been reported in ferrets. However, splenic mast cell tumors can be seen in ferrets, and gastrointestinal signs should be anticipated in affected animals.

#### Physical Examination Findings
• Cutaneous—primarily found in the subcutaneous tissue or dermis; may be papular or nodular, solitary or multiple, and hairy or alopecic or have an ulcerated surface; slight predilection for the head and neck regions
• Tumors may appear to rupture and become covered with a dry, black exudate.
• Alopecia and crusting associated with pruritic masses
• Splenic—splenomegaly is only reported finding

### CAUSES AND RISK FACTORS
Unknown

## DIAGNOSIS

### DIFFERENTIAL DIAGNOSIS
• Any other skin tumor, benign or malignant
• Insect bite or allergic reaction
• Splenic—benign splenomegaly due to extramedullary hematopoiesis; splenic lymphoma

### CBC/BIOCHEMISTRY/URINALYSIS
Usually normal; anemia and mastocythemia seen in other mammals not reported in ferrets

### OTHER LABORATORY TESTS
N/A

### IMAGING
Abdominal radiography—may reveal splenomegaly in animals with rare splenic tumors

### Diagnostic Procedures
• Cytologic examination of fine needle aspirate—most important preliminary diagnostic test; reveals round cells with basophilic cytoplasmic granules that do not form sheets or clumps
• Tissue biopsy—necessary for definitive diagnosis

### PATHOLOGIC FINDINGS
Histopathologic examination—consists of well-differentiated mast cells

## TREATMENT

### APPROPRIATE HEALTH CARE
• Surgery—to excise cutaneous tumor; aggressive surgical excision with wide margins is not necessary since these tumors rarely metastasize or recur.
• Surgical excision is the only effective method for treating pruritic tumors.
• Splenectomy or partial splenectomy—may be necessary for splenic tumor

### NURSING CARE
N/A

### ACTIVITY
N/A

### DIET
N/A

### CLIENT EDUCATION
• Warn client that patient may develop new mast cell tumors.
• Advise client that fine needle aspiration and cytologic examination should be performed as soon as possible on any new mass.

### SURGICAL CONSIDERATIONS
• Complete surgical excision
• Submit excised mass for histologic examination to confirm diagnosis.

## MEDICATIONS

### DRUG(S) OF CHOICE
• Chemotherapy generally unnecessary; if rare case of metastatic mast cell tumor is encountered, consider feline protocols.
• Presurgical treatment with antihistamines usually unnecessary

### CONTRAINDICATIONS
N/A

### PRECAUTIONS
N/A

### POSSIBLE INTERACTIONS
N/A

### ALTERNATIVE DRUGS
N/A

## FOLLOW-UP

### PATIENT MONITORING
Evaluate any new masses cytologically or histologically

### PREVENTION/AVOIDANCE
N/A

### POSSIBLE COMPLICATIONS
• Bleeding
• Appearance of new masses

### EXPECTED COURSE AND PROGNOSIS
• Cutaneous tumors—prognosis excellent; metastasis not reported, but may occur
• Splenic tumor—survival rates not reported

## MISCELLANEOUS

### ASSOCIATED CONDITIONS
N/A

### AGE-RELATED FACTORS
N/A

### ZOONOTIC POTENTIAL
N/A

### PREGNANCY
N/A

### SEE ALSO
• Adrenal disease
• Canine distemper virus
• Dermatophytosis
• Ear mites
• Fleas

### Suggested Reading
Brown SA. Neoplasia. In: Hillyer EV, Quesenberry KE, eds. Ferrets, Rabbits and Rodents: Clinical Medicine and Surgery. Philadelphia: WB Saunders, 1997:99.

Kelleher SA. Skin diseases of the ferret. Vet Clin North Am Exotic Anim Pract 2001;4(2):565–572.

Orcutt C. Dermatologic diseases. In Hillyer EV, Quesenberry KE, eds. Ferrets, Rabbits and Rodents: Clinical Medicine and Surgery. Philadelphia: WB Saunders, 1997:115–125.

Li X, Fox JG. Neoplastic diseases. In: Fox JG, ed. Biology and Diseases of the Ferret. 2nd Ed. Baltimore: Williams & Wilkins, 1998:405–448.

### Portions Adapted From
Elmslie R. Mast Cell Tumor. In: Tilley LP, Smith FWK, Jr., eds. The 5-Minute Veterinary Consult: Canine and Feline, 3rd Ed. Baltimore: Lippincott Williams & Wilkins, 2003.

# BASICS

## DEFINITION
Rather than a single disease entity, megaesophagus refers to esophageal dilation and hypomotility, which may be a primary disorder or secondary to esophageal obstruction or neuromuscular dysfunction.

## PATHOPHYSIOLOGY
• Esophageal motility is decreased or absent, resulting in accumulation and retention of food and liquid in the esophagus.
• Lesions anywhere along the central or peripheral neural pathways, the myoneural junction, or esophageal muscles may result in esophageal hypomotility and distention.
• Sequelae to megaesophagus may include starvation and aspiration pneumonia.

## SYSTEMS AFFECTED
• Gastrointestinal—regurgitation, weight loss/cachexia
• Neuromuscular—may be manifestation of neuromuscular disease
• Respiratory—if aspiration pneumonia occurs

## GENETICS
Congenital idiopathic megaesophagus has not been reported in ferrets, but may exist.

## INCIDENCE/PREVALENCE
True incidence unknown—sporadically seen in clinical practice as a cause of regurgitation or cachexia

## GEOGRAPHIC DISTRIBUTION
N/A

## SIGNALMENT
### Mean Age and Range
• Usually seen in adult ferrets (3–7 years old), implying an acquired form
• Congenital megaesophagus, where signs of regurgitation first appear at weaning, has not been reported in ferrets.

### Predominant Sex
N/A

## SIGNS
### Historical Findings
• May include regurgitation of food and water, dysphagia, gagging, choking, anorexia, weight loss, and hypersalivation
• May see coughing, mucopurulent nasal discharge, and dyspnea with concurrent aspiration pneumonia
• Signs may first be noted days to months prior to presentation.

### Physical Examination Findings
• Related to megaesophagus—regurgitation, weight loss, halitosis, ptyalism, bruxism, bulging of the esophagus at the thoracic inlet, and pain associated with palpation of the cervical esophagus

• Related to the sequelae of megaesophagus—respiratory crackles, tachypnea, and pyrexia with aspiration pneumonia; cachexia, muscle weakness and wasting from starvation; dry mucous membranes and sunken eyes from dehydration.

## CAUSES
• In most cases, the cause is not identified.
• Miscellaneous—esophagitis, toxicosis (lead, thallium, acetylcholinesterase inhibitors)
• Esophageal obstruction—esophageal foreign body, stricture, neoplasia, granuloma
• Neurologic and neuromuscular diseases—botulism, CNS disorders, degenerative, infectious/inflammatory, neoplasia, traumatic disorders of the brainstem and spinal cord, bilateral vagal damage (myasthenia gravis and autoimmune causes have not been identified)

## RISK FACTORS
N/A

# DIAGNOSIS

## DIFFERENTIAL DIAGNOSIS
• Other disorders causing regurgitation.
• Obstructive pharyngeal disease (foreign bodies, inflammation, neoplasia) may produce regurgitation with normal esophageal motility.
• Pharyngeal pain and dysphagia often occur with obstructive pharyngeal disease.
• Distinguish regurgitation from dysphagia and vomition.
• Regurgitation is a passive process with no forceful abdominal contraction, anticipatory salivation, nausea, or retching.
• Bile-stained ingesta suggests vomition.

## CBC/BIOCHEMISTRY/URINALYSIS
• Leukocytosis with secondary aspiration pneumonia; increased PCV with dehydration
• Increased AST and ALT commonly seen; hypoglycemia with starvation and/or concurrent insulinoma

## OTHER LABORATORY TESTS
Blood lead and cholinesterase levels to evaluate for toxicity

## IMAGING
### Survey Thoracic Radiographs
• Esophagus dilated with gas, fluid, or ingesta
• The trachea is often displaced ventrally by the distended esophagus.

### Contrast Esophagram and Fluoroscopy
• An esophagram using either barium liquid or paste may demonstrate contrast pooling and abnormal esophageal motility.
• Abnormal primary and secondary esophageal peristalsis can be visualized with fluoroscopy.

• Contrast studies—not necessary for diagnosing most cases of megaesophagus; use with caution in animal patients with known megaesophagus, because of the risk of aspiration.

## DIAGNOSTIC PROCEDURES
• Endoscopy—can use to visualize a dilated esophagus, foreign bodies, neoplasia, and esophagitis; mucosal biopsy specimens and cytology samples may be obtained; esophageal foreign bodies may be removed. However, the small size of the patient and subsequent limitations on instrument size often limit the use of endoscopy.
• Muscle and nerve biopsies/histopathology—possibly useful to confirm diagnosis of inflammatory and degenerative disorders of muscles and nerves

## PATHOLOGIC FINDINGS
Dilation of both the cervical and thoracic esophagus; inflammation and ulceration of the esophageal mucosa seen with advanced disease

# TREATMENT

## APPROPRIATE HEALTH CARE
Most patients have aspiration pneumonia and/or severe debilitation, requiring hospitalization.

## NURSING CARE
• Correct dehydration with IV fluid therapy (maintenance = 75–100 mL/kg/day) using 0.9% saline or LRS. If hypoglycemic use 2.5% dextrose and 0.45% saline.
• Hospitalize in a warm, quiet location with a hide box to minimize stress.

## ACTIVITY
Restricted due to associated weakness and lethargy

## DIET
• Feed in upright position (45–90° angle to the floor) and maintain position for 10–15 minutes following feeding.
• Feed a high-calorie gruel formulated from meat-based human baby foods, Eukanuba Maximum Calorie diet (Iams Co., Dayton, OH), Feline a/d (Hills Products, Topeka, KS), or moistened ferret pellets supplemented with Nutri-Cal (EVSCO Pharmaceuticals, Buena, NJ), Ensure (Abbot Laboratories, North Chicago, IL), or Clinicare Feline liquid diet (Abbott Laboratories).
• A more liquid consistency may decrease regurgitation but may increase the risk of aspiration pneumonia.
• Resting energy requirements for ferrets have been reported to be 70 kcal/kg body weight per day; sick ferrets have higher requirements.
• Patients with severe regurgitation may need parenteral feeding via gastrotomy tube.

# MEGAESOPHAGUS

## CLIENT EDUCATION

An underlying cause is rarely identified or corrected, and most ferrets are debilitated due to starvation, hepatic lipidosis, and aspiration pneumonia. Advise client of poor prognosis.

## SURGICAL CONSIDERATIONS

• Surgery may be necessary to remove esophageal foreign bodies or neoplasia if identified.
• No surgical procedures improve esophageal motility.

# MEDICATIONS

## DRUG(S) OF CHOICE

• No drugs are commonly used to treat megaesophagus alone; direct treatment at the underlying disease or associated conditions (e.g., aspiration pneumonia).
• Sucralfate (25 mg/kg PO q8h), $H_2$ blockers (e.g., famotidine [0.25–0.5 mg/kg PO, IV q12–24h], cimetidine [5–10 mg/kg PO, SC, IM q8h], or omeprazole [0.7 mg/kg PO q24h]) can be used if reflux esophagitis is present.
• Metoclopramide (0.2–1.0 mg/kg PO, SC, IM q6–8h) speeds gastric emptying, increases gastroesophageal sphincter tone, and is most useful when reflux esophagitis is a contributing or the primary cause; use of metoclopramide for other causes has had limited success.
• Broad-spectrum antibiotics—necessary for patients with aspiration pneumonia; parenteral antibiotics may be required for patients with severe regurgitation. Ideally, based on culture and susceptibility testing from an airway specimen, begin with an antibiotic combination that is broad spectrum and effective against anaerobes (e.g., enrofloxacin 10–20 mg/kg IM q12h plus amoxicillin 10–30 mg/kg IM q12h); alter therapy based on culture/susceptibility results.

## CONTRAINDICATIONS

N/A

## PRECAUTIONS

• Corticosteroids may be necessary to treat conditions causing megaesophagus; use with caution in patients with aspiration pneumonia.
• Cisapride (0.1–0.5 mg/kg PO q8–12h) has been used in dogs to treat megaesophagus, but its use is controversial; it decreases esophageal transit time and increases lower esophageal tone in normal dogs; both of these effects are undesirable when treating megaesophagus; despite this, regurgitation decreases in some patients receiving cisapride; if symptoms of megaesophagus worsen, discontinue cisapride.

## POSSIBLE INTERACTIONS

N/A

## ALTERNATIVE DRUGS

N/A

# FOLLOW-UP

## PATIENT MONITORING

May use repeat thoracic radiographs, esophagrams, and fluoroscopic examinations to follow progression or resolution of megaesophagus.

## PREVENTION/AVOIDANCE

Esophageal obstruction may be prevented if pets are not allowed access to rubber toys, bones, garbage, or other tempting items.

## POSSIBLE COMPLICATIONS

Aspiration pneumonia, hepatic lipidosis

## EXPECTED COURSE AND PROGNOSIS

• Poor to grave, with or without treatment
• Aspiration pneumonia and malnutrition are leading causes of death.

# MISCELLANEOUS

## ASSOCIATED CONDITIONS

• Insulinoma
• Hyperadrenocorticism
• Gastric ulcers

• *Helicobacter mustelae*

## AGE-RELATED FACTORS

Regurgitation at weaning suggests congenital or obstructive megaesophagus but has not been reported in ferrets.

## ZOONOTIC POTENTIAL

Determine rabies vaccination status for all patients.

## PREGNANCY

N/A

## SYNONYMS

N/A

## SEE ALSO

• Dysphagia
• Gastrointestinal foreign bodies
• Pneumonia

## ABBREVIATIONS

• AST = aspartate aminotransferase
• ALT = alanine aminotransferase
• CBC = complete blood count
• LRS = lactated ringer's solution
• PCV = packed cell volume

*Suggested Reading*

Blanco MC, Fox JG, Rosenthal K, et al. Megaesophagus in nine ferrets. J Am Vet Med Assoc 1994; 205;444–447.

Fox JG. Diseases of the gastrointestinal system. In: Fox JG, ed. Biology and Diseases of the Ferret. 2nd Ed. Baltimore: Williams & Wilkins, 1998.

Hoefer HL. Gastrointestinal diseases. In: Hillyer EV, Quesenberry KE, eds. Ferrets, Rabbits and Rodents: Clinical Medicine and Surgery. Philadelphia: WB Saunders, 1997:26–36.

*Portions Adapted From*

Longshore RC. Megaesophagus. In: Tilley LP, Smith FWK, Jr., eds. The 5-Minute Veterinary Consult: Canine and Feline, 3rd Ed. Baltimore: Lippincott Williams & Wilkins, 2003.

## BASICS

### DEFINITION
Presence of digested blood in the feces; appears as green–black, tarry stool

### PATHOPHYSIOLOGY
Usually the result of upper gastrointestinal bleeding; however, melena can also be associated with ingested blood from the oral cavity or upper respiratory tract.

### SYSTEMS AFFECTED
• Gastrointestinal
• Hematopoietic

### SIGNALMENT
No breed or gender predilections

### SIGNS

#### Historical Findings
• Melena may be accompanied by anorexia, weight loss, bruxism, hypersalivation, vomiting, or regurgitation.
• Feces may be formed or diarrheic.
• Question owner about the ferret's chewing habits and possible ingestion of foreign bodies, especially rubber toys, foam rubber or cloth bedding material.
• Exposure to other ferrets or new ferrets in the household

#### Physical Examination Findings
• Pallor of the mucous membranes
• Weight loss—indicates chronic disease
• Poor haircoat or alopecia
• Dehydration
• Fecal staining of the perineum
• Abdominal distention may be due to thickened or fluid-filled intestinal loops, masses, or organomegaly.
• Mesenteric lymph nodes may be palpably enlarged.

### CAUSES
• Bacterial infection—*Helicobacter mustelae* gastritis (most common cause), *Salmonella* sp., *Mycobacterium avium*-intracellulare (rare)
• Viral infection—ECE (common)
• Obstruction—foreign body and neoplasia most common, intussusception
• Neoplasia—lymphoma, adenocarcinoma
• Drugs and toxins—NSAIDs, vaccine reaction
• Infiltrative—lymphoplasmacytic enteritis, eosinophilic enterocolitis
• Ingestion of blood—oropharyngeal, nasal, or sinus lesions (abscess, trauma, neoplasia, mycotic)

#### Other Uncommon Causes
• Metabolic disorders—liver disease, renal disease
• Coagulopathy
• Stress
• Septicemia

### RISK FACTORS
• Unsupervised chewing
• Exposure to other ferrets
• Vaccine reaction

## DIAGNOSIS

### DIFFERENTIAL DIAGNOSIS

#### Differentiating Causes
• Melena and anorexia most common with *H. mustelae* or gastrointestinal foreign body
• Thickened intestinal loops and palpably enlarged mesenteric lymph nodes common with eosinophilic enterocolitis, lymphoplasmacytic enteritis, ECE, or lymphoma
• Bile-stained (green) mucous-covered diarrhea seen most commonly with ECE
• Granular, "bird seed"-like feces seen with maldigestive/malabsorptive disorders.

### CBC/BIOCHEMISTRY
• Regenerative anemia may be seen with chronic gastrointestinal bleeding.
• TWBC elevation with neutrophilia may be seen with bacterial enteritis.
• TWBC elevation with lymphocytosis or normal TWBC with relative lymphocytosis is suggestive of lymphoma.
• Eosinophilia (as high as 35%) in ferrets with eosinophilic enterocolitis
• Serum albumin concentration increased with dehydration
• Hypoalbuminemia may be seen with protein loss from the intestinal tract, especially with proliferative bowel disease.
• Serum biochemistry abnormalities may suggest renal or hepatic disease; ALT elevations usually seen with ECE

### OTHER LABORATORY TESTS
Coagulation studies—may help rule out bleeding disorders; however, very little data on normal values exist. Normal values reported (based on n = 6): APTT 18.4 ± 1.4 seconds; PT 10.3 ± 0.1 seconds; thrombin time 28.8 ± 8.7 seconds; whole blood clotting time 2 ± 0.5 minutes in glass tubes. Normal values for FDP in ferrets have not been reported so results must be interpreted from feline data.

### IMAGING

#### Radiographic Findings
• Survey abdominal radiography may indicate intestinal obstruction, organomegaly, mass, foreign body, or ascites.
• Contrast radiography may indicate thickening of the intestinal wall, mucosal irregularities, mass, severe ileus, foreign body, or stricture.
• Abdominal ultrasonography may demonstrate intestinal wall thickening, gastrointestinal mass, foreign body, ileus, or mesenteric lymphadenopathy. Hyperechogenicity may be seen with hepatic lipidosis or

fibrosis; hypoechoic nodules are suggestive of hepatic necrosis, abscess, or neoplasia.

### OTHER DIAGNOSTIC PROCEDURES
• Fecal cytology—may reveal RBC or fecal leukocytes, which are associated with inflammatory bowel disease or invasive bacterial strains
• Fecal culture should be performed if abnormal bacteria are observed on the fecal Gram's stain or if *Salmonella* is suspected.

#### Surgical Considerations
Exploratory laparotomy and surgical biopsy should be pursued if there is evidence of obstruction or intestinal mass and/or for definitive diagnosis of gastrointestinal inflammatory or infiltrative diseases or *H. mustelae* gastritis.

## TREATMENT
• Treatment must be specific to the underlying cause to be successful.
• Patients with mild disease usually respond to outpatient treatment.
• Patients with moderate to severe disease usually require hospitalization and 24-hour care for parenteral medication and fluid therapy.
• Correct electrolyte and acid-base disturbances.
• Feed high-calorie diets and dietary supplements to emaciated animals in critical condition.
• Easily digestible, high-protein diets such as chicken baby food should be fed to ferrets recovering from ECE or inflammatory bowel disease.
• Exploratory laparotomy to remove foreign bodies or tumors

## MEDICATIONS

### DRUG(S) OF CHOICE

#### Antibiotic Therapy
• Indicated in patients with bacterial inflammatory lesions in the gastrointestinal tract. Also indicated in patients with disruption of the intestinal mucosa evidenced by blood in the feces. Selection should be based on results of culture and susceptibility testing when possible.
• Some choices for empirical use while waiting for culture results include trimethoprim sulfa (15–30 mg/kg q12h), amoxicillin (10–20 mg/kg PO, SC q12h), or enrofloxacin (10–20 mg/kg PO, SC q12h).
• Proliferative bowel disease—chloramphenicol (50 mg/kg, IM, SC, PO q12h)
• Giardiasis, anaerobic bacterial infections—metronidazole (15–20 mg/kg PO q12h)
• *H. mustelae*—amoxicillin (10 mg/kg PO q12h) plus metronidazole (20 mg/kg PO

# MELENA

q12h) and bismuth subsalicylate (17 mg/kg PO q12h) for 2 weeks; or clarithromycin (12.5 mg/kg PO q8h) plus ranitidine bismuth (24 mg/kg q8h) for 2 weeks

### Gastrointestinal Antisecretory Agents
• Are helpful to treat, and possibly prevent, gastritis in anorectic ferrets. Ferrets continually secrete a baseline level of gastric hydrochloric acid and, as such, anorexia itself may predispose to gastric ulceration. Those successfully used in ferrets include omeprazole (0.7 mg/kg PO q24h), famotidine (0.25–0.5 mg/kg PO, IV q12–24h), and cimetidine (5–10 mg/kg PO, SC, IM q8h).
• Intestinal protectants—bismuth subsalicylate (17–20 mg/kg PO q12h or 1 mL/kg of regular strength preparation [262 mg/15 mL] PO q12h); omeprazole (0.7 mg/kg PO q24h)

### Corticosteroids
• Often helpful in treatment of inflammatory bowel diseases (treat underlying disease whenever possible)—prednisone (1.25–2.5 mg/kg PO q24h); when signs resolve, gradually taper the corticosteroid dose to 0.5–1.25 mg/kg every other day.
• Vaccine reaction—diphenhydramine (0.5–2.0 mg/kg IM), dexamethasone (2–4 mg/kg IV), or prednisolone Na succinate (22 mg/kg IV)

### CONTRAINDICATIONS
Do not use corticosteroids if an underlying infectious disease is confirmed or suspected.

### PRECAUTIONS
It is important to determine the cause of diarrhea. A general shotgun antibiotic approach may be ineffective or detrimental.

### POSSIBLE INTERACTIONS
N/A

### ALTERNATE DRUGS
See specific diseases for more detailed description of treatment.

# FOLLOW-UP

### PATIENT MONITORING
• PCV daily until anemia is stabilized, then weekly
• Fecal volume and character, appetite, attitude, and body weight
• If melena does not resolve, consider reevaluation of the diagnosis.

### POSSIBLE COMPLICATIONS
• Septicemia due to bacterial invasion of enteric mucosa
• Dehydration due to fluid loss

# MISCELLANEOUS

### ASSOCIATED CONDITIONS
• Septicemia
• Lymphoma

### AGE-RELATED FACTORS
• Clinical *H. mustelae* more common in ferrets >3 years of age
• Older ferrets demonstrate more severe clinical signs with ECE.
• Proliferative bowel disease seen more commonly in ferrets <1 year of age

### ZOONOTIC POTENTIAL
N/A

### PREGNANCY
N/A

### SEE ALSO
• Epizootic catarrhal enteritis
• Gastric ulcers
• *Helicobacter mustelae*
• Inflammatory bowel disease
• Proliferative bowel disease

### ABBREVIATIONS
• ALT = alanine aminotransferase
• APTT = activated partial thromboplastin time
• FDP = fibrin degradation products
• ECE = epizootic catarrhal enteritis
• NSAID = nonsteroidal antiinflammatory drugs
• PCV = packed cell volume
• PT = prothrombin time
• RBC = red blood cell
• TWBC = total white blood cell count

### Suggested Reading
Finkler MR. Ferret colitis. In: Kirk RW, Bonagura JD, eds. Kirk's Current Veterinary Therapy XI: Small Animal Practice. Philadelphia: WB Saunders, 1992.

Fox JG. Diseases of the gastrointestinal system. In: Fox JG, ed. Biology and Diseases of the Ferret. 2nd Ed. Baltimore: Williams & Wilkins, 1998.

Fox JG, Marini RP. Helicobacter mustelae infection in ferrets: pathogenesis, epizootiology, diagnosis and treatment. Semin Avin Exotic Pet Med 2001;10(1):36–44.

Hoefer HL. Gastrointestinal diseases. In: Hillyer EV, Quesenberry KE, eds. Ferrets, Rabbits and Rodents: Clinical Medicine and Surgery. Philadelphia: WB Saunders, 1997:26–36.

Jenkins JR. Rabbit and ferret liver and gastrointestinal testing. In: Fudge AM, ed. Laboratory Medicine, Avian and Exotic Pets. Philadelphia: WB Saunders, 2000.

### Portions Adapted From
Moore LE, Burrows CF. Melena. In: Tilley LP, Smith FWK, Jr., eds. The 5-Minute Veterinary Consult: Canine and Feline, 3rd Ed. Baltimore: Lippincott Williams & Wilkins, 2003.

# BASICS

## OVERVIEW
• Rare malignant neoplasm of hematopoietic tissue derived from a clonal population of plasma cells, usually in the bone marrow
• Three of four defining features should be present for diagnosis: monoclonal gammopathy; neoplastic plasma cells or bone marrow plasmacytosis; lytic bone lesions; and Bence Jones (light-chain) proteinuria (Bence Jones proteinuria has not been reported in ferrets).
• Neoplasms result in areas of active bone lysis in the skeleton including vertebral column, pelvis, skull, and appendicular bones.
• Neoplastic plasma cells may be present in extraskeletal sites (e.g., liver, spleen, lymph nodes, kidney, pharynx, lung, muscle, and gastrointestinal tract).

## SIGNALMENT
Incidence is unknown; only three reported cases, but many others may go unreported. Sex or age predilections unknown

## SIGNS

### General Comments
Attributed to bone infiltration and lysis, effects of proteins produced by the tumor (e.g., hyperviscosity and nephrotoxicity), and infiltration of organ(s) by neoplastic cells

### Historical Findings
• Depend on location and extent of disease
• Weakness, lameness, pain at the site of the tumor, pathologic fractures, paresis, or paralysis caudal to vertebral tumors

### Physical Examination Findings
• Paresis and paralysis caudal to vertebral tumors
• Other signs such as bleeding, blindness, retinal hemorrhage, lameness, polydipsia, and polyuria have not been reported, but should be considered.

## CAUSES AND RISK FACTORS
Unknown

# DIAGNOSIS

## DIFFERENTIAL DIAGNOSIS
• For caudal paresis or paralysis: metabolic diseases causing anemia (hyperestrogenism, leukemia, CRF); hypoglycemia (insulinomas, gastrointestinal foreign bodies, severe hepatic disease or sepsis); or other spinal disease (IVD extrusion, trauma, discospondylitis, other neoplasms)
• For monoclonal gammopathy—Aleutian disease virus (typically does not affect bone)

## CBC/BIOCHEMISTRY/URINALYSIS
Results not reported in documented cases involving ferrets. In other species: anemia,

neutropenia, thrombocytopenia, eosinophilia, or plasma cell leukemia seen on CBC; high RBC rouleaux formation, high serum viscosity, or high serum total protein with hypoalbuminemia and hyperglobulinemia; high BUN, creatinine, or liver enzymes; urine proteinuria, isosthenuria, cylindruria, pyuria, hematuria, or bacteruria

## OTHER LABORATORY TESTS
• Serum protein electrophoresis—identify monoclonal gammopathy (i.e., protein spike), even if globulin concentration is normal.
• Serum immunoglobulin quantification
• Urine protein electrophoresis—may be used to identify Bence Jones proteins (not documented in ferrets)

## IMAGING
• Radiography—axial and appendicular skeleton; show multifocal, lytic (punched-out) lesions
• Extraskeletal sites may be identified by organomegaly.
• Ultrasonography—detect changes in echotexture of visceral organs (e.g., infiltration)

## DIAGNOSTIC PROCEDURES
Cytologic examination of bone marrow and skeletal and extraskeletal lesions—determine if >20–25% of normal cell population are plasma cells.

## PATHOLOGIC FINDINGS
• Gross appearance—tan to white nodules in bone or soft tissue
• Sheets or isolated discrete round cells with eosinophilic cytoplasm, intracytoplasmic eosinophilic inclusions, and eccentric nuclei

# TREATMENT

## APPROPRIATE HEALTH CARE
• Inpatient—azotemia, dehydration, or anorexia
• Treatments used in other animals such as plasmapheresis and radiotherapy have not been reported in ferrets. Refer to canine and feline references for more information if these modalities are attempted.

## ACTIVITY
Multiple myeloma—treat as immune compromised; take care to prevent bacterial infection.

## DIET
N/A

## CLIENT EDUCATION
• If attempting chemotherapy, radiotherapy, or plasmapheresis, inform client that success rates and treatment protocols for ferrets have not been reported. In dogs and cats these treatments are palliative and long remissions are possible.

• Discuss side effects, which depend on the drugs used.

## SURGICAL CONSIDERATIONS
Areas nonresponsive to chemotherapy or solitary lesions can be removed surgically.

# MEDICATIONS

## DRUG(S) OF CHOICE
Unknown in ferrets; in dogs and cats—melphalan or cyclophosphamide and prednisone have been used to induce remission

## CONTRAINDICATIONS AND POSSIBLE INTERACTIONS
N/A

## PRECAUTIONS
• Melphalan—very bone marrow suppressive, especially to platelets
• Affected animals may have low numbers of neutrophils or nonfunctional lymphocytes; take care to minimize exposure to infectious agents (e.g., viral, bacterial, and fungal).
• Use septic or very clean technique when performing any invasive techniques, even drawing blood.
• Chemotherapy may be toxic; seek advice before initiating any treatment if you are not familiar with cytotoxic drugs.

# FOLLOW-UP

## PATIENT MONITORING
• CBC and platelet counts—to assess bone marrow response
• Protein electrophoresis—until normal levels obtained; monitor periodically for relapse.
• Abnormal skeletal radiographs—to evaluate response to treatment

## PREVENTION/AVOIDANCE
N/A

## POSSIBLE COMPLICATIONS
• Bleeding
• Secondary infections
• Pathologic fractures
• Chemotherapy—may cause leukopenia or thrombocytopenia, anorexia, alopecia, hemorrhagic cystitis, or pancreatitis

## EXPECTED COURSE AND PROGNOSIS
Median survival time is unknown; treatment has not been reported.

# MISCELLANEOUS

## ASSOCIATED CONDITIONS
N/A

# MULTIPLE MYELOMA

### AGE-RELATED FACTORS
N/A

### ZOONOTIC POTENTIAL
N/A

### PREGNANCY
Chemotherapy is contraindicated in pregnant animals.

### SYNONYMS
- Plasma cell myeloma
- Plasmacytoma
- Myelocytoma
- Myelosarcoma
- Plasma cell leukemia
- Lymphocytoma

### ABBREVIATIONS
- BUN = blood urea nitrogen
- CBC = complete blood count
- CRF = chronic renal failure
- IVD = intervertebral disc
- RBC = red blood cell

*Suggested Readings*

Brown SA. Neoplasia. In: Hillyer EV, Quesenberry KE, eds. Ferrets, Rabbits and Rodents: Clinical Medicine and Surgery. Philadelphia: WB Saunders, 1998:109.

Couto, CG. Oncology. In: Sherding RD, ed. The Cat: Diseases and Clinical Management. New York: Churchill Livingstone, 1989:589–647.

Morrison WB. Plasma cell neoplasms. In: Morrison WB, ed. Cancer in Dogs and Cats: Medical and Surgical Management. Baltimore: Williams & Wilkins, 1998:697–704.

Li X, Fox JG. Neoplastic diseases. In: Fox JG, ed. Biology and Diseases of the Ferret. 2nd Ed. Baltimore: Williams & Wilkins.

*Portions Adapted From*

Vonderharr MA. Multiple myeloma. In: Tilley LP, Smith FWK, Jr., eds. The 5-Minute Veterinary Consult: Canine and Feline, 2nd Ed. Baltimore: Lippincott Williams & Wilkins, 2000.

# NASAL DISCHARGE (SNEEZING, GAGGING)

## BASICS

### DEFINITION
• Nasal discharges may be serous, mucoid, mucopurulent, purulent, blood tinged, or frank blood (epistaxis) or contain food debris.
• Sneezing is the reflexive expulsion of air through the nasal cavity and is commonly associated with nasal discharge.
• Gagging and retching are involuntary, reflexive attempts to clear secretions from the pharynx or upper respiratory or gastrointestinal tract.

### PATHOPHYSIOLOGY
• Secretions are produced by mucous cells of the epithelium and glands. Irritation of the nasal mucosa (by mechanical, chemical, or inflammatory stimulation) increases nasal secretion production.
• Mucosal irritation and accumulated secretions are a potent stimulus of the sneeze reflex; sneezing may be the first sign of nasal discharge. Sneezing frequency often decreases with chronic disease.
• Gagging is a protective reflex elicited by oropharyngeal stimulation, usually functioning to clear material from the oropharynx. Gagging often follows a coughing episode as secretions are brought through the larynx into the oropharynx.

### SYSTEMS AFFECTED
• Respiratory—mucosa of the upper respiratory tract, including the nasal cavities, sinuses, and nasopharynx
• Gastrointestinal—these signs may also be observed with extranasal diseases such as swallowing disorders and esophageal or gastrointestinal diseases.
• Hemic/lymphatic/immune—systemic diseases may cause blood-tinged nasal discharge or epistaxis due to hemostasis disorders.

### SIGNALMENT
• Young animals—CDV
• Older animals—nasal tumors, primary dental disease (rare)

### SIGNS

#### Historical Findings
• Nasal discharge and sneezing are commonly reported as concurrent problems. Information concerning both the initial and present character of the discharge and whether it was originally unilateral or bilateral are important historical findings.
• The response to previous antibiotic therapy may be helpful in determining secondary bacterial involvement. Bacterial infection secondary to influenza virus usually responds to treatment; however, bacterial infection secondary to CDV, dental disease, or foreign bodies usually responds initially

to antibiotic therapy but commonly will relapse or progress despite treatment. Nasal tumors and fungal rhinitis typically show little response.

#### Physical Examination Findings
• Secretions or dried discharges on the hair around the muzzle and front limbs
• Concurrent dental disease
• Ocular discharge
• Bony involvement (tumor, fungal infection, tooth abscess) may cause facial swelling or pain secondary to osteomyelitis.
• Regional lymph node enlargement may be present.
• Pyrexia (CDV, influenza, secondary bacterial infections)

### CAUSES
Unilateral discharge often is associated with nonsystemic processes:
• Foreign bodies
• Nasal tumors
• Dental-related disease—abscess, oronasal fistula (rare)
• Fungal infections—cryptococcosis, blastomycosis (occur rarely)
Bilateral discharge is most common with:
• Infectious agents—influenza virus, CDV, secondary bacterial infections
• Nasal tumors may cause unilateral discharge initially then progress to bilateral discharge as the disease extends through the nasal septum.
• Allergies have not been reported as a cause of nasal discharge in the ferret, but should be considered.
Discharge may be unilateral or bilateral with:
• Nasal tumors
• Foreign bodies
• Hypersensitivity reaction
Sneezing without nasal discharge:
Many normal ferrets will sneeze several times a day

### RISK FACTORS
• Exposure to other animals
• Dental disease
• CDV in poorly vaccinated animals
• Immunosuppression

## DIAGNOSIS

### DIFFERENTIAL DIAGNOSIS

#### Differentiating Similar Causes
• Serous discharge associated with mild irritation, viral disorders, acute phase of inflammation, possibly allergies
• Mucoid discharges associated with acute inflammation, early neoplastic conditions
• Purulent (or mucopurulent) discharges are seen with secondary bacterial or mycotic infections, nasal foreign bodies
• Serosanguineous or blood-tinged discharges are seen with destructive processes

(primary nasal tumors) after violent/paroxysmal sneezing episodes (traumatic capillary rupture) associated with coagulopathies.
• The presence of other clinical signs will help to differentiate CDV from other causes. In ferrets with CDV, facial dermatitis (rash, crusts) is usually seen after the onset of nasal discharge. These signs are followed by severe respiratory signs and signs of systemic illness, progressing invariably to death.

### CBC/BIOCHEMISTRY
• Elevated TWBC with inflammatory leukogram is often seen with bacterial or mycotic diseases.
• Although not specific for any particular cause of nasal discharge, a chemistry profile may be valuable for detecting concurrent problems and as part of a thorough evaluation prior to any procedure requiring anesthesia.

### OTHER LABORATORY TESTS
• Fluorescent antibody test for CDV—on conjunctival or mucous membrane scrapings or peripheral blood smears (false negatives possible)
• Coagulation studies (not well described in ferrets)

### IMAGING

#### Radiographic Findings
• Radiography of the nasal cavities can be helpful in cases of chronic nasal discharge, especially to rule out neoplasia, foreign bodies, or associated dental disease. Because of difficulties with overlying structures, the patient should be anesthetized and carefully positioned.
• The lateral view is useful in detecting any periosteal reaction over the nasal bones; for gross changes in the maxillary teeth, nasal cavity, and frontal sinus; and for evaluating the air column of the nasopharynx.
• The open mouth ventro dorsal and the intraoral views (using sheet film) are best for evaluating the nasal cavities and turbinates; disease may be localized to the affected side.
• The lateral oblique views are best for detecting maxillary teeth abnormalities.
• The rostrocaudal view is used to evaluate each frontal sinus (e.g., periosteal reaction, filling).
• CT scans may be helpful in detecting the extent of bony changes associated with nasal tumors and fungal rhinitis.

### OTHER DIAGNOSTIC PROCEDURES
• Rhinoscopy may be indicated in cases of chronic or recurrent nasal discharge; however, the small size of the patient makes this procedure more challenging. Bleeding disorders may be a contraindication.
• Nasal cytology—nonspecific inflammation is most commonly found.
• Cultures may be difficult to interpret due to the presence of normal nasal flora. How-

# NASAL DISCHARGE (SNEEZING, GAGGING)

ever, heavy growth of a single organism is usually significant. Deep cultures obtained by rhinoscopy would be most reliable.
• Biopsy of the nasal cavity is indicated in any animal with chronic nasal discharge in which neoplasia is suspected. Specimens may be obtained by direct endoscopic biopsy or rhinotomy. Multiple samples may be necessary to ensure adequate representation of the disease process.
• Periodontal probing is indicated in animals with dental calculus where tooth root abscess is suspected.

## TREATMENT

• Outpatient treatment is acceptable unless the patient is exhibiting signs of systemic illness in addition to nasal discharge.
• Symptomatic treatment and nursing care are important in the treatment of ferrets with sneezing and nasal discharge. Patient hydration, nutrition, warmth, and hygiene (keeping nares clean) are important.
• Many ferrets with nasal discharge become anorectic; offer high-calorie diets such as Eukanuba Maximum Calorie diet (Iams Co., Dayton, OH), Feline a/d (Hills Products, Topeka, KS), or Clinicare Feline liquid diet (Abbott Laboratories, North Chicago, IL); may also add dietary supplement such as Nutri-Cal (EVSCO Pharmaceuticals, Buena, NJ) to increase caloric content to these foods. Warming the food to body temperature or offering via syringe may increase acceptance. Administer these supplements several times a day.
• Surgery may be necessary to remove foreign bodies, obtain samples for biopsy, or debulk tumors, abscesses, or granulomas.
• Treat associated dental disease—extractions, gingivectomy, flap closure for fistulas—techniques are those used in feline patients.

## MEDICATIONS

### DRUG(S) OF CHOICE

• Nasal secretions clear more easily if the patient is well hydrated; fluid therapy should be considered if hydration is marginal.

• Decongestants or antihistamines may be used in attempt to dry up the nasal secretions (diphenhydramine 0.5–2.0 mg/kg PO q8–12h or chlorpheniramine 1–2mg/kg PO q8–12h).
• Antibiotics for secondary bacterial infections—treat according to culture results. Choices include trimethoprim/sulfonamide (15–30 mg/kg PO, SC q12h); enrofloxacin (10–20 mg/kg PO, SC, IM q12h); or cephalexin (15–25 mg/kg PO q8–12h).
• There are no drugs that palliatively decrease the frequency of sneezing.
• Mycotic rhinitis—amphotericin B (0.4–0.8 mg/kg IV, once per week, not to exceed total dose of 7–25 mg) and ketoconazole (10–30mg/kg PO q12–24h)

### CONTRAINDICATIONS
N/A

### PRECAUTIONS

• Topical or systemic administration of corticosteroids should be used with caution in patients with bacterial or mycotic disease.
• Anorexia, nausea, vomiting, and liver damage are possible with ketoconazole.
• Amphotericin B may cause bone marrow suppression and may be nephrotoxic.

### POSSIBLE INTERACTIONS
N/A

### ALTERNATIVE DRUGS
N/A

## FOLLOW-UP

### PATIENT MONITORING

• Observe nasal discharge; note changes in volume or character.
• Monitor CBC; should return to normal with successful treatment of infectious diseases
• Repeat cytology and cultures to monitor response to treatment.
• If discharge is due to CDV clinical signs will progress, eventually leading to death.

### POSSIBLE COMPLICATIONS

• Loss of appetite
• Extension of primary disease into mouth, eye, or brain
• Dyspnea as a result of nasal obstruction

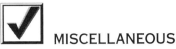

## MISCELLANEOUS

### ASSOCIATED CONDITIONS

• Sinusitis
• CDV
• Influenza
• Dental disease
• Aleutian disease may cause immunosuppression and secondary bacterial infection.

### AGE-RELATED FACTORS
N/A

### ZOONOTIC POTENTIAL
Influenza virus

### PREGNANCY
N/A

### SYNONYMS
N/A

### SEE ALSO

• CDV
• Influenza

### ABBREVIATION

• CBC = complete blood count
• CDV = canine distemper virus
• CT = computed tomography
• TWBC = total white blood cell

*Suggested Reading*

Fox JG. Bacterial and mycoplasmal diseases. In: Fox JG, ed. Biology and Diseases of the Ferret. 2nd Ed. Baltimore: Williams & Wilkins, 1998:321–354.
Kendrick RE. Ferret respiratory diseases. Vet Clin North Am Exotic Anim Pract 2000;3(2):453–464.
Rosenthal KL. Respiratory diseases. In: Hillyer EV, Quesenberry K, eds. Ferrets, Rabbits and Rodents: Clinical Medicine and Surgery. Philadelphia: WB Saunders, 1997:77–84.
Williams BH. Ferret microbiology and virology. In: Fudge AM, ed. Laboratory Medicine Avian and Exotic Pets. Philadelphia: WB Saunders, 2000:335–342.

*Portions Adapted From*

McKiernan BC. Nasal Discharge (Sneezing, Reverse Sneezing). In: Tilley LP, Smith FWK, Jr., eds. The 5-Minute Veterinary Consult: Canine and Feline, 3rd Ed. Baltimore: Lippincott Williams & Wilkins, 2003.

## BASICS

### OVERVIEW
• The most common tumors of the digestive system are functional pancreatic islet cell tumor (insulinoma) and lymphoma. These neoplastic disorders account for a large percentage of all clinical diseases seen in pet ferrets, and are therefore discussed as separate topics.
• Metastatic tumors to the liver are more common than primary tumors, especially lymphoma, islet cell tumors, and pancreatic adenocarcinomas.
• Other digestive system tumors, including tumors of the gastrointestinal tract, liver, pancreas, and salivary gland, occur sporadically in ferrets.
• The incidence of reported digestive system neoplasia in ferrets is low, such that accurate accounts of biologic behavior and response to treatment cannot be assessed.
• Reported tumor types include esophageal, gastric, or intestinal adenocarcinoma, leiomyoma, and leiomyosarcoma; hepatic hemangioma and hemangiosarcoma; hepatocellular or bile duct adenoma and adenosarcoma; bile duct cystadenoma and cystadenocarcinoma; pancreatic adenoma and adenocarcinoma; and salivary gland adenocarcinoma.

### SIGNALMENT
• Age—depends on tumor type; most likely in ferrets 4–7 years old
• Data on sex predilection not available

### SIGNS
• Gastrointestinal tumors—lethargy and weakness (hind limb paresis), anorexia, vomiting, weight loss, diarrhea; gastric mass or distension may be palpable
• Hepatobiliary tumors—lethargy and weakness (hind limb paresis), anorexia, vomiting, weight loss, abdominal distension; ascites, mass, or hepatomegaly may be palpable
• Pancreatic tumors—(nonfunctional tumors) may be asymptomatic if adenomas; adenocarcinomas tend to be aggressive; see weakness, anorexia, vomiting, weight loss, and abdominal distension

### CAUSES AND RISK FACTORS
• Infection with *Helicobacter mustelae* may predispose to gastric adenocarcinoma.
• Other tumors—unknown

## DIAGNOSIS

### DIFFERENTIAL DIAGNOSIS
• Gastrointestinal lymphoma is much more common than other types of neoplasia
• Gastrointestinal foreign body
• Infiltrative or inflammatory bowel diseases
• Infectious causes of vomiting, diarrhea (bacterial, viral, parasitic)
• Chronic cholangiohepatitis
• Hepatic abscess

### CBC/BIOCHEMISTRY/URINALYSIS
• May be normal
• May reflect dehydration or electrolyte disorders from vomiting or diarrhea
• Increased ALT, ALP, bile acids, and bilirubin especially with hepatic or biliary neoplasia
• Anemia with chronic disease; lymphocytosis or lymphopenia reported with lymphoma
• Bilirubinuria with hepatobiliary neoplasia

### OTHER LABORATORY TESTS
N/A

### IMAGING

#### Radiography
• May demonstrate hepatomegaly, a single mass lesion, or apparent asymmetry of hepatic silhouette
• May demonstrate solitary mass or gastric distension
• Positive contrast radiography—may reveal a filling defect (stomach); may note intraluminal space-occupying or annular constriction in the intestines
• Thoracic radiographs—may identify pulmonary metastases

#### Abdominal Ultrasonography
• May reveal a thickened wall of the stomach or bowel
• May reveal discrete mass lesion with variable echogenicity in liver

### DIAGNOSTIC PROCEDURES
• Histopathologic examination—definitive diagnosis
• Suspected hepatic tumor—aspiration cytology using a 23- or 25-gauge 1- to 1.5-inch needle under ultrasonographic guidance
• Exploratory laparotomy—to obtain biopsy samples for definitive diagnosis and to remove tumor when possible. Always evaluate the abdominal lymph nodes, pancreas, and adrenals for evidence of disease, since adrenal disease and insulinomas often occur concurrent with other tumor types.

### PATHOLOGIC FINDINGS
Vary with tumor type

## TREATMENT

### SURGICAL CONSIDERATIONS
• Surgical resection—treatment of choice; may not be curative if complete removal is not possible or metastasis has occurred
• Debulking may provide palliation of obstruction.

• Biopsy of local lymph nodes and normal liver for histologic evaluation is usually indicated to look for metastasis; evaluate adrenal gland and pancreas for evidence of disease.
• When in doubt, follow recommendations for similar tumors in canine or feline patients.

## MEDICATIONS

### DRUG(S) OF CHOICE
Too few reports exist to evaluate effectiveness of chemotherapy; consult an oncologist for recommendations.

### CONTRAINDICATIONS/POSSIBLE INTERACTIONS
N/A

## FOLLOW-UP

### EXPECTED COURSE AND PROGNOSIS
• Gastrointestinal adenocarcinomas tend to metastasize early.
• Pancreatic adenomas are generally benign and may be an incidental finding.
• Pancreatic adenocarcinomas tend to be very aggressive and metastasize early.
• Complete surgical excision—usually curative for discrete, benign masses that can be completely resected

## MISCELLANEOUS

### SEE ALSO
• Adrenal disease
• Hepatomegaly
• Insulinoma
• Lymphosarcoma

### ABBREVIATIONS
• ALP = alkaline phosphatase
• ALT = alanine aminotransferase

*Suggested Reading*

Brown SA. Neoplasia. In: Hillyer EV, Quesenberry KE, eds. Ferrets, Rabbits and Rodents: Clinical Medicine and Surgery. Philadelphia: WB Saunders, 1997:99.

Fox JG, Dangler CA, Sager W, et al. Helicobacter mustelae-associated gastric adenocarcinoma in ferrets (Mustela putorius furo). Vet Pathol 1997;34:225.

Li X, Fox JG. Neoplastic diseases. In: Fox JG, ed. Biology and Diseases of the Ferret. 2nd Ed. Baltimore: Williams & Wilkins.

Li X, Fox JG, Padrid RN. Neoplastic disease in ferrets: 574 cases (1968–1997). J Am Vet Med Assoc 1998;212(9); 1402–1406.

# NEOPLASIA, INTEGUMENTARY

## BASICS

### OVERVIEW
• Integumentary neoplasms are extremely common in ferrets. However, data regarding incidence, biologic behavior, and response to treatment for each tumor type reported is not available.
• Common tumor types reported include mast cell tumor, basal cell tumors, squamous cell carcinomas, and adenocarcinomas.
• Fibromas and fibrosarcomas, hemangioma and hemangiosarcoma, cutaneous lymphoma, myxoma and myxosarcomas, and histiocytomas have been reported less frequently.

### SIGNALMENT
• Common—fourth most common site of neoplasia in ferrets (after adrenal gland, pancreatic, and lymphoma)
• Age—depend on tumor type; most common in ferrets 4–7 years old
• Data on sex predilection not available

### SIGNS
• Mast cell tumors—papular or nodular, solitary or multiple, and hairy or alopecic or have an ulcerated surface; slight predilection for the head and neck regions; tumors may appear to rupture and become covered with a dry black exudate
• Basal cell tumors—well-demarcated firm, alopecic masses, either pedunculated or plaquelike, often pink–beige in color; may occur anywhere on the body
• Adenomas and adenocarcinomas—sebaceous and sweat gland adenoma/adenocarcinoma: may appear anywhere on the body, often firm, raised, multilobulated, or wartlike, tan–brown in color; apocrine gland adenocarcinoma: most found in perineal area (preputial gland, anal gland), ear (ceruminous gland) also reported, often raised red, firm, or ulcerated
• Squamous cell carcinoma—reported on face, feet, and trunk; firm nodules or grey–white plaques described, often ulcerate
• Fibroma and fibrosarcoma—can occur anywhere on the body; well-demarcated firm mass in dermis or subcutaneous tissues
• Hemangioma and hemangiosarcomas—hemangiomas usually dermal and well circumscribed; hemangiosarcoma more common on feet and legs, swollen, red, firm, may have boney involvement

• Cutaneous lymphoma—cutaneous epitheliotropic lymphoma (mycoses fungoides) reported on feet and as generalized alopecia/erythremia; may be pruritic
• Myxoma and myxosarcoma—rarely described; soft, grey–white poorly demarcated masses
• Histiocytoma—rarely described, raised firm dermal masses, may become ulcerated

### CAUSES AND RISK FACTORS
Unknown

## DIAGNOSIS

### DIFFERENTIAL DIAGNOSIS
• Other skin tumors not listed above
• Pyoderma or mycotic dermatitis
• Abscess
• Intradermal cysts

### CBC/BIOCHEMISTRY/URINALYSIS
Normal

### OTHER LABORATORY TESTS
N/A

### IMAGING
Radiographs to look for metastasis (sublumbar or mediastinal lymph nodes) or bony involvement (hemangiosarcoma, fibrosarcoma, ceruminous gland adenocarcinoma, squamous cell carcinoma)

### DIAGNOSTIC PROCEDURES
Histopathologic examination—definitive diagnosis

### PATHOLOGIC FINDINGS
Vary with tumor type

## TREATMENT

### SURGICAL CONSIDERATIONS
• Surgical excision—generally curative for mast cell tumors, basal cell tumors, and some adenomas or hemangiomas
• Wide surgical excision or amputation recommended when possible for hemangiosarcoma, fibrosarcoma, squamous cell carcinoma, and adenocarcinoma; biopsy local lymph nodes when possible to evaluate for metastasis.
• When in doubt, follow recommendations for similar tumors in canine or feline patients.

*Radiotherapy*
• Has been attempted in numerous tumor types, including squamous cell carcinoma, fibrosarcoma, and adenocarcinoma; consult an oncologist for recommendations.

## MEDICATIONS

### DRUG(S) OF CHOICE
Chemotherapy has been attempted in most of the above malignant tumor types. Too few reports exist to evaluate effectiveness; consult an oncologist for recommendations.

### CONTRAINDICATIONS/POSSIBLE INTERACTIONS
N/A

## FOLLOW-UP
• Complete surgical excision—usually curative for mast cell tumors, basal cell tumors, and hemangiomas
• Adenocarcinomas, hemangiosarcomas, fibrosarcomas, and squamous cell carcinomas tend to recur locally, or metastasize, especially to local lymph nodes.

## MISCELLANEOUS

*Suggested Reading*
Brown SA. Neoplasia. In: Hillyer EV, Quesenberry KE, eds. Ferrets, Rabbits and Rodents: Clinical Medicine and Surgery. Philadelphia: WB Saunders, 1997:99.
Fox JG, Dangler CA, Sager W, et al. Helicobacter mustelae-associated gastric adenocarcinoma in ferrets (Mustela putorius furo). Vet Pathol 1997;34:225.
Hamilton TA, Morrison WB. Bleomycin chemotherapy for metastatic squamous cell carcinoma in a ferret. J Am Vet Med Assoc 1991;198:107–108.
Li X, Fox JG. Neoplastic diseases. In: Fox JG, ed. Biology and Diseases of the Ferret. 2nd Ed. Baltimore: Williams & Wilkins, 1998.
Li X, Fox JG, Padrid RN. Neoplastic disease in ferrets: 574 cases (1968–1997). J Am Vet Med Assoc 1998;212(9);1402–1406.

# NEOPLASIA, MUSCULOSKELETAL AND NERVOUS SYSTEM

## BASICS

### OVERVIEW
• Tumors of the musculoskeletal and nervous system are relatively uncommon in ferrets.
• The most common musculoskeletal tumors are chordoma, arising from the notochord remnant, and osteoma; chondroma and chondrosarcoma, fibrosarcoma, rhabdomyosarcoma, and synovial cell sarcoma have also been reported.
• Nervous system tumors have very rarely been reported; schwannoma, neurofibrosarcoma, and ganglioneuromas are reported tumors of the peripheral nervous system; central nervous system tumors reported include granular cell tumors, meningioma, astrocytoma, and glioma.
• The reported incidence of these tumor types in ferrets is low, such that accurate accounts of biologic behavior and response to treatment cannot be assessed.

### SIGNALMENT
Data on age and sex predilection not available

### SIGNS
• Chordoma—most occur on tail, especially the tail tip, appearing as a smooth, round, well-demarcated mass; chordomas of the cervical vertebrae have also been reported, causing spinal cord compression and resultant weakness and ataxia caudal to the mass.
• Osteomas appear as hard, smooth, round masses on the flat bones of the head; other than the mass itself, signs are not apparent unless the mass compresses an adjacent structure.
• Chondroma, chondrosarcoma, and fibroma have all been reported on the vertebrae, intervertebral cartilage, or appendicular skeleton. Clinical signs vary with location.
• Nervous system tumors are rare; schwannomas and ganglioneuromas have been reported in the peritoneal cavity and dermis; tumors of the CNS may cause head tilt, torticollis, ataxia, seizures, and coma.

### CAUSES AND RISK FACTORS
Unknown

## DIAGNOSIS

### DIFFERENTIAL DIAGNOSIS
• For paresis, ataxia—weakness from any metabolic disease is a much more common cause of rear limb paresis.

• For CNS signs—hypoglycemia (insulinoma); viral (CDV, rabies)
• For bone lesions—fungal or bacterial osteomyelitis; metastatic bone lesion from another primary site

### CBC/BIOCHEMISTRY/URINALYSIS
Usually normal

### OTHER LABORATORY TESTS
N/A

### IMAGING

#### Radiography
• Osteoma—dense, bony mass on flat bones of the head
• Fibrosarcoma, chondrosarcoma—bony lysis or proliferation
• Ultrasonography may identify abdominal masses.
• Thoracic radiographs—may identify pulmonary metastases
• Myelography—may establish evidence of spinal cord compression

### DIAGNOSTIC PROCEDURES
• Histopathologic examination—definitive diagnosis
• Cytologic examination of bone aspirate—may yield diagnosis
• Exploratory laparotomy—to obtain biopsy samples for definitive diagnosis and to remove tumor when possible. Always evaluate the abdominal lymph nodes, pancreas, and adrenals for evidence of disease, since adrenal disease and insulinomas often occur concurrent with other tumor types.

## TREATMENT

### SURGICAL CONSIDERATIONS
• Chordoma—usually occurs on the tip of the tail; amputation is generally curative; if in the cervical region surgical resection is indicated, may not be curative if complete removal is not possible or metastasis (rare) has occurred
• Osteoma—treatment is only necessary if causing clinical signs due to compression of adjacent structures, and then surgical resection is indicated
• Fibrosarcoma, osteosarcoma—wide resection or amputation indicated when possible
• When in doubt, follow recommendations for similar tumors in canine and feline patients

## MEDICATIONS

### DRUG(S) OF CHOICE
Too few reports exist to evaluate effectiveness of chemotherapy; consult an oncologist for recommendations.

### CONTRAINDICATIONS/POSSIBLE INTERACTIONS
N/A

## FOLLOW-UP

### EXPECTED COURSE AND PROGNOSIS
• Chordoma—slow growing; good prognosis if confined to tail and amputation is performed
• Osteoma—slow growing and benign; good prognosis
• Fibrosarcoma, osteosarcoma—aggressive; tend to metastasize early
• For other tumors—low numbers reported; follow guidelines for similar tumors in canine or feline patients

## MISCELLANEOUS

### SEE ALSO
• Ataxia
• Insulinoma
• Paresis and paralysis

### ABBREVIATIONS
• CDV = canine distemper virus
• CNS = central nervous system

### Suggested Reading
Brown SA. Neoplasia. In: Hillyer EV, Quesenberry KE, eds. Ferrets, Rabbits and Rodents: Clinical Medicine and Surgery. Philadelphia: WB Saunders, 1997:99.
Li X, Fox JG. Neoplastic diseases. In: Fox JG, ed. Biology and Diseases of the Ferret. 2nd Ed. Baltimore: Williams & Wilkins, 1998.
Li X, Fox JG, Padrid RN. Neoplastic disease in ferrets: 574 cases (1968–1997). J Am Vet Med Assoc 1998;212(9); 1402–1406.

# OBESITY

## BASICS

### DEFINITION
The presence of body fat in sufficient excess to compromise normal physiologic function or predispose to metabolic, surgical, and/or mechanical problems. Obesity has become an extremely common, and often debilitating, problem in pet ferrets.

### PATHOPHYSIOLOGY
• Increased caloric intake and/or decreased activity. Most ferrets are housed in cages that allow minimal exercise.
• Ferrets tend to prefer sweet-tasting treats (e.g., raisins); overfeeding of these treats is the main cause of obesity in pet ferrets. Ferrets are often treated as family members and owners have difficulty denying these treats.
• Ferrets have a short intestinal tract and decreased gastrointestinal transit time (3 hours in an adult) as compared to cats and dogs. Because of this, the feeding of free-choice or multiple small meals is recommended. Generally, free-choice feeding of a high-quality ferret food will not cause obesity if the diet is not supplemented with treats. However, some ferrets will overeat and become obese if the food bowl is left full in the cage all day, due to boredom and lack of exercise.
• Ferrets have a higher protein and fat requirement than dogs or adult cats—for maintenance in normal ferrets, feed a high-quality kitten or ferret chow with animal protein listed as the first ingredient.

### SYSTEMS AFFECTED
• Musculoskeletal—articular and locomotor problems
• Hepatobiliary—hepatic lipidosis may occur
• Cardiovascular

### SIGNALMENT
No age or sex predisposition

### SIGNS
• Excess amounts of body fat for body size; can measure as body condition score >4 on a 1–5 scale in which 1 = cachectic (>20% underweight), 2 = lean (10–20% underweight), 3 = moderate, 4 = stout (20–40% overweight), 5 = obese (>40% overweight)
• Sites of adipose tissue to evaluate during physical examination include the intraabdominal region and inguinal and axillary regions.
• Lethargy and rear limb weakness are common presenting complaints. Due to their elongated body conformation, some severely obese ferrets may have difficulty lifting their body weight with their hind legs.

### CAUSES
Most commonly, excessive access to highly palatable food, often combined with insufficient activity. Owners usually leave food out continuously and supplement by feeding sugary treats and other palatable foods as part of a social activity.

### RISK FACTORS
• Owner lifestyle
• Diet palatability and energy density
• Activity level

## DIAGNOSIS

### DIFFERENTIAL DIAGNOSIS
#### Differentiating Similar Signs
• Normal seasonal weight gain—many normal ferrets will gain weight and develop a thick hair coat in the fall, with subsequent loss in the spring.
• Pregnancy
• Ascites
• Intraabdominal neoplasia or organomegaly (especially splenomegaly)
• The accumulation of fat around peripheral lymph nodes may mimic lymphadenopathy.

#### Differentiating Causes
Similar problems/diseases should be differentiated via history, physical examination, laboratory evaluation, and imaging.

### CBC/BIOCHEMISTRY/URINALYSIS
Normal

### OTHER LABORATORY TESTS
Normal

### IMAGING
Demonstrates excess body fat

### DIAGNOSTIC PROCEDURES
N/A

## TREATMENT
Success is lifelong amelioration of the problem.

### DIET
Discontinue feeding sweet-tasting or high-fat treats and dietary supplements.

### CLIENT EDUCATION
• Most important part of obesity therapy; must be tailored to each particular circumstance
• Discontinue feeding all sweet-tasting or high-fat treats and dietary supplements.
• Most ferrets should have food available free choice if left alone in a cage for the day. Ferrets tend to become hypoglycemic relatively quickly when fasted, and should not go longer than 4–6 hours without food. This is especially true in those with insulinomas.
• If possible, obese ferrets should be released from the cage for exercise and feeding at regular intervals throughout the day, thereby feeding frequent small meals with a reduced total volume of food.
• If the owner's schedule does not allow for this and food is made continuously available in the obese ferret's cage, change to a high-quality feline adult maintenance diet and decrease the amount fed until the desired weight loss is achieved.
• When obesity is caused by owners overfeeding treats as a means of social interaction with the ferret, achieving weight loss can be more challenging. Many of these clients do not seek veterinary help until the ferret is morbidly obese and having difficulty ambulating. At this point, the health risks to the ferret are obvious and clients are more willing to comply.
• Recommended resting energy requirement intake has been reported to be 70 kcal/kg body weight per day. This recommendation may be excessive for a sedentary, cage-bound pet ferret. Optimally, the owners should quantitate exactly the volume of kibble the ferret is eating per day, and caloric content of that volume should be calculated. If the ferret has become obese on a diet containing ≤70 kcal/kg body weight per day, the total volume of food fed per day should be reduced. If treats are fed, the amount of dry kibble fed should be reduced so as to not exceed resting energy requirements. Replace sugary treats with meat-based protein treats.
• Older literature reports that ferrets need a diet containing at least 28% fat. In a sedentary ferret, this may lead to obesity. Current recommendation is a diet containing only 15–20% fat.
• The feeding of high-fiber carbohydrate-based cat foods is not recommended. Ferrets have a short large intestine and a limited ability to properly digest these products.

## MEDICATIONS

### DRUG(S) OF CHOICE
N/A

### CONTRAINDICATIONS
N/A

### PRECAUTIONS
N/A

### POSSIBLE INTERACTIONS
N/A

### ALTERNATIVE DRUGS
N/A

## FOLLOW-UP

### PATIENT MONITORING
• Lifelong follow-up and support are essential to maintain the reduced weight.

• At the initial visit instruct clients to recognize moderate body condition score and to feed the quantity of food necessary to maintain this condition during the changing physiologic and environmental conditions of the pet's life; remind them at checkups.

**POSSIBLE COMPLICATIONS**
N/A

 **MISCELLANEOUS**

**ASSOCIATED CONDITIONS**
• Hepatic lipidosis
• Orthopedic problems
• Insulinoma
• Increased anesthetic risk
• Cardiovascular problems

**AGE-RELATED FACTORS**
N/A

**ZOONOTIC POTENTIAL**
N/A

**PREGNANCY**
Obesity may increase risk of dystocia; however, because of potential risk to the fetus, do not treat pregnant animals.

**SYNONYMS**
N/A

**SEE ALSO**
• Ataxia
• Insulinoma
• Paresis and paralysis

**ABBREVIATIONS**
N/A

*Suggested Reading*
Bell JA. Ferret nutrition. Vet Clin North Am Exotic Anim Pract 1999;2(1):169–192.
Irlbeck NA. Dietary management of ferrets. Proc of The North Am Vet Conf 2001: 877–879.
Williams BH. Therapeutics in ferrets. Vet Clin North Am Exotic Anim Pract 2000; 3(1):131–153.

*Portions Adapted From*
Buffington, CAT. Obesity. In: Tilley LP, Smith FWK, Jr., eds. The 5-Minute Veterinary Consult: Canine and Feline, 2nd Ed. Baltimore: Lippincott Williams & Wilkins, 2000.

# OTITIS EXTERNA AND MEDIA

## BASICS

### OVERVIEW
• Otis externa—inflammation of the external ear canal; rarely seen in ferrets except in animals with ear mites
• Otitis media—inflammation of the middle ear, usually an extension of otitis externa through a ruptured tympanum (extension of otitis externa or through overaggressive cleaning); rarely occurs without a membrane being ruptured; anecdotal reports suggest that neoplasia within the middle ear is common.
• Normal ferrets usually have thick, red-brown or black crusts in the outer ear—may or may not be associated with otitis

### SIGNALMENT
No age or sex predilection; rare disease in ferrets

### SIGNS
• Otitis externa—often a secondary symptom of an underlying disease (mites or overzealous cleaning)
• Infection—purulent and malodorous exudate
• Inflammation—exudation, pain, pruritus, and erythema

#### Historical Findings
• Pain
• Head shaking
• Scratching at the pinnae
• Malodorous ears

#### Physical Examination Findings
• Thick, red-brown or black crusts in the outer ear—may or may not be associated with otitis; this type of material is usually a normal finding in ferret ears.
• Redness and swelling of the external canal
• Exudation—may result in malodor and canal obstruction
• Vestibular signs are extremely rare (head tilt, nystagmus, anorexia, and ataxia), but indicate development of otitis media/interna.

### CAUSES AND RISK FACTORS
• *Otodectes cynotis* mite (ear mites) infestation is common in ferrets.
• Secondary bacterial infections occasionally occur.
• Secondary mycotic infection—*Malassezia* sp. rarely occur.
• Neoplasia of the ear canal (carcinoma, epithelioma) or nearby structures (salivary glands) may predispose.
• Topical drug reaction, irritation, hypersensitivity, and trauma from abrasive cleaning techniques may occur when using topical cleaning solutions.

• Excessive moisture (e.g., from frequent cleanings with improper solutions) can lead to infection; overzealous client compliance with recommendations for ear cleanings may predispose.

## DIAGNOSIS

### DIFFERENTIAL DIAGNOSIS

#### Differentiating Similar Signs
• Normal ferrets often have a dark, red-brown crumbly exudate. This must be differentiated from otitis based on clinical signs, otic examination, and cytology.
• Purulent, odiferous exudate is abnormal and indicates otitis.
• The presence of even normal-appearing exudate in only one ear suggests unilateral disease.
• Alopecia and pruritus around the pinna may be caused by ferret adrenal disease, fleas, sarcoptic mange, or dermatophytes.
• Recurrent, unilateral disease—neoplasia should be strongly suspected.

### CBC/BIOCHEMISTRY/URINALYSIS
May indicate a primary underlying disease

### OTHER LABORATORY TESTS
N/A

### IMAGING
Bullae radiographs—otitis media

### DIAGNOSTIC PROCEDURES
• Microscopic examination of aural exudate—single most important diagnostic tool after complete examination of the ear canal
• Culture of exudate—to assist with antibiotic selection; most important in resistant infection
• Infections within the canal can change with prolonged or recurrent therapy; repeat examination of aural exudate is required in chronic cases.

#### Microscopic Examination
• Preparations—make from both canals (the contents of the canals may not be the same); spread samples thinly on a glass microscope slide; examine both unstained and modified Wright-stained samples.
• Mites—visible with oil preparations or grossly with magnification
• Type(s) of bacteria or yeast—assist in the choice of therapy
• Findings (types of organisms; WBCs)—note in the record; rank the number of organisms and cell types on a scale of 0–4 to allow treatment monitoring.
• WBCs within the exudate—active infection; systemic antibiotic therapy may be warranted.

## TREATMENT

### APPROPRIATE HEALTH CARE
Outpatient, unless severe vestibular signs are noted

### SURGICAL CONSIDERATIONS
• Indicated when neoplasia is diagnosed
• Severe, unresponsive otitis media is extremely rare in ferrets; if diagnosed, a bullae osteotomy may be indicated.

## MEDICATIONS

### DRUG(S) OF CHOICE

#### Systemic
• Antibiotics—useful in severe cases of bacterial otitis externa; mandatory when the tympanum has ruptured; trimethoprim/sulfonamide (15–30 mg/kg PO, SC q12h), enrofloxacin (10–20 mg/kg PO, SC, IM q12h), or cephalexin (15–25 mg/kg PO q8–12h)
• Corticosteroids—reduce swelling and pain; reduce wax production; antiinflammatory dosages of prednisone (0.25–0.5 mg/kg q12h); use sparingly and for short durations only.

#### Topical
• Topical therapy is necessary for resolution and control of otitis externa; however, the small size of the ear canal may hinder client compliance.
• Ivermectin 1% (Ivomec, Merck Agvet)—use parenterally or topically; parenteral: 0.2–0.4 mg/kg SC q14d for three to four doses; topical treatment with ivermectin has shown to be more effective in the treatment of ear mites. Topical: diluted 1:10 in propylene glycol—instill 400 µg/kg divided into each ear topically, repeat in 2 weeks; it is not necessary to clean the ears thoroughly to remove debris prior to topical administration of ivermectin since debris may aid in retention of medication in the canal. Do not use topical and parenteral ivermectin concurrently
• Thiabendazole product (Tresaderm, Merck AgVet) at feline dosages has also been used topically to treat ear mites; however, treatment failures are common due to owner compliance and the small size of the ear canal.
• If secondary bacterial or yeast infection is diagnosed, completely clean the external ear canal of debris.
• Thorough cleaning of the ear daily during initial therapy may be necessary with severe bacterial infections; not recommended routinely or when ear mites alone are diagnosed since cleaners are more likely to irritate the

canal and exacerbate disease; if necessary use mild cleaners for routine cleaning or when the competence of the tympanic membrane is in question; cerumenolytics—dioctyl sodium sulfosuccinate or carbamide peroxide emulsify waxes, facilitating removal.
• Generally, ingredients should be limited to those needed to treat a specific infection (i.e., antibiotics only for a bacterial infection).

### CONTRAINDICATIONS

• Use extreme caution when cleaning the external ear canals of all animals with severe and chronic otitis externa, because the tympanum can easily be ruptured.
• Ivermectin—do not use in pregnant jills.
• Do not use topical and parenteral ivermectin concurrently.
• Ruptured tympanum—use caution with topical cleansers and medications other than sterile saline or dilute acetic acid; potential for ototoxicity is a concern; controversial

### PRECAUTIONS

• All products discussed above are off-label use. Safety and efficacy have not been evaluated in ferrets. Use with caution, especially in young or debilitated animals
• Several topical medications infrequently induce contact irritation or allergic response; reevaluate all worsening cases.

### ALTERNATIVE DRUGS

Selamectin (Revolution) is effective in treating ear mites in dogs and cats, and has been anecdotally used in ferrets; however, safety, efficacy, and dosing have not been evaluated.

 FOLLOW-UP

### PATIENT MONITORING

Repeat exudate examinations can assist in monitoring infection.

### PREVENTION/AVOIDANCE

• Avoid overzealous cleaning of the ear canal.
• Control of underlying diseases

### POSSIBLE COMPLICATIONS

Uncontrolled otitis externa can lead to otitis media, deafness, vestibular disease, cellulitis, facial nerve paralysis, progression to otitis interna, and rarely meningoencephalitis.

### EXPECTED COURSE AND PROGNOSIS

• Otitis due to *Otodectes* mites—prognosis is good; may recur if treated with topical preparations and owner compliance is poor
• Otitis externa—depends on underlying cause; failure to correct underlying primary cause results in recurrence.

 MISCELLANEOUS

### ASSOCIATED CONDITIONS

N/A

### AGE-RELATED FACTORS

N/A

### ZOONOTIC POTENTIAL

Potentially fungal infection

### PREGNANCY

Do not use ivermectin in pregnant jills.

### SYNONYMS

N/A

### SEE ALSO

• Adrenal disease
• Ear mites
• Pruritus

### ABBREVIATION

WBC = white blood cell

*Suggested Reading*

Clyde VL. Practical treatment and control of common ectoparasites in exotic pets. Vet Med 1996;91(7):632–637.

Fox JG. Parasitic diseases. In: Fox JG, ed. Biology and Diseases of the Ferret. 2nd Ed. Baltimore: Williams & Wilkins 1998:375–392.

Kelleher SA. Skin diseases of the ferret. Vet Clin North Am Exotic Anim Pract 2001;4(2):565–572.

Orcutt C. Dermatologic diseases. In: Hillyer EV, Quesenberry KE, eds. Ferrets, Rabbits and Rodents: Clinical Medicine and Surgery. Philadelphia: WB Saunders, 1997:115–125.

*Portions Adapted From*

Werner AA. Otitis Externa and Media. In: Tilley LP, Smith FWK, Jr., eds. The 5-Minute Veterinary Consult: Canine and Feline, 3rd Ed. Baltimore: Lippincott Williams & Wilkins, 2003.

# PARESIS AND PARALYSIS

## BASICS

### DEFINITION
- Paresis—weakness of voluntary movement
- Paralysis—lack of voluntary movement
- Quadriparesis (tetraparesis)—weakness of voluntary movements in all limbs. Mild to moderate generalized weakness (tetraparesis) commonly appears as posterior paresis when due to systemic or metabolic disease. Front limb involvement is more apparent with structural neurologic disorders or with advanced metabolic disease.
- Quadriplegia (tetraplegia)—absence of all voluntary limb movement
- Paraparesis—weakness of voluntary movements in pelvic limbs. Posterior paresis is an extremely common finding in ferrets with systemic disease.
- Paraplegia—absence of all voluntary pelvic limb movement

### PATHOPHYSIOLOGY
- Weakness—may be caused by lesions in the upper or lower motor neuron system. In ferrets, weakness is one of the most common presenting complaints. Weakness, especially paraparesis, is usually due to the effects of systemic or metabolic disease (e.g., hypoglycemia or anemia) or severe obesity. Weakness due to structural damage to the CNS or PNS occurs less commonly.
- Evaluation of limb reflexes—determine which system (upper or lower motor neuron) is involved.
- Upper motor neurons and their axons—inhibitory influence on the large motor neurons of the lower motor neuron system; maintain normal muscle tone and normal spinal reflexes; if injured, spinal reflexes are no longer inhibited or controlled and reflexes become exaggerated or hyperreflexic.
- Lower motor neurons or their processes (peripheral nerves)—if injured, spinal reflexes cannot be elicited (areflexic) or are reduced (hyporeflexic).

### SYSTEMS AFFECTED
*Nervous*
- Endocrine/metabolic—hypoglycemia
- Hemic/lymphatic—anemia

### SIGNALMENT
Any age or gender

### SIGNS

*General Comments*
*Limb Weakness—Acute or Gradual Onset*
- Acute onset generally seen with structural CNS or PNS damage
- Gradual or intermittent weakness seen with systemic or metabolic disease, severe obesity, or sometimes spinal cord damage

*Historical Findings*
- Ferrets with posterior paresis lose the normal arched appearance of the spine when standing or walking—spinal alignment appears flat or parallel to the ground; may progress to dragging the hind limbs, intermittently or continuously
- Weakness may be accompanied by other signs such as lethargy, ptyalism, and stargazing, especially with metabolic diseases.
- Many focal compressive spinal cord diseases begin with ataxia and progress to weakness and finally to paralysis.

*Physical Examination Findings*
- Other than paresis or paralysis, usually normal with structural spinal cord damage
- Often normal in ferrets with insulinomas unless hypoglycemic at the time of physical examination
- If in pain (vertebral disease, disk extrusion), patient may resent handling and manipulation during the examination.
- With systemic or metabolic disease—weight loss, splenomegaly, depression, or dehydration may be seen.
- Severe obesity may cause locomotor difficulty.

*Neurologic Examination Findings*
- Confirm that the problem is weakness or paralysis.
- Localize problem to either lower or upper motor neuron system.
- Paraplegia—bladder may also be paralyzed in ferrets with structural spinal cord damage.

### CAUSES

*Metabolic Disease—Most Common Cause of Posterior Paresis*
- Anemia—seen with hyperestrogenism, blood loss (especially from gastrointestinal tract), leukemia, CRF
- Hypoglycemia—from insulinomas, gastrointestinal foreign bodies, severe hepatic disease, or sepsis
- Cardiac disease
- Severe obesity—due to their elongated body conformation, some severely obese ferrets may have difficulty lifting their body weight with their hind legs.

*Neurologic Disease—CNS or Spinal Cord Disease*
*CNS*
- Neoplastic—any tumor of the CNS (primary or secondary)
- Infectious—CDV, rabies (rear limb ataxia may be the only clinical sign in ferrets with rabies), and any other CNS infection affecting the brain
- Inflammatory, immune-mediated—ADV-induced encephalomyelitis
- Toxic—metronidazole

*Spinal Cord*
- Traumatic—intervertebral disc herniation; fracture or luxation
- Neoplastic—primary bone tumors (especially chondroma, chondrosarcoma); multiple myeloma and metastatic tumors that infiltrate the vertebral body
- Vascular—hematomyelia due to the effects of hyperestrogenism, infarct (rare)
- Infectious—discospondylitis, myelitis (rare)

### RISK FACTORS
N/A

## DIAGNOSIS

### DIFFERENTIAL DIAGNOSIS

*Weak Pelvic Limbs*
- Pain or hyperesthesia elicited at site of spinal cord damage seen with trauma, IVD disease (rare in ferrets), discospondylitis, and some bone tumors. Lack of pain along spinal column—vascular disease (hemorrhage, infarct), some neoplasias, CNS lesions, systemic or metabolic disease
- Acute onset—most common with spinal cord trauma, bone tumors, occasionally CNS disease
- Gradual onset or intermittent weakness—usually systemic or metabolic disease, occasionally seen with IVD extrusion, if extrusion is gradual
- Spinal reflexes—localize weakness to the cervical, thoracolumbar, or lower lumbar cord segments
- Hypoglycemia—intermittent or episodic weakness; often see other signs: ptyalism, star-gazing, tremors, retching or vomiting, diarrhea, poor haircoat, lethargy
- Anemia—pale mucous membranes, petechia or ecchymosis, lethargy, melena, hematemesis, swollen vulva (hyperestrogenism)
- Cardiac disease—murmurs, arrhythmias, collapse with exercise, syncope
- Musculoskeletal disorders—typically produce lameness and a reluctance to move
- Only limbs affected—likely spinal cord dysfunction if all four limbs affected: lesion is in the cervical area or is multifocal to diffuse; only pelvic limbs affected: may be metabolic disease or spinal cord dysfunction; spinal lesion is anywhere below the second thoracic vertebra.

### CBC/BIOCHEMISTRY/URINALYSIS
Usually normal, unless systemic or metabolic diseases involved (e.g., hypoglycemia, electrolyte imbalance, and anemia)

### OTHER LABORATORY TESTS
- Hypoglycemia—simultaneous fasting glucose and insulin determination—may be

helpful in supporting the diagnosis of insulinoma. Be certain that the insulin assay used has been validated for use in ferrets.
• Anemia—differentiate as nonregenerative or regenerative on the basis of the reticulocyte count or bone marrow aspirate.
• Electrolyte imbalance—correct the problem; see if weakness resolves.
• Serum electrophoresis—hypergammaglobulinemia (gammaglobulins >20% of total protein) seen in ferrets with ADV. Perform counterimmunoelectrophoresis (CEP) available through United Vaccines (Madison, WI) as a screening test for ADV.
• Immunofluorescent antibody (IFA) test—to rule out CDV; can be performed on peripheral blood or buffy coat smears or conjunctival or mucous membrane scrapings. False negatives are possible.

### IMAGING
• Spinal radiographs—lesion localized to the spinal cord; may reveal bony tumor, fracture, or luxation; disk herniation and discospondylitis are rare findings.
• Thoracic radiographs—identify neoplasia.
• CT or MRI—if CNS disease suspected; evaluate potential brain disease.
• Abdominal ultrasonography—if hepatic, renal, adrenal, or pancreatic dysfunction suspected
• Echocardiography—if cardiac disease is suspected

### DIAGNOSTIC PROCEDURES
• CSF analysis—do before myelography to detect myelitis and meningitis; if high protein or cell numbers are found, a culture is warranted.
• Myelography—may establish evidence of spinal cord compression. Use 22-gauge spinal needle; infuse iohexol (0.25–0.50 mL/kg)
• Location for CSF tap or myelography—atlanto-occipital region or L5–L6 region

## TREATMENT
• Inpatient—with severe weakness or paralysis
• Activity—restrict until spinal trauma and disk herniation can be ruled out.
• Bedding—move paralyzed patients away from soiled bedding; check and clean frequently to prevent urine scalding and superficial pyoderma; use padded bedding or a waterbed to help prevent decubital ulcer formation.
• Turning—turn quadriplegic patients from side to side four to eight times daily; prevent hypostatic lung congestion and decubital ulcer formation.
• Surgery—for insulinoma, gastrointestinal foreign bodies, fracture, and some neoplasias

## MEDICATIONS

### DRUG(S) OF CHOICE
• Not recommended until the source or cause of the problem is identified
• Methylprednisolone sodium succinate—30 mg/kg IV followed by 15 mg/kg 2 and 6 hours later; may be beneficial for suspected trauma. Other causes (e.g., disk herniation or fibrocartilaginous embolism) are rare.

### CONTRAINDICATIONS
Corticosteroids—do not use with discospondylitis or other infectious causes of paresis/paralysis.

### PRECAUTIONS
Corticosteroids—associated with gastrointestinal ulceration and hemorrhage, delayed wound healing, and heightened susceptibility to infection

### POSSIBLE INTERACTIONS
N/A

### ALTERNATIVE DRUGS
• Dexamethasone—0.5–1 mg/kg q24–48h
• Prednisolone—1–2 mg/kg q12–24h

## FOLLOW-UP

### PATIENT MONITORING
• Neurologic examinations—daily to monitor status
• Bladder—evacuate (via manual expression or catheterization) three to four times a day to prevent overdistension and subsequent bladder atony; once bladder function has returned, patient can be managed at home.

### POSSIBLE COMPLICATIONS
• Urinary tract infection, bladder atony, urine scalding and pyoderma, constipation, decubital ulcer formation
• Spinal cord or neuromuscular disease—progression to weakness and possibly paralysis
• Hypoglycemia—seizures, stupor, coma

## MISCELLANEOUS

### ASSOCIATED CONDITIONS
N/A

### AGE-RELATED FACTORS
N/A

### ZOONOTIC POTENTIAL
Rabies—rare cause of paresis/paralysis in ferrets, but when present has extreme zoonotic potential. Rabies cases must be strictly quarantined and confined to prevent exposure to humans and other animals. Local and state regulations must be adhered to carefully and completely.

### PREGNANCY
N/A

### SEE ALSO
• Gastrointestinal foreign body
• Insulinoma
• Parvovirus Infection (Aleutian disease virus)
• See specific diseases

### ABBREVIATION
• ADV = Aleutian disease virus (parvovirus)
• CDV = Canine distemper virus
• CNS = Central nervous system
• CRF = Chronic renal failure
• CSF = cerebrospinal fluid
• CT = computed tomography
• IVD = Intervertebral disc
• MRI = magnetic resonance imaging
• PNS = peripheral nervous system

*Suggested Reading*
Antinoff N. Musculoskeletal and neurologic diseases. In: Hillyer EV, Quesenberry KE, eds. Ferrets, Rabbits and Rodents: Clinical Medicine and Surgery. Philadelphia: WB Saunders, 1997:126–130.
Caplan ER, Peterson ME, Mulles HS, et al. Diagnosis and treatment of insulin-secreting pancreatic islet cell tumors in ferrets: 57 cases (1986–1994). J Am Vet Med Assoc 1996;209:1741–1745.
de Lahunta A. Veterinary Neuroanatomy and Clinical Neurology. 2nd Ed. Philadelphia: Saunders, 1983.
Hoefer HL. Cardiac disease in ferrets. Proc North Am Vet Conf 1995:577–578.
Oliver JE, Lorenz MD, Kornegay JN. Tetraparesis, hemiparesis, and ataxia. In: Handbook of Veterinary Neurology. 3rd Ed. Philadelphia: Saunders, 1997:173–215.
Weiss CA, Williams BH, Scott MV. Insulinoma in the ferret: clinical findings and treatment comparison of 66 cases. J Am Anim Hosp Assoc 1998;34:471–475.
Withrow SJ. Localization and diagnosis of spinal cord lesions in small animals. Part 1. Compend Contin Educ Pract Vet 1980; 2:464–474.

*Portions Adapted From*
Shell LG. Paralysis. In: Tilley LP, Smith FWK, Jr., eds. The 5-Minute Veterinary Consult: Canine and Feline, 2nd Ed. Baltimore: Lippincott Williams & Wilkins, 2000.

# PARVOVIRUS INFECTION (ALEUTIAN DISEASE VIRUS [ADV])

## BASICS

### DEFINITION
• Aleutian disease virus (ADV) is a parvovirus that can infect mink and ferrets.
• Aleutian mink (mink bred for a grey color dilution) are exquisitely susceptible to ADV, and severe illness is seen in these animals. Other color varieties of mink show varying degrees of illness. Ferrets are also susceptible to ADV; the extent of illness is dependent on the strain of virus and host immunity.
• ADV-F is a strain of ADV recently isolated from clinically ill ferrets. It is genetically very similar, but not identical to strains of ADV isolated from mink. Other strains of ADV have not yet been characterized, but likely exist.
• ADV is a chronic systemic illness characterized by wasting and nervous system signs.
• Not all ferrets infected with ADV will become clinically ill.
• Ferrets may be persistently infected but remain asymptomatic, be persistently infected and develop clinical disease (sometimes months to years after infection), or eliminate the virus with or without showing clinical signs.

### PATHOPHYSIOLOGY
• Although the exact mode of natural transmission has not been documented in ferrets, it is presumed to have both aerosol and oral routes (similar to CDV in mink). The virus may be transmitted by direct contact with urine, saliva, blood, or feces, or through fomites.
• Unlike parvoviral infections in dogs and cats, disease is caused by the long-term effects of immune-complex deposition, not by the cytotoxic effect of the virus.
• Exposure to the virus causes an antibody response and subsequent plasma cell proliferation; however, the antibody response is not protective.
• Virus-antibody complex deposition results in glomerulonephritis, arteritis, and lymphoplasmacytic infiltrates in the liver, kidneys, spleen, lymph nodes, gastrointestinal tract, and nervous tissues.
• The course of the disease is usually protracted, extending over 18–24 months.
• It is presumed that ferrets with antibody titers to ADV are shedding the virus; however, the mode or duration of viral shedding is currently unknown.

### SYSTEMS AFFECTED
• Hemic/lymphatic/immune—hypergammaglobulinemia; thymus, lymph nodes, spleen: plasmacytic infiltration
• Renal—membranoproliferative glomerulonephritis, lymphoplasmacytic nephritis
• Hepatobiliary—bile duct hyperplasia, portal lymphoplasmacytic hepatitis

• Nervous—nonsuppurative encephalomyelitis, nonsuppurative meningitis
• Gastrointestinal—lymphoplasmacytic enteritis
• Cardiovascular—lymphoplasmacytic arteritis
• Respiratory—interstitial pneumonia, pleural effusion
• Ophthalmic—anterior uveitis

### GENETICS
Unknown

### INCIDENCE/PREVALENCE
• Most common in breeding facilities, animal shelters, and pet stores
• Limited data available for prevalence rates; rates within individual colonies of ferrets from 42 to 60% have been reported, based on serum antibody titers.

### GEOGRAPHIC DISTRIBUTION
Worldwide

### SIGNALMENT
No age or sex predilection

### SIGNS

#### General Comments
Suspect ADV infection in ferrets with chronic wasting, other nonspecific signs (lethargy, intermittent anorexia), or neurologic signs combined with hypergammaglobulinemia.

#### Historical Findings
• Chronic, progressive weight loss
• Nonspecific signs: lethargy, anorexia, poor haircoat, collapse
• Neurologic signs include: rear limb paresis, which may progress cranially, fecal and/or urinary incontinence, and head tremors
• Melena or frank hemorrhage from the gastrointestinal tract
• Coughing, dyspnea

#### Physical Examination Findings
• Emaciation and muscle wasting are consistent features.
• Rear limb paresis, muscle atrophy in the rear limbs
• Head tremors
• Splenomegaly may be palpated.
• Occasionally, enlarged mesenteric lymph nodes are palpable.
• Pale mucous membranes with anemic animals
• Signs of dehydration

### RISK FACTORS
• Exposure to mink
• Exposure to ADV-positive ferrets
• Crowding and poor sanitation increases the risk of infection.
• Copathogens such as parasites, viruses, and certain bacterial species hypothesized to exacerbate illness; ferrets with ADV are presumed to be immunosuppressed, and therefore more susceptible to other pathogens.

## DIAGNOSIS

### GENERAL COMMENTS
Definitive diagnosis of ADV requires viral isolation or detection in tissue samples. A presumptive diagnosis can be made based on the presence of supportive clinical signs, hypergammaglobulinemia, positive serologic testing, and exclusion of other causes.

### DIFFERENTIAL DIAGNOSIS
• For chronic wasting—gastrointestinal foreign bodies, *Helicobacter mustelae*, infiltrative bowel disease (eosinophilic gastroenteritis, lymphoplasmacytic enteritis, lymphosarcoma), neoplasia, estrogen-induced anemia
• For rear limb paresis and tremors—spinal cord disease, insulinoma, heavy metal toxicosis, CDV, rabies

### CBC/BIOCHEMISTRY/URINALYSIS
• Serum protein electrophoresis—the hallmark of ADV is hypergammaglobulinemia. Gammaglobulins usually represent >20% of total protein; hypoalbuminemia may also be seen.
• Leukopenia and/or anemia—occasionally seen
• Increased BUN and creatinine with severe renal disease
• Increased liver enzymes in ferrets with hepatic involvement

### OTHER LABORATORY TESTS

#### Serologic Testing
• Counterimmunoelectrophoresis (CEP), available through United Vaccines (Madison, WI), can be used as a screening test. Positive test indicates exposure to virus and the presence of antibodies. Not all ferrets with positive titers will develop the disease. A positive test, coupled with clinical signs and hypergammaglobulinemia, supports, but does not confirm, the diagnosis of ADV. The results are reported only as positive or negative. Therefore, a rise in titer, indicating ongoing infection, cannot be detected.
• An ADV antibody ELISA test is available through Avecon Diagnostics, Inc. (Perkasic, PA) that detects antibody in either saliva or blood. Likewise, a positive result indicates exposure to virus; not all ferrets that have been exposed will develop the disease. A positive result, combined with clinical data, supports, but does not confirm, the diagnosis of ADV.
• Immunofluorescent antibody (IFA) test, available through Diagnostic Laboratory, Division of Comparative Medicine, Massachusetts Institute of Technology (Cambridge, MA), can be used to detect a rise in titer, suggesting active infection. A positive titer, coupled with clinical signs and hypergammaglobulinemia, supports, but does not confirm, the diagnosis of ADV.

## PARVOVIRUS INFECTION (ALEUTIAN DISEASE VIRUS [ADV])

### IMAGING
• Abdominal radiographs are usually normal, but may reveal splenomegaly and either an increase or decrease in the size of the kidneys. Thoracic radiographs may demonstrate pleural effusion or an interstitial pattern in animals with pneumonia (rare).
• Radiographs may be helpful to rule out other causes of rear limb paresis, such as vertebral disorders.

### DIAGNOSTIC PROCEDURES
• PCR-enhanced DNA probe can be used to detect virus in tissue samples.
• Virus may be identified in tissue samples by electron microscopy.

### PATHOLOGIC FINDINGS
• Gross changes are often absent, other than emaciation and muscle wasting. Other reported changes include enlarged spleen, enlarged mesenteric lymph nodes, small kidneys, pleural effusion, hemorrhagic pneumonia, lung lobe consolidation, cardiomegaly, and frank hemorrhage into the small intestinal lumen.
• Histopathology demonstrates immune complex deposition and lymphoplasmacytic infiltration including portal and periportal lymphoplasmacytic hepatitis, membranoproliferative glomerulonephritis, interstitial lymphoplasmacytic nephritis, nonsuppurative encephalomyelitis, perivascular accumulations of plasmacytes and astrocytic hypertrophy in spinal cord, hemorrhagic intersitial pneumonia, and multifocal arteritis (may include cardiac muscle)

### TREATMENT

### APPROPRIATE HEALTH CARE
• Symptomatic and supportive only—there is no specific treatment for ADV.
• Intensity depends on the severity of signs on examination.
• Proper, strict isolation procedures are essential. Exercise care to prevent spread of ADV, a very stable virus.

### NURSING CARE
Symptomatic therapy includes attention to fluid and electrolyte derangements, reduction in environmental stressors, and modification of the diet to improve palatability.

### ACTIVITY
N/A

### DIET
• Most ferrets will accept high-calorie dietary supplements such as Nutri-Cal (EVSCO Pharmaceuticals, Buena, NJ), Ensure (Abbott Laboratories, North Chicago, IL), or Clinicare Feline (Abbott Laboratories, North Chicago, IL). Administer these supplements several times a day.  Some anorectic ferrets will accept meat-based human baby foods or moistened ferret pellets, especially if these foods are warmed to body temperature.
• Reported resting energy requirement for healthy ferrets is 70 k/cal/kg body weight per day.

### CLIENT EDUCATION
Inform about the need for thorough disinfection, especially if other ferrets are on the premises. See prevention.

### SURGICAL CONSIDERATIONS
N/A

### MEDICATIONS

### DRUG(S) OF CHOICE
• Treat secondary or opportunistic infections with the appropriate antibiotic or antiparasitic agent.
• Prednisone (1.25–2.5 mg/kg PO q24h) may decrease the progression of the immune-mediated effects of ADV in some ferrets.

### CONTRAINDICATIONS
N/A

### PRECAUTIONS
Use caution with prednisone treatment in animals with concurrent infectious diseases.

### POSSIBLE INTERACTIONS
N/A

### ALTERNATIVE DRUGS
Cyclophosphamide (10 mg/kg IP 3 times weekly for 13 weeks) has been shown to be effective in decreasing the immune-mediated effects of ADV in mink. Use in ferrets has not been reported. Side effects were serious and included anorexia, cyanosis, and leukopenia.

### FOLLOW-UP

### PATIENT MONITORING
N/A

### PREVENTION/AVOIDANCE
• Vaccines are not available and would be contraindicated due to the immune-mediated effects of this disease.
• The virus can survive for months, especially in the presence of gross debris. Thoroughly clean all organic debris and apply a 1:30 dilution of bleach (5% sodium hypochlorite).
• It is assumed that all serologically positive ferrets are capable of shedding the virus. Serologically positive animals should not be housed in the same home as serologically negative animals.

### POSSIBLE COMPLICATIONS
Secondary bacterial, parasitic, or viral infections

### EXPECTED COURSE AND PROGNOSIS
• Prognosis is good to guarded in asymptomatic ferrets testing positive on serology. These ferrets may never develop clinical disease. If clinical disease eventually develops, the prognosis depends on the strain of virus and organ system affected.
• Prognosis is guarded in severely affected ferrets and ferrets demonstrating neurologic signs. Signs may or may not progress, and there are no predictive diagnostic tests available.

### MISCELLANEOUS

### ASSOCIATED CONDITIONS
N/A

### AGE-RELATED FACTORS
N/A

### ZOONOTIC POTENTIAL
N/A

### PREGNANCY
No in utero infections have been reported in ferrets.

### SYNONYMS
Mink parvovirus

### SEE ALSO
• Paresis and paralysis
• Weight loss and cachexia

### ABBREVIATIONS
• BUN = blood urea nitrogen
• CDV = canine distemper virus
• ELISA = enzyme-linked immunosorbent assay
• PCR = polymerase chain reaction

*Suggested Reading*

Fox JG, Pearson RC, Gorham JR. Viral diseases. In: Fox JG, ed. Biology and Diseases of the Ferret. 2nd Ed. Baltimore: Williams & Wilkins, 1998.

McCrackin Stevenson MA, Murray J, Gates L, et al. Aleutian mink disease parvovirus: implications for companion ferrets. Compend Contin Edu Pract Vet 2001;23(2):178–185.

Palley LS. Parvovirus-associated syndrome (Aleutian disease) in two ferrets. J Am Vet Med Assoc 1992;201:100–106.

Une Y, Wakimoto Y, Kakano Y, et al. Spontaneous Aleutian disease in a ferret. J Vet Med Sci 2000;62(5):553–555.

Williams BH. Ferret microbiology and virology. In: Fudge AM, ed. Laboratory Medicine, Avian and Exotic Pets. Philadelphia: WB Saunders, 2000:334–342.

# PETECHIA/ECCHYMOSIS/BRUISING

## BASICS

### DEFINITION
Disorders of primary hemostasis (platelet- or vessel-wall–mediated) that result in bleeding into the skin or mucous membranes to a degree out of proportion to the trauma

### PATHOPHYSIOLOGY
• Thrombocytopenia is the most common cause of petechia or ecchymosis in ferrets. Defective platelet function causing impaired primary hemostasis (i.e., failure of platelet plug formation) has not been reported in ferrets but should be considered since little is known about hemostasis in ferrets.
• Thrombocytopenia—caused by impaired thrombopoiesis, shortened platelet life span, or platelet sequestration
• Acquired platelet function deficits (not reported in ferrets, but should be considered)—may be associated with uremia, drugs (e.g., aspirin), dysproteinemia, or myeloproliferative disease

### SYSTEMS AFFECTED
• Hemic/lymph/immune
• Skin/exocrine—petechia/ecchymosis/bruising
• Respiratory—epistaxis
• Renal/urologic—hematuria
• Gastrointestinal—melena

### SIGNALMENT
• Seen most commonly in intact females with hyperestrogenism
• Other causes of thrombocytopenia and platelet function defects are not associated with age or sex predisposition.

### SIGNS
• Hyperestrogenism—large vulva, serous or purulent vaginal discharge
• Bilaterally symmetric alopecia, usually beginning at the tail base and progressing cranially with ferret adrenal disease
• Splenomegaly

### CAUSES

#### Thrombocytopenia
• Low platelet production—hyperestrogenism (sustained estrus in intact females or ferret adrenal disease), myelophthisis
• Sequestration of platelets in a large spleen, liver, or other sizable mass of microvasculature usually does not lead to bleeding.
• Increase in platelet use or destruction—consumptive coagulopathy
• Immune-mediated disease—not yet reported in ferrets but should be considered

#### Thrombocytopathy
Acquired platelet function disorders (not described, but possible in ferrets in a similar manner as dogs and cats)—uremia, DIC, liver disease, myeloproliferative and lymphoproliferative disease, and treatment with NSAIDs

### RISK FACTORS
• Hyperestrogenism—failure to breed intact females, ovarian remnant in neutered females, ferret adrenal disease, estrogen-secreting adrenal tumors. Evidence suggests that ferret adrenal disease may be related to neutering at an early age.
• Previous administration of aspirin or other NSAIDs

## DIAGNOSIS

### DIFFERENTIAL DIAGNOSIS
• Usually are not mistaken for anything else; however, injuries causing an expected amount of bleeding or bruising must be ruled out by history and physical examination.
• Evidence of any of the diseases mentioned (see causes) should raise suspicion that it may be the underlying cause of petechiae or bruising.

### CBC/BIOCHEMISTRY/URINALYSIS
• Platelets are low either by estimation on a well-made blood smear or by a direct count in patients with thrombocytopenia; normal platelet count in ferrets (n = 5) 300,000 +/− 46,000/μL
• RBC fragmentation suggests DIC or other vascular disease.
• Patients with myeloproliferative and lymphoproliferative diseases may be leukemic or cytopenic.
• Biochemical analysis—rule out hepatic or renal causes

### OTHER LABORATORY TESTS
Coagulation studies—may help rule out DIC; however, very little data on normal values exist. Normal values (based on n = 6): APTT 18.4 ± 1.4 seconds; PT 10.3 ± 0.1 seconds; thrombin time 28.8 ± 8.7 seconds; whole blood clotting time 2 ± 0.5 minutes in glass tubes; normal values for FDP in ferrets have not been reported, so results must be interpreted from feline data.

### IMAGING
Abdominal radiography or ultrasonography may help identify splenomegaly or hepatomegaly.

### DIAGNOSTIC PROCEDURES
• The buccal mucosa bleeding time—long in patients with most of the thrombopathies in addition to thrombocytopenia; normal range in ferrets not reported, but presumed to be similar to dogs and cats (<4 minutes in dogs and <2 minutes in cats)
• Most invasive procedures are contraindicated in patients with bleeding disorders.
• Bone marrow examination—indicated if cytopenia is detected

## TREATMENT
Usually as inpatient until a definitive diagnosis is made

### NURSING CARE
• Discontinue any medications that may alter platelet function (e.g., aspirin and other NSAIDs).
• Indications for whole blood transfusion are the same as those for dogs or cats. In general, most ferrets will benefit from a transfusion when the PCV falls below 15%, depending on clinical signs. Identifiable blood groups have not been demonstrated in ferrets, and transfusion reactions are unlikely. However, administration of dexamethasone sodium phosphate 4–6 mg/kg IV once prior to transfusion has been recommended as a precaution. Healthy, large males with a normal PCV are the most appropriate blood donors. Up to 0.6% of donor's body weight can be safely collected (usually, 6–12 mL, depending on the size of the ferret and volume required). Collect blood from anesthetized donor ferret via the anterior vena cava or jugular vein into a syringe with 1 mL acid-citrate-dextrose anticoagulant per 6 mL of blood. (Volume of blood to be transfused is estimated in the same manner as for cats.) Ideally, blood should be filtered during administration to the recipient. Administer blood slowly with a 21- to 22-gauge catheter into a large vein such as the jugular or via an interosseous catheter if a vein is not accessible. Follow transfusion with IV administration of 0.9% NaCl to meet maintenance and dehydration needs.
• Supportive care, such as fluid therapy, warmth, and adequate nutrition

### ACTIVITY
Minimize activity to reduce the risk of even minor trauma.

### DIET
Anorectic ferrets may be willing to eat chicken baby foods, canned cat foods, or commercial nutritional supplements.

## MEDICATIONS

### DRUG(S) OF CHOICE
Vary with the cause of the bruising

### CONTRAINDICATIONS
N/A

### PRECAUTIONS
Aspirin and other NSAIDs should be avoided.

### POSSIBLE INTERACTIONS
N/A

### ALTERNATIVE DRUGS
N/A

## FOLLOW-UP

### PATIENT MONITORING
In patients with thrombocytopenia, conduct a daily platelet count until a response is noted; see specific diseases for details.

### POSSIBLE COMPLICATIONS
• Death or morbidity caused by hemorrhage into the brain or other vital organs
• Shock caused by hemorrhagic hypovolemia

## MISCELLANEOUS

### ASSOCIATED CONDITIONS
N/A

### AGE-RELATED FACTORS
None

### ZOONOTIC POTENTIAL
None

### PREGNANCY
N/A

### SYNONYMS
• Hemorrhagic diatheses
• Bleeding

### SEE ALSO
• Adrenal Disease
• Hyperestrogenism

### ABBREVIATIONS
• APTT = activated partial thromboplastin time
• DIC = disseminated intravascular coagulation
• FDP = fibrin degradation product
• NSAIDs = nonsteroidal antiinflammatory drugs
• PCV = packed cell volume
• PT = prothrombin time
• RBC = red blood cell

### Suggested Reading
Benson KG, Paul-Murphy J, Ramer JC. Evaluating and stabilizing the critical ferret: basic diagnostic and therapeutic techniques. Compend Contin Edu Pract Vet 2000;22:490–497.

Green RA. Hemostatic disorders: coagulopathies and thrombotic disorders. In: Ettinger SJ, ed. Textbook of Veterinary Internal Medicine. Philadelphia: Saunders, 1989:2246–2264.

Orcutt CJ. Fluids and critical care in small mammals. Proc North Am Vet Conf 2001; 886.

Ryland LM. Remission of estrus associated anemia following hysterectomy and multiple blood transfusions in a ferret. J Am Vet Med Assoc 1982;181:820–822.

Williams BH. Therapeutics in ferrets. Vet Clin North Am Exotic Anim Pract 2000;3(1):131–153.

*Portions Adapted From*

Boon GD. Petechia/Ecchymosis/Bruising. In: Tilley LP, Smith FWK, Jr., eds. The 5-Minute Veterinary Consult: Canine and Feline, 2nd Ed. Baltimore: Lippincott Williams & Wilkins, 2000.

# PLEURAL EFFUSION

 **BASICS**

## OVERVIEW
- Abnormal accumulation of fluid within the pleural cavity
- May be due to increased production or decreased resorption of fluid
- Alterations in hydrostatic and oncotic pressures or vascular permeability and lymphatic function may contribute to fluid accumulation.

## INCIDENCE/PREVALENCE
Common finding in clinical practice

## SIGNALMENT
Varies with underlying cause

## SIGNS

### General Comments
Depend on the fluid volume, rapidity of fluid accumulation, and the underlying cause

### Historical Findings
- Weakness, often manifested as rear limb paresis or paralysis
- Dyspnea
- Tachypnea
- Open-mouth breathing
- Cyanosis
- Lethargy
- Inappetence
- Cough

### Physical Examination Findings
- Dyspnea—respirations often shallow and rapid
- Muffled or inaudible heart and lung sounds ventrally
- Preservation of breath sounds dorsally

## CAUSES AND RISK FACTORS

### High Hydrostatic Pressure
- CHF—most common cause
- Intrathoracic neoplasia—(mediastinal lymphosarcoma, thymoma) very common cause
- Overhydration

### Vascular or Lymphatic Abnormality
- Infectious—bacterial, viral, or fungal
- Neoplasia (e.g., mediastinal lymphosarcoma, metastatic disease)
- Chylothorax (e.g., from CHF, cranial vena cava obstruction, neoplasia, fungal, diaphragmatic hernia, and trauma)
- Hemothorax (e.g., from trauma, neoplasia, and coagulopathy)
- Diaphragmatic hernia (rare)

### Low Oncotic Pressure
Hypoalbuminemia—less common cause of pleural effusion in ferrets; protein-losing enteropathy, protein-losing nephropathy, and liver disease

 **DIAGNOSIS**

## DIFFERENTIAL DIAGNOSIS
- Historical or physical evidence of external trauma—consider hemothorax or diaphragmatic hernia.
- Fever suggests an inflammatory, infectious, or neoplastic cause.
- Murmurs, gallops, or arrhythmias combined with jugular venous distension or pulsation suggest an underlying cardiac cause.
- Decreased compressibility of the cranial thorax suggests a cranial mediastinal mass, especially lymphoma.
- Concurrent ascites suggests CHF; severe hypoalbuminemia, diaphragmatic hernia, and disseminated neoplasia are unusual causes.

### Fluid Analysis
Should include physical characteristics (i.e., color, clarity, odor, clots), pH, glucose, total protein, total nucleated cell count, and cytologic examination to aid in differentiating causes:
- Transudate—early CHF, hypoalbuminemia (rare)
- Modified transudate—CHF, neoplasia
- Nonseptic exudate—neoplasia, ADV, diaphragmatic hernia (rare)
- Septic Exudate—pyothorax
- Hemorrhage—neoplasia, trauma, coagulopathy

## CBC/BIOCHEMISTRY/URINALYSIS
- Hemogram results may be abnormal in patients with pyothorax or neoplasia.
- Severe hypoalbuminemia (generally <1 g/dL to cause effusion) suggests protein-losing enteropathy, protein-losing nephropathy, or liver disease.
- Hyperglobulinemia (monoclonal) suggests ADV.

## OTHER LABORATORY TESTS
- Cardiac disease suspected—perform heartworm testing.
- Infection suspected—do a bacterial culture and sensitivity test and consider special stains. (e.g., Gram and acid-fast stains) of the fluid.
- Chyle suspected—do an ether clearance test or Sudan stain of the pleural fluid, and triglyceride and cholesterol evaluations of the fluid and serum.

## IMAGING

### Radiographic Findings
- Used to confirm pleural effusion; should not be performed until after thoracocentesis in dyspneic patients with evidence of pleural effusion on physical examination
- Evidence of pleural effusion includes separation of lung borders away from the thoracic wall and sternum by fluid density in the pleural space, fluid-filled interlobar fissure lines, loss or blurring of the cardiac and diaphragmatic borders, blunting of the lung margins at the costophrenic angles (ventrodorsal view), and widening of the mediastinum (ventrodorsal view).
- Unilateral effusion—consider chylothorax, pyothorax; hemothorax, pulmonary neoplasia, diaphragmatic hernias, and lung lobe torsion.
- Evaluate postthoracocentesis radiographs carefully for cardiomegaly, intrapulmonary lesions, mediastinal masses, diaphragmatic hernia, lung lobe torsion, and evidence of trauma (e.g., rib fractures).

### Echocardiographic Findings
- Ultrasonographic evaluation of the thorax is recommended whenever cardiac disease, a diaphragmatic hernia, or cranial mediastinal mass is suspected.
- Echocardiography is easiest to perform before thoracocentesis, provided the patient is stable.

## DIAGNOSTIC PROCEDURES

### Thoracocentesis
Allows characterization of the fluid type and determination of potential underlying cause. The following parameters were extrapolated from canine and feline data:

#### Transudate
- Clear and colorless to pale yellow
- Protein <1.5 g/dL
- Specific gravity <1.018
- Cells <1000/mm³—mostly mesothelial cells

#### Modified Transudate
- Yellow or pink; may be slightly cloudy
- Protein 2.5–5.0 g/dL
- Specific gravity >1.018
- Cells 1,000–7,000 /mm³ (LSA up to 100,000)—macrophage, mesothelial cell predominant cell type; few non-degenerate neutrophils erythrocytes, and lymphocytes; may contain neoplastic cells

#### Exudate (Nonseptic)
- Yellow or pink; cloudy; fibrin may be present
- Protein 3.0–8.0 g/dL
- Specific gravity >1.018
- Cells 5,000–20,000/mm3 (LSA up to 100,000)—nondegenerate neutrophil and macrophage predominant cell type; lymphocytes and neoplastic cells may be seen

#### Exudate (Septic)
- Yellow to red-brown; cloudy to opaque; may contain fibrin
- Protein. 3.0–7.0 g/dL
- Specific gravity >1.018

## PLEURAL EFFUSION

• Cells 5,000–300,000/mm³—degenerate neutrophil and macrophage predominant cell type; bacteria

*Hemorrhage*
• Red; spun supernatant clear and sediment red
• Protein >3.0 g/dL
• Specific gravity 1.007–1.027
• Cells consistent with peripheral blood, may see macrophages with erythrophagocytosis
• Does not clot

*Chyle*
• Milky white; opaque
• Protein 2.5–6.0 g/dL
• Cells 1,000–20,000/mm³—lymphocytes, neutrophils, and macrophages

### *Exploratory Thoracotomy*
To obtain biopsy specimens of lung, lymph nodes, or pleura, if indicated

## TREATMENT
• First, thoracocentesis to relieve respiratory distress. When performing thoracocentesis be aware that the heart is located much more caudally within the thorax in the ferret as compared to dogs and cats. Sedation (midazolam 0.3–1.0 mg/kg IM, SC or ketamine 10–20 mg/kg IM plus diazepam 1–2 mg/kg IM) or anesthesia with isoflurane by mask may be necessary.
• If the patient is stable after thoracocentesis, outpatient treatment may be possible for some diseases. Most patients are hospitalized because they require intensive management.
• Preventing fluid reaccumulation requires treatment based on a definitive diagnosis.
• Surgery may be indicated for management of some neoplasias; other indications such as diaphragmatic hernia repair, foreign body removal, and lung lobectomy for lung lobe torsion are rare in ferrets.

## MEDICATIONS

### DRUG(S) OF CHOICE
• Treatment varies with specific disease.
• Diuretics generally reserved for patients with diseases causing fluid retention and volume overload (e.g., CHF)

### CONTRAINDICATIONS
N/A

### PRECAUTIONS
• Drugs that depress respirations or decrease blood pressure
• Inappropriate use of diuretics predisposes the patient to dehydration and electrolyte disturbances without eliminating the effusion.

### POSSIBLE INTERACTIONS
N/A

### ALTERNATIVE DRUGS
N/A

## FOLLOW-UP

### PATIENT MONITORING
Radiographic evaluation key to assessment of treatment in most patients

### PREVENTION/AVOIDANCE
N/A

### POSSIBLE COMPLICATIONS
Death due to respiratory compromise

### EXPECTED COURSE AND PROGNOSIS
Varies with underlying cause, but usually guarded to poor

## MISCELLANEOUS

### SEE ALSO
• Congestive heart failure
• Heartworm disease
• Lymphosarcoma

### ABBREVIATIONS
• ADV = Aleutian disease virus
• CHF = congestive heart failure
• LSA = lymphosarcoma

*Suggested Reading*
Benson KG, Paul-Murphy J, Ramer JC. Evaluating and stabilizing the critical ferret: basic diagnostic and therapeutic techniques. Compend Contin Edu Pract Vet 2000;22:490–497.
Brown SA. Neoplasia. In: Hillyer EV, Quesenberry KE, eds. Ferrets, Rabbits and Rodents: Clinical Medicine and Surgery. Philadelphia: WB Saunders, 1997:99.
Hoefer HL. Thoracic disease rule-outs in the ferret. Proc North Am Vet Conf 2001;867–868.
Kendrick RE. Ferret respiratory diseases. Vet Clin North Am Exotic Anim Pract 2000;3(2):453–464.
Rosenthal K. Management of cardiac disease in ferrets. Waltham/OSU Symp Treatment Sm Anim Dis 1997;Sept.
Rosenthal K. Respiratory diseases. In: Hillyer EV, Quesenberry KE, eds. Ferrets, Rabbits and Rodents: Clinical Medicine and Surgery. Philadelphia: WB Saunders, 1997:77–84.
Stamoulis ME, Miller MS, Hillyer EV. Cardiovascular diseases part 1. In: Hillyer EV, Quesenberry KE, eds. Ferrets, Rabbits and Rodents: Clinical Medicine and Surgery. Philadelphia: WB Saunders, 1997:63–70.

*Portions Adapted From*
Lehmkuhl LB, Smith FWK, Jr. Pleural Effusion. In: Tilley LP, Smith FWK, Jr., eds. The 5-Minute Veterinary Consult: Canine and Feline, 2nd Ed. Baltimore: Lippincott Williams & Wilkins, 2000.

# PNEUMONIA, ASPIRATION

## BASICS

### OVERVIEW
• Inflammation of the lungs caused by inhaled material (e.g., oral ingesta, regurgitated material, and vomitus) and subsequent pulmonary dysfunction; develops when laryngeal reflexes function improperly or are overwhelmed and is thus a consequence of an underlying problem
• Pulmonary dysfunction—caused by a combination of factors: (1) obstruction—large particles obstruct large airways, causing acute respiratory distress; particulates cause direct obstruction of small airways and indirect obstruction from bronchospasm and the production of mucous and exudate; (2) aspiration of gastric acid—results in marked damage to the respiratory epithelium; (3) bacterial pneumonia—common component in regurgitated material, food, or pharyngeal flora; may initiate an immediate infection or a secondary infection occurring later in the course of disease

### SIGNALMENT
No age or sex predilection

### SIGNS
• May be peracute, acute, or chronic
• Dyspnea, tachypnea
• Fever
• Cyanosis
• Weakness, lethargy—often manifested as rear limb paresis
• Nasal discharge
• Coughing is an unusual finding in ferrets with pneumonia.

### CAUSES AND RISK FACTORS
#### Esophageal Abnormalities
• Megaesophagus
• Esophageal obstruction—mass, foreign body, stricture
#### Altered Consciousness
• Sedation
• Anesthesia—during or recovery from
• Postictus
• Severe metabolic disturbance (eg., hypoglycemia)
#### Iatrogenic Causes
• Forced feeding
• Tube feeding—improper technique, misplacement of tube
• Mineral oil administration

## DIAGNOSIS

### DIFFERENTIAL DIAGNOSIS
• Mediastinal mass—especially mediastinal lymphoma in young ferrets

• Bacterial pneumonia—component of disease; may develop for reasons other than the overt aspiration of foreign material
• Lung lobe abscess—consolidated appearance radiographically; may be a sequela to aspiration pneumonia, bacterial pneumonia, or foreign body

### CBC/BIOCHEMISTRY/URINALYSIS
• Neutrophilic leukocytosis with a left shift
• WBC count—may be normal
• Nonregenerative anemia associated with inflammatory disease

### OTHER LABORATORY TESTS
N/A

### IMAGING
Thoracic radiography—bronchoalveolar pattern most severe in the gravity-dependent lung lobes (cranial, ventral); may take up to 24 hours for pattern to develop after acute aspiration; scrutinize for evidence of esophageal or mediastinal disease.

### DIAGNOSTIC PROCEDURES
• Tracheal wash—collect material for bacterial culture and sensitivity testing; collect before administering antibiotics; infection often caused by multiple organisms with unpredictable susceptibility. Submit specimen for cytologic examination, bacterial (aerobic and anaerobic), and mycotic culture.
• Bronchoscopy—suspected large airway obstruction based on breathing pattern, auscultation, or radiographic findings
• Appropriate tests to investigate underlying causes

## TREATMENT
• Oxygen—respiratory distress; if distress persists, provide ventilatory support.
• Intravenous fluids—indicated for shock or dehydration
• Cage rest—for respiratory distress
• Do not allow patient to remain laterally recumbent on one side for more than 2 hours.
• Once stable, mild exercise may assist in productive cough and airway clearance.
• Nebulization and coupage—recommended for consolidation or if resolution is proceeding slowly
• Airway suction—indicated only if aspiration is observed (e.g., during recovery from anesthesia)
• Lavage—contraindicated; forces material deeper into lungs; any gastric acid neutralized in seconds

## MEDICATIONS
### DRUG(S) OF CHOICE
• Antibiotic therapy—ideally, withhold until an airway specimen is collected; begin with an antibiotic combination that is broad spectrum and effective against anaerobes (eg., enrofloxacin 10 mg/kg IM q12h plus amoxicillin 10 mg/kg IM q12h); alter therapy based on culture/susceptibility results, and continue for 10 days after resolution of clinical and radiographic signs.
• Bronchodilators (e.g., theophylline 4.25 mg/kg PO q8–12h)—may improve breathing with acute aspiration and with auscultated wheezing
• Short-acting corticosteroids—may be administered once to combat inflammation with peracute life-threatening aspiration

### CONTRAINDICATIONS/POSSIBLE INTERACTIONS
• Diuretics—contraindicated
• Corticosteroids—avoid; predisposes patient to infection
• Theophylline-derivative bronchodilators—use cautiously when combined with fluoroquinolone antibiotics and chloramphenicol; these antibiotics may prolong clearance of bronchodilators, resulting in signs of toxicity.

## FOLLOW-UP
### PATIENT MONITORING
• Radiographs and clinical signs—monitor response to treatment.
• Radiographs—evaluate every 3–7 days initially to determine appropriateness of treatment, then every 1–2 weeks.
• Signs do not resolve or suddenly worsen—possible recurrence of aspiration or a secondary infection; repeat diagnostic evaluation, including examination of tracheal wash.

### PREVENTION/AVOIDANCE
The underlying cause must be identified and managed.

### POSSIBLE COMPLICATIONS
• Secondary infection common
• Abscess or foreign body granuloma

### EXPECTED COURSE AND PROGNOSIS
• Prognosis—depends on severity of signs when patient is examined and the ability to correct the underlying problem
• Acute, severe aspiration—can be fatal
• Recurrence—likely if underlying cause is not or cannot be addressed

## MISCELLANEOUS

**SEE ALSO**
- Lymphosarcoma
- Megaesophagus
- Pneumonia, bacterial

**ABBREVIATION**
WBC = white blood cell

*Suggested Reading*

Antinoff N. Musculoskeletal and neurologic diseases. In: Hillyer EV, Quesenberry KE, eds. Ferrets, Rabbits and Rodents: Clinical Medicine and Surgery. Philadelphia: WB Saunders, 1997:126–130.

Benson KG, Paul-Murphy J, Ramer JC. Evaluating and stabilizing the critical ferret: basic diagnostic and therapeutic techniques. Compend Contin Edu Pract Vet 2000;22:490–497.

Blanco MC, Fox JG, Rosenthal K, et al. Megaesophagus in nine ferrets. J Am Vet Med Assoc 1994;205:444–447.

Fox JG. Bacterial and mycoplasmal diseases. In: Fox JG, ed. Biology and Diseases of the Ferret. 2nd Ed. Baltimore: Williams & Wilkins, 1998:321–354.

Hoefer HL. Gastrointestinal diseases. In: Hillyer EV, Quesenberry KE, eds. Ferrets, Rabbits and Rodents: Clinical Medicine and Surgery. Philadelphia: WB Saunders, 1997:26–36.

Hoefer HL. Thoracic disease rule-outs in the ferret. Proc North Am Vet Conf 2001:867–868.

Kendrick RE. Ferret respiratory diseases. Vet Clin North Am Exotic Anim Pract 2000;3[2]:453–464.

Rosenthal KL: Respiratory diseases. In: Hillyer EV, Quesenberry KE, eds. Ferrets, Rabbits and Rodents: Clinical Medicine and Surgery. Philadelphia: WB Saunders, 1997:77–84.

Williams BH. Therapeutics in ferrets. Vet Clin North Am: Exotic Anim Pract 2000; 3(1):131–153.

*Portions Adapted From*

Hawkins EC. Pneumonia, Aspiration. In: Tilley LP, Smith FWK, Jr., eds. The 5-Minute Veterinary Consult: Canine and Feline, 2nd Ed. Baltimore: Lippincott Williams & Wilkins, 2000.

# PNEUMONIA, BACTERIAL

## BASICS

### OVERVIEW
- Bacterial pneumonia is relatively uncommon in ferrets, but when present is generally a serious, life-threatening disease.
- Usually occurs secondary to viral infection or aspiration of foreign material
- Bacteria—enter the lower respiratory tract primarily by the inhalation or aspiration routes; enter less commonly by the hematogenous route; infections incite an overt inflammatory reaction.
- Respiratory infection—development depends on the complex interplay of many factors: size, inoculation site, number of organisms and their virulence, and resistance of the host.

### SIGNALMENT
Unusual disease in pet ferrets; no data available on age or sex predilection

### SIGNS

#### Historical Findings
- Weakness, lethargy often manifested as rear limb paresis
- Anorexia and weight loss
- Labored breathing
- Nasal discharge
- Fever
- Sudden death
- Cough (rare)

#### Physical Examination Findings
- Fever
- Dyspnea
- Abnormal breath sounds on auscultation—increased intensity or bronchial breath sounds, crackles, and wheezes
- Weight loss
- Serous or mucopurulent nasal discharge
- Lethargy
- Dehydration

### CAUSES
- Bacterial pathogens—poorly documented; *Streptococcus zooepidemicus, Escherichia coli, Klebsiella pneumoniae, Pseudomonas aeruginosa, Bordetella bronchiseptica*, and *Mycoplasma* spp. have been reported.
- Isolates—most thought to be opportunistic invaders
- Anaerobic bacteria—found in pulmonary abscesses and aspiration pneumonia

### RISK FACTORS
- Exposure to CDV in unvaccinated animals
- Exposure to people or ferrets with influenza virus
- Regurgitation, dysphagia, or vomiting
- Reduced level of consciousness—stupor, coma, and anesthesia
- Thoracic trauma or surgery
- Immunosuppressive therapy—chemotherapy; perhaps high-dose, long-term glucocorticoids
- Severe metabolic disorders—uremia, diabetes mellitus
- Protein-calorie malnutrition

## DIAGNOSIS

### DIFFERENTIAL DIAGNOSIS
- Viral pneumonia—CDV and influenza virus; possibly ADV
- Fungal pneumonia—histoplasmosis, blastomycosis, coccidioidomycosis, and cryptococcosis
- Metastatic neoplasia
- Bacterial or fungal rhinitis
- Mediastinal lymphoma
- Pulmonary abscess
- Pleural infection—pyothorax

### CBC/BIOCHEMISTRY/URINALYSIS
Inflammatory leukogram—neutrophilic leukocytosis with or without a left shift; absence does not rule out the diagnosis.

### OTHER LABORATORY TESTS
Immunofluorescent antibody (IFA) test for CDV—can be performed on peripheral blood or buffy coat smears or conjunctival or mucous membrane scrapings. Vaccination will not affect the results.

### IMAGING

#### Thoracic Radiography
Alveolar pattern characterized by increased pulmonary densities (margins indistinct; air bronchograms or lobar consolidation); patchy or lobar alveolar pattern with a cranial ventral lung lobe distribution

### DIAGNOSTIC PROCEDURES
- Microbiologic and cytologic examinations—aspirates or washings; definitive diagnosis
- Samples—transtracheal washing, bronchoalveolar lavage, or fine needle lung aspiration
- Septic inflammation with degenerate neutrophils predominates
- Recent antibiotic administration—nonseptic inflammation likely
- Bacteria—may be visible microscopically; always culture specimens, even if no bacteria are seen on cytologic examination.

## TREATMENT

### APPROPRIATE HEALTH CARE
Inpatient—recommended with multisystemic signs (e.g., anorexia, high fever, weight loss, and lethargy)

### NURSING CARE
- Maintain normal systemic hydration—important to aid mucociliary clearance and secretion mobilization
- Nebulization with bland aerosols—results in more rapid resolution if used in conjunction with physiotherapy and antibacterials
- Physiotherapy—chest wall coupage; always do immediately after nebulization; avoid allowing the patient to lie in one position for a prolonged time.
- Oxygen therapy—for respiratory distress

## MEDICATIONS

### DRUG(S) OF CHOICE
Antibiotic therapy—ideally, withhold until an airway specimen is collected; begin with an antibiotic combination that is broad spectrum and effective against anaerobes (eg., enrofloxacin 10 mg/kg IM q12h plus amoxicillin 10 mg/kg IM q12h); alter therapy based on culture/susceptibility results, and continue for 10 days after resolution of clinical and radiographic signs.

### CONTRAINDICATIONS
Anticholinergics and antihistamines—may thicken secretions and inhibit mucokinesis and exudate removal from airways

### PRECAUTIONS
Antitussives—use with caution and only for short intervals to control intractable cough; potent, centrally acting agents may inhibit mucokinesis and exudate removal from airways.

### POSSIBLE INTERACTIONS
N/A

## FOLLOW-UP

### PATIENT MONITORING
- Auscultate patient thoroughly several times daily.
- Thoracic radiographs—improve more slowly than the clinical appearance

### PREVENTION/AVOIDANCE
Vaccination—against CDV

### EXPECTED COURSE AND PROGNOSIS
Prognosis—good to guarded with aggressive antibacterial and supportive therapy; more guarded in young animals, patients with immunodeficiency, and patients that are debilitated or have severe underlying disease

## MISCELLANEOUS

**ASSOCIATED CONDITIONS**
N/A

**AGE-RELATED FACTORS**
N/A

**ZOONOTIC POTENTIAL**
Influenza virus can be transmitted to humans.

**PREGNANCY**
N/A

**SEE ALSO**
• Canine distemper virus
• Influenza virus
• Pneumonia, aspiration

**ABBREVIATIONS**
• ADV = Aleutian disease virus
• CDV = canine distemper virus

*Suggested Reading:*

Benson KG, Paul-Murphy J, Ramer JC. Evaluating and stabilizing the critical ferret: basic diagnostic and therapeutic techniques. Compend Contin Edu Pract Vet 2000;22:490–497.

Fox JG. Bacterial and mycoplasmal diseases. In: Fox JG, ed. Biology and Diseases of the Ferret. 2nd Ed. Baltimore: Williams & Wilkins, 1998:321–354.

Hoefer HL. Thoracic disease rule-outs in the ferret. Proc North Am Vet Conf 2001:867–868.

Kendrick RE. Ferret respiratory diseases. Vet Clin North Am Exotic Anim Pract 2000;3(2):453–464.

Rosenthal KL. Respiratory diseases. In: Hillyer EV, Quesenberry KE, eds. Ferrets, Rabbits and Rodents: Clinical Medicine and Surgery. Philadelphia, WB Saunders, 1997:77–84.

Williams BH. Therapeutics in ferrets. Vet Clin North Am: Exotic Anim Pract 2000;3(1):131–153.

*Portions Adapted From*

Roudebush P. Pneumonia, Bacterial. In: Tilley LP, Smith FWK, Jr., eds. The 5-Minute Veterinary Consult: Canine and Feline, 3rd Ed. Baltimore: Lippincott Williams & Wilkins, 2003.

# PNEUMONIA, MYCOTIC

## BASICS

### OVERVIEW
• Fungal pneumonia is rarely diagnosed in ferrets; ferrets rarely housed outside are less likely to be exposed to fungal elements.
• Mycelial fungal elements—inhaled from contaminated soil; organisms then colonize the lungs.
• Dimorphic fungi—grow in the yeast phase at body temperature
• Cell-mediated immunity—important response to fungal infection; leads to pyogranulomatous inflammation

### Systems Affected
• Depend on the specific fungal disease; since very few cases of fungal pneumonia have been reported in ferrets, data on organ system involvement are unavailable.
• Blastomycosis—few existing reported cases describe granulomatous pneumonia.
• Histoplasmosis—diffuse interstitial pneumonia and lymphadenopathy reported anecdotally
• Coccidioidomycosis—diffuse interstitial or bronchial pneumonia with dissemination to bones, CNS, abdominal organs, and heart have been reported.
• Cryptococcosis—nasal cavity, lungs, and CNS involvement reported

### Geographic Distribution
• Blastomycosis—U.S. Southeast and Midwest along the Mississippi, Ohio, Missouri, and Tennessee rivers and southern Great Lakes; also in southern Mid-Atlantic states
• Histoplasmosis—similar to but more widely distributed than blastomycosis; pockets of disease in Texas, Oklahoma, and California
• Coccidioidomycosis—U.S. Southwest from Texas to California
• Cryptococcosis—sporadically throughout the United States

### SIGNALMENT
Rare disease in pet ferrets; no data available on age or sex predilection

### SIGNS

#### General Comments
• Depend primarily on the organ systems involved
• Multisystemic illness may be apparent.

#### Historical Findings
• Chronic weight loss and inappetence
• Fever
• Oculonasal discharge
• Coughing—seen inconsistently in ferrets, even with marked pulmonary disease of any kind
• Dyspnea

• Acute blindness or blepharospasm—possible; however, ocular involvement not reported in ferrets
• Cutaneous nodules—uncommon; anecdotal reports exist.
• Lameness—if osteomyelitis develops

#### Physical Examination Findings
• Depression and emaciation—may note in chronically affected patients
• Fever
• Harsh, loud breath sounds or crackles on auscultation

### CAUSES
• Blastomyces dermatitidis
• Histoplasma capsulatum
• Coccidioides immitis
• Cryptococcus neoformans

### RISK FACTORS
• Blastomycosis, histoplasmosis, and cryptococcosis—environmental exposure to soils rich in organic matter; exposure to bird droppings or other fecal matter possible risk factor
• Coccidioidomycosis—environmental exposure to sandy, alkaline soil after periods of rainfall; outdoor activities
• Immunosuppression
• Antineoplastic chemotherapy

## DIAGNOSIS

### DIFFERENTIAL DIAGNOSIS
• Metastatic neoplasia
• Bacterial pneumonia
• Chronic bronchial disease
• Pulmonary edema

### CBC/BIOCHEMISTRY/URINALYSIS
• Depend on the systems affected
• No consistent findings reported in ferrets due to small number of cases. In other mammals may see moderate leukocytosis with or without a left shift; lymphopenia, thrombocytopenia, and nonregenerative anemia; hyperglobulinemia and hypoalbuminemia

### OTHER LABORATORY TESTS
• Cytologic or histologic identification of the organism—definitive diagnosis
• Culture—not usually necessary; may be difficult
• Serologic testing—usefulness in ferrets undetermined
• Latex agglutination test—for cryptococcosis capsular antigen; usefulness in ferrets undetermined

### IMAGING
• Thoracic radiography—diffuse nodular interstitial and peribronchial infiltrates; nodular densities may coalesce to granulomatous masses with indistinct edges;

tracheobronchial lymphadenopathy possible; large focal granulomas possible
• Appendicular or axial skeleton radiography—if bony involvement: osteolysis with periosteal proliferation; soft tissue swelling
• Abdominal ultrasonography—to look for granulomas or large lymph nodes
• Ocular ultrasonography—to look for retrobulbar mass

### DIAGNOSTIC PROCEDURES
• Impression smear or aspirate of a skin nodule
• Fine needle aspirate of the lung—more likely to be diagnostic than transtracheal aspirate or bronchoalveolar lavage specimen
• Lymph node aspirate or biopsy
• CSF tap—with cryptococcosis
• Examination of bone marrow or splenic aspirate—with histoplasmosis
• Biopsy—may be needed; expected findings include pyogranulomatous inflammation and possibly organisms. In other species, organisms are usually seen with blastomycosis, histoplasmosis, and cryptococcosis; sometimes difficult to find coccidioidomycosis

## TREATMENT

### APPROPRIATE HEALTH CARE
• Inpatient evaluation and treatment—dehydration, anorexia, and severe hypoxia
• Administration of fluids, oxygen, and antibiotics as needed

### CLIENT EDUCATION
• Warn client that treatment is expensive and will probably be necessary for at least 2 months; prognosis is guarded to poor.
• Advise client to clean areas in the environment with high organic matter or feces.

### SURGICAL CONSIDERATIONS
None

## MEDICATIONS

### DRUG(S) OF CHOICE
All treatment protocols have been extrapolated from feline dosages as follows:
• Itraconazole—5–10 mg/kg PO daily (cats); most often used first; must be given with food
• Amphotericin B—0.25 mg/kg (cats) IV three times a week to a total dose of 8 mg/kg if used alone or 4 mg/kg if used with an azole drug (e.g., itraconazole); administer in 200–500 mL of $D_5W$; best used with itraconazole or ketoconazole for severely affected patients

• Amphotericin B—alternative: 0.5–0.8 mg/kg two to three times per week (cats); to reduce nephrotoxicity, may give subcutaneously diluted in 400 mL of 0.45% saline/2.5% dextrose solution
• Fluconazole—10 mg/kg PO q12h; drug of choice in cats with cryptococcosis and CNS or urinary tract involvement

## PRECAUTIONS/POSSIBLE INTERACTIONS

• All antifungal drug dosages listed above are feline dosages. Use of these medications has only anecdotally been used in ferrets; their safety and efficacy have not been evaluated.
• Avoid corticosteroid use.
• Azole drugs—do not use with severe liver disease.
• Amphotericin B—do not use in azotemic or dehydrated patients; stop use if serum BUN and creatinine concentrations increase.
• Itraconazole and the other azole drugs—anorexia, increase in liver enzymes, cutaneous vasculitis seen in other mammalian species
• Antacids and anticonvulsants—may lower the blood concentration of itraconazole

## FOLLOW-UP

### PATIENT MONITORING

• Liver enzymes—evaluate monthly while patient is on itraconazole, fluconazole, or ketoconazole.
• BUN and creatinine—measure before each dose of amphotericin B.

• Thoracic radiographs—reevaluate before discontinuing treatment.

### PREVENTION/AVOIDANCE

Monitor for signs of recurrence

### POSSIBLE COMPLICATIONS

Renal failure from amphotericin B

### EXPECTED COURSE AND PROGNOSIS

• Generally poor to guarded prognosis; however, data are not available.
• Treatment recommendations for feline/canine patients: blastomycosis—requires a minimum of 2 months of treatment; 60–70% of dogs are cured by itraconazole; those not cured usually relapse; others—continued until 1 month past remission
• Relapse—may occur up to 1 year after treatment

## MISCELLANEOUS

### ASSOCIATED CONDITIONS

None

### ZOONOTIC POTENTIAL

Infections in people—primarily from a common environmental source; no direct transmission from animals to humans, except by penetrating wounds contaminated by the organism

### PREGNANCY

Azole antifungals—teratogenic; do not use in pregnant animals.

### SEE ALSO

• Dyspnea and tachypnea
• Pneumonia, bacterial

### ABBREVIATIONS

• BUN = blood urea nitrogen
• CNS = central nervous system
• CSF = cerebrospinal fluid

*Suggested Reading*

Benson KG, Paul-Murphy J, Ramer JC. Evaluating and stabilizing the critical ferret: basic diagnostic and therapeutic techniques. Compend Contin Edu Pract Vet 2000;22:490–497.

Fox JG. Mycotic diseases. In: Fox JG, ed. Biology and Diseases of the Ferret. 2nd Ed. Baltimore: Williams & Wilkins, 1998:393–403.

Hoefer HL. Thoracic disease rule-outs in the ferret. Proc North Am Vet Conf 2001:867–868.

Kendrick RE. Ferret respiratory diseases. Vet Clin North Am Exotic Anim Pract 2000;3(2):453–464.

Rosenthal KL. Respiratory diseases. In: Hillyer EV, Quesenberry KE, eds. Ferrets, Rabbits and Rodents: Clinical Medicine and Surgery. Philadelphia: WB Saunders, 1997:77–84.

Williams BH. Therapeutics in ferrets. Vet Clin North Am Exotic Anim Pract 2000;3(1):131–153.

Wolf AM, Troy GC. Deep mycotic diseases. In: Ettinger SJ, Feldman EC, eds. Textbook of Veterinary Internal Medicine. 4th Ed. Philadelphia: Saunders, 1995:439–463.

*Portions Adapted From*

Taboada J. Pneumonia, Fungal. In: Tilley LP, Smith FWK, Jr., eds. The 5-Minute Veterinary Consult: Canine and Feline, 2nd Ed. Baltimore: Lippincott Williams & Wilkins, 2000.

# PODODERMATITIS AND NAIL BED DISORDERS

## BASICS

### DEFINITION
Inflammation of the feet, including foot pads, nail beds, and interdigital spaces

### PATHOPHYSIOLOGY
• Depends on the underlying cause
• Causes include infectious, allergic, neoplastic, and environmental diseases; autoimmune and endocrine or metabolic causes have not been described in ferrets.
• Nails and nailfolds—subject to trauma, infection, neoplasia, and dystrophy
• Psychogenic dermatoses not reported

### SYSTEMS AFFECTED
Skin/exocrine—primary or secondary infection (bacterial, fungal, or parasitic); neoplasia

### INCIDENCE/PREVALENCE
Uncommon presenting complaint in pet ferrets

### SIGNALMENT
No age or sex predilection

### SIGNS

#### Historical Findings
• History—extremely important; determine environment and general husbandry (e.g., unsanitary conditions, other pets affected, trauma, contact irritants, and vaccination status).
• Lesions elsewhere on the body—may aid in diagnosis of cause
• Licking
• Lameness
• Pain
• Swelling, erythema, exudate, or hyperkeratosis
• Deformity or sloughing of nail

### CAUSES
• Viral—CDV is a common cause of pododermatitis in unvaccinated ferrets, usually causing hyperkeratosis.
• Parasitic—sarcoptic mange: (relatively common) two forms recognized, one involving primarily the feet, another more generalized or localized to other areas of the body; *Demodex*—very rare in ferrets
• Neoplastic—epitheliotropic lymphoma, mast cell tumor, hemangioma/hemangiopericytoma, squamous cell carcinoma
• Bacterial—pyoderma, abscess (unusual cause)
• Mycotic—dermatomycosis (relatively common)
• Trauma
• Immunologic—contact dermatitis has been anecdotally reported in ferrets. Cutaneous lesions resembling urticaria or histologic lesions characteristic of allergic reactions in other species have also been anecdotally reported; however, there are no confirmed cases of atopy, food allergy, or other allergic dermatitis in ferrets.

### RISK FACTORS
• Infection—trauma, unsanitary conditions
• CDV—contact of nonimmunized animals with CDV-infected animals (ferrets, dogs, or wild carnivores)

## DIAGNOSIS

### DIFFERENTIAL DIAGNOSIS
• CDV—pododermatitis usually follows a catarrhal phase characterized by naso-ocular discharge, depression, and anorexia, followed by a characteristic, erythematous, pruritic rash on the chin and lips, and spreads caudally to the inguinal area; pododermatitis is characterized by hyperkeratinization of the footpads, erythema, and swelling. CDV is uniformly fatal, and signs other than pododermatitis alone will be seen.
• Sarcoptic mange—foot lesions characterized by severe inflammation and crusting that can progress to nail and skin sloughing if untreated; generally extremely pruritic/painful
• Neoplastic—in most tumor types only one foot affected; lymphoma may affect multiple feet; can be nodular, inflamed, swollen, or ulcerative, depending on tumor type. Mast cell tumors—raised alopecic nodules; may become ulcerated or covered with a thick black crust; may be single or multiple. Squamous cell carcinoma—usually firm and ulcerated. Hemangioma/hemangiopericytoma—swelling, red/purple discoloration
• Bacterial—swelling, diffuse or localized depending on underlying cause (e.g., cellulitis vs. abscess), inflammation, may be ulcerated
• Mycotic—dermatophytes rarely involve feet; partial to complete alopecia with scaling; with or without erythema; not always ringlike; may begin as small papules
• Trauma—depends on underlying cause; usually only one digit or foot; chronic interdigital inflammation, ulceration, pyogranulomatous abscesses, draining tracts, or swelling; with or without pruritus
• Hypersensitivity/contact irritant—uncommon cause; dermatitis of the ventral interdigital surfaces is usually worse, although the whole paw may be involved; feet appear erythematous and alopecic, secondary to pruritus

### CBC/BIOCHEMISTRY/URINALYSIS
• Depend on the underlying cause
• Rarely used in the initial workup

### OTHER LABORATORY TESTS
CDV—immunofluorescent antibody (IFA) test—can be performed on peripheral blood or buffy coat smears or conjunctival or mucous membrane scrapings. Vaccination will not affect the results.

### IMAGING
• Radiographs and ultrasound—rarely used in the initial workup
• Neoplastic—depending on the underlying cause, may be necessary to confirm system disease or stage tumors

### DIAGNOSTIC PROCEDURES
• Skin scrapings, fungal culture, and cytologic examination of stained smear of any exudate or pustule contents
• Biopsy or FNA—histopathology, rule out neoplasia
• Wood's lamp—do not use as the sole means of diagnosing or excluding dermatomycosis, owing to false negatives and misinterpretations of fluorescence
• Trial therapy—to rule out scabies; can be difficult to diagnose; skin scrapes often negative; trial course (ivermectin) may be necessary to rule out

## TREATMENT

### APPROPRIATE HEALTH CARE
Outpatient, unless surgery is indicated

### NURSING CARE
Foot soaks, hot packing, and/or bandaging may be necessary, depending on cause.

### ACTIVITY
Depends on severity of the lesions and the underlying cause

### SURGICAL CONSIDERATIONS
• Neoplasia—may require surgical excision or amputation, depending on tumor type
• Infectious—abscess: lance and drain exudate; severe infections/necrosis: may benefit from surgical debridement of devitalized tissue before medical therapy

## MEDICATIONS

### DRUG(S) OF CHOICE
• CDV—supportive care only, uniformly fatal
• Sarcoptic mites—ivermectin 0.2–0.4 mg/kg SC q14d for three to four doses
• Neoplasia—depends on tumor type (e.g., lymphoma may respond to prednisone or other chemotherapeutic protocols)
• Bacterial pododermatitis, abscess, cellulitis—systemic antibiotics based on culture and sensitivity; trimethoprim/sulfonamide (15–30 mg/kg PO, SC q12h) or enrofloxacin (10–20 mg/kg PO, SC, IM q12h) pending culture result
• Dermatomycosis—lime sulfur dip q7d has been used to successfully; may be antipru-

ritic; has antiparasitic, antibacterial, and antifungal properties; disadvantages are bad odor and staining; miconazole cream for focal lesions
• Hypersensitivity/contact irritant—wash feet to remove substance; antihistamines: hydroxyzine 2mg/kg PO q8h; diphenhydramine 0.5–2.0 mg/kg PO q8–12h; chlorpheniramine 1–2 mg/kg PO q8–12h; corticosteroids: prednisone 0.25–1.0 mg/kg q 24h PO divided

### CONTRAINDICATIONS
N/A

### PRECAUTIONS
• Depend on the treatment protocol selected for the underlying cause; see specific drugs and their precautions.
• Ivermectin—anecdotally associated with birth defects when used in pregnant jills

### POSSIBLE INTERACTIONS
Depend on the underlying cause and treatment protocol selected

### ALTERNATIVE DRUGS
N/A

# FOLLOW-UP

### PATIENT MONITORING
Depends on the underlying cause and treatment protocol selected

### PREVENTION/AVOIDANCE
• Vaccination for CDV
• Environmental causes—good husbandry and preventative medical practices should avoid recurrence.

### POSSIBLE COMPLICATIONS
Depend on the underlying cause and treatment protocol selected

### EXPECTED COURSE AND PROGNOSIS
• Success of therapy depends on finding the underlying cause.
• Sarcoptes—prognosis is good to guarded depending on severity of lesions at presentation.
• Bacterial—usually good; however, treatment may be prolonged.
• Onychomycosis and onychorrhexis—may require amputation of the third phalanx for resolution
• Dermatophytes—prognosis is good.
• Neoplasia—some can be totally excised or removed; others are highly malignant and may have already spread by the time of diagnosis.

# MISCELLANEOUS

### ASSOCIATED CONDITIONS
N/A

### AGE-RELATED FACTORS
N/A

### ZOONOTIC POTENTIAL
Some causes (e.g., sarcoptic mange)

### PREGNANCY
Avoid ivermectin

### SYNONYMS
N/A

### SEE ALSO
• Alopecia
• Canine distemper virus
• Lymphosarcoma
• Pruritus
• Sarcoptic mange

### ABBREVIATIONS
• CDV = canine distemper virus
• FNA = fine needle aspirate

*Suggested Reading*

Fox JG. Parasitic diseases. In: Fox JG, ed. Biology and Diseases of the Ferret. 2nd Ed. Baltimore: Williams & Wilkins, 1998: 375–392.

Fox JG, Pearson RC, Gorham JR. Viral diseases. In: Fox JG, ed. Biology and Diseases of the Ferret. 2nd Ed. Baltimore: Williams & Wilkins, 1998.

Kelleher SA. Skin diseases of the ferret. Vet Clin North Am Exotic Anim Pract 2001; 4(2):565–572.

Orcutt C: Dermatologic diseases. In: Hillyer EV, Quesenberry KE, eds. Ferrets, Rabbits and Rodents: Clinical Medicine and Surgery. Philadelphia: WB Saunders, 1997:115–125.

Williams BH. Ferret microbiology and virology. In: Fudge AM, ed. Laboratory Medicine, Avian and Exotic Pets. Philadelphia: WB Saunders, 2000:334–342.

*Portions Adapted From*

Murphy KM. Pododermatitis. In: Tilley LP, Smith FWK, Jr., eds. The 5-Minute Veterinary Consult: Canine and Feline, 2nd Ed. Baltimore: Lippincott Williams & Wilkins, 2000.

# POLYURIA AND POLYDIPSIA

## BASICS

### DEFINITION
• Polyuria is defined as greater than normal urine production, and polydipsia as greater than normal water consumption. Assessment may be more subjective in ferrets since an extremely wide range of urine production has been reported, ranging from 8 to 140 mL/24 hours (mean, 26–28 mL/24 hours); normal water consumption volumes has been reported to be 75–100 mL/kg/24 hours.
• Polyuria and polydipsia are uncommon clinical complaints in ferrets.

### PATHOPHYSIOLOGY
• Urine production and water consumption (thirst) are controlled by interactions between the kidneys, pituitary gland, and hypothalamus.
• Usually, polydipsia occurs as a compensatory response to polyuria to maintain hydration. The patient's plasma becomes relatively hypertonic and activates thirst mechanisms. Occasionally, polydipsia may be the primary process and polyuria is the compensatory response. Then, the patient's plasma becomes relatively hypotonic because of excessive water intake, and ADH secretion is reduced, resulting in polyuria.

### SYSTEMS AFFECTED
• Renal/urologic—kidneys
• Endocrine/metabolic—pituitary gland and hypothalamus
• Cardiovascular—alterations in "effective" circulating volume

### SIGNALMENT
• More likely to be seen in middle-aged to older ferrets.
• No sex predilection

### SIGNS
N/A

### CAUSES
• Primary polyuria due to impaired renal response to ADH—renal failure, pyelonephritis, pyometra, hepatic failure, hypercalcemia, hypokalemia, drugs
• Primary polyuria caused by osmotic diuresis—diabetes mellitus, postobstructive diuresis, some diuretics (e.g., mannitol and furosemide), ingestion or administration of large quantities of solute (e.g., sodium chloride or glucose)
• Primary polyuria due to ADH deficiency(not reported in ferrets, but should be considered)—traumatic, neoplastic; some drugs (e.g., alcohol)

• Primary polydipsia—such as behavioral problems, pyrexia, or pain; organic disease of the anterior hypothalamic thirst center of neoplastic, traumatic, or inflammatory origin—not reported in ferrets but should be considered

### RISK FACTORS
• Renal disease or liver disease
• Selected electrolyte disorders
• Administration of diuretics and anticonvulsants

## DIAGNOSIS

### DIFFERENTIAL DIAGNOSIS
#### Differentiating Similar Signs
• Differentiate polyuria from an abnormal increase in the frequency of urination (pollakiuria). Pollakiuria is often associated with dysuria, stranguria, or hematuria. Patients with polyuria void large quantities of urine; patients with pollakiuria typically void small quantities of urine.
• Measuring urinary-specific gravity may provide evidence of adequate urine-concentrating ability (1.030), which rules out polyuria/polydipsia.

#### Differentiating Causes
• If associated with progressive weight loss—consider renal failure, diabetes mellitus, hepatic failure, pyometra, and pyelonephritis.
• If associated with polyphagia—consider diabetes mellitus (rare).
• If associated with bilateral alopecia and other cutaneous problems—consider concurrent adrenal disease (abscessed urogenital cysts, prostatic abscess or pyometra secondary to adrenal disease).
• If associated with signs of nausea such as anorexia, pawing at the mouth, and bruxism (occasionally vomiting)—consider renal failure, pyelonephritis, hepatic failure, hypercalcemia, hypokalemia, and diabetes mellitus.
• If associated with recent estrus in an intact female—consider pyometra.
• If associated with abdominal distention—consider hepatic failure.
• If associated with behavioral or neurologic disorder—consider hepatic failure, primary polydipsia, or concurrent insulinoma.

### CBC/BIOCHEMISTRY/URINALYSIS
• Serum sodium concentration may help differentiate primary polyuria from primary polydipsia. Plasma osmolarity has been reported to be 328 ± 1 mOsm/kg, rising to 366 ± 11 following 24 hours of water deprivation for normal ferrets.

• Relative hypernatremia or high serum osmolarity suggests primary polyuria.
• Hyponatremia or low serum osmolarity suggests primary polydipsia.
• Azotemia is consistent with renal causes for polyuria/polydipsia but may also indicate dehydration resulting from inadequate compensatory polydipsia. Increased BUN may be seen more commonly than increases in serum creatinine in ferrets with renal disease.
• Unexpectedly low BUN concentrations suggest hepatic failure.
• High hepatic enzyme activities are consistent hepatic failure, pyometra, and diabetes mellitus.
• Persistent hyperglycemia is consistent with diabetes mellitus.
• Hyperkalemia, particularly if associated with hyponatremia, suggests possible iatrogenic hypoadrenocorticism or therapy with potassium-sparing diuretics.
• Hypercalcemia and hypokalemia can cause, or occur in association with, other diseases that cause polyuria/polydipsia (e.g., chronic renal failure may be associated with both).
• Hypoalbuminemia supports renal or hepatic causes of polyuria/polydipsia.
• Neutrophilia is consistent with pyelonephritis, pyometra, or hepatitis.
• Glucosuria (rare in ferrets) supports a diagnosis of diabetes mellitus or renal glucosuria; pyuria, white blood cell casts, and/or bacteriuria should prompt consideration of pyelonephritis or paraurethral cysts.

### OTHER LABORATORY TESTS
• Urine culture—chronic pyelonephritis cannot be conclusively ruled out by absence of pyuria or bacteriuria.
• Cytologic examination of lymph node aspirate or biopsy may provide evidence of lymphosarcoma, which induces polyuria by direct infiltration of renal tissues (hypercalcemic nephrotoxicity has not been reported in ferrets with lymphoma).

### IMAGING
Abdominal survey radiography and ultrasonography may provide additional evidence of renal (e.g., primary renal diseases and urinary obstruction), hepatic (e.g., microhepatica, hepatic infiltrate), or uterine (e.g., pyometra) disorders that can contribute to polyuria/polydipsia.

### DIAGNOSTIC PROCEDURES
N/A

## TREATMENT

• Serious medical consequence for the patient is rare if patient has free access to water and is willing and able to drink. Until the mechanism of polyuria is understood, discourage owners from limiting access to water. Direct treatment at the underlying cause.
• Provide polyuric patients with free access to water unless they are vomiting. If polyuric patients are vomiting, give replacement maintenance fluids parenterally. Also provide fluids parenterally when other conditions limit oral intake or dehydration persists despite polydipsia.
• Base fluid selection on knowledge of the underlying cause for fluid loss. In most patients, lactated Ringer's solution is an acceptable replacement fluid.
• Primary polydipsia—treat by limiting water intake to a normal daily volume. Monitor the patient closely to avoid iatrogenic dehydration.

## MEDICATIONS

### DRUG(S) OF CHOICE
Vary with underlying cause

### CONTRAINDICATIONS
N/A

### PRECAUTIONS
Until renal and hepatic failure have been excluded as potential causes for polyuria/polydipsia, use caution in administering any drug eliminated via these pathways.

### POSSIBLE INTERACTIONS
N/A

### ALTERNATIVE DRUGS
N/A

## FOLLOW-UP

### PATIENT MONITORING
• Hydration status by clinical assessment of hydration and serial evaluation of body weight
• Fluid intake and urine output—provide a useful baseline for assessing adequacy of hydration therapy.

### POSSIBLE COMPLICATIONS
Dehydration

## MISCELLANEOUS

### ASSOCIATED CONDITIONS
• Bacterial urinary tract infection
• Ferret adrenal disease

### AGE-RELATED FACTORS
N/A

### ZOONOTIC POTENTIAL
N/A

### PREGNANCY
N/A

### SYNONYMS
N/A

### SEE ALSO
• Diabetes mellitus
• Dysuria and hematuria
• Pyometra and stump pyometra

• Renal failure
• Urinary tract obstruction

### ABBREVIATIONS
• ADH = antidiuretic hormone
• BUN = blood urea nitrogen

*Suggested Reading*

Antinoff N. Urinary disorders in ferrets. Semin Avian Exotic Pet Med 1998;7(2): 89–92.

Esteves MI, Marini RP, Ryden EB, et al. Estimation of glomerular filtration rate and evaluation of renal function in ferrets. Am J Vet Res 1994;55:166–172.

Fox JG, Pearson RC, Bell JA. Diseases of the genitourinary system. In: Fox JG, ed. Biology and Diseases of the Ferret. 2nd Ed. Baltimore: Williams & Wilkins, 1998:247–272.

Hillyer EV. Urogenital diseases. In: Hillyer EV, Quesenberry KE, eds. Ferrets, Rabbits and Rodents: Clinical Medicine and Surgery. Philadelphia: WB Saunders, 1997:44–52.

Meric SM. Polyuria and polydipsia. In: Ettinger SJ, Feldman EC, eds. Textbook of Veterinary Internal Medicine. Philadelphia: Saunders, 1995:159–163.

*Portions Adapted From*

Polzin DJ. Polyuria and Polydipsia. In: Tilley LP, Smith FWK, Jr., eds. The 5-Minute Veterinary Consult: Canine and Feline, 3rd Ed. Baltimore: Lippincott Williams & Wilkins, 2003.

# PREGNANCY TOXEMIA

## BASICS

### OVERVIEW
• A life-threatening condition to both the jill and kits caused by a negative energy balance in late pregnancy
• Usually develops in the last week of gestation
• Occurs during periods of inadvertent food deprivation or anorexia, or with large litter size

### SIGNALMENT
Usually seen in primiparous jills

### SIGNS
#### Historical Findings
• Poor diet fed during pregnancy
• Sudden changes in diet—may cause jill to refuse food
• Accidental food deprivation
• Anorexia
• Sudden onset of profound lethargy and depression

#### Physical Examination Findings
• Lethargy, depression
• Profound weakness
• Abnormal mentation (star-gazing)
• Melena
• Dehydration
• Hair easily epilates
• Large litter size (>10 fetuses)

### CAUSES AND RISK FACTORS
• Inadequate caloric intake during late gestation results in negative energy balance. This may occur by feeding of a poor diet, inadequate access to food, diet changes, or anorexia.
• Even short periods of anorexia or food deprivation (<24 hours) may cause toxemia.
• Excessive calorie demands caused by a large litter size (>10 fetuses)
• Most affected jills have hepatic lipidosis; the severity of lipidosis may strongly influence the outcome.

## DIAGNOSIS

### DIFFERENTIAL DIAGNOSIS
• Hypoglycemia—usually concurrent; history of food deprivation or large litter size to differentiate
• Sepsis—distinguished by signalment and history
• Hypocalcemia—rare in ferrets, may see muscle rigidity; differentiated by signalment; calcium concentration diagnostic

### CBC/BIOCHEMISTRY/URINALYSIS
• Hypoglycemia—serum glucose concentration <50 g/dL

• Increased BUN—prerenal azotemia
• Anemia often present—PCV <30%
• Dehydration—may cause increase total protein, albumin
• May detect ketonuria

### IMAGING
Radiographs or ultrasound to detect large litter size

### OTHER LABORATORY TESTS
N/A

### DIAGNOSTIC PROCEDURES
N/A

## TREATMENT
• Emergency inpatient
• An emergency cesarean section is often necessary to save the life of the jill, but the kits will not be viable if delivered at <40 days gestation.
• If toxemia occurs prior to the 40th day of gestation and viable kits are desired, intensive supportive care may keep the jill alive until a cesarean section can be performed. Supportive care alone carries a poorer prognosis than surgical treatment.

#### Supportive Care
• Administer IV fluid therapy containing 2.5% dextrose.
• Correct any electrolyte imbalances.
• Offer high-quality ferret food, containing >35% protein and 20% fat.
• Supplement diet with high-calorie supplements such as Nutri-Cal (EVSCO Pharmaceuticals, Buena, NJ) or Clinicare Feline liquid diet (Abbott Laboratories, North Chicago, IL). Administer these supplements several times a day.
• If the ferret will not accept ferret kibble, offer canned chicken human baby foods and Eukanuba Maximum Calorie diet (Iams Co., Dayton, OH) along with the dietary supplement. Warming the food to body temperature or offering via syringe may increase acceptance.
• Resting energy requirement for ferrets is reported to be 70 kcal/kg body weight per day. Clinicare Feline contains 1 kcal/mL; Eukanuba Maximum Calorie diet contains 2 kcal/mL.

## MEDICATIONS

### DRUG(S) OF CHOICE
• Isoflurane anesthesia for cesarean section
• For gastric ulceration—famotidine (0.25–0.5 mg/kg PO, IV q12–24h), ranitidine HCl (3.5 mg/kg PO q12h), cimetidine (5–10 mg/kg PO, SC, IV q8h), or omeprazole (0.7 mg/kg PO q24h); sucralfate sus-

pension (25 mg/kg PO q8h) may be added to protect ulcerated tissue by binding to ulcer sites.

### CONTRAINDICATIONS/POSSIBLE INTERACTIONS
N/A

## FOLLOW-UP

### PATIENT MONITORING
• If no improvement is seen with supportive care alone, perform a cesarean section.
• Following cesarean section, monitor jill for evidence of lactation.
• To prevent toxemia in the future—feed a diet consisting of at least 35% protein and 20% fat; ensure that food is available 24 hours a day; monitor the volume of food remaining in the feed dishes to be certain the jill is eating; do not attempt a diet change during pregnancy.

### POSSIBLE COMPLICATIONS
• Some jills will not lactate following treatment; hand rearing of kits is difficult and carries a poor survival rate.
• Death

### EXPECTED COURSE AND PROGNOSIS
Prognosis—good with immediate cesarean section; poor with delayed treatment

### ABBREVIATIONS
• BUN = blood urea nitrogen
• PCV = packed cell volume

## MISCELLANEOUS

*Suggested Reading*

Bell JA. Periparturient and neonatal diseases. In: Hillyer EV, Quesenberry KE, eds. Ferrets, Rabbits and Rodents: Clinical Medicine and Surgery. Philadelphia: WB Saunders, 1997:53–62.

Fox JG, Pearson RC, Bell JA. Diseases of the genitourinary system. In: Fox JG, ed. Biology and Diseases of the Ferret. 2nd Ed. Baltimore: Williams & Wilkins, 1998:247–272.

Harrenstein L. Critical care of ferrets, rabbits and rodents. Semin Avian Exotic Pet Med 1994;3(4):217–228.

Hillyer EV. Urogenital diseases. In: Hillyer EV, Quesenberry KE, eds. Ferrets, Rabbits and Rodents: Clinical Medicine and Surgery. Philadelphia: WB Saunders, 1997:44–52.

# BASICS

## OVERVIEW
• Proliferative bowel disease (PBD) is a characteristic infection of the distal colon caused by the spiral bacteria *Lawsonia intracellularis*. The organism is closely related to the bacterium that causes proliferative enteritis in hamsters and swine.
• The disease is characterized by large bowel diarrhea and rectal prolapse in young ferrets.

## SIGNALMENT
• A relatively uncommon disease
• Seen primarily in ferrets 12 weeks to 6 months of age; stressed, immunosuppressed older animals also may be affected.
• May be a higher incidence in males

## SIGNS

### Historical Findings
• Large bowel diarrhea—may be profuse and watery, but more often green in color with mucous; fresh blood usually present; small scant stools with green mucous; tenesmus and crying out when defecating
• Rectal prolapse—highly suggestive of PBD
• Severe weight loss
• Ataxia, weakness, muscle tremors
• Anorexia, abdominal discomfort, or generalized unthriftiness

### Physical Examination Findings
• Distal colon may be palpably thickened; mesenteric lymph nodes may be enlarged.
• Emaciation, muscle wasting
• Fecal and urine staining of perineum
• Partial to complete rectal prolapse
• Weakness, ataxia, and dehydration may be noted.

## CAUSES AND RISK FACTORS
Stress, poor hygiene, concurrent disease

# DIAGNOSIS
Presumptive diagnosis is often made on signalment, signs, and response to treatment; definitive diagnosis requires colonic biopsy.

## DIFFERENTIAL DIAGNOSIS
• ECE and Coccidia are more common causes of diarrhea in young ferrets.
• Consider all causes of diarrhea, including systemic or metabolic disease, as well as specific intestinal disorders.
• Blood and mucous in stool is also seen with Coccidia, clostridia, *Campylobacter*, and *Salmonella*. These organisms all can cause disease alone or be copathogens with *Lawsonia intracellularis*.
• Wasting, thickened gastrointestinal tract, and palpable mesenteric lymph nodes—consider ECE, clostridia, *Campylobacter*, and lymphoma.

## CBC/BIOCHEMISTRY/URINALYSIS
• Leukocytosis usually seen; differential count often demonstrates neutrophilia with a left shift.
• Hypoproteinemia
• Dehydration—elevated PCV, TP, and azotemia

## OTHER LABORATORY TESTS
Fecal direct examination, fecal flotation, and zinc sulfate centrifugation may demonstrate gastrointestinal parasites.

### Microbiology
• Aerobic and anaerobic fecal cultures rule out clostridia or *Salmonella.*
• Cultures for *Lawsonia intracellularis* are not useful, since they are intracellular organisms not usually shed in the feces.
• Fecal cytology may demonstrate clostridia or other organisms and increased WBC or RBC numbers

## IMAGING
• Survey abdominal radiographs—usually normal
• Barium contrast studies—rarely reveal mucosal abnormalities or thickened bowel loops; generally not helpful in establishing a definitive diagnosis; can be normal even in individuals with severe disease

## DIAGNOSTIC PROCEDURES
• Colonic biopsy needed for definitive diagnosis. Organisms are intracellular and are demonstrated histologically using silver stains. Exploratory laparotomy may be useful rule out gastrointestinal foreign bodies, neoplasia, and intestinal inflammatory diseases.
• Since this is an expensive, invasive procedure, diagnosis may be attempted based on response to empirical treatment. However, other disease or copathogens, if present, are unlikely to respond, necessitating definitive diagnosis.
• Abdominocentesis and cytology may help determine if perforation and subsequent peritonitis has occurred.

## PATHOLOGIC FINDINGS
Grossly thickened and segmented distal colon. Histopathology—mucosal cell proliferation; epithelial hyperplasia; hypertrophy of the tunica muscularis; organisms demonstrated in epithelium using silver stains

# TREATMENT

## APPROPRIATE HEALTH CARE
• Most patients with mild to moderate diarrhea can be treated as outpatients.
• Hospitalize when diarrhea is severe, resulting in dehydration and electrolyte imbalance; administer supportive fluids on the basis of hydration status.

## DIET
Anorectic ferrets may refuse kibble, but are often willing to eat canned cat foods, meat baby foods, or high-calorie liquid or paste dietary supplements.

## SURGICAL CONSIDERATIONS
• Rectal prolapse should be replaced and sutured with a purse-string closure until feces return to a normal consistency.
• Owners should be advised to monitor the ferret to be sure defecation occurs while the sutures are in place.

# MEDICATIONS

## DRUG(S) OF CHOICE

### Antibiotics
• Most patients respond well to chloramphenicol 50 mg/kg IM, SC, PO q12h for a minimum of 14 days.
• Metronidazole (15–20 mg/kg PO q12h × 10–14 days) may also be effective
• Relapses may occur when antibiotics are discontinued, requiring prolonged antibiotic therapy.

## CONTRAINDICATIONS
N/A

## PRECAUTIONS
N/A

## POSSIBLE INTERACTIONS
N/A

## ALTERNATIVE DRUGS
N/A

# FOLLOW-UP

## PATIENT MONITORING
• Monitor patients for reoccurrence of diarrhea or concurrent diseases such as gastrointestinal ulceration or enteric copathogens.
• Response to therapy supports the diagnosis; repeat diagnostics are rarely necessary.

## PREVENTION/AVOIDANCE
Avoid stress and unsanitary conditions.

## POSSIBLE COMPLICATIONS
Colonic ulceration, necrosis, or rupture may occur, leading to septic peritonitis

## EXPECTED COURSE AND PROGNOSIS
Most animals with mild to moderate disease respond well to chloramphenicol therapy; chronic patients may require long-term therapy; failure to respond suggests concurrent disease; further diagnostic evaluation is indicated.

# PROLIFERATIVE BOWEL DISEASE

## MISCELLANEOUS

### ASSOCIATED CONDITIONS
- Other enteric disease
- Rectal prolapse

### AGE-RELATED FACTORS
N/A

### ZOONOTIC POTENTIAL
N/A

### PREGNANCY
N/A

### SYNONYMS
Proliferative colitis

### SEE ALSO
- Coccidia
- ECE Epizootic Catarrhal Enteritis
- Gastrointestinal foreign body
- Inflammatory bowel disease

### ABBREVIATIONS
- ECE = epizootic catarrhal enteritis
- PCV = packed cell volume
- RBC = red blood cell
- TP = total protein
- WBC = white blood cell

### Suggested Reading

Finkler MR. Ferret colitis. In: Kirk RW, Bonagura JD, eds. Kirk's Current Veterinary Therapy XI: Small Animal Practice. Philadelphia: WB Saunders, 1992.

Fox JG. Diseases of the gastrointestinal system. In: Fox JG, ed. Biology and Diseases of the Ferret. 2nd Ed. Baltimore: Williams & Wilkins, 1998.

Hoefer HL. Gastrointestinal diseases. In: Hillyer EV, Quesenberry KE, eds. Ferrets, Rabbits and Rodents: Clinical Medicine and Surgery. Philadelphia: WB Saunders, 1997:26–36.

Jenkins JR: Rabbit and ferret liver and gastrointestinal testing. In: Fudge AM, ed. Laboratory Medicine, Avian and Exotic Pets. Philadelphia: WB Saunders, 2000.

# BASICS

## OVERVIEW

The prostate is a fusiform structure surrounding the dorsal aspect of the proximal urethra. Bacterial prostatitis and prostatic abscesses are usually secondary to urogenital cystic disease. Urogenital cystic disease (prostatic and paraprostatic cysts) is caused by ferret adrenal disease and the resultant excessive production of androgens. Accumulation of prostatic secretions within these cysts can become secondarily infected, resulting in chronic bacterial prostatitis or prostatic abscess. Bacteria usually gain access to the prostate gland and prostatic cysts by ascending the urethra and overcoming the lower urinary tract host defense mechanisms. Frequently, abscesses or cysts will impinge on the urethra causing partial or complete obstruction.

## SIGNALMENT

Seen primarily in neutered males, 3–7 years old

## CAUSES AND RISK FACTORS

• Evidence suggests that ferret adrenal disease and subsequent urogenital cysts and prostatitis may be related to neutering at an early age.
• Most ferrets with bacterial urinary tract infection have the same bacteria present in the prostate gland. However, ferrets may have a prostatic infection without evidence of bacteria or inflammation in their urine.

## SIGNS

• Pollakiuria, tenesmus, dysuria, including intense straining and crying out when urinating
• With complete obstruction, ferrets will have signs of uremia, including depression, lethargy, and anorexia.
• Bilaterally symmetric alopecia or pruritus due to adrenal disease
• Abdominal distension
• Cysts and abscesses are often palpable and may be larger than the urinary bladder.
• Weight loss, depression, anorexia
• Purulent preputial discharge

# DIAGNOSIS

## DIFFERENTIAL DIAGNOSIS

• For stranguria—urolithiasis, neoplasia of the bladder neck or urethra, or urethral stricture
• For mass detected in area of prostate—urogenital cysts, prostatic neoplasia, or other abdominal mass: neoplasia, abscess, or granuloma

## CBC/BIOCHEMISTRY/URINALYSIS

• Usually normal
• Hemogram may show nonregenerative anemia and leukocytosis.
• Hypoglycemia may be present—usually due to concurrent insulinoma
• Urinalysis may be helpful to diagnose urolithiasis (usually struvite) or bacterial cystitis. However, prostatic or paraprostatic abscesses may drain into the urinary bladder or urethra, resulting in thick purulent exudate mixed with urine in the bladder. In rare cases, this exudate can be thick enough to cause urethral blockage.

## OTHER LABORATORY TESTS

• Elevations of plasma estradiol, androstenedione, and 17-hydroxyprogesterone combined are most diagnostic (available through the University of Tennessee Clinical Endocrinology Laboratory, Department of Comparative Medicine).
• Elevation in plasma estrogens alone in males is diagnostic of adrenal disease.
• Examination of fluid from abscess—thick, greenish purulent exudate
• Bacterial culture of fluid from abscess

## IMAGING

• Survey radiographs often reveal what appear to be two or more urinary bladders, as abscesses can be as large as or larger than the urinary bladder.
• Ultrasonography is often useful for demonstrating adrenal gland enlargement. Ideally, the affected gland should be identified prior to surgery.

## OTHER DIAGNOSTIC PROCEDURES

N/A

# TREATMENT

• Surgical removal of the affected adrenal gland(s), coupled with complete surgical excision of any abscess (if possible) or marsupialization of abscesses. Both of these procedures require special surgical expertise, especially if the right adrenal gland is diseased. Proximity of the right adrenal to the vena cava and the potential for vena cava invasion by malignant tumors make complete excision a high-risk procedure. Referral to a surgeon or clinician with experience is recommended when possible.
• Several techniques for adrenalectomy have been advocated, and problems may be associated with each surgical option, depending on the surgeon's expertise. Refer to suggested reading list for a more detailed description of surgical procedures.
• Many practitioners advocate debulking rather than removal of the right adrenal as a procedure carrying less risk of life-threatening complications. If this method is chosen, signs of clinical disease will return,

necessitating repeat surgery or medical therapy alone.
• Removal of the affected adrenal gland(s) will cause a significant reduction in the size of prostatic tissue, usually within a few days.
• If the bladder is full of purulent exudate, a cystotomy may be indicated to remove accumulated material.
• If the urethra is partially or completely obstructed, catheterization is indicated. Once the urinary bladder is reached, suture the catheter in place and maintain for 1–3 days postoperatively.
• Alternatively, adrenal disease may be treated medically (see alternative drugs, below). Medical treatment has been anecdotally reported to cause a significant reduction in the size of prostatic tissue within as little as 2–3 days. Surgical debridement of prostatic abscess is still necessary.

# MEDICATIONS

## DRUG(S) OF CHOICE

Antibiotic therapy should be based on results of culture and susceptibility testing. Choose antibiotics that are able to enter the prostatic lumen, such as trimethoprim/sulfonamide (15–30 mg/kg PO, SC q12h) or enrofloxacin (10–20 mg/kg PO, SC, IM q12h). A minimum of 4–6 weeks of antimicrobial administration is usually necessary.

## CONTRAINDICATIONS/POSSIBLE INTERACTIONS

N/A

## ALTERNATIVE MEDICATIONS

• Large prostatic cysts or abscesses are unlikely to respond to medical treatment alone; surgical debulking or drainage is generally necessary.
• Successful treatment of prostatic hyperplasia has been anecdotally reported using leuprolide acetate, a GNRH analog. This is a potent inhibitor of gonadotropin secretion used to inhibit ovarian and testicular steroidogenesis. It is available as a 1- or 4-month depot injection and has been anecdotally reported to alleviate the dermal and reproductive organ signs of adrenal disease in ferrets. Significant reduction in prostate size has anecdotally been reported to occur in as little as 2–3 days. Reported dosages: Lupron 30-day depot, 100–200 µg/kg IM q4w until signs resolve, then q4–8w prn, lifelong. This drug has no effect on adrenal tumor growth or metastasis. Large prostatic cysts or abscesses are unlikely to respond to medical treatment alone; surgical debulking or drainage is generally necessary. Side effects include dyspnea, lethargy, and local injection site irritation.
• Flutamide (10 mg/kg PO q12h) inhibits androgen uptake and binding in target tis-

# PROSTATITIS AND PROSTATIC ABSCESSES

sues and is used in the treatment of androgen-responsive prostatic tumors in humans. It has been used to reduce the size of prostatic tissue and treat alopecia in ferrets with adrenal disease. This drug has no effect on adrenal tumor growth or metastasis. Large prostatic cysts or abscesses are unlikely to respond to medical treatment alone; surgical debulking or drainage is generally necessary. Side effects may include gynomastia and hepatic injury; monitor liver enzyme concentrations during therapy.

## FOLLOW-UP

• The prognosis is poor when large prostatic abscesses are found, because complete removal may be difficult and the response to antibiotic therapy is variable.
• Monitor for signs of peritonitis, such as pyrexia, anorexia, lethargy, and abdominal distension.
• Following unilateral adrenalectomy or subtotal adrenalectomy, monitor for return of clinical signs, because tumor recurrence and subsequent prostatic disease is common.
• Ultrasonographic examination at 2- to 4-week intervals after adrenalectomy may be used to follow resolution of abscesses.

## MISCELLANEOUS

**SEE ALSO**
• Adrenal disease
• Dysuria and pollakiuria
• Urogenital cystic disease

**ABBREVIATIONS**
• GNRH = gonadotropin-releasing hormone

*Suggested Reading*

Antinoff N. Urinary disorders in ferrets. Semin Avian Exotic Pet Med 1998;7(2):89–92.
Beeber NL. Abdominal surgery in ferrets. Vet Clin North Am Exot Anim Pract 2000;3(3):647–662.
Brown SA. Neoplasia. In: Hillyer EV, Quesenberry KE, eds. Ferrets, Rabbits and Rodents: Clinical Medicine and Surgery. Philadelphia: WB Saunders, 1997:99.
Fox JG, Marini RP. Diseases of the endocrine system. In: Fox JG, ed. Biology and Diseases of the Ferret. 2nd Ed. Baltimore: Williams & Wilkins, 1998.
Hillyer EV. Urogenital diseases. In: Hillyer EV, Quesenberry KE, eds. Ferrets, Rabbits and Rodents: Clinical Medicine and Surgery. Philadelphia: WB Saunders, 1997:44–52.

Li X, Fox JG, Erdman SE, et al. Cystic urogenital anomalies in ferrets (Mustela putorius furo). Vet Pathol 1996;33:150–158.
Marini RP, Esteves MI, Fox JG. A technique for catheterization of the urinary bladder in the ferret. Lab Anim 1994;28:155–157.
Quesenberry KE, Rosenthal KL. Endocrine disease. In: Hillyer EV, Quesenberry KE, eds. Ferrets, Rabbits and Rodents: Clinical Medicine and Surgery. Philadelphia: WB Saunders, 1997.
Weiss CA, Scott MV. Clinical aspects and surgical treatment of hyperadrenocorticism in the domestic ferret: 94 cases (1994–1996). J Am Anim Hosp Assoc 1997;33:487–493.
Wheeler J, Bennet RA. Ferret abdominal surgical procedures. Part I. Adrenal gland and pancreatic beta-cell tumors. Compend Contin Educ Pract Vet 1999;21(9):815–822.

*Portions Adapted From*

Cowan LA. Prostatitis and Prostatic Abscesses. In: Tilley LP, Smith FWK, Jr., eds. The 5-Minute Veterinary Consult: Canine and Feline, 2nd Ed. Baltimore: Lippincott Williams & Wilkins, 2000.

# BASICS

## DEFINITION
- Abnormally large prostate gland determined by abdominal palpation or by abdominal radiography or prostatic ultrasonography
- In ferrets, the prostate is a fusiform structure surrounding the dorsal aspect of the proximal urethra.
- Enlargement is usually due to urogenital, prostatic, or periprostatic cysts; cystic structures found on the dorsal aspect of the urinary bladder or surrounding the proximal urethra in male and (rarely) female ferrets. These structures likely arise from remnants of the mesonephric or paramesonephric ducts, from the prostate, or from periprostatic tissues.
- Cysts can become very large, may be single or multiple, and often cause partial or complete obstruction of the urethra.
- Secondary bacterial infections within the cystic fluid are extremely common.

## PATHOPHYSIOLOGY
- Prostatic hyperplasia and cyst formation are associated with ferret adrenal disease and the resultant excessive production of androgens.
- Enlargement can result from epithelial cell hyperplasia or hypertrophy, cystic change within the prostatic or periprostatic tissues, neoplasia of prostatic epithelium or stroma, or inflammatory cell infiltration (e.g., acute and chronic bacterial prostatitis and prostatic abscess).
- Obstruction of the urethra may occur due to extraluminal compression by the cyst or hyperplastic tissue or, with bacterial infection, may become obstructed by thick, tenacious exudate in the urine.

## SYSTEMS AFFECTED
- Renal/urologic—obstruction of the urethra, secondary bacterial cystitis
- Gastrointestinal—ferrets with large cysts may have tenesmus.
- Peritoneum—focal or generalized peritonitis can develop in animals with bacterial infection of cystic fluid or abscesses.

## SIGNALMENT

### Predominant Sex
Seen primarily in neutered males; female ferrets may be affected (enlargement of periurethral tissues), although quite rare.

### Mean Age and Range
Middle-aged animals, 3–7 years old

## SIGNS

### Historical and Physical Examination Findings
- Presenting complaint is typically stranguria due to urethral obstruction by cysts, hyperplastic prostatic tissue, or thick exudate blocking the urethra.
- Pollakiuria, tenesmus, dysuria, including intense straining and crying out when urinating
- Stranguria may be confused with constipation.
- With complete urethral obstruction, ferrets will have signs of uremia, including depression, lethargy, and anorexia.
- Weight loss, depression, and anorexia may be seen with secondary bacterial infections (abscesses).
- Purulent preputial discharge with abscesses
- Bilaterally symmetric alopecia or pruritus due to adrenal disease
- Abdominal distension
- Firm mass near bladder; may contain multiple cysts of varying size
- Fluid-filled cysts are often palpable and may be larger than the urinary bladder.

## CAUSES
- Prostatic hyperplasia, urogenital (prostatic, periprostatic) cysts—caused by excessive androgen production due to functional adrenal hyperplasia, adenoma, or carcinomas
- Neoplasia—adenocarcinoma, sarcoma, metastatic neoplasia (rare)

## RISK FACTORS
Evidence suggests that ferret adrenal disease and subsequent urogenital cysts may be related to neutering at an early age.

# DIAGNOSIS

## DIFFERENTIAL DIAGNOSIS
- For stranguria—urolithiasis, neoplasia of the bladder neck or urethra, or urethral stricture
- For mass detected in area of prostate—prostatic hyperplasia, prostatic neoplasia, or other abdominal mass: neoplasia, abscess, or granuloma

## CBC/BIOCHEMISTRY/URINALYSIS
- CBC normal in patients with sterile cysts or prostatic hyperplasia
- Leukocytosis in patients with prostatic abscess and prostatic neoplasia (occasionally)
- Urinalysis may be helpful to diagnose urolithiasis (usually struvite) or bacterial cystitis. However, secondary bacterial infections leading to abscess formation in many prostatic or paraprostatic cysts may drain into the urinary bladder or urethra, resulting in thick purulent exudate mixed with urine in the bladder. In some cases, this exudate can be thick enough to cause urethral blockage.

## OTHER LABORATORY TESTS
- Elevations in plasma estradiol, androstenedione, and 17-hydroxyprogesterone to rule out ferret adrenal disease (available through the University of Tennessee Clinical Endocrinology Laboratory, Department of Comparative Medicine)
- Examination of cyst fluid—gross appearance can range from clear yellow, or more commonly, thick, greenish, foul-smelling fluid; cytologic examination ranges from serosanguinous fluid to purulent exudate (more common).
- Culture the fluid for bacteria.

## IMAGING

### Radiographic Findings
- Abdominal radiographs reveal prostatomegaly.
- Ultrasonography reveals large prostate with single to multiple fluid-filled cysts of varying size; uniform parenchymal echogenicity seen in some ferrets
- Ultrasonography may be useful for demonstrating adrenal gland enlargement.
- Prostatomegaly

## DIAGNOSTIC PROCEDURES
Ultrasound—guided aspiration of cystic structures; take care to avoid rupturing a prostatic abscess.

# TREATMENT
- Ferret adrenal disease may be treated with adrenalectomy or managed medically. The decision as to which form of treatment is appropriate is multifactorial; which gland is affected (left vs. right), surgeon's experience and expertise, severity of clinical signs, age of the animal, concurrent diseases, and financial issues should be considered.
- Removal of the affected adrenal gland(s) and drainage of the cysts at the time of surgery is often curative in ferrets with mild prostatomegaly, sterile cysts, or small abscessed cyst. These procedures require special surgical expertise, especially if the right adrenal gland is diseased. Proximity of the right adrenal gland to the vena cava and the potential for vena cava invasion by malignant tumors make complete excision a high-risk procedure. Referral to a surgeon or clinician with experience is recommended when possible.
- Large or multiple cysts that are abscessed or infection with resistant bacterial pathogens may require prolonged treatment; prognosis is poorer for complete resolution as compared to sterile cysts.
- Always submit samples of prostatic tissue and removed adrenal gland for histologic examination.
- Fluid therapy, either subcutaneous or intravenous, depending on the state of hydration. Ferrets that are uremic require intravenous fluid therapy. Correct any acid-base disturbances as indicated by the serum biochemistry profile.

# PROSTATOMEGALY

• Postoperative fluid therapy should continue for 24–48 hours.
• If the urethra is partially or completely obstructed, catheterize prior to surgery and maintain catheter in place for 2–3 days postoperatively.

## MEDICATIONS

### DRUG(S) OF CHOICE
• Successful treatment of prostatic hyperplasia has been anecdotally reported using leuprolide acetate, a GNRH analog. This is a potent inhibitor of gonadotropin secretion used to inhibit ovarian and testicular steroidogenesis. It has been anecdotally reported to alleviate the dermal and reproductive organ signs of adrenal disease in ferrets. Significant reduction in prostate size has anecdotally been reported to occur in as little as 2–3 days. Reported dosages: Lupron 30-day depot, 100–200 μg/kg IM q4w until signs resolve, then q4–8w prn, lifelong. This drug has no effect on adrenal tumor growth or metastasis. Side effects include dyspnea, lethargy, and local injection site irritation. Large prostatic cysts or abscesses are unlikely to respond to medical treatment alone.
• If secondary bacterial infection or abscess is evident, antibiotic therapy should be based on results of culture and susceptibility testing. Choose antibiotics that are able to enter the prostatic lumen, such as trimethoprim/sulfonamide (15–30 mg/kg PO, SC q12h), enrofloxacin (10–20 mg/kg PO, SC, IM q12h), or chloramphenicol (50 mg/kg PO, SC q12h). A minimum of 4–6 weeks of antimicrobial administration is usually necessary.

### CONTRAINDICATIONS
N/A

### PRECAUTIONS
N/A

### POSSIBLE INTERACTIONS
N/A

### ALTERNATIVE DRUGS
Flutamide (10 mg/kg PO q12h) inhibits androgen uptake and binding in target tissues and is used in the treatment of androgen-responsive prostatic tumors in humans. It has been used to reduce the size of prostatic tissue and treat alopecia in ferrets with adrenal disease. This drug has no effect on adrenal tumor growth or metastasis. Side effects may include gynecomastia and hepatic injury; monitor liver enzyme concentrations during therapy.

## FOLLOW-UP

### PATIENT MONITORING
• Following adrenalectomy, prostatic tissue should decrease in size within 1–3 days. If urethral obstruction persists, a second adrenal tumor may be present.
• With medical therapy, reduction in prostate size has been anecdotally reported to occur in as little as 2–3 days, but reports of weeks to months for a response also exist.
• Abdominal radiographs or prostatic ultrasonography to assess efficacy of treatment
• Urine culture to access efficacy of treatment in patients with abscessed cysts and bacterial cystitis

### POSSIBLE COMPLICATIONS
• Urethral obstruction
• Peritonitis
• Return of prostatomegaly if all hyperfunctioning adrenal tissue is not removed

## MISCELLANEOUS

### ASSOCIATED CONDITIONS
Insulinoma, lymphoma, and/or congestive heart failure are often seen concurrently.

### AGE-RELATED FACTORS
N/A

### ZOONOTIC POTENTIAL
N/A

### PREGNANCY
N/A

### SYNONYMS
• Paraurethral cysts
• Periprostatic cysts
• Prostatic cysts

### SEE ALSO
• Adrenal disease
• Prostatitis and prostatic abscess
• Urogenital cystic disease

### ABBREVIATIONS
• CBC = complete blood count
• GNRH = gonadotropin-releasing hormone

*Suggested Reading*

Antinoff N. Urinary disorders in ferrets. Semin Avian Exotic Pet Med 1998;7(2):89–92.

Beeber NL. Abdominal surgery in ferrets. Vet Clin North Am Exot Anim Pract 2000;3(3):647–662.

Brown SA. Neoplasia. In: Hillyer EV, Quesenberry KE, eds. Ferrets, Rabbits and Rodents: Clinical Medicine and Surgery. Philadelphia: WB Saunders, 1997:99.

Fox JG, Marini RP. Diseases of the endocrine system. In: Fox JG, ed. Biology and Diseases of the Ferret. 2nd Ed. Baltimore: Williams & Wilkins, 1998.

Hillyer EV. Urogenital diseases. In: Hillyer EV, Quesenberry KE, eds. Ferrets, Rabbits and Rodents: Clinical Medicine and Surgery. Philadelphia: WB Saunders, 1997:44–52.

Li X, Fox JG, Erdman SE, et al. Cystic urogenital anomalies in ferrets (Mustela putorius furo). Vet Pathol 1996;33:150–158.

Marini RP, Esteves MI, Fox JG. A technique for catheterization of the urinary bladder in the ferret. Lab Anim 1994;28:155–157.

Quesenberry KE, Rosenthal KL. Endocrine disease. In: Hillyer EV, Quesenberry KE, eds. Ferrets, Rabbits and Rodents: Clinical Medicine and Surgery. Philadelphia: WB Saunders, 1997.

Weiss CA, Scott MV. Clinical aspects and surgical treatment of hyperadrenocorticism in the domestic ferret: 94 cases (1994–1996). J Am Anim Hosp Assoc 1997;33:487–493.

Wheeler J, Bennet RA. Ferret abdominal surgical procedures. Part I. Adrenal gland and pancreatic beta-cell tumors. Compend Contin Educ Pract Vet 1999;21(9):815–822.

*Portions Adapted From*

Klausner JS, Root-Kustritz MV. Prostatomegaly. In: Tilley LP, Smith FWK, Jr., eds. The 5-Minute Veterinary Consult: Canine and Feline, 3rd Ed. Baltimore: Lippincott Williams & Wilkins, 2003.

# BASICS

## DEFINITION
The sensation that provokes the desire to scratch, rub, chew, or lick; often an indicator of inflamed skin

## PATHOPHYSIOLOGY
• Pruritus, or itching, is a primary cutaneous sensation that may be elicited from the epidermis, dermis, or mucous membranes.
• The mediators of pruritus in the ferret are unknown. In other mammalian species, histamines and proteolytic enzymes are believed to be the primary mediators. Proteolytic enzymes are released by bacteria, fungi, and mast cells and can be released by damage to epidermal cells, inflammatory infiltrate, and capillary dilation.

## SYSTEMS AFFECTED
• Skin/exocrine
• Endocrine/metabolic

## SIGNALMENT
Variable; depends on the underlying cause

## SIGNS
• The act of scratching, licking, biting, or chewing
• Evidence of self-trauma and cutaneous inflammation is often present.
• Alopecia often seen

## CAUSES
• Endocrine—pruritus, sometimes severe, occurs in approximately 30% of ferrets with adrenal disease.
• Parasitic—fleas and sarcoptic mange: usually pruritic; *Otodectes cyanotis* (ear mites) occasionally pruritic; *Demodex*—very rare in ferrets, may be pruritic
• Neoplastic—cutaneous epitheliotropic lymphoma; mast cell tumor
• Bacterial/fungal—pyoderma, dermatomycosis
• Immunologic—contact dermatitis has been anecdotally reported in ferrets. Cutaneous lesions resembling urticaria or histologic lesions characteristic of allergic reactions in other species have also been anecdotally reported; however, there are no confirmed cases of atopy, food allergy, or other allergic dermatitis in ferrets.

## RISK FACTORS
N/A

# DIAGNOSIS

## DIFFERENTIAL DIAGNOSIS
• Alopecia—diffuse/symmetrical: over 95% of neutered ferrets with bilaterally symmetric alopecia have adrenal disease. Hair loss often begins in late winter or early spring; hair initially may regrow later in the year, followed by progressive alopecia the following spring. Alopecia typically begins in the tail region and progresses cranially. In severe cases, the ferret will become completely bald. In most cases, the skin has a normal appearance, although 30% of affected ferrets are pruritic and secondary pyoderma is occasionally seen. Other signs related to adrenal disease, such as a swollen vulva in spayed females, may be seen.
• Alopecia—focal: in most cases, a clear history of pruritus is noted; some animals may excessively lick themselves without the owner's knowledge; ear mites, scabies, dermatomycosis, bacterial pyoderma, and some cutaneous neoplasms may all cause alopecia with varying degrees of inflammation and pruritus.

### Distribution of Lesions
• Ear mites—most ferrets with ear mites are not pruritic. In pruritic animals, one will see partial to complete alopecia caudal to the ears, waxy brown aural discharge, and excoriations around pinna.
• Fleas—patchy alopecia at tail base and in cervical and dorsal thoracic region; excoriations; secondary pyoderma sometimes seen
• Sarcoptic mange—two forms reported: generalized form with diffuse alopecia and intense pruritus and local form affecting the feet with secondary pododermatitis
• Bacterial dermatitis—usually secondary infection: localized or multifocal areas of alopecia depending on primary cause; lesions may appear ulcerated
• Dermatomycosis—partial to complete alopecia with scaling; with or without erythema; not always ringlike; may begin as small papules
• Mast cell tumors—raised alopecic nodules; may become ulcerated or covered with a thick black crust; may be single or multiple; usually found on neck and trunk
• History—gradual onset of alopecia and pruritus seen with adrenal disease and neoplasia; acute onset more commonly seen with infectious diseases

## CBC/BIOCHEMISTRY/URINALYSIS
N/A

## OTHER LABORATORY TESTS
Ferret adrenal disease—elevations in serum estradiol, androstenedione, and 17-hydroxyprogesterone combined are most diagnostic (available through the University of Tennessee Clinical Endocrinology Laboratory, Department of Comparative Medicine).

## IMAGING
Ultrasonography—evaluate adrenal glands for evidence of ferret adrenal disease.

## DIAGNOSTIC PROCEDURES
• Skin scrapes, epidermal cytology, and dermatophyte cultures (with microscopic identification)—identify primary or coexisting diseases caused by parasites or other microorganisms
• Microscopic examination of ear exudate placed in mineral oil—usually a very effective means of identifying ear mites
• Wood's lamp—do not use as the sole means of diagnosing or excluding dermatomycosis, owing to false negatives and misinterpretations of fluorescence.
• Skin biopsy or fine needle aspirate—useful to diagnose cutaneous neoplasms
• Trial therapy—to rule out scabies; can be difficult to diagnose; skin scrapes often negative; trial course (ivermectin) may be necessary to rule out.

# TREATMENT
More than one disease may be contributing to the itching; if treatment for an identified condition does not result in improvement, consider other causes.

## SURGICAL CONSIDERATIONS
Adrenalectomy may be the preferred treatment for adrenal disease in ferrets. Consider age of ferret, concurrent diseases, and owner financial considerations when determining if medical or surgical treatment is most appropriate.

# MEDICATIONS

## DRUG(S) OF CHOICE
### Topical Therapy
• Symptomatic therapy—the efficacy of topical sprays, lotions, creams, and shampoos used in dogs and cats have not been evaluated in ferrets. Colloidal oatmeal and steroids have been anecdotally reported as most useful topical medications.

# PRURITUS

• Dermatomycosis—lime sulfur dip q7d has been used successfully; may be antipruritic; has antiparasitic, antibacterial, and antifungal properties; disadvantages are bad odor and staining; miconazole cream for focal lesions
• Fleas—fipronil (Frontline, Rhone Merieux) 1/5–1/2 of cat pipette applied topically q60d; imidacloprid (Advantage, Bayer) 1 cat dose divided onto two to three spots topically q30d; selamectin (Revolution, Pfizer) topical application of the cat dosage has been anecdotally reported to be effective; 5% carbaryl powders applied topically q7d × 3–6 treatments; topical pyrethrin products safe for use in puppies and kittens applied topically q7d
• Ear mites—ivermectin 1% (Ivomec, Merck Agvet) diluted 1:10 in propylene glycol: instill 400 µg/kg divided into each ear topically; repeat in 2 weeks—do not use topical and parenteral ivermectin concurrently; selamectin (Revolution, Pfizer) topical application of the cat dosage has been anecdotally reported to be effective; thiabendazole product (Tresaderm, Merck AgVet) at feline dosages has also been used topically, but treatment failures are common due to owner compliance and the small size of the ear canal.
• Demodex—rarely occurs; the use of amitraz (Mitaban, Upjohn) applied topically to affected area three to six times q14d has been reported.

### Systemic Therapy
*Symptomatic*
• Symptomatic therapy—corticosteroids—most effective in controlling itching: prednisone (0.25–1.0 mg/kg q 24h PO divided)
• Antihistamines—use is anecdotal, generally not as effective as steroids: hydroxyzine (2 mg/kg PO q8h); diphenhydramine (0.5–2.0 mg/kg PO q8–12h); chlorpheniramine (1–2 mg/kg PO q8–12h)
• Adrenal disease—leuprolide acetate, an LHRH agonist, is a potent inhibitor of gonadotropin secretion used to inhibit ovarian and testicular steroidogenesis. It is available as a 1- or 4-month depot injection and has been anecdotally reported to alleviate the dermal and reproductive organ signs of adrenal disease in ferrets. Reported dosages: Lupron 30-day depot, 100–200 µg/kg IM q4w until signs resolve, then q4–8w prn, lifelong. This drug has no effect on adrenal tumor growth or metastasis. Side effects include dyspnea, lethargy, and local injection site irritation.
• *Sarcoptes* and *Otodectes* mites—ivermectin 0.2–0.4 mg/kg SC q14d for three to four doses; topical treatment with ivermectin has been shown to be more effective in the treatment of ear mites.

## CONTRAINDICATIONS
Sometimes the application of anything topically, including water and products containing alcohol, iodine, and benzoyl peroxide, can exacerbate itching; cool water may be soothing.

## PRECAUTIONS

### Ivermectin
Anecdotally associated with birth defects when used in pregnant jills

### Topical Antiparasitic Agents
• Fipronil, imidacloprid, and selamectin—off-label use; no reports of toxicity; however, use is not widespread and safety has not been evaluated; use with caution.
• Flea shampoos, sprays, or powders—use cautiously and sparingly to minimize ingestion during grooming.

### Steroids
• Most well-known drug used to control itching
• Used wisely, usually safe
• Avoid long-term daily administration of oral corticosteroids.
• Short-term use seldom causes serious problems.
• In ferrets with concurrent infectious diseases, use corticosteroids with caution.

## POSSIBLE INTERACTIONS
N/A

## ALTERNATIVE DRUGS
N/A

 FOLLOW-UP

## PATIENT MONITORING
• Monitor for alleviation of itching and hair regrowth.
• Following unilateral adrenalectomy or subtotal bilateral adrenalectomy, monitor for return of clinical signs because tumor recurrence is common.

## POSSIBLE COMPLICATIONS
• Client frustration owing to the chronic nature of pruritus
• Recurrence of tumor or development of tumor in the remaining gland in patients with unilateral or subtotal bilateral adrenalectomies

 MISCELLANEOUS

## ASSOCIATED CONDITIONS
*Demodex* may be associated with chronic high dose corticosteroid administration.

## AGE-RELATED FACTORS
N/A

## ZOONOTIC POTENTIAL
Some causes (e.g., sarcoptic mange)

## PREGNANCY
N/A

## SEE ALSO
• Adrenal disease
• Canine distemper virus
• Dermatophytosis
• Ear mites
• Fleas and Flea Infestation
• Sarcoptic mange

## ABBREVIATION
LHRH = luteinizing hormone–releasing hormone

*Suggested Reading*
Clyde VL. Practical treatment and control of common ectoparasites in exotic pets. Vet Med 1996;91(7):632–637.
Fox JG, Marini RP. Diseases of the endocrine system. In: Fox JG, ed. Biology and Diseases of the Ferret. 2nd Ed. Baltimore: Williams & Wilkins, 1998.
Kelleher SA. Skin diseases of the ferret. Vet Clin North Am Exotic Anim Pract 2001;4(2):565–572.
Orcutt C. Dermatologic diseases. In: Hillyer EV, Quesenberry KE, eds. Ferrets, Rabbits and Rodents: Clinical Medicine and Surgery. Philadelphia: WB Saunders, 1997.
Patterson MM, Kirchain SM. Comparison of three treatments for control of ear mites in ferrets. Lab Anim Sci 1999;49(6): 655–657.
Rosenthal KL. Endocrine disorders of ferrets: insulinoma and adrenal gland disease. 21st Annu Waltham/OSU Symp Treat Small Anim Dis Exotics 1997: 35–38.
Rosenthal KL. Ferret and rabbit endocrine disease diagnosis. In: Fudge AM, ed. Laboratory Medicine, Avian and Exotic Pets. Philadelphia: WB Saunders, 2000.
Scott D. Dermatoses of pet rodents, rabbits and ferrets. In: Scott D, Miller W, Ariffen C, eds. Small Animal Dermatology. 5th Ed. Philadelphia: WB Saunders, 1995.

*Portions Adapted From*
Gram WB, Williamson N. Pruritus. In: Tilley LP, Smith FWK, Jr., eds. The 5-Minute Veterinary Consult: Canine and Feline, 3rd Ed. Baltimore: Lippincott Williams & Wilkins, 2003.

# BASICS

## DEFINITION
• Excessive production of saliva
• Pseudoptyalism is the excessive release of saliva that has accumulated in the oral cavity.

## PATHOPHYSIOLOGY
• Ptyalism is an extremely common complaint in ferrets and usually associated with nausea.
• Saliva is constantly produced and secreted into the oral cavity from the salivary glands.
• Salivation increases because of excitation of the salivary nuclei in the brainstem.
• Stimuli that lead to this are taste and tactile sensations involving the mouth and tongue.
• Higher centers in the CNS can also excite or inhibit the salivary nuclei.
• Lesions involving either the CNS or the oral cavity can cause excessive salivation.
• Diseases that affect the pharynx, esophagus, and stomach also stimulate excessive production of saliva.
• Normal saliva production may appear excessive in patients with an anatomic abnormality that allows saliva to dribble out of the mouth or a condition that affects swallowing (pseudoptyalism).

## SYSTEMS AFFECTED
N/A

## SIGNALMENT
• Young animals are more likely to have ptyalism caused by ingestion of a toxin, caustic agent, or foreign body.
• Older animals are more likely to have ptyalism due to nausea from gastrointestinal or metabolic disease (eg., insulinoma)

## SIGNS

### Historical Findings
• Pawing at the face or muzzle—frequently accompanies ptyalism; common sign of nausea; can also occur in patients with oral discomfort or pain
• Anorexia—seen most often in patients with oral lesions, gastrointestinal disease, and systemic disease
• Teeth grinding—seen with oral or gastrointestinal pain
• Vomiting—secondary to gastrointestinal or systemic disease
• Diarrhea or melena—seen with gastrointestinal tract disease
• Eating behavior changes—patients with oral disease may refuse to eat hard food, not chew with the affected side (patients with unilateral lesions), hold the head in an unusual position while eating, or drop prehended food.
• Other behavioral changes—irritability, aggressiveness, and reclusiveness are common,

especially in patients with a painful condition.
• Dysphagia—may be seen if inability to swallow
• Regurgitation—in patients with esophageal disease
• Neurologic signs—patients that have been exposed to causative drugs or toxins, insulinomas and (rarely) hepatic encephalopathy

### Physical Examination Findings
• May be normal in many ferrets with insulinomas or gastrointestinal tract diseases
• Weight loss, muscle wasting—with gastrointestinal or metabolic disease
• Abdominal palpation—may reveal gastrointestinal foreign body, mesenteric lymphadenopathy, thickened intestinal tract, or splenomegaly
• Periodontal disease—inflammation may cause ptyalism
• Stomatitis, lesions of the tongue or oropharynx—ulceration and inflammation of many different causes is associated with ptyalism.
• Mass in the oral cavity
• Halitosis—usually caused by oral cavity disease, but also by esophageal and gastric disease
• Facial pain—caused by oral cavity or pharyngeal disease
• Dysphagia—caused by oral cavity, pharyngeal, or neuromuscular disease or abnormally large retropharyngeal lymph nodes
• Salivary gland problem—inflamed, necrotic, or painful salivary glands can cause ptyalism (rare).

## CAUSES

### Metabolic Disorders
• Insulinoma—very common cause; hypoglycemia causes nausea characterized by ptyalism and pawing at the mouth.
• Uremia
• Hepatoencephalopathy—hepatic failure

### Gastrointestinal Disorders
• Gastric ulcer—very common cause
• Gastrointestinal foreign body—very common cause
• Infiltrative gastroenteritis—also common in ferrets; eosinophilic gastroenteritis, lymphoplasmacytic gastroenteritis, gastrointestinal lymphoma
• Infectious or parasitic gastroenteritis— ECE, salmonellosis, *Giardiasis*

### Esophageal Disorders
• Esophageal foreign body
• Esophageal neoplasm
• Esophagitis—secondary to ingestion of a caustic agent or poisonous plant
• Megaesophagus

### Oral and Pharyngeal Diseases
• Foreign body
• Neoplasm
• Gingivitis or stomatitis—secondary to periodontal disease, uremia, ingestion of a

caustic agent, poisonous plant, or burns (e.g., those from biting on an electrical cord)

### Salivary Gland Diseases
Sialocele (ranula)

### Neurologic Disorders
• Canine distemper virus
• Rabies
• Botulism
• Disorders that cause seizures—during a seizure, ptyalism may occur because of autonomic discharge or reduced swallowing of saliva and may be exacerbated by chomping of the jaws
• Nausea associated with vestibular disease

### Drugs and Toxins
• Those that are caustic (e.g., household cleaning products and some common house plants)
• Those with a disagreeable taste—many antibiotics and anthelminthics
• Those that induce hypersalivation, including organophosphate compounds, cholinergic drugs, insecticides containing boric acid, pyrethrin and pyrethroid insecticides, caffeine, and illicit drugs such as amphetamines, cocaine, and opiates

## RISK FACTORS
N/A

# DIAGNOSIS

## DIFFERENTIAL DIAGNOSIS
• Differentiating causes of ptyalism and pseudoptyalism requires a thorough history, including possible foreign body exposure, current medications, and possible toxin exposure.
• May be able to distinguish salivation associated with nausea (signs of depression, pawing at the mouth, and anorexia) from dysphagia by observing the patient.
• Complete physical examination (with special attention to the oral cavity and neck) and neurologic examination are critical; wear examination gloves when rabies exposure is possible.

## CBC/BIOCHEMISTRY/URINALYSIS
• CBC—often normal; leukocytosis in patients with infectious disease; lymphocytosis in ferrets with lymphoma; eosinophilia in ferrets with eosinophilic gastroenteritis
• Biochemical analysis—hypoglycemia in ferrets with insulinoma; azotemia with renal disease; elevated hepatic enzyme activities with hepatic disease and ECE

## OTHER LABORATORY TESTS
• Fecal flotation—to screen for gastrointestinal parasitism
• For *Helicobacter*—culture usually requires gastric biopsy and specialized isolation techniques and media; success rates are low.

# PTYALISM

• Postmortem fluorescent antibody testing of the brain if rabies is suspected

### IMAGING
• Survey radiography of the oral cavity, neck, and thorax when foreign body or neoplasm is suspected
• Perform abdominal radiography and abdominal ultrasonography to identify hidden conditions such as gastrointestinal tract disease, hepatic disease, insulinoma, or lymphoma. Consider thoracic radiography to rule out cardiac or pulmonary disease.
• The need for further diagnostic imaging varies with the underlying condition suspected (see other topics on specific diseases).

### DIAGNOSTIC PROCEDURES
• Cytologic examination of oral lesions or fine needle aspiration of oral mass
• Biopsy and histopathology of oral lesion, salivary gland, or mass
• To establish a causal relationship between infection with *Helicobacter* and clinical signs, a gastric biopsy is needed. Biopsy is performed via laparotomy. Evidence of characteristic histologic lesions combined with documentation of the organism is needed to support *Helicobacter* infection as the cause of clinical disease. Exploratory laparotomy is also useful to evaluate the extent of gastric pathology and to rule out gastrointestinal foreign bodies, neoplasia, and intestinal inflammatory diseases. Alternatively, a presumptive diagnosis of *Helicobacter* may be based on a favorable response to treatment.
• Consider esophagoscopy or gastroscopy if lesions distal to the oral cavity are suspected. Use is limited in ferrets due to small patient size.

# TREATMENT
Treat the underlying cause (refer to sections pertaining to specific conditions).

# MEDICATIONS

### DRUG(S) OF CHOICE
• Hypoglycemia may usually be alleviated by administering honey or syrups orally, taking care to avoid being bitten.
• Antiemetics/histamine $H_2$-receptor antagonists for animals with gastritis or gastric ulcers—famotidine (0.25–0.5 mg/kg PO, IV q12–24h), ranitidine HCl (3.5 mg/kg

PO q12h), cimetidine (5–10 mg/kg PO, SC, IV q8h), or omeprazole (0.7 mg/kg PO q24h)
• Astringent solutions applied for 10 minutes q8–12h—can be used to treat areas of moist dermatitis secondary to hypersalivation
• Crystalloid fluids—give IV or SC to treat dehydration in anorectic animals with metabolic disease.

### CONTRAINDICATIONS
N/A

### PRECAUTIONS
N/A

### POSSIBLE INTERACTIONS
N/A

### ALTERNATIVE DRUGS
N/A

# FOLLOW-UP

### PATIENT MONITORING
• Depends on the underlying cause (see causes)
• Continually monitor hydration, serum electrolytes, and nutritional status, especially in dysphagic or anorectic animals.

### POSSIBLE COMPLICATIONS
• Dehydration
• Moist dermatitis

# MISCELLANEOUS

### ASSOCIATED CONDITIONS
N/A

### AGE-RELATED FACTORS
N/A

### ZOONOTIC POTENTIAL
Rabies

### PREGNANCY
N/A

### SYNONYMS
• Hypersalivation
• Drooling
• Sialorrhea

### SEE ALSO
• Gastroduodenal ulcers
• Gastrointestinal foreign body
• Insulinoma

### ABBREVIATIONS
• CBC = complete blood count
• ECE = epizootic catarrhal enteritis

### Suggested Reading
Caplan ER, Peterson ME, Mulles HS, et al. Diagnosis and treatment of insulin-secreting pancreatic islet cell tumors in ferrets: 57 cases (1986–1994). J Am Vet Med Assoc 1996;209:1741–1745.

DeBowes LJ. Ptyalism. In: Ettinger SJ, ed. Veterinary Internal Medicine. 4th Ed. Philadelphia: Saunders, 1995:125–128.

Fox JG. Bacterial and mycoplasmal diseases. In: Fox JG, ed. Biology and Diseases of the Ferret. 2nd Ed. Baltimore: Williams & Wilkins, 1998.

Fox JG. Diseases of the gastrointestinal system. In: Fox JG, ed. Biology and Diseases of the Ferret. 2nd Ed. Baltimore: Williams & Wilkins, 1998.

Fox JG, Marini RP. Helicobacter mustelae infection in ferrets: pathogenesis, epizootiology, diagnosis and treatment. Semin Avin Exotic Pet Med 2001;10(1):36–44.

Hoefer HL. Gastrointestinal diseases. In: Hillyer EV, Quesenberry KE, eds. Ferrets, Rabbits and Rodents: Clinical Medicine and Surgery. Philadelphia: WB Saunders, 1997:26–36.

Jenkins C, Bassett JR. Helicobacter infection. Compend Contin Edu Pract Vet 1997;19(3):267–279.

Quesenberry KE, Rosenthal KL. Endocrine disease. In: Hillyer EV, Quesenberry KE, eds. Ferrets, Rabbits and Rodents: Clinical Medicine and Surgery. Philadelphia: WB Saunders, 1997.

Weiss CA, Williams BH, Scott MV. Insulinoma in the ferret: clinical findings and treatment comparison of 66 cases. J Am Anim Hosp Assoc 1998;34:471–475.

Wheeler J, Bennett RA. Ferret abdominal surgical procedures. Part II. Gastrointestinal foreign bodies, splenomegaly, liver biopsy, cystotomy and ovariohysterectomy. Compend Contin Edu Pract Vet 1999;21(11):1049–1057.

Williams BH. Ferret microbiology and virology. In: Fudge Am, ed. Laboratory Medicine, Avian and Exotic Pets. Philadelphia: WB Saunders, 2000.

### Portions Adapted From
Crandall J. Ptyalism. In: Tilley LP, Smith FWK, Jr., eds. The 5-Minute Veterinary Consult: Canine and Feline, 3rd Ed. Baltimore: Lippincott Williams & Wilkins, 2003.

# PYOMETRA AND STUMP PYOMETRA

# BASICS

## DEFINITION
• Pyometra—a life-threatening uterine infection that develops when bacterial invasion of the endometrium leads to intraluminal accumulation of purulent exudate
• Stump pyometra—infection of the uterine remnant, usually secondary to hormonal disorders seen with ferret adrenal disease or in ferrets with ovarian remnant

## PATHOPHYSIOLOGY
• Normal reproductive cycle—ferrets are seasonally polyestrous (breeding season March–August) and induced ovulators. Ovulation, followed by a pregnancy or pseudopregnancy lasting 41–43 days, is induced by stimulation of the cervix by mating or artificial means. Approximately half of unbred females will remain in estrus. Serum estrogen concentration will remain elevated for the remainder of the breeding season (6 months or more) in females that are not bred.
• Pyometra is most likely to develop in pseudopregnant jills, postpartum jills, or ferrets with hyperestrogenism due to a prolonged estrus. Ferrets with hyperestrogenism and resultant pancytopenia are immunocompromised and predisposed to the development of pyometra.
• Stump pyometra may be seen in ferrets with hormonal disorders caused by adrenal disease or from a uterine remnant.
• Bacteria—uterine secretions provide excellent media for growth. Bacteria (normal vaginal flora) ascend from the vagina through the partially open cervix.

## SYSTEMS AFFECTED
• Reproductive
• Renal/urologic
• Hemic/lymphatic/immune
• Hepatobiliary

## INCIDENCE/PREVALENCE
• Pyometra is seen most commonly in breeding jills. However, a low overall incidence exists since most pet ferrets are spayed at a very young age, prior to sale.
• In spayed ferrets, stump pyometra may occur secondary to ferret adrenal disease or an ovarian remnant.

## GEOGRAPHIC DISTRIBUTION
N/A

## SIGNALMENT

### Mean Age and Range
Sexually mature females (>8–12 months of age)

## SIGNS

### Historical Findings
• Signs of estrus within the previous month

• Open cervix—vaginal discharge, usually mucopurulent, pink to brown tinged, followed by signs of systemic illness
• Closed cervix—signs of systemic illness, progressing to signs of septicemia and shock

### Physical Examination Findings
• Swollen vulva
• Uterus—palpably large with pyometra in intact jills; careful palpation may allow determination of size; overly aggressive palpation may induce rupture; with open cervix, may not be palpably large; stump pyometra often not palpable
• Pain on palpation of the caudal abdomen
• Vaginal discharge—depends on cervical patency; usually mucopurulent
• Depression and lethargy
• Anorexia
• Pyrexia
• Symmetric alopecia in ferrets with adrenal disease
• Abdominal distension
• Vomiting

## CAUSES
Common pathogens include *Escherichia coli*, *Staphylococcus*, *Streptococcus*, and *Corynebacterium*.

## RISK FACTORS
• Pyometra—pseudopregnancy caused by fertilization failure or induction of ovulation by artificial stimulation of the cervix; estrogen-induced pancytopenia due to failure to breed females in estrus
• Stump pyometra—ovarian remnant or ferret adrenal disease

# DIAGNOSIS

## DIFFERENTIAL DIAGNOSIS
For purulent vaginal discharge:
• Urogenital cystic disease in ferrets with adrenal disease—although relatively rare in females, urogenital cysts can occur in a similar physical location as stump pyometra; cysts can become secondarily infected and fill with purulent exudate; solitary, abscessed cysts can be distinguished from stump pyometra on gross and histologic examination.
• Primary vaginitis
• Secondary vaginitis—from foreign body, urinary tract infection, vaginal neoplasia, and fetal death
• Perivulvar dermatitis
For enlarged uterus in intact females:
• Pregnancy
• Fetal death
• Postpartum metritis

## CBC/BIOCHEMISTRY/URINALYSIS
• Neutrophilia—may be seen in ferrets with pyometra that do not have estrogen-induced pancytopenia

• Nonregenerative anemia, thrombocytopenia, and leukopenia in ferrets with hyperestrogenism
• Hyperglobulinemia and hyperproteinemia

## OTHER LABORATORY TESTS
• Cytologic examination of vaginal discharge—regenerative polymorphonuclear cells and bacteria; may be indistinguishable from the purulent discharge associated with vaginal disease (e.g., vaginitis, vaginal mass) or abscessed urogenital cysts
• Bacterial culture and sensitivity test of vaginal discharge—not helpful in confirming diagnosis (bacteria cultured are usually normal vaginal flora); is useful in determining appropriate antibiotic use
• Elevations in serum estradiol, androstenedione, and 17-hydroxyprogesterone combined are most diagnostic for ferret adrenal disease (available through the University of Tennessee Clinical Endocrinology Laboratory, Department of Comparative Medicine).

## IMAGING

### Radiography
• Rule out pregnancy
• Pyometra—uterus may appear as a distended, tubular structure in the caudal ventral abdomen.

### Ultrasonography
• Assess size of uterus and nature of uterine contents.
• Rule out pregnancy—20–24 days after ovulation
• Normal uterine wall—not visible as a distinct entity
• Pyometra associated with a thickened uterine wall and intraluminal fluid
• Demonstrate adrenal gland enlargement in ferrets with adrenal disease.
• May see single or multiple cysts in ferrets with urogenital cystic disease secondary to adrenal disease

## DIAGNOSTIC PROCEDURES
N/A

## PATHOLOGIC FINDINGS
• Endometrial surface—covered by malodorous, mucopurulent exudate; thickened because of increased endometrial gland size and cystic gland distension
• Glands may be filled with degenerating neutrophils; endometrium—mixed inflammatory cell, focal abscess formation

# TREATMENT

## APPROPRIATE HEALTH CARE
• Inpatient—pyometra is a life-threatening condition, especially in ferrets with estrogen-induced pancytopenia resulting in anemia and hemorrhage due to thrombocytopenia.

# Pyometra and Stump Pyometra

• Surgery is usually the treatment of choice; if the ferret is clinically stable and a valuable breeding animal, medical treatment may be attempted.

## NURSING CARE

• Immediate, intravenous fluid administration and antibiotics are usually necessary in the treatment of pyometra.
• Estrogen-induced pancytopenia—ovariohysterectomy is the treatment of choice. This is usually a relatively safe procedure in ferrets with PCV >30. Ferrets with PCV <30 will usually require a blood transfusion prior to surgery (see surgical considerations, below)
• Indications for whole blood transfusion are the same as those for dogs or cats. Identifiable blood groups have not been demonstrated in ferrets, and transfusion reactions are unlikely. However, administration of dexamethasone sodium phosphate 4–6 mg/kg IV once prior to transfusion has been recommended as a precaution. Healthy, large males with a normal PCV are the most appropriate blood donors. Up to 0.6% of a donor's body weight can be safely collected (usually 6–12 mL, depending on the size of the ferret and volume required). Collect blood from the anesthetized donor ferret via the anterior vena cava or jugular vein into a syringe with 1 mL of acid-citrate-dextrose anticoagulant per 6 mL of blood. (Volume of blood to be transfused is estimated in the same manner as for cats.) Ideally, blood should be filtered during administration to the recipient. Administer blood slowly with a 21- to 22-gauge catheter into a large vein such as the jugular or via an interosseous catheter if a vein is not accessible. Follow transfusion with IV administration of 0.9% NaCl to meet maintenance and dehydration needs.
• Ferrets that are extremely anemic, thrombocytopenic, and with secondary infections are poor surgical risks and should be stabilized if possible prior to surgery (transfusion as needed and medical treatment with hCG—see below)

## ACTIVITY

N/A

## DIET

If the ferret has been anorectic or is emaciated, feed high-calorie diets such as Eukanuba Maximum Calorie diet (Iams Co., Dayton, OH), Feline a/d (Hills Products, Topeka, KS), or Clinicare Feline liquid diet (Abbott Laboratories, North Chicago, IL); may also add dietary supplement such as Nutri-Cal (EVSCO Pharmaceuticals, Buena, NJ) to increase caloric content of these foods. Warming the food to body temperature or offering via syringe may increase acceptance. Administer these supplements several times a day.

## CLIENT EDUCATION

• Inform client that ovariohysterectomy is the preferred treatment.
• Ferrets with estrogen-induced pancytopenia are poor surgical candidates and require aggressive supportive care prior to and following surgery.
• Recommend medical treatment only for valuable breeding animals.
• Warn client that medical treatment of closed-cervix pyometra can be associated with uterine rupture and peritonitis.

## SURGICAL CONSIDERATIONS

Pyometra in intact females:
• Pyometra (open and closed cervix)—ovariohysterectomy preferred treatment
• Closed-cervix pyometra—use caution during ovariohysterectomy; enlarged uterus may be friable.
• Uterine rupture or leakage of purulent material from the uterine stump—repeated lavage of the peritoneal cavity with sterile saline
• Patients with pancytopenia due to hyperestrogenism—stabilize patient prior to surgery; terminate estrus by administering hCG; administer antibiotic therapy, fluid therapy, and blood transfusions if necessary
Spayed females with stump pyometra:
• Usually good surgical candidates
• Perform celiotomy in ferrets with ovarian remnant. Ovarian tissue may be small and is located at the caudolateral pole of the kidney. These ferrets are usually not severely anemic presurgery, but a blood transfusion may be required if intraoperative hemorrhage is extensive.
• Perform a celiotomy in ferrets with stump pyometra secondary to adrenal disease. The adrenal glands should be examined for evidence of adrenal disease and the uterine stump removed. The affected adrenal gland may be removed, or adrenal disease may be managed medically. The decision as to which form of treatment is appropriate is multifactorial; which adrenal gland is affected (left vs. right), surgeon's experience and expertise, severity of clinical signs, age of the animal, concurrent diseases, and financial issues should be considered.
• Always explore the entire abdominal cavity during surgery since concurrent disease (e.g., insulinoma, lymphoma) is extremely common.
• Obtain samples from the uterus for culture and susceptibility testing during surgery.
• Supportive care, such as fluid therapy, warmth, and adequate nutrition are required for recovery.

 **MEDICATIONS**

## DRUG(S) OF CHOICE

### Antibiotics

• All patients with pyometra
• Empirical, pending results of bacterial culture and sensitivity test
• Common choices—enrofloxacin (10–20 mg/kg PO, SC, IM q12h); trimethoprim/sulfonamide (15–30 mg/kg PO, SC q12h)

### Termination of Estrus

For ferrets with estrogen-induced pancytopenia—administer hCG, 100 IU per ferret IM, to stimulate ovulation and terminate estrus prior to surgery. Signs of estrus (particularly vulvar swelling) should diminish within 3–4 days. If signs are still apparent 1 week posttreatment, repeat the injection. Treatment is only effective after day 10 of estrus.

### Medical Treatment of Valuable Breeding Animals

• PGF2α (Lutalyse, Pharmacia & Upjohn Animal Health) causes disruption of the corpus luteum in postpartum or pseudopregnant jills.
• 0.5–1.0 mg/animal (0.1–0.2 mL/animal)
• If uterine distension is noted 24 hours following treatment with PGF2α, a second course of treatment with PGF2α may be necessary.
• Flunixin meglumine (0.5–2.0 mg/kg IM, IV, PO q24h) may be administered following expulsion of all uterine contents and continued for up to 3 days for analgesia. Flunixin is a powerful prostaglandin antagonist and will block the effects of PGF2α; therefore, do not administer until the uterine contents have been expelled.

## CONTRAINDICATIONS

• PGF2α with closed-cervix pyometra—strong myometrial contractions may cause uterine rupture or force purulent exudate through the uterine tubes, causing secondary peritonitis.
• PGF2α in a valuable breeding animal—always rule out pregnancy before administering.

## PRECAUTIONS

• PGF2α—not approved for use in ferrets
• Side effects of PGF2α—referable to contraction of smooth muscle; hypersalivation, emesis, defecation
• Flunixin meglumine—may cause severe gastric ulceration, especially when administered for >72 hours.

## POSSIBLE INTERACTIONS

N/A

## ALTERNATIVE DRUGS

Antibiotics—not efficacious as sole treatment

 **FOLLOW-UP**

### PATIENT MONITORING

• Antibiotics—administration continued for 3–4 weeks
• Repeat CBC 1–2 weeks posttreatment to monitor bone marrow response in patients with estrogen-induced pancytopenia.

### PREVENTION/AVOIDANCE

• Ovariohysterectomy—recommended for all pet ferrets
• Treat with an appropriate antibiotic for 3 weeks.

### POSSIBLE COMPLICATIONS

• Uterine rupture and peritonitis in ferrets treated medically
• Death due to blood loss and anemia during or following surgery. This is particularly a risk in severely anemic and thrombocytopenic patients with estrogen-induced pancytopenia.

### EXPECTED COURSE AND PROGNOSIS

• Good with surgical treatment of pseudo-pregnant jills
• Good with surgical treatment of patients with hyperestrogenism if not significantly anemic
• Fair to poor with surgical treatment of severely anemic patients with hyperestrogenism
• Fair with medical treatment of pseudo-pregnant jills

 **MISCELLANEOUS**

### ASSOCIATED CONDITIONS

• Ferret adrenal disease
• Ovarian remnant
• Pancytopenia

### AGE-RELATED FACTORS

N/A

### ZOONOTIC POTENTIAL

N/A

### PREGNANCY

PGF2α—always rule out pregnancy before administration to valuable breeding animals; effective pregnancy-terminating agent

### SEE ALSO

• Adrenal disease
• Hyperestrogenism
• Urogenital cystic disease

### ABBREVIATIONS

• CBC = complete blood count
• hCG = human chorionic gonadotropin
• PCV = packed cell volume
• PGF2α = prostaglandin F2-alpha

### Suggested Reading

Bell JA. Periparturient and neonatal diseases. In: Hillyer EV, Quesenberry KE, eds. Ferrets, Rabbits and Rodents: Clinical Medicine and Surgery. Philadelphia: WB Saunders, 1997:53–62.

Benson KG, Paul-Murphy J, Ramer JC. Evaluating and stabilizing the critical ferret: basic diagnostic and therapeutic techniques. Compend Contin Edu Pract Vet 2000;22:490–497.

Fox JG, Pearson RC, Bell JA. Diseases of the genitourinary system. In: Fox JG, ed. Biology and Diseases of the Ferret. 2nd Ed. Baltimore: Williams & Wilkins, 1998.

Hillyer EV. Ferret endocrinology. In: Kirk RW, ed. Current Veterinary Therapy XI. Philadelphia: WB Saunders, 1992.

Hillyer EV. Urogenital diseases. In: Hillyer EV, Quesenberry KE, eds. Ferrets, Rabbits and Rodents: Clinical Medicine and Surgery. Philadelphia: WB Saunders, 1997:44–52.

Marini RP, Jackson LR, Esteves MI, et al. The effect of isoflurane on hematologic variables in ferrets. Am J Vet Res 1994;55:1497.

Orcutt CJ. Fluids and critical care in small mammals. Proc North Am Vet Conf 2001:886–886.

Ryland LM. Remission of estrus associated anemia following hysterectomy and multiple blood transfusions in a ferret. J Am Vet Med Assoc 1982;181:820–822.

Wheeler J, Bennett RA. Ferret abdominal surgical procedures. Part II. Gastrointestinal foreign bodies, splenomegaly, liver biopsy, cystotomy and ovariohysterectomy. Compend Contin Edu Pract Vet 1999;21(11):1049–1057.

Williams BH. Therapeutics in ferrets. Vet Clin North Am Exotic Anim Pract 2000;3(1):131–153.

### Portions Adapted From

Root-Kustritz MV. Pyometra and Cystic Endometrial Hyperplasia. In: Tilley LP, Smith FWK, Jr., eds. The 5-Minute Veterinary Consult: Canine and Feline, 3rd Ed. Baltimore: Lippincott Williams & Wilkins, 2003.

# RABIES

## BASICS

### DEFINITION
A severe, invariably fatal, viral polioencephalitis of warm-blooded animals, including humans

### PATHOPHYSIOLOGY
Virus—enters body through a wound (usually from a bite of rabid animal) or via mucous membranes; replicates in myocytes; spreads to the neuromuscular junction and neurotendinal spindles; travels to the CNS via intraaxonal fluid within peripheral nerves; spreads throughout the CNS; finally spreads centrifugally within peripheral, sensory, and motor neurons

### SYSTEMS AFFECTED
• Nervous—clinical encephalitis
• Salivary glands—in ferrets infected with the raccoon rabies variant (the most common variant causing infection in ferrets), infectious virus particles are contained in the salivary glands and shed in saliva.

### GENETICS
None

### INCIDENCE/PREVALENCE
• Incidence of disease within infected animals, high (approaches 100%)
• Prevalence—overall, low; <20 cases reported in the United States since 1954; only two reports exist in the United States since 1992.

### GEOGRAPHIC DISTRIBUTION
• Worldwide
• Exceptions—British Isles, Australia, New Zealand, Hawaii, Japan, and parts of Scandinavia

### SIGNALMENT

*Species*
• All warm-blooded animals, including dogs, cats, and humans
• United States—four strains endemic within fox, raccoon, skunk, and bat populations; all four strains can be transmitted to ferrets.

*Breed Predilections*
None

*Mean Age and Range*
None

*Predominant Sex*
None

### SIGNS

*General Comments*
The clinical signs of rabies in ferrets are usually mild and include anxiety, lethargy, and posterior paresis. These signs are very similar to many common diseases in ferrets. The furious form of rabies seen in other carnivores is unusual in ferrets. However, consider rabies as a differential diagnosis in any ferret displaying neurologic signs.

*Historical Findings*
• Change in attitude—apprehension, nervousness, anxiety, unusual shyness or aggressiveness
• Disorientation
• Muscular—rear limb paresis, incoordination, seizures, paralysis
• Erratic behavior—biting or snapping, biting at cage, wandering and roaming, excitability, irritability, viciousness (rarely reported in ferrets)

*Physical Examination Findings*
All or some of the historical findings

### CAUSES
Rabies virus—a single-stranded RNA virus, genus Lyssavirus, family Rhabdoviridae

### RISK FACTORS
• Lack of adequate vaccination against rabies
• Use of modified live virus rabies vaccine
• Exposure to wildlife, especially skunks, raccoons, bats, and foxes—this exposure rarely occurs in ferrets since most are indoor pets.
• Bite or scratch wounds from unvaccinated dogs, cats, or wildlife
• Exposure to aerosols in bat caves

## DIAGNOSIS

### DIFFERENTIAL DIAGNOSIS
• Must seriously consider rabies for any ferret showing unusual mood or behavior changes or exhibiting any unaccountable neurologic signs; caution: handle with considerable care to prevent possible transmission of the virus to individuals caring for or treating the animal.
• For rear limb paresis—spinal cord damage, ADV, insulinoma, weakness from chronic systemic illness
• CDV—neurologic signs may be seen without an early catarrhal phase.

### CBC/BIOCHEMISTRY/URINALYSIS
No characteristic hematologic or biochemical changes

### OTHER LABORATORY TESTS
N/A

### IMAGING
N/A

### DIAGNOSTIC PROCEDURES
DFA test of nervous tissue—rapid and sensitive test; collect brain, head, or entire body of animal that has died or has been euthanatized; chill sample immediately; submit to a state-approved laboratory for rabies diagnosis; caution: use extreme care when collecting, handling, and shipping these specimens.

### PATHOLOGIC FINDINGS
• Gross changes—generally absent, despite dramatic neurologic disease
• Histopathologic changes—acute to chronic polioencephalitis; large neurons within the brain may contain the classic intracytoplasmic inclusions (Negri bodies).

## TREATMENT

### APPROPRIATE HEALTH CARE
Strictly inpatient

### NURSING CARE
Administer with extreme caution.

### ACTIVITY
• Confine to secured quarantine area with clearly posted signs indicating suspected rabies.
• Runs or cages should be locked; only designated people should have access.
• Feed and water without opening the cage or run door.

### DIET
N/A

### CLIENT EDUCATION
• Thoroughly inform client of the seriousness of rabies to the animal and the zoonotic potential.
• Ask client about any human exposure (e.g., contact, bite) and strongly urge client to see a physician immediately.
• Local public health official must be notified.

### SURGICAL CONSIDERATIONS
None

## MEDICATIONS

### DRUG(S) OF CHOICE
• No treatment
• If the diagnosis is strongly suspected, euthanasia is indicated.

### CONTRAINDICATIONS
None

### PRECAUTIONS
N/A

### POSSIBLE INTERACTIONS
N/A

### ALTERNATIVE DRUGS
N/A

## FOLLOW-UP

### PATIENT MONITORING
• All suspected rabies patients should be securely isolated and monitored for any development of mood change, attitude

change, or clinical signs that might suggest the diagnosis.
• An apparently healthy ferret that bites or scratches a person should be monitored for a period of 10 days regardless of vaccination status; contact local public health regulatory agency for instructions on quarantining ferrets inflicting bite wounds.
• If the ferret dies during quarantine, the head should be submitted for testing as outlined above.
• An unvaccinated ferret that is bitten or exposed to a known rabid animal must be euthanized or quarantined for up to 6 months or according to local or state regulations.

## PREVENTION/AVOIDANCE
• Vaccines—vaccinate according to standard recommendations and state and local requirements; all ferrets should be vaccinated at 12 weeks of age, then annually thereafter using an approved killed virus vaccine. Only use a killed vaccine approved in ferrets; MLV vaccines have caused disease in ferrets.
• Disinfection—any contaminated area, cage, food dish, or instrument must be thoroughly disinfected; use a 1:32 dilution (4 ounces per gallon) of household bleach to quickly inactivate the virus.

## POSSIBLE COMPLICATIONS
N/A

## EXPECTED COURSE AND PROGNOSIS
Prognosis—grave; almost invariably fatal

## MISCELLANEOUS

## ASSOCIATED CONDITIONS
None

## AGE-RELATED FACTORS
None

## ZOONOTIC POTENTIAL
• Extreme
• Humans must avoid being bitten by a rabid animal or an asymptomatic animal that is incubating the disease.
• Rabies cases must be strictly quarantined and confined to prevent exposure to humans and other animals.
• Local and state regulations must be adhered to carefully and completely.

## PREGNANCY
Infection during pregnancy will be fatal to dam.

## SYNONYMS
N/A

## ABBREVIATIONS
• ADV = Aleutian disease virus
• CDV = canine distemper virus
• DFA = direct immunofluorescent antibody
• MLV = modified live virus

*Suggested Reading*
Antinoff N. Musculoskeletal and neurologic diseases. In: Hillyer EV, Quesenberry KE, eds. Ferrets Rabbits and Rodents: Clinical Medicine and Surgery. Philadelphia: WB Saunders, 1997:126–130.
Fox JG, Pearson RC, Gorham JR. Viral diseases. In: Fox JG, ed. Biology and Diseases of the Ferret. 2nd Ed. Baltimore: Williams & Wilkins, 1998.
Hoover JP, Baldwin CA, Rupprecht CE. Serologic response of domestic ferrets (Mustela putorius furo) to canine distemper and rabies virus vaccines. J Am Vet Med Assoc 1989;194(2):234–238.
Williams BH. Ferret microbiology and virology. In: Fudge AM, ed. Laboratory Medicine, Avian and Exotic Pets. Philadelphia: WB Saunders, 2000:334–342.

*Portions Adapted From*
Scott FW. Rabies. In: Tilley LP, Smith FWK, Jr., eds. The 5-Minute Veterinary Consult: Canine and Feline, 3rd Ed. Baltimore: Lippincott Williams & Wilkins, 2003.

# RECTAL AND ANAL PROLAPSE

## BASICS

### OVERVIEW
• An anal prolapse (partial prolapse) is a protrusion of rectal mucosa through the external anal orifice.
• A double layer of the rectum that protrudes through the anal canal is a rectal prolapse (complete prolapse).

### SIGNALMENT
• Usually young ferrets, 2–6 months of age
• Rarely occurs in adult ferrets

### SIGNS
• Persistent tenesmus, may cry out when defecating
• Tubular hyperemic mass protruding from the anus

### CAUSES AND RISK FACTORS
• Coccidiosis—most common cause of anal prolapse in young ferrets
• Anal sacculectomy—most ferrets purchased from pet shops have had the anal sacs removed by the breeding facility at a very young age; excessive removal of the anal sphincter or damage to nerves supplying the anus may cause anal or rectal prolapse.
• Proliferative bowel disease (PBD)—caused by *Campylobacter*-like organism *(Lawsonia intracellularis)*; is a relatively uncommon disease, but when occurring is likely to cause anal/rectal prolapse
• Prostatomegaly and resultant straining to urinate or defecate may cause prolapse.
• Chronic diarrhea—from epizootic catarrhal enteritis, lymphoma, infiltrative bowel diseases, *Giardia*, or other bacterial or parasitic causes
• Gastrointestinal foreign body
• Rectal or anal tumors (rare)
• Tenesmus following perineal or urogenital surgery

## DIAGNOSIS

### DIFFERENTIAL DIAGNOSIS
• Coccidia, *Giardia*, PBD, and prolapse secondary to anal sac removal are seen in younger ferrets.
• Chronic diarrhea, prostatomegaly, and neoplasia are more likely to cause prolapse in older ferrets.

### CBC/BIOCHEMISTRY/URINALYSIS
• Usually normal
• May reflect underlying cause (e.g., inflammatory leukogram with infectious disease)

### OTHER LABORATORY TESTS
Fecal examination may confirm parasitism.

### IMAGING
• Abdominal radiography and ultrasonography—usually normal in young ferrets with coccidia, PBD, or prolapse postanal gland excision
• Abdominal radiography—may demonstrate foreign body, prostatomegaly
• Contrast radiography may indicate thickening of the intestinal wall, mucosal irregularities, mass, severe ileus, foreign body, or stricture.
• Abdominal ultrasonography may demonstrate intestinal wall thickening, gastrointestinal mass, foreign body, ileus, or mesenteric lymphadenopathy, prostatomegaly, or intussusception.

### DIAGNOSTIC PROCEDURES
Exploratory laparotomy and surgical biopsy should be pursued if there is evidence of obstruction or intestinal mass and/or for definitive diagnosis of gastrointestinal inflammatory or infiltrative diseases.

### PATHOLOGIC FINDINGS
Assess viability of the prolapsed tissue by surface appearance and tissue temperature—vital tissue appears swollen and hyperemic, and red blood exudes from the cut surface; devitalized tissue appears dark purple or black, and dark cyanotic blood exudes from the cut surface; ulcerations may be present.

## TREATMENT

### APPROPRIATE HEALTH CARE
• If prolapse is mild and does not cause straining, treating the underlying cause without replacing the mucosa may be sufficient; keep tissues moist by use of a lubricant until underling problem resolves.
• Must identify and treat underlying cause
• Conservative medical management—gently replace prolapsed tissue through the anus with the use of lubricants; osmotic agents may help if severe swelling exists.
• Adjunctive use of a purse-string suture may aid in retention and prevent postreduction recurrence; place the suture to allow room for defecation.
• Colopexy via left paramedian approach recommended for recurrent viable prolapses—procedure is that used for dogs and cats.
• If prolapse is devitalized (rare), amputation and rectal anastomosis are recommended—procedure is that used for dogs and cats.

## MEDICATIONS

### DRUG(S) OF CHOICE
• Appropriate anesthetic/analgesics as needed

• Topical agents to aid in reduction—50% dextrose solution and KY Jelly
• Specific treatment for the underlying cause

### CONTRAINDICATIONS/POSSIBLE INTERACTIONS
N/A

## FOLLOW-UP

### PATIENT MONITORING
Purse-string removal in 5–7 days

### POSSIBLE COMPLICATIONS
Recurrence—especially if uncontrolled underlying problem exists

## MISCELLANEOUS

### ASSOCIATED CONDITIONS
See causes

### SEE ALSO
• Coccidiosis
• Diarrhea
• Dyschezia and hematochezia

*Suggested Reading*

Burrows CF, Ellison GE. Recto anal disease. In: Ettinger SJ, Feldman EC, eds. Textbook of Veterinary Internal Medicine. 3rd Ed. Philadelphia: Saunders, 1989:1559–1568.

Fox JG. Parasitic diseases. In: Fox JG, ed. Biology and Diseases of the Ferret. 2nd Ed. Baltimore: Williams & Wilkins, 1998:375–392.

Fox JG. Diseases of the gastrointestinal system. In: Fox JG, ed. Biology and Diseases of the Ferret. 2nd Ed. Baltimore: Williams & Wilkins, 1998:273–290.

Hoefer HL. Gastrointestinal diseases. In: Hillyer EV, Quesenberry KE, eds. Ferrets, Rabbits and Rodents: Clinical Medicine and Surgery. Philadelphia: WB Saunders, 1997:26–36.

Finkler MR. Ferret colitis. In: Kirk RW, Bonagura JD, eds. Kirk's Current Veterinary Therapy XI: Small Animal Practice. Philadelphia: WB Saunders, 1992.

Rosenthal K. Update on ECE disease in ferrets. Proc North Am Vet Conf 2000:1017–1018.

*Portions Adapted From*

Pope ER. Rectal and Anal Prolapse. In: Tilley LP, Smith FWK, Jr., eds. The 5-Minute Veterinary Consult: Canine and Feline, 3rd Ed. Baltimore: Lippincott Williams & Wilkins, 2003.

# BASICS

## DEFINITION
Expulsion of undigested food from the esophagus through the oral cavity
- Usually implies dysphagia
- Most commonly associated with the esophageal stage of swallowing
- Regurgitation is a rare clinical presentation in ferrets.

## PATHOPHYSIOLOGY
Swallowing consists of a series of sequential, well-coordinated events that transport food and liquids from the mouth to the stomach. This process is divided into three major phases: oropharyngeal, esophageal, and gastroesophageal. Altered motility of food from the mouth to the stomach allows food to accumulate in the esophagus, and eventually it is regurgitated out the oral cavity.

## SYSTEMS AFFECTED
- Gastrointestinal
- Respiratory—aspiration pneumonia

## SIGNALMENT
- Younger animals—esophageal foreign body
- Middle-aged to older ferrets—megaesophagus, esophagitis, neoplasia
- No sex predilection

## SIGNS

### Historical Findings
- Often mistaken for vomiting
- Take a thorough history to differentiate vomiting (forceful abdominal contractions) from regurgitation (passive).
- The character of the expelled ingesta and the time interval from ingestion to expulsion may also help differentiate vomiting and regurgitation.
- There may be a ravenous appetite; food may be dropped from the mouth.
- Weight loss may be profound.
- Ptyalism is common.
- Dysphagia, choking, or distress shortly after eating may be noted.
- Coughing and/or dyspnea may be the complaint when aspiration pneumonia is present.

### Physical Examination Findings
- Emaciation and weakness are common.
- The cervical esophagus may bulge on expiration or with compression of the thorax.
- Fever and abnormal lung sounds on auscultation may be present in those with aspiration pneumonia.

## CAUSES
- All are rare
- Idiopathic megaesophagus
- Megaesophagus—secondary to systemic illness or toxin

- Esophagitis
- Esophageal foreign body
- Esophageal stricture

## RISK FACTORS
N/A

# DIAGNOSIS

## DIFFERENTIAL DIAGNOSIS

### Differentiating Similar Signs
- Must distinguish from vomiting
- Signs of nausea, such as ptyalism, licking the lips, pawing at the mouth and backing up, are usually seen just prior to vomiting or retching.
- Forceful retching and involuntary abdominal contractions associated with the expulsion of digested and bile-stained ingesta or liquid support vomiting.
- Effortless expulsion of foam, liquid, or partially digested or undigested food supports regurgitation.

## CBC/BIOCHEMISTRY
- Results normal in most patients
- TWBC elevation with aspiration pneumonia or esophagitis
- ALT elevation with secondary hepatic lipidosis

## OTHER LABORATORY TESTS
Blood lead and cholinesterase levels to evaluate for toxicity if suspected (rare)

## IMAGING

### Radiographic Findings
- Survey thoracic radiographs—may reveal an esophagus dilated with gas, fluid, or ingesta (in patients with megaesophagus) or may be within normal limits; may also reveal pulmonary infiltrates consistent with aspiration pneumonia
- Contrast esophagram (with liquid barium and/or barium-coated food) may confirm obstructive disorders (foreign bodies, strictures, neoplasia, or granulomas)
- Fluoroscopy can detect pharyngeal dysfunction and esophageal motility disorders.

## OTHER DIAGNOSTIC PROCEDURES
Esophagoscopy—can be useful with obstructive disorders of the esophagus and esophagitis; usually unrewarding with megaesophagus; difficult due to small patient size.

# TREATMENT

## APPROPRIATE HEALTH CARE
- For causes other than primary idiopathic megaesophagus, aim treatment at the primary cause.
- If no known underlying cause, treatment goals include minimizing risk of aspiration

pneumonia and providing and maintaining adequate nutrition.
- Most patients with megaesophagus have aspiration pneumonia and/or severe debilitation requiring hospitalization.
- Hospitalize in a warm, quiet location with a hide box to minimize stress.

## NURSING CARE
- If the patient is dehydrated, a balanced electrolyte solution may be indicated.
- Correct dehydration with IV fluid therapy (maintenance = 75 mL/kg/day) using 0.9% saline or LRS. If hypoglycemic use 2.5% dextrose and 0.45% saline.

## ACTIVITY
Restricted due to associated weakness and lethargy

## DIET
- Feed in upright position (45–90° angle to the floor) and maintain position for 10–15 minutes following feeding.
- Feed a high-calorie gruel formulated from meat-based human baby foods, Eukanuba Maximum Calorie diet (Iams Co., Dayton, OH), Feline a/d (Hills Products, Topeka, KS) or moistened ferret pellets supplemented with Nutri-Cal (EVSCO Pharmaceuticals, Buena, NJ), Ensure (Abbot Laboratories, North Chicago, IL), or Clinicare Feline liquid diet (Abbott Laboratories).
- A more liquid consistency may decrease regurgitation, but may increase the risk of aspiration pneumonia.
- Reported resting energy requirement for ferrets is 70 kcal/kg body weight per day.
- Patients with severe regurgitation may need parenteral feeding via gastrotomy tube.

## CLIENT EDUCATION
If an underlying cause is not identifiable or corrected, most animals become debilitated due to starvation, hepatic lipidosis, and aspiration pneumonia. Advise client of poor prognosis.

## SURGICAL CONSIDERATIONS
- Surgery may be necessary to remove esophageal foreign bodies or neoplasia if identified.
- No surgical procedures improve esophageal motility.

# MEDICATIONS

## DRUG(S) OF CHOICE
- Specific medications are recommended if regurgitation is secondary to identifiable, treatable disorders.
- Sucralfate (25 mg/kg PO q8h), $H_2$ blockers (e.g., famotidine 0.25–0.5 mg/kg PO, IV q12–24h), cimetidine (5–10 mg/kg PO, SC, IM q8h), or omeprazole (0.7 mg/kg PO q24h) can be used if reflux esophagitis is present.

# REGURGITATION

• Metoclopramide (0.2–1.0 mg/kg PO, SC, IM q6–8h) speeds gastric emptying, increases gastroesophageal sphincter tone, and is most useful when reflux esophagitis is a contributing or the primary cause; use of metoclopramide for other causes has had limited success.
• Broad-spectrum antibiotics—necessary for patients with aspiration pneumonia; parenteral antibiotics may be required for patients with severe regurgitation. Ideally, based on culture and susceptibility testing from an airway specimen; begin with an antibiotic combination that is broad-spectrum and effective against anaerobes (e.g., enrofloxacin 10 mg/kg IM q12h plus amoxicillin 10 mg/kg IM q12h); alter therapy based on culture/susceptibility results.

## CONTRAINDICATIONS
N/A

## PRECAUTIONS
• Corticosteroids may be necessary to treat conditions causing megaesophagus; use with caution in patients with aspiration pneumonia.
• Cisapride (0.1–0.5 mg/kg PO q8–12h) has been used in dogs to treat megaesophagus, but its use is controversial; it decreases esophageal transit time and increases lower esophageal tone in normal dogs; both of these effects are undesirable when treating megaesophagus; despite this, regurgitation decreases in some patients receiving cisapride; if symptoms of megaesophagus worsen, discontinue cisapride.

## POSSIBLE INTERACTIONS
N/A

## ALTERNATE DRUGS
N/A

 FOLLOW-UP

## PATIENT MONITORING
Monitor for the development of aspiration pneumonia. Obtain thoracic radiographs if aspiration pneumonia is suspected—fever, cough, nasal discharge

## POSSIBLE COMPLICATIONS
• Aspiration pneumonia
• Esophageal stricture following tumor or foreign body removal
• Hepatic lipidosis

## EXPECTED COURSE AND PROGNOSIS
• Depends on the underlying cause
• If a cause is not identified, the prognosis is poor to grave, with or without treatment.
• Aspiration pneumonia and malnutrition are likely causes of death.

 MISCELLANEOUS

## ASSOCIATED CONDITIONS
• Insulinoma
• Hyperadrenocorticism
• Gastric ulcers
• *Helicobacter mustelae*

## AGE-RELATED FACTORS
N/A

## ZOONOTIC POTENTIAL
Determine rabies vaccination status for all patients.

## PREGNANCY
N/A

## SEE ALSO
• Dysphagia
• Gastrointestinal and esophageal foreign bodies
• Pneumonia, aspiration

## ABBREVIATIONS
• ALT = Alanine aminotransferase
• LRS = lactated Ringer's solution
• TWBC = total white blood cell count

*Suggested Reading*

Blanco MC, Fox JG, Rosenthal K, et al. Megaesophagus in nine ferrets. J Am Vet Med Assoc 1994;205;444–447.
Fox JG. Diseases of the gastrointestinal system. In: Fox JG, ed. Biology and Diseases of the Ferret. 2nd Ed. Baltimore: Williams & Wilkins, 1998.
Hoefer HL. Gastrointestinal diseases. In: Hillyer EV, Quesenberry KE, eds. Ferrets, Rabbits and Rodents: Clinical Medicine and Surgery. Philadelphia: WB Saunders, 1997:26–36.

*Portions Adapted From*

Jones BD. Regurgitation. In: Tilley LP, Smith FWK, Jr., eds. The 5-Minute Veterinary Consult: Canine and Feline, 1st Ed. Baltimore: Lippincott Williams & Wilkins, 1997.

# BASICS

## DEFINITION
• Azotemia and urine specific gravity <1.030
• Acute renal failure (ARF) is a syndrome characterized by sudden onset of filtration failure by the kidneys, accumulation of uremic toxins, and dysregulation of fluid, electrolyte, and acid-base balance.
• Chronic renal failure (CRF) results from primary renal disease that has persisted for months to years; it is characterized by irreversible renal dysfunction that tends to deteriorate progressively.

## PATHOPHYSIOLOGY
Reduction in functional renal mass results in impaired urine-concentrating ability (leading to polyuria and polydipsia [PU/PD]) and retention of nitrogenous waste products of protein catabolism (leading to azotemia). With chronicity, decreased erythropoietin and calcitriol production by the kidneys results in hypoproliferative anemia

## SYSTEMS AFFECTED
• Renal/urologic—impaired renal function leading to PU/PD and signs of uremia
• Nervous, gastrointestinal, musculoskeletal, and other body systems—secondarily affected by uremia
• Hemic/lymph/immune—anemia

## GENETICS
N/A

## INCIDENCE /PREVALENCE
Not well documented; however, renal failure is a common sequela to many conditions affecting ferrets (see below).

## SIGNALMENT
Animals of any age can be affected, but prevalence increases with increasing age.

### Predominant Sex
None

## SIGNS

### General Comments
Clinical signs are related to the severity of renal dysfunction and presence or absence of complications.

### Historical Findings
• ARF—sudden onset of anorexia, listlessness, vomiting (+/− blood), diarrhea (+/− blood), halitosis, ataxia, seizures, known toxin exposure, recent medical or surgical conditions, and oliguria/anuria or polyuria
• CRF—PU/PD, anorexia, ptyalism, diarrhea, vomiting, weight loss, lethargy, poor hair coat, ataxia seizures or coma seen in late stages. Asymptomatic animals with stable CRF may decompensate, resulting in a uremic crisis.

### Physical Examination Findings
• ARF—depression, dehydration (sometimes overhydration), hypothermia, fever, tachypnea, bradycardia, nonpalpable urinary bladder if oliguric
• CRF—small, irregular kidneys (or enlarged kidneys secondary to cystic kidneys or lymphoma), dehydration, cachexia, mucous membrane pallor

## CAUSES
• Shock, heart failure, prolonged anesthesia, or septicemia can cause ARF.
• ARF or CRF—glomerulonephritis, amyloidosis, pyelonephritis, cystic kidneys, nephroliths, chronic urinary obstruction, drugs (e.g., aminoglycoside, sulfonamides, chemotherapeutic agents), heavy metals, lymphoma, hypercalcemia, ADV, and, possibly, diabetes mellitus

## RISK FACTORS
• ARF—preexisting renal disease, dehydration, hypovolemia, hypotension, advanced age, concurrent disease, prolonged anesthesia or surgery, and administration of nephrotoxic drugs
• CRF—aging, uroliths, cystic kidneys, urinary tract infection, diabetes mellitus

# DIAGNOSIS

## DIFFERENTIAL DIAGNOSIS
• For PU/PD—pyometra, hepatic failure, hypercalcemia, diabetes mellitus, postobstructive diuresis, some diuretics (e.g., mannitol and furosemide), ingestion or administration of large quantities of solute (e.g., sodium chloride or glucose), behavioral
• For renomegaly—renal neoplasia (lymphoma), cystic kidneys, hydronephrosis
• Prerenal azotemia—(decreased renal perfusion) characterized by azotemia with concentrated urine (specific gravity >1.030); correctable with fluid repletion
• Postrenal azotemia—characterized by azotemia with obstruction or rupture of the excretory system

## CBC/BIOCHEMISTRY/URINALYSIS
• Nonregenerative anemia with CRF, normal or high PCV with ARF
• BUN elevation seen more commonly than elevation in creatinine; normal creatinine concentration in ferrets is lower than in dogs and cats (0.4–0.6 mg/dL)
• Electrolyte and acid-base abnormalities similar to those seen in other small animals
• Inability to concentrate urine, mild to moderate proteinuria, glucosuria, WBCs, RBCs; variable bacteriuria and crystalluria

may be seen depending on the underlying cause.

## OTHER LABORATORY TESTS
• Urinary protein:creatinine ratio may be useful to determine the magnitude of proteinuria; however, reference values have not been established for ferrets.
• The value of using microalbuminuria assays to screen for glomerular injury has not been evaluated in ferrets.
• Serum lead or zinc concentration
• Plasma electrophoresis—elevated globulins in ferrets with ADV

## IMAGING
• Abdominal radiographs may demonstrate small kidneys (or large kidneys secondary to cystic kidneys or lymphoma) in animals with CRF.
• Ultrasound reveals anechoic cavitating lesions characterized by sharply marginated smooth walls and distal enhancement in patients with cystic kidneys.
• Animals with lymphoma often have renomegaly with hypoechoic renal parenchyma.

## DIAGNOSTIC PROCEDURES
• Direct or indirect blood pressure determination is indicated to monitor for hypertension (how commonly this occurs in ferrets is unknown), and to monitor ferrets on ACE inhibitor therapy (see below).
• Evaluation of ultrasound-guided fine needle aspirates of the kidney may allow differentiation of cystic kidneys from other diseases that cause renomegaly.
• Renal biopsy may be helpful in selected patients to document underlying cause.

## PATHOLOGIC FINDINGS
• Gross findings—small kidneys with a lumpy or granular surface seen in many ferrets with CRF; large, irregular kidneys with cystic kidneys or lymphoma
• Histopathologic findings—frequently nonspecific; chronic generalized nephropathy or end-stage kidneys; findings are specific for diseases causing CRF in some patients; nephrosis or nephritis seen in ferrets with ARF

# TREATMENT

## APPROPRIATE HEALTH CARE
Patients with compensated CRF may be managed as outpatients; patients in ARF or uremic crisis should be managed as inpatients.

## NURSING CARE
• Patients in ARF or uremic crisis—correct estimated fluid deficits with normal (0.9%) saline or balanced polyionic solution within

# RENAL FAILURE

4–6 hours to prevent additional renal injury from ischemia; once the patient is hydrated, ongoing fluid requirements are provided by 5% dextrose or balanced electrolyte solution (approximately 75–100 mL/kg/ day).
• Patients in CRF—subcutaneous fluid therapy (daily or every other day) may benefit patients with moderate to severe CRF.

## ACTIVITY
Unrestricted

## DIET
• Dietary protein restriction is difficult to achieve in ferrets.
• If anorectic or normal diet of kibble is refused, most ferrets will accept high-calorie diets such as Eukanuba Maximum Calorie diet (Iams Co., Dayton, OH), Feline a/d (Hills Products, Topeka, KS) or Clinicare Feline liquid diet (Abbott Laboratories, North Chicago, IL); may also add dietary supplement such as Nutri-Cal (EVSCO Pharmaceuticals, Buena, NJ) to increase caloric content to these foods. Warming the food to body temperature or offering via syringe may increase acceptance. Administer these foods several times a day.
• Reported resting energy requirement for ferrets is 70 kcal/kg body weight per day. Clinicare Feline contains 1 kcal/mL; Eukanuba Maximum Calorie diet contains 2 kcal/mL.
• Allow free access to fresh water at all times.

## CLIENT EDUCATION
• CRF—tends to progress over months, possibly to years
• ARF—inform of the poor prognosis for complete recovery, potential for morbid complications of treatment (e.g., fluid overload, sepsis, and multiple organ failure), expense of prolonged hospitalization.

## SURGICAL CONSIDERATIONS
Avoid hypotension during anesthesia to prevent additional renal injury.

## MEDICATIONS

### DRUG(S) OF CHOICE

#### Inadequate Urine Production (Anuric or Oliguric Renal Failure)
• Ensure patient is fluid-volume-replete; provide additional isonatric fluid to achieve mild (3–5%) volume expansion; failure to induce diuresis by fluid replacement indicates severe parenchymal damage or underestimation of fluid deficit.
• Furosemide and dopamine—follow feline/canine treatment protocols.
• If these treatments fail to induce diuresis within 4–6 hours, the prognosis is grave.

### Uremic Crisis
• If vomiting—NPO until vomiting subsides
• Reduce gastric acid production—cimetidine (5–10 mg/kg PO, SC, IM q8h) or omeprazole (0.7 mg/kg PO q24h)
• Mucosal protectant—sucralfate (25 mg/kg PO q6–8h)
• Antiemetics—metoclopramide (0.2–1.0 mg/kg PO, SC, IM q6–8h)
• Potassium chloride IV as needed to correct hypokalemia (based on cat dosages)

### Compensated CRF
• Famotidine (0.25–0.5 mg/kg PO, IV q12–24h) or cimetidine (5–10 mg/kg PO, SC, IM q8h)
• Potassium gluconate to correct hypokalemia and/or intestinal phosphate binders if hyperphosphatemic—use feline dosage protocols.
• Erythropoietin has been used to treat chronic anemia in ferrets (100 U/kg three times per week until the PCV is stable, then 1–2 times a week). Monitor the PCV and titrate dose as needed.
• The usefulness of ACE inhibitors (enalapril or benazepril) has not been evaluated in ferrets with renal failure. However, ferrets are more sensitive to the hypotensive effects of ACE inhibitors and may become hypotensive (weak, lethargic). This effect may be mitigated by using a lower dose or longer dosage interval. Reported dosage in ferrets is 0.25–0.5 mg/kg q24–48h.

### CONTRAINDICATIONS
Avoid nephrotoxic agents.

### PRECAUTIONS
• Modify dosages of all drugs that require renal metabolism or elimination.
• Use ACE inhibitors with caution; monitor for lethargy, weakness, or worsening of azotemia or proteinuria.

### POSSIBLE INTERACTIONS
Metoclopramide may impair the effects of dopamine.

### ALTERNATIVE DRUGS
Control of vomiting—chlorpromazine (0.5 mg/kg IM q6–12h) can be used to treat vomiting but is associated with CNS depression, vasodilatation, and hypotension.

### PATIENT MONITORING
• ARF—fluid, electrolyte, and acid-base balances; body weight; urine output; and clinical status; daily
• CRF—monitor at 1- to 3-month intervals, depending on therapy and severity of disease.

### POSSIBLE COMPLICATIONS
• ARF—seizures, gastrointestinal bleeding, cardiac arrhythmias, congestive heart failure, pulmonary edema, hypovolemic shock, coma, cardiopulmonary arrest, and death

• CRF—uremic stomatitis, gastroenteritis, anemia

### PREVENTION/AVOIDANCE
Anticipate the potential for ARF in patients that are hemodynamically unstable, receiving nephrotoxic drugs, have multiple organ failure, or are undergoing prolonged anesthesia and surgery; maintenance of hydration and/or mild saline volume expansion may be preventive.

### EXPECTED COURSE AND PROGNOSIS
• Nonoliguric ARF—milder than oliguric; recovery may occur, but the prognosis remains guarded to unfavorable.
• Oliguric ARF—extensive renal injury, is difficult to manage, and has a poor prognosis for recovery
• Anuric ARF—generally fatal
• CRF—short-term prognosis depends on severity; long-term prognosis guarded to poor because CRF tends to be progressive

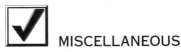

## MISCELLANEOUS

### ASSOCIATED CONDITIONS
• Urolithiasis
• Urogenital cysts
• Splenomegaly
• Pyometra
• Lymphoma

### AGE-RELATED FACTORS
Increased incidence in older animals; normal renal function decreases with aging.

### ZOONOTIC POTENTIAL
Leptospirosis is extremely rare in pet ferrets, but may have zoonotic potential.

### PREGNANCY
ARF is a rare complication of pregnancy in animals; promoted by acute metritis, pyometra, and postpartum sepsis or hemorrhage

### SYNONYMS
Kidney failure

### SEE ALSO
• Polydipsia and Polyuria
• Urinary Tract Obstruction

### ABBREVIATIONS
• ACE = angiotensin converting enzyme
• ADV = Aleutian disease virus
• BUN = blood urea nitrogen
• CNS = central nervous system
• NPO = nothing by mouth
• PCV = packed cell volume
• PU/PD = polyuria/polydipsia
• RBC = red blood cell
• WBC = white blood cell

*Suggested Reading*

Antinoff N. Urinary disorders in ferrets. Semin Avian Exotic Pet Med 1998;7(2):89–92.

Esteves MI, Marini RP, Ryden EB, et al. Estimation of glomerular filtration rate and evaluation of renal function in ferrets. Am J Vet Res 1994;55:166–172.

Fox JG, Pearson RC, Bell JA. Diseases of the genitourinary system. In: Fox JG, ed. Biology and Diseases of the Ferret. 2nd Ed. Baltimore: Williams & Wilkins, 1998.

Hillyer EV. Urogenital diseases. In: Hillyer EV, Quesenberry KE, eds. Ferrets, Rabbits and Rodents: Clinical Medicine and Surgery. Philadelphia: WB Saunders, 1997.

Hoefer HL. Rabbit and ferret renal disease diagnosis. In: Fudge Am, ed. Laboratory Medicine, Avian and Exotic Pets. Philadelphia: WB Saunders, 2000.

*Portions Adapted From*

Cowgill LD. Renal Failure—Acute. Adams LG. Renal Failure—Chronic. In: Tilley LP, Smith FWK, Jr., eds. The 5-Minute Veterinary Consult: Canine and Feline, 3rd Ed. Baltimore: Lippincott Williams & Wilkins, 2003.

# RENOMEGALY

## BASICS

### OVERVIEW
• One or both kidneys are abnormally large as detected by abdominal palpation or radiography.
• The kidneys may become abnormally large because of the development of renal cysts or pseudocysts, abnormal cellular infiltration (e.g., inflammation, infection, and neoplasia), urinary tract obstruction, or acute tubular necrosis.

### SIGNALMENT
Renomegaly is a somewhat common physical examination finding, especially in middle-aged to older ferrets.

### SIGNS
• One or both kidneys palpably large
• If significant renal disease is present, owners may report lethargy, loss of appetite, weight loss, polyuria and polydipsia, diarrhea, vomiting, or abdominal distension.
• With significant renal disease, may detect dehydration, pale mucous membranes, and cachexia
• Renal cysts often remain undetected until they become large and numerous enough to contribute to renal failure or abdominal enlargement; thus, patients typically are clinically normal during initial stages of cyst formation and growth.
• May detect bosselated (lumpy) kidneys by abdominal palpation
• Most renal cysts are not painful when palpated
• Abnormally large abdomen

### CAUSES
• Renal cysts—very common; can be unilateral or bilateral; affected kidney often irregularly shaped
• Neoplasia—lymphoma most common renal tumor; may cause bilateral or unilateral renomegaly and often bosselated kidneys; other (rarely) reported tumors include renal carcinoma and cystadenocarcinoma.
• Hydronephrosis—can cause unilateral or bilateral renomegaly; develops secondarily to ureteral obstruction (e.g., abscess, ligation, neoplasia, and urolithiasis)
• Infection/inflammation—ADV, renal abscess
• Hematoma—can occur secondarily to trauma; rare

### RISK FACTORS
• The stimuli for renal cyst formation remain obscure.
• Any cause of ureteral obstruction including uroliths; neoplasia; prostatic disease; retroperitoneal abscess, cysts, hematoma, or other mass; inadvertent ureteral ligation during ovariohysterectomy

• A viral etiology for lymphoma has been proposed; exposure to other ferrets with lymphoma may increase risk; exposure to ferrets with ADV

## DIAGNOSIS

### DIFFERENTIAL DIAGNOSIS
• Must distinguish from other abdominal masses
• Confirmation may require diagnostic imaging procedures or exploratory celiotomy.

### CBC/BIOCHEMISTRY/URINALYSIS
• Results usually unremarkable unless patient has renal insufficiency
• Nonregenerative anemia secondary to chronic renal failure in some
• Azotemia, hyperphosphatemia, and low urine specific gravity in patients with renal failure
• Leukocytosis expected in patients with infectious, inflammatory, and neoplastic causes of renomegaly
• Neoplastic cells rarely observed in urine of patients with renal neoplasia

### OTHER LABORATORY TESTS
Cytologic examination and bacterial culture of cyst fluid

### IMAGING

#### Radiographic Findings
• Abdominal radiographs to confirm renomegaly
• Can use excretory urography to confirm presence of renomegaly, hydronephrosis, and space-occupying masses of the kidneys
• Thoracic radiography indicated to detect metastases in patients with renal neoplasia

#### Ultrasonographic Findings
Helpful to confirm diagnosis and identify potential causes such as renal cysts, neoplastic mass, abscess, and subcapsular hematoma

### DIAGNOSTIC PROCEDURES
• Examination of fine needle aspirate can confirm presence of renal cyst, abscess, and neoplasia (especially lymphoma).
• If no definitive diagnosis is made by cytologic evaluation of renal aspirates, renal biopsy may be indicated.

## TREATMENT
• Diagnose and treat underlying cause if possible.
• None for renal cysts. Ultrasound-guided aspiration of cystic fluid may temporarily decrease size; however, fluid is likely to reform. Spontaneous resolution of cysts is not documented in ferrets; with time, most cysts increase in size and may compress

adjacent normally functioning renal parenchyma.
• Specific treatment for hydronephrosis depends on the cause and whether there is concurrent renal failure or other disease process (e.g., neoplasia, abscess). If obstruction is removable and sufficient renal function remains, removal of the affected kidney is not necessary.
• Treatment for renal failure may be necessary.

## MEDICATIONS

### DRUG(S) OF CHOICE
Vary with the cause

### CONTRAINDICATIONS
Avoid nephrotoxic drugs.

### PRECAUTIONS
N/A

### POSSIBLE INTERACTIONS
N/A

### ALTERNATIVE DRUGS
N/A

## FOLLOW-UP

### PATIENT MONITORING
• Renal cysts—perform physical examination and monitor size of cysts through ultrasound.
• Monitor for signs of renal failure.

### POSSIBLE COMPLICATIONS
• Renal failure, depending on underlying cause of renomegaly
• Metastasis of renal tumor

## MISCELLANEOUS

### ASSOCIATED CONDITIONS
• Ferret adrenal disease
• Insulinoma

### AGE-RELATED FACTORS
N/A

### ZOONOTIC POTENTIAL
N/A

### PREGNANCY
N/A

### SYNONYMS
None

### SEE ALSO
• Hydronephrosis
• Lymphosarcoma
• Polydipsia and polyuria
• Renal Failure

### ABBREVIATION
ADV = Aleutian disease virus

*Suggested Reading*

Antinoff N. Urinary disorders in ferrets. Semin Avian Exotic Pet Med 1998;7(2):89–92.

Beeber NL. Abdominal surgery in ferrets. Vet Clin North Am Exot Anim Pract 2000;3(3):647–662.

Brown SA. Neoplasia. In: Hillyer EV, Quesenberry KE, eds. Ferrets, Rabbits and Rodents: Clinical Medicine and Surgery. Philadelphia: WB Saunders, 1997:99.

Esteves MI, Marini RP, Ryden EB, et al. Estimation of glomerular filtration rate and evaluation of renal function in ferrets. Am J Vet Res 1994;55:166–172.

Fox JG, Pearson RC, Bell JA. Diseases of the genitourinary system. In: Fox JG, ed. Biology and Diseases of the Ferret. 2nd Ed. Baltimore: Williams & Wilkins, 1998.

Hillyer EV. Urogenital diseases. In: Hillyer EV, Quesenberry KE, eds. Ferrets, Rabbits and Rodents: Clinical Medicine and Surgery. Philadelphia: WB Saunders, 1997.

*Portions Adapted From*

Forrester SD. Renomegaly. In: Tilley LP, Smith FWK, Jr., eds. The 5-Minute Veterinary Consult: Canine and Feline, 3rd Ed. Baltimore: Lippincott Williams & Wilkins, 2003.

# SALMONELLOSIS

## BASICS

### OVERVIEW
• A bacterial disease that causes enteritis and sometimes septicemia; disease may be caused by many different serotypes of *Salmonella*
• Salmonella—a Gram-negative bacterium; colonizes the small intestine; adheres to and invades enterocytes; eventually enters and multiplies in the lamina propria and local mesenteric lymph nodes; cytotoxins and enterotoxins are produced resulting in secretory diarrhea and mucosal sloughing
• Uncomplicated gastroenteritis—organisms are stopped at the mesenteric lymph node stage; patient has only gastrointestinal tract signs.
• Bacteremia and septicemia following gastroenteritis—more serious disease

### SIGNALMENT
• Salmonellosis is an unusual cause of gastrointestinal tract disease in pet ferrets. Most reports are of outbreaks occurring in breeding or research colonies or in ferrets eating undercooked meats or poultry products.
• No age or sex predilections

### SIGNS

#### General Comments
Disease severity varies from subclinical to mild, moderate, and severe clinical disease
• Asymptomatic carrier states—no clinical signs (rare)
• Gastroenteritis—diarrhea, often with fresh blood and/or mucous; malaise/lethargy; anorexia; vomiting; progressive dehydration; abdominal pain; tenesmus; pale mucous membranes; mesenteric lymphadenopathy; weight loss
• Gastroenteritis with bacteremia and septicemia, septic shock, or endotoxemia—pale mucous membranes, weakness, cardiovascular collapse, tachycardia, tachypnea

### CAUSES AND RISK FACTORS
• Anecdotal reports have been associated with feeding uncooked meats and poultry products.
• Salmonella serotype—virulence factors, infectious dose, and route of exposure determines course of disease; *Salmonella hadar, S. enteritidis, S. newport,* and *S. typhimurium* reported
• Host factors that increase susceptibility—neonatal/young ferrets, immature immune system, debilitation, other concurrent disease

## DIAGNOSIS

### DIFFERENTIAL DIAGNOSIS
*Salmonella* is relatively rare in household ferrets. Diseases that are much more likely to cause clinical gastroenteritis include:
• ECE—most common infectious cause
• Gastrointestinal foreign body
• *Helicobacter mustelae* gastroenteritis
• Inflammatory bowel disease—lympho-plasmacytic gastroenteritis, eosinophilic gastroenteritis
• Neoplasia, especially lymphoma, occasionally adenocarcinoma or other gastrointestinal tract tumors
Also consider these less common causes of gastrointestinal tract disease in pet ferrets:
• Other bacterial infections—*Campylobacter* spp., *Clostridium* spp., *Lawsonia intracellularis, Mycobacterium avium-intracellulare.*
• Parasitic diseases—*Giardia,* coccidia, *Cryptosporidium* spp.

### CBC/BIOCHEMISTRY/URINALYSIS
• CBC—variable; depends on stage of illness; nonregenerative anemia or lymphopenia sometimes seen
• Hypoalbuminemia

### OTHER LABORATORY TESTS
N/A

### IMAGING
N/A

### DIAGNOSTIC PROCEDURES
• Fecal culture—special media needed; may require multiple samples
• Fecal leukocytes may be present.
• Subclinical carrier states—chronic; intermittent fecal culture positive
• NOTE: use of antimicrobials in a patient before sampling may produce false-negative cultures.

### PATHOLOGIC FINDINGS
• Gross lesions—only in severely affected patients
• Cultures of ileum, mesenteric lymph nodes

## TREATMENT

### APPROPRIATE HEALTH CARE
• Outpatient—uncomplicated gastroenteritis (without bacteremia) and carrier states
• Inpatient—with bacteremia/septicemia and for gastroenteritis in animals that are rapidly debilitated by diarrhea

### NURSING CARE
Varies according to severity of illness—assess percentages of dehydration, body weight, ongoing fluid loss, shock, PCV/total protein, electrolytes, and acid-base status.

#### Uncomplicated Gastroenteritis
• Supportive care—fluid and electrolyte replacement
• Parenteral, balanced, isotonic solution (lactated Ringer's)

### SURGICAL CONSIDERATIONS
N/A

## MEDICATIONS

### DRUG(S) OF CHOICE
• Antimicrobial therapy—indicated; culture and susceptibility testing/MIC necessary to assess drug-resistance problems
• Trimethoprim-sulfa—15–30 mg/kg PO, SC q12h
• Enrofloxacin—10–20 mg/kg PO, SC, IM q12h
• Chloramphenicol—30–50 mg/kg PO, SC, IM q12h

### CONTRAINDICATIONS AND POSSIBLE INTERACTIONS
N/A

## FOLLOW-UP

### PATIENT MONITORING
• Fecal culture—repeat monthly for a few months to assess development of carrier state.
• Other animals—monitor for secondary spread of infection.
• Advise client to contact veterinarian if patient shows signs of recurring disease.

### PREVENTION/AVOIDANCE
Keep animals healthy—proper nutrition; no raw meat; clean and disinfect cages and food and water dishes frequently; store food and feeding utensils properly.

### POSSIBLE COMPLICATIONS
• Spread of infection possible within household to other animals or humans
• Development of chronic infection with diarrhea
• Recurrence of disease with stress

## MISCELLANEOUS

**ASSOCIATED CONDITIONS**
N/A

**ZOONOTIC POTENTIAL**
• High potential, especially in children, elderly, immunosuppressed, and antimicrobial drug users
• Acutely ill animals may shed large numbers of salmonellae in stool.
• Isolation is needed.

**PREGNANCY**
• May complicate disease
• Abortion—may be a sequela to infection
• Antimicrobial therapy—take into account the effect on the fetus.

**SYNONYMS**
N/A

**ABBREVIATIONS**
• CBC = complete blood count
• ECE = epizootic catarrhal enteritis
• MIC = minimal inhibitory concentration
• PCV = packed cell volume

*Suggested Reading*

Fox JG. Bacterial and mycoplasmal diseases. In: Fox JG, ed. Biology and Diseases of the Ferret. 2nd Ed. Baltimore: Williams & Wilkins, 1998.

Fox JG. Diseases of the gastrointestinal system. In: Fox JG, ed. Biology and Diseases of the Ferret. 2nd Ed. Baltimore: Williams & Wilkins, 1998.

Hoefer HL. Gastrointestinal diseases. In: Hillyer EV, Quesenberry KE, eds. Ferrets, Rabbits and Rodents: Clinical Medicine and Surgery. Philadelphia: WB Saunders, 1997.

Marini RP, Adkins JA, Fox JG. Proven or potential zoonotic disease of ferrets. J Am Vet Med Assoc 1989;195:990–993.

Williams BH. Ferret microbiology and virology. In: Fudge AM, ed. Laboratory Medicine, Avian and Exotic Pets. Philadelphia: WB Saunders, 2000.

*Portions Adapted From*

McDonough PL. Salmonellosis. In: Tilley LP, Smith FWK, Jr., eds. The 5-Minute Veterinary Consult: Canine and Feline, 3rd Ed. Baltimore: Lippincott Williams & Wilkins, 2003.

# SARCOPTIC MANGE

## BASICS

### OVERVIEW
• An uncommon, contagious parasitic skin disease of ferrets caused by infestation with the mite *Sarcoptes scabiei*
• Two forms reported—local form affecting the feet with intense pruritus and secondary pododermatitis and generalized form with diffuse or focal alopecia and pruritus
• Mites are transmissible from dogs to ferrets or ferret to ferret.

### SIGNALMENT
• Uncommon disease of ferrets
• No age or sex predilection

### SIGNS
• Foot lesions characterized by severe inflammation, swelling, and crusting that can progress to nail and skin sloughing if untreated; generally extremely pruritic/painful
• Alopecia and erythematous rash may appear in any area of the body, either focal lesions or more generalized coalescent lesions
• Nonseasonal, usually intense pruritus
• Secondary crusts, excoriations, and pyoderma may occur.
• Possible peripheral lymphadenopathy
• Multiple pet households—more than one animal (ferrets or dogs) may show signs.

### CAUSES AND RISK FACTORS
• Exposure to a carrier animal before development of symptoms
• Residence in breeding colonies
• Residence at animal shelter
• Boarding

## DIAGNOSIS

### DIFFERENTIAL DIAGNOSIS

#### Differentiating Causes
• Ferret adrenal disease—bilaterally symmetric alopecia. Hair loss often begins in late winter or early spring; hair initially may regrow later in the year, followed by progressive alopecia the following spring. Alopecia begins in the tail region and progresses cranially. In severe cases, the ferret will become completely bald. In most cases, the skin has a normal appearance; 30% of affected ferrets are pruritic and secondary pyoderma is occasionally seen. Other signs related to adrenal disease, such as a swollen vulva in spayed females, may be seen.
• Seasonal flank alopecia—not pruritic; seen in intact animals (or females with ovarian remnant); bilaterally symmetric alopecia begins at the tail base and progresses throughout the breeding season (March–August for females, December–July for males).

• CDV—pododermatitis usually follows a catarrhal phase characterized by naso-ocular discharge, depression, and anorexia, followed by a characteristic, erythematous, pruritic rash on the chin and lips, and spreads caudally to the inguinal area; pododermatitis is characterized by hyperkeratinization of the footpads, erythema, and swelling. CDV is uniformly fatal, and signs other than pododermatitis alone will be seen.
• Neoplasia—lesions may occur on feet; however, with most tumor types only one foot is affected; lymphoma may affect multiple feet; can be nodular, inflamed, swollen, or ulcerative, depending on tumor type. Mast cell tumors—raised alopecic nodules; may become ulcerated or covered with a thick black crust; may be single or multiple, usually pruritic and found on neck and trunk
• Ear mites—most ferrets with ear mites are not pruritic. In pruritic animals, one may see partial to complete alopecia caudal to the ears; waxy brown aural discharge; excoriations around pinna; differentiate by otic examination and skin scrape.
• Fleas—patchy alopecia at tail base and in cervical and dorsal thoracic region; excoriations; secondary pyoderma sometimes seen
• Bacterial dermatitis—usually secondary infection; localized or multifocal areas of alopecia depending on primary cause; lesions may appear ulcerated; pruritus sometimes seen; may be concurrent with scabies
• Dermatomycosis—partial to complete alopecia with scaling; with or without erythema; not always ringlike; may begin as small papules; not usually pruritic
• Demodicosis—extremely rare, has been reported in association with corticosteriod use; mites will be present on skin scrape
• Hypersensitivity/contact irritant—uncommon cause; dermatitis localized to area of contact with irritant

### CBC/BIOCHEMISTRY/URINALYSIS
N/A

### OTHER LABORATORY TESTS
• CDV—immunofluorescent antibody (IFA) test—can be performed on peripheral blood or buffy coat smears or conjunctival or mucous membrane scrapings. Vaccination will not affect the results.
• Ferret adrenal disease—elevations in serum estradiol, androstenedione, and 17-hydroxyprogesterone combined are most diagnostic (available through the University of Tennessee Clinical Endocrinology Laboratory, Department of Comparative Medicine).

### IMAGING
N/A

### DIAGNOSTIC PROCEDURES
• Superficial skin scrapings—mites are not always seen.
• Favorable response to scabicidal treatment—common method for tentative diagnosis
• Biopsy or FNA—histopathology, rule out neoplasia
• Wood's lamp, fungal culture, and cytologic examination of stained smear of any exudate or pustule contents—rule out mycotic or bacterial infection

## TREATMENT

• All in-contact ferrets or dogs—should be treated, even those with no clinical signs; may be asymptomatic carriers
• Thoroughly clean and treat environment; *Sarcoptes* mites can survive for up to 3 weeks.

## MEDICATIONS

### DRUG(S) OF CHOICE
• Ivermectin—highly effective; 0.2–0.4 mg/kg SC q14d for three to four doses
• Whole-body lime sulfur dip q7d may be used but less effective due to lack of owner compliance; disadvantages are bad odor and staining.
• Selamectin (Revolution; Pfizer)—topical application of the cat dosage has been anecdotally reported to be effective; use with caution—not labeled for use in ferrets
• Systemic antibiotics—may be needed to resolve any secondary pyoderma
• Symptomatic therapy to relieve pruritus—prednisone 0.25–1.0 mg/kg q 24h PO divided or antihistamines—use is anecdotal, generally not as effective as steroids. Hydroxyzine (Atarax, Roerig) 2 mg/kg PO q8h; diphenhydramine (Benadryl, Parke-Davis) 0.5–2.0 mg/kg PO q8–12h; chlorpheniramine (Chlor-Trimeton, Squibb) 1–2 mg/kg PO q8–12h
• Milbemycin (Interceptor) and amitraz (Mitaban) dip have not been used to treat *Sarcoptes* in ferrets.

### CONTRAINDICATIONS/POSSIBLE INTERACTIONS
Ivermectin—anecdotally associated with birth defects when used in pregnant jills

## FOLLOW-UP

• Topical treatments are prone to failure, owing to incomplete application of the treatment solution.

• Reinfection can occur if the contact with infected animals continues.

## MISCELLANEOUS

### ASSOCIATED CONDITIONS
N/A

### ZOONOTIC POTENTIAL
People who come in close contact with an affected ferret may develop a pruritic, papular rash on their arms, chest, or abdomen; human lesions are usually transient and should resolve spontaneously after the affected animal has been treated; if the lesions persist, clients should seek advice from their dermatologist.

### ABBREVIATIONS
• CDV—canine distemper virus
• FNA—fine needle aspirate

### SEE ALSO
• Adrenal disease
• Canine distemper virus
• Dermatophytosis
• Ear mites
• Fleas and flea infestation
• Pododermatitis and nailbed disorders

### Suggested Reading

Clyde VL. Practical treatment and control of common ectoparasites in exotic pets. Vet Med 1996;91(7):632–637.

Fox JG, Marini RP. Diseases of the endocrine system. In: Fox JG, ed. Biology and Diseases of the Ferret. 2nd Ed. Baltimore: Williams & Wilkins, 1998.

Kelleher SA. Skin diseases of the ferret. Vet Clin North Am Exotic Anim Pract 2001;4(2):565–572.

Orcutt C. Dermatologic diseases. In: Hillyer EV, Quesenberry KE, eds. Ferrets, Rabbits and Rodents: Clinical Medicine and Surgery. Philadelphia: WB Saunders, 1997.

Patterson MM, Kirchain SM. Comparison of three treatments for control of ear mites in ferrets. Lab Anim Sci 1999;49(6):655–657.

Rosenthal KL. Endocrine disorders of ferrets: insulinoma and adrenal gland disease. 21st Annu Waltham/OSU Symp Treat Small Anim Dis Exotics 1997:35–38.

Rosenthal KL. Ferret and rabbit endocrine disease diagnosis. In: Fudge Am, ed. Laboratory Medicine, Avian and Exotic Pets. Philadelphia: WB Saunders, 2000.

Scott D. Dermatoses of pet rodents, rabbits and ferrets. In: Scott D, Miller W, Ariffen C, eds. Small Animal Dermatology. 5th Ed. Philadelphia: WB Saunders, 1995.

### Portions Adapted From

Smith MO. Sarcoptic Mange. In: Tilley LP, Smith FWK, Jr., eds. The 5-Minute Veterinary Consult: Canine and Feline, 3rd Ed. Baltimore: Lippincott Williams & Wilkins, 2003.

# SPLENOMEGALY

## BASICS

### DEFINITION
Enlargement of the spleen; characterized as either diffuse or nodular

### PATHOPHYSIOLOGY
• The spleen will often gradually increase in size with age in apparently normal ferrets; the cause of this is unknown.
• Function of the spleen included removal of senescent and abnormal erythrocytes; filtration and phagocytosis of antigenic particles; production of lymphocytes and plasma cells; reservoir for erythrocytes and platelets; and hematopoiesis, as required.
• Splenomegaly is an extremely common finding in ferrets and reflects splenic functions.
• Hypersplenism is a syndrome in which red or white blood cells are removed at an abnormally high rate by the spleen, resulting in one or more cytopenias. Hypersplenism is a rare cause of splenomegaly in ferrets.

#### Diffuse
General pathologic mechanisms include:
• Lymphoreticular hyperplasia—most common cause of splenomegaly; hyperplasia of mononuclear phagocytes and lymphoid elements (in response to antigens); accelerated erythrocyte destruction
• Infiltration—involves cellular invasion of the spleen or deposition of abnormal substances
• Inflammatory (splenitis)—associated with infectious agents; rarely seen in ferrets

#### Nodular
Associated with neoplastic (tumor) or non-neoplastic disorders (hemorrhage, infection, or inflammation)

### SYSTEMS AFFECTED
N/A

### SIGNALMENT
No age or sex predilection

### SIGNS

#### General Comments
• Reflect the underlying disease rather than splenic enlargement
• Often nonspecific

#### Historical Findings
Reflect underlying disease

#### Physical Examination Findings
• Enlarged spleen on abdominal palpation—enlarged spleen may occupy up to one-third of the abdominal cavity and cause abdominal distension and discomfort.
• Usually diffuse, uniform enlargement palpable

• Nodular, irregular enlargement suggests neoplasia or infiltrative disease.
• Infiltrative or inflammatory disease—implied by hepatomegaly, thickened intestines, and/or enlarged mesenteric lymph nodes
• Lymphosarcoma—suggested by concurrent peripheral lymphadenopathy

### CAUSES

#### Diffuse
*Infiltration*
• Extramedullary hematopoiesis—chronic inflammation, infectious disease, estrogen-induced pancytopenia, chronic anemia, malignancy, insulinoma, adrenal disease
• Lymphoid hyperplasia—chronic antigenic stimulation
• Neoplasia—lymphosarcoma
*Hyperplasia*
• Congestion—anesthetic agents, portal hypertension, right-sided heart failure
• Infection—bacterial endocarditis, other systemic infection
*Inflammation (Splenitis)*
Rare in ferrets, but may see eosinophilic splenitis with eosinophilic gastroenteritis, lymphoplasmacytic with lymphoplasmacytic enteritis, or granulomatous with mycobacteriosis

#### Nodular
• Neoplastic—malignant: hemangiosarcoma, lymphosarcoma, metastatic insulinoma, fibrosarcoma, leiomyosarcoma; benign: hemangioma, myelolipoma, leiomyoma, metastatic carcinoma
• Nonneoplastic—hematoma, abscess, rarely extramedullary hematopoiesis

### RISK FACTORS
N/A

## DIAGNOSIS

### DIFFERENTIAL DIAGNOSIS
Other cranial organomegaly or masses

### CBC/BIOCHEMISTRY/URINALYSIS
• Leukocytosis with a left shift—may indicate infectious and inflammatory conditions
• Lymphocytosis—suggests lymphoma
• Leukopenia—may be seen with hypersplenism
• Thrombocytopenia—from increased consumption secondary to hemangiosarcoma, increased destruction or sequestration (hypersplenism), or decreased production (estrogen toxicity)
• Regenerative anemia and splenomegaly—may indicate blood loss
• Eosinophilia—suggests hypereosinophilic syndrome

• Hyperglobulinemia—from ADV, chronic inflammation
• Serum glucose concentration decreased with insulinoma

### OTHER LABORATORY TESTS
Elevations in serum estradiol, androstenedione, and 17-hydroxyprogesterone diagnostic of hyperadrenocorticism

### IMAGING

#### Abdominal Radiography
• Confirm or detect splenomegaly
• May provide evidence for the underlying cause—gastrointestinal tract disease, adrenal disease, insulinoma
• Effusion—may indicate hemorrhage from splenic rupture (hemangiosarcoma, hematoma); rare in ferrets

#### Thoracic Radiography
Right and left lateral views—screen for metastasis and underlying disease

#### Abdominal Ultrasonography
• Distinguishes between diffuse and nodular
• Diffuse enlargement with normal parenchyma—may be noted with congestion or cellular infiltration
• Reduced echogenicity—may be seen with lymphosarcoma
• Nodular abnormalities easily identified
• Complex, mixed echogenic pattern—hemangiosarcoma
• Can identify concurrent abdominal diseases affecting liver, kidneys, intestines, and lymph nodes

### DIAGNOSTIC PROCEDURES

#### Fine Needle Aspiration
• Contraindicated if hemangiosarcoma is suspected—fatal hemorrhage may occur. Rule out hemangiosarcoma (rare in ferrets) on abdominal ultrasound.
• Procedure—place patient in right lateral or dorsal recumbency; use a 23- or 25-gauge (1- to 1.5-in) needle and 5 mL syringe; diffuse: may aspirate without ultrasonography; nodular: requires ultrasound guidance; anesthesia or tranquilization may be required.
• Specimens—identify the predominant inflammatory cell type.
• Neoplastic infiltrates—classified as hematopoietic, lymphatic, carcinoma, or sarcoma

#### Bone Marrow Aspiration
• Indicated with cytopenias before splenectomy (spleen may be the main source of circulating blood cells)
• Marrow may be normal or hypercellular with hypersplenism.

## TREATMENT

Depends on underlying cause; supportive nursing care as needed—the spleen is rarely the cause of disease.

### SURGICAL CONSIDERATIONS

*Splenectomy*
• Indicated only for hypersplenism, splenic rupture, and splenic neoplasia
• Occasionally, the spleen may become large enough to cause abdominal discomfort—partial splenectomy may alleviate discomfort. The need for total splenectomy should be carefully evaluated, especially in anemic animals, since EMH in the spleen may be a major source of hematopoiesis.
• Perform bone marrow aspirate first in ferrets with anemia or leukopenia—rule out bone marrow aplasia; spleen may be providing hematopoietic activity.
• Exploratory celiotomy—permits direct evaluation of all abdominal organs for diagnosis and treatment of underlying causes of splenomegaly.

## MEDICATIONS

### DRUG(S) OF CHOICE
Depend on underlying disease

### CONTRAINDICATIONS
N/A

### PRECAUTIONS
N/A

### POSSIBLE INTERACTIONS
N/A

### ALTERNATIVE DRUGS
N/A

## FOLLOW-UP

### POSSIBLE COMPLICATIONS
• Postoperative sepsis—uncommon complication after surgery
• Antibiotics—indicated in patients that are receiving immunosuppressive therapy

## MISCELLANEOUS

### ASSOCIATED CONDITIONS
• Hyperadrenocorticism
• Insulinoma

### AGE-RELATED FACTORS
The spleen may gradually enlarge with age in normal ferrets.

### ZOONOTIC POTENTIAL
N/A

### PREGNANCY
N/A

### SEE ALSO
• Hypersplenism
• Infiltrative bowel disease
• Lymphosarcoma

### ABBREVIATIONS
• ADV = Aleutian disease virus
• EMH = extramedullary hematopoiesis

*Suggested Reading*

Brown SA. Neoplasia. In: Hillyer EV, Quesenberry KE, eds. Ferrets, Rabbits and Rodents: Clinical Medicine and Surgery. Philadelphia: WB Saunders, 1997:99.

Hillyer EV. Cardiovascular diseases. Part II, other diseases. In Hillyer EV, Quesenberry KE, eds. Ferrets, Rabbits and Rodents: Clinical Medicine and Surgery. Philadelphia: WB Saunders, 1997:71–76.

Hillyer EV. Working up the ferret with a large spleen. Proc North Am Vet Conf 1994:819–821.

Wheeler J, Bennett RA. Ferret abdominal surgical procedures. Part II. Gastrointestinal foreign bodies, splenomegaly, liver biopsy, cystotomy and ovariohysterectomy. Compend Contin Edu Pract Vet 1999;21(11):1049–1057.

*Portions Adapted From*

Cornetta AM, Balkman CE. Splenomegaly. In: Tilley LP, Smith FWK, Jr., eds. The 5-Minute Veterinary Consult: Canine and Feline, 3rd Ed. Baltimore: Lippincott Williams & Wilkins, 2004.

# URINARY TRACT OBSTRUCTION

 **BASICS**

## DEFINITION
Restricted flow of urine from the kidneys through the urinary tract to the external urethral orifice

## PATHOPHYSIOLOGY
• Excess resistance to urine flow through the urinary tract develops because of lesions affecting the excretory pathway, which cause increased pressure in the urinary space proximal to the obstruction and may cause abnormal distension of this space with urine. Ensuing pathophysiologic consequences depend on the site, degree, and duration of obstruction. Complete obstruction produces a pathophysiologic state equivalent to oliguric acute renal failure.
• Perforation of the excretory pathway with extravasation of urine is functionally equivalent.

## SYSTEMS AFFECTED
• Renal/urologic
• Gastrointestinal, cardiovascular, nervous, and respiratory systems as uremia develops

## SIGNALMENT
More common in males than females

## SIGNS

### Historical Findings
• Pollakiuria
• Intense straining and crying out when urinating
• Urine staining in the perineal area
• Urine dribbling
• Bilaterally symmetric alopecia in ferrets with adrenal disease
• Gross hematuria
• Signs of uremia develop when urinary tract obstruction is complete (or nearly complete): lethargy, dull attitude, reduced appetite, and vomiting

### Physical Examination Findings
• Excessive (i.e., overly large or turgid) or inappropriate (i.e., remains after voiding efforts), palpable distension of the urinary bladder
• Palpably enlarged prostate or urogenital cysts near the bladder; cysts may be as large as or larger than the urinary bladder.
• Uroliths may sometimes be palpated in the urinary bladder.
• Purulent preputial discharge with prostatic abscesses
• Occasionally, palpable renomegaly is discovered in an animal with chronic partial ureteral obstruction, especially when the lesion is unilateral.
• Signs of severe uremia—dehydration, weakness, hypothermia, stupor, or coma occurring terminally, tachycardia

• Signs of perforation of the excretory pathway—leakage of urine into the peritoneal cavity causes abdominal pain and distension; fever

## CAUSES

### Intraluminal Causes
• Solid or semisolid structures including uroliths, purulent exudate (with prostatic abscesses or urogenital cysts), urethral plugs, blood clots, and sloughed tissue fragments very common cause
• Most common site—the urethra

### Intramural Causes
• Urogenital cysts (common cause)
• Prostatomegaly—hyperplasia, abscesses, or neoplasia (common)
• Neoplasia of the bladder neck or urethra (uncommon)
• Fibrosis at a site of prior injury or inflammation can cause stricture or stenosis, which may impede urine flow or may be a site where intraluminal debris becomes lodged.
• Edema, hemorrhage, or spasm of muscular components can occur at sites of intraluminal (e.g., urethral) obstruction and contribute to persistent or recurrent obstruction to urinary flow after removal of the intraluminal material. Tissue changes might develop because of injury inflicted by the obstructing material, by the manipulations used to remove the obstructing material, or both.
• Ruptures, lacerations, and punctures—usually caused by traumatic incidents

## RISK FACTORS
• Hyperadrenocorticism may cause urogenital cysts, prostatic hyperplasia, or prostatic cysts.
• Feeding of dog foods may lead to the development of urolithiasis.

 **DIAGNOSIS**

## DIFFERENTIAL DIAGNOSIS
• Repeated unproductive squatting in the litter box can be misinterpreted as constipation.
• Animals whose efforts to urinate are not observed by their owners can be examined because of signs referable to uremia without a history of possible obstruction.
• Evaluation of any patient with azotemia should include consideration of possible postrenal causes (e.g., urinary obstruction).
• Ferrets with hyperadrenocorticism and secondary urogenital cysts or prostatomegaly generally have other clinical signs such as bilaterally symmetric alopecia and vulvar swelling in females.
• Once existence of urinary obstruction is recognized, diagnostic efforts focus on de-

tecting the presence and evaluating the magnitude of abnormalities secondary to obstruction, and identifying the location, cause, and completeness of the impediment(s) to urine flow.

## CBC/BIOCHEMISTRY/URINALYSIS
• Results of a hemogram are usually normal, but a stress leukogram may be seen.
• Hemogram may show nonregenerative anemia or leukocytosis due to secondary bacterial infection of cysts in ferrets with urogenital cystic disease.
• Biochemistry analysis may reveal azotemia, hyperphosphatemia, metabolic acidosis, and hyperkalemia proportional to the duration of complete obstruction.
• Alkaline urine (pH 6.5–7.0) and magnesium ammonium phosphate crystals seen in most ferrets with struvite urolithiasis
• In ferrets with adrenal disease, urogenital cysts may become secondarily infected, leading to abscess formation. Cysts/abscesses may drain into the urinary bladder or urethra, resulting in thick purulent exudate mixed with urine in the bladder. In some cases, this exudate can be thick enough to cause urethral blockage.

## OTHER LABORATORY TESTS
• Elevations in serum estradiol, androstenedione, and 17-hydroxyprogesterone are seen in ferrets with adrenal disease and associated urogenital cystic disease or prostatomegaly (available through the University of Tennessee Clinical Endocrinology Laboratory, Department of Comparative Medicine).
• Uroliths passed or retrieved should be sent for crystallographic analysis to determine their composition.

## IMAGING

### Abdominal Radiography
• Struvite uroliths are radiodense and may be detected by survey radiography.
• In ferrets with urogenital cysts, survey radiographs may reveal what appear to be two or more urinary bladders, as the cysts can be as large as or larger than the urinary bladder; contrast urocystography can be used to delineate the cyst(s).

### Abdominal Ultrasonography
Ultrasonography may be useful for demonstrating adrenal gland enlargement and large urogenital cysts.

## DIAGNOSTIC PROCEDURES
• Urinary catheterization has diagnostic and therapeutic value. As the catheter is inserted, the location and nature of obstructing material may be determined. Some or all of the obstructing material (e.g., small uroliths and urethral plugs) may be induced to pass out of the urethra distally for identification and analysis. Retrograde irrigation of the urethral lumen may propel intraluminal debris toward the bladder.

• Cytologic evaluation of specimens obtained from the urinary tract with the assistance of catheters may be diagnostic, particularly for carcinoma of the urethra or bladder and some prostatic cysts or abscesses.
• Ultrasound-guided aspiration of cystic structures; take care to avoid rupturing a prostatic abscess.

## TREATMENT

### APPROPRIATE HEALTH CARE
• Complete obstruction is a medical emergency that can be life-threatening; treatment should usually be started immediately.
• Partial obstruction—not necessarily an emergency, but these patients may be at risk for developing complete obstruction; may cause irreversible urinary tract damage if not treated promptly
• Treat as an inpatient until the patient's ability to urinate has been restored.
• Long-term management and prognosis depend on the cause of the obstruction.
• Treatment has three major components: combating the metabolic derangements associated with postrenal uremia (e.g., dehydration, hypothermia, acidosis, hyperkalemia, and azotemia); restoring and maintaining a patent pathway for urine outflow; and implementing specific treatment for the underlying cause of urine retention.

### SURGICAL CONSIDERATIONS
• If the urethra is blocked with calculi or debris and retrograde urohydropropulsion is unsuccessful, attempt anterograde flushing of the urethra via cystotomy (see nursing care, below).
• Immovable urethroliths may require urethrostomy. Ferrets have an os penis that extends from the tip of the penis to the ventral rim of the pelvis. Therefore, the urethrostomy site should be approximately 1 cm below the anus.
• Obstruction caused by urogenital cysts or prostatomegaly secondary to adrenal disease may be treated with adrenalectomy and debulking of cysts or managed medically. The decision as to which form of treatment is appropriate is multifactorial; which gland is affected (left vs. right), surgeon's experience and expertise, severity of clinical signs, age of the animal, concurrent diseases, and financial issues should be considered.
• If the cysts or prostatomegaly are not causing life-threatening urethral obstruction, medical treatment (see alternative medications, below) may cause a sufficient reduction in prostate size to alleviate clinical signs. Depending on the circumstances medical treatment may be preferred; however, medical treatment is not curative, must

be administered lifelong, and has no effect on adrenal tumor size or potential metastasis.
• Surgical removal of the affected adrenal gland(s), often coupled with intraoperative aspiration of sterile cysts or debulking of infected cysts, is generally necessary to treat large prostatic cysts causing life-threatening urethral obstruction. These procedures may require special surgical expertise, especially if the right adrenal gland is diseased.
• Large prostatic abscesses require surgical resection and/or marsupialization, require special surgical expertise, and carry a poor prognosis.
• If the bladder is full of purulent exudate, a cystotomy may be indicated to remove accumulated material.

### NURSING CARE
• Give fluid therapy to patients with dehydration or azotemia. Give fluids intravenously if systemic derangements are moderately severe or worse. Lactated Ringer's solution is the fluid of choice, except for patients with severe hyperkalemia, in which the fluid of choice is 0.45% saline and 2.5% dextrose solution with addition of sodium bicarbonate to correct acidosis.
• Relieve urethral obstruction by performing urinary catheterization. Without experience, one may find catheterization of male ferrets to be more difficult than male cats; the urethra is much smaller in diameter, the urethral opening is often difficult to visualize, and ferrets have a j-shaped os penis that extends to the tip of the penis. With practice, however, catheterization can be easily mastered. Catheterization should be performed under isoflurane anesthesia. A 3.5 Fr. red rubber catheter or a 3 Fr. ferret urethral catheter (Cook Veterinary Products) is used to flush the urethra. Both of these catheters are flexible and long enough to reach the urinary bladder. If catheterization is difficult using either of these catheters, attempt to dislodge the calculus using a 24-gauge over the needle intravenous catheter or 20- to 22-gauge jugular catheter (each with stylet removed). Administration of 1–2 mg/kg diazepam IM and infusion of 0.02–0.3 mL of 1% or 2% lidocaine locally into the urethra may aid in urethral dilation and passage of the catheter. Flush with saline as the catheter is advanced. Advance the catheter slowly and carefully, since the urethra is fragile and may easily tear. If catheterization is initially unsuccessful, decompress the bladder via cystocentesis and make a second attempt. Handle the bladder carefully and perform the cystocentesis under anesthesia or rupture may occur. Once the obstruction is cleared, suture the catheter in place using a tape butterfly. Most ferrets with indwelling urinary catheters require an Elizabethan collar.

## MEDICATIONS

### DRUG(S) OF CHOICE
• Procedures for relief of obstruction often require, or are facilitated by, giving sedatives or anesthetics. When substantial systemic derangements exist, start fluid administration and other supportive measures first. Careful decompression of the bladder by cystocentesis may be performed before anesthesia and catheterization. Calculate the dosage of sedative or anesthetic drug using the low end of the recommended range or give only to effect. Isoflurane is the anesthetic of choice.
• If bacterial cystitis is evident, begin oral administration of appropriate antibiotics, chosen on the basis of bacterial culture and antimicrobial susceptibility tests.
• If bacterial prostatitis or abscess is evident, choose antibiotics that are able to enter the prostatic lumen, such as trimethoprim/sulfonamide (15–30 mg/kg PO, SC q12h) or enrofloxacin (10–20 mg/kg PO, SC, IM q12h). A minimum of 4–6 weeks of antimicrobial administration is usually necessary.

### CONTRAINDICATIONS
Avoid intramuscular ketamine in patients with complete obstruction, because it is excreted through the kidneys. If the obstruction cannot be eliminated, prolonged sedation may result.

### PRECAUTIONS
Avoid drugs that reduce blood pressure or induce cardiac dysrhythmia until dehydration and hyperkalemia are resolved.

### POSSIBLE INTERACTIONS
N/A

### ALTERNATIVE DRUGS
• Successful treatment of prostatic hyperplasia has been anecdotally reported using leuprolide acetate, a GNRH analog. This is a potent inhibitor of gonadotropin secretion used to inhibit ovarian and testicular steroidogenesis. It is available as a 1- or 4-month depot injection, and has been anecdotally reported to alleviate the dermal and reproductive organ signs of adrenal disease in ferrets. Significant reduction in prostate size has anecdotally been reported to occur in as little as 2–3 days. Reported dosages: Lupron 30-day depot, 100–200 µg/kg IM q4w until signs resolve, then q4-8w prn, lifelong. This drug has no effect on adrenal tumor growth or metastasis. Side effects include dyspnea, lethargy, and local injection site irritation. Large prostatic cysts or abscesses are unlikely to respond.
• Flutamide (10 mg/kg q12h or q24h) inhibits androgen uptake and binding in target tissues and is used in the treatment of

# URINARY TRACT OBSTRUCTION

androgen-responsive prostatic tumors. It has been used to reduce the size of prostatic cysts or hyperplasia in ferrets with adrenal disease. This drug has no effect on adrenal tumor growth or metastasis. Side effects include gynecomastia and hepatic injury; monitor liver enzyme concentrations during therapy.

 FOLLOW-UP

## PATIENT MONITORING
• Assess urine production and hydration status frequently and adjust fluid administration rate accordingly.
• Verify ability to urinate adequately or use urinary catheterization to combat urine retention.

## POSSIBLE COMPLICATIONS
• Death
• Injury to the excretory pathway while trying to relieve obstruction
• Hypokalemia during postobstruction diuresis
• Recurrence of obstruction

 MISCELLANEOUS

## ASSOCIATED CONDITIONS
• Ferret adrenal disease
• Insulinoma
• Bacterial cystitis

## AGE-RELATED FACTORS
N/A

## ZOONOTIC POTENTIAL
N/A

## PREGNANCY
N/A

## SYNONYMS
Urethral obstruction

## SEE ALSO
• Adrenal disease
• Prostatomegaly
• Urogenital cystic disease
• Urolithiasis

## ABBREVIATION
GNRH = gonadotropin-releasing hormone

*Suggested Reading*

Antinoff N. Urinary disorders in ferrets. Semin Avian Exotic Pet Med 1998;7(2):89–92.
Beeber NL. Abdominal surgery in ferrets. Vet Clin North Am Exot Anim Pract 2000;3(3):647–662.
Fox JG, Pearson RC, Bell JA. Diseases of the genitourinary system. In: Fox JG, ed. Biology and Diseases of the Ferret. 2nd Ed. Baltimore: Williams & Wilkins, 1998.
Hillyer EV. Urogenital diseases. In: Hillyer EV, Quesenberry KE, eds. Ferrets, Rabbits and Rodents: Clinical Medicine and Surgery. Philadelphia: WB Saunders, 1997.
Li X, Fox JG, Erdman SE, et al. Cystic urogenital anomalies in ferrets (Mustela putorius furo). Vet Pathol 1996;33:150–158.
Marini RP, Esteves MI, Fox JG. A technique for catheterization of the urinary bladder in the ferret. Lab Anim 1994;28:155–157.
Palmore WP, Bartos KD. Food intake and struvite crystalluria in ferrets. Vet Res Commun 1987;11:519–526.
Quesenberry KE, Rosenthal KL. Endocrine disease. In: Hillyer EV, Quesenberry KE, eds. Ferrets, Rabbits and Rodents: Clinical Medicine and Surgery. Philadelphia: WB Saunders, 1997.
Weiss CA, Scott MV. Clinical aspects and surgical treatment of hyperadrenocorticism in the domestic ferret: 94 cases (1994–1996). J Am Anim Hosp Assoc 1997;33:487–493.
Wheeler J, Bennet RA. Ferret abdominal surgical procedures. Part I. Adrenal gland and pancreatic beta-cell tumors. Compend Contin Educ Pract Vet 1999;21(9):815–822.

*Portions Adapted From*

Lees GE. Urinary Tract Obstruction. In: Tilley LP, Smith FWK, Jr., eds. The 5-Minute Veterinary Consult: Canine and Feline, 3rd Ed. Baltimore: Lippincott Williams & Wilkins, 2003.

# UROGENITAL CYSTIC DISEASE (PARAURETHRAL CYSTS)

## BASICS

### DEFINITION
Cystic structures found on the dorsal aspect of the urinary bladder or surrounding the proximal urethra in male and (rarely) female ferrets. These structures likely arise from remnants of the mesonephric or para-mesonephric ducts, from the prostate, or from paraprostatic tissues. Cysts are usually large, may be single or multiple, and often cause partial or complete obstruction of the urethra. Secondary bacterial infections within the cystic fluid are extremely common.

### PATHOPHYSIOLOGY
• Urogenital cysts are associated with ferret adrenal disease and the resultant excessive production of androgens. Excessive sex steroid production is believed to cause hyperplasia of mesonephric or para-mesonephric ductal tissue remnants in both sexes and prostatic or paraprostatic tissues in males.
• True prostatic cysts secondary to inflammation or neoplasia are rare.
• Severe secondary bacterial infections may occur and cause chronic abscesses or prostatitis.
• Obstruction of the urethra often occurs due to extraluminal compression by the cyst or hyperplastic tissue or, with bacterial infection, may become obstructed by thick, tenacious exudate in the urine.

### SYSTEMS AFFECTED
• Urinary—obstruction of the urethra, secondary bacterial cystitis
• Gastrointestinal—ferrets with large urogenital cysts may have tenesmus.
• Peritoneum—focal or generalized peritonitis can develop in animals with bacterial infection of cystic fluid or abscesses.

### Genetics
Unknown; however, genetics may play a role in the development of ferret adrenal disease.

### INCIDENCE/PREVALENCE
• Urogenital cystic disease is a common cause of dysuria in ferrets.
• This disease is seen more commonly in the spring, but may occur any time of the year.

### GEOGRAPHIC DISTRIBUTION
Urogenital cystic disease and ferret adrenal disease is seen more commonly in ferrets in North America as compared to those in Europe. This may be due to genetics, early neutering practices, or differing husbandry practices.

### SIGNALMENT

#### Predominant Sex
Seen primarily in neutered males; female ferrets may be affected (enlargement of peri-urethral tissues), although quite rare.

#### Mean Age and Range
Middle-aged animals, 3–7 years old

### SIGNS

#### Historical and Physical Examination Findings
• Presenting complaint is typically stranguria due to urethral obstruction by cysts, hyperplastic prostatic tissue, or thick exudate blocking the urethra.
• Pollakiuria, tenesmus, and dysuria, including intense straining and crying out when urinating
• With complete obstruction, ferrets will have signs of uremia, including depression, lethargy, and anorexia.
• Weight loss, depression, and anorexia may be seen with secondary bacterial infections (abscesses).
• Purulent preputial discharge with abscesses
• Bilaterally symmetric alopecia or pruritus due to adrenal disease
• Abdominal distension
• Firm mass near bladder; may contain multiple cysts of varying size
• Fluid-filled cysts are often palpable and may be larger than the urinary bladder.

### CAUSES
• Excessive estrogen or androgen production due to functional adrenal hyperplasia, adenoma, or carcinomas
• Rarely, prostatic cysts are secondary to prostatic neoplasia.

### RISK FACTORS
Evidence suggests that ferret adrenal disease and subsequent urogenital cysts may be related to neutering at an early age.

## DIAGNOSIS

### DIFFERENTIAL DIAGNOSIS
• For stranguria—urolithiasis, neoplasia of the bladder neck or urethra, or urethral stricture
• For mass detected in area of prostate—prostatic hyperplasia, prostatic neoplasia, or other abdominal mass: neoplasia, abscess, or granuloma
• Radiography and results of cytologic examination of fluid and ultrasonographic examination usually rule out these diseases. Many cysts become secondarily infected.

### CBC/BIOCHEMISTRY/URINALYSIS
• Usually normal
• Hemogram may show nonregenerative anemia or leukocytosis due to secondary bacterial infection of cysts.
• Hypoglycemia may be present—usually due to concurrent insulinoma
• Urinalysis may support a diagnosis of urolithiasis (usually struvite) or bacterial cystitis. Secondary bacterial infections leading to abscess formation in many prostatic or paraprostatic cysts may drain into the urinary bladder or urethra, resulting in thick purulent exudate mixed with urine in the bladder. In some cases, this exudate can be thick enough to cause urethral blockage.

### OTHER LABORATORY TESTS
• Elevations in plasma estradiol, androstenedione, and 17-hydroxyprogesterone combined are most diagnostic (available through the University of Tennessee Clinical Endocrinology Laboratory, Department of Comparative Medicine).
• Elevation in plasma estrogens alone in males is diagnostic of adrenal gland disease.
• Examination of cyst fluid—gross appearance can range from clear yellow (rarely) or, more commonly, thick, greenish, foul-smelling fluid; cytologic examination ranges from serosanguinous fluid (rarely) to purulent exudate (most common).
• Culture the fluid for bacteria.

### IMAGING
• Survey radiographs may reveal soft tissue density in the area of the prostate.
• Radiographs may demonstrate what appear to be two or more urinary bladders, as the cysts can be as large as or larger than the urinary bladder.
• Contrast urocystography can be used to delineate the cyst(s). Initially, both the cyst and urinary bladder will fill with contrast medium. After urinating, the cyst will retain the contrast media.
• Ultrasonography may be useful for demonstrating adrenal gland enlargement and urogenital cysts.

### OTHER DIAGNOSTIC PROCEDURES
Ultrasound-guided aspiration of cystic structures; take care to avoid rupturing a prostatic abscess.

### PATHOLOGIC FINDINGS
• Gross examination reveals single or multiple cysts—may be bi- or multilobulated
• Histologic examination—cyst walls usually consist of three layers: epithelium, muscle, and serosa lined with squamous epithelial cells. Areas of multifocal ulceration and necrosis are common, as is infiltration by inflammatory cells.

# UROGENITAL CYSTIC DISEASE (PARAURETHRAL CYSTS)

• Adrenal disease is always present—gross enlargement with irregular surface or discoloration of the affected gland, cysts, or differences in texture within the affected gland. Histologically, see adrenal hyperplasia, adenomas, or adenocarcinomas.

## TREATMENT

### APPROPRIATE HEALTH CARE
• Ferret adrenal disease and secondary urogenital cysts may be treated with adrenalectomy or managed medically. The decision as to which form of treatment is appropriate is multifactorial; which gland is affected (left vs. right), surgeon's experience and expertise, severity of clinical signs, age of the animal, concurrent diseases, and financial issues should be considered.
• If the prostatomegaly is not causing life-threatening urethral obstruction, medical treatment (see alternative medications, below) may cause a sufficient reduction in prostate size to alleviate clinical signs. Depending on the circumstances, medical treatment may be preferred; however, medical treatment is not curative, must be administered lifelong, and has no effect on adrenal tumor size or potential metastasis.
• Surgical removal of the affected adrenal gland(s), often coupled with intraoperative aspiration of sterile cysts or debulking of infected cysts, is generally necessary to treat large prostatic cysts causing life-threatening urethral obstruction. These procedures may require special surgical expertise, especially if the right adrenal gland is diseased.
• If the urethra is partially or completely obstructed, hospitalization is necessary for urethral catheterization (see below).

### NURSING CARE
• Fluid therapy, either subcutaneous or intravenous depending on the state of hydration. Ferrets that are uremic require intravenous fluid therapy. Correct any acid-base disturbances as indicated by the serum biochemistry profile.
• Postoperative fluid therapy should continue for 24–48 hours.
• If the urethra is partially or completely obstructed, catheterize prior to surgery. Without experience, one may find catheterization of male ferrets to be more difficult than male cats; the urethra is smaller in diameter, the urethral opening can be difficult to visualize, and ferrets have a j-shaped os penis that extends to the tip of the penis. With practice, however, catheterization can be easily mastered. Catheterization should be performed under isoflurane anesthesia. A 3.5 Fr. red rubber catheter or a 3 Fr. ferret urethral catheter (Cook Veterinary Prod-

ucts) is used to flush the urethra. Both of these catheters are flexible and long enough to reach the urinary bladder. Administration of 1–2 mg/kg diazepam IM and infusion of 0.02–0.3 mL of 1% or 2% lidocaine locally into the urethra may aid in urethral dilation and passage of the catheter. Flush with saline as the catheter is advanced. Advance the catheter slowly and carefully, since the urethra is fragile and may easily tear. If catheterization is initially unsuccessful, decompress the bladder via cystocentesis and make a second attempt. Handle the bladder carefully and perform the cystocentesis under anesthesia or rupture may occur. Once the catheter reaches the urinary bladder, suture the catheter in place using a tape butterfly. Maintain urinary catheter in place for 1–3 days postoperatively. Ferrets with indwelling urinary catheters often require an Elizabethan collar.

### ACTIVITY
Activity should be limited postoperatively.

### DIET
No dietary changes are necessary.

### CLIENT EDUCATION
• Removal of the affected adrenal gland(s) and drainage of the cysts at the time of surgery is often curative in ferrets with mild prostatomegaly, sterile cysts, or small abscessed cyst.
• Large or multiple cysts that are abscessed or infection with resistant bacterial pathogens may require prolonged treatment; prognosis is poorer for complete resolution as compared to sterile cysts.

### SURGICAL CONSIDERATIONS
• Surgical removal of the affected adrenal gland(s) will cause a significant reduction in the size of hypertrophied paraurethral or prostatic tissue, usually within a few days.
• Surgical removal of the affected adrenal gland(s) is often coupled with intraoperative aspiration of sterile cysts or debulking of infected cysts. These procedures require special surgical expertise, especially if the right adrenal gland is diseased. Proximity of the right adrenal gland to the vena cava and the potential for vena cava invasion by malignant tumors make complete excision a high-risk procedure. Referral to a surgeon or clinician with experience is recommended when possible.
• Several techniques for adrenalectomy have been advocated, and problems may be associated with each surgical option, depending on the surgeon's expertise. Refer to suggested reading list for more detailed descriptions of surgical procedures.
• Many practitioners advocate debulking rather than removal of the right adrenal as a procedure carrying less risk of life-threaten-

ing complications. If this method is chosen, signs of clinical disease will return, necessitating repeat surgery or medical therapy alone.
• Sterile cysts may be drained intraoperatively, using needle aspiration. Submit aspirated fluid for bacterial culture and susceptibility testing. For large, sterile cysts, it may be necessary to create an incision into the cyst wall and to suture omentum into the incision to absorb any fluid produced postoperatively.
• Resect or drain as many prostatic abscesses as possible; pack off the cystic tissue prior to draining/debriding and flush abdomen well. Large abscesses may require marsupialization and carry a poorer prognosis.
• Some ferrets may develop peritonitis following surgery for abscesses, requiring longer-term medical management.
• If the bladder is full of purulent exudate, a cystotomy may be indicated to remove accumulated material.

## MEDICATIONS

### DRUG(S) OF CHOICE
Medical treatment of adrenal disease:
• Successful treatment of prostatic hyperplasia has been anecdotally reported using leuprolide acetate, a GNRH analog. This is a potent inhibitor of gonadotropin secretion used to inhibit ovarian and testicular steroidogenesis. It has been anecdotally reported to alleviate the dermal and reproductive organ signs of adrenal disease in ferrets. Significant reduction in prostate size has anecdotally been reported to occur in as little as 2–3 days. Reported dosages: Lupron 30-day depot, 100–200 µg/kg IM q4w until signs resolve, then q4–8w prn, lifelong. This drug has no effect on adrenal tumor growth or metastasis. Side effects include dyspnea, lethargy, and local injection site irritation. Large prostatic cysts or abscesses are unlikely to respond.
If surgical treatment is opted:
• If a combination of left and subtotal right adrenalectomy is performed, administer prednisone 0.25–0.5 mg/kg PO q12h for 1 week, then gradually tapering the dose over 1–2 weeks.
• If bilateral adrenalectomy is performed, long-term treatment with glucocorticoids is often necessary. The dosage is titrated to the individual patient and tapered to the lowest dosage interval necessary to prevent clinical signs of hypoadrenocorticism. Many ferrets have accessory adrenal tissue, and some may be weaned from exogenous steroids completely if carefully monitored. However, some ferrets do become critically ill due to

# UROGENITAL CYSTIC DISEASE (PARAURETHRAL CYSTS)

hypoadrenocorticism even with prednisone supplementation, and treatment with mineralocorticoid may also be required. Treatment is initiated based on clinical signs and electrolyte status (signs typically occur within days to weeks postoperatively). Dosages have been extrapolated from feline dose; 0.05–0.1 mg/kg Florinef (fludrocortisone acetate) PO q24h or divided q12h.
• If secondary bacterial infection or abscess is evident, antibiotic therapy should be based on results of culture and susceptibility testing. Choose antibiotics that are able to enter the prostatic lumen, such as trimethoprim/sulfonamide (15–30 mg/kg PO, SC q12h), enrofloxacin (10–20 mg/kg PO, SC, IM q12h), or chloramphenicol (50 mg/kg PO, SC q12h). A minimum of 4–6 weeks of antimicrobial administration is usually necessary.

## CONTRAINDICATIONS
N/A

## PRECAUTIONS
N/A

## ALTERNATIVE DRUGS
Flutamide (10 mg/kg PO q12h) inhibits androgen uptake and binding in target tissues and is used in the treatment of androgen-responsive prostatic tumors in humans. It has been used to reduce the size of prostatic tissue and treat alopecia in ferrets with adrenal disease. This drug has no effect on adrenal tumor growth or metastasis. Side effects may include gynomastia and hepatic injury; monitor liver enzyme concentrations during therapy.

## FOLLOW-UP

### PATIENT MONITORING
• With surgical therapy, a reduction in cyst size may be seen in as little as 2–3 days, relieving urethral obstruction.
• Response to therapy is evident by remission of clinical signs, particularly hair regrowth and reduction in the size of paraurethral cysts.
• Following unilateral adrenalectomy or subtotal adrenalectomy, monitor for return of clinical signs since tumor recurrence is common. Clinical signs typically develop 1 year postoperatively.

• In ferrets with bilateral adrenalectomy, monitor for the development of Addison's disease.
• Ultrasonographic examination at 2- to 4-week intervals after adrenalectomy may be used to follow resolution of cysts.
• With medical therapy, reduction in prostate size may gradually occur over a period of weeks to months.

### PREVENTION/AVOIDANCE
Neutering at an older age may decrease the incidence of disease.

### POSSIBLE COMPLICATIONS
• Peritonitis
• Recurrence of cysts if all hyperfunctioning adrenal tissue is not removed
• Rupture of the bladder

### EXPECTED COURSE/PROGNOSIS
• Sterile cysts—following adrenalectomy, prostatic tissue should decrease in size within 1–3 days. If urethral obstruction persists, a second adrenal tumor may be present.
• Medical therapy has shown promising results in reducing the size of prostatic tissue in ferrets with adrenal disease. Anecdotal reports suggest that significant reduction in size may occur in as little as 2–3 days. Insufficient data exists to predict the outcome of long-term therapy.
• The prognosis is poor when large prostatic abscesses are found, because complete removal is difficult and the response to antibiotic therapy is variable.

## MISCELLANEOUS

### ASSOCIATED CONDITIONS
• Ferret adrenal disease—always
• Insulinomas
• Splenomegaly
• Lymphoma

### AGE-RELATED FACTORS
N/A

### ZOONOTIC POTENTIAL
N/A

### PREGNANCY
N/A

## SYNONYMS
• Paraurethral cysts
• Paraprostatic cysts
• Prostatic cysts

## SEE ALSO
• Adrenal disease
• Prostatitis and prostatic abscesses
• Prostatomegaly

## ABBREVIATION
GNRH = gonadotropin-releasing hormone

*Suggested Reading*
Antinoff N. Urinary disorders in ferrets. Semin Avian Exotic Pet Med 1998;7(2):89–92.
Beeber NL. Abdominal surgery in ferrets. Vet Clin North Am Exot Anim Pract 2000;3(3):647–662.
Brown SA. Neoplasia. In: Hillyer EV, Quesenberry KE, eds. Ferrets, Rabbits and Rodents: Clinical Medicine and Surgery. Philadelphia: WB Saunders, 1997:99.
Fox JG, Marini RP. Diseases of the endocrine system. In: Fox JG, ed. Biology and Diseases of the Ferret. 2nd Ed. Baltimore: Williams & Wilkins, 1998.
Hillyer EV. Urogenital diseases. In: Hillyer EV, Quesenberry KE, eds. Ferrets, Rabbits and Rodents: Clinical Medicine and Surgery. Philadelphia: WB Saunders, 1997:44–52.
Li X, Fox JG, Erdman SE, et al. Cystic urogenital anomalies in ferrets (Mustela putorius furo). 1996;Vet Pathol 1996;33:150–158.
Marini RP, Esteves MI, Fox JG. A technique for catheterization of the urinary bladder in the ferret. Lab Anim 1994;28:155–157.
Quesenberry KE, Rosenthal KL. Endocrine disease. In: Hillyer EV, Quesenberry KE, eds. Ferrets, Rabbits and Rodents: Clinical Medicine and Surgery. Philadelphia: WB Saunders, 1997
Weiss CA, Scott MV. Clinical aspects and surgical treatment of hyperadrenocorticism in the domestic ferret: 94 cases (1994–1996). J Am Anim Hosp Assoc 1997;33:487–493.
Wheeler J, Bennet RA. Ferret abdominal surgical procedures. Part I. Adrenal gland and pancreatic beta-cell tumors. Compend Contin Educ Pract Vet 1999;21(9):815–822.

# UROLITHIASIS

## BASICS

### DEFINITION
Formation of polycrystalline concretions (i.e., uroliths, calculi, or stones), usually composed of MAP, or struvite, in the urinary tract

### PATHOPHYSIOLOGY

#### Sterile Struvite
• Occurs more commonly than infection-induced struvite. Dietary or metabolic factors may be involved in the genesis of sterile struvite, as calculi are seen in ferrets fed diets containing plant-based proteins or dog foods and poor-quality cat foods containing insufficient dietary protein.
• Ferrets fed a diet containing plant-based protein (especially corn) will produce alkaline urine (pH of 6.5–7), whereas ferrets fed a high-quality animal-based protein diet will produce a more acidic urine (pH near 6). The formation of MAP crystals occurs when the urine pH is above 6.4.
• In addition to urinary pH, the specific type of protein fed appears to affect crystal formation. Research has demonstrated that ferrets with urinary pH of 6–7 were less likely to form struvite uroliths when fed animal based proteins as compared to ferrets with the same urinary pH but fed diets with corn-based proteins.
• Microbial urease is not involved in formation of sterile struvite uroliths.

#### Infection-Induced Struvite
• Urine must be supersaturated with MAP for struvite uroliths to form. MAP supersaturation of urine may be associated with several factors, including urinary tract infections with urease-producing microbes, alkaline urine, diet, and possibly a genetic predisposition.
• Urinary tract infections caused by urease-producing microbes (especially species of *Staphylococcus* or *Proteus* spp.) and urine containing sufficient urea favors the formation of struvite uroliths.
• Consumption of plant-based dietary protein results in alkaluria, which favors stone formation.
• Metabolic and anatomic abnormalities may indirectly induce struvite uroliths by predisposing to urinary tract infections.

#### Uroliths of Other Mineral Composition
Anecdotal reports exist of urolithiasis due to cysteine; however, the pathophysiology is unknown.

### SYSTEMS AFFECTED
Renal/urologic

### GENETICS
Unknown

### INCIDENCE/PREVALENCE
• The incidence of struvite urolithiasis is declining since most ferret owners have become aware of the need to feed appropriate diets. In one study struvite uroliths were found in 14% of necropsies performed on ferrets fed dog foods.
• Stranguria in male ferrets is more likely to be caused by prostatomegaly or urogenital cysts than by uroliths.

### GEOGRAPHIC DISTRIBUTION
Ubiquitous

### SIGNALMENT

#### Species or Breed Predilections
N/A

#### Mean Age and Range
• Most common in middle-aged to older ferrets, 3–7 years of age
• Most uroliths in younger ferrets are infection- induced struvite.

#### Predominant Sex
Urethral obstruction is more common in males, but can occur in females. Bacterial cystitis is more common in females.

### SIGNS

#### General Comments
Signs depend on location, size, and number of uroliths.

#### Historical Findings
• Typical signs of urocystoliths include pollakiuria, dysuria, hematuria, urine straining in the perineal area, and urine dribbling.
• Typical signs of urethroliths include pollakiuria and dysuria, including intense straining and crying out when urinating. With complete obstruction, ferrets will have signs of uremia, including depression, lethargy, and anorexia.
• Nephroliths are rare but may be associated with signs of renal insufficiency. Obstruction to urine outflow with bacterial urinary tract infection may result in generalized pyelonephritis and septicemia.

#### Physical Examination Findings
• Uroliths may sometimes be palpated in the urinary bladder.
• Obstruction of the urethra may cause enlargement of the urinary bladder.
• Obstruction of a ureter may cause enlargement of the associated kidney.
• Complete urine outflow obstruction—depression, dehydration, lethargy, or coma
• Complete urine outflow obstruction combined with bacterial infection may cause ascending urinary tract infection, signs of renal failure, and signs of septicemia.

### CAUSES
• Alkaline urine decreases the solubility of struvite, resulting in formation of calculi.
• Urinary tract disorders that predispose to infections with urease-producing bacteria

### RISK FACTORS
• Feeding dog foods, poor-quality cat foods, or diets with plant-based proteins
• Abnormal retention of urine

## DIAGNOSIS

### DIFFERENTIAL DIAGNOSIS
• Uroliths mimic other causes of pollakiuria, dysuria, hematuria, and/or outflow obstruction, the most common of which is urogenital cystic disease (paraurethral cysts).
• Ferrets with urogenital cysts usually have other signs of adrenal disease, especially bilaterally symmetric alopecia.
• Differentiate from other causes by urinalysis, urine culture, radiography, and ultrasonography.

### CBC/BIOCHEMISTRY/URINALYSIS
• Complete urinary outflow obstruction can cause postrenal azotemia (e.g., high BUN, creatinine, and phosphorus).
• Pyuria (normal value 0–1 WBC/hpf), hematuria (normal value 0–3 RBC/hpf), and proteinuria (normal value 0–33 mg/dL) indicate urinary tract inflammation, but these are nonspecific findings that may result from infectious and noninfectious causes of lower urinary tract disease.
• Some urogenital or periprostatic cysts may become secondarily infected, forming abscesses that drain into the urinary bladder or urethra. Thick, purulent exudate from theses abscesses may mix with urine in the bladder, resulting in significant pyuria and bacteriuria. In some cases, this exudate can be thick enough to cause urethral blockage.
• Identification of bacteria in urine sediment suggests that urinary tract infection is causing or complicating lower urinary tract disease or may be seen in ferrets with abscessed urogenital cysts. If small numbers of bacteria are seen, consider contamination of urine during collection and storage when interpreting urinalysis results.
• Alkaline urine (pH 6.5–7) seen in most ferrets with struvite urolithiasis
• Magnesium ammonium phosphate crystals typically appear as colorless, orthorhombic (having three unequal axes intersecting at right angles), coffinlike prisms. They may have three to six or more sides and often have oblique ends.

## OTHER LABORATORY TESTS

• Quantitative bacterial culture of urine, preferably collected by cystocentesis
• Bacterial culture of inner portions of infection-induced struvite uroliths
• Quantitative mineral analysis of uroliths retrieved via cystotomy

## IMAGING

• Struvite uroliths are radiodense and may be detected by survey radiography.
• Ultrasonography—can detect uroliths, but provides no information about their density or shape. Ultrasonography is useful to rule out other causes of stranguria, such as paraurethral cysts or masses within the urinary bladder.

## DIAGNOSTIC PROCEDURES

N/A

## PATHOLOGIC FINDINGS

N/A

# TREATMENT

## APPROPRIATE HEALTH CARE

Retrograde urohydropropulsion to eliminate urethral stones and/or surgery require hospitalization.

## NURSING CARE

• Fluid therapy, either subcutaneous or intravenous depending on the state of hydration. Ferrets that are uremic require intravenous fluid therapy. Correct any acid-base disturbances as indicated by the serum biochemistry profile.
• Postoperative fluid therapy should continue for 34–48 hours.
• Attempt retrograde urohydropropulsion in ferrets with urethral calculi or plugs. Without experience, one may find catheterization of male ferrets to be more difficult than male cats; the urethra is much smaller in diameter, the urethral opening is often difficult to visualize, and ferrets have a j-shaped os penis that extends to the tip of the penis. With practice, however, catheterization can be easily mastered. Catheterization should be performed under isoflurane anesthesia. A 3.5 Fr. red rubber catheter or a 3 Fr. ferret urethral catheter (Cook Veterinary Products) is used to flush the urethra. Both of these catheters are flexible and long enough to reach the urinary bladder. If catheterization is difficult using either of these catheters, attempt to dislodge the calculus using a 24-gauge over the needle intravenous catheter or 20- to 22-gauge jugular catheter (each with stylet removed). Administration of 1–2 mg/kg diazepam IM and infusion of 0.02–0.3 mL of 1% or 2% lidocaine locally into the urethra may aid in

urethral dilation and passage of the catheter. Flush with saline as the catheter is advanced. Advance the catheter slowly and carefully, since the urethra is fragile and may easily tear. If catheterization is initially unsuccessful, decompress the bladder via cystocentesis and make a second attempt. Handle the bladder carefully and perform the cystocentesis under anesthesia or rupture may occur. Once the obstruction is cleared, suture the catheter in place using a tape butterfly. Most ferrets with indwelling urinary catheters require an Elizabethan collar.

## ACTIVITY

Activity should be limited postoperatively.

## DIET

• Place affected ferrets on a high-quality cat or ferret food. Feeding of this diet will usually prevent recurrence of calculi. Dietary acidifying agents are not necessary since this diet will produce acidic urine.
• Calculolytic diet (Prescription Diet Canine s/d; Hills Pet Nutrition) are not palatable and are poorly accepted by ferrets. Successful dissolution is sometimes possible, but these diets do not contain sufficient protein for long-term use.

## CLIENT EDUCATION

Feeding of high-quality ferret or cat foods will usually prevent recurrence.

## SURGICAL CONSIDERATIONS

• If the urethra is blocked and retrograde urohydropropulsion is unsuccessful, attempt anterograde flushing of the urethra via cystotomy.
• Immovable urethroliths may require urethrostomy. Ferrets have an os penis that extends from the tip of the penis to the ventral rim of the pelvis. Therefore, the urethrostomy site should be approximately 1 cm below the anus.
• Calculi located within the bladder should be removed via cystotomy. This procedure is similar to that performed on cats.

# MEDICATIONS

## DRUG(S) OF CHOICE

If bacterial cystitis is evident, begin oral administration of appropriate antibiotics, chosen on the basis of bacterial culture and antimicrobial susceptibility tests.

## CONTRAINDICATIONS

N/A

## PRECAUTIONS

N/A

## ALTERNATIVE DRUGS

N/A

# FOLLOW-UP

## PATIENT MONITORING

Monitor for licking and chewing at incision site; Elizabethan collars may be often necessary.

## PREVENTION/AVOIDANCE

• Infection-induced struvite urolithiasis may be prevented by eradicating and controlling infections by urease-producing bacteria.
• Recurrent sterile struvite uroliths may be prevented by feeding a high-quality ferret or cat food.

## POSSIBLE COMPLICATIONS

• Rupture of the bladder
• Urethral tear
• Pyelonephritis and septicemia with urethral obstruction and bacterial cystitis
• Recurrence of uroliths if diet is not improved

## EXPECTED COURSE AND PROGNOSIS

• Following surgical removal and appropriate antimicrobial therapy, calculi within the bladder are unlikely to recur.
• Treatment of urethroliths carries a good to guarded prognosis. If urohydropropulsion via urethral catheterization is successful in removing the obstruction, the prognosis is good. Urohydropropulsion via urethral catheterization can sometimes be difficult to successfully perform, and emergency procedures such as cystotomy for anterograde urohydropropulsion or perineal urethrostomy may be necessary to relieve the obstruction. Complications such as bladder or urethral rupture may occur.
• Nephroliths are usually asymptomatic if the ureters remain unobstructed and often respond to dietary changes alone.

# MISCELLANEOUS

## ASSOCIATED CONDITIONS

Any disease that predisposes to bacterial urinary tract infection

## AGE-RELATED FACTORS

Infection-induced struvite is the most common form of urolith in younger ferrets.

## ZOONOTIC POTENTIAL

None

## PREGNANCY

In pregnant jills close to parturition, a caesarean section should be performed at the same time as cystotomy to prevent straining and dehiscence during parturition.

# UROLITHIASIS

## SYNONYMS
- Phosphate calculi
- Triple-phosphate stones

## SEE ALSO
- Adrenal disease
- Lower urinary tract infection
- Prostatomegaly
- Urogenital cysts

## ABBREVIATIONS
- BUN = blood urea nitrogen
- MAP = magnesium ammonium phosphate
- RBC = red blood cell
- WBC = white blood cell

*Suggested Reading*

Antinoff N. Urinary disorders in ferrets. Semin Avian Exotic Pet Med 1998;7(2):89–92.

Bell JA. Ferret nutrition. Vet Clin North Am Exoti Anim Pract 1999;2(1):169–192.

Fox JG, Pearson RC, Bell JA. Diseases of the genitourinary system. In: Fox JG, ed. Biology and Diseases of the Ferret. 2nd Ed. Baltimore: Williams & Wilkins, 1998.

Hoefer HL. Rabbit and ferret renal disease diagnosis. In: Fudge AM, ed. Laboratory Medicine, Avian and Exotic Pets. Philadelphia: WB Saunders, 2000.

Li X, Fox JG, Erdman SE, et al. Cystic urogenital anomalies in ferrets (Mustela putorius furo). Vet Pathol 1996;33:150–158.

Marini RP, Esteves MI, Fox JG. A technique for catheterization of the urinary bladder in the ferret. Lab Anim 1994;28:155–157.

Palmore WP, Bartos KD. Food intake and struvite crystalluria in ferrets. Vet Res Commun 1987;11:519–526.

Wheeler J, Bennett RA. Ferret abdominal surgical procedures. Part II. Gastrointestinal foreign bodies, splenomegaly, liver biopsy, cystotomy and ovariohysterectomy. Compend Contin Edu Pract Vet 1999;21(11):1049–1057.

*Portions Adapted From*

Osborne CA, Lulich JP, Pozlin DJ. Uroliths, Struvite—Dogs. In: Tilley LP, Smith FWK, Jr., eds. The 5-Minute Veterinary Consult: Canine and Feline, 3rd Ed. Baltimore: Lippincott Williams & Wilkins, 2003.

# BASICS

## DEFINITION
Any substance emanating from the vulvar labia

## PATHOPHYSIOLOGY
May originate from several distinct sources, depending in part on the age and reproductive status of the patient or presence of underlying diseases (e.g., adrenal disease); from urinary tract, uterus, vagina or perivulvar skin; may be normal or abnormal

## SYSTEMS AFFECTED
- Reproductive
- Endocrine
- Renal/urologic
- Skin/exocrine

## SIGNALMENT
- Estrual and postpartum females—bloody discharge not normally visible with estrus; postpartum discharge may be normal.
- Postestrual, pregnant, and postpartum or spayed females—may be more serious

## SIGNS

### Historical Findings
- Sexually mature females (>8–12 months old)
- Swollen vulva
- Bilaterally symmetric alopecia
- Attracting males
- Parturition—with postpartum discharge
- Recent estrus—with pyometra or vaginitis

### Physical Examination Findings
- Discharge may appear serosanguinous, sanguinous, clear, mucoid, or purulent.
- Alopecia
- Swollen vulva
- Pruritus

## CAUSES

### Serosanguineous
- Urinary tract infection
- Foreign body
- Vaginal neoplasia
- Vaginal trauma
- Fetal death
- Vaginal hematoma

### Purulent Exudate
- Primary vaginitis
- Secondary vaginitis—from foreign body, urinary tract infection, vaginal neoplasia, and fetal death
- Pyometra or stump pyometra
- Embryonic and fetal death
- Postpartum metritis
- Perivulvar dermatitis

### Other
Acquired perivulvar dermatitis can also be mistaken for vaginal discharge.

## RISK FACTORS
- Adrenal disease—may predispose to vaginitis or stump pyometra
- Prolonged estrus in unbred females—hyperestrogenism predisposes patient to pyometra.
- Small litter size—litters of <3 kits may be insufficient to stimulate parturition, resulting in fetal death.

# DIAGNOSIS

## DIFFERENTIAL DIAGNOSES
- History and signalment—establish hormonal influences (e.g., prolonged estrus, adrenal disease, pregnancy, and parturition).
- Source and type of the discharge—must be identified by appropriate diagnostics
- Rule out adrenal disease—usually seen in ferrets >2 years of age and associated with bilaterally symmetric alopecia. Secretion of sex steroids may cause vulvar swelling, discharge, vaginitis, pyometra, or stump pyometra.
- Rule out hyperestrogenism—in unbred females remaining in estrus for >1 month: may cause vaginitis, pyometra, or bleeding disorders due to the toxic effects of estrogen on bone marrow
- Rule out ovarian remnant in spayed females—may also cause estrogen toxicity; may predispose patient to vaginitis or stump pyometra

## CBC/BIOCHEMISTRY/URINALYSIS
- Nonregenerative anemia, pancytopenia—in ferrets with hyperestrogenism
- Leukocytosis with a left shift—with pyometra or metritis
- High BUN and creatinine—with pyometra
- Urinary tract infection—may be noted

## OTHER LABORATORY TESTS
- Examination of vaginal cytology may reveal numerous cornified cells or purulent exudate in ferrets with pyometra.
- Elevations in serum estradiol, androstenedione, and 17-hydroxyprogesterone to diagnose adrenal disease as underlying cause of discharge (available through the University of Tennessee Clinical Endocrinology Laboratory, Department of Comparative Medicine)
- High serum estrogen (estradiol) concentration to help confirm hyperestrogenism

## IMAGING
- Radiography—detect a large uterus in patients with pyometra or later stages of fetal death
- Ultrasonography—determine pregnancy as early as 12 days postbreeding; may be used to detect pyometra or stump pyometra or to identify affected adrenal gland in ferrets with adrenal disease

## DIAGNOSTIC PROCEDURES
- hCG challenge test in spayed females with swollen vulva, to differentiate ovarian remnant from adrenal disease; 100 IU of hCG IM once at least 2 weeks following onset of vulvar swelling. If swelling subsides 3–4 days postinjection, an ovarian remnant is most likely. Some ovarian remnants do not respond to a single injection of hCG, requiring a second injection 2 weeks later. If the vulva remains swollen, adrenal disease is most likely the cause.
- Vaginal bacterial culture—via guarded culturette; perform before doing any other vaginal procedure.
- Vaginal cytologic examination—determine if the discharge is sanguinous, serosanguineous, or purulent; extent of cornification helps establish whether the jill is in proestrus or estrus.
- Cystocentesis and bacterial culture—help rule out urinary tract infection
- Biopsy of vaginal mass—rule out neoplasia

# TREATMENT
- Outpatient, unless pyometra or hyperestrogenism
- Hospitalization is required for ferrets exhibiting clinical signs related to anemia or hemorrhage due to hyperestrogenism or for pyometra patients exhibiting anorexia, dehydration, or weakness. Supportive care, such as fluid therapy, warmth, and adequate nutrition are required for recovery in these patients.
- Blood transfusions may be required in patients with pancytopenia due to hyperestrogenism.
- Ovariohysterectomy is the treatment of choice in patients with pyometra or hyperestrogenism. This is a relatively safe procedure in ferrets with PCV >30 and no evidence of bleeding disorders. Ferrets with PCV <30 usually benefit from a blood transfusion prior to surgery. Ferrets that are extremely anemic, thrombocytopenic, and with secondary infections such as pneumonia or pyometra are poor surgical risks, and should be stabilized if possible prior to surgery (transfusion as needed and medical treatment with hCG, see below).
- Perform celiotomy in ferrets with ovarian remnant. Ovarian tissue may be small and is located at the caudolateral pole of the kidney.
- Adrenalectomy is the treatment of choice for most ferrets with adrenal disease.
- Remove or treat any other inciting causes—foreign body, neoplasia, urinary tract infection

# VAGINAL DISCHARGE

## MEDICATIONS

### DRUG(S) OF CHOICE
• Hyperestrogenism—administer hCG 100 IU per ferret IM to stimulate ovulation and end estrus. Signs of estrus (particularly vulvar swelling) should diminish within 3–4 days. If signs are still apparent 1 week post-treatment, repeat the injection. Treatment is only effective after day 10 of estrus.
• Metritis or primary vaginitis—systemic antibiotics such as trimethoprim-sulfa combinations (SMZ-TMP 15–30 mg/kg PO q12h), enrofloxacin (10–20 mg/kg PO, IM, SC q12h), or a cephalosporin (cephalexin 15–25 mg/kg PO q8–12h)

### CONTRAINDICATIONS
Many antibiotics are contraindicated during pregnancy.

### PRECAUTIONS
N/A

### POSSIBLE INTERACTIONS
N/A

### ALTERNATIVE DRUGS
N/A

## FOLLOW-UP

### PATIENT MONITORING
Ultrasonography or radiography—determine uterine size and contents with pyometra or metritis.

### POSSIBLE COMPLICATIONS
Toxic shock—with severe pyometra or metritis

## MISCELLANEOUS

### ASSOCIATED CONDITIONS
• Insulinoma
• Adrenal disease

### AGE-RELATED FACTORS
N/A

### ZOONOTIC POTENTIAL
N/A

### PREGNANCY
Many antibiotics are contraindicated during pregnancy.

### SEE ALSO
• Adrenal disease
• Hyperestrogenism
• Pyometra

### ABBREVIATIONS
• BUN = blood urea nitrogen
• hCG = human chorionic gonadotropin
• PCV = packed cell volume

### *Suggested Reading*
Antinoff N. Urinary disorders in ferrets. Semin Avian Exotic Pet Med 1998;7(2):89–92.
Bell JA. Periparturient and neonatal diseases. In: Hillyer EV, Quesenberry KE, eds. Ferrets, Rabbits and Rodents: Clinical Medicine and Surgery. Philadelphia: WB Saunders, 1997:53–62.
Brown SA. Neoplasia. In: Hillyer EV, Quesenberry KE, eds. Ferrets, Rabbits and Rodents: Clinical Medicine and Surgery. Philadelphia: WB Saunders, 1997:99.

Fox JG, Marini RP. Diseases of the endocrine system. In: Fox JG, ed. Biology and Diseases of the Ferret. 2nd Ed. Baltimore: Williams & Wilkins, 1998.
Fox JG, Pearson RC, Bell JA. Diseases of the genitourinary system. In: Fox JG, ed. Biology and Diseases of the Ferret. 2nd Ed. Baltimore: Williams & Wilkins, 1998:247–272.
Hillyer EV. Urogenital diseases. In: Hillyer EV, Quesenberry KE, eds. Ferrets, Rabbits and Rodents: Clinical Medicine and Surgery. Philadelphia: WB Saunders, 1997:44–52.
Quesenberry KE, Rosenthal KL. Endocrine disease. In: Hillyer EV, Quesenberry KE, eds. Ferrets, Rabbits and Rodents: Clinical Medicine and Surgery. Philadelphia: WB Saunders, 1997.
Weiss CA, Scott MV. Clinical aspects and surgical treatment of hyperadrenocorticism in the domestic ferret: 94 cases (1994–1996). J Am Anim Hosp Assoc 1997;33:487–493.
Wheeler J, Bennet RA. Ferret abdominal surgical procedures. Part I. Adrenal gland and pancreatic beta-cell tumors. Compend Contin Educ Pract Vet 1999;21(9):815–822.

### *Portions Adapted From*
Eilts BE. Vaginal Discharge. In: Tilley LP, Smith FWK, Jr., eds. The 5-Minute Veterinary Consult: Canine and Feline, 3rd Ed. Baltimore: Lippincott Williams & Wilkins, 2003.

# BASICS

## DEFINITION
A complex reflex that results in the expulsion of food or fluid from the alimentary tract through the oral cavity

## PATHOPHYSIOLOGY
Vomiting can be caused by diseases of the alimentary tract or can occur secondary to toxic, neurologic, metabolic, infectious, and noninfectious causes. Vomiting is seen less frequently in ferrets as compared to dogs and cats with similar diseases and, when seen, usually indicates serious disease. Vomiting occurs when the vomiting center, located in the brain, is stimulated by input from various receptor sites throughout the body. Vomiting can be stimulated by peripheral receptors located in the gastrointestinal tract or in various organs. Vomiting can also be initiated directly by stimulation of the receptors in the vomiting center in animals with CNS disease. Stimulation of the chemoreceptor trigger zone by metabolic or bacterial toxins, drugs, motion sickness, or vestibulitis will also trigger vomiting.

## SYSTEMS AFFECTED
• Endocrine/metabolic—electrolyte abnormalities, prerenal azotemia, dehydration
• Gastrointestinal—reflux esophagitis
• Respiratory—aspiration pneumonia
• Nervous—altered mental attitude

## SIGNALMENT
N/A

## SIGNS

### Historical Findings
• Signs of nausea, such as ptyalism, licking the lips, pawing at the mouth, and backing up are usually seen just prior to vomiting or retching.
• Change in diet or access to spoiled foods or garbage
• Exposure to other ferrets
• Chewing habits—missing toys, chewing on furniture (especially foam rubber)
• Changes in appetite
• Weight loss

### Physical Examination Findings
• Weight loss with loss of fat stores and musculature—indicates chronic disease
• Poor haircoat—seen with chronic disease (infiltrative intestinal disease, hepatic disease, metabolic disorders)
• Thickened bowel loops, masses, or pain on abdominal palpation
• Diarrhea or melena
• Dry, pale mucous membranes if the ferret is dehydrated

## CAUSES
• Bacterial infection—*Helicobacter mustelae* (common), *Campylobacter* spp., *Salmonella* sp., *Clostridium* spp.
• Viral infection—ECE: very common cause, rotavirus, parvovirus less common
• Obstruction—very common foreign body most common cause, followed by foreign body, intussusception rare
• Infiltrative—lymphocytic/plasmacytic enteritis, eosinophilic enterocolitis (common diseases, occasionally cause vomiting)
• Neoplasia—lymphoma, adenocarcinoma, insulinoma; all very common
• Parasitic causes—*Giardia*, Coccidia (both may be primary pathogens or secondary to ECE), *Cryptosporidium* spp.
• Metabolic disorders—liver disease, renal disease, pancreatitis, metabolic acidosis, and electrolyte abnormalities (e.g., hypokalemia, hyperkalemia, hyponatremia, and hypercalcemia)
• Dietary—diet changes, eating spoiled food, dietary intolerance
• Drugs and toxins—vaccine reaction (causes acute onset of vomiting), chemotherapeutic agents, plant toxins, isoflurane anesthesia
• Nervous—cerebral edema, CNS tumor encephalomeningitis, otitis media/interna

## RISK FACTORS
• Exposure to other ferrets (ECE, other infectious diseases)
• Unsupervised chewing (foreign bodies)
• Stress, debility (predisposes to *Helicobacter*-induced gastritis)
• Feeding raw meat products (bacterial enteritis, cryptosporidiosis)
• Vaccine reaction
• Dietary changes

# DIAGNOSIS

## DIFFERENTIAL DIAGNOSIS

### Differentiating Similar Signs
• Differentiate primary alimentary tract disease from disease of other organ systems.
• It is important to distinguish vomiting from regurgitation, since regurgitation is usually caused by esophageal disease. Vomiting is often preceded by restlessness, pawing at the mouth, hypersalivating, licking the lips, backing up, and retching. Vomitus may be digested food, mucous, or liquid with bile staining; fresh or digested blood may be present, especially with gastrointestinal ulceration. Regurgitation is a passive act that results in the expulsion of food into the oral cavity. The contents may be tubular in shape and typically composed of undigested food. Esophageal disorders are

relatively rare in ferrets, but can occur concurrently with diseases of the stomach and small intestine.
• Diarrhea, abnormal stool, or significant weight loss is more suggestive of intestinal disease.
• Vomiting is an uncommon clinical sign in ferrets; when seen, a thorough diagnostic workup is indicated.

## CBC/BIOCHEMISTRY/URINALYSIS
• Hemogram may be normal or reveal nonregenerative anemia secondary to chronic disease.
• Increased hematocrit and serum protein concentration seen with dehydration
• Regenerative anemia may be seen with chronic gastrointestinal bleeding.
• TWBC elevation with neutrophilia occasionally seen with bacterial enteritis.
• TWBC elevation with lymphocytosis or normal TWBC with relative lymphocytosis may be suggestive of lymphoma.
• Eosinophilia (as high as 35%) may be seen in ferrets with eosinophilic enterocolitis
• Hypoalbuminemia may be seen with protein loss from the intestinal tract, especially with proliferative or infiltrative bowel disease.
• Serum biochemistry abnormalities may suggest renal or hepatic disease; ALT elevations usually seen with ECE

## OTHER LABORATORY TESTS
• Fecal direct examination, fecal flotation, and zinc sulfate centrifugation may demonstrate gastrointestinal parasites.
• Fecal cytology—may reveal RBC or fecal leukocytes, which are associated with inflammatory bowel disease or invasive bacterial strains
• Fecal culture should be performed if abnormal bacteria are observed on the fecal Gram's stain or if *Salmonella* is suspected.

## IMAGING

### Radiographic Findings
• Survey abdominal radiography may indicate intestinal obstruction, organomegaly, mass, foreign bodies, or ascites.
• Contrast radiography may indicate thickening of the intestinal wall, mucosal irregularities, mass, severe ileus, foreign body, or stricture.
• Abdominal ultrasonography may demonstrate intestinal wall thickening, gastrointestinal mass, foreign body, ileus, or mesenteric lymphadenopathy. Hyperechogenicity may be seen with hepatic lipidosis or fibrosis; hypoechoic nodules are suggestive of hepatic necrosis, abscess, or neoplasia.

## OTHER DIAGNOSTIC PROCEDURES
• Gastroscopy to detect and remove small foreign bodies or to identify and biopsy

# VOMITING

mucosal lesions. Endoscopy is superior to radiography in evaluating inflammation, erosions, and ulcers. However, the small size of the patient and subsequent limitations on instrument size often limit the use of endoscopy.
• Exploratory laparotomy and surgical biopsy should be pursued if there is evidence of obstruction or intestinal mass and/or for definitive diagnosis of gastrointestinal inflammatory or infiltrative diseases or *H. mustelae*–induced gastritis.

## TREATMENT

• Treatment must be specific to the underlying cause to be successful.
• Patients with mild disease usually respond to outpatient treatment.
• Patients with moderate to severe disease usually require hospitalization and 24-hour care for parenteral medication and fluid therapy.
• Correct electrolyte and acid-base disturbances.
• Ferrets rarely have intractable vomiting where holding NPO for long periods is necessary. If holding NPO, monitor ferrets carefully for hypoglycemia. A fast of greater than 4 hours can be dangerous. Insulinomas are extremely common in middle-aged ferrets and may be the cause of signs of gastritis or may occur simultaneously with other causes of gastritis.
• Once vomiting has subsided, offer a bland diet such as canned chicken baby foods. If the patient has been anorectic, offer high-calorie diets such as Eukanuba Maximum Calorie diet (Iams Co., Dayton, OH), Feline a/d (Hills Products, Topeka, KS), or Clinicare Feline liquid diet (Abbott Laboratories, North Chicago, IL); may also add dietary supplement such as Nutri-Cal (EVSCO Pharmaceuticals, Buena, NJ) to increase caloric content to these foods. Warming the food to body temperature or offering via syringe may increase acceptance. Administer these foods several times a day.

## MEDICATIONS

### DRUG(S) OF CHOICE

• Depend on the cause of vomiting; see specific diseases for more detailed treatment options.
• Antibiotic therapy—indicated in patients with bacterial inflammatory lesions in the gastrointestinal tract. Also indicated in patients with disruption of the intestinal mucosa evidenced by blood in the feces. Se-

lection should be based on results of culture and susceptibility testing when possible. For empirical treatment, use broad-spectrum antibiotics such as trimethoprim sulfa (15–30 mg/kg q12h), amoxicillin (20–30 mg/kg PO, SQ q12h), or enrofloxacin (10–20 mg/kg PO, SQ q12h).
• *H. mustelae*—amoxicillin (10–20 mg/kg PO q12h) plus metronidazole (20 mg/kg PO q12h) and bismuth subsalicylate (17 mg/kg PO q12h) for at least 2 weeks.
• Gastrointestinal antisecretory agents are helpful to treat, and possibly prevent, gastritis in anorectic ferrets. Ferrets continually secrete a baseline level of gastric hydrochloric acid and, as such, anorexia itself may predispose to gastric ulceration. Those successfully used in ferrets include omeprazole (0.7 mg/kg PO q24h), famotidine (0.25–0.5 mg/kg PO, IV q12–24h), and cimetidine (5–10 mg/kg PO, SC, IM q8h).
• Sucralfate suspension (25 mg/kg PO q8h) protects ulcerated tissue (cytoprotection) by binding to ulcer sites.
• Inflammatory enterocolitis—prednisolone 1.25–2.5 mg/kg PO q 24h initially; gradually taper dose.
• Antiemetics should be reserved for patients with refractory vomiting that have not responded to treatment of the underlying disease. Options include chlorpromazine (0.2–0.4 mg/kg IM, SC q6–12h) and metoclopramide (0.2–1.0 mg/kg PO, SC, IM q6–8h) .

### CONTRAINDICATIONS

• Alpha-adrenergic blockers such as chlorpromazine should not be used in dehydrated patients, since they can cause hypotension.
• Metoclopramide is contraindicated in patients with gastrointestinal obstruction and is associated with signs of restlessness and depression.

### PRECAUTIONS

Antiemetics such as chlorpromazine may cause severe drowsiness and should be avoided when possible since they can mask an underlying problem.

### POSSIBLE INTERACTIONS
N/A

### ALTERNATE DRUGS
N/A

## FOLLOW-UP

### PATIENT MONITORING

Continued vomiting, fecal volume and character, appetite, attitude, and body condition

### POSSIBLE COMPLICATIONS

• Reflux esophagitis
• Aspiration pneumonia
• Dehydration due to fluid loss

## MISCELLANEOUS

### ASSOCIATED CONDITIONS
N/A

### AGE-RELATED FACTORS

• Foreign body or lymphoma may be seen in any age ferret.
• *H. mustelae* more common in ferrets <3 years of age
• Older ferrets demonstrate more severe clinical signs with ECE
• Kits 4–6 weeks of age more susceptible to rotavirus

### ZOONOTIC POTENTIAL

• Cryptosporidiosis
• *Giardia*

### PREGNANCY
N/A

### SEE ALSO

• Epizootic catarrhal enteritis
• Gastrointestinal foreign bodies
• *Helicobacter mustelae*
• Inflammatory bowel disease

### ABBREVIATIONS

• ALT = alanine transferase
• CNS = central nervous system
• ECE = epizootic catarrhal enteritis
• NPO = nothing by mouth
• RBC = red blood cell
• TWBC = total white blood cell count

*Suggested Reading*

Finkler MR. Ferret colitis. In: Kirk RW, Bonagura JD, eds. Kirk's Current Veterinary Therapy XI: Small Animal Practice. Philadelphia: WB Saunders, 1992.

Fox JG. Diseases of the gastrointestinal system. In: Fox JG, ed. Biology and Diseases of the Ferret. 2nd Ed. Baltimore: Williams & Wilkins, 1998.

Hoefer HL. Gastrointestinal diseases. In: Hillyer EV, Quesenberry KE, eds. Ferrets, Rabbits and Rodents: Clinical Medicine and Surgery. Philadelphia: WB Saunders, 1997:26–36.

Jenkins JR. Rabbit and ferret liver and gastrointestinal testing. In: Fudge AM, ed. Laboratory Medicine, Avian and Exotic Pets. Philadelphia: W.B Saunders, 2000.

*Portions Adapted From*

Jenkins CC, DeNovo RC. Vomiting—Chronic. In: Tilley LP, Smith FWK, Jr., eds. The 5-Minute Veterinary Consult: Canine and Feline, 1st Ed. Baltimore: Lippincott Williams & Wilkins, 1997.

# WEIGHT LOSS AND CACHEXIA

## BASICS

### DEFINITION
• Weight loss is considered clinically important when it exceeds 10% of the normal body weight and is not associated with fluid loss.
• Cachexia is defined as the state of extreme poor health and is associated with anorexia, weight loss, weakness, and mental depression.

### PATHOPHYSIOLOGY
• Weight loss can result from many different pathophysiologic mechanisms that share a common feature—insufficient caloric intake or availability to meet metabolic needs.
• Insufficient caloric intake can be caused by (1) a high energy demand (e.g., that characteristic of a hypermetabolic state); (2) inadequate energy intake, including insufficient quantity or quality of food, or inadequate nutrient assimilation (e.g., with anorexia, dysphagia, regurgitation, or malabsorptive disorders); and (3) excessive loss of nutrients or fluid, which can occur in patients with gastrointestinal losses, glucosuria, or proteinuria.

### SYSTEMS AFFECTED
Any can be affected by weight loss, especially if severe or the result of systemic disease.

### SIGNALMENT
No age or sex predilection

### SIGNS

#### Historical Findings
• Clinical signs of particular diagnostic value in patients with weight loss are whether the appetite is normal, increased, decreased, or absent.
• Historical information is very important, especially regarding type of diet; environment (chewing habits and access to potential gastrointestinal foreign bodies); signs of gastrointestinal disease, including dysphagia, regurgitation, vomiting, and diarrhea; or signs of any specific disease.

#### Physical Examination Findings
Seek signs of systemic disease, gastrointestinal disease, neoplasia, cardiac disease, and neuromuscular disorders.

### CAUSES

#### Malabsorptive Disorders
• Infiltrative and inflammatory bowel disease—very common
• Gastric foreign body—very common
• Gastritis and gastroduodenal ulcers
• Epizootic catarrhal enteritis
• Severe intestinal parasitism (rare)

#### Metabolic Disorders
• Organ failure—cardiac failure, hepatic failure, and renal failure
• Insulinoma
• Cancer cachexia—lymphoma, adrenal neoplasia
• Aleutian disease virus—parvovirus

#### Excessive Nutrient Loss
• Protein-losing enteropathy (secondary to infectious or infiltrative diseases)—common
• Protein-losing nephropathy
• Diabetes mellitus (rare)

#### Anorexia and Pseudoanorexia
• Inability to smell, prehend, or chew food
• Dysphagia
• Regurgitation
• Vomiting

#### Dietary Causes
• Insufficient quantity
• Poor quality
• Inedible food—decreased palatability

#### Neuromuscular Disease
• Lower motor neuron disease—rare
• CNS disease—usually associated with anorexia or pseudoanorexia

#### Excessive Use of Calories
• Increased physical activity
• Pregnancy or lactation
• Increased catabolism—fever, inflammation, cancer; very common cause

### RISK FACTORS
See causes (above).

## DIAGNOSIS
• First confirm weight loss by comparing the current weight to previous weights.
• If previous weights are not available, subjectively assess the patient for cachexia, emaciation, dehydration, or other clues that would confirm the owner's complaint of weight loss.
• After weight loss is confirmed, seek the underlying cause.

### DIFFERENTIAL DIAGNOSIS
• First categorize the weight loss as occurring with a normal, increased, or decreased appetite.
• The list of likely differential diagnoses for a patient with weight loss despite a normal or increased appetite is much different and much shorter than that for patients with decreased appetite or anorexia.
• Determine what the patient's appetite was at the onset of weight loss; any condition can lead to anorexia if it persists long enough for the patient to become debilitated.

• The patient's age may provide a clue as to the underlying cause (e.g., gastrointestinal foreign body or *Helicobacter* gastritis in a young ferret and neoplasia or insulinoma in a middle-aged or older ferret).
• Also seek causes of pseudoanorexia (e.g., loss of sense of smell, dysphagia, and disorders of the oral cavity, head, and neck).
• Fever suggests that the underlying cause may be infectious or inflammatory.

### CBC/BIOCHEMISTRY/URINALYSIS
• Help identify infectious, inflammatory, and metabolic diseases including organ failure.
• Especially helpful when the history and physical examination do not provide much useful information

### OTHER LABORATORY TESTS
• Determined by the clinician's list of most likely differential diagnoses on the basis of the specific findings of the history and physical examination
• Fecal direct examination, fecal flotation, and zinc sulfate centrifugation to rule out gastrointestinal parasites, especially in patients with diarrhea
• Fecal cytology—may reveal RBC or fecal leukocytes, which are associated with inflammatory bowel disease or invasive bacterial strains

### IMAGING
• If underlying disease is suspected but no abnormalities are revealed by the physical examination or minimum database, perform abdominal radiography and abdominal ultrasonography to identify hidden conditions such as gastrointestinal tract disease, hepatic disease, insulinoma, or lymphoma. Consider thoracic radiography to rule out cardiac or pulmonary disease.
• The need for further diagnostic imaging varies with the underlying condition suspected (see other topics on specific diseases).

#### Diagnostic Procedures
• Vary depending on initial diagnostic findings and the suspected underlying cause of weight loss
• If gastrointestinal disease is probable but unconfirmed, examine biopsy specimens taken from the indicated portions of the gastrointestinal tract via exploratory laparotomy.
• Many indications for exploratory laparotomy exist—obtain multiple biopsy specimens from the suspected organ or organs as well as from other routinely biopsied abdominal organs such as liver, gastrointestinal tract, pancreas, and mesenteric lymph nodes.

# WEIGHT LOSS AND CACHEXIA

## TREATMENT

- The most important treatment principle is to treat the underlying cause of the weight loss.
- Symptomatic therapy includes attention to fluid and electrolyte derangements, reduction in environmental stressors, and modification of the diet to improve palatability.
- Most ferrets will accept high-calorie diets such as Eukanuba Maximum Calorie diet (Iams Co., Dayton, OH), Feline a/d (Hills Products, Topeka, KS), or Clinicare Feline liquid diet (Abbott Laboratories, North Chicago, IL); may also add dietary supplement such as Nutri-Cal (EVSCO Pharmaceuticals, Buena, NJ) to increase caloric content to these foods. Warming the food to body temperature or offering via syringe may increase acceptance. Administer these supplements several times a day.
- Reported resting energy requirement for ferrets is 70 kcal/kg body weight per day (sick ferrets have higher requirements). Clinicare Feline contains 1 kcal/mL; Eukanuba Maximum Calorie diet contains 2 kcal/mL.
- Techniques for providing enteral nutrition include force-feeding or placement of nasogastric, esophagostomy, gastrostomy, or jejunostomy tubes.
- Parenteral nutrition may be provided via infusion through a polyurethane jugular catheter using a syringe pump.

## MEDICATIONS

### DRUG(S) OF CHOICE

- Depend on the underlying cause of the weight loss; see specific topic for each condition, including anorexia.
- See other sections regarding specific disorders or problems.

### CONTRAINDICATIONS
N/A

### PRECAUTIONS
N/A

### POSSIBLE INTERACTIONS
N/A

### ALTERNATIVE DRUGS
N/A

## FOLLOW-UP

### PATIENT MONITORING
The necessity for frequent patient monitoring and the methods required depend on the underlying cause of the weight loss; however, the patient should be weighed regularly and often.

### POSSIBLE COMPLICATIONS
See causes.

## MISCELLANEOUS

### ASSOCIATED CONDITIONS
See causes.

### AGE-RELATED FACTORS
N/A

### ZOONOTIC POTENTIAL
N/A

### PREGNANCY
Pregnancy and lactation can be associated with weight loss due to increased calorie expenditure.

### SYNONYMS
N/A

### SEE ALSO
- Epizootic Catarrhal Enteritis
- Eosinophilic gastroenteritis
- Gastroduodenal ulcers
- Gastrointestinal foreign bodies
- Insulinoma
- Lymphoplasmacytic gastroenteritis
- Lymphosarcoma

### ABBREVIATIONS
- CNS = central nervous system
- ECE = epizootic catarrhal enteritis
- RBC = red blood cell

### Suggested Reading

Brown SA. Neoplasia. In: Hillyer EV, Quesenberry KE, eds. Ferrets, Rabbits and Rodents: Clinical Medicine ans Surgery. Philadelphia: WB Saunders, 1998:109.

Caplan ER, Peterson ME, Mulles HS, et al. Diagnosis and treatment of insulin-secreting pancreatic islet cell tumors in ferrets: 57 cases (1986–1994). J Am Vet Med Assoc 1996;209:1741–1745.

Fox JG. Diseases of the gastrointestinal system. In: Fox JG, ed. Biology and Diseases of the Ferret. 2nd Ed. Baltimore: Williams & Wilkins, 1998.

Fox JG, Marini RP. Helicobacter mustelae infection in ferrets: pathogenesis, epizootiology, diagnosis and treatment. Semin Avin Exotic Pet Med 2001;10(1):36–44.

Hoefer HL. Cardiac disease in ferrets. Proc North Am Vet Conf 1995:577–578.

Hoefer HL. Gastrointestinal diseases. In: Hillyer EV, Quesenberry KE, eds. Ferrets, Rabbits and Rodents: Clinical Medicine and Surgery. Philadelphia: WB Saunders, 1997:26–36.

Stamoulis ME, Miller MS, Hillyer EV. Cardiovascular diseases part 1. In: Hillyer EV, Quesenberry KE, eds. Ferrets, Rabbits and Rodents: Clinical Medicine and Surgery. Philadelphia: WB Saunders, 1997:63–70.

Li X, Fox JG. Neoplastic diseases. In: Fox JG, ed. Biology and Diseases of the Ferret. 2nd Ed. Baltimore: Williams & Wilkins, 1998:405–448.

### Portions Adapted From

Harrington DP, Meyers NC, III. Weight Loss and Cachexia. In: Tilley LP, Smith FWK, Jr., eds. The 5-Minute Veterinary Consult: Canine and Feline, 2nd Ed. Baltimore: Lippincott Williams & Wilkins, 2000.

# RABBIT

# ABSESSATION

 BASICS

## DEFINITION
An abscess is a localized collection of purulent exudate contained within a fibrous capsule. Abscesses are an extremely common finding in rabbits.

## PATHOPHYSIOLOGY
• Unlike cats and dogs, abscesses in rabbits do not often rupture and drain. Rabbit abscesses are filled with a thick, caseous exudate, surrounded by a fibrous capsule. They can be either slow growing or become large very quickly, and often extend aggressively into surrounding soft tissue and bone. Abscesses with bony involvement (facial, plantar, joints) can be extremely difficult to treat, requiring surgical intervention and prolonged medical care. Prognosis is fair to poor depending on the severity and location.
• Abscesses in rabbits are usually associated with an underlying cause. Identification and correction of the underlying cause is paramount for successful treatment.
• Abscesses occur most commonly on the face and are almost always caused by dental disease; occasionally they may be secondary to upper respiratory infections, otitis, or trauma.
• Abscesses on the trunk or extremities are usually caused by trauma, puncture or bite wounds, abrasions, foreign bodies, furunculosis, or osteomyelitis.
• Hepatic abscessation is often secondary to corticosteroid use.
• Abscessation secondary to bacteremia may occur anywhere on the body, including internal organs; often the original source cannot be identified.
• Affected rabbits often appear to not be in pain, unless osteomyelitis or dental disease is present. However, assessment of pain in rabbits is often difficult for owners, as compared to predatory species such as dogs and cats.

## SYSTEMS AFFECTED
• Skin/exocrine—percutaneous
• Skeletal—especially skull and plantar abscesses
• Ophthalmic—periorbital tissues
• Hepatobiliary—liver parenchyma
• Respiratory—lung parenchyma, nasal turbinates, sinuses
• Reproductive—mammary gland

## INCIDENCE/PREVALENCE
Extremely common in pet rabbits. Most common cause of subcutaneous swelling

## SIGNALMENT
• No age or sex predilection for most abscesses

• Dwarf and lop-eared rabbits are predisposed to abscesses secondary to dental disease.

## SIGNS
### General Comments
• Determined by organ system and/or tissue affected
• Associated with a combination of inflammation (pain, swelling, loss of function), tissue destruction, and/or organ system dysfunction caused by accumulation of exudate

### Historical Findings
• Facial abscesses—history of dental disease, ptyalism, nasal or ocular discharge, exophthalmos, and otitis externa, interna, or media
• Anorexia, depression—seen with dental disease, pain from skeletal abscesses. Intrathoracic or hepatic abscesses—often the only clinical signs until abscess is large enough to cause space-occupying effects
• Lameness, reluctance to move—plantar or digital abscesses; pain
• Occasionally history of traumatic insult or previous infection
• Dyspnea with large or multiple intrathoracic abscesses
• A rapidly appearing, variably painful swelling if affected area is visible

### Physical Examination Findings
Determined by the organ system or tissue affected
• Mandibular, cheeks, nasal rostrum, retrobulbar—usually caused by dental disease. Palpable mass of fluctuant to firm consistency, usually attached to and involving underlying bone. Findings may include ptyalism, anorexia, nasal discharge, ocular discharge, exophthalmia. Always perform a thorough oral examination under anesthesia, including skull radiographs. Occasionally, mass is freely movable within the subcutaneous tissues and not attached to bone—more likely caused by external trauma, better prognosis
• Anorectic rabbits—may show signs of gastrointestinal hypomotility: scant, dry feces; dehydration; firm stomach or cecal contents; gas-filled intestinal loops
• Ears—mass occasionally palpable arising from ear canal; vestibular signs (torticollis, ataxia, rolling, nystagmus) with extension into inner ear or brain
• Limbs—lameness; single or multiple palpable masses, especially on plantar or interdigital surfaces; hair loss; cellulitis (erythema, swelling); may rupture and form scabs with caseous exudate underneath
• Superficial abscess—variable size mass; firm or fluctuant; nonpainful; freely movable unless attached to underlying tissues; occasionally large areas of necrotic skin (may slough)

• Intrathoracic abscesses—dull or absent lung sounds on thoracic auscultation; dyspnea; anorexia; depression

## CAUSES
• Pyogenic bacteria—odontogenic abscesses—*Pasteurella* generally not present; common isolates from dental-related abscesses include anaerobic bacteria such as *Fusobacterium nucleatum*, *Prevotella* spp., *Peptostreptococcus micros*, *Actinomyces israelii*, and *Arcanobacterium haemolyticum*. *Streptococcus* spp. may also be cultured from odontogenic abscesses. Other abscesses—may culture *Pasteurella multocida*, *Staphylococcus aureus*, *Pseudomonas* spp., *Escherichia coli*, b-hemolytic *Streptococcus* spp., *Proteus* spp., and *Bacteroides* spp.
• Dental disease—periapical or tooth root abscesses, food lodged between teeth and/or gingival mucosa, malocclusion causing sharp points on crowns that penetrate oral mucosa
• Foreign objects

## RISK FACTORS
• Mandibular, cheeks—elongated cheek teeth and incisor malocclusion often caused by feeding of diets containing inadequate roughage
• Periorbital—dental disease; elongated maxillary tooth roots penetrating into nasal passages most common cause
• Brain—otitis interna, sinusitis; often caused by chronic nasal pasteurellosis extending via eustachian tube or into sinuses; may be extension of otitis externa/media
• Percutaneous—abrasions, puncture (bite) wounds, sepsis
• Plantar/digital—improper surfaces (wire cages, nonpadded surfaces), urine scald, sitting on soiled bedding material, abrasions, furunculosis, trauma, puncture wounds, foreign bodies, immobility from pain, obesity
• Liver—use of topical or systemic corticosteroids, sepsis
• Lung—sepsis, bacterial pneumonia, foreign object aspiration
• Mammary gland—mastitis
• Immunosuppression—systemic or topical corticosteroid use, immunosuppressive chemotherapy, underlying predisposing disease (e.g., chronic renal failure)

 DIAGNOSIS

## DIFFERENTIAL DIAGNOSIS
### Mass Lesions
• Granuloma—generally firmer without fluctuant center
• Neoplasia—variable growth; variably painful
• Cyst—lack of white caseous exudate

• Fibrous scar tissue—firm; nonpainful; does not enlarge
• Hematoma/seroma—nonencapsulated; unattached to surrounding tissues; fluctuant and fluid-filled initially but more firm with organization
• Cuterebra

## CBC/BIOCHEMISTRY/URINALYSIS
• CBC—often normal; TWBC elevations generally do not occur; instead the neutrophil:lymphocyte ratio shifts to a relative neutrophilia and lymphopenia.
• Urinalysis and serum chemistry profile—depend on system affected
• Liver—slight to moderate increases in liver enzymes if hepatic involvement

## OTHER LABORATORY TESTS
Serology for *Pasteurella*—usefulness is severely limited and generally not helpful in the diagnosis of pasteurellosis in pet rabbits. An ELISA is available, and results are reported as negative, low positive, or high positive. Positive results, even when high, only indicate prior exposure to *Pasteurella* and the development of antibodies, and do not confirm active infection. Low-positive results may occur due to cross-reaction with other, nonpathogenic bacteria (false positive). False-negative results are common with immunosuppression or early infection. No evidence exists to support correlation of titers to the presence or absence of disease.

## IMAGING
• Radiography—to determine the extent of bone involvement; essential in guidance of treatment plan and expected prognosis; osteomyelitis carries poorer prognosis, prolonged treatment
• Thoracic and abdominal radiographs may help identify and determine the extent of internal abscesses
• Skull radiographs—essential to identify type and extent of dental disease in rabbits with facial abscesses; perform under general anesthesia; five views are recommend for thorough assessment including ventral–dorsal, lateral, two lateral obliques, and rostral–caudal.
• Ultrasonography—determine organ system affected, extent of disease
• Echocardiography—helpful for diagnosis of pericardial abscess
• CT or MRI—more accurate than radiographs for assessment of facial abscesses, bullae involvement, or brain abscess

## DIAGNOSTIC PROCEDURES
A thorough oral examination under sedation to look for dental disease is crucial in the diagnosis and treatment of all rabbits with facial abscesses.

### Aspiration
• Reveals a thick, creamy to caseous, white exudate
• High nucleated cell count; primarily degenerative neutrophils with lesser numbers of macrophages and lymphocytes
• Pyogenic bacteria—may be seen in cells; higher number in wall of abscess; Gram's stain to direct antibiotic therapy

### Biopsy
• To rule out neoplasia, granuloma, and other causes of masses
• Sample should contain both normal and abnormal tissue in the same specimen.
• Tissue submitted for histopathologic examination and culture

### Culture
• Affected tissue and/or exudate—aerobic and anaerobic bacteria; lack of growth is common, especially with anaerobic infections or fastidious bacterial infections
• If anaerobic culture is not possible, diagnosis is often presumed
• Growth may be more likely if wall or capsule is sampled; bacteria deep within exudate are often nonviable
• Bacterial susceptibility testing to direct antibiotic therapy

## PATHOLOGIC FINDINGS
• Exudate—large numbers of neutrophils in various stages of degeneration, other inflammatory cells, necrotic tissue
• Surrounding tissue congested, fibrin, large number of neutrophils, variable number of lymphocytes, plasma cells, macrophages, fibrous connective tissue
• Causative agent variably detectable, especially with anaerobic infections

 TREATMENT

## APPROPRIATE HEALTH CARE
• Simple lancing, flushing, and draining are not adequate to treat rabbits' abscesses. Thick exudates do not drain well, and the abscess will recur. It is crucial to remove/correct the underlying cause for long-term success.
• Depends on location of abscess and treatment required
• Outpatient—smaller, well-demarcated subcutaneous abscesses
• Inpatient—sepsis, extensive surgical procedures, treatment requiring extended hospitalization
• Surgical removal of abscess, nidus of infection (e.g., teeth), or foreign object is necessary.
• Institution of long-term antimicrobial therapy

## NURSING CARE
• Depends on location of abscess and type of surgical repair (see below)
• Use protective bandaging and/or Elizabethan collars as needed.
• Sepsis or peritonitis—aggressive fluid therapy and support

## ACTIVITY
Restrict until the abscess has resolved and adequate healing of tissues has taken place.

## DIET
• It is absolutely imperative that the rabbit continue to eat during and following treatment. Anorexia will often cause gastrointestinal hypomotility, derangement of the gastrointestinal microflora, and overgrowth of intestinal bacterial pathogens.
• Offer a large selection of fresh, moistened greens such as cilantro, romaine lettuce, parsley, carrot tops, dandelion greens, spinach, collard greens, etc., and good-quality grass hay. Many rabbits will begin to eat these foods, even if they were previously anorectic. Also, try offering the rabbit's usual pelleted diet.
• If the patient refuses these foods, syringe feed a gruel such as Critical Care for Herbivores (Oxbow Pet Products, Murdock, NE) 10–15 mL/kg PO q6–8h. Larger volumes and more frequent feedings are often accepted; feed as much as the rabbit will readily accept. Alternatively, pellets can be ground and mixed with fresh greens, vegetable baby foods, water, or juice to form a gruel. If sufficient volumes of food are not accepted in this manner, nasogastric intubation is indicated.
• High-carbohydrate, high-fat nutritional supplements should be avoided.
• Encourage oral fluid intake by offering fresh water and wetting leafy vegetables.

## CLIENT EDUCATION
• Discuss need to correct or prevent risk factors.
• Abscesses of the head and those involving bone have a guarded to poor prognosis for complete resolution. Most will require extensive surgery, sometimes multiple surgeries and multiple follow-up visits. Recurrences in the same or other locations are common. Clients must be aware of the monetary and time investment.

## SURGICAL CONSIDERATIONS
### Superficial Abscesses (Not Involving Bone or Teeth)
• En bloc excision of entire abscess, leaving wide margins (similar to excision of malignant sarcoma in dogs or cats); exercise care not to rupture capsule.
• If entire abscess cannot be removed en bloc, lance, remove exterior wall, curette all

## ABSCESSATION

exudates, and leave wound to heal via second intention. Irrigate wound with dilute antiseptic solution (chlorhexidine or iodine) two to three times daily until healthy granulation bed forms, followed by antibiotic cream until reepithelialization occurs; long-term antibiotic therapy
• Remove any foreign objects(s), necrotic tissue, or nidus of infection.
• Placement of Penrose or similar drains are contraindicated; they do not facilitate drainage and may serve as an avenue for further infection.
• Place on long-term antibiotic therapy.

### Facial Abscesses
• Remove, in entirety, all teeth involved in the abscess.
• Remove the abscess, abscess capsule, and affected bone, in entirety, whenever possible.
• If all affected tissues cannot be removed entirely, remove abscess at the level of the bone and curette/debride all grossly abnormal bone, teeth, and soft tissue. Flush copiously to remove exudates.
• Depending on location of abscess, either leave open to heal by second intention as described above, or fill the defect with antibiotic-impregnated polymethyl methacrylate (AIPMMA) beads.
• In rabbits with extensive head abscesses, aggressive debridement of bone is often indicated, and special expertise may be required. Given the expense and pain involved in these procedures, the author recommends referral to a specialist if surgical expertise or AIPMMA beads are not available.
• AIPMMA beads release a high concentration of antibiotic into local tissues for several months. Selection of antibiotic is limited to those known to elute appropriately from bead to tissues, and should be based on culture and susceptibility testing. AIPMMA beads are not commercially available, but can be made using PMMA by Surgical Simplex Bone Cement (Howmedica, Rutherford, NJ) or Bone Cement (Zimmer, Charlotte, NC). Antibiotics successfully used include cephalothin, cefazolin, or ceftiofur (2 g/20 g PMMA); gentamicin or tobramycin (1 g/2 g PMMA); or amikacin (1.25 g/2 g PMMA). Antibiotic is added to the copolymer powder before adding the liquid and formed into small, spherical beads. Beads must be manufactured and inserted aseptically, and unused bead should be gas sterilized prior to future use. Beads should be left in the incision site for at least 2 months, but can be left in indefinitely.
• Place on long-term antibiotic therapy; appropriate pain management

### Abscesses Involving Joints or Feet
• As above, remove as much abscess en bloc as possible, using care not to rupture the abscess and further contaminate the incision site.

• Debride/curette all visible abnormal tissue; flush copiously.
• Treat as open wound—flush, debride would daily initially, followed by twice weekly to weekly debridement as healing occurs. Follow debridement with application of soft bandages. Bandages must be changed immediately if they become wet.
• When feasible, AIPMMA beads may be placed in the defect as described above. If placed in a joint space, remove beads after 4–6 weeks.
• Severe osteomyelitis may require amputation.
• Correct underlying cause—provide soft bedding; improve husbandry; weight loss
• Place on long-term antibiotic therapy; appropriate pain management

### Internal Abscesses
• Thoracic abscess—occasionally may be amenable to surgical excision via thoracotomy; if not excised, treat with supportive care and long-term antibiotics.
• Abdominal abscesses—surgical removal when possible, followed by long-term antibiotic therapy

## MEDICATIONS

### DRUG(S) OF CHOICE

#### Antibiotics
Antimicrobial drugs effective against the infectious agent; gain access to site of infection. Choice of antibiotic is ideally based on results of culture and susceptibility testing. Depending on the severity of infection, long-term antibiotic therapy is required (4–6 weeks minimum to several months or years). Use broad-spectrum antibiotics such as enrofloxacin (5–20 mg/kg PO, SC, IM q12–24h), trimethoprim sulfa (30 mg/kg PO q12h), or chloramphenicol (50 mg/kg PO q8h). Most facial or dental abscesses contain anaerobic bacteria; use antibiotics effective against anaerobes such as azithromycin (30 mg/kg PO q24h); can be used alone or combined with metronidazole (20 mg/kg PO q12h). Alternatively, use penicillin g (40,000–60,000 IU/kg SC q2–7d). Combine with topical treatment (surgical debridement, AIPPMA beads) listed above.

#### Acute Pain Management
• Butorphanol (0.1–1.0 mg/kg SC, IM, IV q4–6h)—may cause profound sedation; short-acting
• Buprenorphine (0.01–0.05 mg/kg SC, IM IV q8–12h)—less sedating, longer acting than butorphanol
• Morphine (2–5 mg/kg SC IM q2–4h) or oxymorphone (0.05–0.2 mg/kg SC IM q8–12h)—use with caution; more than one to two doses may cause gastrointestinal stasis.

• Meloxicam (0.2 mg/kg SC, IM q24h)
• Carprofen (1–4 mg/kg SC q12h)

#### Long-Term Pain Management
• NSAIDs—have been used for short- or long-term therapy to reduce pain and inflammation; meloxicam (0.2–0.5 mg/kg PO q24h); carprofen (2.2 mg/kg PO q12–24)
• For sedation—light sedation with midazolam (0.5–2 mg/kg IM) or diazepam (1–2 mg/kg IM); for deeper sedation and longer procedures the author prefers ketamine (15–20 mg/kg IM) plus midazolam (0.5–1.0 mg/kg IM); many other sedation protocols exist.

### CONTRAINDICATIONS
• Oral administration of most antibiotics effective against anaerobes will cause a fatal gastrointestinal dysbiosis in rabbits. Do not administer penicillins, macrolides, lincosamides, and cephalosporins by oral administration.
• The use of corticosteroids (systemic or topical in otic preparations) can severely exacerbate abscesses.
• Placement of Penrose or similar drains
• The placement of calcium hydroxide paste in the defect following debridement is contraindicated, as extensive tissue necrosis may occur.

### PRECAUTIONS
• Chloramphenicol—avoid human contact with chloramphenicol due to potential blood dyscrasia. Advise owners of potential risks.
• Meloxicam—use with caution in rabbits with compromised renal function.
• Oral administration of any antibiotic may potentially cause enteric dysbiosis; discontinue use if diarrhea or anorexia occurs.

### POSSIBLE INTERACTIONS
N/A

### ALTERNATIVE DRUGS
• If AIPPMA beads are not available, packing the postdebridement deficit with antibiotic-laden gauze has been used as an alternative. The choice of antibiotic is based on culture and susceptibility testing. Antibiotics used include penicillin (80,000 IU/kg), ampicillin (20mg/kg), cefazolin (25 mg/kg), and metronidazole (50 mg/kg). Oral antibiotic therapy is used simultaneously during the entire treatment period. The wounds are evaluated and the gauze is removed and repacked every 7 days under general anesthesia, until complete resolution occurs. Effectiveness varies, depending on severity of disease and owner compliance.
• 50% dextrose-soaked gauze has been anecdotally used with success as a topical abscess treatment following surgical debridement. Dextrose has bactericidal properties and promotes granulation bed formation. The abscess cavity is filled with dextrose-laden

gauze and replaced daily until a healthy granulation bed appears. Honey has been used in a similar manner. Effectiveness varies, depending on the severity of disease and owner compliance.

## FOLLOW-UP

### PATIENT MONITORING
Monitor for progressive decrease in exudate, resolution of inflammation, and improvement of clinical signs.

### PREVENTION/AVOIDANCE
• Prevent progressive dental disease by selecting pets without congenital predisposition (when possible), providing high-fiber foods and good-quality hay, and periodically trimming of overgrown crowns.
• Prevent joint or feet abscess by providing clean, solid surfaces, appropriate surface substrates; prevent obesity.
• Treating otitis or upper respiratory infections in early stages may prevent otitis media and/or brain abscesses.
• Prevent fighting between rabbits.

### POSSIBLE COMPLICATIONS
• Severe deformation of face with chronic facial abscesses
• Compromise of organ function
• Sepsis
• Peritonitis/pleuritis if intraabdominal or intrathoracic abscess ruptures
• Recurrence, chronic pain, or extensive tissue destruction warranting euthanasia due to poor quality of life

### EXPECTED COURSE AND PROGNOSIS
Depend on organ system involved and amount of tissue destruction
• Superficial abscess—good to fair prognosis; recurrence locally or in other sites likely

• Facial abscesses, osteomyelitis—depend on severity of bone involvement and location. Rabbits with abscesses in the nasal passages or with exophthalmos, multiple or severe maxillary abscesses, or brain abscesses have a guarded to poor prognosis. Multiple surgeries and follow-up treatments are usually required, and recurrence rates are high. Euthanasia may be warranted if rabbits are in pain and quality of life is unacceptable.
• Internal abscesses—fair to grave prognosis depending on location
• Without surgical treatment—many facial abscesses are slow growing. If surgical treatment is not elected, continue antibiotic treatment long term. Many rabbits will live for months in comfort, even with relatively large abscesses.

## MISCELLANEOUS

### ASSOCIATED CONDITIONS
• Immunosuppression
• Gastrointestinal hypomotility

### AGE-RELATED FACTORS
N/A

### ZOONOTIC POTENTIAL
N/A

### PREGNANCY
N/A

### SEE ALSO
• Arthritis—septic
• Cheek teeth (molar and premolar) malocclusion and elongation
• Otitis externa
• Rhinitis and sinusitis
• Ulcerative pododermatitis (sore hocks)

### ABBREVIATIONS
• CBC = complete blood count
• CT = computed tomography

• ELISA = enzyme-linked immunosorbent assay
• MRI = magnetic resonance imaging
• NSAIDs = nonsteroidal antiinflammatory drugs
• TWBC = total white blood cell

*Suggested Reading*
Bennett RA. Treatment of abscesses in the head of rabbits. Proc North Am Vet Conf 1999;821–823.
Crossley DA, Aiken S. Small mammal dentistry. In: Quesenberry KE, Carpenter JW, eds. Ferrets, Rabbits and Rodents: Clinical Medicine and Surgery. 2nd Ed. Philadelphia: WB Saunders, 2004:370–382.
DeLong D, Manning PJ. Bacterial diseases. In: Manning P, Ringler DH, Newcomer CE, eds. The Biology of the Laboratory Rabbit. Orlando, FL: Academic Press, 1994:129–170.
Ethell MT, Bennett RA, Brown MP, et al. In vitro elution of gentamicin, amikacin, and ceftiofur from polymethylmethacrylate and hydroxyapatite cement. Vet Surg 2000;29:375–382.
Jenkins JR. Soft tissue surgery. In: Quesenberry KE, Carpenter JW, eds. Ferrets, Rabbits and Rodents: Clinical Medicine and Surgery. 2nd Ed. Philadelphia: WB Saunders, 2004:221–230.
Langan GP, Schaeffer DO. Rabbit microbiology and virology. In: Fudge AM, ed. Laboratory Medicine: Avian and Exotic Pets. Philadelphia: WB Saunders, 2000:325–333.
Lukehart SA, Fohn MJ, Baker-Zander SA. Efficacy of azithromycin for therapy of active syphilis in the rabbit model. J Antimicrob Chemother. 1990;25 Suppl A:91–99.
Tyrell KC, Citron DM, Jenkins JR, et al. Periodontal bacteria in rabbit mandibular and maxillary abscesses. J Clin Microbiol 2002;40(3):1044–1047.

# ALOPECIA

## BASICS

### DEFINITION
- Common disorder in rabbits
- Characterized by a complete or partial lack of hair in areas where it is normally present
- May be associated with a multifactorial cause
- May be the primary problem or only a secondary phenomenon

### PATHOPHYSIOLOGY
- Multifactorial causes
- All of the disorders represent a disruption in the growth of the hair follicle from infection, trauma, immunologic attack, mechanical "plugging," or blockage of the receptor sites for stimulation of the cycle.

### SYSTEMS AFFECTED
Skin/exocrine

### SIGNALMENT
No specific age, breed, or sex predilection

### SIGNS
- The pattern and degree of hair loss are important for establishing a differential diagnosis.
- Multifocal patches of alopecia—most frequently associated with folliculitis from parasitic, mycotic, or bacteria infection
- Large diffuse areas of alopecia—indicate a follicular dysplasia or metabolic component; not reported in rabbits
- May be acute in onset or slowly progressive

### CAUSES
- Normal shedding pattern—some breeds, especially dwarf, miniature lop, and angora rabbits, lose hair in patches when shedding, leaving well-demarcated areas of short hair.
- Behavioral—barbering—dominant cage mates may chew or pull out hair of submissive rabbit, especially on flanks.
- Parasitic—*Cheyletiella*, ear mites, fleas
- Endocrine—pregnant or pseudopregnant females will pull hair from chest and abdomen to line nest.
- Infectious—bacterial pyoderma, dermatophytosis; most often a secondary problem, especially moist dermatitis
- Neoplastic—cutaneous lymphoma, mast cell tumor
- Immunologic—contact dermatitis
- Nutrition—particularly protein deficiencies
- Trauma—foot pad alopecia

### RISK FACTORS
N/A

## DIAGNOSIS

### DIFFERENTIAL DIAGNOSIS

#### Differentiating Causes
Pattern and degree—important features for formulating a differential diagnosis

#### Symmetrical
Barbering—hair loss along the flanks, face, nape of neck, and/or body wall. Close examination reveals broken hairs. Dominant cage mate pulls/chews hairs on submissive rabbit; owners may not observe this behavior.

#### Multifocal to Focal
- *Cheyletiella* sp. (or less commonly, *Leporacarus gibbus*)—lesions are usually located in the intrascapular or tail base region and associated with copious amounts of large, white scale. Mites are readily identified in skin scrapes or acetate tape preparations under low magnification.
- Ear mites—alopecia around ear base, pinna; may extend to face, neck, abdomen, perineal region; intense pruritus; brown, beige, crusty exudate in the ear canal and pinna
- Fleas—patchy alopecia; finding flea dirt will help to differentiate; secondary pyoderma sometimes seen
- Other ectoparasites—*Sarcoptes scabiei* and *Notoedres cati* rarely infest rabbits. Lesions are located around the head and neck and are intensely pruritic.
- Injection reactions—alopecia, scabs, scale, erythema, usually in the intrascapular region as this is a common site of subcutaneous injections
- Normal shedding pattern—some breeds, especially dwarf, miniature lop, and angora rabbits, lose hair in patches when shedding, leaving well-demarcated alopecic areas.
- Lack of grooming—may cause alopecia and an accumulation of scale in intrascapular or tail base regions
- Contact dermatitis—alopecia with or without erythema; scale on ventral abdomen or other contact areas
- Moist dermatitis—alopecia, with or without erythema, scale, or ulceration. Facial—associated with epiphora or ptyalism; perineal/ventrum—associated with urinary disease, diarrhea, or uneaten cecotrophs
- Dermatophytosis—partial to complete alopecia with scaling, with or without erythema; not always ringlike; may begin as small papules
- *Treponema cuniculi* (rabbit syphilis)—alopecia; crusts at mucocutaneous junctions, especially nose, lips, and genitalia

- Neoplasia—cutaneous lymphoma, cutaneous epitheliotropic lymphoma (mycoses fungoides), or mast cell tumors—rare in rabbits; focal or diffuse truncal alopecia; scaling and erythema; may see plaque formation

### CBC/BIOCHEMISTRY/URINALYSIS
To identify underlying disease, especially in rabbits with perineal dermatitis or urine scald

### OTHER LABORATORY TESTS
Serologic testing for *Treponema cuniculi* if consistent lesions are identified

### IMAGING
Radiographs—skull/dental to identify underlying dental disease in rabbits with moist dermatitis secondary to chronic epiphora or ptyalism; whole body radiographs may be helpful in identifying spinal/orthopedic, gastrointestinal, or renal diseases contributing to perineal or ventral moist dermatitis.

### DIAGNOSTIC PROCEDURES
- Fungal culture
- Skin scraping; acetate tape preparation
- Cytology
- Skin biopsy (silver staining to identify *Treponema cuniculi*)

## TREATMENT
- Treatment must be specific to the underlying cause to be successful.
- Moist dermatitis—identify and correct underlying cause (dental disease in facial or dewlap dermatitis; urinary, gastrointestinal, or musculoskeletal disease in perineal/ventral dermatitis).
- Separate from dominant rabbits if barbering is suspected.

## MEDICATIONS

### DRUG(S) OF CHOICE
Varies with specific cause
- Ear mites—ivermectin 1% (0.4 mg/kg SC q10–14d) for two to three doses or selamectin. (Revolution, Pfizer) (6–12 mg/kg) applied topically q30d. Treat all affected animals; clean the environment.
- *Cheyletiella*—ivermectin 1% (0.4 mg/kg SC q10–14d) for two to three doses or selamectin (Revolution, Pfizer) (6–12 mg/kg) applied topically q30d. Treat all affected animals; clean the environment.

• Fleas—imidacloprid (Advantage, Bayer) one dose for cats less than 9 lbs. divided onto two to three spots topically q30d (anecdotal dosage) or selamectin (Revolution, Pfizer) (6–12 mg/kg) applied topically q30d. Treat all affected animals; clean the environment.

• Sarcoptic mange—ivermectin (0.2–0.4 mg/kg SC q14d) for three to four doses

• Bacterial folliculitis—antibiotic therapy, preferably based on culture and susceptibility testing; good initial choices include enrofloxacin (5–20 mg/kg PO q12–24h) and trimethoprim sulfa (30 mg/kg PO q12h).

• Dermatophytosis—lime sulfur dip q7d has been used successfully; lime sulfur is odiferous and can stain; dipping is often difficult to perform on rabbits; 1% clotrimazole cream for focal lesions; itraconazole (5 mg/kg PO q24h) for 4–6 weeks or griseofulvin (25 mg/kg PO q24h) for 4–6 weeks for refractory cases

• Treponema cuniculi—penicillin g, benzathine (42,000–84,000 IU/kg IM q7d) for three treatments. Treat all affected rabbits.

• Neoplasia—various chemotherapy protocols

## CONTRAINDICATIONS

• Oral administration of antibiotics that select against Gram-positive bacteria (penicillins, macrolides, lincosamides, and cephalosporins) can cause fatal enteric dysbiosis and enterotoxemia.

• The use of corticosteroids (systemic or topical) can severely exacerbate infectious causes of alopecia. Corticosteroid use is associated with gastrointestinal ulceration and hemorrhage, delayed wound healing, and heightened susceptibility to infection.

• Do not use fipronil on rabbits.

• Do not use flea collars on rabbits.

• Do not use organophosphate-containing products on rabbits.

• Do not use straight permethrin sprays or permethrin spot-ons on rabbits.

## PRECAUTIONS

• Use extreme caution when dipping or bathing rabbits due to the high risk of skeletal fractures and excessive chilling with inexperienced owners.

• Most flea-control products discussed above are off-label use. Safety and efficacy

has not been evaluated in rabbits. Use with caution, especially in young or debilitated animals.

• Prevent rabbits or their cage mates from licking topical spot-on products before they are dry.

• Toxicity—if any signs are noted, the animal should be bathed thoroughly to remove any remaining chemicals and treated appropriately.

• Topical flea preparation for use in dogs and cats, such as permethrins and pyrethrins, are less effective and may be toxic to rabbits.

• Griseofulvin—bone marrow suppression reported in dogs and cats as an idiosyncratic reaction or with prolonged therapy; not yet reported in rabbits but may occur; weekly or biweekly CBC is recommended. Neurologic side effects reported in dogs and cats—monitor for this possibility in rabbits; do not use during the first two trimesters of pregnancy; it is teratogenic.

• Oral administration of any antibiotic may potentially cause enteric dysbiosis; discontinue use if diarrhea or anorexia occurs.

## POSSIBLE INTERACTIONS

None

## ALTERNATIVE DRUGS

Ketoconazole (10–15 mg/kg PO q24h) for dermatophytes—efficacy and safety in rabbits is unknown. Hepatopathy reported in dogs and cats can be quite severe.

 **FOLLOW-UP**

### PATIENT MONITORING

Varies with cause

### POSSIBLE COMPLICATIONS

N/A

 **MISCELLANEOUS**

### ASSOCIATED CONDITIONS

• Dental disease
• Musculoskeletal disease
• Obesity

### AGE-RELATED FACTORS

N/A

### ZOONOTIC POTENTIAL

Dermatophytosis and *Cheyletiella* can cause skin lesions in people.

### PREGNANCY

Avoid griseofulvin and ivermectin in pregnant animals.

### SYNONYMS

None

### SEE ALSO

• Cheyletiellosis
• Dermatophytosis
• Ear mites
• Epiphora
• Fleas
• Ptyalism

### ABBREVIATION

CBC = complete blood count

*Suggested Reading*

Clyde VL. Practical treatment and control of common ectoparasites in exotic pets. Vet Med 1996;91(7):632–637.

Harcourt-Brown F. Skin diseases. In: Harcourt-Brown F, ed. Textbook of Rabbit Medicine. Oxford: Butterworth-Heinemann, 2002:224–248.

Hess L. Dermatologic diseases. In: Quesenberry KE, Carpenter JW, eds. Ferrets, Rabbits and Rodents: Clinical Medicine and Surgery. 2nd Ed. Philadelphia: WB Saunders, 2004:194–202.

Jenkins JR. Skin disorders of the rabbit. Vet Clin North Am Exotic Anim Pract 2001;4(2):543–563.

*Portions Adapted From*

Rhodes KH. Alopecia. In: Tilley LP, Smith FWK, Jr., eds. The 5-Minute Veterinary Consult: Canine and Feline, 3rd Ed. Baltimore: Lippincott Williams & Wilkins, 2004.

# ANOREXIA AND PSEUDOANOREXIA

 BASICS

## DEFINITION
• The lack or loss of appetite for food; appetite is psychologic and depends on memory and associations, compared with hunger, which is physiologically aroused by the body's need for food; the existence of appetite in animals is assumed.
• The term pseudoanorexia is used to describe animals that have a desire for food, but are unable to eat because they cannot prehend, chew, or swallow food. Pseudoanorexia due to dental disease is one of the most common causes of lack of food intake in rabbits.

## PATHOPHYSIOLOGY
• Anorexia is most often associated with systemic disease but can be caused by many different mechanisms.
• The control of appetite is a complex interaction between the CNS and the periphery.
• The regulation of food intake also depends on the peripheral control of appetite.
• The gastric distension theory suggests that gastric distension promotes satiety, which is probably hormonally mediated.
• Beyond the stomach, satiety can be induced by placing food in the small intestine.
• Inflammatory, infectious, metabolic, or neoplastic diseases can cause inappetence, probably as a result of the release of a variety of chemical mediators.
• Pseudoanorexia is commonly associated with oral pain or inability to chew due to dental disease.

## SYSTEMS AFFECTED
All body systems are affected; breakdown of the intestinal mucosal barrier and enteric dysbiosis are particularly important in sick patients.

## SIGNALMENT
Depends on the underlying cause

## SIGNS

### Historical Findings
• Refusal to eat is a common complaint presented by rabbit owners, because owners often associate a poor appetite with illness.
• Clinical signs in true anorexia vary and are related to the underlying cause.
• Fecal pellets often become scant and small in size.
• Rabbits with gastrointestinal tract disease (especially gastrointestinal tract hypomotility) often initially stop eating pellets but continue to eat treats, followed by complete anorexia.
• Signs of pain, such as teeth grinding, a hunched posture, and reluctance to move, are extremely common in rabbits with oral disease or gastrointestinal hypomotility.

• Patients with disorders causing dysfunction or pain of the face, neck, oropharynx, and esophagus may display an interest in food but be unable to complete prehension and swallowing (pseudoanorexia).
• Pseudoanorectic patients commonly display weight loss, excessive drooling, difficulty in prehension and mastication of food, halitosis, dysphagia, and odynophagia (painful eating). This may be preceded by a preference for softer foods such as lettuce.

### Physical Examination Findings
• Reluctance to eat may be the only abnormality identified after an evaluation of the patient history and physical examination; this is typical in rabbits with gastrointestinal tract diseases or pseudoanorexia from oral disease prior to thorough examination of the oral cavity.
• Most underlying causes of pseudoanorexia can be identified by a thorough examination of the face, mandible, teeth, neck, oropharynx, and esophagus for dental disease, ulceration, traumatic lesions, masses, foreign bodies, and neuromuscular dysfunction.
• A thorough examination of the oral cavity, including the incisors, molars and buccal and lingual mucosa, is necessary to rule out dental disease. Use of an otoscope or speculum may be useful in identifying severe abnormalities; however, many problems will be missed by using this method alone. A thorough examination of the cheek teeth requires heavy sedation or general anesthesia and specialized equipment. Use a focused, directed light source and magnification (or a rigid endoscope, if available) to provide optimal visualization. Use a rodent mouth gag and cheek dilators (Jorgensen Laboratories, Inc., Loveland, CO) to open the mouth and pull buccal tissues away from teeth surfaces to allow adequate exposure. Identify cheek teeth elongation, irregular crown height, spikes, curved teeth, oral ulceration, or abscesses.
• Significant tooth root abnormalities may be present despite normal-appearing crowns. Skull films are required to identify apical disorders.
• Abdominal palpation is an extremely valuable tool in the diagnosis of gastrointestinal hypomotility or stasis disorders. The presence of hair and ingesta is normal and should be palpable in the stomach of a healthy rabbit. The normal stomach should be easily deformable, feel soft and pliable, and not remain pitted on compression. A firm, noncompliant stomach or stomach contents that remain pitted on compression is an abnormal finding.
• Gas distension of the intestines or cecum is common in rabbits with gastrointestinal tract disease

• Abdominal palpation may also reveal the presence of organomegaly, masses, or gastrointestinal foreign bodies.
• Auscultation of the thorax may reveal cardiac murmurs, arrhythmias, or abnormal breath sounds.
• Auscultation of the abdomen may reveal decreased or absent borborygmus in rabbits with gastrointestinal hypomotility. Borborygmus may be increased in rabbits with acute intestinal obstruction.

## CAUSES

### Anorexia
• Almost any systemic disease process
• Gastrointestinal disease is one of the most common causes—especially problems related to gastrointestinal hypomotility or stasis; gastric ulceration may also contribute.
• Pain—especially in rabbits with dental disease, orthopedic disorders, or urolithiasis
• Metabolic disease—especially hepatic or renal disease
• Neoplasia involving any site
• Cardiac failure
• Infectious disease
• Respiratory disease
• Neurologic disease
• Psychologic—unpalatable diets, alterations in routine or environment, stress
• Toxicosis and drugs
• Musculoskeletal disorders
• Acid-base disorders
• Miscellaneous—high environmental temperature, etc.

### Pseudoanorexia
• Any disease process that interferes with the swallowing reflex
• Diseases causing painful prehension and mastication are extremely common, especially dental disease (e.g., malocclusion, dental abscess, molar impaction); stomatitis, glossitis, gingivitis (e.g., physical agents, caustics, bacterial infections, foreign bodies, uremia), retrobulbar abscess, oral or glossal neoplasia (e.g., squamous cell carcinoma), musculoskeletal disorders (mandible fracture or subluxation)
• Diseases causing oropharyngeal dysphagia (uncommon); glossal disorders (neurologic, neoplastic), pharyngitis, pharyngeal neoplasia, retropharyngeal disorders (lymphadenopathy, abscess, hematoma), neuromuscular disorders (CNS lesions, botulism)
• Diseases of the esophagus (rare)—esophagitis, neoplasia, and neuromuscular disorders

## RISK FACTORS
• Rabbits on a diet containing inadequate amounts of long-stem hay are at risk for developing disease related to gastrointestinal hypomotility and dental disease.
• Rabbits with limited exercise or mobility (cage restriction, orthopedic disorders, obe-

sity) are at higher risk of developing gastrointestinal motility disorders and hypercalciuria.

• Anesthesia and surgical procedures commonly cause temporary anorexia.

## DIAGNOSIS

### DIFFERENTIAL DIAGNOSIS

• Gastrointestinal hypomotility and stasis disorders are the most common causes of anorexia in rabbits, followed by pseudoanorexia from dental disease. Gastrointestinal hypomotility can be the result of improper diet or secondary to any disease process.

• Obtain a minimum database (CBC, biochemistry, whole-body radiographs) to help delineate underlying medical disorders.

• Questioning about the patient's interest in food and ability to prehend, masticate, and swallow food, along with a thorough examination of the animal's teeth, oropharynx, face, and neck, will help identify pseudoanorexia; if the owners are poor historians the patient should be observed while eating.

• A thorough history regarding the animal's environment, and diet, other animals and people in the household, and any recent changes involving any of these helps identify psychologic anorexia.

• A thorough history regarding the rabbit's diet, food and water consumption, and physical activity, as well as volume and character of fecal production will aid in the diagnosis of gastrointestinal motility disorders.

• Any abnormalities detected in the physical examination or historical evidence of illness mandates a diagnostic workup for the identified problem.

### CBC/BIOCHEMISTRY/URINALYSIS

Abnormalities vary with different underlying diseases and causes of pseudoanorexia and anorexia.

### OTHER LABORATORY TESTS

Special tests may be necessary to rule out specific diseases suggested by the history, physical examination, or minimum database (see other topics on specific diseases).

### IMAGING

• If underlying disease is suspected but no abnormalities are revealed by the physical examination or minimum database, perform abdominal radiography and abdominal ultrasonography to identify hidden conditions such as gastrointestinal tract disease, hepatic disease, urolithiasis, orthopedic disease, or neoplasia. Consider thoracic radiography to rule out cardiac or pulmonary disease.

• Skull films may identify the presence of and extent of dental disease.

• The need for further diagnostic imaging varies with the underlying condition suspected (see other topics on specific diseases).

### DIAGNOSTIC PROCEDURES

Vary with underlying condition suspected (see other topics regarding specific diseases)

## TREATMENT

• Treat underlying cause.

• Symptomatic therapy includes attention to fluid and electrolyte derangements, reduction in environmental stressors, and modification of the diet.

• Most rabbits that are anorectic have also refused water and are dehydrated to some degree. Lack of oral intake of fluid also contributes to desiccation of intestinal contents, gastrointestinal hypomotility, and further anorexia. The route of fluid therapy depends on the degree of dehydration, but most anorectic rabbits will benefit from oral or subcutaneous fluids. Intravenous or intraosseous fluids are required in patients that are severely dehydrated or depressed; maintenance fluid requirements are estimated at 100 mL/kg/day.

• It is absolutely imperative that the rabbit begin eating as soon as possible, regardless of the underlying cause. Continued anorexia will exacerbate gastrointestinal hypomotility and cause further derangement of the gastrointestinal microflora and overgrowth of intestinal bacterial pathogens.

• Offer a large selection of fresh, moistened greens such as cilantro, romaine lettuce, parsley, carrot tops, dandelion greens, spinach, collard greens, etc., and good-quality grass hay. Many rabbits will begin to eat these foods, even if they were previously anorectic. Also offer the rabbit's usual pelleted diet, because the initial goal is to get the rabbit to eat.

• If the patient refuses these foods, syringe feed a gruel such as Critical Care for Herbivores (Oxbow Pet Products, Murdock, NE) 10–15 mL/kg PO q6–8h. Larger volumes and more frequent feedings are often accepted; feed as much as the rabbit will readily accept. Alternatively, pellets can be ground and mixed with fresh greens, vegetable baby foods, water, or juice to form a gruel. The addition of canned pumpkin to this gruel is a palatable source of fiber and calories. If sufficient volumes of food are not accepted in this manner, nasogastric intubation is indicated.

• High-carbohydrate, high-fat nutritional supplements are contraindicated.

• The diet should be permanently modified to include sufficient amounts of roughage and long-stemmed hay.

• Parenteral nutrition may be provided via infusion through a polyurethane jugular catheter using a syringe pump.

• Encourage exercise for 10- to 15-minute intervals every 6–8 hours, unless contraindicated by underlying condition.

## MEDICATIONS

### DRUG(S) OF CHOICE

• Depends on the underlying cause

• Anorexia, regardless of the cause, contributes to or causes gastrointestinal tract hypomotility. The use of promotility agents, such as metoclopramide (0.2–0.5 mg/kg PO, SC q6–8h) or cisapride (0.5 mg/kg PO q8–12h) may be helpful in regaining normal motility; cisapride is available through many compounding pharmacies.

• $H_2$-receptor antagonists may ameliorate or prevent gastric ulceration—cimetidine (5–10 mg/kg PO, SC, IM, IV q6–12h) or ranitidine (2 mg/kg IV q24h or 2–5 mg/kg PO q12h)

• Analgesics such as buprenorphine (0.01–0.05 mg/kg SC, IM, IV q8–12h) or meloxicam (0.2–0.5 mg/kg PO q24h). Pain is common in rabbits with orthopedic disorders, dental disease, and intestinal distention; pain impairs mobility and decreases appetite and may severely inhibit recovery.

### CONTRAINDICATIONS

Avoid promotility agents if gastrointestinal obstruction is present or suspected.

### PRECAUTIONS

Meloxicam—use with caution in rabbits with compromised renal function.

### POSSIBLE INTERACTIONS

N/A

### ALTERNATIVE DRUGS

N/A

## FOLLOW-UP

### PATIENT MONITORING

Body weight, production of fecal pellets, and hydration can be used to determine if management is effective.

### POSSIBLE COMPLICATIONS

• Dehydration, malnutrition, and cachexia are most likely; these exacerbate the underlying disease.

• Hepatic lipidosis is a possible complication of anorexia, especially in obese rabbits.

• Breakdown of the intestinal mucosal barrier is a concern in debilitated patients.

• Anorexia may cause enteric dysbiosis and subsequent enterotoxemia.

# ANOREXIA AND PSEUDOANOREXIA

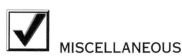 MISCELLANEOUS

**ASSOCIATED CONDITIONS**
See causes.

**AGE-RELATED FACTORS**
N/A

**ZOONOTIC POTENTIAL**
N/A

**PREGNANCY**
N/A

**SYNONYMS**
Inappetence

**SEE ALSO**
• Abscesses
• Cheek teeth malocclusion and elongation

• Gastrointestinal hypomotility
• Hypercalciuria
• Trichobezoars

**ABBREVIATIONS**
• CBC = complete blood count
• CNS = central nervous system

*Suggested Reading*
Brown SA, Rosenthal KL. The anorexic rabbit. Proc North Am Vet Conf 1997:788.
Crossley DA, Aiken S. Small mammal dentistry. In: Quesenberry KE, Carpenter JW, eds. Ferrets, Rabbits and Rodents: Clinical Medicine and Surgery. 2nd Ed. Philadelphia: WB Saunders, 2004:370–382.
Donoghue S. Nutrition and pet rabbits. In: Rosenthal KL, ed. Practical Exotic Animal Medicine: The Compendium Collection.

Trenton, NJ: Veterinary Learning Systems, 1997:107.
Jenkins JR. Gastrointestinal diseases. In: Quesenberry KE, Carpenter JW, eds. Ferrets, Rabbits and Rodents: Clinical Medicine and Surgery. 2nd Ed. Philadelphia: WB Saunders, 2004:161–171
Paul-Murphy JA, Ramer JC. Urgent care of the pet rabbit. Vet Clin North AM Exot Anim Pract 1998;1(1):127–152.

*Portions Adapted From*
Walker MC. Anorexia. In: Tilley LP, Smith FWK, Jr., eds. The 5-Minute Veterinary Consult: Canine and Feline, 2nd Ed. Baltimore: Lippincott Williams & Wilkins, 2004.

# ANTERIOR UVEITIS

## BASICS

### DEFINITION
Inflammation of the iris and/or ciliary body

### PATHOPHYSIOLOGY
• Common theme from all causes—tissue destruction secondary to breakdown of the blood–aqueous barrier
• Iridal abscesses, corneal stromal abscesses, and phacoclastic uveitis secondary to *Encephalitozoon cuniculi* and ulcerative keratitis are most common causes in rabbits.
• Associated most commonly with cellular infiltration, iridal congestion, aqueous flare, and hypopyon; keratic precipitates and corneal edema occasionally seen

### SYSTEMS AFFECTED
• Ophthalmic
• Others—if cause is a systemic disease

### GENETICS
N/A

### INCIDENCE/PREVALENCE
• Common
• True incidence unknown

### GEOGRAPHIC DISTRIBUTION
N/A

### SIGNALMENT
• *E. cuniculi*—more common in young, dwarf breeds
• Other causes—no age, breed, or gender predilection

### SIGNS

#### Historical Findings
• Usually owner complains of a change in appearance of the affected eye(s).
• May have history of respiratory disease, dental disease, abscesses, or CNS signs, depending on the underlying cause.

#### Physical Examination Findings
• Iridal swelling, white or pink nodule on the iris—common, especially in rabbits with *E. cuniculi* or iridal bacterial abscesses. Rabbits are often presented for evaluation of an intraocular white "mass," with the remainder of the eye appearing relatively quiet.
• Ocular discomfort—suggested by photophobia, blepharospasm, and epiphora. Rabbits are less likely to show discomfort, but pain is more difficult to assess in rabbits because they are "prey" species and less likely to outwardly demonstrate pain.
• Conjunctival hyperemia—common; nonspecific indication of ocular irritation
• Fibrinous exudation—severe disease; may cause fibrin clot formation within the anterior chamber
• Intraocular pressure—usually low with anterior uveitis; depends on severity and dura-

tion of disease; may be high with severe disease and secondary glaucoma
• Miosis—pupillary constriction; subtle miosis best observed in a darkened room by simultaneously examining both eyes with retroillumination
• Hypopyon (accumulation of WBCs in the anterior chamber)—develops with extreme breakdown of blood–aqueous barrier; cellular components typically settle homogeneously in the ventral anterior chamber; common finding in rabbits with iridal or corneal stromal abscesses and with ocular *E. cuniculi* infection
• Ciliary flush—may be observed in the limbal region; result of hyperemia of the perilimbal anterior ciliary vessels; along with conjunctival hyperemia, may contribute to red eye
• Aqueous flare—increased turbidity of aqueous humor; occasionally seen, but less common than in dogs and cats. It is not uncommon to have a large iris stromal abscess or granuloma present without seeing significant flare.
• Keratic precipitates—occasionally seen on the corneal endothelial surface; indicates active or previous disease
• Corneal edema—not as common as in dogs or cats
• Hyphema (accumulation of RBCs in the anterior chamber)—common with intraocular tumors and systemic hypertension

### CAUSES
Most common causes are bacterial iridal or corneal stromal abscesses, phacoclastic uveitis from *E. cuniculi*, or ulcerative keratitis.
• Bacterial—iridial or corneal stromal abscess most often seen; either hematogenous spread (iridial abscess) or secondary to keratitis (corneal stromal abscess); caused by any systemic bacterial disease (*Pasteurella* most common) or underlying dental or respiratory disease (corneal stromal abscess)
• *E. cuniculi*—in utero infection, vertical transmission of organism into the developing lens. Replication of spores within the lens of young rabbits results in cataract formation with a thin anterior portion, or lens rupture, resulting in phacoclastic uveitis with focal granuloma formation at site of rupture.
• Ulcerative keratitis—common cause, secondary to trauma, chronic dacryocystitis, conjunctivitis, or environmental irritants
• Other infectious agents—fungal, protozoan, or viral not well described in rabbits
• Traumatic—blunt or penetrating injuries common
• Immune mediated—cataracts (lens-induced uveitis); lens trauma (rupture of lens capsule)
• Neoplastic (primary or secondary)—primary uncommon in rabbits; lymphoma

and metastasis from other neoplasia (e.g., uterine adenocarcinoma) more likely
• Metabolic—not described in rabbits

### RISK FACTORS
Immunosuppression—stress, poor diet, dental disease, and glucocorticoid therapy, especially rabbits with bacterial infection or *E. cuniculi*

## DIAGNOSIS

### DIFFERENTIAL DIAGNOSIS
• Conjunctivitis—clinical signs (hyperemia, chemosis, ocular discharge, and pain) vary, depending on the duration and severity; normal intraocular pressure and intraocular examination
• Glaucoma—pupil usually dilated; clinical signs may be identical; must measure intraocular pressure to distinguish
• Ulcerative keratitis—may be accompanied by anterior uveitis
• Horner syndrome—may have similar appearance because the pupil is miotic and upper lid ptosis creates the impression of blepharospasm; normal intraocular pressure; no aqueous flare; conjunctiva not injected or mildly injected

### CBC/BIOCHEMISTRY/URINALYSIS
CBC, serum biochemistry, and urinalysis—usually unremarkable; may reflect underlying systemic disease

### OTHER LABORATORY TESTS
• Serologic testing for *E. cuniculi*—many tests are available, but usefulness is extremely limited since a positive titer indicates only exposure and does not confirm *E. cuniculi* as the cause of uveitis. *E. cuniculi* can only be definitively diagnosed by finding organisms and resultant lesions on ocular histopathology or by positive DNA probe on removed lens material. Antibody titers usually become positive by 2 weeks postinfection, but generally do not continue to rise with active infection or decline with treatment. No correlation exits between antibody titers and shedding of organism and presence or severity of disease. It is unknown if exposed rabbits eventually become seronegative. Available tests include ELISA, indirect IFA, and carbon immunoassay.
• Serology for *Pasteurella*—usefulness is severely limited and generally not helpful in the diagnosis of pasteurellosis in pet rabbits. An ELISA is available and results reported as negative, low positive, or high positive. Positive results, even when high, only indicate prior exposure to *Pasteurella* and the development of antibodies and do not confirm active infection. Low-positive results may occur due to cross-reaction with other, nonpathogenic bacteria (false positive).

# ANTERIOR UVEITIS

False-negative results are common with immunosuppression or early infection. No evidence exists to support correlation of titers to the presence or absence of disease.

## IMAGING
• Skull radiographs—rule out underlying dental disease and nasal, sinus, or maxillary bone lesions
• CT—superior to radiographs to identify underlying dental disease and nasal, sinus, or maxillary bone lesions
• Thoracic radiographs—rule out neoplastic (and possibly fungal) diseases or abscesses
• Abdominal radiographs and ultrasound—for palpable abdominal mass
• Ocular ultrasonography—for trauma; rule out penetrating wounds and foreign bodies not obviously visible; when the ocular media are too opaque to allow complete examination of the eye

## DIAGNOSTIC PROCEDURES
• Aqueous humor paracentesis—seldom helpful
• Tonometry—usually reveals low intraocular pressure unless primary or secondary glaucoma is present. Normal intraocular pressure reported as 10–20 mm Hg when measured by applanation tonometry
• Nasolacrimal duct flush—identifies patients with dacryocystitis
• Fluorescein stain—rule out ulcerative keratitis; corneal epithelium usually intact with corneal stromal abscess; test for nasolacrimal function.
• Thorough adnexal examination—rule out lid abnormalities, lash abnormalities, and foreign bodies in cul-de-sacs or under nictitans.

## PATHOLOGIC FINDINGS
• *E. cuniculi*—phacoclastic uveitis secondary to lens rupture; leakage results in inflammation and granuloma formation, usually on the iris surrounding the rupture. Histologically may see *E. cuniculi* organisms in lens material or may detect using DNA probe
• Eye—conjunctival hyperemia, ciliary flush, aqueous flare, miosis, variable vision
• Iridal abscesses—often walled off; composed of accumulations of degenerate neutrophils, lymphocytes, and plasma cells

# TREATMENT

## APPROPRIATE HEALTH CARE
• Inpatient—severe disease and/or high intraocular pressure; for initial diagnostic workup and medical management
• Outpatient—mild to moderate disease

## NURSING CARE
N/A

## ACTIVITY
No restrictions

## DIET
Make sure that the rabbit continues to eat to avoid secondary gastrointestinal disorders.

## CLIENT EDUCATION
• Discuss the need for early aggressive medical management and a thorough diagnostic workup to identify the cause.
• Warn client of the adverse sequelae, including blindness, cataracts, endophthalmitis or panophthalmitis, lens luxation, phthisis bulbi, posterior synechiae with iris bombé, and secondary glaucoma.

## SURGICAL CONSIDERATIONS
• Lens removal by phacoemulsification is recommended in rabbits with ocular *E. cuniculi*. Spontaneous lens regeneration can occur in rabbits; insertion of prosthetic lens post–lens removal is not recommended. May recur following treatment, requiring medical treatment or enucleation
• Enucleation may be indicated in rabbits with iridal abscess, severe phacoclastic uveitis, or panophthalmitis when medical therapy is not successful or rabbit is painful. Enucleation can be more difficult than for dogs or cats due to the presence of a large orbital venous plexus that increases the risk of hemorrhage.

# MEDICATIONS

## DRUG(S) OF CHOICE

### Topically Applied Agents
• Frequency of treatment depends on the severity of disease.
• NSAIDs—0.03% flurbiprofen (Ocufen) or 1% diclofenac; q6h daily to control inflammation
• Mydriatic-cycloplegic drugs—1% atropine q12h for acute disease; to dilate the pupil, minimize posterior synechia and paralyze the ciliary muscle (cycloplegia); reduces ocular pain. May not be effective in all rabbits, since some species of rabbits produce atropinase; addition of 10% phenylephrine may facilitate mydriasis in these rabbits.
• Topical antibiotics, chloramphenicol, or ciprofloxacin first choice for corneal stromal abscess, dacryocystitis, keratitis; alternatively, triple antibiotic or gentamicin q6–12h, depending on organism isolated and severity of infection.

• Corticosteroids—1% prednisolone acetate; q6–12h with severe disease; use with extreme caution in rabbits (see precautions).

### Systemic Medications
• Systemic antibiotics—indicated in rabbits with iridal or corneal stromal abscess or to treat underlying bacterial disease. Choice of antibiotic is ideally based on results of culture and susceptibility testing. Use broad-spectrum antibiotics such as enrofloxacin (5–20 mg/kg PO, SC, IM q12–24h), trimethoprim sulfa (30 mg/kg PO q12h), or chloramphenicol (50 mg/kg PO q8h). Most facial or dental abscesses contain anaerobic bacteria; use antibiotics effective against anaerobes such as azithromycin (30 mg/kg PO q24h); can be used alone or combined with metronidazole (20 mg/kg PO q12h)
• Pain management—NSAIDs have been used for short- or long-term therapy to reduce pain and inflammation in rabbits with ocular pain: meloxicam (0.2–0.5 mg/kg PO q24h) and carprofen (2.2 mg/kg PO q12–24h)
• *E. cuniculi*—benzimidazole anthelmintics are effective against *E. cuniculi* in vitro and have been shown to prevent experimental infection in rabbits. However, efficacy in rabbits with clinical signs is unknown. Anecdotal reports suggest a response to treatment in rabbits with *E. cuniculi*–associated phacoclastic uveitis. Published treatments include albendazole (20–30 mg/kg q24h × 30 days, then 15 mg/kg PO q24h for 30 days) and fenbendazole (20 mg/kg q24h × 5–28 days). A 7- to 10-day course of treatment may be sufficient in rabbits with ocular disease only.

## CONTRAINDICATIONS
• Topical corticosteroids—never use if the cornea retains fluorescein stain, if abscesses are present, or if bacterial infection is suspected.
• Oral administration of most antibiotics effective against anaerobes will cause a fatal gastrointestinal dysbiosis in rabbits. Do not administer penicillins, macrolides, lincosamides, and cephalosporins by oral administration.
• Atropine in rabbits with glaucoma

## PRECAUTIONS
• Topical corticosteroids or antibiotic–corticosteroid combinations—avoid; associated with gastrointestinal ulceration and hemorrhage, iatrogenic diabetes mellitus, delayed wound healing, and heightened susceptibility to infection; rabbits are very sensitive to the immunosuppressive effects of both topic and systemic corticosteroids; use may exacerbate subclinical bacterial infection.

• Albendazole has been associated with bone marrow toxicity in dogs and cats; toxicity in rabbits is unknown; however, anecdotal reports of pancytopenia leading to death in rabbits exist.
• Topical aminoglycosides—may be irritating; may impede reepithelialization if used frequently or at high concentrations
• Topical solutions—are preferable to ointments if corneal perforation is possible
• Topical antibiotics—may lead to enteric dysbiosis if excessive ingestion occurs during grooming
• Atropine—may exacerbate KCS and glaucoma
• Topical atropine—may cause salivation

**POSSIBLE INTERACTIONS**
N/A

**ALTERNATIVE DRUGS**
N/A

 **FOLLOW-UP**

**PATIENT MONITORING**
• Complete ocular examination—repeated 5–7 days after initiation of treatment for severe disease
• Intraocular pressure—monitored for secondary glaucoma
• Reevaluation—every 2–3 weeks, depending on response to treatment

**PREVENTION/AVOIDANCE**
N/A

**POSSIBLE COMPLICATIONS**
• Adverse sequelae—blindness; cataracts; endophthalmitis or panophthalmitis; iris atrophy; lens luxation; phthisis bulbi; rubeosis iridis; posterior synechiae with iris bombé; secondary glaucoma
• Secondary glaucoma—frequent complication; tends to be recalcitrant to medical treatment

**EXPECTED COURSE AND PROGNOSIS**
• Regardless of the initial response to treatment, treat for at least 2 months with decreasing frequency because the blood–aqueous barrier remains disrupted for about 8 weeks after an insult.

• *E. cuniculi* associated uveitis—depends on severity and chronicity of infection and presence of secondary bacterial infections—if cannot treat surgically, prognosis for viability of the affected eye is guarded as most will progress to glaucoma.
• Iridal abscesses—often do not respond well to medical treatment; enucleation may be necessary.
• Corneal stromal abscess—good to fair prognosis when treated early and aggressively with topical and systemic antibiotics; with advanced disease and panophthalmitis—poor prognosis for viability of affected eye; enucleation may be required.
• Secondary to a systemic disease—prognosis usually determined by the systemic disease rather than by the anterior uveitis
• Prognosis for resolution of inflammation without deleterious sequelae—depends on severity of the disease at initial examination and on the response to aggressive medical treatment

 **MISCELLANEOUS**

**ASSOCIATED CONDITIONS**
N/A

**AGE-RELATED FACTORS**
*E. cuniculi*–related anterior uveitis seen most often in young rabbits <2 years old

**ZOONOTIC POTENTIAL**
*E. cuniculi*—unlikely, but possible in immunosuppressed humans. Modes of transmission and susceptibility in humans are unclear.

**PREGNANCY**
• Systemic steroids—do not use in pregnant animals if at all avoidable.
• Topical steroids—use with caution; systemic absorption occurs.

**SYNONYM**
Iridocyclitis

**SEE ALSO**
• *E. cuniculi*
• Pasteurellosis
• Red eye
• Tooth root abscess

**ABBREVIATIONS**
• CBC = complete blood count
• CNS = central nervous system
• CT = computed tomography
• ELISA = enzyme-linked immunosorbent assay
• IFA = immunofluorescence assay
• KCS = keratoconjunctivitis sicca
• NSAIDs = nonsteroidal antiinflammatory drugs
• WBC = white blood cell

*Suggested Reading*
Andrew SE. Corneal disease of rabbits. Vet Clin Noth AM: Exotic Anim Pract 2002;5(2):341–356.
Felchle LM, Sigler RL. Phacoemulsification for the management of *Encephalitozoon cuniculi*-induced phacoclastic uveitis in a rabbit. *Vet Ophthalmol* 2002;5(3):211–215.
Munger RJ, Langevin JP. Spontaneous cataracts in laboratory rabbits. Vet Ophthalmol 2002;5(3):177–181.
Stiles J, Dider E, Ritchie B, et al. *Encephalitozoon cuniculi* in the lens of a rabbit with phacoclastic uveitis: confirmation and treatment. Vet Comp Ophthalmol 1997;7(4):233–238.
Van der Woerdt A. Ophthalmologic disease in small pet animals. In: Quesenberry KE, Carpenter JW, ed. Ferrets, Rabbits and Rodents: Clinical Medicine and Surgery. 2nd Ed. Philadelphia: WB Saunders, 2004:421–428.
Williams DL. Laboratory animal ophthalmology. In: Gelatt KN, ed. Veterinary ophthalmology. 3rd Ed. Philadelphia: Lippincott Williams & Wilkins, 1999:151–181.

*Portions Adapted From*
Ringle MJ. Anterior Uveitis—Cats. In: Tilley LP, Smith FWK, Jr., eds. The 5-Minute Veterinary Consult: Canine and Feline, 2nd Ed. Baltimore: Lippincott Williams & Wilkins, 2000.

# ANTICOAGULANT RODENTICIDE POISONING

## BASICS

### OVERVIEW
• Coagulopathy caused by reduced vitamin K1–dependent clotting factors in the circulation after ingestion of anticoagulant rodenticides
• Relatively common toxicosis in rabbits—many baits are sold over the counter and widely used in homes.
• Variable susceptibility to poisoning—some laboratory rabbits have demonstrated genetically determined resistance to warfarin toxicosis; however, all rabbits ingesting or suspected to have ingested toxin should be treated.
• Secondary toxicosis by consumption of poisoned rodents does not occur in rabbits.

### SIGNALMENT
• No breed, age, or sex predilections
• More common in rabbits allowed to free-roam in the house or outdoors

### SIGNS

#### General Comments
• Clinical signs may not begin for several days postingestion, depending on the dose of toxin ingested and the amount of circulating clotting factors present in the rabbit.
• May be slightly more prevalent in the spring and fall when rodenticide products are used

#### Historical Findings
• Use of anticoagulant rodenticides
• Dyspnea
• Bleeding
• Hematuria or hematochezia

#### Physical Examination Findings
• Hematomas—often ventral and at venipuncture sites
• Muffled heart or lung sounds
• Pale mucous membranes
• Lethargy
• Depression
• Swollen joints

### CAUSES AND RISK FACTORS
• Exposure to anticoagulant rodenticide products
• Small doses over several days more dangerous than a single large dose; either type of exposure may cause toxicosis.
• First-generation coumarin anticoagulants (e.g., warfarin, pindone)—largely replaced by more potent second-generation anticoagulants
• Second-generation anticoagulants (e.g., brodifacoum, bromadiolone, diphacinone, and chlorphacinone)—generally more toxic and persist much longer before excretion than first-generation agents

• Difenthialone (D-Cease)—highly toxic to rats and mice

## DIAGNOSIS

### DIFFERENTIAL DIAGNOSES
• DIC—especially secondary to endotoxin; rabbits are more susceptible to endotoxin-induced intravascular coagulation than many other mammalian species.
• Congenital clotting factor deficiencies—not well described in rabbits
• Chronic, severe hepatopathy

### CBC/BIOCHEMISTRY/URINALYSIS
Anemia—with marked hemorrhage

### OTHER LABORATORY TESTS
• Bleeding time—prolongation supports coagulopathy. Normal values not well described. One report of normal time for cut made on the marginal ear vein was 2.91 +/− 0.85 minutes (n = 6).
• Prolonged PT and PTT—support exposure to rodenticide; PT affected earlier than is PTT. Normal values not well described in rabbits. May simultaneously obtain a coagulation profile from a normal rabbit to use as control. One study reported PT range of 7.5 +/− 1.5 seconds to 14.6 +/− 4.3 seconds (n = 12). APTT values were 32.8 +/− 4.5 seconds (n = 6).
• Analysis of blood or liver—confirms exposure to a specific product

### IMAGING
Thoracic radiography—may detect hemothorax or hemopericardium

### DIAGNOSTIC PROCEDURES
Thoracentesis—dyspneic patients; may confirm hemothorax

### PATHOLOGIC FINDINGS
• Free blood in the thoracic cavity, lungs, and abdominal cavity
• Hemorrhage into the cranial vault, gastrointestinal tract, and urinary tract

## TREATMENT

### APPROPRIATE HEALTH CARE
• Inpatient—acute crisis
• Outpatient—consider once the coagulopathy is stabilized or treating patients with history of exposure prior to the onset of clinical signs.
• Treatment immediately postingestion (24–48 hours)—administer activated charcoal; apply an Elizabethan collar to prevent ingestion of cecotrophs for 3 days postingestion.

• Have the owner bring the package from the product ingested to the veterinary hospital to identify the specific type of rodenticide ingested. Duration of therapy is dependent of type of toxin ingested.

### NURSING CARE
• Cannot induce vomition
• Fresh whole blood or plasma transfusion—may be required with hemorrhaging; provides immediate access to vitamin K–dependent clotting factors; whole blood may be preferred with severe anemia from acute or chronic blood loss. Perform in-house crossmatch prior to administration; transfusion reactions not described for rabbits

### ACTIVITY
Confine patient during the early stages; activity enhances blood loss.

### DIET
Be sure the rabbit continues to eat; anorexia is a significant risk factor in the development of gastrointestinal hypomotility, stasis, and potentially fatal dysbiosis.

## MEDICATIONS

### DRUG(S) OF CHOICE
• Vitamin K1—2.5 mg/kg PO q24h for 10–30 days (depending on the specific product); the injectable form may be administered orally; bioavailability enhanced by the concurrent feeding of a small amount of fat; has also been administered IM (2–10 mg/kg PRN), however anaphylactic reactions have been reported anecdotally with IV or SC administration.
• Vitamin K1 administration—continued for 14 days following warfarin exposure, for 21 days following bromadiolone exposure, and for 30 days following exposure to brodifacoum and other second-generation anticoagulants
• Activated charcoal—after acute ingestion (24–48 hours postingestion); does not detoxify but prevents absorption if properly used. Dosage—1–3 g/kg body weight in a concentration of 1 g charcoal/5–10 mL water. Dosage may need to be repeated. Administer via syringe (when possible) or via orogastric tube.

### CONTRAINDICATIONS
• Cannot induce vomition
• Vitamin K3—not efficacious in the treatment of anticoagulant rodenticide toxicosis; contraindicated
• Intravenous vitamin K1—reported anaphylactic reactions; avoid this route of administration.

# ANTICOAGULANT RODENTICIDE POISONING

## PRECAUTIONS
• Subcutaneous vitamin K1 administration—anaphylactic reactions anecdotally reported
• Avoid unnecessary surgical procedures and parenteral injections.
• Use the smallest possible needle when giving an injection or collecting samples.
• Activated charcoal—monitor rabbit for signs of gastrointestinal hypomotility and treat accordingly for several days after treatment.

## POSSIBLE INTERACTIONS
Sulfonamides and phenylbutazone—may displace anticoagulant rodenticides from plasma-binding sites, leading to more free toxicant and toxicosis

## ALTERNATIVE DRUGS
None

## FOLLOW-UP

### PATIENT MONITORING
PT—assess efficacy of therapy; monitoring continued 3–5 days after discontinuation of treatment

## MISCELLANEOUS

### ABBREVIATIONS
• APTT = activated partial thromboplastin time
• DIC = disseminated intravascular coagulation
• PPT = partial thromboplastin time
• PT = prothrombin time

*Suggested Reading*
Dodds WJ. Rabbit and ferret hemostasis. In: Fudge AM, ed. Laboratory Medicine, Avian and Exotic Pets. Philadelphia: WB Saunders, 2000.
Murphy M, Gerken D. The anticoagulant rodenticides. In: Kirk RW, Bonagura J, eds. Current Veterinary Therapy X. Philadelphia: Saunders, 1989:143–146.
Paul-Murphy JA, Ramer JC. Urgent care of the pet rabbit. Vet Clin North Am Exot Anim Pract 1998;1(1):127–152.

*Portions Adapted From*
Murphy MJ. Anticoagulant Rodenticide Poisoning. In: Tilley LP, Smith FWK, Jr., eds. The 5-Minute Veterinary Consult: Canine and Feline, 3rd Ed. Baltimore: Lippincott Williams & Wilkins, 2004.

# ARTHRITIS—OSTEOARTHRITIS

 BASICS

## OVERVIEW
• Progressive deterioration of articular cartilage found in diarthrodial joints
• Degenerative joint disease—more appropriate term in veterinary medicine

## SIGNALMENT
• No breed or gender predilection
• Actual incidence not reported
• Hereditary or developmental disorders—young animals
• Trauma/infection induced—any age

## SIGNS

### General Comments
Radiographic severity may not correlate with clinical severity.

### Historical Findings
• Lameness or stiff gait; may be intermittent; slowly becomes more severe and frequent; may have history of previous joint trauma (fracture, ligament injury, dislocation), osteochondral disease, or developmental disorder
• Restricted motion, inability to hop (may be intermittent)
• Signs referable to an inability to properly groom or attain a normal stance while urinating due to stiffness or pain may be seen. Affected rabbits may not be able to groom the intrascapular, perineal, or tail head region, or may be unable to consume cecotrophs from the rectum resulting in feces or cecotrophs pasted to perineum. If unable to attain a normal stance while urinating, urine may soak the ventrum, resulting in urine scald.
• May be exacerbated by exercise, long periods of recumbency

### Physical Examination Findings
• Stiffness of gait
• Lameness
• Decreased range of motion
• Crepitus
• Joint swelling and pain
• Joint instability (ligament tear, subluxation), depending on the duration of disease
• Signs referable to inability to groom, depending on which joints are involved—feces pasted to perineum, flaky skin, urine scald, unkempt haircoat
• Obesity

## CAUSES AND RISK FACTORS
• Primary—thought to be the result of long-term use combined with aging; no identifiable predisposing cause
• Secondary—results from an initiating cause: joint instability, trauma, joint incongruity

 DIAGNOSIS

## DIFFERENTIAL DIAGNOSIS
• Septic arthritis
• Neoplasia
• Spondylosis deformans
• Urolithiasis
• Pododermatitis

## CBC/BIOCHEMISTRY/URINALYSIS
• CBC/biochemistry profile usually normal
• Urinalysis may reflect hypercalciuria or urinary tract infection secondary to insufficient voiding

## OTHER LABORATORY TESTS
N/A

## IMAGING
Radiographic changes—joint capsular distension; osteophytosis; soft tissue thickening; soft tissue mineralization; narrowed joint spaces. Oblique views of the spine may be helpful in delineating spinal arthritis.

## DIAGNOSTIC PROCEDURES
• Arthrocentesis and synovial fluid analysis—may support the diagnosis; slight increase in mononuclear cells; large numbers of neutrophils likely the result of infectious arthritis
• Bacterial culture and sensitivity—synovial fluid
• Biopsy of synovial tissue—helps rule out other arthritides or neoplasia

 TREATMENT

## APPROPRIATE HEALTH CARE
Treat as outpatient with limited exercise and analgesic administration.

## NURSING CARE
• Keep perineum clean, dry, and free of fecal matter
• Use soft bedding; keep bedding clean and dry to prevent dermatitis or bed sores
• Physical therapy—may be beneficial in enhancing limb function and general well-being; range-of-motion exercises, combination heat and cold therapy

## ACTIVITY
Limited to a level that minimizes aggravation of clinical signs

## DIET
• Weight reduction for obese patients—decreases stress placed on affected joints
• Rabbits in pain may be reluctant to eat. It is absolutely imperative that the rabbit continue to eat during and following treatment. Anorexia will often cause gastrointestinal hypomotility, derangement of the gastroin-

testinal microflora, and overgrowth of intestinal bacterial pathogens.
• Offer a large selection of fresh, moistened greens such as cilantro, romaine lettuce, parsley, carrot tops, dandelion greens, spinach, collard greens, etc., and good-quality grass hay. Many rabbits will begin to eat these foods, even if they were previously anorectic. Also try offering pelleted diets.
• If the patient refuses these foods, syringe feed a gruel such as Critical Care for Herbivores (Oxbow Pet Products, Murdock, NE) 10–15 mL/kg PO q8–12h. Larger volumes and more frequent feedings are often accepted; feed as much as the rabbit will accept. Alternatively, pellets can be ground and mixed with fresh greens, vegetable baby foods, water, or juice to form a gruel. If sufficient volumes of food are not accepted in this manner, nasogastric intubation is indicated.
• High-carbohydrate, high-fat nutritional supplements should be avoided.
• Encourage oral fluid intake by offering fresh water and wetting leafy vegetables.

## CLIENT EDUCATION
• Inform client that medical therapy is palliative and the condition is likely to progress.
• Discuss treatment options, activity level, and diet.

## SURGICAL CONSIDERATIONS
• Arthrotomy—to treat underlying causes (osteochondral diseases)
• Reconstructive procedures—to eliminate joint instability
• Arthroplasty procedures—femoral head ostectomy as salvage procedure
• Arthrodesis—for selected chronic cases and for joint instability

 MEDICATIONS

## DRUG(S) OF CHOICE
NSAIDs—have been used for short- or long-term therapy to reduce pain and inflammation in rabbits with musculoskeletal disease: meloxicam (0.2–0.5 mg/kg PO q24h; 0.2 mg/kg SC, IM q24h); carprofen (2.2 mg/kg PO q12–24); use only when the patient is exhibiting signs.

## CONTRAINDICATIONS
Corticosteroids—associated with gastrointestinal ulceration and hemorrhage, delayed wound healing, and heightened susceptibility to infection; rabbits are very sensitive to the immunosuppressive effects of both topical and systemic corticosteroids; use may exacerbate subclinical bacterial infection.

## PRECAUTIONS
Meloxicam—use with caution in rabbits with compromised renal function.

## ALTERNATIVE DRUGS
• Chondroitin sulfate (Cosequin, Nutramax) has been used anecdotally using feline dosage protocols; polysulfate glycosaminoglycan (Adequan, Luitpold) 2.2 mg/kg SC, IM q3d × 21–28 days, then q14d.
• Acupuncture may be effective for rabbits with chronic pain.

## FOLLOW-UP

## PATIENT MONITORING
Clinical deterioration—indicates need to change drug selection or dosage; may indicate need for surgical intervention

## PREVENTION/AVOIDANCE
Early identification of predisposing causes and prompt treatment—help reduce progression of secondary condition

## POSSIBLE COMPLICATIONS
• Gastrointestinal hypomotility or stasis
• Dermatitis, urine scald, ulcerative pododermatitis (sore hocks)
• Hypercalciuria

## EXPECTED COURSE AND PROGNOSIS
• Slow progression of disease likely
• Some form of medical or surgical treatment usually allows a good quality of life.

## MISCELLANEOUS

## ASSOCIATED CONDITIONS
N/A

## AGE-RELATED FACTORS
N/A

## ZOONOTIC POTENTIAL
N/A

## PREGNANCY
N/A

## SYNONYMS
Degenerative joint disease

## SEE ALSO
• Arthritis—septic
• Dysuria and pollakiuria
• Ulcerative pododermatitis

## ABBREVIATIONS
• CBC = complete blood count
• NSAIDs = nonsteroidal antiinflammatory drugs

*Suggested Reading*

Deeb BJ, Carpenter JW. Neurologic and musculoskeletal diseases. In: Quesenberry KE, Carpenter JW, eds. Ferrets, Rabbits and Rodents: Clinical Medicine and Surgery. 2nd Ed. Philadelphia: WB Saunders, 2004:203–210.

Harcourt-Brown F. Neurological and locomotor diseases. In: Harcourt-Brown F, ed. Textbook of Rabbit Medicine. Oxford: Butterworth-Heinemann, 2002:307–323.

Kapatkin A. Orthopedics in small mammals. Quesenberry KE, Carpenter JW, eds. Ferrets, Rabbits and Rodents: Clinical Medicine and Surgery. 2nd Ed. Philadelphia: WB Saunders, 2004:383–391.

*Portions Adapted From*

Beale BS. Arthritis—Osteoarthritis. In: Tilley LP, Smith FWK, Jr., eds. The 5-Minute Veterinary Consult: Canine and Feline, 2nd Ed. Baltimore: Lippincott Williams & Wilkins, 2000.

# ARTHRITIS—SEPTIC

## BASICS

### OVERVIEW
• Definition—pathogenic microorganisms within the closed space of one or more synovial joints
• Usually caused by the hematogenous spread of microorganisms from a distant septic focus; contamination associated with traumatic injury (e.g., a direct penetrating injury such as bite wounds or cage injury); the extension of a primary osteomyelitis, especially on the plantar/palmar surfaces of the feet; or a contaminated surgery
• Sources of infection—abscesses; dental disease; upper respiratory infection; skin; wounds; sometimes not identified

### SIGNALMENT
No age, breed, or gender predilection

### SIGNS

#### General Comments
Consider the diagnosis in patients with lameness associated with soft tissue swelling, heat, and pain.

#### Historical Findings
• Lameness
• Lethargy, anorexia
• History of upper respiratory infection, dental disease, abscess
• May report previous trauma—bite wound, penetrating injury

#### Physical Examination Findings
• Joint pain and swelling
• Localized joint heat
• Decreased range of motion
• Signs of concurrent infection—URI, dental disease, ulcerative pododermatitis, abscess

### CAUSES AND RISK FACTORS
• Pyogenic bacteria—especially staphylococci, *Pasteurella,* and anaerobic bacteria
• Predisposing factors—immunosuppression, chronic bacterial infection, penetrating trauma to the joint

## DIAGNOSIS

### DIFFERENTIAL DIAGNOSIS
• Lameness affecting one limb—fracture, soft tissue injury, abscess, ulcerative pododermatitis, neoplasia
• Lameness affecting multiple limbs—spinal trauma, spondylosis, disc disease, *Encephalitozoon cuniculi*

### CBC/BIOCHEMISTRY/URINALYSIS
• Hemogram—normal or lymphopenia; inflammatory left shift not usually seen in rabbits; may see mild anemia
• Other results normal

### OTHER LABORATORY TESTS
• Serologic testing for *E. cuniculi*—many tests are available, but usefulness is extremely limited since a positive titer indicates only exposure and does not confirm *E. cuniculi* as the cause of clinical signs. *E. cuniculi* can only be definitively diagnosed by finding organisms and resultant lesions on histopathology. Antibody titers usually become positive by 2 weeks postinfection, but generally do not continue to rise with active infection or decline with treatment. No correlation exists between antibody titers and shedding of organism and presence or severity of disease. It is unknown if exposed rabbits eventually become seronegative. Available tests include ELISA, indirect IFA, and carbon immunoassay.
• Serology for *Pasteurella*—usefulness is severely limited and generally not helpful in the diagnosis of pasteurellosis in pet rabbits. An ELISA is available, and results are reported as negative, low positive, or high positive. Positive results, even when high, only indicate prior exposure to *Pasteurella* and the development of antibodies and do not confirm active infection. Low-positive results may occur due to cross-reaction with other, nonpathogenic bacteria (false positive). False-negative results are common with immunosuppression or early infection. No evidence exists to support correlation of titers to the presence or absence of disease.

### IMAGING

#### Radiography
Similar to lesions found in dogs and cats—may reveal thickened periarticular tissues; evidence of synovial effusion; bone destruction, osteolysis, irregular joint space, erosions, and periarticular osteophytosis

### DIAGNOSTIC PROCEDURES

#### Synovial Fluid Analysis
• Increased volume
• Turbid fluid
• Elevated WBC count—predominate neutrophils
• Bacteria in the synovial fluid or within neutrophils

#### Synovial Fluid Culture
• Must be collected aseptically; requires heavy sedation or general anesthesia
• Submit fluid samples for aerobic and anaerobic culture; bacterial susceptibility testing to direct antibiotic therapy

## TREATMENT

### APPROPRIATE HEALTH CARE
• It is essential to remove/correct the underling cause for long-term success.
• Inpatient—for initial stabilization or surgical debridement

• Outpatient—for long-term management

### NURSING CARE
• Depends on severity of disease
• Bandage changes postarthrotomy
• Anorectic rabbits require forced alimentation
• Soft bedding; daily bedding changes

### ACTIVITY
Restricted until resolution of symptoms

### DIET
• It is absolutely imperative that the rabbit continue to eat during and following treatment. This condition is often painful, resulting in anorexia. Anorexia will often cause gastrointestinal hypomotility, derangement of the gastrointestinal microflora, and overgrowth of intestinal bacterial pathogens.
• Offer a large selection of fresh, moistened greens such as cilantro, romaine lettuce, parsley, carrot tops, dandelion greens, spinach, collard greens, etc., and good-quality grass hay. Many rabbits will begin to eat these foods, even if they were previously anorectic. Also, try offering the rabbit's usual pelleted diet.
• If the patient refuses these foods, syringe feed a gruel such as Critical Care for Herbivores (Oxbow Pet Products, Murdock, NE) 10–15 mL/kg PO q6–8h. Larger volumes and more frequent feedings are often accepted; feed as much as the rabbit will accept. Alternatively, pellets can be ground and mixed with fresh greens, vegetable baby foods, water, or juice to form a gruel. If sufficient volumes of food are not accepted in this manner, nasogastric intubation is indicated.
• High-carbohydrate, high-fat nutritional supplements are contraindicated.
• Encourage oral fluid intake by offering fresh water and wetting leafy vegetables.

### CLIENT EDUCATION
• Warn client about the need for long-term antibiotics and the likelihood of residual degenerative joint disease.
• Severe disease, especially with multiple joint involvement, carries a guarded to poor prognosis for complete resolution. Most will require surgical debridement, sometimes multiple surgeries and multiple follow-up visits. Recurrences are common, especially if the underlying cause cannot be corrected. Clients must be aware of the monetary and time investment.

### SURGICAL CONSIDERATIONS
• Open arthrotomy with debridement of the synovium; debride all visibly necrotic tissue.
• Simple lancing and draining is not adequate. In rabbits, septic joints usually contain thick exudates that do not drain well. Instead of draining, curette all visible

exudates and flush copiously with warmed physiologic saline.
• Joints that are extensively diseased or abscessed often respond well to implantation of antibiotic-impregnated polymethyl methacrylate (AIPMMA) beads into the joint.
• AIPMMA beads release a high concentration of antibiotic into local tissues for several months. Selection of antibiotic is limited to those known to elute appropriately from bead to tissues and should be based on culture and susceptibility testing. AIPMMA beads are not commercially available, but can be made using PMMA by Surgical Simplex Bone Cement (Howmedica, Rutherford, NJ) or Bone Cement (Zimmer, Charlotte, NC). Antibiotics successfully used include cephalothin, cefazolin, or ceftiofur (2 g/20 g PMMA); gentamicin or tobramycin (1 g/2 g PMMA); or amikacin (1.25 g/2 g PMMA). Antibiotic is added to the copolymer powder before adding the liquid and formed into small, spherical beads. Beads must be inserted aseptically, and unused bead should be gas sterilized prior to future use. Beads should be removed from the joint space in 4–6 weeks.
• Given the expense and pain involved in these procedures, the author recommends referral to a specialist if surgical expertise or AIPMMA beads are not available.
• Place on long-term systemic antibiotic therapy; appropriate pain management
• Severe infection that is not responsive to debridement, AIPMMA bead therapy, and systemic antibiotic therapy may require amputation. Most rabbits tolerate amputation of a single front or hind limb well.

## MEDICATIONS

### DRUG(S) OF CHOICE
• Use antimicrobial drugs effective against the infectious agent; gain access to site of infection. Choice of antibiotic is based on results of culture and susceptibility testing. Depending on the severity of infection, long-term antibiotic therapy is required (4–6 weeks minimum to several months). Use broad-spectrum antibiotics such as enrofloxacin (5–20 mg/kg PO, SC, IM q12–24h) or trimethoprim sulfa (30 mg/kg POq12h); if anaerobic infections are suspected, use chloramphenicol (50 mg/kg PO q8h), metronidazole (20 mg/kg PO q12h), or azithromycin (30 mg/kg PO q24h); can be used alone or combined with metronidazole. Alternatively, use penicillin g (40,000–60,000 IU/kg SC q2–7d). Combine with topical treatment (surgical debridement, AIPPMA beads) listed above.

• For pain management—meloxicam (0.2–0.5 mg/kg PO q24h) or carprofen 2.2 mg/kg PO q12h may be used long term. Postsurgical, buprenorphine 0.01–0.05 mg/kg SC or IM q6–8h is effective.

### CONTRAINDICATIONS
• Oral administration of antibiotics that select against Gram-positive bacteria (penicillins, macrolides, lincosamides, and cephalosporins) can cause fatal enteric dysbiosis and enterotoxemia.
• The use of corticosteroids (systemic or topical preparations) can severely exacerbate septic arthritis.

### PRECAUTIONS
• Failure to respond to conventional antibiotic therapy—may indicate anaerobic disease or other unusual cause (fungal, spirochete)
• Oral administration of any antibiotic can potentially cause intestinal dysbiosis. Discontinue use if anorexia or diarrhea occurs.

### POSSIBLE INTERACTIONS
N/A

### ALTERNATIVE DRUGS
N/A

 FOLLOW-UP

### PATIENT MONITORING
• Duration of antibiotic therapy—4–8 weeks or longer; depends on clinical signs and pathogenic organism
• Monitor for progressive decrease in exudate, resolution of inflammation, and improvement of clinical signs.

### PREVENTION/AVOIDANCE
N/A

### POSSIBLE COMPLICATIONS
• Chronic disease—severe degenerative joint disease
• Recurrence of infection
• Limited joint range of motion
• Generalized sepsis
• Osteomyelitis

### EXPECTED COURSE AND PROGNOSIS
• Acutely diagnosed disease—good to fair prognosis with aggressive treatment
• Advanced disease, multiple joint involvement or resistant or highly virulent organisms—guarded to poor prognosis

 MISCELLANEOUS

### ASSOCIATED CONDITIONS
• Immunosuppression
• Dental disease
• Rhinitis/sinusitis

• Hypercalciuria
• Ulcerative pododermatitis
• Moist pyoderma

### AGE-RELATED FACTORS
N/A

### ZOONOTIC POTENTIAL
N/A

### PREGNANCY
N/A

### SYNONYMS
Infectious arthritis

### SEE ALSO
• Abscessation
• Ulcerative pododermatitis

### ABBREVIATIONS
• ELISA = enzyme-linked immunosorbent assay
• IFA = immunofluorescent assay
• URI = Upper respiratory infection
• WBC = white blood cell

*Suggested Reading*

Bennet RA. Treatment of abscesses in the head of rabbits. Proc North Am Vet Conf 1999;821–823.

Deeb BJ, Carpenter JW. Neurologic and musculoskeletal diseases. In: Quesenberry KE, Carpenter JW, eds. Ferrets, Rabbits and Rodents: Clinical Medicine and Surgery. 2nd Ed. Philadelphia: WB Saunders, 2004:203–210.

Ethell MT, Bennett RA, Brown MP, et al. In vitro elution of gentamicin, amikacin, and ceftiofur from polymethylmethacrylate and hydroxyapatite cement. Vet Surg 2000;29:375–382.

Harcourt-Brown F. Neurological and locomotor diseases. In: Harcourt-Brown F, ed. Textbook of Rabbit Medicine. Oxford: Butterworth-Heinemann, 2002:307–323.

Kapatkin A. Orthopedics in small mammals. In: Quesenberry KE, Carpenter JW, eds. Ferrets, Rabbits and Rodents: Clinical Medicine and Surgery. 2nd Ed. Philadelphia: WB Saunders, 2004: 383–391.

Lukehart SA, Fohn MJ, Baker-Zander SA. Efficacy of azithromycin for therapy of active syphilis in the rabbit model. J Antimicrob Chemother 1990;25 Suppl A:91–99.

Paul-Murphy JA, Ramer JC. Urgent care of the pet rabbit. Vet Clin North Am Exot Anim Pract 1998;1(1):127–152.

*Portions Adapted From*

Taylor RA. Arthritis—Septic. In: Tilley LP, Smith FWK, Jr., eds. The 5-Minute Veterinary Consult: Canine and Feline, 2nd Ed. Baltimore: Lippincott Williams & Wilkins, 2000.

## ATAXIA

## BASICS

### DEFINITION
- A sign of sensory dysfunction that produces incoordination of the limbs, head, and/or trunk
- Three clinical types—sensory (proprioceptive), vestibular, and cerebellar; all produce changes in limb coordination, but vestibular and cerebellar ataxia also produce changes in head and neck movement.

### PATHOPHYSIOLOGY

#### Sensory
- Proprioceptive pathways in the spinal cord relay limb and trunk position to the brain.
- When the spinal cord is slowly compressed, proprioceptive deficits are usually the first signs observed, because these pathways are located more superficially in the white matter and their larger-sized axons are more susceptible to compression than are other tracts.
- Generally accompanied by weakness owing to early concomitant upper motor neuron involvement; weakness not always obvious early in the course of the disease

#### Vestibular
- Changes in head and neck position are relayed through the vestibulocochlear nerve to the brainstem.
- Diseases that affect the vestibular receptors, the nerve in the inner ear, or the nuclei in the brainstem cause various degrees of disequilibrium with ensuing vestibular ataxia.
- Affected animal leans, tips, falls, or even rolls toward the side of the lesion; accompanied by head tilt

#### Cerebellar
- The cerebellum regulates, coordinates, and smooths motor activity.
- Proprioception is normal, because the ascending proprioceptive pathways to the cortex are intact; weakness does not occur, because the upper motor neurons are intact.
- Inadequacy in the performance of motor activity; strength preservation; no proprioceptive deficits

### SYSTEMS AFFECTED
Nervous—spinal cord (and brainstem); cerebellum; vestibular system

### SIGNALMENT
Any age, breed, or sex

### SIGNS
- Important to define the type of ataxia to localize the problem
- Only one limb involved—consider a lameness problem.

- Only hindlimbs affected—likely a spinal cord disorder
- All or both ipsilateral limbs affected—cerebellar
- Head tilt—vestibular
- Nasal/ocular discharge—likely vestibular; spread of upper respiratory infection to inner/middle ear
- Urine scald, perineal dermatitis, alopecia in the intrascapular region—seen in rabbits with spinal disease due to inability to maintain normal stance while urinating or inability to properly groom

### CAUSES

#### Neurologic

*Cerebellar and CNS Vestibular*
- Infectious—bacterial most common, especially central erosion caused by otitis media and interna; encephalitis due to *Pasteurella* spp. or other bacteria; listeriosis (rare); *Encephalitozoon cuniculi* reportedly common; aberrant baylisascariasis migration (unusual cause); rabies virus and herpes virus (rare)
- Toxin ingestion—lead most common
- Degenerative and anomalous—not yet described in rabbits
- Neoplastic—any tumor of the CNS (primary or secondary) localized to the cerebellum
- Inflammatory, idiopathic, immune-mediated—granulomatous meningoencephalomyelitis is a common postmortem finding in rabbits both with and without antemortem neurologic signs; has been attributed to *E. cuniculi* infection, but organisms not always found; similar lesions can be found on postmortem examination of rabbits in the absence of clinical signs.

*Vestibular—PNS*
- Infectious—otitis media interna the most common cause; *Pasteurella multocida, Staphylococcus aureus, Pseudomonas aeruginosa, Escherichia coli,* and *Listeria monocytogenes* most often cultured
- Idiopathic—not well described in rabbits; however, a definitive diagnosis is often not found, and many rabbits with vestibular signs improve with supportive care.
- Neoplastic—not well described in rabbits
- Traumatic

#### Spinal Cord
- Traumatic—fracture or luxation, very common in pet rabbits; intervertebral disc herniation—anecdotally reported
- Degenerative—spondylosis, common in older rabbits
- Anomalous—kyphosis, lordosis, hemivertebrae
- Infectious—diskospondylitis; *E. cuniculi* spinal cord and nerve route lesions anecdotally reported
- Vascular and neoplastic diseases—uncommon, not well described in rabbits

#### Metabolic
- Anemia
- Electrolyte disturbances—hypokalemia and hypoglycemia

#### Miscellaneous
- Respiratory compromise
- Cardiac compromise

### RISK FACTORS
- Otitis media/interna—chronic upper respiratory infection, immunosuppression (stress, corticosteroid use, concurrent disease)
- Spinal fractures, luxations, or intervertebral disk disease—improper restraint, possibly disuse atrophy from confinement
- *E. cuniculi*—immunosuppression (stress, corticosteroid use, concurrent disease)
- Baylisascariasis—outdoor housing, exposure to raccoon feces
- Spondylosis—unknown, possibly related to small caging, lack of exercise

## DIAGNOSIS

### DIFFERENTIAL DIAGNOSIS
- Differentiate the types of ataxia
- Differentiate from other disease processes that can affect gait—musculoskeletal, metabolic, cardiovascular, respiratory
- Musculoskeletal disorders—typically produce lameness and a reluctance to move
- Systemic illness, cardiovascular, and metabolic disorders—can cause intermittent ataxia, especially of the pelvic limbs; fever, weight loss, murmurs, arrhythmias, or collapse with exercise: suspect a nonneurologic cause; obtain minimum data from hemogram, biochemistry analysis, and urinalysis.
- Head tilt or nystagmus—likely vestibular
- Intention tremors of the head or hypermetria—likely cerebellar
- Only limbs affected—likely spinal cord dysfunction; all four limbs affected: lesion is in the cervical area or is multifocal to diffuse; only pelvic limbs affected: lesion is anywhere below the second thoracic vertebra
- Upper respiratory disease—likely vestibular; spread of infection to inner/middle ear or brainstem

### CBC/BIOCHEMISTRY/URINALYSIS
Normal unless metabolic cause (e.g., hypoglycemia, electrolyte imbalance, and anemia)

### OTHER LABORATORY TESTS
- Electrolyte imbalance—correct the problem; see if ataxia resolves.
- Serologic testing for *E. cuniculi*—many tests are available, but usefulness is extremely limited since a positive titer indicates only exposure and does not con-

firm *E. cuniculi* as the cause of neurologic signs. *E. cuniculi* can only be definitively diagnosed by finding organisms and resultant lesions on histopathologic examination in areas that anatomically correlate with observed clinical signs. Antibody titers usually become positive by 2 weeks postinfection but generally do not continue to rise with active infection or decline with treatment. No correlation exists between antibody titers and shedding of organism and presence or severity of disease. It is unknown if exposed rabbits eventually become seronegative. Available tests include ELISA, indirect IFA, and carbon immunoassay.

• Serology for *Pasteurella*—usefulness is severely limited and generally not helpful in the diagnosis of pasteurellosis in pet rabbits. An ELISA is available and results are reported as negative, low positive, or high positive. Positive results, even when high, only indicate prior exposure to *Pasteurella* and the development of antibodies but do not confirm active infection. Low-positive results may occur due to cross-reaction with other, nonpathogenic bacteria (false positive). False-negative results are common with immunosuppression or early infection. No evidence exists to support correlation of titers to the presence or absence of disease.

• Bacterial culture and sensitivity testing—from ear exudate or nasal discharge

### IMAGING
• Spinal radiographs—if spinal cord dysfunction suspected; referral for myelogram may be indicated
• Bullae radiographs—if peripheral vestibular disease suspected; CT or MRI scans superior; many rabbits with bullae disease have normal-appearing radiographs.
• Thoracic radiographs—identify heart disease, neoplasia
• CT or MRI—if cerebellar disease suspected; evaluate potential brain disease
• Abdominal ultrasonography—if underlying metabolic disease (renal, hepatic) is suspected

### DIAGNOSTIC PROCEDURES
• Otoscopic examination—in rabbits with otitis externa, thick, white, creamy exudate may be found in the horizontal and/or vertical canals. Otitis interna/media may occur in the absence of otitis externa via extension through the eustachian tube; may see bulging tympanum. Some rabbits with otitis interna have no visible otoscopic abnormalities.
• CSF—may aid in confirming nervous system causes

## TREATMENT
• Usually outpatient, depending on the severity and acuteness of clinical signs
• Exercise—decrease or restrict if spinal cord disease suspected; if vestibular signs—restrict (e.g., avoid stairs and slippery surfaces) according to the degree of disequilibrium; encourage return to activity as soon as safely possible; activity may enhance recovery of vestibular function

### DIET
• It is absolutely imperative that the rabbit continue to eat during and following treatment. Anorexia will often cause gastrointestinal hypomotility, derangement of the gastrointestinal microflora, and overgrowth of intestinal bacterial pathogens.
• Offer a large selection of fresh, moistened greens such as cilantro, romaine lettuce, parsley, carrot tops, dandelion greens, spinach, collard greens, etc., and good-quality grass hay. Many rabbits will begin to eat these foods, even if they were previously anorectic. Also, try offering the rabbit's usual pelleted diet, as the initial goal is to get the rabbit to eat. Bring the food to the rabbit if nonambulatory or offer food by hand.
• If the patient refuses these foods, syringe feed a gruel such as Critical Care for Herbivores (Oxbow Pet Products, Murdock, NE) 10–15 mL/kg PO q6–8h. Larger volumes and more frequent feedings are often accepted; feed as much as the rabbit will readily accept. Alternatively, pellets can be ground and mixed with fresh greens, vegetable baby foods, water, or juice to form a gruel.
• High-carbohydrate, high-fat nutritional supplements are contraindicated.
• Encourage oral fluid intake by offering fresh water, wetting leafy vegetables, or flavoring water with vegetable juices. CAUTION: Be aware of aspiration secondary to abnormal body posture in patients with severe head tilt and vestibular disequilibrium or brainstem dysfunction.
• Client should monitor gait for increasing dysfunction or weakness; if paresis worsens or paralysis develops, other testing is warranted.

## MEDICATIONS

### DRUG(S) OF CHOICE
Not recommended until the source or cause of the problem is identified

### CONTRAINDICATIONS AND PRECAUTIONS
• Oral administration of antibiotics that select against Gram-positive bacteria (penicillins, macrolides, lincosamides, and cephalosporins) can cause fatal enteric dysbiosis and enterotoxemia.
• Topical and systemic corticosteroids—rabbits are very sensitive to the immunosuppressive effects of corticosteroids; use may exacerbate subclinical bacterial infection. Use is contraindicated unless intervertebral disc disease is demonstrated by myelography.

### POSSIBLE INTERACTIONS
N/A

### ALTERNATIVE DRUGS
N/A

## FOLLOW-UP

### PATIENT MONITORING
Periodic neurologic examinations to assess condition

### POSSIBLE COMPLICATIONS
• Spinal cord or neuromuscular disease—progression to weakness and possibly paralysis
• Cerebellar disease—head tremors, severe torticollis, rolling, anorexia

## MISCELLANEOUS

### ASSOCIATED CONDITIONS
N/A

### AGE-RELATED FACTORS
N/A

### ZOONOTIC POTENTIAL
N/A

### PREGNANCY
N/A

### SYNONYMS
N/A

### SEE ALSO
• Head tilt (vestibular disease)
• Paresis and paralysis
• See specific diseases

### ABBREVIATIONS
• CSF = cerebrospinal fluid
• CT = computed tomography
• ELISA = enzyme-linked immunosorbent assay
• IFA = immunofluorescence assay
• MRI = magnetic resonance imaging
• PNS = peripheral nervous system

## ATAXIA

*Suggested Reading*

Deeb BJ, Carpenter JW. Neurologic and musculoskeletal diseases. In: Quesenberry KE, Carpenter JW, eds. Ferrets, Rabbits and Rodents: Clinical Medicine and Surgery. 2nd Ed. Philadelphia: WB Saunders, 2004:203–210.

de Lahunta A. Veterinary neuroanatomy and clinical neurology. 2nd Ed. Philadelphia: Saunders, 1983.

Harcourt-Brown F. Neurological and loco-motor diseases. In: Harcourt-Brown F, ed. Textbook of Rabbit Medicine. Oxford: Butterworth-Heinemann, 2002:307–323.

Oliver JE, Lorenz MD. Handbook of Veterinary Neurologic Diagnosis. 2nd Ed. Philadelphia: Saunders, 1993.

Paul-Murphy J, Ramer JC. Urgent care of the pet rabbits. Vet Clin North Am Exotic Anim Pract 1998;1(1):127–152.

Rosenthal KR. Torticollis in rabbits. Proc North Am Vet Conf 2005;1378–1379.

*Portions Adapted From*

Shell LG. Ataxia. In: Tilley LP, Smith FWK, Jr., eds. The 5-Minute Veterinary Consult: Canine and Feline, 3rd Ed. Baltimore: Lippincott Williams & Wilkins, 2004.

# BASICS

## OVERVIEW
• Opacification of the lens
• Term cataract—may refer to an entire lens that is opaque or to a opacity within the lens; does not imply cause
• Basic mechanism—thought to be cross-linking of lens protein
• Most common causes—congenital cataracts reported; *Encephalitozoon cuniculi* in utero infection with vertical transmission of organism into the developing lens; replication of spores within the lens of young rabbits results in cataract formation, thin anterior portion, or lens rupture resulting in phacoclastic uveitis with focal granuloma formation at site of rupture.
• Other causes (nutritional deficiency; elevated blood glucose; toxins; altered composition of the aqueous humor caused by uveitis) not well described in rabbits
• Traditional terminology—immature (only part of the lens is involved); mature (entire lens is opaque); hypermature (lens liquefaction has occurred); implies progressive condition

## SIGNALMENT
• *E. cuniculi*—most common in dwarf breeds <2 years old
• Spontaneous juvenile cataracts—one study demonstrated an incidence of 4.3% in laboratory New Zealand white rabbits
• No breed predilection described for congenital cataracts

## SIGNS
• Opacification of lens
• Liquefied lens material leaking from the lens—seen most often with *E. cuniculi*
• Iridal swelling, white nodule on the iris—common in rabbits with *E. cuniculi*; consists of granulomatous reaction to leakage of lens material. Rabbits are often presented for evaluation of an intraocular white "mass," with the remainder of the eye appearing relatively quiet.
• Associated with uveitis—typically see hypopyon and low intraocular pressure

### Choroid Reflection
• Easiest method of detection
• Obstruction of light by lenticular opacities (retroillumination)
• Appear as black or gray spots
• Cloudiness owing to sclerosis—will not detect discreet foci of obstruction

## CAUSES AND RISK FACTORS
• Congenital
• In utero infection with *E. cuniculi*

• Spontaneous—unknown cause; senile or degenerative cataracts have not been well described
• Uveitis—secondary to synechia formation or altered aqueous humor composition
• Diabetes mellitus—not reported in rabbits

# DIAGNOSIS

## DIFFERENTIAL DIAGNOSIS
For white mass protruding from iris—iridal abscess (common); neoplasia

## CBC/BIOCHEMISTRY/URINALYSIS
Routine hematology and blood chemistry profiles—screen for infectious diseases when associated with uveitis.

## OTHER LABORATORY TESTS
Serologic testing for *E. cuniculi*—many tests are available, but usefulness is limited since a positive titer indicates only exposure and does not confirm *E. cuniculi* as the cause of uveitis. Can only be definitively diagnosed by finding organism on ocular histopathology or positive DNA probe on removed lens material. Antibody titers usually become positive by 2 weeks postinfection but generally do not continue to rise with active infection or decline with treatment. No correlation exits between antibody titers and shedding of organism or severity of disease. It is unknown if exposed rabbits eventually become seronegative. Available tests include ELISA, indirect IFA, and carbon immunoassay.

## IMAGING
N/A

## DIAGNOSTIC PROCEDURES
N/A

# TREATMENT

## APPROPRIATE HEALTH CARE
Rabbits undergoing surgery—inpatient

## NURSING CARE
N/A

## ACTIVITY
N/A

## DIET
Make certain that the rabbit continues to eat to avoid secondary gastrointestinal disorders.

## CLIENT EDUCATION
• Inform client that surgery can be performed on congenital or spontaneous cataract that is causing or is anticipated to cause vision loss if no other ocular pathol-

ogy is present. However, spontaneous regeneration of the lens following phacoemulsification has been reported in rabbits.
• Warn client that the prognosis for surgery is better if it is done early in the course of cataract development, before hypermaturity, lens-induced uveitis, and retinal detachment occur.
• Phacoemulsification may offer best prognosis for cataracts caused by *E. cuniculi*.

## SURGICAL CONSIDERATIONS
• Phacoemulsification—ultrasonic lens fragmentation; procedure of choice
• Intraocular lenses—not recommended because spontaneous lens regeneration has been reported in rabbits; insertion of prosthetic lens post–lens removal is not recommended.
• *E. cuniculi*—may recur following surgery, requiring medical treatment or enucleation

# MEDICATIONS

## DRUG(S) OF CHOICE
• Topical NSAIDs—0.03% flurbiprofen (Ocufen) or 1% diclofenac; q6h daily to control inflammation
• 1% prednisolone acetate—has been used q6h to prevent and control lens-induced uveitis; use with extreme caution in rabbits (see precautions).
• *E. cuniculi*—benzimidazole anthelmintics are effective against *E. cuniculi* in vitro and have been shown to prevent experimental infection in rabbits. However, efficacy in rabbits with clinical signs is unknown. Anecdotal reports suggest a response to treatment in rabbits with *E. cuniculi*–associated phacoclastic uveitis. Published treatments include albendazole (20–30 mg/kg q24h × 30 days, then 15 mg/kg PO q24h for 30 days) and fenbendazole (20 mg/kg q24h × 5–28 days). A 7- to 10-day course of treatment may be sufficient in rabbits with ocular disease only.

## CONTRAINDICATIONS
Topical corticosteroids—never use if the cornea retains fluorescein stain.

## PRECAUTIONS
• Topical corticosteroids or antibiotic–corticosteroid combinations—avoid; associated with gastrointestinal ulceration and hemorrhage, delayed wound healing, and heightened susceptibility to infection; rabbits are very sensitive to the immunosuppressive effects of both topic and systemic corticosteroids; use may exacerbate subclinical bacterial infection.

## CATARACTS

• Albendazole has been associated with bone marrow toxicity in dogs and cats; toxicity in rabbits is unknown; however, anecdotal reports of pancytopenia leading to death in rabbits exist.

### POSSIBLE INTERACTIONS
N/A

### ALTERNATIVE DRUGS
N/A

## FOLLOW-UP

### PATIENT MONITORING
• All patients—monitored carefully for progression
• Intraocular pressure—monitored for secondary glaucoma in rabbits with *E. cuniculi*. Normal intraocular pressure reported as 10–20 mm Hg when measured by applanation tonometry

### POSSIBLE COMPLICATIONS
Complete cataracts—potential to cause lens-induced uveitis, secondary glaucoma, and retinal detachment

### EXPECTED COURSE AND PROGNOSIS
• Congenital or spontaneous cataracts—insufficient data available on prognosis following phacoemulsification or progression to uveitis
• *E. cuniculi*–associated uveitis—depends on severity and chronicity of infection and presence of secondary bacterial infections. If cannot treat surgically, prognosis for viability of the affected eye is guarded, as most will progress to glaucoma; enucleation may be indicated.

## MISCELLANEOUS

### ASSOCIATED CONDITIONS
N/A

### AGE-RELATED FACTORS
*E. cuniculi*–related anterior uveitis seen most often in young rabbits <2 years old

### ZOONOTIC POTENTIAL
*E. cuniculi*—unlikely, but possible in immunosuppressed humans. Modes of transmission and susceptibility in humans are unclear.

### PREGNANCY
• Systemic steroids—do not use in pregnant animals if at all avoidable.
• Topical steroids—use with caution; systemic absorption occurs.

### SYNONYM
Iridocyclitis

### SEE ALSO
• *E. cuniculi*
• Red eye

### ABBREVIATIONS
• ELISA = enzyme-linked immunosorbent assay
• IFA = immunofluorescence assay

*Suggested Reading*

Andrew SE. Corneal disease of rabbits. Vet Clin Noth Am Exotic Anim Pract 2002;5:341–356.

Felchle LM, Sigler RL. Phacoemulsification for the management of *Encephalitozoon cuniculi*-induced phacoclastic uveitis in a rabbit. Vet Ophthalmol 2002;5(3):211–215.

Munger RJ, Langevin JP. Spontaneous cataracts in laboratory rabbits. Vet Ophthalmol 2002;5(3):177–181.

Stiles J, Dider E, Ritchie B, et al. *Encephalitozoon cuniculi* in the lens of a rabbit with phacoclastic uveitis: confirmation and treatment. Vet Comp Ophthalmol 1997;7(4):233–238.

Van der Woerdt A. Ophthalmologic disease in small pet animals. In: Quesenberry KE, Carpenter JW, eds. Ferrets, Rabbits and Rodents: Clinical Medicine and Surgery. 2nd Ed. Philadelphia: WB Saunders, 2004:421–428.

Williams DL. Laboratory animal ophthalmology. In: Gelatt KN, ed. Veterinary Ophthalmology. 3rd Ed. Philadelphia: Lippincott Williams & Wilkins, 1999:151–181.

*Portions Adapted From*

Nasisse MP. Cataract. In: Tilley LP, Smith FWK, Jr., eds. The 5-Minute Veterinary Consult: Canine and Feline, 3rd Ed. Baltimore: Lippincott Williams & Wilkins, 2004.

# CHEEK TEETH (MOLAR AND PREMOLAR) MALOCCLUSION AND ELONGATION

## BASICS

### DEFINITION
• Cheek teeth—normal dentition: a total of six incisors, including two sets (lower and upper) of large incisor teeth and two small peg teeth located lingual to the upper incisors. No canine teeth, but instead a large diastema followed by the cheek teeth. The premolars and molars are aligned as one functional unit and are therefore referred to as cheek teeth. Cheek teeth consist of three upper premolars, three upper molars, two lower premolars, and three lower molars on each side.
• Cheek teeth elongation—occurs when normal wear or occlusion does not occur
• Malocclusion of the cheek teeth—can occasionally be caused by congenital skeletal malocclusion or by trauma, but acquired malocclusion is more common

### PATHOPHYSIOLOGY
• All teeth are open-rooted and grow continuously at a rate of approximately 3 mm per week, with growth originating from the germinal bud located at the apex of the tooth.
• The rate of normal wear should equal the rate of eruption, approximately 3 mm per week. Normal wear requires proper occlusion with the opposing set of teeth and a highly abrasive diet to grind coronal surfaces.
• The cause of acquired cheek teeth elongation is likely multifactorial and not completely known. The most significant contributing or exacerbating factor is feeding diets that contain inadequate amounts of coarse roughage food material required to properly grind coronal surfaces. Malocclusion may also be an inherited or congenital defect.
• Cheek teeth are naturally slightly curved. When erupted crowns are a normal length, they will contact the opposing set of cheek teeth at an angle such that the teeth will occlude with a flat grinding surface. If normal wear does not occur and teeth overgrow, the exposed coronal surfaces will curve away from the opposing set of teeth, contact at an abnormal angle, and cause the formation of sharp spikes.
• Spikes on the cheek teeth can become very long and penetrate into adjacent soft tissues or, in some cases, entrap the tongue. Secondary bacterial infections are common.
• Cheek teeth that do not occlude normally will continue to elongate into the oral cavity until normal jaw tone arrests upward growth. At this point, pressure from the

opposing set of cheek teeth will cause the teeth to grow in an apical direction (ventrally into the mandible or upward into the maxilla) such that the apices intrude into cortical bone.
• Poor skull mineralization due to nutritional secondary hyperparathyroidism has also been proposed to be a contributing factor. The mechanism and incidence of this proposed disorder have not been well defined.
• Most incisor overgrowth and malocclusion are caused by overgrown cheek teeth. Elongation of the cheek teeth prohibits complete closure of the mouth, preventing the upper incisors from contacting the lower incisors, which allows unopposed growth of the incisors.

### SYSTEMS AFFECTED
• Oral cavity
• Ocular—nasolacrimal duct obstruction, retroorbital invasion of tooth roots
• Respiratory—apical (tooth root) invasion of the sinuses
• Musculoskeletal—weight loss, muscle wasting

### GENETICS
Unknown

### INCIDENCE/PREVALENCE
One of the most common presenting complaints in pet rabbits

### GEOGRAPHIC DISTRIBUTION
N/A

### SIGNALMENT
• Usually seen in middle-aged or older rabbits—acquired cheek tooth elongation
• Young animals—congenital malocclusion
• Dwarf and lop breeds—congenital malocclusion
• No breed or gender predilection for acquired cheek tooth elongation

### SIGNS

#### General Comments
• Owners generally notice incisor overgrowth first, as these teeth are readily visible. In nearly all cases, incisor overgrowth is also a symptom of cheek teeth elongation and generalized dental disease.
• Always perform a thorough oral examination under sedation or general anesthesia to examine the cheek teeth. Rabbits have a long, narrow mouth; use of a directed light source and magnification (or endoscope), a nasal speculum, cheek dilators and mouth gag, are needed to thoroughly examine the teeth.
• Significant cheek teeth apical abnormalities may be present despite normal-appearing crowns. Skull films are required to identify apical (root) disorders.

#### Historical Findings
• Inability to prehend food; dropping food out of the mouth; preference for soft feeds
• Weight loss
• Anorexia or decreased appetite; often show an interest in food, but unable to eat; may be anorectic from pain with advanced disease
• Preference for a water bowl over a sipper bottle
• Excessive drooling
• Nasal discharge
• Tooth grinding
• Excessive tear production
• Facial asymmetry or exophthalmos in rabbits with tooth root abscesses
• Signs of pain—reluctance to move, depression, lethargy, hiding, hunched posture
• Unkempt haircoat, lack of grooming

#### Physical Examination Findings
*Oral Examination*
• A thorough examination of the cheek teeth requires heavy sedation or general anesthesia and specialized equipment. A cursory examination using an otoscope for illumination and visualization is insufficient for rabbits with dental disease.
• A focused, directed light source and magnification will provide optimal visualization.
• Use a rodent mouth gag and cheek dilators (Jorgensen Laboratories, Inc., Loveland, CO) to open the mouth and pull buccal tissues away from teeth surfaces to allow adequate exposure. Use a cotton swab or tongue depressor to retract the tongue from lingual surfaces.
• Normal cheek teeth—do not have a flat surface, but small vertical cusps; normal crown length for maxillary cheek teeth: approximately 1 mm (maximum 2 mm); normal crown length for mandibular cheek teeth: approximately 3 mm (maximum 5 mm)
• Identify cheek teeth abnormalities—elongation, irregular crown height, spikes, curved teeth, discolored teeth, missing teeth, purulent exudate, odor, impacted food, oral ulceration, or abscesses
• Identify incisor abnormalities—overgrown incisors, horizontal ridges or grooves, malformation, discoloration, fractures, increased or decreased curvature, loose teeth; malocclusion: bite appears level or mandibular incisors rostral to maxillary incisors.
• Buccal or lingual mucosa and lip margins—ulceration, abrasions, secondary bacterial infection, or abscess formation if incisors or cheek teeth spikes have damaged soft tissues

# CHEEK TEETH (MOLAR AND PREMOLAR) MALOCCLUSION AND ELONGATION

### Other Findings
• Ptyalism causing secondary moist pyoderma and alopecia around the mouth, neck, and dewlap areas
• A scalloped edge or single bony protrusion may be palpable on the ventral rim of the mandible in rabbits in which the cheek teeth have intruded into and distorted surrounding bone.
• Soft tissue swelling, abscesses most commonly located on the mandible or below the eye
• Exophthalmus in rabbits with retrobulbar abscesses from periapical cheek tooth abscesses
• Weight loss, emaciation
• Nasal discharge—tooth root invasion into the sinuses; tooth root abscesses
• Ocular discharge—blocked nasolacrimal duct from diseased tooth roots (usually the second upper premolar); pressure on the eye from retrobulbar abscess or overgrown molar roots
• Signs of gastrointestinal hypomotility—scant feces, intestinal pain, diarrhea
• Dental tartar, carries, and periodontal disease infrequently seen

### CAUSES
• Congenital skeletal malocclusion—most likely in young, dwarf, or lop-eared breeds
• Acquired cheek teeth elongation—likely multiple etiologies; inadequate fibrous, tough foods or foods containing silicates (grasses) to properly grind teeth such that coronal surfaces cannot wear normally
• Elongation may be part of normal aging. Pet rabbits often live significantly longer than production rabbits or wild rabbits, so teeth grow for longer periods of time than would occur within a natural lifespan.

### RISK FACTORS
• Feeding pelleted diets and simple carbohydrate treats—these diets lack sufficient abrasive material to properly wear teeth; small, calorically dense food requires less chewing, less wear on teeth
• Breeding rabbits with congenital malocclusion

 DIAGNOSIS

### DIFFERENTIAL DIAGNOSIS
• For epiphora—upper respiratory tract disease, blocked nasolacrimal duct (exudate, scarring, stricture), primary ocular disease
• For ptyalism—wet dewlap from water bowls, oral trauma or abscess not related to tooth disease, oral neoplasia, rabies (rare), swallowing disorders (rare)

### CBC/BIOCHEMISTRY/URINALYSIS
Usually normal even when oral or facial abscess occur; may see abnormalities in liver enzymes in rabbits with hepatic lipidosis secondary to anorexia

### OTHER LABORATORY TESTS
N/A

### IMAGING
#### Skull Radiographs
• Mandatory to identify type and extent of dental disease, to plan treatment strategies, and to monitor progression of treatment.
• Perform under general anesthesia
• Five views are recommend for thorough assessment—ventral–dorsal, lateral, two lateral obliques, and rostral–caudal
• With early disease—elongation of the crowns and roots, loss of normal coronal occlusal pattern, mild radiolucency around tooth roots, enlargement of germinal bud, lysis of bone
• Moderate to severe disease—crooked teeth, reduction in the diameter or obliteration of the pulp cavity, widening of the interdental space, apical radiolucency and bony lysis, penetration of the tooth roots into surrounding cortical bone
• Periapical abscess—severe lysis of cortical bone, bony proliferation
• CT—superior to radiographs to evaluate the extent of dental disease and bony destruction

### DIAGNOSTIC PROCEDURES
• Fine needle aspiration of facial swelling—may be helpful to identify abscess
• Bacterial culture of affected tissue and/or exudate—aerobic and anaerobic bacteria; growth more likely if wall or capsule is sampled; bacteria deep within exudate are often nonviable.
• Culture results often yield no growth with anaerobic infections; anaerobic infection is often presumed based on evidence derived from previous studies of odontogenic abscesses in rabbits.
• Bacterial susceptibility testing to direct antibiotic therapy
• Rabbits with epiphora—instill fluorescein stain into the affected eye to determine patency of the nasolacrimal duct or perform nasolacrimal duct irrigation.

 TREATMENT

### APPROPRIATE HEALTH CARE
• Outpatient—patients with mild to moderate dental disease requiring coronal reduction

• Inpatient—patients with periapical or facial abscess, patients requiring extraction, or debilitated patients

### NURSING CARE
Keep fur around face clean and dry.

### ACTIVITY
N/A

### DIET
• It is absolutely imperative that the rabbit continue to eat during and following treatment. Many rabbits with dental disease will become anorectic. Rabbits may be unable to eat solid food following radical coronal reduction, extractions, or surgical treatment of abscesses. Anorexia will cause or exacerbate gastrointestinal hypomotility, derangement of the gastrointestinal microflora, and overgrowth of intestinal bacterial pathogens.
• Syringe feed a gruel such as Critical Care for Herbivores (Oxbow Pet Products, Murdock, NE) 10–15 mL/kg PO q8–12h. Larger volumes and more frequent feedings are often accepted; feed as much as the rabbit will readily accept. Alternatively, pellets can be ground and mixed with fresh greens, vegetable baby foods, water, or juice to form a gruel.
• Most rabbits will require assisted feeding for 36–48 hours postoperatively; following coronal reduction, assisted feeding may be needed for several weeks.
• High-carbohydrate, high-fat nutritional supplements are contraindicated.
• Return the rabbit to a solid-food diet as soon as possible to encourage normal occlusion and wear. Increase the amount of tough, fibrous foods and foods containing abrasive silicates such as hay and wild grasses; avoid pelleted food and soft fruits or vegetables.
• Encourage oral fluid intake by offering fresh water or wetting leafy vegetables.

### CLIENT EDUCATION
• Early tooth elongation may sometimes be corrected by sequential coronal reduction and diet change.
• By the time clinical signs of cheek teeth elongation are noted, disease is usually advanced. Lifelong treatment, consisting of periodic coronal reduction (teeth trimming), is required, usually every 1–3 months.
• Severe dental disease, especially with tooth root abscesses and severe bony destruction, carries a guarded to poor prognosis for complete resolution. Most will require extensive surgery, sometimes multiple surgeries and multiple follow-up visits. Recurrences in the same or other locations are common. Clients must be aware of the monetary and time investment.

# CHEEK TEETH (MOLAR AND PREMOLAR) MALOCCLUSION AND ELONGATION

• With severe disease, euthanasia may be the most humane option, especially in rabbits with intractable pain or those that cannot eat

## SURGICAL CONSIDERATIONS

### Trimming of Cheek Teeth (Coronal Reduction)

• Trimming of spurs and sharp points alone will be of little benefit for most rabbits; in most cases the crowns all of the cheek teeth are elongated and maloccluded and will need to be reduced.
• Always perform under general anesthesia—premedicate with buprenorphine (plus ketamine and diazepam in nervous patients); induce with isoflurane via mask, moving the mask over nose to maintain anesthesia (rabbits are obligate nasal breathers); or intubate.
• Use a focused, directed light source and magnification (e.g., lighted magnification loop).
• Adequate exposure of the teeth and protection of soft tissues are crucial. Use a rodent mouth gag and cheek dilators (Jorgensen Laboratories, Inc., Loveland, CO) to open the mouth and pull buccal tissues away from teeth surfaces. Protect soft tissues by using dental spatulas to protect the tongue and buccal tissues and a bur guard while trimming the teeth.
• Trim using a straight, low-speed dental handpiece with an appropriate bur and bur guard to protect soft tissues. Burs with long shanks made specifically for use in rabbits are available. Alternatively, a dremel tool with a diamond bit can be used.
• Avoid "floating" the teeth with a rasp or file or clipping the points whenever possible. These procedures can traumatize the teeth and gums.
• Rabbits with severe malocclusion—grinding the teeth down to the level of gums every 4–8 weeks, combined with dietary correction, may realign occlusal surfaces, preventing or slowing elongation in selected cases. However, owner compliance is essential; most rabbits undergoing this treatment require prolonged assisted feeding.

### Molar Extraction

• Indicated in rabbits with loose molars, significantly misdirected teeth, or tooth root abscesses
• Because rabbits have very long, deeply embedded and curved tooth roots, extraction per os can be extremely time consuming and labor intensive as compared to with dogs and cats. If the germinal bud is not completely removed, the teeth may regrow or an abscess may form. If not experienced with tooth extraction in rabbits, the author

recommends referral to a veterinarian with special expertise whenever feasible.
• Extraction of multiple cheek teeth in a single procedure can be extremely traumatic; some rabbits may not recover.
• Large tooth root abscesses should be removed via a cutaneous approach. All material within the abscess should be removed with the capsule intact until bone is reached. All teeth associated with the abscess must be removed. All bone involved in abscess must be thoroughly debrided. Long-term topical treatment, using antibiotic-impregnated polymethyl methacrylate (AIPMMA) beads or other topical therapy, is necessary to prevent recurrence. If not experienced with facial abscesses in rabbits, the author recommends referral to a veterinarian with special expertise whenever feasible.

## MEDICATIONS

### DRUG(S) OF CHOICE

#### Antibiotics

Indicated in rabbits with periapical abscesses. Choice of antibiotic is ideally based on results of culture and susceptibility testing. Depending on the severity of infection, long-term antibiotic therapy is required (3 months minimum to several months or years). Most facial or dental abscesses are caused by anaerobic bacteria; use antibiotics effective against anaerobes such as azithromycin (30 mg/kg PO q24h); can be used alone or combined with metronidazole (20 mg/kg PO q12h). Alternatively, use penicillin g (40,000–60,000 IU/kg SC q2–7d) or chloramphenicol (50 mg/kg PO q8h). Combine with topical treatment (surgical debridement, AIPPMA beads). If aerobic bacteria are isolated, use broad-spectrum antibiotics such as enrofloxacin (5–20 mg/kg PO, SC, IM q12–24h) or trimethoprim sulfa (30 mg/kg PO q12h).

#### Acute Pain Management

• Buprenorphine (0.01–0.05 mg/kg SC, IM, IV q8–12h)—use preoperatively for extractions, coronal reduction, or surgical abscess treatment.
• Butorphanol (0.1–1.0 mg/kg SC, IM, IV q4–6h)—may cause profound sedation; short-acting
• Morphine (2–5 mg/kg SC, IM q2—4h) or oxymorphone (0.05–0.2 mg/kg SC, IM q8–12h)—use with caution; more than one to two doses may cause gastrointestinal stasis.
• Meloxicam (0.2 mg/kg SC, IM q24h)
• Carprofen (1–4 mg/kg SC q12h)

### Long-Term Pain Management

• NSAIDs have been used for short- or long-term therapy to reduce pain and inflammation—meloxicam (0.2–0.5 mg/kg PO q24h) or carprofen (2.2 mg/kg PO q12–24)
• Sedation for oral examination—ketamine (15–20 mg/kg IM) plus midazolam (0.5–1.0 mg/kg IM); many other sedation protocols exist; alternatively, administer general anesthesia with isoflurane.

### CONTRAINDICATIONS

• Oral administration of most antibiotics effective against anaerobes will cause a fatal gastrointestinal dysbiosis in rabbits. Do not administer penicillins, macrolides, lincosamides, and cephalosporins by oral administration.
• Corticosteroids—associated with gastrointestinal ulceration and hemorrhage, delayed wound healing, and heightened susceptibility to infection; rabbits are very sensitive to the immunosuppressive effects of both topical and systemic corticosteroids; use may exacerbate subclinical bacterial infection.

### PRECAUTIONS

• Chloramphenicol—avoid human contact with chloramphenicol due to potential blood dyscrasia. Advise owners of potential risks.
• Meloxicam—use with caution in rabbits with compromised renal function.

### POSSIBLE INTERACTIONS
N/A

### ALTERNATIVE DRUGS
N/A

## FOLLOW-UP

### PATIENT MONITORING

• Reevaluate, and trim as needed, every 4–8 weeks. Evaluate the entire oral cavity and the skull with each recheck and repeat skull radiographs at least every 3–6 months to monitor progression.
• Perform a thorough oral examination and radiograph frequently to monitor for regrowth of extracted cheek teeth if germinal buds have not been completely removed.
• Monitor for signs of apical abscess or invasion of the tooth roots into surrounding bone or sinuses (epiphora, nasal discharge, facial swelling).

### PREVENTION/AVOIDANCE

• In rabbits with acquired dental disease, prevention is not possible once clinical signs of malocclusion are present. With periodic coronal reduction and appropriate diet,

# CHEECK TEETH (MOLAR AND PREMOLAR) MALOCCLUSION AND ELONGATION

progression of disease may be arrested, but treatment is lifelong.
• To help prevent acquired dental disease, discontinue or limit the feeding of pellets and soft fruits or vegetables; provide adequate tough, fibrous foods such as hay and grasses to encourage normal wear of teeth.
• Do not breed rabbits with congenital malocclusion.

### POSSIBLE COMPLICATIONS
• Periapical abscesses, recurrence, chronic pain, or extensive tissue destruction warranting euthanasia due to poor quality of life
• Hepatic lipidosis with prolonged anorexia
• Chronic epiphora with nasolacrimal duct occlusion

### EXPECTED COURSE AND PROGNOSIS
• Mild to moderate disease—good to fair prognosis with regular trimming and appropriate diet change, depending on severity of disease; lifelong trimming may be required.
• Periapical or facial abscesses, osteomyelitis—depend on severity of bone involvement and location. Rabbits with abscesses in the nasal passages, exophthal-

mos, or multiple or severe maxillary abscesses have a guarded to poor prognosis. Euthanasia may be warranted with severe or advanced disease, especially in rabbits that are in pain or cannot eat.

## MISCELLANEOUS

### ASSOCIATED CONDITIONS
N/A

### AGE-RELATED FACTORS
N/A

### ZOONOTIC POTENTIAL
N/A

### PREGNANCY
N/A

### SYNONYMS
N/A

### SEE ALSO
• Abscessation
• Epiphora
• Incisor malocclusion and overgrowth

*Suggested Reading*
Crossley DA. Oral biology and disorders of lagomorphs. Vet Clin North Am Exotic Anim Pract 2003;6(3):629–659.
Crossley DA, Aiken S. Small mammal dentistry. In: Quesenberry KE, Carpenter JW, eds. Ferrets, Rabbits and Rodents: Clinical Medicine and Surgery. 2nd Ed. Philadelphia:WB Saunders, 2004:370–382.
Harcourt-Brown F. Dental disease. In: Harcourt-Brown F, ed. Textbook of Rabbit Medicine. Oxford: Butterworth-Heinemann, 2002:165–205.
Lukehart SA, Fohn MJ, Baker-Zander SA. Efficacy of azithromycin for therapy of active syphilis in the rabbit model. J Antimicrob Chemother 1990;25 Suppl A:91–99.
Tyrell KC, Citron DM, Jenkins JR, et al. Periodontal bacteria in rabbit mandibular and maxillary abscesses. J Clin Microbiol 2002;40(3):1044–1047.

# CHEYLETIELLOSIS (FUR MITES)

## BASICS

### OVERVIEW
• A highly contagious parasitic skin disease of rabbits, dogs, and cats, caused by infestation with *Cheyletiella* spp. mites
• Nonburrowing mite lives on the epidermal keratin layer
• Life cycle is approximately 35 days; entire cycle is spent on the host.
• Many rabbits are asymptomatic—disease occurs in young animals, debilitated animals, or those with underlying diseases that prohibit adequate grooming.
• Signs of scaling and pruritus can mimic other diseases
• Often referred to as "walking dandruff," because of the large mite size and excessive scaling
• Human (zoonotic) lesions can occur.
• Lesions may less commonly be caused by the fur mite *Leporacarus gibbus*

### SIGNALMENT
• Seen in any-aged rabbit
• Most common in young animals, debilitated animals, or those with underlying diseases that prohibit adequate grooming to remove keratin and mites
• May see in otherwise healthy rabbits with heavy infestation.
• May be more common in long-haired rabbits

### SIGNS

#### Historical Findings
• Pruritus—none to severe, depending on the individual's response to infestation
• Alopecia, most commonly in the intrascapular region
• May have history of dental disease, obesity, or underlying musculoskeletal disease

#### Physical Examination Findings
• Scaling—most important clinical sign. Copious amounts of large, white flakes of scale are seen. Most often focal, beginning in intrascapular region; may become diffuse; most severe in chronically infested and debilitated animals
• Lesions—dorsal location, either between the scapulae or at the tail base most common. Some rabbits are unable to adequately groom these regions, especially obese animals or those with dental or musculoskeletal disease. Lesions are most commonly found in these regions, where lack of grooming allows proliferation of mites.
• Underlying skin irritation may be minimal. With chronic infestation, the underlying skin may become thickened.
• Alopecia occurs along with excessive scaling. Alopecia is generally located centrally within the lesion.

• A thorough oral examination is indicated to rule out underlying dental disease.
• Ataxia, proprioceptive deficits, paresis; pain on palpation or manipulation of the spine may be found in rabbits with underlying musculoskeletal disease.
• Facial or perineal dermatitis may be seen in rabbits with underlying skeletal disease, due to an inability to groom these areas or an inability to maintain a normal posture while urinating.
• Obesity—may be an underlying cause

### CAUSES AND RISK FACTORS
• Healthy rabbits with normal grooming habits often remain asymptomatic.
• Disease is more common in young animals and those with underlying diseases that prohibit adequate grooming.
• Inability to adequately reach the intrascapular or tail base regions for grooming contributes to the formation of lesions in these areas.
• Common sources of initial infestation—pet stores, animal shelters, breeders

## DIAGNOSIS

### DIFFERENTIAL DIAGNOSIS
• Cheyletiellosis should be considered in every animal that has scaling, with or without pruritus.
• Also consider ear mite (*Psoroptes cuniculi*) infestation, *Sarcoptes scabiei*, and *Notoedres cati* (rare), flea hypersensitivity dermatitis, dermatophytes, and bacterial dermatitis.
• In some rabbits, lack of grooming alone may cause an accumulation of scale, without the presence of mites.
• Injection reactions—the intrascapular region is a common site of subcutaneous injections (including fluids); reaction to irritating substances (especially enrofloxacin) in this region may mimic Cheyletiellosis
• Sebaceous adenitis—very similar appearance; usually begins around the head and neck. Differentiate by skin biopsy and histologic examination.

### CBC/BIOCHEMISTRY/URINALYSIS
N/A

### OTHER LABORATORY TESTS
N/A

### IMAGING
Spinal or dental radiographs to rule out underlying dental or musculoskeletal disease

### DIAGNOSTIC PROCEDURES
• Examination of epidermal debris—very effective in diagnosing infestation
• Collection of debris—flea combing (most effective), skin scraping, and acetate tape preparation

• Cheyletiella mites are large—scales and hair may be examined under low magnification; staining is not necessary.
• A thorough physical examination, including oral, orthopedic, and neurologic, is indicated to rule out underlying cause.
• Skin biopsy with histologic examination to rule out sebaceous adenitis

## TREATMENT
• Identification and correction of any underlying disease that may prohibit normal grooming behavior is essential to ensure complete resolution.
• Treat all animals in the household, including cats and dogs.
• Comb daily with a fine-toothed comb to remove scale.
• Bathing is also effective in removing scale, but often difficult to perform on rabbits. Bathing can be dangerous in nervous rabbits with inexperienced owners and can result in spinal fractures and excessive chilling. Sudden death has also been reported following bathing.
• Lime-sulfur rinses have been effective, but are difficult to use in rabbits. Apply such rinses with caution, as stated in bathing, above.
• Environmental treatment with frequent cleaning—extremely important for eliminating infestation, adult mites can live up to 10 days off of the host. Remove and discard all organic material from cage (wood or paper products, bedding); replace bedding with shredded paper bedding that can be discarded and the cage thoroughly cleaned every day during the treatment period.
• Combs, brushes, and grooming utensils—discard or thoroughly disinfect before reuse.
• Zoonotic lesions—self-limiting after eradication of the mites from household animals

## MEDICATIONS

### DRUG(S) OF CHOICE
• Ivermectin and selamectin—more safe and effective when compared to topical therapy
• Ivermectin—usually effective: 400 μg/kg SC three times at 2-week intervals
• Selamectin—6–12 mg/kg applied topically; retreatment in 2–4 weeks may be required.

### ALTERNATIVE DRUGS
Carbaryl powder (5%) applied topically once weekly; may also be used to treat the environment

## CHEYLETIELLOSIS (FUR MITES)

### CONTRAINDICATIONS/POSSIBLE INTERACTIONS

- Do not use fipronil on rabbits.
- Do not use flea collars on rabbits.
- Do not use organophosphate-containing products on rabbits.
- Do not use straight permethrin sprays or spot-ons on rabbits.
- Topical flea preparation for use in dogs and cats, such as permethrins and pyrethrins, are less effective and may be toxic to rabbits.
- Use extreme caution when dipping or bathing rabbits due to the high risk of skeletal fractures and excessive chilling with inexperienced owners. Sudden death has also been reported during or after bathing rabbits.
- Ivermectin and selamectin—not FDA approved for this use in rabbits; client disclosure and consent are paramount before administration, although no adverse reactions have been reported.
- Topical medications may be accidentally ingested during self-grooming or grooming by cage mates.

### FOLLOW-UP

- Treatment failure necessitates reevaluation for other causes of pruritus and scaling.
- Reinfestation may indicate contact with an asymptomatic carrier or the presence of an unidentified source of mites (e.g., untreated bedding).

### MISCELLANEOUS

#### ZOONOTIC POTENTIAL

A pruritic papular rash may develop in areas of contact with the pet. This rash is self-limiting with removal of the mite from pets and the environment.

#### SYNONYMS

- Fur mites
- Walking dandruff

#### ABBREVIATIONS

N/A

#### SEE ALSO

- Dermatophytosis
- Ear mites
- Fleas
- Pruritus

#### Suggested Reading

Clyde VL. Practical treatment and control of common ectoparasites in exotic pets. Vet Med 1996;91(7):632–637.

Harcourt-Brown, F. Skin diseases. In: Harcourt-Brown F. ed. Textbook of Rabbit Medicine. Oxford: Butterworth-Heinemann, 2002:224–248.

Hess L. Dermatologic diseases. In: Quesenberry KE, Carpenter JW, eds. Ferrets, Rabbits and Rodents: Clinical Medicine and Surgery. 2nd Ed. Philadelphia: WB Saunders, 2004:194–202.

Jenkins, JR. Skin disorders of the rabbit. Vet Clin North Am Exotic Anim Pract 2001;4(2):543–563.

McTier TL, Hair A, Walstrom DJ, et al. Efficacy and safety of topical administration of selamectin for treatment of ear mite infestation in rabbits. J Am Vet Med Assoc 2003;223(3):322–324.

#### Portions Adapted From

Werner AH. Cheyletiellosis. In: Tilley LP, Smith FWK, Jr., eds. The 5-Minute Veterinary Consult: Canine and Feline, 3rd Ed. Baltimore: Lippincott Williams & Wilkins, 2004.

# CLOSTRIDIAL ENTERITIS/ENTEROTOXICOSIS

## BASICS

### OVERVIEW
• Clostridial enteritis and enterotoxicosis is common in rabbits. The usual syndrome is characterized by acute diarrhea, anorexia, lethargy, dehydration, and death due to enterotoxin production by *Clostridium spiroforme.*
• Some rabbits appear to suffer from a milder form of subacute to chronic enteritis. In these patients, clinical signs are mild to moderate. Clostridia-like organisms can be identified on fecal cytology, and disease often resolves with appropriate treatment.
• Young, weaning-aged rabbits (5–8 weeks old) are more susceptible to acute enteric colonization by *C. spiroforme*. This is likely due to incomplete enteric colonization by commensal bacteria, allowing rapid colonization by *C. spiroforme* from the environment. This may cause either a profuse, watery diarrhea or mucoid diarrhea (mucoid enteritis) with cecal colonization. Disease is acute and severe, usually causing death in 1–3 days.
• Older rabbits require one or more predisposing factors to allow enteric colonization of clostridial species. These include stress, inappropriate diet, and inappropriate antibiotic use. Colonization may cause acute, often fatal disease as seen in neonates, or a milder form of disease that is more amenable to treatment.
• In any-aged rabbit, diets containing high-carbohydrate concentrations provide excessive fermentable by-products that can lead to an overgrowth of intestinal clostridia organisms.
• In any-aged rabbit, antibiotic usage can cause severe, acute, often fatal diarrhea due to alteration of normal gut flora. Diarrhea follows the oral administration of antibiotics that are effective against Gram-positive bacteria and some Gram-negative anaerobes, such as lincomycin, clindamycin, erythromycin, ampicillin, amoxicillin, cephalosporins, and penicillins. These antibiotics should never be orally administered to rabbits.

### SIGNALMENT
• Common cause of diarrhea in pet rabbits
• Weaning-aged rabbits—acute, often fatal disease
• Older rabbits—variable severity of disease

### SIGNS

#### General Comments
Clinical syndromes are associated with either an acute, watery diarrhea; chronic intermittent diarrhea; or serious, life-threatening disease associated with enterotoxemia.

#### Historical Findings
• Most common—acute onset of watery diarrhea, depression, anorexia, and listlessness; owners may describe a foul-smelling diarrhea.
• Mucoid enteritis—acute onset of mucoid diarrhea, depression, and anorexia in weaning-aged rabbits
• Diarrhea may be described as soft and sticky, mucous covered or watery in adults; may be intermittent
• In adults—history of diets low in roughage and long-stem hay, diets high in simple carbohydrates (pellets, excessive fruits, or sugary vegetables, cereal "treats," grain or bread products, sugars; infrequent feeding of good-quality long stemmed hay and fresh leafy greens)
• In adults—history of recent stress or fearful stimuli (surgery, hospitalization, illness, diet change, environmental change)
• History of antibiotic use—especially those with a Gram-positive spectrum (clindamycin, lincomycin, penicillin, ampicillin, amoxicillin)

#### Physical Examination Findings
*Mild to Moderate Diarrhea*
• Abdominal discomfort and gas- or fluid-filled intestines or cecum may be detected on palpation.
• May be evidence of fecal staining of perineum
• Abdominal pain characterized by a hunched posture, reluctance to move, or bruxism
*Acute, Severe Diarrhea; Enterotoxic Shock*
• Dehydration and depression
• Abdominal distension; tympanic abdomen
• Tachycardia or bradycardia
• Tachypnea
• Signs of hypovolemic shock (e.g., pale mucous membranes, decreased capillary refill time, weak pulses)
• Hypothermia—body temperature is usually low in rabbits that are in shock. Incomplete insertion of the thermometer into the rectum is a common cause of falsely low body temperature measurement. Be certain that the thermometer is completely inserted into the rectum (approximately 3 cm) to register an accurate body temperature.

### CAUSES AND RISK FACTORS
• Low-fiber, high-carbohydrate diet
• Improper antibiotic use
• Stress
• Dirty environment

## DIAGNOSIS

### DIFFERENTIAL DIAGNOSIS
• Diarrhea should be differentiated from cecotrophs (or night feces). Cecotrophs are formed in the cecum, are rich in nutrients, and are usually eliminated once daily. Normally, cecotrophs are not observed because rabbits will ingest them directly from the rectum. Occasionally, rabbits are unable to consume the cecotroph, which may be mistaken for diarrhea. Cecotrophs are dark in color, have a soft consistency, tend to clump together, and are covered with mucous.
• Weaning-aged rabbits—Coccidia, other bacterial pathogens (*Escherichia coli, Salmonella*), *C. pilforme* (Tyzzer's disease), rotavirus, coronavirus
• Adult rabbits—other bacterial pathogens (*E. coli, Salmonella, Campylobacter*), intussusception, partial gastrointestinal tract obstruction; chronic disease can sometimes present as acute diarrhea; systemic illness may also result in diarrhea as a secondary event.

### CBC/BIOCHEMISTRY/URINALYSIS
• With mild to moderate diarrhea—usually normal
• With acute severe diarrhea—expect hemogram abnormalities consistent with acute inflammation and hemoconcentration/shock; electrolyte abnormalities and acid-base alterations may be seen.

### OTHER LABORATORY TESTS
Fecal direct examination, fecal flotation, and zinc sulfate centrifugation to rule out gastrointestinal parasites

#### Microbiology
Anaerobic fecal cultures may demonstrate clostridia organisms, but occasionally are negative due to the fastidious nature of the organism.

#### Fecal Cytology
• Large numbers of large, Gram-positive, endospore-producing bacteria can usually be found in the feces in patients with clinical disease. Low numbers of spore-producing bacteria are a normal finding.
• Gram's stain—preferred stain; allows identification of concurrent overgrowth of Gram-negative bacteria.
• Must differentiate from normal enteric yeast (*Saccharomyces* spp. or *Cyniclomyces guttulatus*)—much larger than enteric bacteria

### IMAGING
• Gas-filled intestinal tract is the most common finding in rabbits with clostridial enterotoxicosis.
• May be helpful to rule out other causes of diarrhea (foreign body, neoplasia, intussusception)

### DIAGNOSTIC PROCEDURES
N/A

### PATHOLOGIC FINDINGS
• With bloat syndrome, grossly dilated, thin-walled stomach and intestines; diffuse necrosis of mucosa on histologic examination.

# CLOSTRIDIAL ENTERITIS/ENTEROTOXICOSIS

• With enterotoxemia, gross or histologic intestinal lesions may be absent.

## TREATMENT

### APPROPRIATE HEALTH CARE
• Most adult rabbits with mild diarrhea that are otherwise bright and alert can be treated as outpatients. These patients can usually be successfully treated with oral or subcutaneous fluid therapy, dietary modification, and metronidazole.
• Hospitalize rabbits with signs of lethargy, depression, dehydration, or shock, even if diarrhea is mild or absent.
• Hospitalize when diarrhea is profuse, resulting in dehydration and electrolyte imbalance.
• Hospitalize rabbits <5 months of age, regardless of the severity of diarrhea.

### NURSING CARE
• Fluid therapy and correction of electrolyte imbalances are the mainstays of treatment in most cases.
• Can give crystalloid fluid therapy orally, subcutaneously, or intravenously, as required
• Aim to return the patient to proper hydration status (over 12–24 hours) and replace any ongoing losses.
• Severe volume depletion can occur with acute diarrhea; aggressive shock fluid therapy may be necessary.
• Fluid choice for intravenous or subcutaneous use should take into consideration the electrolyte and hydration status.

### DIET
• It is imperative that the rabbit continue to eat during and following treatment. Continued anorexia will exacerbate gastrointestinal motility disorders and cause further derangement of the gastrointestinal microflora and overgrowth of intestinal bacterial pathogens.
• Offer a good-quality grass hay and a large selection of fresh, moistened greens such as cilantro, romaine lettuce, parsley, carrot tops, dandelion greens, spinach, collard greens, etc. Many rabbits will begin to eat these foods, even if they were previously anorectic.
• In some rabbits, addition of leafy greens may exacerbate diarrhea. For these patients, offer good-quality grass hay alone.
• If the patient refuses these foods, syringe feed a gruel such as Critical Care for Herbivores (Oxbow Pet Products, Murdock, NE) 10–15 mL/kg PO q6–8h. Larger volumes and more frequent feedings are often accepted; feed as much as the rabbit will readily accept. Alternatively, pellets can be ground and mixed with fresh greens, veg-

etable baby foods, water, or juice to form a gruel. If sufficient volumes of food are not accepted in this manner, nasogastric intubation is indicated.
• High-carbohydrate, high-fat nutritional supplements are contraindicated.
• The diet should be permanently modified to include sufficient amounts of roughage and long-stemmed hay. Offer high-quality fresh hay (grass or timothy preferred; commercially available hay cubes are not sufficient) and an assortment of washed, fresh leafy greens. These foods should always constitute the bulk of the diet. Pellets should be limited (one-quarter cup pellets per 5 lb. body weight, if offered at all) and foods high in simple carbohydrates prohibited or limited to the occasional treat.

### CLIENT EDUCATION
• Warn clients that in rabbits with acute, severe diarrhea, death may occur despite treatment. Young rabbits (<6 months old) and rabbits showing signs of depression and shock also have a guarded prognosis with treatment, even when diarrhea is mild.
• Emphasize the importance of permanent dietary modification (described above) in surviving rabbits.

## MEDICATIONS

### DRUG(S) OF CHOICE
• Antibiotics for *Clostridium* spp.—metronidazole (20 mg/kg PO, IV q12h for 3 weeks)
• Cholestyramine (Questran, Bristol Laboratories) is an ion-exchange resin that binds clostridial iota toxins. A dose of 2 g in 20 mL of water administered by gavage q24h for up to 18–21 days has been reported to be effective in preventing death in rabbits with acute clostridia enterotoxemia.
• Analgesics such as buprenorphine (0.01–0.05 mg/kg SC, IM, IV q8–12h), or meloxicam (0.2 mg/kg SC, IM q24h) may be beneficial for rabbits with intestinal pain. Intestinal pain from gas distention and ileus impairs mobility and decreases appetite, and may severely inhibit recovery.

### CONTRAINDICATIONS
• Antibiotics that are generally effective against clostridia in other species, such as clindamycin or penicillins, are contraindicated in rabbits. Do not administer lincomycin, clindamycin, erythromycin, ampicillin, amoxicillin cephalosporins, and penicillins orally to rabbits.
• Do not use corticosteroids in the treatment of shock in rabbits.

### PRECAUTIONS
N/A

### POSSIBLE INTERACTIONS
N/A

### ALTERNATIVE DRUGS
N/A

## FOLLOW-UP

### PATIENT MONITORING
• Response to therapy supports the diagnosis; repeat diagnostics are rarely necessary.
• Monitor body temperature, appetite, hydration, fecal production, and serial fecal Gram's stain for a positive response to therapy.

### PREVENTION/AVOIDANCE
• Feed a diet consisting of good-quality grass hay, fresh leafy greens, and minimal pellets. Avoid fruit-, vegetable-, or cereal-based treats.
• Do not administer oral antibiotics that are primarily Gram positive in spectrum (penicillins, cephalosporins, macrolides, and lincosamides).
• Infection in weaning-aged rabbits is associated with environmental contamination; disinfection is difficult.

### POSSIBLE COMPLICATIONS
Death due to continued diarrhea, dehydration, electrolyte imbalances, or enterotoxic shock

### EXPECTED COURSE AND PROGNOSIS
• Most animals with mild to moderate disease respond well to therapy.
• The prognosis is fair to grave in rabbits with acute, severe, watery diarrhea, depending on the extent of infection and time elapsed to treatment.
• The prognosis is poor to grave in rabbits demonstrating signs of shock (hypothermia, bradycardia, lethargy) and young rabbits (<6 months old) even with treatment.

## MISCELLANEOUS

### ASSOCIATED CONDITIONS
Frequently other enteric disease

### AGE-RELATED FACTORS
• Young, weaning-aged rabbits develop acute, watery diarrhea or mucoid diarrhea; prognosis is poorer.
• Adult rabbits require predisposing factors (poor diet, stress, antibiotic usage); and usually carry a better prognosis

### ZOONOTIC POTENTIAL
Unknown

### PREGNANCY
N/A

## CLOSTRIDIAL ENTERITIS/ENTEROTOXICOSIS

**SYNONYMS**
- Mucoid enteritis
- Enterotoxemia

**SEE ALSO**
- Diarrhea, acute
- Gastrointestinal hypomotility

**ABBREVIATIONS**
N/A

*Suggested Reading*

Brown SA, Rosenthal KL. The anorexic rabbit. Proc North Am Vet Conf 1997:788.

Donoghue S. Nutrition and pet rabbits. In: Rosenthal KL, ed. Practical Exotic Animal Medicine: The Compendium Collection. Trenton, NJ: Veterinary Learning Systems, 1997:107.

Jenkins JR. Feeding recommendations for the house rabbit. Vet Clin Noth Am Exotic Anim Pract 1999;2(1):143–151.

Jenkins JR. Gastrointestinal diseases. In: Quesenberry KE, Carpenter JW, eds. Ferrets, Rabbits and Rodents: Clinical Medicine and Surgery. 2nd Ed. Philadelphia: WB Saunders, 2004:161–171.

Langan GP, Schaeffer DO, Rabbit microbiology and virology. In: Fudge AM, ed. Laboratory Medicine: Avian and Exotic Pets. Philadelphia: WB Saunders, 2000:325–333.

Paul-Murphy JA, Ramer JC. Urgent care of the pet rabbits. Vet Clin North Am Exotic Anim Pract 1998;1(1):127–152.

Rees Davies R, Rees Davies JAE. Rabbit gastrointestinal physiology. Vet Clin North Am Exotic Anim Pract 2003;6(1):139–153.

# COCCIDIOSIS

 BASICS

## OVERVIEW
• An enteric or hepatic infection, associated with *Eimeria* spp.
• Twelve different species of Coccidia have been reported to infect the rabbit intestinal tract. Many rabbits that are clinically ill have more than one species of Coccidia.
• Only one species, *E. stiedae,* infects the liver.
• Strictly host-specific (i.e., no cross-transmission)
• Asexual multiplication occurs in intestinal epithelial cells and causes cellular damage and disease.
• Following asexual multiplication, sexual reproduction results in shedding of oocysts in the feces.
• Oocysts become infective 1–4 days after being shed in the feces.
• Immunity naturally develops against each *Eimeria* species following exposure; however, no cross-protection exists. Therefore, young or adult rabbits can become clinically ill following exposure to a species that they have not developed immunity to.
• Disease severity depends on the species of *Eimeria*, the immune status of the rabbit (including age and environmental stressors), and the number of oocysts ingested.
• Infection may predispose to bacterial enteritis.

## SIGNALMENT
• Usually a disease of young and recently weaned rabbits, 4–16 weeks of age—causes moderate to severe clinical disease
• Occasionally causes clinical disease in adult rabbits, especially when debilitated or exposed to large numbers of oocysts of an *Eimeria* species to which they have no immunity
• The hepatic form can occur in any-aged rabbit.

## SIGNS
• Often asymptomatic
• Watery to mucoid, sometimes blood-tinged, diarrhea with intestinal form
• Diarrhea may be intermittent.
• Tenesmus with intestinal form
• Weakness, lethargy, dehydration, and weight loss with heavy infections, especially in young rabbits; may cause intussusception and death
• With hepatic involvement, may see anorexia, weight loss, depression, abdominal enlargement, cranial abdominal pain, diarrhea, or acute death

## CAUSES AND RISK FACTORS
• Infected rabbits contaminating environment with oocysts of *Eimeria* spp. Screen rabbits for shedding of oocysts and separate those shedding from young rabbits.
• Poor sanitation—sanitation is critical for control, especially within rabbit colonies or multirabbit homes. Routinely disinfect food bowls, water bottles, and cages.
• Stress, debility, and concurrent disease may predispose older animals to infection.

 DIAGNOSIS

## DIFFERENTIAL DIAGNOSIS
• Consider all causes of diarrhea, including systemic or metabolic disease, as well as specific intestinal disorders.
• Blood and mucous in stool is also seen with bacterial dysbiosis, especially overgrowth of clostridia or *Escherichia coli*; differentiate by fecal cytology.
• Fluid-filled, blood-tinged, or mucous-covered diarrhea—usually associated with Coccidia or bacterial enteritis in young rabbits; in older rabbits—associated with bacterial enteritis following antibiotic use, severe systemic illness, or intestinal obstruction/intussusception; less often Coccidia
• Anorexia, hepatomegaly, and jaundice—consider other causes of hepatitis, hepatic lipidosis, or neoplasia.

## CBC/BIOCHEMISTRY/URINALYSIS
• Usually normal; may be hemoconcentrated if dehydrated
• Increased liver enzymes (even mild increases can be significant) or bilirubin with hepatic involvement

## OTHER LABORATORY TESTS
N/A

## IMAGING
Hepatomegaly or ascites may be seen in rabbits with hepatic coccidiosis; often unremarkable in rabbits with intestinal coccidiosis.

## DIAGNOSTIC PROCEDURES
• Fecal examination for oocysts using routine fecal floatation or fecal wet mount
• Oocysts range in size from 15–40 μm
• Organisms can be identified from intestinal mucosal scrapings on necropsy or on histologic examination of intestinal specimens.

 TREATMENT

• Usually treated as an outpatient
• Patients with moderate to severe disease usually require hospitalization and 24-hour care for parenteral medication and fluid therapy.

• Fluid therapy and correction of electrolyte imbalances are the mainstays of treatment in most cases.
• Can give crystalloid fluid therapy orally, subcutaneously, or intravenously, as required
• Aim to return the patient to proper hydration status (over 12–24 hours) and replace any ongoing losses.
• Severe volume depletion can occur with acute diarrhea; aggressive shock fluid therapy may be necessary.
• Fluid choice for intravenous or subcutaneous use should take into consideration the electrolyte and hydration status.

## DIET
• It is imperative that the rabbit continue to eat during and following treatment. Continued anorexia will exacerbate gastrointestinal motility disorders and cause further derangement of the gastrointestinal microflora and overgrowth of intestinal bacterial pathogens.
• Offer a large selection of fresh, moistened greens such as cilantro, romaine lettuce, parsley, carrot tops, dandelion greens, spinach, and collard greens and good-quality grass hay. Many rabbits will begin to eat these foods, even if they were previously anorectic. Also offer the rabbit's normal pelleted diet.
• If the patient refuses these foods, syringe feed a gruel such as Critical Care for Herbivores (Oxbow Pet Products, Murdock, NE) 10–15mL/kg PO q6–8h. Larger volumes and more frequent feedings are often accepted; feed as much as the rabbit will accept. Alternatively, pellets can be ground and mixed with fresh greens, vegetable baby foods, water, or juice to form a gruel. The addition of canned pumpkin to this gruel is a palatable source of fiber and calories. If sufficient volumes of food are not accepted in this manner, nasogastric intubation is indicated.
• High-carbohydrate, high-fat nutritional supplements are contraindicated.
• The diet should be permanently modified to include sufficient amounts of indigestible fiber. Initially, feed only grass or timothy hay and washed fresh greens. These foods should always constitute the bulk of the diet. Pellets should be limited (if offered at all) and high-carbohydrate foods strictly prohibited.

 MEDICATIONS

## DRUG(S) OF CHOICE
• Coccidiostats—only slow multiplication of organisms until host immunity develops. Adult animals with subclinical infections will develop natural immunity and may not require medication.

• Sulfadimethoxine—50mg/kg PO first dose, then 25 mg/kg q24h for 10–20 days
• Trimethoprim/sulfamethoxazole—30 mg/kg PO q12h for 10 days
• Antibiotics—if secondary gastrointestinal bacterial infection is present. If indicated, use only broad-spectrum antibiotics such as trimethoprim sulfa (30 mg/kg PO q12h) or enrofloxacin (5–20 mg/kg PO, SC, IM q12h–24). For *Clostridium* spp.— metronidazole (20 mg/kg PO, IV q12h for up to 3 weeks)

### CONTRAINDICATIONS
The use of antibiotics that are primarily Gram positive in spectrum is contraindicated in rabbits. Use of these antibiotics will suppress the growth of commensal flora, allowing overgrowth of enteric pathogens and often a fatal enterotoxemia. Do not orally administer lincomycin, clindamycin, erythromycin, ampicillin, amoxicillin cephalosporins, or penicillins.

### ALTERNATE DRUGS
Coccidia—amprolium 9.6% in drinking water (0.5 mL per 500 mL); not consistently effective as water consumption is variable.

## FOLLOW-UP
Fecal examination for oocysts 1–2 weeks following treatment

### EXPECTED COURSE AND PROGNOSIS
• Intestinal coccidiosis—variable, depending on severity of infection, dehydration age, and immunocompetency of the rabbit
• Hepatic coccidiosis—guarded to poor in rabbits with heavy infestation, and signs of hepatic failure are present on presentation

## MISCELLANEOUS

### AGE-RELATED FACTORS
Disease usually in young patients 4–16 weeks old

### SEE ALSO
• Clostridia enterotoxemia
• Diarrhea, acute

### ABBREVIATIONS
N/A

*Suggested Reading*
Brown SA, Rosenthal KL. The anorexic rabbit. Proc North Am Vet Conf 1997:788.
Donoghue S. Nutrition and pet rabbits. In: Rosenthal KL, ed. Practical Exotic Animal Medicine: The Compendium Collection. Trenton, NJ: Veterinary Learning Systems, 1997:107.
Jenkins JR. Gastrointestinal diseases. In: Quesenberry KE, Carpenter JW, eds. Ferrets, Rabbits and Rodents: Clinical Medicine and Surgery. Philadelphia: WB Saunders, 2004:161–171.
Murphy JA, Ramer JC. Urgent care of the pet rabbit. Vet Clin North Am Exot Anim Pract 1998;1(1):127–152.
Tynes VV. Managing common gastrointestinal disorder in pet rabbits. Vet Med 2001;96(3):226–233.

# CONGESTIVE HEART FAILURE

 **BASICS**

## DEFINITION
• Left-sided congestive heart failure (L-CHF)—failure of the left side of the heart to advance blood at a sufficient rate to meet the metabolic needs of the patient or to prevent blood from pooling within the pulmonary venous circulation
• Right-sided congestive heart failure (R-CHF)—Failure of the right side of the heart to advance blood at a sufficient rate to meet the metabolic needs of the patient or to prevent blood from pooling within the systemic venous circulation

## PATHOPHYSIOLOGY
• CHF in rabbits may be due to cardiomyopathy, tricuspid or mitral insufficiency, and, less commonly, congenital heart disease.
• Rabbits have limited collateral myocardial circulation and may therefore be more prone to myocardial ischemia.
• L-CHF—low cardiac output causes lethargy, exercise intolerance, syncope, and prerenal azotemia. High hydrostatic pressure causes leakage of fluid from pulmonary venous circulation into pulmonary interstitium and alveoli. When fluid leakage exceeds ability of lymphatics to drain the affected areas, pulmonary edema develops.
• R-CHF—high hydrostatic pressure leads to leakage of fluid from venous circulation into the pleural and peritoneal space and interstitium of peripheral tissue. When fluid leakage exceeds ability of lymphatics to drain the affected areas, pleural effusion, ascites, and peripheral edema develop.

## SYSTEMS AFFECTED
All organ systems can be affected by either poor delivery of blood or the effects of passive congestion from backup of venous blood.

## INCIDENCE/PREVALENCE
Although anecdotally reported as common, very little published information on rabbit heart disease is available.

## SIGNALMENT
Little information is available; cardiomyopathy may be more common in giant breeds.

## SIGNS

### General Comments
Signs vary with underlying cause.

### Historical Findings
• Weakness, lethargy, exercise intolerance
• Anorexia or inappetence, weight loss
• Dyspnea or tachypnea
• Syncope
• Abdominal distension with ascites

### Physical Examination Findings
*L-CHF*
• Tachypnea (normal respiratory rate is 30–60 breaths/min)
• Inspiratory and expiratory dyspnea when animal has pulmonary edema
• Pulmonary crackles and wheezes
• Prolonged capillary refill time
• Possible murmur
• Possible arrhythmia (normal heart rate is 180–330 beats/min)
• Weak, irregular pulses
*R-CHF*
• Hepatomegaly
• Splenomegaly
• Ascites
• Possible murmur
• Muffled heart sounds if animal has pleural or pericardial effusion
• Rapid, shallow respiration if animal has pleural effusion
• Possible jugular venous distention or jugular pulses

## CAUSES AND RISK FACTORS

### Pump (Muscle) Failure of Left or Right Ventricle
• Idiopathic cardiomyopathy—most common reported cause
• Myocarditis secondary to *Pasteurella multocida*, *Salmonella* sp, coronavirus, or *Encephalitozoon cuniculi*

### Pressure Overload to Left Heart
Causes reported in other mammals, such as systemic hypertension, subaortic stenosis, or left ventricular tumors, have not yet been reported in rabbits. However, these causes should be considered since there is no reason that these diseases should not occur, and they may be underreported.

### Pressure Overload to Right Heart
Causes reported in other mammals, such as chronic obstructive pulmonary disease, pulmonary thromboembolism, pulmonic stenosis, right ventricular tumors, or primary pulmonary hypertension, have not yet been reported in rabbits. However, these causes should be considered since there is no reason that these diseases should not occur.

### Volume Overload of Left Heart
• Mitral valve insufficiency
• Aortic insufficiency
• Ventricular septal defect anecdotally reported; other congenital defects have not been reported.

### Impediment to Filling of Left Heart
• Hypertrophic cardiomyopathy
• Pericardial effusion with tamponade
• Restrictive pericarditis
• Left atrial masses (e.g., tumors and thrombus), pulmonary thromboembolism, and mitral stenosis have not yet been reported in rabbits. However, these causes should be considered since there is no reason that

these diseases should not occur, and they may be underreported.

### Impediment to Right Ventricular Filling
• Pericardial effusion
• Restrictive pericarditis
• Right atrial or caval masses and tricuspid stenosis have not yet been reported in rabbits. However, these causes should be considered since there is no reason that these diseases should not occur, and they may be underreported.

### Rhythm Disturbances
• Respiratory sinus arrhythmia is not considered normal in rabbits.
• Little information is available.
• Atrial fibrillation, atrial tachycardia, and ventricular premature beats and ventricular tachycardia anecdotally reported

 **DIAGNOSIS**

## DIFFERENTIAL DIAGNOSIS
• Must differentiate from other causes of dyspnea and weakness; generally requires a complete diagnostic workup including CBC, biochemistry profile, thoracocentesis or abdominocentesis with fluid analysis, and thoracic and abdominal ultrasound
• Pleural effusion—thymoma or lymphoma, other neoplasia, abscess
• Dyspnea—rhinitis or sinusitis (rabbits are obligate nasal breathers) and primary pulmonary disease (abscess, pneumonia) most common; neoplasia (thymoma or lymphoma, heart-based tumors, metastatic neoplasia), pleural effusion; trauma resulting in diaphragmatic hernia, pulmonary hemorrhage, pneumothorax; airway obstruction due to foreign body or laryngeal edema
• Ascites, abdominal distension—consider hypoproteinemia, severe liver disease, ruptured bladder, peritonitis, abdominal neoplasia, and abdominal hemorrhage.

## CBC/BIOCHEMISTRY/URINALYSIS
• CBC usually normal
• Mild to moderately high alanine transaminase, aspartate transaminase, and serum alkaline phosphatase with R-CHF
• Prerenal azotemia in some animals

## OTHER LABORATORY TESTS
N/A

## IMAGING

### Radiographic Findings
• Generalized cardiomegaly—bear in mind that the thoracic cavity is smaller in rabbits compared to other mammals; heart may be large relative to thoracic cage.
• Soft tissue density cranial to heart—normal to some degree due to thymus (does not regress in rabbits) and intrathoracic fat

# CONGESTIVE HEART FAILURE

• Pulmonary edema (L-CHF), pleural effusion, or both in some animals
• Hepatomegaly or ascites may be seen (R-CHF)
• Different forms of cardiomyopathy cannot be differentiated by radiography.

### Echocardiography
• Echocardiography is the diagnostic modality of choice to differentiate forms of cardiomyopathy, cardiac masses, pericardial effusion, and valvular insufficiency.
• Findings vary markedly with cause.
• Normal findings have been reported (see suggested reading list).

## DIAGNOSTIC PROCEDURES

### Electrocardiographic Findings
• Often are normal and therefore not helpful in the diagnosis
• Rabbits resist attachment of alligator clips; use padded clips or file the teeth from the clips.
• Respiratory sinus arrhythmias are not normal findings in rabbits.
• The ECG of normal rabbits differs from the feline ECG in that p, R, and T waves are shorter in lead II; reported normal ranges exist on a limited number of rabbits (see suggested reading list).
• Both ventricular and supraventricular arrhythmias can be seen.
• May show atrial or ventricular enlargement patterns

### Abdominocentesis
Ascites is rare; analysis of ascitic fluid in patients with R-CHF generally reveals modified transudate.

### Pleural Effusion Analysis
Pleural effusion typically is a modified transudate with total protein <4.0 g/dL and nucleated cell counts <2500/mL (these values have been extrapolated from other mammalian species to be used as a guideline). Analysis of the pleural effusion is important to rule out other causes of pleural effusion; can be both diagnostic and therapeutic

## PATHOLOGIC FINDINGS
Cardiac findings vary with disease

## TREATMENT

### APPROPRIATE HEALTH CARE
• Severely dyspneic, weak, or anorectic rabbits in CHF should be treated as inpatients.
• Mildly affected animals can be treated as outpatients.

### NURSING CARE
• Supplemental oxygen therapy is extremely important for dyspneic rabbits. Face mask delivery of oxygen can be very stressful to rabbits; oxygen cage should be used if available.

• Minimize handling of critically dyspneic animals. Stress can kill!
• Thoracocentesis is both therapeutic and diagnostic. If there is significant pleural effusion, drain each hemithorax with a 20-gauge butterfly catheter after the rabbit is stable enough to be handled. Sedation or anesthesia with isoflurane by mask may be necessary.
• If hypothermic, external heat (incubator or heating pad) is recommended. Monitor temperature carefully, as rabbits are extremely sensitive to heat stress.

## ACTIVITY
Restrict activity.

## DIET
• Provide adequate nutrition. It is imperative that the rabbit continue to eat during and following treatment. Anorexia will often cause gastrointestinal hypomotility, derangement of the gastrointestinal microflora, and overgrowth of intestinal bacterial pathogens.
• If the patient refuses food, syringe feed a gruel such as Critical Care for Herbivores (Oxbow Pet Products, Murdock, NE), giving approximately 10–15 mL/kg PO q8–12h. Alternatively, pellets can be ground and mixed with fresh greens, vegetable baby foods, water, or juice to form a gruel.
• Encourage oral fluid intake by offering fresh water, wetting leafy vegetables, or flavoring water with vegetable juices.

## CLIENT EDUCATION
CHF is not curable and will progress.

## SURGICAL CONSIDERATIONS
N/A

## MEDICATIONS

### DRUG(S) OF CHOICE

#### Diuretics
• Furosemide is recommended at the lowest effective dose to eliminate pulmonary edema and pleural effusion. If the rabbit is in fulminant cardiac failure, administer furosemide at 1–4 mg/kg q8–12h IM or IV. Initially, furosemide should be administered parenterally. Long-term therapy should be continued at a dose of 1–2 mg/kg q8–12h PO. The pediatric elixir may be well accepted.
• Predisposes the patient to dehydration, pre-renal azotemia, and electrolyte disturbances

#### Venodilators
• Nitroglycerin (2% ointment) 1/16–1/8 inch applied topically to the inner pinna can be used in conjunction with diuretics in the acute management of CHF to further reduce preload. Nitroglycerin may lower the dose of furosemide and is

particularly useful in patients with hypothermia or dehydration.
• May be useful in animals with chronic L-CHF when used intermittently

### Digoxin
• Digoxin is used in animals with dilated cardiomyopathy (myocardial failure) at a dose of 0.005–0.01 mg/kg PO q24–48h. Use the low end of dosage range initially, and increase gradually. Monitor for signs of digoxin toxicity (anorexia) and monitor serum digoxin concentrations (see below).
• Digoxin also indicated to treat supraventricular arrhythmias (e.g., sinus tachycardia, atrial fibrillation, and atrial or junctional tachycardia) in patients with CHF

### ACE Inhibitors
Enalapril is recommended for long-term maintenance to reduce afterload and preload. A dose of 0.25–0.5 mg/kg PO q24–48h has been anecdotally used. Enalapril can be compounded into a suspension by a compounding pharmacy for ease of administration.

### Other Medications
• Beta-blockers may be beneficial in patients with hypertropic cardiomyopathy; doses have not been reported in rabbits; extrapolate from cat or ferret doses. Beneficial effects may include slowing of sinus rate and correcting atrial and ventricular arrhythmias. Role in asymptomatic patients is unresolved.
• Calcium channel blockers may also be beneficial in the treatment of hypertropic cardiomyopathy; doses have not been reported in rabbits; extrapolate from cat or ferret doses. Beneficial effects may include slower sinus rate, resolution of supraventricular arrhythmias, improved diastolic relaxation, and peripheral vasodilation, but these have not been documented in rabbits.

## CONTRAINDICATIONS
Positive inotropic drugs should be avoided in patients with HCM.

## PRECAUTIONS
• Rabbits may become anorectic with enalapril administration. If anorexia occurs, decrease the dosage and/or frequency of administration.
• ACE inhibitors and digoxin must be used cautiously in patients with renal disease.
• Overzealous diuretic therapy may cause dehydration and hypokalemia.

## POSSIBLE INTERACTIONS
• The use of a calcium channel blocker in combination with a beta-blocker should be avoided as clinically significant bradyarrhythmias can develop in other small animals and are likely to also occur in rabbits.
• Combination of high-dose diuretics and ACE inhibitor may alter renal perfusion and cause azotemia.

# CONGESTIVE HEART FAILURE

## ALTERNATIVE DRUGS
• Other vasodilators, including hydralazine, may be used instead of or in addition to an ACE inhibitor. Dosages have been anecdotally extrapolated from feline dosages; however, their use is not widespread, and efficacy and safety are unknown (beware of hypotension).
• Other beta-blockers, such as atenolol, carvedilol, or metoprolol, can be used instead of propranolol to help control ventricular response rate in atrial fibrillation. Dosages have been anecdotally extrapolated from feline dosages; however, their use is not widespread, and efficacy and safety are unknown.
• Patients unresponsive to furosemide, vasodilators, and digoxin (if indicated) may benefit from combination diuretic therapy by adding spironolactone. Dosages have been anecdotally extrapolated from feline dosages; however, their use is not widespread, and efficacy and safety are unknown.
• Potassium supplementation if animal has hypokalemia—use potassium supplements cautiously in animals receiving an ACE inhibitor or spironolactone.

## FOLLOW-UP

### PATIENT MONITORING
• Monitor radiographs, echocardiography, renal status, electrolytes, hydration, respiratory rate and effort, heart rate, body weight, and abdominal girth.

• If azotemia develops, reduce the dosage of diuretic. If azotemia persists and the animal is also on an ACE inhibitor, reduce or discontinue the ACE inhibitor. Use digoxin with caution if azotemia develops.
• Monitor ECG if arrhythmias are suspected.
• Check digoxin concentration periodically. Therapeutic range (as extrapolated from dogs and cats) is between 1–2 ng/dL 8–12 hours postpill.

### PREVENTION/AVOIDANCE
Minimize stress and exercise in patients with heart disease.

### POSSIBLE COMPLICATIONS
• Sudden death due to arrhythmias
• Iatrogenic problems associated with medical management (see above)

### EXPECTED COURSE AND PROGNOSIS
Prognosis varies with underlying cause; little data exist for rabbits.

## MISCELLANEOUS

### ASSOCIATED CONDITIONS
N/A

### AGE-RELATED FACTORS
Degenerative heart conditions generally seen in middle-aged to old animals

### ZOONOTIC POTENTIAL
N/A

### PREGNANCY
N/A

### SYNONYMS
N/A

### SEE ALSO
Dyspnea and tachypnea

### ABBREVIATIONS
• ACE = angiotensin-converting enzyme
• CBC = complete blood count
• ECG = electrocardiogram
• HCM = hypertrophic cardiomyopathy

*Suggested Reading*

Harcourt-Brown F. Cardiorespiratory diseases. In: Harcourt-Brown F, ed. Textbook of Rabbit Medicine. Oxford: Butterworth-Heinemann, 2002:325–334.
Huston SM, Quesenberry KE. Cardiovascular and lymphoproliferative diseases. In: Quesenberry KE, Carpenter JW, eds. Ferrets, Rabbits and Rodents: Clinical Medicine and Surgery. 2nd Ed. Philadelphia: WB Saunders, 2004:211–220.
Paul-Murphy JA, Ramer JC. Urgent care of the pet rabbit. Vet Clin North Am Exot Anim Pract 1998:1(1):127–152.
Redrobe S. Imaging techniques in small mammals. Semin Avian Exotic Pet Med 2001;10:195.

*Portions Adapted From*

Smith FWK, Keene BW. Congested Heart Failure. In: Tilley LP, Smith FWK, Jr., eds. The 5-Minute Veterinary Consult: Canine and Feline, 2nd Ed. Baltimore: Lippincott Williams & Wilkins, 2000.

# BASICS

## DEFINITION
Inflammation of the conjunctiva, the vascularized mucous membrane that covers the anterior portion of the globe (bulbar portion) and lines the lids and third eyelid (palpebral portion)

## PATHOPHYSIOLOGY
• Primary—infectious, environmental, KCS
• Secondary to an underlying ocular or systemic disease—tooth root disorders, glaucoma, uveitis, neoplasia

## SYSTEMS AFFECTED
• Ophthalmic—ocular with occasional lid involvement (e.g., blepharoconjunctivitis)
• Respiratory
• Oral cavity

## GENETICS
N/A

## INCIDENCE/PREVALENCE
Common

## GEOGRAPHIC DISTRIBUTION
N/A

## SIGNALMENT
• Acquired cheek tooth elongation causing blockage of nasolacrimal duct or intrusion into the retrobulbar space—usually seen in middle-aged rabbits
• Young animals—congenital tooth malocclusion, congenital eyelid deformities
• Dwarf and lop breeds—congenital tooth malocclusion
• Dwarf and Himalayan breeds—glaucoma more common
• Rex and New Zealand White breeds—entropion and trichiasis more common

### Mean Age and Range
N/A

### Predominant Sex
N/A

## SIGNS

### Historical Signs
• History of previous treatment for dental disease
• History of nasal discharge or previous upper respiratory infection
• Facial asymmetry, masses, or exophthalmos in rabbits with tooth root abscesses
• Signs of pain—reluctance to move, depression, lethargy, hiding, hunched posture in rabbits with painful ocular conditions or underlying dental disease
• Unilateral or bilateral alopecia, crusts, and matted fur in periocular area, cheeks, and/or nasal rostrum

### Physical Examination Findings
• Blepharospasm
• Conjunctival hyperemia

• Ocular discharge—serous, mucoid, or mucopurulent
• Thick, white exudate accumulation in medial canthus in rabbits with dacryocystitis
• Corneal ulcers associated with dacryocystitis are usually superficial and ventrally located; ulcers secondary to exposure keratitis are usually central and may be superficial or deep.
• Chemosis
• Excessive conjunctival tissue—may partially or completely occlude the cornea
• Facial pyoderma—alopecia, erythema, and matted fur in periocular area, cheeks, and/or nasal rostrum; due to constant moisture in rabbits with epiphora
• A thorough examination of the oral cavity is indicated in every rabbit with epiphora to rule out dental disease. Use of an otoscope or speculum may be useful in identifying severe abnormalities; however, many problems will be missed by using this method alone. A thorough examination of the cheek teeth requires heavy sedation or general anesthesia and specialized equipment. Use a focused, directed light source and magnification (or a rigid endoscope, if available) to provide optimal visualization. Use a rodent mouth gag and cheek dilators (Jorgensen Laboratories, Inc., Loveland, CO) to open the mouth and pull buccal tissues away from teeth surfaces to allow adequate exposure. Use a cotton swab or tongue depressor to retract tongue from lingual surfaces.
• Identify cheek teeth elongation, irregular crown height, spikes, curved teeth, tooth discoloration, tooth mobility, missing teeth, purulent exudate, oral ulceration, or abscesses.
• Incisors—may see overgrowth, horizontal ridges or grooves, malformation, discoloration, fractures, malocclusion, increased or decreased curvature
• Significant tooth root abnormalities may be present despite normal-appearing crowns. Skull radiographs are required to identify apical disorders.

## CAUSES

### Bacterial
• Primary condition (i.e., not secondary to another condition such as dacryocystitis or KCS)—rare
• Secondary infection—*Staphylococcus* spp., *Pseudomonas* spp., *Moraxella* spp., *Pasteurella multocida, Neisseria* spp., and *Bordetella* spp. frequently cultured; usually secondary to URI or dental disease

### Secondary to Adnexal Disease
• Secondary to obstruction of the outflow of the nasolacrimal duct or dacryocystitis—one of the most common causes—obstruction usually secondary to tooth root elongation or tooth root abscesses blocking outflow or

due to the presence of thick exudates, scarring, or inflammation of the duct from chronic upper respiratory tract infection
• Secondary to maxillary tooth root elongation—irritation to the globe due to impingement of overgrown tooth roots or abscesses into the retrobulbar space
• Lid diseases (e.g., entropion, ectropion) and lash diseases (e.g., distichiasis, ectopic cilia)—may lead to clinical signs of conjunctivitis
• Aqueous tear film deficiency (KCS); often secondary to facial nerve paralysis

### Secondary to Trauma or Environmental Causes
• Conjunctival foreign body
• Irritation—dust, chemicals, or ophthalmic medications

### Secondary to Other Ocular Diseases
• Ulcerative keratitis—trauma most common; exposure keratitis following anesthesia, facial nerve paralysis; corneal abrasion in rabbits with torticollis
• Anterior uveitis—most commonly bacterial or *Encephalitozoon cuniculi*
• Glaucoma

### Viral Causes
Myxomatosis—unusual

### Neoplastic Causes
Tumors involving conjunctiva—rare

### Aberrant Conjunctival Overgrowth
Cause not completely understood; may occur as congenital disorder, idiopathic or secondary to trauma or inflammation. Conjunctiva grows from the limbus, is nonadherent to the cornea, and may completely cover the cornea; does not appear to be painful; may not be associated with significant inflammation in patients with congenital or idiopathic disease

## RISK FACTORS
• Dental disease
• Upper respiratory disease
• Immunosupression—systemic or topical corticosteriod use; stress, debility
• Poor husbandry—inappropriate diet, dirty environment

# DIAGNOSIS

## DIFFERENTIAL DIAGNOSIS
• Primary—must distinguish from condition that is secondary to other ocular diseases
• Differentiate between conjunctival vessels (freely mobile and will blanch with sympathomimetic) and episcleral (deep) vessels (immobile and do not blanch with sympathomimetics), because episcleral congestion indicates intraocular disease, whereas conjunctival hyperemia may be a sign of primary conjunctivitis or intraocular disease.

# CONJUNCTIVITIS

• Unilateral condition with ocular pain (blepharospasm)—usually indicates a tooth root disorder, foreign body, or corneal injury
• Chronic, bilateral condition—usually due to chronic upper respiratory tract infection (scarring, inflammation of duct); can indicate a congenital problem; bilateral tooth root disorders also seen
• Acute, bilateral condition with severe eyelid edema—consider myxomatosis.
• Facial pain, swelling, nasal discharge, or sneezing—seen with tooth root elongation or abscess; may indicate nasal or sinus infection; may indicate obstruction from neoplasm
• White discharge confined to the medial canthus—usually indicates dacryocystitis

## CBC/BIOCHEMISTRY/URINALYSIS
Normal, except with systemic disease

## OTHER LABORATORY TESTS
N/A

## IMAGING
• Skull radiographs are mandatory to identify dental disease and nasal, sinus, or maxillary bone lesions and, if present, to plan treatment strategies and to monitor progression of treatment.
• Perform under general anesthesia
• Five views are recommend for thorough assessment—ventral–dorsal, lateral, two lateral obliques, and rostral–caudal.
• CT—superior to radiographs to localize nasolacrimal duct obstruction and characterize associated lesions
• Orbital ultrasonography—helpful in defining the retrobulbar abscess or neoplasia and extent of the lesion
• Dacryocystorhinography—radiopaque contrast material to help localize nasolacrimal duct obstruction

## DIAGNOSTIC PROCEDURES
• Complete ophthalmic examination
• Schirmer tear test—rule out KCS. Average values reported as 5 mm/min; however, even lower values can be seen in normal rabbits.
• Fluorescein stain—rule out ulcerative keratitis; test for nasolacrimal function; dye flows through the nasolacrimal system and reaches the external nares in approximately 10 seconds in normal rabbits.
• Intraocular pressures—rule out glaucoma.
• Examine for signs of anterior uveitis (e.g., hypotony, aqueous flare, and miosis).
• Thorough adnexal examination—rule out lid abnormalities, lash abnormalities, and foreign bodies in cul-de-sacs or under nictitans.
• Perform a nasolacrimal flush—rule out nasolacrimal disease; may dislodge foreign

material. Topical administration of an ophthalmic anesthetic is generally sufficient for this procedure; nervous rabbits may require mild sedation. Rabbits have only a single nasolacrimal punctum located in the ventral eyelid at the medial canthus. A 23-gauge lacrimal cannula or a 24-gauge Teflon intravenous catheter can be used to flush the duct. Irrigation will generally produce a thick, white exudate from the nasal meatus.
• Aerobic bacterial culture and sensitivity—consider with mucopurulent discharge; ideally specimens taken before anything is placed in the eye (e.g., topical anesthetic, fluorescein, and flush) to prevent inhibition or dilution of bacterial growth; not routinely indicated for KCS and a mucopurulent discharge (secondary bacterial overgrowth almost certain). Often, only normal organisms are isolated (*Bacillus subtilis*, *Staphylococcus aureus*, *Bordetella* spp.).
• Conjunctival cytology—may reveal a cause (rare); may see degenerate neutrophils and intracytoplasmic bacteria, which indicate bacterial infection
• Conjunctival biopsy—may be useful with mass lesions and immune-mediated disease; may help with chronic disease for which a definitive diagnosis has not been made
• Rhinoscopy—with or without biopsy or bacterial culture; may be indicated if previous tests suggest a nasal or sinus lesion

 TREATMENT

## APPROPRIATE HEALTH CARE
• Primary—often outpatient
• Secondary to other diseases (e.g., tooth root elongation or abscess)—may require hospitalization while the underlying problem is diagnosed and treated

## NURSING CARE
• Nasolacrimal duct irrigation—as described above if obstruction is diagnosed; if blocked or inflamed, irrigation of the duct often needs to be repeated, either daily for 2–3 consecutive days, or once every 3–4 days until irrigation produces a clear fluid. Failure to keep ducts patent may result in scarring or permanent obstruction.
• Keep fur around face clean and dry

## DIET
### Anorexia
• Many rabbits with ocular disease, especially those with underlying dental disease, are in pain and may become inappetent. It is absolutely imperative that the rabbit con-

tinue to eat during and following treatment. Anorexia will cause or exacerbate gastrointestinal hypomotility, derangement of the gastrointestinal microflora, and overgrowth of intestinal bacterial pathogens.
• Syringe feed a gruel such as Critical Care for Herbivores (Oxbow Pet Products, Murdock, NE) 10–15 mL/kg PO q8–12h. Alternatively, pellets can be ground and mixed with fresh greens, vegetable baby foods, water, or juice to form a gruel.
• High-carbohydrate, high-fat nutritional supplements are contraindicated.
• Encourage oral fluid intake by offering fresh water or wetting leafy vegetables.

### Rabbits With Underlying Dental Disease
Encourage normal occlusion and wear by increasing the amount of tough, fibrous foods and foods containing abrasive silicates such as hay and wild grasses; avoid pelleted food and soft fruits or vegetables.

## CLIENT EDUCATION
• If copious discharge is noted, instruct the client to clean the eyes before giving treatment.
• If solutions and ointments are both prescribed, instruct the client to use the solution(s) before the ointment(s).
• If several solutions are prescribed, instruct the client to wait several minutes between treatments.
• Instruct the client to call for instructions if the condition worsens, which indicates that the condition may not be responsive or may be progressing or that the animal may be having an adverse reaction to a prescribed medication.
• Inform client that an Elizabethan collar should be placed on the patient if self-trauma occurs.

## SURGICAL CONSIDERATIONS
• Irritation of the globe or blocked nasolacrimal duct due to elongation of cheek tooth roots—trimming of cheek teeth (coronal reduction) may correct or control progression of root elongation
• Tooth extraction—because rabbits have very long, deeply embedded, and curved tooth roots, extraction per os can be extremely time consuming and labor intensive as compared to for dogs and cats. If the germinal bud is not completely removed, the teeth may regrow or a new abscess may form. If not experienced with tooth extraction in rabbits, the author recommends referral to a veterinarian with special expertise whenever feasible.
• In rabbits with extensive tooth root abscesses—aggressive debridement is

indicated, and special expertise may be required. Maxillary and retrobulbar abscesses can be particularly challenging. If not experienced with facial abscesses in rabbits, the author recommends referral to a veterinarian with special expertise whenever feasible.
• Aberrant conjunctival overgrowth—surgical excision of the excessive conjunctiva; often only palliative, may reform; to minimize recurrence, the cut edge may be sutured to the limbus. Immunomodulating agents may prevent reformation.
• Chronic corneal ulcers not responsive to medical treatment—may require debridement of loose epithelium, punctate or grid keratotomy, or conjunctival flap. Procedures are similar to those performed in cats and dogs.

## MEDICATIONS

### DRUG(S) OF CHOICE

*Bacterial*
• Based on bacterial culture and sensitivity results
• Initial treatment—broad-spectrum topical antibiotic or based on results of cytologic examination while awaiting culture results; may try empirical treatment, performing a culture only if patient is refractory to treatment
• Topical triple antibiotic, chloramphenicol, gentamicin, or ciprofloxacin—q6–12h, depending on severity
• Systemic antibiotics—indicated in rabbits with tooth root abscess or upper respiratory infection as the cause of conjunctivitis
• Topical NSAIDs—0.03% flurbiprofen or 1% diclofenac may help reduce inflammation and irritation associated with nasolacrimal duct flushes.
• Artificial tears and lubricant ointments—for alleviation of keratoconjunctivitis sicca; must be applied frequently; only transiently relieve dryness
• Cyclosporine A has also been used in rabbits to increase tear production (0.2% ointment instilled q12h). Use with discretion—information on use in rabbits is limited; be aware that Schirmer tear test results can be very low in normal rabbits.
• Sedation for nasolacrimal duct flushing or oral examination—light sedation with midazolam (0.5–2 mg/kg IM) or diazepam (1–2 mg/kg IM); oral examinations or longer procedures require deeper sedation; the author prefers ketamine (15–20 mg/kg IM) plus midazolam (0.5–1.0 mg/kg IM);

many other sedation protocols exist. Alternatively, administer general anesthesia with isoflurane.
• Long-term pain management—indicated in rabbits with dental disease. NSAIDs have been used for short- or long-term therapy to reduce pain and inflammation: meloxicam (0.2–0.5 mg/kg PO q24h) or carprofen (2.2 mg/kg PO q12–24)

### CONTRAINDICATIONS
• Topical corticosteroids—never use if the cornea retains fluorescein stain. Never use in face of evidence of local or systemic bacterial infection.
• Oral administration of most antibiotics effective against anaerobes will cause a fatal gastrointestinal dysbiosis in rabbits. Do not administer penicillins, macrolides, lincosamides, and cephalosporins by oral administration.

### PRECAUTIONS
• Topical corticosteroids or antibiotic–corticosteroid combinations—avoid; associated with gastrointestinal ulceration and hemorrhage, delayed wound healing, and heightened susceptibility to infection; rabbits are very sensitive to the immunosuppressive effects of both topical and systemic corticosteroids; use may exacerbate subclinical bacterial infection.
• Aggressive flushing of the nasolacrimal duct may cause temporary swelling of the periocular tissues. Swelling using resolves within 12–48 hours.
• Topical aminoglycosides—may be irritating
• Topical antibiotics—may lead to enteric dysbiosis if excessive ingestion occurs during grooming

### POSSIBLE INTERACTIONS
N/A

### ALTERNATIVE DRUGS
N/A

## FOLLOW-UP

### PATIENT MONITORING
Recheck shortly after beginning treatment (i.e., 5–7 days); then recheck as needed.

### PREVENTION/AVOIDANCE
Treat any underlying disease that may be exacerbating the condition (e.g., dental disease, eyelid disorders, KCS).

### POSSIBLE COMPLICATIONS
N/A

### EXPECTED COURSE AND PROGNOSIS
• Warn client that recurrence is common in patients with nasolacrimal obstruction. The nasolacrimal duct may become completely obliterated in rabbits with severe infection or tooth root disease (abscesses, elongation, neoplasia). Epiphora may be lifelong. Home management, including keeping the face clean and dry, is crucial to prevent secondary pyoderma. In many cases, acquisition of a second rabbit can be beneficial if the second rabbit grooms discharges from the face.
• Rabbits with aberrant conjunctival overgrowth—recurrence is common; more than one surgery may be required.
• Mild conjunctivitis as part of upper respiratory tract infection—prognosis is good, although recurrence is common.
• Rabbits with cheek tooth root elongation—by the time clinical signs are noted, disease is usually advanced. Lifelong treatment, consisting of periodic coronal reduction (teeth trimming), is required, usually every 1–3 months.
• Severe dental disease, especially in rabbits with tooth root abscesses and severe bony destruction, carries a guarded to poor prognosis for complete resolution. Most will require extensive surgery, sometimes multiple surgeries and multiple follow-up visits. Recurrences in the same or other locations are common. Clients must be aware of the monetary and time investment.

## MISCELLANEOUS

### ASSOCIATED CONDITIONS
• Moist dermatitis ventral to the medial canthus
• Nasal discharge

### AGE-RELATED FACTORS
N/A

### ZOONOTIC POTENTIAL
N/A

### PREGNANCY
• Use systemic antibiotics and corticosteroids with caution, if at all, in pregnant animals.
• Consider absorption of topically applied medications; weigh benefits of treatment against possible complications.

### SEE ALSO
• Cheek tooth malocclusion and elongation
• Facial nerve paresis/paralysis
• Incisor malocclusion and overgrowth
• Red eye
• Tooth root abscesses

## CONJUNCTIVITIS

### ABBREVIATIONS
- CT = computed tomography
- KCS = keratoconjunctivitis sicca
- NSAIDs = nonsteroidal antiinflammatory drugs
- URI = upper respiratory infection

*Suggested Reading*

Andrew SE. Corneal disease of rabbits. Vet Clin Noth Am Exotic Anim Pract 2002;5:341–356.

Crossley DA. Oral biology and disorders of lagomorphs. Vet Clin Noth Am Exotic Anim Pract 2003;6:629–659.

Felchle LM, Sigler RL. Phacoemulsification for the management of *Encephalitozoon cuniculi*-induced phacoclastic uveitis in a rabbit. Vet Ophthalmol 2002;5(3):211–215.

Munger RJ, Langevin JP. Spontaneous cataracts in laboratory rabbits. Vet Ophthalmol 2002;5(3):177–181.

Stiles J, Dider E, Ritchie B, et al. *Encephalitozoon cuniculi* in the lens of a rabbit with phacoclastic uveitis: confirmation and treatment. Vet Comp Ophthalmol 1997;7(4):233–238.

Van der Woerdt A. Ophthalmologic disease in small pet animals. In: Quesenberry KE, Carpenter JW, eds. Ferrets, Rabbits and Rodents: Clinical Medicine and Surgery. 2nd Ed. Philadelphia: WB Saunders, 2004:421–428.

Williams DL. Laboratory animal ophthalmology. In: Gelatt KN, ed. Veterinary Ophthalmology. 3rd Ed. Philadelphia: Lippincott Williams & Wilkins, 1999:151–181.

*Portions Adapted From*

Champagne ES. Conjunctivitis—Dogs and Cats. In: Tilley LP, Smith FWK, Jr., eds. The 5-Minute Veterinary Consult: Canine and Feline, 3rd Ed. Baltimore: Lippincott Williams & Wilkins, 2004.

# CONSTIPATION (LACK OF FECAL PRODUCTION)

## BASICS

### DEFINITION
• Constipation—infrequent, incomplete, or difficult defecation with passage of scant, small, hard, or dry fecal pellets
• Constipation and obstipation, in which the colon is filled with large amounts of hard, dry feces, generally do not occur in rabbits. The exception to this is a very distal colonic outflow obstruction (neoplasia, abscess, stricture or anal atresia).
• Scant fecal production or lack of fecal production is usually the result of anorexia and/or gastrointestinal motility dysfunction (gastrointestinal hypomotility)

### PATHOPHYSIOLOGY
• Rabbits are hind-gut fermenters and are extremely sensitive to alterations in diet.
• Proper hind-gut fermentation and gastrointestinal tract motility are dependent on the ingestion of large amounts of roughage and long-stemmed hay. If adequate amounts of roughage are ingested and gastrointestinal tract motility is normal, fur ingested as a result of normal grooming behavior will pass through the gastrointestinal tract with the ingesta.
• Diets that contain inadequate amounts of long-stemmed, coarse fiber (such as the feeding of only commercial pelleted food without hay or grasses) cause cecocolonic hypomotility that may lead to accumulation of ingesta, including fur and other material, in the gastrointestinal tract.
• Affected rabbits suddenly or gradually refuse food. As motility slows, ingesta accumulates proximal to the colon (stomach, cecum); fecal pellets become small and scant; water is removed from fecal pellets in the colon, making the fecal pellets drier than normal.
• Cecocolonic hypomotility also causes alterations in cecal fermentation, pH, and substrate production, resulting in alteration of enteric microflora populations. Diets low in coarse fiber typically contain high simple carbohydrate concentrations, which provide a ready source of fermentable products and promote the growth of bacterial pathogens such as *Escherichia coli* and *Clostridium* spp. Bacterial dysbiosis can cause acute diarrhea, enterotoxemia, ileus, or chronic intermittent diarrhea.
• Anorexia due to infectious or metabolic disease, pain, stress, or starvation may cause or exacerbate gastrointestinal hypomotility

### SYSTEMS AFFECTED
Gastrointestinal

### INCIDENCE/PREVALENCE
Gastrointestinal hypomotility, resulting in scant or lack of feces, chronic intermittent diarrhea, abdominal pain, and ill-thrift, is one of the most common clinical problems seen in the rabbit.

### SIGNALMENT
• More commonly seen in older rabbits on inappropriate diets, but can occur in any-aged rabbit
• No breed or gender predilections

### SIGNS
#### Historical Findings
• Scant or no production of fecal pellets
• Small, hard, dry feces
• Infrequent defecation
• Inappetence or anorexia; rabbits often initially stop eating pellets, but continue to eat treats, followed by complete anorexia.
• Signs of pain, such as teeth grinding, a hunched posture, and reluctance to move, are extremely common.
• History of inappropriate diet (e.g., cereals, grains, commercial pellets only, sweets, large quantities of fruits, lack of feeding long-stemmed hay)
• Recent history of illness or stressful event
• Weight loss in rabbits with underlying or chronic disease
• Obesity in rabbits on diets consisting of mainly commercial pellets
• Patients are usually bright and alert, except those with enterotoxemia or acute small intestinal obstruction (gastric dilation), who are depressed, lethargic, or shocky.

#### Physical Examination Findings
• Small, hard fecal pellets or absence of fecal pellets palpable in the colon
• Cecum may be filled with gas, fluid, or firm, dry contents, depending on the underlying cause.
• Palpation of the stomach is an extremely valuable tool in the diagnosis of abnormal retention of stomach contents. Ingesta normally should be palpable in the stomach of a healthy rabbit. The normal stomach should be easily deformable, feel soft and pliable, and not remain pitted on compression. Rabbits with early gastrointestinal hypomotility will have a firm, often enlarged stomach that remains pitted when compressed. With complete gastrointestinal stasis, severe dehydration, or prolonged hypomotility, the stomach may be severely distended, hard, and nondeformable.
• The presence of firm ingesta in the stomach of a rabbit that has been anorectic for 1–3 days is compatible with the diagnosis of gastrointestinal hypomotility.

• With acute small intestinal or pyloric outflow obstruction, the stomach is severely distended, tympanic, and full of gas and/or fluid. Patients are usually presented in shock, and emergency decompression is indicated.
• Little or no borborygmus is heard on abdominal auscultation in rabbits with gastrointestinal hypomotility. With acute small intestinal or pyloric outflow obstruction, borborygmus may be increased.
• Occasionally, large amounts of hard, dry feces are palpable in the distal colon, similar to constipation or obstipation in dogs and cats. This may be caused by a very distal colonic outflow obstruction (neoplasia, abscess, stricture or anal atresia).
• Other physical examination findings depend on the underlying cause; perform a complete physical examination, including a thorough oral examination.

### CAUSES
#### Dietary and Environmental Causes
• In the majority of cases, gastrointestinal hypomotility is caused by feeding diets with insufficient roughage, such as grasses and long-stemmed hay, and/or excessive simple carbohydrate content. Examples of improper diets include a diet consisting primarily of commercial pellets, especially those containing seeds, oats, or other high-carbohydrate treats; feeding of cereal products (bread, crackers, breakfast cereals); and feeding large amounts of fruits containing simple carbohydrates. Proper hind-gut fermentation and gastrointestinal motility rely on large quantities of indigestible coarse fiber, as found in long-stemmed hay and grasses. Most commercial pelleted diets contain inadequate roughage, coarse fiber, and excessive calories. This high-caloric content often contributes to obesity and hepatic lipidosis, both of which may exacerbate intestinal disease.
• Hair—excessive consumption (barbering) may contribute; a craving for fiber due to a fiber-deficient diet may contribute to barbering. However, ingestion of hair is normal in rabbits and, if the gastrointestinal tract is functioning normally, hair will pass uneventfully. Consumption of a whole, large hair mat may act as a small intestinal foreign body.
• Foreign material—ingestion of cloth (towels, carpeting, etc.) may cause gastrointestinal tract obstruction; scoopable cat litters can cause severe cecal impaction.
• Change of environment—hospitalization, boarding; can cause significant stress and contribute to gastrointestinal hypomotility
• New animals in the household; social stress; fighting

# CONSTIPATION (LACK OF FECAL PRODUCTION)

• Lack of exercise (cage confinement, obesity)—often a significant contributing factor

### Drugs
• Anesthetic agents may cause or exacerbate gastrointestinal hypomotility
• Anticholinergics
• Opioids
• Barium sulfate, Kapectolin, or sucralfate
• Diuretics

### Painful Defecation
• Anorectal disease—abscess, perineal moist dermatitis, myiasis, anal stricture, rectal foreign body, rectal prolapse
• Trauma—fractured pelvis, fractured limb, dislocated hip, perianal bite wound or laceration, perineal abscess

### Mechanical Obstruction
• Extraluminal—intraabdominal abscess, intrapelvic neoplasia, intraabdominal adhesions
• Intraluminal and intramural—colonic or rectal neoplasia or polyp, rectal stricture, rectal foreign body, rectal prolapse, and congenital defect (atresia ani)

### Neuromuscular Disease
• Central nervous system—paraplegia, spinal trauma, intervertebral disk disease, cerebral disease (lead toxicity, *Baylisascaris*, abscess, *Encephalitozoon cuniculi*)
• Peripheral nervous system—sacral nerve trauma

### Metabolic and Dental Disease
• Conditions that result in inappetence or anorexia may also cause gastrointestinal hypomotility. Common causes of anorexia include dental disease (malocclusion, molar elongation, tooth root abscesses), metabolic disease (renal disease, liver disease), pain (oral, trauma, postoperative pain, adhesions), neoplasia (gastrointestinal, uterine), and toxins.
• Debility—general muscle weakness, dehydration, neoplasia

## RISK FACTORS
• Diets with inadequate indigestible coarse fiber content
• Inactivity due to pain, obesity, cage confinement
• Anesthesia and surgical procedures
• Unsupervised chewing behavior
• Underlying dental, gastrointestinal tract, or metabolic disease

## DIAGNOSIS

### DIFFERENTIAL DIAGNOSIS
• Dyschezia and tenesmus—may be mistaken for constipation by owners; associated with increased frequency of attempts to defecate and frequent production of small amounts of liquid feces containing blood and/or mucous

• Stranguria (e.g., caused by hypercalciuria)—may be mistaken for constipation by owners; can be associated with abnormal findings on urinalysis; rabbits with calciuria may produce thick, sandlike urine that can be mistaken for feces.

### CBC/BIOCHEMISTRY/URINALYSIS
• Usually normal
• May be used to identify underlying causes of gastrointestinal hypomotility
• PCV and TS elevation in dehydrated patients
• Serum ALT or ALP elevation in rabbits with liver disease, especially lipidosis

### OTHER LABORATORY TESTS
N/A

### IMAGING
• Rabbits should not be fasted prior to taking radiographs.
• Gastric contents (primarily food and hair) are normally present and visible radiographically, even if the rabbit has been inappetent. The presence of ingesta (including hair) in the stomach is a normal finding.
• Distension of the stomach with ingesta is usually visible with gastrointestinal hypomotility. In some rabbits with gastrointestinal stasis, a halo of gas can be observed around the inspissated stomach contents. Gas distension is also common throughout the intestinal tract, including the cecum in rabbits with gastrointestinal hypomotility or stasis.
• Cecal distention with ingesta and/or gas may be seen.
• Severe distention of the stomach with fluid and/or gas is usually seen with acute small intestinal obstructions.
• Abdominal ultrasound can be useful for documenting an intestinal foreign body; may be difficult to interpret when large amounts of gas are present within the intestinal tract; may help define extraluminal mass
• Abdominal radiography may reveal colonic or rectal foreign body, colonic or rectal mass, spinal fracture, fractured pelvis, or dislocated hip.

### DIAGNOSTIC PROCEDURES
N/A

## TREATMENT
• Remove or ameliorate any underlying cause if possible.
• Rabbits that have not produced feces or have been anorectic for 1–3 days should be evaluated and treated as soon as possible.
• Rabbits that have not produced feces or have been anorectic for >3 days should be seen on an emergency basis.

## NURSING CARE

### Fluid Therapy
• Fluid therapy is an essential component of the medical management of all patients with gastrointestinal hypomotility. Administer both oral and parenteral fluids. Oral fluid administration will aid in the rehydration of inspissated gastric contents. Mildly affected rabbits will usually respond well to oral and subcutaneous fluid administration, dietary modification described below, and in some cases, treatment with intestinal motility modifiers and analgesics
• Intravenous or intraosseous fluids are required in patients that are severely dehydrated or depressed. Maintenance fluid requirements are estimated at 100 mL/kg/day.
• Rehydration is essential to treatment success in severely ill rabbits. Initially, a balanced fluid (e.g., lactated Ringer's solution) may be used.
• A warm, quiet environment should be provided.

## ACTIVITY
If patient is not debilitated, encourage exercise (hopping) for at least 10–15 minutes every 6–8 hours as activity promotes gastric motility.

## DIET
• It is absolutely imperative that the rabbit continue to eat during and following treatment. Continued anorexia will exacerbate gastrointestinal hypomotility and cause further derangement of the gastrointestinal microflora and overgrowth of intestinal bacterial pathogens.
• Offer a large selection of fresh, moistened greens such as cilantro, romaine lettuce, parsley, carrot tops, dandelion greens, spinach, collard greens, etc., and good-quality grass hay. Many rabbits will begin to eat these foods, even if they were previously anorectic. Also offer the rabbit's usual pelleted diet, as the initial goal is to get the rabbit to eat.
• If the patient refuses these foods, syringe feed a gruel such as Critical Care for Herbivores (Oxbow Pet Products, Murdock, NE) 10–15 mL/kg PO q6–8h. Larger volumes and more frequent feedings are often accepted; feed as much as the rabbit will readily accept. Alternatively, pellets can be ground and mixed with fresh greens, vegetable baby foods, water, or juice to form a gruel. If sufficient volumes of food are not accepted in this manner, nasogastric intubation is indicated. (NOTE: Assisted or forced feeding is contraindicated in rabbits with acute small intestinal obstruction.)
• High-carbohydrate, high-fat nutritional supplements are contraindicated.
• Encourage oral fluid intake by offering fresh water, wetting leafy vegetables, or flavoring water with vegetable juices.

# CONSTIPATION (LACK OF FECAL PRODUCTION)

• The diet should be permanently modified to include sufficient amounts of indigestible, coarse fiber. Offer long-stemmed grass or timothy hay (commercially available hay cubes are not sufficient) and an assortment of washed, fresh leafy greens. These foods should always constitute the bulk of the diet. Pellets should be limited (if offered at all) and foods high in simple carbohydrates prohibited or limited to the occasional treat.

### CLIENT EDUCATION
• Discuss possible complications prior to treatment, especially if surgery is required.
• Discuss the importance of dietary modification.
• Advise owners to regularly monitor food consumption and fecal output; seek veterinary attention with a noticeable decrease in either.

### SURGICAL CONSIDERATIONS
• Gastrointestinal hypomotility—accumulation of inspissated gastric contents (including ingested hair) will usually pass with medical treatment alone; surgery is generally contraindicated in rabbits with gastrointestinal hypomotility. Surgical manipulation of the intestinal tract, hypothermia, anesthetic agents, and pain all exacerbate gastrointestinal hypomotility; gastrointestinal stasis is often worse postoperatively. The combination of these factors results in a significantly worsened prognosis with surgical treatment.
• Ingested foreign material—surgery may be indicated to remove foreign material such as cloth from the stomach; in rare cases, inspissated ingesta forms a concretion in the stomach that does not respond to medical treatment.
• Gastric dilation due to small intestinal or pyloric foreign body—a surgical emergency; patients usually present in shock and require decompression prior to surgery.
• Surgery is also indicated in rabbits with extraluminal compression of the gastrointestinal tract and intestinal neoplasia.
• If surgery is performed, the entire gastrointestinal tract and liver should be assessed and biopsy specimens collected when indicated.

## MEDICATIONS
Use parenteral medications in animals with severely compromised intestinal motility; oral medications may not be properly absorbed; begin oral medication when intestinal motility begins to return (fecal production, return of appetite, radiographic evidence).

### DRUG(S) OF CHOICE
• Motility modifiers may be helpful in rabbits with gastrointestinal hypomotility. Cisapride (0.5 mg/kg PO q8–12h) enhances gastric emptying and is available through many compounding pharmacies.
• Analgesics such as buprenorphine (0.01–0.05 mg/kg SC, IM, IV q8–12h), or meloxicam (0.2 mg/kg SC, IM q24h or 0.2–0.5 mg/kg PO q24h) are essential to treatment of most rabbits with gastrointestinal hypomotility. Intestinal pain, either postoperative or from gas distention and ileus, impairs mobility and decreases appetite and may severely inhibit recovery.
• Antibiotic therapy—indicated in patients with bacterial overgrowth that sometimes occurs secondary to gastrointestinal hypomotility; more common in patients that have been anorectic for several days; indicated in patients with diarrhea, abnormal fecal cytology, and disruption of the intestinal mucosa (evidenced by blood in the feces)
• When antibiotics are indicated, always use broad-spectrum antibiotics such as trimethoprim sulfa (30 mg/kg PO q12h) or enrofloxacin (5–20 mg/kg PO, SC, IM q12–24h)
• If secondary overgrowth of *Clostridium* spp. is evident, use metronidazole (20 mg/kg PO q12h)
• Simethicone 65–130 mg/rabbit q1h for two to three treatments may be helpful in alleviating painful intestinal gas.

### CONTRAINDICATIONS
• The use of antibiotics that are primarily Gram positive in spectrum is contraindicated in rabbits. Use of these antibiotics will suppress the growth of commensal flora, allowing overgrowth of enteric pathogens. Do not orally administer lincomycin, clindamycin, erythromycin, ampicillin, amoxicillin cephalosporins, or penicillins.
• The use of gastrointestinal motility enhancers is contraindicated in rabbits with complete gastrointestinal tract obstruction due to the possibility of intestinal rupture.

### PRECAUTIONS
• Meloxicam—use with caution in rabbits with compromised renal function.
• Oral administration of any antibiotic may potentially cause enteric dysbiosis; discontinue use if diarrhea or anorexia occurs.

### POSSIBLE INTERACTIONS
N/A

### ALTERNATIVE DRUGS
• Metoclopramide (0.2–0.5 mg/kg PO, SC q6–8h) has also been used as a gastrointestinal promotility agent; efficacy is questionable.

• Enzymatic digestion of small trichobezoars with fresh pineapple juice, papaya extract, or pancreatic enzymes has been advocated. However, these substances should be used with caution (or preferably, not at all), as they may exacerbate gastric mucosal ulceration/erosions and may contribute to gastric rupture. Additionally, these substances do nothing to treat the underlying cause of trichobezoars and gastrointestinal hypomotility.
• Intestinal lubricants such as cat laxatives are unlikely to aid in the passage of trichobezoars as they simply lubricate the intestinal contents and do nothing to treat the underlying motility disorder.
• The addition of psyllium-based food supplements is not an adequate source of fiber for rabbits.

## FOLLOW-UP

### PATIENT MONITORING
Monitor the appetite and production of fecal pellets. Rabbits that are successfully treated will regain a normal appetite and begin to produce normal volumes of feces. Initially the fecal pellets are sometimes expelled bound together with hair.

### PREVENTION/AVOIDANCE
• Strict feeding of diets containing adequate amounts of indigestible coarse fiber (long-stemmed hay) and low simple carbohydrate content along with access to fresh water will often prevent episodes.
• Be certain that postoperative patients are eating and passing feces prior to release.

### POSSIBLE COMPLICATIONS
• Death due to gastric rupture, hypovolemic or endotoxic shock
• Postoperative gastrointestinal stasis
• Overgrowth of bacterial pathogens

### EXPECTED COURSE AND PROGNOSIS
• Early medical management of animals with gastrointestinal hypomotility usually carries a good to excellent prognosis.
• The prognosis following surgical removal of foreign material or acute small intestinal obstructions is guarded to poor.
• Prognosis for other causes varies.

## MISCELLANEOUS

### ASSOCIATED CONDITIONS
• Dental disease
• Hypercalciuria
• Hepatic lipidosis

### AGE-RELATED FACTORS
Older rabbits on a poor diet are more likely to develop gastrointestinal hypomotility.

## CONSTIPATION (LACK OF FECAL PRODUCTION)

**ZOONOTIC POTENTIAL**
N/A

**PREGNANCY**
N/A

**SYNONYMS**
N/A

**SEE ALSO**
- Clostridial enterotoxicosis
- Diarrhea, chronic
- Gastric dilation
- Gastrointestinal hypomotility

**ABBREVIATIONS**
- ALT = alanine aminotransferase
- ALP = alkaline phosphatase
- PCV = packed cell volume

- TS = total solids

*Suggested Reading*
Brown SA, Rosenthal KL. The anorexic rabbit. Proc North Am Vet Conf 1997:788.
Cheeke PR. Rabbit Feeding and Nutrition. Orlando, FL: Academic Press, 1987.
Donoghue S. Nutrition and pet rabbits. In: Rosenthal KL, ed. Practical Exotic Animal Medicine: The Compendium Collection. Trenton, NJ: Veterinary Learning Systems, 1997:107.
Jenkins JR. Feeding recommendations for the house rabbit. Vet Clin Noth Am Exotic Anim Pract 1999;2(1):143–151.
Jenkins JR. Gastrointestinal diseases. In: Quesenberry KE, Carpenter JW, eds. Ferrets, Rabbits and Rodents: Clinical Medicine and Surgery. 2nd Ed. Philadelphia: WB Saunders, 2004:161–171.
Paul-Murphy JA, Ramer JC. Urgent care of the pet rabbits. Vet Clin North Am Exotic Anim Pract 1998;1(1):127–152.
Rees Davies R, Rees Davies JAE. Rabbit gastrointestinal physiology. Vet Clin North Am: Exotic Anim Pract 2003;6(1):139–153.

BASICS

## OVERVIEW
• A cutaneous fungal infection affecting the cornified regions of hair, nails, and occasionally the superficial layers of the skin
• Isolated organisms most commonly include *Trichophyton mentagrophytes*, *Microsporum canis*, and *M. gypseum*.
• Exposure to or contact with a dermatophyte does not necessarily result in an infection.
• Dermatophytes—grow in the keratinized layers of hair, nail, and skin; do not thrive in living tissue or persist in the presence of severe inflammation
• Rabbits can be asymptomatic carriers.

## SIGNALMENT
• Uncommon disease of rabbits
• More common in young or debilitated animals

## SIGNS

### Historical Findings
• Lesions often begin as alopecia and dry, scaly skin.
• A history of previously confirmed infection or exposure to an infected animal or environment is a useful but not consistent finding.
• Variable pruritus

### Physical Examination Findings
• Often begins as focal areas of alopecia
• Classic circular alopecia may be seen
• Scales, crust, erythema—variable, usually in more advanced cases
• Lesions most commonly begin on the face, head, and feet, but may occur anywhere on the body.
• Variable pruritus

## CAUSES AND RISK FACTORS
• Exposure to affected animals, including other rabbits, cats, and dogs
• Poor management practices—overcrowding, poor ventilation, dirty environment, poor nutrition
• As in other species, immunocompromising diseases or immunosuppressive medications may predispose to infection, but this has not been clearly demonstrated in rabbits.

 DIAGNOSIS

## DIFFERENTIAL DIAGNOSIS

### Differentiating Causes
• Fur mites—*Cheyletiella* spp., or less commonly, *Leporacarus gibbus*; may be concurrent with dermatophytosis. Fur mite lesions are usually located in the intrascapular or tail base region and associated with copious amounts of large, white scale. Mites are readily identified in skin scrapes or acetate tape preparations under low magnification.
• Ear mites (*Psoroptes cuniculi*)—usually intensely pruritic; lesions typically localized to areas inside pinnae, surrounding ears, face, and neck. Skin thickening and exudative crusts form with chronic infestation. Mites can be seen with unaided eye or with microscopic examination under low power.
• Other ectoparasites—*Sarcoptes scabiei* and *Notoedres cati* rarely infest rabbits. Lesions are located around the head and neck and are intensely pruritic.
• Fleas—patchy alopecia usually appears in other areas in addition to head and feet; finding flea dirt will help to differentiate.
• Demodicosis—extremely rare, may occur in association with corticosteriod use; mites will be present on skin scrape.
• Contact dermatitis—usually ventral distribution of lesions; acute onset
• Barbering—by cage mates or self-inflicted—causes hair loss alone without pruritus, scale, or skin lesions
• Lack of grooming due to obesity or underlying dental or musculoskeletal disease may cause an accumulation of scale, especially in the intrascapular region.
• Injection site reactions—especially with irritating substances such as enrofloxacin, may cause alopecia and crusting

## CBC/BIOCHEMISTRY/URINALYSIS
May be useful to identify underlying disease.

## OTHER LABORATORY TESTS
N/A

## IMAGING
N/A

## DIAGNOSTIC PROCEDURES

### Fungal Culture
• Best means of confirming diagnosis
• Hairs that exhibit a positive apple-green fluorescence under Wood's lamp examination are considered ideal candidates for culture (*M. canis* only).
• Pluck hairs from the periphery of an alopecic area; do not use a random pattern.
• Test media—change to red when they becomes alkaline; dermatophytes typically produce this color during the early growing phase of their culture; saprophytes, which also produce this color, do so in the late growing phase; thus, it is important to examine DTM media daily.
• Positive culture—indicates existence of a dermatophyte; however, it may have been there only transiently, as may occur when the culture is obtained from the feet, which are likely to come in contact with a geophilic dermatophyte.

### Wood's Lamp Examination
Not a very useful screening tool; many pathogenic dermatophytes do not fluoresce; false fluorescence is common; lamp should warm up for a minimum of 5 minutes and then be exposed to suspicious lesions for up to 5 minutes; a true positive reaction associated with *M. canis* consists of apple-green fluorescence of the hair shaft; keratin associated with epidermal scales and sebum will often produce a false-positive fluorescence.

### Skin Biopsy
• Can be helpful in confirming true invasion and infection
• Can be helpful to rule out other causes of alopecia

 TREATMENT

## APPROPRIATE HEALTH CARE
• May resolve spontaneously with no treatment
• Consider quarantine owing to the infective and zoonotic nature of the disease.
• Environmental treatment, including fomites, is important, especially in recurrent cases; dilute bleach (1:10) is a practical and relatively effective means of providing environmental decontamination; concentrated bleach and formalin (1%) are more effective at killing spores, but their use is not as practical in many situations; chlorhexidine was ineffective in pilot studies.

 MEDICATIONS

## DRUG(S) OF CHOICE
• Topical therapy—lime sulfur dip q7d has been used successfully; lime sulfur is odiferous and can stain; dipping is often difficult to perform on rabbits. Dipping and bathing can be dangerous with nervous rabbits and inexperienced owners, and can result in serious consequences such as spinal fractures or excessive chilling.
• Topical therapy—1% clotrimazole cream (applied to lesions q12h) or miconazole cream or lotion (applied to lesions q24h × 14–28 days). Wear glove while applying.
• Itraconazole (5 mg/kg PO q24h × 3–4 weeks)—for treatment of refractory cases or severely affected animals
• Griseofulvin—for treatment of refractory cases or severely affected animals; less effective than itraconazole; 25 mg/kg PO q24h for 4–6 weeks
• Treat all in-contact animals.

## CONTRAINDICATIONS
The use of corticosteroids (systemic or topical) can severely exacerbate dermatophytosis.

## PRECAUTIONS

### Griseofulvin
• Bone marrow suppression (anemia,

## DERMATOPHYTOSIS

pancytopenia, and neutropenia) reported in dogs and cats as an idiosyncratic reaction or with prolonged therapy; not yet reported in rabbits but may occur; weekly or biweekly CBC is recommended.
• Neurologic side effects reported in dogs and cats—monitor for this possibility in rabbits.
• Do not use during the first two trimesters of pregnancy; it is teratogenic.

### Bathing, Dipping
Use extreme caution when dipping or bathing rabbits due to the high risk of skeletal fractures and excessive chilling with inexperienced owners.

### POSSIBLE INTERACTIONS
N/A

### ALTERNATIVE DRUGS
Ketoconazole (10—15 mg/kg PO q24h)—efficacy and safety in rabbits is unknown. Hepatopathy reported in dogs and cats can be quite severe.

## FOLLOW-UP

### PATIENT MONITORING
Repeat fungal cultures toward the end of the treatment regimen and continue treatment until at least one culture result is negative.

### PREVENTION/AVOIDANCE
• Initiate a quarantine period and obtain dermatophyte cultures of all animals

entering the household to prevent reinfection from other animals.
• Avoid infective soil if a geophilic dermatophyte is involved.

### POSSIBLE COMPLICATIONS
False-negative dermatophyte cultures

### EXPECTED COURSE AND PROGNOSIS
• Many animals will "self-clear" a dermatophyte infection over a period of a few months.
• Treatment for the disease hastens clinical cure and helps reduce environmental contamination.

## MISCELLANEOUS

### ASSOCIATED CONDITIONS
N/A

### AGE-RELATED FACTORS
N/A

### ZOONOTIC POTENTIAL
Dermatophytosis is zoonotic.

### PREGNANCY
• Griseofulvin is teratogenic.
• Ketoconazole can affect steroidal hormone synthesis, especially testosterone.

### SYNONYMS
Ringworm

### SEE ALSO
• Cheyletiellosis
• Ear mites

• Fleas
• Pruritus

### ABBREVIATIONS
• CBC = complete blood count
• DTM = dermatophyte test media

### Suggested Reading
Donnelly TM, Rush EM, Lackner PA. Ringworm in small exotic pets. Semin Avian Exotic Pet Med 2000;9:82–93.
Harkness JE, Wagner JE. The Biology and Medicine of Rabbits and Rodents. 3rd Ed. Baltimore: Williams & Wilkins, 1989.
Harcourt-Brown F. Skin diseases. In: Harcourt-Brown F, ed. Textbook of Rabbit Medicine. Oxford: Butterworth-Heinemann, 2002:224–248.
Hess L. Dermatologic diseases. In: Quesenberry KE, Carpenter JW, eds. Ferrets, Rabbits and Rodents: Clinical Medicine and Surgery. 2nd Ed. Philadelphia: WB Saunders, 2004:194–202.\
Jenkins JR. Skin disorders of the rabbit. Vet Clin North Am Exotic Anim Pract 2001;4(2):543–563.

### Portions Adapted From
Gram WD. Dermatophytosis. In: Tilley LP, Smith FWK, Jr., eds. The 5-Minute Veterinary Consult: Canine and Feline, 3rd Ed. Baltimore: Lippincott Williams & Wilkins, 2004.

# BASICS

## DEFINITION
Abrupt or recent onset of abnormally frequent discharge and fluid content of fecal matter

## PATHOPHYSIOLOGY
• Caused by imbalance in the absorptive, secretory, and motility actions of the intestines
• May or may not be associated with inflammation of the intestinal tract (enteritis)
• Normally, the intestinal epithelium secretes fluid and electrolytes to aid in the digestion, absorption, and propulsion of food. In disease states this secretion can overwhelm the absorptive activity and produce a secretory diarrhea. Many of the infectious causes of diarrhea are related to increased secretion.
• Rabbits are hind-gut fermenters and are extremely sensitive to alterations in diet. Proper hind-gut fermentation and gastrointestinal tract motility are dependent on the ingestion of large amounts of roughage and long-stemmed hay. Diets that contain inadequate amounts of coarse fiber (such as the feeding of only commercial pelleted food without hay or grasses) cause cecocolonic hypomotility and produce diarrhea due to motility changes and secondary decreases in absorption.
• A common predisposing cause of diarrhea in rabbits is disruption of enteric commensal flora. Flora may be altered by antibiotic usage, stress, or, more commonly, poor nutrition. Cecocolonic hypomotility can cause alterations in cecal fermentation, pH, and substrate production and alter enteric microflora populations. Diets low in coarse fiber typically contain high simple carbohydrate concentrations, which provide a ready source of fermentable products and promote the growth of bacterial pathogens such as *Escherichia coli* and *Clostridium sp.* Bacterial dysbiosis can cause acute diarrhea, enterotoxemia, ileus, or chronic intermittent diarrhea
• Antibiotic usage can cause severe, acute, often fatal diarrhea due to alteration of normal gut flora. Diarrhea follows the oral administration of antibiotics that are effective against Gram-positive bacteria and some Gram-negative anaerobes, such as lincomycin, clindamycin, erythromycin, ampicillin, amoxicillin cephalosporins, and penicillins. These antibiotics should not be orally administered to rabbits.
• Diarrhea can result from a combination of factors.

## SYSTEMS AFFECTED
• Gastrointestinal
• Endocrine/metabolic—fluid, electrolyte, and acid-base imbalances

## SIGNALMENT
No specific age or gender predilection

## SIGNS

### General Comments
• Diarrhea can occur with or without systemic illness.
• Signs can vary from diarrhea in an apparently healthy patient to severe systemic signs.
• The choice of diagnostic and therapeutic measures depends on the severity of illness.
• Patients that are not systemically ill have normal hydration and minimal systemic signs.
• Signs of more severe illness (e.g., anorexia, weight loss, abdominal pain, blood in the diarrhea, severe dehydration, depression, and shock) should prompt more aggressive diagnostic and therapeutic measures.

### Historical Findings
• Can range from a history of soft, formed stool to liquid consistency
• Owner may report fecal accidents, changes in fecal consistency and volume, blood or mucous in the feces, or straining to defecate.
• History of diet change or diets containing inadequate amounts of long-stemmed hay or grasses and excessive simple carbohydrates (e.g., feeding only pellets, excessive fruits, sugary vegetables, sweets, or grain products)
• Inappropriate chewing habits—barbering or chewing on fabrics, carpet, etc.
• Antibiotic usage—the use of antibiotics that are primarily Gram positive in spectrum will suppress the growth of commensal flora, allowing overgrowth of enteric pathogens.
• Stress—hospitalization, environmental changes, and concurrent illness may contribute to alterations in intestinal commensal flora.

### Physical Examination Findings
• Vary with the severity of disease
• Dehydration, depression, or lethargy often present to some degree.
• Abdominal pain characterized by a hunched posture, reluctance to move, bruxism, or pain on palpation
• Fever
• Signs of hypotension and weakness may occur in more severely affected individuals.
• Hypothermia in rabbits in enterotoxemic shock
• Fecal staining of the perineum

• Abdominal distention may be due to thickened or fluid-filled intestinal loops, cecal impaction, masses, or organomegaly.
• Fluid or gas is often palpable within the cecum

## CAUSES
• Dietary—high simple carbohydrate, low coarse-fiber diets, diet changes—most common cause
• Bacterial infection/enterotoxemia—*E. coli, Clostridium spiroforme, C. piliforme* (Tyzzer's disease), *Salmonella* spp., *Pseudomonas* spp., *Campylobacter* spp.
• Obstruction—neoplasia, small intestinal foreign body (usually cloth or mat of fur), intussusception
• Drugs and toxins—oral administration of lincomycin, clindamycin, erythromycin, ampicillin, amoxicillin cephalosporins, and penicillins; plant toxins
• Metabolic disorders—liver disease, renal disease
• Viral infection—coronavirus (3- to 10-week-old rabbits), rotavirus (usually a copathogen with coronavirus); seen in neonates
• Parasitic causes—Coccidia (*Eimeria* spp., hepatic or intestinal); usually young rabbits.
• Chronic disease can sometimes present as acute diarrhea.
• Systemic illness may also result in diarrhea as a secondary event.
• Neoplasia—adenocarcinoma, leiomyosarcoma, leiomyoma, papilloma

## RISK FACTORS
• Diets with inadequate indigestible coarse fiber content and high simple carbohydrate content
• Improper antibiotic usage
• Unsupervised chewing

# DIAGNOSIS

## DIFFERENTIAL DIAGNOSIS

### Differentiating Similar Signs
• Diarrhea should be differentiated from normal cecotrophs (or night feces). Cecotrophs are formed in the cecum, are rich in nutrients, and are usually eliminated during the early morning hours. Normally, cecotrophs are not observed because rabbits will ingest them directly from the anus. Occasionally rabbits are unable to consume cecotrophs (due to orthopedic or neuromuscular disorders, application of Elizabethan collars), which may be mistaken for diarrhea. Cecotrophs are dark in color, have a soft consistency, tend to clump together, and are covered with mucous.

## DIARRHEA, ACUTE

• Fluid-filled, blood-tinged diarrhea—usually associated with Coccidia or bacterial enteritis in young rabbits; in older rabbits—associated with bacterial enteritis (especially *Clostridia* sp., *E. coli*, or *Salmonella* sp.), severe systemic illness, or intestinal obstruction/intussusception
• Severe depression, lethargy, hypothermia, and signs of shock—usually associated with acute small intestinal obstruction or clostridial enterotoxicosis
• Soft stool, sticky or pasty consistency—usually associated with inappropriate diet or diet changes

### CBC/BIOCHEMISTRY
• Often normal with mild illness
• More severe illness should prompt a more complete evaluation.
• Increased hematocrit and serum protein concentration seen with dehydration
• Anemia may be seen with gastrointestinal bleeding.
• TWBC elevations may be seen with bacterial enteritis, but this rarely occurs.
• Electrolytes are commonly abnormal because of intestinal losses (hypokalemia, hypochloremia, hyponatremia).
• Altered protein levels because of intestinal loss (decreased) or dehydration (increased)
• Serum glucose concentration may be elevated due to stress.
• Altered renal values with dehydration or gastrointestinal hemorrhage (prerenal azotemia) or with renal disease
• Liver enzymes can be elevated with disease in these organ systems.

### OTHER LABORATORY TESTS
N/A

### IMAGING
#### Radiographic Findings
• Rabbits should not be fasted prior to taking radiographs.
• Gastric contents (primarily food and hair) are normally present and visible radiographically, even if the rabbit has been inappetent. The presence of ingesta (including hair) in the stomach is a normal finding in healthy rabbits.
• Distension of the stomach due to abnormal retention of ingesta is usually visible with gastrointestinal hypomotility. In some rabbits with gastrointestinal stasis, a halo of gas can be observed around the inspissated stomach contents. Gas distension is also common throughout the intestinal tract, including the cecum in rabbits with gastrointestinal hypomotility or overgrowth of *Clostridium* sp.
• Cecal distension with ingesta and/or gas may be seen.
• Severe distention of the stomach with fluid and/or gas is usually seen with acute small intestinal obstructions. In most cases, this is an acute, life-threatening finding.
• Abdominal ultrasound can be useful for documenting an intestinal foreign body; may be difficult to interpret when large amounts of gas are present within the intestinal tract; may help define extraluminal mass. Hyperechogenicity may be seen with hepatic lipidosis or fibrosis; hypoechoic nodules are suggestive of hepatic necrosis, abscess, or neoplasia.

### OTHER DIAGNOSTIC PROCEDURES
#### Fecal Examination
• Fecal direct examination, fecal flotation, and zinc sulfate centrifugation may demonstrate gastrointestinal parasites.
• Fecal Gram's stain—may demonstrate large numbers of spore-forming bacteria consistent with *Clostridia* spp. or excessive numbers of Gram-negative bacteria. Yeast (*Saccharomyces* spp. or *Cyniclomyces guttulatus*) can be mistaken for *Clostridia* spp. on Gram's stain or direct smear, but can generally be differentiated based on size (*Saccharomyces* are three to four times larger than bacteria).
• Fecal cytology—may reveal RBC or fecal leukocytes, which are associated with inflammatory disease or invasive bacterial strains.
• Fecal culture may be difficult to interpret since *E. coli* and clostridia may be present in small numbers in normal rabbits. A heavy growth of these bacteria is considered significant. Fecal culture should be performed if other bacterial infections, such as with *Salmonella* sp., is suspected.
• Fecal occult blood testing—in patients with dark brown–black stool to confirm melena

## TREATMENT

### APPROPRIATE HEALTH CARE
• Treatment must be specific to the underlying cause to be successful.
• Most adult rabbits with mild diarrhea that are otherwise bright and alert can be treated as outpatients.
• Hospitalize rabbits with signs of lethargy, depression, dehydration, or shock, even if diarrhea is mild or absent.
• Hospitalize when diarrhea is profuse, resulting in dehydration and electrolyte imbalance.
• Hospitalize rabbits under 5 months of age, regardless of the severity of diarrhea.
• Rabbits with mild, intermittent diarrhea, characterized by the production of soft, pasty stool and lack of other clinical signs, may respond to dietary correction alone. Often, these rabbits will have a few soft stools each day, with the remainder of the feces normally formed pellets. See "diarrhea, chronic" for details.

### NURSING CARE
• Fluid therapy and correction of electrolyte imbalances are the mainstays of treatment in most cases.
• Can give crystalloid fluid therapy orally, subcutaneously, or intravenously, as required
• Aim to return the patient to proper hydration status (over 12–24 hour) and replace any ongoing losses.
• Severe volume depletion can occur with acute diarrhea; aggressive shock fluid therapy may be necessary.
• Fluid choice for intravenous or subcutaneous use should take into consideration the electrolyte and hydration status.

### DIET
• It is imperative that the rabbit continue to eat during and following treatment. Continued anorexia will exacerbate gastrointestinal motility disorders and cause further derangement of the gastrointestinal microflora and overgrowth of intestinal bacterial pathogens.
• Offer a good-quality grass hay and a large selection of fresh, moistened greens such as cilantro, romaine lettuce, parsley, carrot tops, dandelion greens, spinach, collard greens, etc. Many rabbits will begin to eat these foods, even if they were previously anorectic.
• In some rabbits, addition of leafy greens may exacerbate diarrhea. For these patients, offer good-quality grass hay alone.
• If the patient refuses these foods, syringe feed a gruel such as Critical Care for Herbivores (Oxbow Pet Products, Murdock, NE) 10–15 mL/kg PO q6–8h. Larger volumes and more frequent feedings are often accepted; feed as much as the rabbit will readily accept. Alternatively, pellets can be ground and mixed with fresh greens, vegetable baby foods, water, or juice to form a gruel. If sufficient volumes of food are not accepted in this manner, nasogastric intubation is indicated. (NOTE: Assisted or forced feeding is contraindicated in rabbits with acute small intestinal obstruction or shock.)
• High-carbohydrate, high-fat nutritional supplements are contraindicated.
• The diet should be permanently modified to include sufficient amounts of roughage and long-stemmed hay. Offer high-quality, fresh hay (grass or timothy preferred; commercially available hay cubes are not sufficient) and an assortment of washed, fresh leafy greens. These foods should always constitute the bulk of the diet. Pellets should be limited (one-quarter cup pellets per 5 lb body weight, if offered at all) and foods high in simple carbohydrates prohibited or limited to the occasional treat.

# MEDICATIONS

### DRUG(S) OF CHOICE
• Antibiotic therapy—indicated in patients with abnormal fecal cytology and disruption of the intestinal mucosa (evidenced by blood in the feces). Selection should be based on results of culture and susceptibility testing when possible.
• When antibiotics are indicated, always use broad-spectrum antibiotics such as trimethoprim sulfa (30 mg/kg PO q12h) or enrofloxacin (5–20 mg/kg PO, SC, IM q12–24h)
• *Clostridium* spp.—metronidazole (20 mg/kg PO, IV q12h for 2–3 weeks)
• Coccidia—sulfadimethoxine (50 mg/kg PO first dose, then 25 mg/kg q24h for 10–20 days) or trimethoprim sulfa (30 mg/kg PO q12h × 10 days)
• Cholestyramine (Questran, Bristol Laboratories) is an ion-exchange resin that binds clostridial iota toxins. A dose of 2 g in 20 mL of water administered by gavage q24h for up to 18–21 days has been reported to be effective in preventing death in rabbits with acute clostridia enterotoxemia.
• Analgesics such as buprenorphine (0.01–0.05 mg/kg SC, IM q6–12h), meloxicam (0.2–0.5 mg/kg PO q24h), or carprofen (2.2 mg/kg PO q12–24h) may be beneficial for rabbits with intestinal pain. Intestinal pain from gas distention and ileus impairs mobility and decreases appetite and may severely inhibit recovery.

### CONTRAINDICATIONS
• The use of antibiotics that are primarily Gram positive in spectrum is contraindicated in rabbits. Use of these antibiotics will suppress the growth of commensal flora, allowing overgrowth of enteric pathogens and often a fatal enterotoxemia. Do not orally administer lincomycin, clindamycin, erythromycin, ampicillin, amoxicillin cephalosporins, or penicillins.

• Administration of corticosteroids may cause immunosuppression and should not be used in rabbits with infectious causes of diarrhea. Corticosteroid use is associated with gastrointestinal ulceration and hemorrhage, delayed wound healing, and heightened susceptibility to infection.

### PRECAUTIONS
• Meloxicam—use with caution in rabbits with compromised renal function.
• Oral administration of any antibiotic may potentially cause enteric dysbiosis; discontinue use if diarrhea or anorexia occurs.

### POSSIBLE INTERACTIONS
N/A

### ALTERNATE DRUGS
Coccidia—amprolium 9.6% in drinking water (0.5 mL per 500 mL)

# FOLLOW-UP

### PATIENT MONITORING
• Fecal volume and character, fecal cytology, appetite, attitude, and body weight
• If diarrhea does not resolve, consider reevaluation of the diagnosis.

### POSSIBLE COMPLICATIONS
• Septicemia due to bacterial invasion of enteric mucosa
• Dehydration due to fluid loss
• Shock, death from clostridial enterotoxicosis

# MISCELLANEOUS

### ASSOCIATED CONDITIONS
• Gastrointestinal hypomotility
• Hypercalciuria

### AGE-RELATED FACTORS
*E. coli, Clostridia* sp., coccidia, and viral-related diarrhea more severe in neonates

### ZOONOTIC POTENTIAL
*Salmonella*

### PREGNANCY
N/A

### SEE ALSO
• Chronic intermittent diarrhea
• Clostridial enteritis/enterotoxicosis
• Gastrointestinal hypomotility

### ABBREVIATIONS
• RBC = red blood cell
• TWBC = total white blood cell

*Suggested Reading*
Brown SA, Rosenthal KL. The anorexic rabbit. Proc North AmVet Conf 1997:788.
Cheeke PR. Rabbit Feeding and Nutrition. Orlando, FL: Academic Press, 1987.
Donoghue S. Nutrition and pet rabbits. In: Rosenthal KL, ed. Practical Exotic Animal Medicine: The Compendium Collection. Trenton, NJ: Veterinary Learning Systems, 1997:107.
Jenkins JR. Feeding recommendations for the house rabbit. Vet Clin Noth Am Exotic Anim Pract 1999;2(1):143–151.
Jenkins JR. Gastrointestinal diseases. In: Quesenberry KE, Carpenter JW, eds. Ferrets, Rabbits and Rodents: Clinical Medicine and Surgery. Philadelphia: WB Saunders, 2004:161–171.
Paul-Murphy JA, Ramer JC. Urgent care of the pet rabbits. Vet Clin North Am Exotic Anim Pract 1998;1(1):127–152.

*Portions Adapted From*
Duval DS. Diarrhea—Acute. In: Tilley LP, Smith FWK, Jr., eds. The 5-Minute Veterinary Consult: Canine and Feline, 2nd Ed. Baltimore: Lippincott Williams & Wilkins, 2000.

# DIARRHEA, CHRONIC

## BASICS

### DEFINITION
A change in the frequency, consistency, and volume of feces for weeks to months, or with a pattern of episodic recurrence

### PATHOPHYSIOLOGY
In rabbits, the most common predisposing cause of chronic diarrhea is disruption of enteric commensal flora. Flora may be altered by antibiotic usage, stress, or, more commonly, poor nutrition. Rabbits are hind-gut fermenters and are extremely sensitive to alterations in diet. Proper hind-gut fermentation and gastrointestinal tract motility are dependent on the ingestion of large amounts of roughage and long-stemmed hay. Diets that contain inadequate amounts of coarse fiber (such as the feeding of only commercial pelleted food without hay or grasses) cause cecocolonic hypomotility and produce diarrhea due to motility changes and secondary decreases in absorption. Cecocolonic hypomotility can also cause alterations in cecal fermentation, pH, and substrate production alter enteric microflora populations. Diets low in coarse fiber typically contain high simple carbohydrate concentrations, which provide a ready source of fermentable products and promote the growth of bacterial pathogens such as *Escherichia coli* and *Clostridium* sp. Bacterial dysbiosis can cause acute diarrhea, enterotoxemia, ileus, or chronic intermittent diarrhea

### SYSTEMS AFFECTED
• Gastrointestinal
• Endocrine/metabolic—fluid, electrolyte, and acid-base imbalances

### SIGNALMENT
No specific age or gender predilection

### SIGNS

#### General Comments
Patients can be placed into categories according to the severity of their illness. The extent of diagnostic workup and treatment are determined by the category. Mild illness—patients are alert and active and have no other clinical signs; moderate illness—patients remain alert and active, but have other clinical signs such as anorexia or weight loss; severe illness—patients are depressed, dehydrated, or listless and may also show signs listed under moderate illness.

#### Historical Findings
• Owners describe soft, pasty stools that stick together; these are usually interspersed with normal, dry fecal pellets.
• Frequency of abnormal stools may vary from several times a day to weekly.

• History of diet change or diets containing inadequate amounts of long-stemmed hay or grasses and excessive simple carbohydrates (e.g., feeding only pellets, excessive fruits, sugary vegetables, sweets, or grain products)
• Inappropriate chewing habits—barbering or chewing on fabrics, carpet, towels, etc.
• Antibiotic usage—the use of antibiotics that are primarily Gram positive in spectrum will suppress the growth of commensal flora, allowing overgrowth of enteric pathogens.
• Stress—hospitalization, environmental changes, and concurrent illness may contribute to alterations in intestinal commensal flora.

#### Physical Examination Findings
• Vary with the severity of disease
• Diarrhea can occur with or without systemic illness.
• Signs can vary from diarrhea in an apparently healthy patient to severe systemic signs.
• Weight loss
• Dehydration, depression, or lethargy may be present to some degree.
• Abdominal pain characterized by a hunched posture, reluctance to move, bruxism, or pain on palpation
• Poor haircoat
• Signs of hypotension and weakness may occur in more severely affected individuals.
• Fecal staining of the perineum
• Abdominal distention may be due to thickened or fluid-filled intestinal loops, cecal impaction, masses, or organomegaly.
• Fluid or gas is often palpable within the cecum.

### CAUSES
• Dietary—the most common cause of chronic, intermittent diarrhea (especially in patients that appear otherwise normal) is inappropriate diet. Diets that are high in simple carbohydrates (yogurt drops or other sweets, commercial pellets, sugary fruits and vegetables, bread and grain products) and low in coarse, indigestible fiber such as long-stemmed hay cause chronic gastrointestinal hypomotility and disruption of normal gastrointestinal flora and function.
• Bacterial infection/enterotoxemia—*E. coli, Clostridium spiroforme, Salmonella* sp., *Pseudomonas* sp., *Campylobacter* sp. These patients are typically fed a diet consisting of commercial pellets only or pellets supplemented with sugary fruits and vegetables, grains, or bread products.
• Lack of exercise (cage confinement, obesity, neuromuscular or skeletal disorders)—often a significant contributing factor to the development of gastrointestinal hypomotility
• Neoplasia—adenocarcinoma, leiomyosarcoma, leiomyoma, papilloma

• Partial obstruction—foreign body (especially cloth or cat litters), neoplasia
• Drugs and toxins—especially antibiotics, lead
• Metabolic disorders—liver disease, renal disease
• Inflammatory bowel disease and dietary intolerance has not been described in rabbits.

### RISK FACTORS
• Diets with inadequate indigestible coarse fiber content and high simple carbohydrate content—most prominent risk factor
• Inactivity due to pain, obesity, cage confinement
• Stress
• Dietary changes
• Unsupervised chewing

## DIAGNOSIS

### DIFFERENTIAL DIAGNOSIS

#### Differentiating Similar Signs
• Diarrhea should be differentiated from normal cecotrophs (or night feces). Cecotrophs are formed in the cecum, are rich in nutrients, and are usually eliminated in the early morning hours. Normally, cecotrophs are not observed because rabbits will ingest them directly from the anus. Occasionally, rabbits are unable to consume the cecotroph, which may be mistaken for diarrhea. Cecotrophs are dark in color, have a soft consistency, tend to clump together, and are covered with mucous.
• Intermittent, soft, sticky feces—most commonly associated with improper diet, especially in rabbits with little or no other clinical signs
• Anorexia, hunched posture, and bruxism—often associated with chronic partial obstruction as seen with gastrointestinal hypomotility, gastrointestinal foreign bodies or enteric dysbiosis
• Lethargy, anorexia, and weight loss—often associated with enteric dysbiosis, chronic metabolic disease, or gastrointestinal hypomotility
• Severe depression, lethargy, hypothermia, and signs of shock—usually seen in rabbits with acute diarrhea, acute small intestinal obstruction, or clostridial enterotoxicosis

### CBC/BIOCHEMISTRY
• Increased hematocrit and serum protein concentration seen with dehydration
• Anemia may be seen with gastrointestinal bleeding.
• TWBC elevations may be seen with bacterial enteritis, but this is uncommon.
• Serum biochemistry abnormalities may suggest renal or hepatic disease.

**OTHER LABORATORY TESTS**
N/A

**IMAGING**

*Radiographic Findings*
• Most otherwise healthy rabbits with chronic, intermittent soft stools will respond to diet change alone; radiographs may not initially be necessary.
• Rabbits should not be fasted prior to taking radiographs.
• Often no abnormalities are noted. Gastric contents (primarily food and hair) are normally present and visible radiographically, even if the rabbit has been inappetent. The presence of ingesta (including hair) in the stomach is a normal finding in healthy rabbits.
• Distension of the stomach due to abnormal retention of ingesta is usually visible in rabbits with gastrointestinal hypomotility. In some rabbits with gastrointestinal stasis, a halo of gas can be observed around the inspissated stomach contents. Gas distension is also common throughout the intestinal tract, including the cecum in rabbits with gastrointestinal hypomotility or overgrowth of *Clostridium* sp.
• Cecal distention with ingesta and/or gas may be seen.
• Severe distention of the stomach with fluid and/or gas is usually seen with acute small intestinal obstructions.
• Abdominal ultrasound can be useful for documenting an intestinal foreign body; may be difficult to interpret when large amounts of gas are present within the intestinal tract; may help define extraluminal mass. Hyperechogenicity may be seen with hepatic lipidosis or fibrosis; hypoechoic nodules are suggestive of hepatic necrosis, abscess, or neoplasia.

**OTHER DIAGNOSTIC PROCEDURES**

*Fecal Examination*
• Fecal direct examination, fecal flotation, and zinc sulfate centrifugation may demonstrate gastrointestinal parasites.
• Fecal Gram's stain—may demonstrate large numbers of spore-forming bacteria consistent with *Clostridia* spp. or excessive numbers of Gram-negative bacteria. Yeast (*Saccharomyces* spp. or *Cyniclomyces guttulatus*) can be mistaken for *Clostridia* spp. on Gram's stain or direct smear, but can generally be differentiated based on size.(*Saccharomyces* are 3–4x larger than bacteria)
• Fecal cytology—may reveal RBC or fecal leukocytes, which are associated with inflammatory disease or invasive bacterial strains
• Fecal culture may be difficult to interpret since *E. coli* and *Clostridia* may be present in small numbers in normal rabbits. A heavy growth of these bacteria is considered

significant. Fecal culture should be performed if other bacterial infections, such as with *Salmonella* sp., is suspected.
• Fecal occult blood testing—in patients with dark brown–black stool to confirm melena

**TREATMENT**
• Rabbits with mild, intermittent diarrhea, characterized by the production of soft, pasty stool and lack of other clinical signs, usually respond to dietary correction alone (see diet, below). Often, these rabbits will have a few soft stools each day, with the remainder of the feces being normally formed pellets.
• Patients with mild disease usually respond to outpatient treatment.
• Patients with moderate to severe disease usually require hospitalization and 24-hour care for parenteral medication and fluid therapy. Correct electrolyte and acid-base disturbances.
• Treatment must be specific to the underlying cause to be successful.

**DIET**
Patients with intermittent soft stool and no other clinical signs:
• Dietary modification is the mainstay of treatment of chronic, intermittent soft stools (diarrhea). It may take days to weeks for these dietary recommendations to change intestinal flora. Allow sufficient time on strict dietary modification for diarrhea to resolve. Warn clients not to give up if a change is not noted immediately; sometimes diarrhea may worsen slightly before improving. Strict client compliance is essential to successful treatment.
• First eliminate all fruit-, vegetable-, or grain-based treats (oats, crackers, breads, cereal) and sugary treats (yogurt drops, candy). Offer high-quality, fresh, long-stemmed hay (grass or timothy preferred; commercially available hay cubes are not sufficient). Gradually add a large selection of fresh, moistened greens such as cilantro, romaine lettuce, parsley, carrot tops, dandelion greens, spinach, collard greens, etc., eventually feeding these free-choice every day. Offer only a limited amount (one-quarter cup pellets per 5 lb body weight) of high-fiber timothy-based pellet (Oxbow Pet Products, Murdock, NE). Some rabbits will respond to this change alone.
• If intermittent soft stool is still seen following dietary modification and the rabbit is otherwise normal, try eliminating all pellets from the diet in addition to eliminating sugary treats, fruits, vegetables, and grain. Most rabbits will respond to this diet change.

• A few rabbits cannot tolerate fresh leafy greens or pelleted foods in the diet. If intermittent soft stool is still seen and the rabbit is otherwise normal, feed a diet consisting of good-quality hay and grasses alone.
• The addition of psyllium-based food supplements is not an adequate source of fiber for rabbits.
Anorectic, systemically ill patients:
• Patients with chronic, intermittent diarrhea are rarely anorectic. If anorexia is present, it is imperative that the rabbit receive oral nutrition during and following treatment. Continued anorexia will exacerbate gastrointestinal motility disorders and cause further derangement of the gastrointestinal microflora and overgrowth of intestinal bacterial pathogens.
• Sometimes offering hay and leafy greens alone may entice anorectic rabbits to eat.
• If the patient refuses these foods, syringe feed a gruel such as Critical Care for Herbivores (Oxbow Pet Products, Murdock, NE) 10–15 mL/kg PO q6–8h. Larger volumes and more frequent feedings are often accepted; feed as much as the rabbit will readily accept. Alternatively, pellets can be ground and mixed with fresh greens, vegetable baby foods, water, or juice to form a gruel. If sufficient volumes of food are not accepted in this manner, nasogastric intubation is indicated.
• High-carbohydrate, high-fat nutritional supplements are contraindicated.
• The diet should be permanently modified to include sufficient amounts of indigestible coarse fiber, as described above.

**MEDICATIONS**

**DRUG(S) OF CHOICE**
• Antibiotic therapy—is usually not indicated in rabbits with chronic intermittent soft stool; may be indicated in patients with abnormal bacterial flora found on Gram's stain and fecal culture and those with signs of severe intestinal disease. Selection should be based on results of culture and susceptibility testing when possible.
• When antibiotics are indicated, always use broad-spectrum antibiotics such as trimethoprim sulfa (30 mg/kg PO q12h) or enrofloxacin (5–20 mg/kg PO, SC, IM q12–24h).
• *Clostridium* spp.—metronidazole (20 mg/kg PO q12h)
• Analgesics such as buprenorphine (0.01–0.05 mg/kg SC, IM, IV q8–12h), meloxicam (0.2–0.5 mg/kg PO q24h), or carprofen (2.2 mg/kg PO q12–24) may be beneficial for rabbits with intestinal pain. Intestinal pain from gas distention and ileus

# DIARRHEA, CHRONIC

impairs mobility and decreases appetite, and may severely inhibit recovery.

## CONTRAINDICATIONS
• The use of antibiotics that are primarily Gram positive in spectrum is contraindicated in rabbits. Use of these antibiotics will suppress the growth of commensal flora, allowing overgrowth of enteric pathogens and often a fatal enterotoxemia.
• Administration of corticosteroids may cause immunosuppression and should not be used in rabbits with infectious causes of diarrhea. Corticosteroid use is associated with gastrointestinal ulceration and hemorrhage, delayed wound healing, and heightened susceptibility to infection.

## PRECAUTIONS
• Oral administration of any antibiotic may potentially cause enteric dysbiosis; discontinue use if diarrhea or anorexia occurs.
• Meloxicam—use with caution in rabbits with compromised renal function.

## POSSIBLE INTERACTIONS
N/A

## ALTERNATE DRUGS
N/A

# FOLLOW-UP

## PATIENT MONITORING
• It often takes days to weeks for dietary modification for resolution of diarrhea.

Owners must be diligent in feeding only the recommended diet.
• Monitor fecal volume and character, appetite, attitude, and body weight.
• If diarrhea does not resolve, consider reevaluation of the diagnosis.

## POSSIBLE COMPLICATIONS
• Septicemia due to bacterial invasion of enteric mucosal
• Dehydration due to fluid loss
• Shock, death from clostridial enterotoxicosis

# MISCELLANEOUS

## ASSOCIATED CONDITIONS
• Gastrointestinal hypomotility
• Hypercalciuria

## AGE-RELATED FACTORS
• Infectious causes of diarrhea more severe in neonates
• Inappropriate diet is more commonly a cause of chronic intermittent diarrhea in older rabbits.

## ZOONOTIC POTENTIAL
N/A

## PREGNANCY
N/A

## SEE ALSO
• Clostridial enteritis/enterotoxemia
• Diarrhea, acute
• Gastrointestinal hypomotility

## ABBREVIATIONS
• RBC = red blood cell
• TWBC = total white blood cell

*Suggested Reading*

Brown SA, Rosenthal KL. The anorexic rabbit. Proc North Am Vet Conf 1997:788.

Donoghue S. Nutrition and pet rabbits. In: Rosenthal KL, ed. Practical Exotic Animal Medicine: The Compendium Collection. Trenton, NJ: Veterinary Learning Systems, 1997:107.

Jenkins JR. Feeding recommendations for the house rabbit. Vet Clin Noth Am Exotic Anim Pract 1999;2(1):143–151.

Jenkins JR. Gastrointestinal diseases. In: Quesenberry KE, Carpenter JW, ed: Ferrets, Rabbits and Rodents: Clinical Medicine and Surgery. 2nd Ed. Philadelphia: WB Saunders, 2004:161–171.

Paul-Murphy JA, Ramer JC. Urgent care of the pet rabbits. Vet Clin North Am Exotic Anim Pract 1998;1(1):127–152.

*Portions Adapted From*

Grooters AM. Diarrhea—Chronic. In: Tilley LP, Smith FWK, Jr., eds. The 5-Minute Veterinary Consult: Canine and Feline, 2nd Ed. Baltimore: Lippincott Williams & Wilkins, 2004.

# BASICS

## DEFINITION
- Dyspnea is the distressful feeling associated with difficult or labored breathing, tachypnea is rapid breathing (not necessarily labored), and hyperpnea is deep breathing. In animals, the term dyspnea often is applied to labored breathing that appears to be uncomfortable.
- Open-mouthed breathing is a poor prognostic sign in rabbits. Open-mouth breathing occurs with severe upper or lower respiratory tract disease. Rabbits are obligate nasal breathers. The rim of the epiglottis is normally situated dorsal to the elongated soft palate to allow air passage from the nose to the trachea during normal respiration. With complete obstruction of the nasal passages, rabbits may attempt open-mouth breathing.

## PATHOPHYSIOLOGY
- Nonrespiratory causes of dyspnea may include abnormalities in pulmonary vascular tone (CNS disease, shock), pulmonary circulation (CHF), oxygenation (anemia), or ventilation (obesity, ascites, abdominal organomegaly, musculoskeletal disease).
- Primary respiratory diseases may be divided into upper and lower respiratory tract problems.

## SYSTEMS AFFECTED
- Respiratory
- Cardiovascular
- Nervous (secondary to hypoxia)

## SIGNALMENT
Any

## SIGNS

### Historical Findings
- Orthopnea (recumbent dyspnea), restlessness, and poor sleeping may occur in rabbits with pleural space disease (effusions, abscesses) or CHF.
- Exercise intolerance may occur with upper respiratory tract disease (rabbits are obligatory nasal breathers), lower respiratory tract disease, or CHF.
- Sneezing or nasoocular discharge, facial abscess, dental disease, and ptyalism may be seen with upper respiratory infections.
- Anorexia and lethargy are often the only historical complaint in rabbits with LRT disease
- Coughing is not often observed in this species.

### Physical Examination Findings
- Upper airway obstruction-stridor, stertor, open-mouth breathing
- Serous or mucopurulent nasal discharge, ocular discharge, facial abscess, dental disease, ptyalism with URT disease

- Pneumonia—harsh inspiratory and expiratory bronchovesicular sounds sometimes auscultated
- Pulmonary abscesses—absent lung sounds over site of abscess
- Pleural effusion—absent lung sounds ventrally, harsh lung sounds dorsally
- Pulmonary edema—fine inspiratory crackles
- Pyrexia (viral or bacterial infections)
- Weight loss and poor haircoat in rabbits with chronic respiratory disease
- Anorectic rabbits—may show signs of gastrointestinal hypomotility; scant, dry feces; dehydration; firm stomach or cecal contents; gas-filled intestinal loops

## CAUSES

### Nonrespiratory Causes
- Pain, fever, heat stroke, obesity, anxiety
- Neuromuscular disease—severe CNS disease (trauma, abscess, neoplasia, inflammation), spinal disease (trauma, *Encephalitozoon cuniculi*)
- Hematologic—anemia
- Metabolic disease—acidosis, uremia
- Cardiac disease—CHF, severe arrhythmias, cardiogenic shock
- Abdominal distension—organomegaly, ascites, pregnancy, gastric dilation

### Respiratory Causes
*Upper Respiratory Tract*
- Nasal obstruction—rhinitis/sinusitis (usually bacterial, mycotic is rare), dental disease (periapical abscess, elongated maxillary tooth roots penetrating into nasal passages), granuloma, foreign body, neoplasia
- Laryngotracheal obstruction—laryngeal edema following traumatic intubation, foreign body, abscess, neoplasia
- Traumatic airway rupture
- Extraluminal tracheal compression—abscess (pasteurellosis), neoplasia
*Lower Respiratory Tract*
- Extraluminal tracheal compression—abscess (pasteurellosis), mediastinal mass
- Pneumonia (bacterial most common; myomatosis and mycotic are rare), pulmonary contusion (trauma), neoplasia (primary, metastatic), intrathoracic tracheal disease (foreign body, neoplasia, abscess), pulmonary edema (cardiogenic and noncardiac), pneumonitis (allergic)

### Plural Space Disease
- Mediastinal masses (abscess or thymoma most common)
- Pneumothorax, hemothorax, pleural effusion caused by cardiac or pericardial disease
- Diaphragmatic hernia (rare)

## RISK FACTORS
- Dental disease—periapical or tooth root abscesses, malocclusion
- Dysphagia, aspiration
- Trauma, bite wounds

- Poor husbandry—dirty, urine-soaked bedding (high ammonia concentrations); poor ventilation, dusty cat litter; diets too low in fiber content may predispose to dental disease.
- Bleach, smoke, or other inhaled irritants
- Stress
- Immunosuppression, corticosteroid use

# DIAGNOSIS

## DIFFERENTIAL DIAGNOSIS

### Differentiating Causes
- Tachypnea without dyspnea may be a physiologic response to fear, physical exertion, anxiety, fever, pain, or acidosis.
- Pneumonia usually presents with signs of systemic disease (emaciation, anorexia, depression).
- URT dyspnea is often more pronounced on inspiration; nasal discharge, facial abscesses, or signs of dental disease usually present
- LRT dyspnea is more often associated with expiratory effort.
- Primary cardiac disease often presents with a constellation of other signs (e.g., heart murmur, arrhythmias).
- Tracheal mass or foreign body may cause both inspiratory and expiratory dyspnea and orthopnea.
- Pleural space disease often presents as exaggerated thoracic excursions that generate only minimal airflow at the mouth or nose.

## CBC/BIOCHEMISTRY/URINALYSIS
- Hemogram—TWBC elevations are usually not seen with bacterial diseases. A relative neutrophilia and/or lymphopenia are more common.
- Biochemistry panel—may help to define underlying cause with metabolic diseases; increased liver enzyme activity or bile acids (liver disease), increased CK (muscle wasting, heart disease) uremia

## OTHER LABORATORY TESTS
Serology for *Pasteurella*—usefulness is severely limited and generally not helpful in the diagnosis of pasteurellosis in pet rabbits. An ELISA is available and results are reported as negative, low positive, or high positive. Positive results, even when high, only indicate prior exposure to *Pasteurella* and the development of antibodies but do not confirm active infection. Low-positive results may occur due to cross-reaction with other, nonpathogenic bacteria (false positive). False-negative results are common with immunosuppression or early infection. No evidence exists to support correlation of titers to the presence or absence of disease.

## DYSPNEA AND TACHYPNEA

### IMAGING

#### Radiography
• Skull—nasal obstructions, sinusitis, bone destruction from tooth root abscesses, neoplasia, mycotic or severe bacterial infections. CT scans or MRI is much more useful in the diagnosis of URT disease, but availability may be limited.
• Thoracic—pulmonary disease (small airway disease, pulmonary edema and pneumonia), pleural space disease (effusions, mediastinal mass, pneumothorax)
• Cardiac shadow—cardiomegaly
• Abdominal—gas-filled stomach due to aerophagia, organomegaly, ascites

#### Ultrasonography
• Echocardiography to evaluate pericardial effusion, cardiomyopathy, congenital defects, and valvular disease
• Thoracic ultrasound may be beneficial in some animals with mediastinal mass lesions, but the beam is often greatly attenuated by any air in surrounding lung lobes.
• Abdominal ultrasound may be used to evaluate masses or organomegaly.

### OTHER DIAGNOSTIC PROCEDURES
• Microbiologic and cytologic examinations—LRT samples—transtracheal washing and bronchoalveolar lavage are difficult procedures in rabbits due to the location of glottis; fine needle lung aspiration can be performed under ultrasound guidance; URT samples—nasal swab or flush rarely yields diagnostic sample; nonspecific inflammation is most commonly found.
• Cultures—may be difficult to interpret, since commonly isolated bacteria (e.g., *Bordetella* sp., *Pasteurella* sp.) often represent only commensal organisms or opportunistic pathogens. A heavy growth of a single organism is usually significant. Deep cultures obtained by inserting a mini-tipped culturette 2–4 cm into each nostril are sometimes reliable
• A lack of growth does not rule out *Pasteurella*, since the infection may be in an inaccessible, deep area of the nasal cavity or sinuses, and *Pasteurella* is sometimes difficult to grow on culture.
• Rhinoscopy—valuable to visualize nasal abnormalities, retrieve foreign bodies, or obtain biopsy samples
• Laryngopharyngoscopy—to evaluate for laryngeal trauma, foreign bodies, or neoplasia
• Biopsy of the nasal cavity is indicated in any animal with chronic nasal discharge in which neoplasia is suspected.
• Thoracocentesis—fluid analysis and culture

## TREATMENT
• Breathing—supply $O_2$ enrichment ($O_2$ cage or induction chamber) in a quiet environment.
• Maintain normal systemic hydration—important to aid mucociliary clearance and secretion mobilization; use a balanced multielectrolyte solution.
• Nebulization with bland aerosols—may contribute to a more rapid resolution if used in conjunction with antibacterials
• Keep nares clear of nasal discharges in rabbits with URT disease.
• Chest tap—may be both diagnostic and therapeutic in animals with pleural space disease. In acutely dyspneic animals, perform tap prior to radiography. A negative tap for air or fluid suggests solid pleural space (mass, abscess, or hernia), primary pulmonary, or cardiac disease.
• Surgery may be necessary to remove foreign bodies, to obtain samples for biopsy, or to debulk tumors, abscesses, or granulomas; however, maintaining adequate ventilation can be challenging.

### DIET
• Provide adequate nutrition. It is imperative that the rabbit continue to eat during and following treatment. Anorexia will often cause gastrointestinal hypomotility, derangement of the gastrointestinal microflora, and overgrowth of intestinal bacterial pathogens. If the patient refuses these foods, syringe feed a gruel such as Critical Care for Herbivores (Oxbow Pet Products, Murdock, NE), giving approximately 10–15 mL/kg PO q6–8h. Alternatively, pellets can be ground and mixed with fresh greens, vegetable baby foods, water, or juice to form a gruel.
• Encourage oral fluid intake by offering fresh water, wetting leafy vegetables, or flavoring water with vegetable juices.

## MEDICATIONS

### DRUG(S) OF CHOICE
• Oxygen is the single most useful drug in the treatment of acute severe dyspnea.
• See primary disorder for definitive therapy.

### CONTRAINDICATIONS
• Oral administration of antibiotics that select against Gram-positive bacteria (penicillins, macrolides, lincosamides, and cephalosporins) can cause fatal enteric dysbiosis and enterotoxemia.

• The use of corticosteroids (systemic or topical in otic preparations) can severely exacerbate bacterial infection; use is almost never indicated in rabbits.
• In animals with CHF and blunt chest trauma, iatrogenic fluid overload and pulmonary edema is a potential problem. Intravenous administration of crystalloids should be used judiciously.
• Respiratory rate and effort should be monitored carefully and frequently in these patients

### PRECAUTIONS
N/A

### POSSIBLE INTERACTIONS
N/A

### ALTERNATE DRUGS
N/A

## FOLLOW-UP

### PATIENT MONITORING
• Repeat any abnormal tests.
• Radiographs—monitor response to therapy in animals with pulmonary disease. Pulmonary edema should be visibly improved within 12 hours of therapy, if effective therapy is used. Monitor the recurrence of pleural effusion, based upon how quickly effusion accumulates. Pneumonia—radiographic lesions improve more slowly than the clinical appearance; may not improve with pulmonary abscesses
• Cardiac ultrasound—3–12 weeks, depending on the condition

### POSSIBLE COMPLICATIONS
• Depends on the underlying disease
• Relapse, progression of disease, and death are common.

## MISCELLANEOUS

### ASSOCIATED CONDITIONS
• Dental disease
• Gastrointestinal hypomotility

### ZOONOTIC POTENTIAL
N/A

### PREGNANCY
N/A

### SYNONYMS
N/A

**SEE ALSO**
- Cheek teeth malocclusion and elongation
- Congestive heart failure
- Pasteurellosis
- Pneumonia
- Rhinitis and sinusitis

**ABBREVIATIONS**
- CHF = congestive heart failure
- CK = creatine kinase
- CNS = central nervous system
- CT = computed tomography
- ELISA = enzyme-linked immunosorbent assay
- MRI = magnetic resonance imaging
- URT = upper respiratory tract
- LRT = lower respiratory tract

*Suggested Reading*

Burglof A, Norlander T, Feinstein R, et al. Association of bronchopneumonia with sinusitis due to *Bordetella bronchiseptica* in an experimental rabbit model. Am J Rhinol 2000;43:255–232.

Crossley DA. Oral biology and disorders of lagomorphs. Vet Clin Noth Am Exotic Anim Pract 2003;6(3):629–659.

Crossley DA, Aiken S. Small mammal dentistry. In: Quesenberry KE, Carpenter JW, eds. Ferrets, Rabbits and Rodents: Clinical Medicine and Surgery. 2nd ed. Philadelphia: WB Saunders, 2004:370–382.

Deeb BJ. Respiratory disease and pasteurellosis. In: Quesenberry KE, Carpenter JW, eds. Ferrets, Rabbits and Rodents: Clinical Medicine and Surgery. 2nd Ed. Philadelphia: WB Saunders, 2004:172–182.

Deeb BJ, DiGiacomo RF. Respiratory diseases of rabbits. Vet Clin North Am Exotic Anim Pract 2000;3(2):465–480.

Harcourt-Brown F. Cardiorespiratory disease. In: Harcourt-Brown F, ed. Textbook of Rabbit Medicine. Oxford: Butterworth-Heinemann, 2002:324–334.

Paul-Murphy J, Ramer JC. Urgent care of the pet rabbits. Vet Clin North Am Exotic Anim Pract 1998;1(1):127–152.

*Portions Adapted From*

Mason RA. Dyspnea, Tachypnea, and Panting. In: Tilley LP, Smith FWK, Jr., eds. The 5-Minute Veterinary Consult: Canine and Feline, 2nd Ed. Baltimore: Lippincott Williams & Wilkins, 2000.

# DYSURIA AND POLLAKIURIA

## BASICS

### DEFINITION
• Dysuria—difficult or painful urination
• Pollakiuria—voiding small quantities of urine with increased frequency

### PATHOPHYSIOLOGY
The urinary bladder normally serves as a reservoir for storage and periodic release of urine. Inflammatory and noninflammatory disorders of the lower urinary tract may decrease bladder compliance and storage capacity by damaging structural components of the bladder wall or by stimulating sensory nerve endings located in the bladder or urethra. Sensations of bladder fullness, urgency, and pain stimulate premature micturition and reduce functional bladder capacity. Dysuria and pollakiuria are caused by lesions of the urinary bladder and/or urethra and provide evidence of lower urinary tract disease; these clinical signs do not exclude concurrent involvement of the upper urinary tract or disorders of other body systems.

### SYSTEMS AFFECTED
Renal/urologic—bladder, urethra

### SIGNALMENT
N/A

### SIGNS

#### Historical Findings
• Frequent trips to the litter box, urination outside of the litter box
• Urinating when picked up by owners
• Hematuria
• Thick, white- or tan-appearing urine
• Urine staining in the perineum
• Anorexia, weight loss, lethargy, tooth grinding, tenesmus, and a hunched posture in rabbits with chronic or obstructive lower urinary tract disease

#### Physical Examination Findings
• May be normal
• Abdominal palpation may demonstrate urocystoliths; failure to palpate uroliths does not exclude them from consideration.
• In rabbits with crystalluria, the bladder palpates as a soft, doughy mass.
• A large urinary bladder may be palpable in patients with partial or complete urethral obstruction, or in rabbits with chronic hypercalciuria.
• Manual expression of the bladder may reveal thick, beige- to brown-colored urine. Manual expression of the bladder may expel thick, brown urine even in rabbits that have normal-appearing voided urine.

## CAUSES

### Urinary Bladder
• Hypercalciuria—most common cause
• Urinary tract infection—bacterial; sometimes accompanies hypercalciuria
• Urolithiasis—often accompanies hypercalciuria
• Neoplasia
• Trauma
• Iatrogenic—for example, catheterization, overdistension of the bladder during contrast radiography, and surgery

### Urethra
• Urinary tract infection
• Urethrolithiasis—occasionally seen with hypercalciuria
• Urethral plugs—consisting of calcium precipitates
• Trauma—especially bite wounds
• Neoplasia (rare)

### Reproductive
• Endometrial hyperplasia
• Uterine adenoma or adenocarcinoma

### RISK FACTORS
• Feeding diets high in bioavailable calcium such as alfalfa pellets and alfalfa hay alone may predispose to hypercalciuria and cystic calculi.
• Obese, sedentary rabbits are prone to hypercalciuria.
• Intact females likely to develop uterine disease
• Diseases, diagnostic procedures, or treatments that (1) alter normal host urinary tract defenses and predispose to infection, (2) predispose to formation of uroliths, or (3) damage the urothelium or other tissues of the lower urinary tract
• Mural or extramural diseases that compress the bladder or urethral lumen

## DIAGNOSIS

### DIFFERENTIAL DIAGNOSIS

#### Differentiating From Other Abnormal Patterns of Micturition
• Rule out polyuria—increased frequency and volume of urine
• Rule out urethral obstruction—stranguria, anuria, overdistended urinary bladder, signs of postrenal uremia

#### Differentiate Causes of Dysuria and Pollakiuria
• Rule out urinary tract infection—hematuria; bacteruria; painful, thickened bladder
• Rule out hypercalciuria—thick, white to beige urine, sometimes streaked with fresh blood; radiopaque bladder
• Rule out urolithiasis—hematuria, palpable uroliths in bladder, radiopaque bladder
• Rule out neoplasia—hematuria; palpable masses in urethra or bladder possible; radiographs and ultrasound may differentiate
• Rule out neurogenic disorders—flaccid bladder wall; residual urine in bladder lumen after micturition; other neurologic deficits to hind legs, tail, perineum, and anal sphincter
• Rule out iatrogenic disorders—history of catheterization, reverse flushing, contrast radiography, or surgery
• Rule out uterine disease—female rabbits; rabbits with uterine disease often strain and expel blood when urinating. Blood may mix with urine and be mistaken for hematuria.

### CBC/BIOCHEMISTRY/URINALYSIS
• Results may be normal.
• Elevated serum calcium concentration seen both in rabbits with hypercalciuria and in normal rabbits
• Lower urinary tract disease complicated by urethral obstruction may be associated with azotemia.
• Patients with concurrent pyelonephritis may have impaired urine-concentrating capacity, leukocytosis, and azotemia.
• Disorders of the urinary bladder are best evaluated with a urine specimen collected by cystocentesis.
• Pyuria (normal value 0–1 WBC/hpf), hematuria (normal value 0–1 RBC/hpf), and proteinuria (normal value 0–33 mg/dL) indicate urinary tract inflammation, but these are nonspecific findings that may result from infectious and noninfectious causes of lower urinary tract disease.
• Identification of bacteria in urine sediment suggests that urinary tract infection is causing or complicating lower urinary tract disease.
• Identification of neoplastic cells in urine sediment indicates urinary tract neoplasia (rare).
• Most normal rabbits have numerous crystals in the urine. The most common types are calcium oxalate and calcium carbonate.

### OTHER LABORATORY TESTS
Quantitative urine culture—the most definitive means of identifying and characterizing bacterial urinary tract infection; negative urine culture results suggest a noninfectious cause.

## IMAGING
Survey abdominal radiography, contrast cystography, and urinary tract and uterine ultrasonography are important means of identifying and localizing causes of dysuria and pollakiuria.

## DIAGNOSTIC PROCEDURES
N/A

# TREATMENT
• Patients with nonobstructive lower urinary tract diseases are typically managed as outpatients; diagnostic evaluation may require brief hospitalization.
• Dysuria and pollakiuria associated with systemic signs of illness (e.g., pyrexia, depression, anorexia, and dehydration) or laboratory findings of azotemia or leukocytosis warrant aggressive diagnostic evaluation and initiation of supportive and symptomatic treatment.
• Treatment depends on the underlying cause and specific sites involved. See specific chapters describing diseases listed in section on causes.

# MEDICATIONS

## DRUG(S) OF CHOICE
• Depend on the underlying cause
• If bacterial cystitis is demonstrated, begin treatment with a broad-spectrum antibiotic such as enrofloxacin (5–20 mg/kg PO, SC, IM q12–24h) or trimethoprim sulfa (30 mg/kg PO q12h). Modify antibacterial treatment based on results of urine culture and susceptibility testing.
• Symptomatic rabbits with hypercalciuria are sometimes in pain and therefore reluctant to urinate. Pain management may aid in urination and promote appetite and water consumption. NSAIDS reduce pain and may decrease inflammation in the bladder: meloxicam (0.2–0.5 mg/kg PO q24h) or carprofen (2.2 mg/kg PO q12–24h)

## CONTRAINDICATIONS
• Glucocorticoids or other immunosuppressive agents

• Oral administration of antibiotics that select against Gram-positive bacteria (penicillins, macrolides, lincosamides, and cephalosporins) can cause fatal enteric dysbiosis and enterotoxemia.
• Potentially nephrotoxic drugs (e.g., aminoglycosides, NSAIDs) in patients who are febrile, dehydrated, or azotemic or who are suspected of having pyelonephritis, septicemia, or preexisting renal disease.

## PRECAUTIONS
N/A

## POSSIBLE INTERACTIONS
N/A

## ALTERNATIVE DRUGS
N/A

# FOLLOW-UP

## PATIENT MONITORING
• Response to treatment by clinical signs, serial physical examinations, laboratory testing, and radiographic and ultrasonic evaluations appropriate for each specific cause
• Refer to specific chapters describing diseases listed in section on causes.

## POSSIBLE COMPLICATIONS
Refer to specific chapters describing diseases listed in section on causes.

# MISCELLANEOUS

## ASSOCIATED CONDITIONS
• Obesity
• Gastrointestinal hypomotility
• Pyoderma (urine scald)

## AGE-RELATED FACTORS
N/A

## ZOONOTIC POTENTIAL
N/A

## PREGNANCY
N/A

## SYNONYMS
N/A

## SEE ALSO
• Hypercalciuria
• Lower urinary tract infection
• Urinary tract obstruction

## ABBREVIATIONS
• NSAIDs = nonsteroidal antiinflammatory drugs
• RBC = red blood cell
• WBC = white blood cell

*Suggested Reading*

Brown SA. Rabbit urinary tract disease. Proc North Am Vet Conf 1997:785–787.
Cheeke PR, Amberg JW. Comparative calcium excretion by rats and rabbits. J Anim Sci 1973;37:450–454.
Donoghue S. Nutrition and pet rabbits. In: Rosenthal KL, ed. Practical Exotic Animal Medicine: The Compendium Collection. Trenton, NJ: Veterinary Learning Systems, 1997:107.
Garibaldi BA, Pecquet-Goad ME. Hypercalcemia with secondary nephrolithiasis in a rabbit. Lab Anim Sci 1988;38:331–333.
Harkness JE, Wagner JE. The Biology and Medicine of Rabbits and Rodents. 3rd Ed. Baltimore: Williams & Wilkins, 1989.
Harcourt-Brown F. Urogenital disease. In: Harcourt-Brown F, ed. Textbook of Rabbit Medicine. Oxford: Butterworth-Heinemann, 2002:335–351.
Kampheus J. Calcium metabolism of rabbits as an etiological factor for urolithiasis. J Nutr 1991;121:595–596.
Pare JA, Paul-Murphy J. Disorders of the reproductive and urinary systems. In: Quesenberry KE, Carpenter JW, eds. Ferrets, Rabbits and Rodents: Clinical Medicine and Surgery. 2nd Ed. Philadelphia: WB Saunders, 2004:183–193.
Paul-Murphy J, Ramer JC. Urgent care of the pet rabbits. Vet Clin North Am Exotic Anim Pract 1998;1(1):127–152.
Redrobe S. Calcium metabolism in rabbits. Semin Avian Exotic Pet Med 2002;11(2):94–101.

*Portions Adapted From*

Kruger JM. Dysuria and Pollakiuria. In: Tilley LP, Smith FWK, Jr., eds. The 5-Minute Veterinary Consult: Canine and Feline, 3rd Ed. Baltimore: Lippincott Williams & Wilkins, 2004.

# EAR MITES

## BASICS

### OVERVIEW
• *Psoroptes cuniculi* mite infestation is seen occasionally in rabbits. Most affected rabbits are intensely pruritic and in pain, although early infestations may be asymptomatic or only mildly pruritic.
• Mites are spread to other areas of the body during grooming. Lesions may be seen around the head, abdomen, and perineal regions.
• *P. cuniculi* are nonburrowing mites and spend their entire 3-week life cycle on the host; eggs hatch within 4 days.

### SIGNALMENT
Can be seen in any-aged rabbit; no gender predilection

### SIGNS
• Mild to moderate pruritus around the pinna, head, and neck in mildly affected or subclinical rabbits
• Intense pruritus (more common) primarily located around the ears, head, and neck; occasionally generalized. Head shaking and scratching exacerbate lesions. Affected areas may become extremely painful.
• Thick, brown to beige crusty exudate in the ear canal, eventually spreading to cover the pinna. With severe infestations, thick crust layer can develop a foliated appearance that is pathognomonic for ear mites in rabbits.
• Occasionally, brown to beige crusting and pruritus occur on the pinna and feet only.
• Alopecia and excoriations around the pinnae may occur, owing to the intense pruritus.
• Mites and lesions may extend to the face, neck, abdomen, perineal region, and even feet via grooming.
• Signs of otitis interna/media such as head tilt and vestibular signs may occur with secondary infections and chronic disease.

### CAUSES AND RISK FACTORS
• Exposure to affected rabbits—pet stores, shelters, multirabbit households
• Exposure to fomites—hay, grass, straw, or wood chip bedding

## DIAGNOSIS

### DIFFERENTIAL DIAGNOSIS
#### Exudate in the Ear Canal
• Normal wax—most rabbits normally have a light yellow–beige, waxy exudate in the ear canal. Exudate normally does not extend onto the pinnae, as seen in ear mite infestations.

• Bacterial or mycotic otitis externa—more common than ear mite infestation in pet rabbits; exudate is usually thick, white, creamy, and limited to the external canal; differentiate by microscopic examination of exudate.

#### Pruritus/Alopecia
• Fur mites—*Cheyletiella* sp. or, less commonly, *Leporacarus gibbus*. May be concurrent with ear mite infestation. Fur mite lesions are usually located in the intrascapular or tail base region and associated with copious amounts of large white scale. Mites are readily identified in skin scrapes or acetate tape preparations under low magnification. There is no exudate in ear canals.
• Other ectoparasites—*Sarcoptes scabiei* and *Notoedres cati* rarely infest rabbits. Lesions are located around the head and neck and are intensely pruritic. Exudate in ear canals is not seen.
• Fleas—patchy alopecia usually appears in other areas in addition to the head; finding flea dirt will help to differentiate.

### CBC/BIOCHEMISTRY/URINALYSIS
Normal

### OTHER LABORATORY TESTS
N/A

### IMAGING
N/A

### DIAGNOSTIC PROCEDURES
• Ear swabs placed in mineral oil and examined under low magnification—usually a very effective means of identification
• Skin scrapings—identify mites, if signs are generalized.
• Otoscopic examination—to visualize mites
• Mites are also visible to the unaided eye

## TREATMENT
• Contagious; important to treat all in-contact rabbits
• Thoroughly clean and treat the environment; extremely important for eliminating infestation; mites can live on exfoliated crusts in the environment up to 21 days, depending on conditions. Remove and discard all organic material from cage (wood or paper products, bedding); replace bedding with shredded paper bedding that can be discarded, and the cage should be thoroughly cleaned every day during the treatment period.
• Combs, brushes, and grooming utensils—discard or thoroughly disinfect before reuse.
• Cleaning of the ear canal does not enhance treatment and can be very painful and traumatize the ear canal. Treat first with

ivermectin or selamectin. Most crusts and lesions will resolve rapidly without the need for manually removing crusts.

## MEDICATIONS

### DRUG(S) OF CHOICE
• Ivermectin 1%—0.4 mg/kg SC q10–14d for two to three doses. It is not necessary and may be detrimental to clean the ears to remove debris during this treatment period.
• Selamectin (Revolution, Pfizer)—monthly spot treatment for cats and dogs; appears to be safe and effective at 6–12 mg/kg applied topically q30d
• Topical otic antibiotic or antifungal medications are usually not required. Secondary bacterial and/or yeast otitis is usually the result of overzealous cleaning of the pinnae and/or ear canals.

### CONTRAINDICATIONS
• Avoid overzealous cleaning of the ear canals; do not attempt to manually remove crusts.
• Ivermectin—do not use in pregnant animals.
• Do not use topical and parenteral ivermectin concurrently.
• Do not use fipronil on rabbits.
• Do not use flea collars on rabbits.
• Do not use organophosphate-containing products on rabbits.
• Do not use straight permethrin sprays or permethrin spot-ons on rabbits.

### PRECAUTIONS
• All products discussed above are off-label use. Safety and efficacy have not been evaluated in rabbits. Use with caution, especially in young or debilitated animals.
• Topical otic medications containing corticosteroids should be avoided in rabbits.
• Prevent rabbits or their cage mates from licking topical spot-on products before they are dry.

### ALTERNATIVE DRUGS
N/A

## FOLLOW-UP
• An ear swab and physical examination should be done 1 month after therapy commences.
• For most patients, prognosis is excellent.
• Infestation is more likely to recur or fail to respond to treatment with topical thiabendazole or if the environment is not thoroughly cleaned.

## MISCELLANEOUS

**ZOONOTIC POTENTIAL**

N/A

**SEE ALSO**

• Cheyletiellosis
• Dermatophytosis
• Fleas
• Pruritus

*Suggested Reading*

Harcourt-Brown F. Skin diseases. In: Harcourt-Brown F, ed. Textbook of Rabbit Medicine. Oxford: Butterworth-Heinemann, 2002:224–248.

Hess L. Dermatologic diseases. In: Quesenberry KE, Carpenter JW, eds. Ferrets, Rabbits and Rodents: Clinical Medicine and Surgery. 2nd Ed. Philadelphia: WB Saunders, 2004:194–202.

Jenkins JR. Skin disorders of the rabbit. Vet Clin North Am Exotic Anim Pract 2001;4(2):543–563.

McTier TL, Hair A, Walstrom DJ, et al. Efficacy and safety of topical administration of selamectin for treatment of ear mite infestation in rabbits. J Am Vet Med Assoc 2003;223(3):322–324.

# ENCEPHALITOZOONOSIS

 BASICS

## DEFINITION
*Encephalitozoon cuniculi*—an obligate intracellular microsporidian parasite that infects rabbits, mice, guinea pigs, hamsters, dogs, cats, primates, and humans; most are opportunistic infections in immunocompromised hosts.

## PATHOPHYSIOLOGY
• Infection—ingestion of spores in urine-contaminated food; spores spread to extraintestinal organs via reticuloendothelial system; rupture of intracellular spore-filled vacuoles results in granulomatous inflammation.
• In normal life cycle—localizes in renal tubular epithelial cells, resulting in spores shed in urine 6 weeks after infection; shedding peaks 2 months postinfection and ends 3 months postinfection.
• In utero infection—vertical transmission of organism into the developing lens; replication of spores within the lens of young rabbits results in cataract formation, lens rupture, uveitis, and glaucoma.
• The prevalence of *E. cuniculi* as a cause of CNS disease is controversial since definitive antemortem diagnosis is not possible and postmortem lesions do not always correlate well with clinical disease.
• Severity and manifestation—depend on location and degree of tissue injury; most infections are asymptomatic or remain asymptomatic until the rabbit becomes immunocompromised (stress, debility, age); renal compromise is uncommon.
• Myocarditis, vasculitis, pneumonitis, hepatitis, splenitis, and spinal nerve root inflammation have also been reported.
• Clinical disease—most likely occurs in older or immunosuppressed animals

## SYSTEMS AFFECTED
• Renal—lesions typically incidental finding; may cause renal compromise if severe
• Ophthalmic—cataract formation and phacoclastic uveitis from in utero infections
• CNS—granulomatous encephalitis, spinal nerve root inflammation

## GENETICS
N/A

## INCIDENCE/PREVALENCE
• Many rabbits (up to 80% of those tested) in the United States and Europe are serologically positive for *E. cuniculi*. Most are exposed in utero or at birth.
• Most animals are asymptomatic.
• The true incidence of clinical disease is unknown.

## GEOGRAPHIC DISTRIBUTION
Worldwide

## SIGNALMENT
• No sex predilection
• Phacoclastic uveitis seen in young animals; dwarf breeds more commonly affected
• CNS disease anecdotally more likely in older animals

## SIGNS

### General Comments
• Determined mainly by site and extent of tissue damage; ocular and CNS signs most commonly reported
• Most infections are asymptomatic.
• The extent to which *E. cuniculi* causes neurologic disease in rabbits is controversial. Many rabbits with CNS signs demonstrate postmortem histologic CNS lesions compatible with *E. cuniculi*, but the organism itself is often not identified in tissues. On the other hand, many rabbits have similar postmortem lesions (and sometimes, organism identified) in the absence of neurologic signs.

### Historical Findings
• Ocular—photophobia, hypopyon, intraocular abscess, cataract; usually unilateral
• Neurologic—vestibular signs (with head tilt, nystagmus, anorexia, ataxia, and rolling) predominate; seizures; tremors; paresis/paralysis also reported anecdotally
• Renal compromise (unusual)—nonspecific signs of lethargy, depression, anorexia, and weight loss

### Physical Examination Findings
• Renal disease—irregular, pitted kidneys (usually incidental finding); if renal compromise (unusual)—depression, dehydration, cachexia, evidence of gastrointestinal hypomotility
• Neurologic—vestibular signs predominate (ataxia, head tilt, nystagmus, torticollis); tremors, paresis, paralysis, seizures, stiff rear limb gait, and incontinence also reported
• Ocular signs (postnatal infections)—often unilateral, iridal abscess, cataract, lens rupture, uveitis (aqueous flare, hyphema, mydriasis); hypopyon
• Cardiac or hepatic involvement—occurs; usually not clinically apparent

## CAUSES
*E. cuniculi*

## RISK FACTORS
Immunosuppression—predisposes to clinical disease: stress, poor diet, concurrent disease, and glucocorticoid or antitumor chemotherapy. Asymptomatic rabbits with subclinical infections often demonstrate clinical signs following one or more of these events.

 DIAGNOSIS

## GENERAL COMMENTS
Antemortem diagnosis is usually presumed based on clinical signs, exclusion of other diagnoses, positive antibody titers, and sometimes, response to treatment. Definitive antemortem diagnosis is problematic, since a positive antibody titer indicates exposure only, rabbits often respond minimally or not at all to treatment, and many rabbits will improve with no treatment at all. Definitive diagnosis requires identification of organisms and characteristic inflammation in affected tissues, generally acquired at postmortem examination.

## DIFFERENTIAL DIAGNOSIS
• Neurologic—vestibular signs—otitis interna/media most common cause. Many rabbits with otitis interna/media lack exudate in external canal or other signs of otitis externa. Bulla disease is not always visible on skull radiographs and often requires CT or MRI to diagnose. Every attempt should be made to rule out otic disease prior to assuming *E. cuniculi* infection. Other causes—CNS abscess, neoplasia, trauma; parasitic (toxoplasmosis, aberrant migration of *Baylisascaris* sp.). Rear limb weakness/ataxia—spinal disease, lead toxicosis, generalized weakness from metabolic disease, orthopedic disease
• Intraocular disease (anterior uveitis)—bacterial; trauma; lens-induced; corneal ulceration with reflex uveitis

## CBC/BIOCHEMISTRY/URINALYSIS
• CBC usually unremarkable; increased PCV with dehydration possible secondary to renal disease or anorexia
• Biochemistry—increased BUN and creatinine with renal disease (rare)

## OTHER LABORATORY TESTS
Serologic testing—many tests are available, but usefulness is limited in pet rabbits since a positive titer indicates only exposure and does not confirm *E. cuniculi* as the cause of clinical signs. *E. cuniculi* can only be definitively diagnosed by finding organisms and resultant lesions on histopathologic examination in areas that anatomically correlate with observed clinical signs. Antibody titers usually become positive by 2 weeks postinfection, but generally do not continue to rise with active infection or decline with treatment. No correlation exists between antibody titers and shedding of organism or severity of disease. It is unknown if exposed rabbits eventually become seronegative. Available tests include ELISA, indirect IFA, and carbon immunoassay.

## IMAGING
• Radiographs—skull films to rule out otitis interna/media; spinal films to rule out spinal disease/trauma; may see small, malformed kidneys with severe renal involvement
• CT or MRI—to rule out bulla disease, CNS neoplasia, abscess

## DIAGNOSTIC PROCEDURES
Urine sedimentation—Gram's stain may demonstrate spores, oval $2.5 \times 1.5\ \mu m$ in diameter. Spores are only passed for up to 3 weeks following infection and generally are not present in urine when neurologic, ophthalmologic, or renal signs are present.

## PATHOLOGIC FINDINGS
• CNS—multifocal nonsuppurative granulomatous meningoencephalomyelitis; astrogliosis; perivascular lymphocytic infiltration; lymphocytic meningitis. Spores $(1.5 \times 2.5\ mm)$ stain positive with Gram's and carbol fuchsin stains.
• Kidneys—gross: multifocal, depressed areas of fibrosis pitting the surface of the kidney—usually an incidental finding; histologic with active disease—lymphohistiocytic tubulointerstitial nephritis, interstitial nephrosis, renal tubular necrosis. Protozoa may be identified with Gram's stain.
• Ocular—lens capsule rupture with anterior uveitis; organisms may be identified on histologic examination of the liquefied lens; iridal abscesses or hypopyon with secondary bacterial infection

# TREATMENT

## APPROPRIATE HEALTH CARE
• Usually outpatient
• Inpatient—severe disease; patient cannot maintain adequate nutrition or hydration.
• Many rabbits improve with supportive care alone.

## NURSING CARE
• Dehydration—intravenous fluids or subcutaneous fluids
• Assist-feed anorectic animals.

## ACTIVITY
Restrict or confine—patients with neurologic signs; provide padded cages for rabbits that are severely ataxic, having seizures, or rolling

## DIET
• It is absolutely imperative that the rabbit continue to eat during and following treatment. Anorexia will often cause gastrointestinal hypomotility, derangement of the gastrointestinal microflora, and overgrowth of intestinal bacterial pathogens.
• Offer a large selection of fresh, moistened greens such as cilantro, romaine lettuce, parsley, carrot tops, dandelion greens, spinach, collard greens, etc., and good-quality grass hay. Many rabbits will begin to eat these foods, even if they were previously anorectic. Also, try offering the rabbit's usual pelleted diet.
• If the patient refuses these foods, syringe feed a gruel such as Critical Care for Herbivores (Oxbow Pet Products, Murdock, NE) 10–15 mL/kg PO q6–8h. Larger volumes and more frequent feedings are often accepted; feed as much as the rabbit will accept. Alternatively, pellets can be ground and mixed with fresh greens, vegetable baby foods, water, or juice to form a gruel. (CAUTION: Be aware of aspiration secondary to abnormal body posture in patients with severe head tilt and vestibular disequilibrium or brainstem dysfunction.)
• High-carbohydrate, high-fat nutritional supplements are contraindicated.
• Encourage oral fluid intake by offering fresh water, wetting leafy vegetables, or flavoring water with vegetable juices.

## CLIENT EDUCATION
• Prognosis guarded in patients needing therapy; response to therapy inconsistent
• Long-term home nursing care (assisted feeding, padded bedding in recumbent animals) may be required; residual neurologic signs common in rabbits that partially recover; a waxing and waning course of progression is seen in some rabbits.

## SURGICAL CONSIDERATIONS
Phacoclastic uveitis—phacoemulsification has been successfully performed. Rabbits with glaucoma secondary to *E. cuniculi* may require enucleation.

# MEDICATIONS

## DRUG(S) OF CHOICE
• Benzimidazole anthelmintics are effective against *E cuniculi* in vitro and have been shown to prevent experimental infection in rabbits. However, efficacy in rabbits with clinical signs is unknown. Anecdotal reports suggest a response to treatment; however, many rabbits with neurologic signs improve with or without treatment. Long-term treatment has been recommended, as treatment only prevents replication rather than kills the parasite. Published treatments include oxibendazole (20–30 mg/kg PO q24h × 7–14 days, then reduce to 15 mg/kg q24h × 30–60 days); albendazole (20–30 mg/kg q24h × 30 days, then 15 mg/kg PO q24h × 30 days); and fenbendazole (20 mg/kg q24h × 5–28 days).
• Phacoclastic uveitis—1% prednisolone acetate drops every 6–12 hours for 5 days; use concurrently with benzimidazole anthelmintics.

• Severe vestibular signs (rolling, torticollis) or seizures—diazepam 1–2 mg/kg IM or midazolam 1–2 mg/kg IM
• Vestibular signs—meclizine 2–12 mg/kg PO q24h may reduce clinical signs, control nausea, and induce mild sedation.

## CONTRAINDICATIONS
N/A

## PRECAUTIONS
• Topical and systemic corticosteroids—topical corticosteroids may be indicated to decrease ocular inflammation, progression of uveitis, and development of glaucoma. However, the use of either topical or systemic corticosteroids in rabbits with *E. cuniculi* is controversial. Rabbits are very sensitive to the immunosuppressive effects of corticosteroids; use may exacerbate signs of *E. cuniculi* or subclinical bacterial infection.
• Albendazole has been associated with bone marrow toxicity in dogs and cats. Toxicity in rabbits is unknown; however, anecdotal reports of pancytopenia leading to death in rabbits exist.

## POSSIBLE INTERACTIONS
None

## ALTERNATIVE DRUGS
Systemic corticosteroids have been advocated by some practitioners for treatment of *E. cuniculi*–induced CNS granulomatous inflammation. Most recommend a single dose of a short-acting corticosteroid at immunosuppressive doses, followed by antiinflammatory doses only if necessary. Use of corticosteroids is controversial. Rabbits are very sensitive to the immunosuppressive effects of corticosteroids; immunosuppression may exacerbate subclinical bacterial or *E. cuniculi* infection.

# FOLLOW-UP

## PATIENT MONITORING
• Uveitis—monitor for progression of uveitis and development of glaucoma.
• Monitor for progression of neurologic signs.

## PREVENTION/AVOIDANCE
• Most infections occur when rabbits are young (i.e., doe to offspring). Rabbits with CNS, ocular, or renal signs are no longer shedding spores. Clean environment daily; spores are inactivated by most common disinfectants. Select serologically negative rabbits for breeding, when possible.
• Some practitioners advocate serologic testing prior to purchase or addition of a new rabbit and excluding seropositive rabbits. Antibody titers usually develop within 2 weeks of infection; however, infected rabbits

## ENCEPHALITOZOONOSIS

will only shed spores for 3 weeks following infection. After this period, rabbits with chronic or subclinical disease are not contagious. No correlation has been demonstrated between antibody titers, shedding of spores, or clinical signs. Antibody titers may be helpful in the development of SPF colonies.

### POSSIBLE COMPLICATIONS
N/A

### EXPECTED COURSE AND PROGNOSIS
• Prognosis—guarded; varied response to drug treatment; many rabbits improve with supportive care alone.
• Acute, severe neurologic signs or renal insufficiency—guarded to poor prognosis; some improve with supportive care.
• Residual deficits (especially neurologic) cannot be predicted until after a course of therapy.
• Ocular disease—variable response to medical therapy; removal of the lens by phacoemulsion may prevent progression to glaucoma; ocular disease is not expected to progress to CNS or renal disease.
• Severe muscular or neurologic disease—usually chronic debility

## MISCELLANEOUS

### ASSOCIATED CONDITIONS
• Pasteurellosis
• Gastrointestinal hypomotility

### AGE-RELATED FACTORS
N/A

### ZOONOTIC POTENTIAL
Unlikely, but possible in immunosuppressed humans. Mode of transmission and susceptibility in humans is unclear.

### PREGNANCY
Placental transmission possible

### ABBREVIATIONS
• BUN = blood urea nitrogen
• CNS = central nervous system
• CT = computed tomography
• ELISA = enzyme-linked immunosorbent assay
• IFA = immunofluorescence assay
• MRI = magnetic resonance imaging
• PCV = packed cell volume
• SPF = specific pathogen free

### Suggested Reading
Cox JC. Altered immune responsiveness associated with *Encephalitozoon cuniculi* in rabbits. Lab Anim 2000;34:281–289.

Deeb BJ, Carpenter JW. Neurologic and musculoskeletal diseases. In: Quesenberry KE, Carpenter JW, eds. Ferrets, Rabbits and Rodents: Clinical Medicine and Surgery. 2nd Ed. Philadelphia: WB Saunders, 2004:194–210.

Felchle LM, Sigler RL. Phacoemulsification for the management of *Encephalitozoon cuniculi*-induced phacoclastic uveitis in a rabbit. Vet Ophthalmol 2002;5(3):211–215.

Harcourt-Brown F. Neurological and locomotor diseases. In Harcourt-Brown F, ed. Textbook of Rabbit Medicine. Oxford: Butterworth-Heinemann, 2002:307–323.

Rosenthal KR. Torticollis in rabbits. Proc North Am Vet Conf 2005;1378–1379.

Stiles J, Dider E, Ritchie B, et al. *Encephalitozoon cuniculi* in the lens of a rabbit with phacoclastic uveitis: confirmation and treatment. Vet Comp Ophthalmol 1997;7(4):233–238.

Van der Woerdt A. Ophthalmologic disease in small pet animals. In: Quesenberry KE, Carpenter JW, eds. Ferrets, Rabbits and Rodents: Clinical Medicine and Surgery. 2nd Ed. Philadelphia: WB Saunders, 2004:421–428.

# ENCEPHALITIS AND MENINGOENCEPHALITIS

## BASICS

### DEFINITION
• Encephalitis—inflammation of the brain that may be accompanied by spinal cord and/or meningeal involvement
• Meningoencephalitis—inflammation of the meninges and brain

### PATHOPHYSIOLOGY
• Inflammation—caused by an infectious agent or by the patient's own immune system
• Bacterial infection of the CNS by extension of an infected extraneural site, especially ears or sinuses (most common) or by hematogenous route
• Immune-mediated—cause of immune system derangement generally unknown

### SYSTEMS AFFECTED
• Nervous
• Multisystemic signs—may be noted in patients with infectious diseases

### INCIDENCE/PREVALENCE
Common problem in pet rabbits; exact incidence unknown

### GEOGRAPHIC DISTRIBUTION
Varies with the cause or agent implicated

### SIGNALMENT
• Lop-eared rabbits may be more likely to show signs of otitis with subsequent meningeal/brain involvement.
• Dwarf breeds and older and immunosuppressed rabbits may be more predisposed to signs due to infectious causes.

### SIGNS

#### Historical Findings
• Usually a preacute to acute onset of clinical signs
• History of upper respiratory infection, dental disease, and otitis externa/interna in rabbits with bacterial meningoencephalitis or brain abscesses
• History of grazing outdoors consistent with parasitic encephalitis (Baylisascariasis, toxoplasmosis)

#### Physical Examination Findings
• Head tilt accompanied by other vestibular signs often seen in rabbits with brain abscess; similar signs also reported in rabbits with encephalitozoonosis
• In rabbits with otitis externa, thick, white, creamy exudate may be found in the horizontal and/or vertical canals. Otitis interna/media may occur in the absence of otitis externa via extension through the eustachian tube; may see bulging tympanum. Some rabbits with otitis interna have no visible otoscopic abnormalities.

#### Neurologic Examination Findings
• Determined by the portion of the brain most affected
• Forebrain—seizures, personality change, decreasing level of responsiveness
• Brainstem—depression, head tilt, rolling, abnormal nystagmus, facial paresis/paralysis, incoordination

### CAUSES
• Bacterial—very common, especially secondary to local extension from infection of the ears, eyes, sinuses, and nasal passages caused by Pasteurella spp. or other bacteria
• Protozoal—Encephalitozoon cuniculi: reportedly common. How often E. cuniculi is truly the cause of neurologic signs is controversial, since antemortem definitive diagnosis is not possible and postmortem changes often do not correlate well with clinical disease; toxoplasmosis: sporadic cause
• Inflammatory, idiopathic, immune-mediated—granulomatous meningoencephalomyelitis, common postmortem finding in rabbits both with and without antemortem neurologic signs; has been attributed to E. cuniculi infection, but organisms not always found
• Parasite migration—sporadic; Baylisascaris (raccoon roundworm)
• Viral—rare; rabies virus and herpes reported
• Mycotic—not yet reported in rabbits

### RISK FACTORS
• Bacterial—otitis interna/media, dental disease, chronic upper respiratory infection, immunosuppression (stress, corticosteroid use, concurrent disease)
• E. cuniculi—immunosuppression (stress, corticosteroid use, concurrent disease)
• Toxoplasma sp., Baylisascaris sp.—grazing outdoors, exposure to feed contaminated with cat or raccoon feces
• Injury involving the CNS or adjacent structures

## DIAGNOSIS

### DIFFERENTIAL DIAGNOSIS
• Bacterial diseases—usually preceded by history of, or accompanied by, signs of upper respiratory disease, dental disease, or otitis. Not all rabbits with otitis interna/media have signs of otitis externa, since bacterial extension via the eustachian tube is common.
• Encephalitozoonosis—diagnosis of exclusion; first rule out other causes of encephalitis, especially bacterial.
• Primary CNS neoplasia—rare in rabbits; signs may be similar to encephalitis.
• Metabolic or toxic encephalopathy—bilateral, symmetrical neurologic abnormalities that relate to the cerebrum

• Trauma—history and physical evidence of injury

### CBC/BIOCHEMISTRY/URINALYSIS
• Hemogram—frequently normal
• Serum chemistry—to rule out metabolic disease

### OTHER LABORATORY TESTS
• Serologic testing for E. cuniculi—may be helpful in ruling out encephalitozoonosis; however, usefulness is limited in pet rabbits, since a positive titer indicates only exposure and does not confirm E. cuniculi as the cause of neurologic signs. E. cuniculi can only be definitively diagnosed by finding organisms and resultant lesions on histopathologic examination in areas that anatomically correlate with observed clinical signs. Antibody titers usually become positive by 2 weeks postinfection but generally do not continue to rise with active infection or decline with treatment. No correlation exists between antibody titers and shedding of organism and presence or severity of disease. It is unknown if exposed rabbits eventually become seronegative. Available tests include ELISA, indirect IFA, and carbon immunoassay.
• Serology for Pasteurella—usefulness is severely limited and generally not helpful in the diagnosis of pasteurellosis in pet rabbits. An ELISA is available and results are reported as negative, low positive, or high positive. Positive results, even when high, only indicate prior exposure to Pasteurella and the development of antibodies and do not confirm active infection. Low-positive results may occur due to cross-reaction with other, nonpathogenic bacteria (false positive). False-negative results are common with immunosuppression or early infection. No evidence exists to support correlation of titers to the presence or absence of disease.
• Serologic testing for toxoplasmosis—anecdotal reports of using serum antibody titers available for testing in dogs and cats to diagnose infection in rabbits exist.

### IMAGING
• Tympanic bullae and skull radiography—may help rule out otitis interna/media; however, normal radiographs do not rule out bulla disease.
• CT and MRI—valuable for confirming bulla lesions and CNS extension from otitis or to document localized tumor, granuloma, and extent of inflammation

### DIAGNOSITIC PROCEDURES
• Bacterial culture and sensitivity testing in rabbits with concurrent otitis—sample from myringotomy or surgical drainage of tympanic bulla is most accurate.
• Culture of the nasal cavity—may be helpful to direct antibiotic therapy in rabbits with intact tympanum and evidence of concurrent respiratory infection if extension of

# ENCEPHALITIS AND MENINGOENCEPHALITIS

URI is suspected. To obtain a sample, a mini-tip culturette (#4 Calgiswab) is inserted 1–4 cm inside the nares near the nasal septum. Sedation and appropriate restraint are required to obtain a deep, meaningful sample. The nasal cavity is extremely sensitive, and rabbits that appear sedated may jump or kick when the nasal mucosa is touched. Inadequate sedation or restraint may result in serious spinal or other musculoskeletal injury.

• CSF analysis—sample from the cerebellomedullary cistern; may be valuable for evaluating central disease; detect inflammatory process; sample collection may put the patient at risk for herniation if there is a mass or high intracranial pressure.

## PATHOLOGIC FINDINGS

The lesions are a function of the brain response to the infectious agent or other cause.

## TREATMENT

### APPROPRIATE HEALTH CARE

Inpatient—diagnosis and initial therapy

### NURSING CARE

Supportive fluids—replacement or maintenance fluids (depend on clinical state); may be required in the acute phase when disorientation and nausea preclude oral intake

### ACTIVITY

Restrict (e.g., avoid stairs and slippery surfaces) according to the degree of disequilibrium; encourage return to activity as soon as safely possible; activity may enhance recovery of vestibular function.

### DIET

• It is absolutely imperative that the rabbit continue to eat during and following treatment. Anorexia will often cause gastrointestinal hypomotility, derangement of the gastrointestinal microflora, and overgrowth of intestinal bacterial pathogens.

• Offer a large selection of fresh, moistened greens such as cilantro, romaine lettuce, parsley, carrot tops, dandelion greens, spinach, collard greens, etc., and good-quality grass hay. Many rabbits will begin to eat these foods, even if they were previously anorectic. Also, try offering the rabbit's usual pelleted diet, as the initial goal is to get the patient to eat.

• If the rabbit refuses these foods, syringe feed a gruel such as Critical Care for Herbivores (Oxbow Pet Products, Murdock, NE) 10–15 mL/kg PO q6–8h. Larger volumes and more frequent feedings are often accepted; feed as much as the rabbit will accept. Alternatively, pellets can be ground and mixed with fresh greens, vegetable baby foods, water, or juice to form a gruel.

• High-carbohydrate, high-fat nutritional supplements are contraindicated.

• Encourage oral fluid intake by offering fresh water, wetting leafy vegetables, or flavoring water with vegetable juices.

CAUTION: Be aware of aspiration secondary to abnormal body posture in patients with severe head tilt and vestibular disequilibrium or brainstem dysfunction.

### CLIENT EDUCATION

• Inform client that the condition is life threatening if left untreated.

• Emphasize the importance of the diagnostic workup.

• Inform client that antiseizure treatment is only symptomatic and may not consistently help unless a primary cause can be identified and treated.

## MEDICATIONS

### DRUG(S) OF CHOICE

• Apply specific therapy once diagnosis is reached or highly suspected.

• Seizures—control may be erratic unless the encephalitis can be treated: diazepam (1–5 mg/kg IV, IM; begin with 0.5–1.0 mg/kg IV bolus); may repeat if gross seizure activity has not stopped within 5 minutes; can be administered rectally if IV access cannot be obtained; may diminish or stop the gross motor seizure activity to allow IV catheter placement; constant rate infusion protocols used in dogs and cats have been anecdotally used.

• Severe vestibular signs (continuous rolling, torticollis)—diazepam (1–2 mg/kg IM) or midazolam (1–2 mg/kg IM); meclizine (2–12 mg/kg PO q24h) may reduce clinical signs, control nausea, and induce mild sedation.

• Bacterial meningoencephalitis, abscess—antibiotics; choice is ideally based on results of culture and susceptibility testing when possible (otitis, extension from sinuses). Long-term antibiotic therapy is generally required (4–6 weeks minimum to several months). Use broad-spectrum antibiotics such as enrofloxacin (5–20 mg/kg PO, SC, IM q12–24h) or trimethoprim sulfa (30 mg/kg PO q12h); if anaerobic infections are suspected, use chloramphenicol (50 mg/kg PO q8h) or parenteral penicillin g (40,000–60,000 IU/kg SC q2–7d).

• Encephalitozoonosis—benzimidazole anthelmintics are effective against E. cuniculi in vitro and have been shown to prevent experimental infection in rabbits. However, efficacy in rabbits with clinical signs is unknown. Anecdotal reports suggest a response to treatment; however, many rabbits with neurologic signs improve with or without treatment. Published treatments include oxibendazole (20 mg/kg PO q24h × 7–14 days, then reduce to 15 mg/kg q24h × 30–60 days), albendazole (20–30 mg/kg q24h × 30 days, then 15 mg/kg PO q24h × 30 days), and fenbendazole (20 mg/kg q24h × 5–28 days).

• Toxoplasmosis—trimethoprim sulfa (15–30 mg/kg PO q12h); sulfadiazine in combination with pyrimethamine for 2 weeks has also been recommended.

### CONTRAINDICATIONS

• Dexamethasone—contraindicated in patients with infectious diseases, but may help decrease brain edema when impending brain herniation or life-threatening edema is suspected

• Oral administration of clindamycin and other antibiotics that select against Gram-positive bacteria (penicillins, macrolides, lincosamides, and cephalosporins) can cause fatal enteric dysbiosis and enterotoxemia.

### PRECAUTIONS

• Topical and systemic corticosteroids—rabbits are very sensitive to the immunosuppressive effects of corticosteroids; use may exacerbate subclinical bacterial or E. cuniculi infection.

• Albendazole has been associated with bone marrow toxicity in dogs and cats. Toxicity in rabbits is unknown; however, anecdotal reports of pancytopenia leading to death in rabbits exist.

### POSSIBLE INTERACTIONS

N/A

### ALTERNATIVE DRUGS

Systemic corticosteroids have been advocated by practitioners for treatment of E. cuniculi–induced CNS granulomatous inflammation. Use of corticosteroids is controversial. Although clinical improvement has been anecdotally reported, rabbits are very sensitive to the immunosuppressive effects of corticosteroids; immunosuppression may exacerbate subclinical bacterial or E. cuniculi infection.

## FOLLOW-UP

### PATIENT MONITORING

• Repeat the neurologic examination at a frequency dictated by the underlying cause.

• Head tilt or other neurologic signs may persist.

### POSSIBLE COMPLICATIONS

• Progression of disease with deterioration of mental status

• CSF collection or natural course of the disease—tentorial herniation and death

### EXPECTED COURSE AND PROGNOSIS

• Resolution of signs—generally gradual (2–8 weeks)

• Prognosis—guarded depending on underlying cause; viral, parasitic migration—almost always progress to death; protozoal—course varies greatly, response to treatment erratic; many improve with supportive care; bacterial—depends on extent of infection, may improve with long-term antibiotic care
• Following acute episodes of vestibular signs, head tilt often persists. Most rabbits adapt well to this, will ambulate, eat well, and appear to live comfortable lives. Recurrence of acute episodes may occur.
• Residual neurologic deficits cannot be predicted.

 **MISCELLANEOUS**

### ASSOCIATED CONDITIONS
• Dental disease
• Upper respiratory infections
• Facial abscesses
• Gastrointestinal hypomotility

### AGE-RELATED FACTORS
Encephalitozoonosis and bacterial disease may be more common in older, especially immunosuppressed animals.

### ZOONOTIC POTENTIAL
• Rabies—consider in endemic areas if the patient is an outdoor animal that has rapidly progressive encephalitis.
• Encephalitozoonosis—unlikely, but possible in immunosuppressed humans. Modes of transmission and susceptibility in humans are unclear.

### PREGNANCY
N/A

### SYNONYMS
N/A

### SEE ALSO
• Ataxia
• Head tilt
• Seizures

### ABBREVIATIONS
• CNS = central nervous system
• CSF = cerebrospinal fluid
• CT = computed tomography
• ELISA = enzyme-linked immunosorbent assay
• IFA = immunofluorescent assay
• MRI = magnetic resonance imaging
• URI = upper respiratory infection

*Suggested Reading*

Cox JC. Altered immune responsiveness associated with *Encephalitozoon cuniculi* in rabbits. Lab Anim 2000;34:281–289.

Deeb BJ, Carpenter JW. Neurologic and musculoskeletal diseases. In: Quesenberry KE, Carpenter JW, eds. Ferrets, Rabbits and Rodents: Clinical Medicine and Surgery. 2nd Ed. Philadelphia: WB Saunders, 2004:203–210.

Harcourt-Brown F. Neurological and locomotor diseases. In: Harcourt-Brown F, ed. Textbook of Rabbit Medicine. Oxford: Butterworth-Heinemann, 2002:307–323.

Paul-Murphy J, Ramer JC. Urgent care of the pet rabbits. Vet Clin North Am Exotic Anim Pract 1998;1(1):127–152.

Rosenthal KR. Torticollis in rabbits. Proc North Am Vet Conf 2005;1378–1379.

*Portions Adapted From*

Sisson A. Encephalitis. In: Tilley LP, Smith FWK, Jr., eds. The 5-Minute Veterinary Consult: Canine and Feline, 3rd Ed. Baltimore: Lippincott Williams & Wilkins, 2004.

# ENCEPHALITIS SECONDARY TO PARASITIC MIGRATION

## BASICS

### OVERVIEW
• Aberrant migration of worms (helminthiasis) or fly larvae (myasis) into the CNS
• Only raccoon roundworm, *Baylisascaris procyonis,* has been reported in rabbits; myasis common in other anatomic locations.
• *Baylisascaris*—eggs in raccoon feces contaminate vegetation and hay; remain infective for 1 year; rabbits allowed to graze outdoors or fed hay stored outdoors are susceptible.
• Access to CNS—*Baylisascaris*: larvae ingested, migrate to CNS

### SIGNALMENT
• Rare and sporadic
• Animals exposed to an outside environment

### SIGNS
• Vary with the portion of CNS affected
• Likely asymmetrical
• May suggest a mass lesion or multifocal disease process

### CAUSES AND RISK FACTORS
Housing or grazing in area previously occupied by raccoons

## DIAGNOSIS

### DIFFERENTIAL DIAGNOSIS
• Other, more common causes of (focal) encephalopathy—infectious diseases most common, especially bacterial (brain abscess, extension from otitis interna/media, meningoencephalitis) or protozoal (encephalitozoonosis); viral, fungal rare in rabbits; brain tumor, ischemic encephalopathy also rare
• Physical examination findings helpful in diagnosing more common problems—nasal/ocular discharge: historical or current common with spread of upper respiratory infection to inner/middle ear; otitis: thick, white, creamy exudate may be found in the horizontal and/or vertical canals
• Definitive diagnosis is usually made on necropsy, because the disease is difficult to diagnose antemortem.

### CBC/BIOCHEMISTRY/URINALYSIS
Normal unless the parasite also affects non-neural tissues

### OTHER LABORATORY TESTS
• Serologic testing for *Encephalitozoon cuniculi*—may be helpful in ruling out encephalitozoonosis; however, usefulness is limited in pet rabbits since a positive titer indicates only exposure and does not confirm *E. cuniculi* as the cause of neurologic signs. *E. cuniculi* can only be definitively diagnosed by finding organisms and resultant lesions on histopathologic examination

in areas that anatomically correlate with observed clinical signs. Antibody titers usually become positive by 2 weeks postinfection, but generally do not continue to rise with active infection or decline with treatment. No correlation exists between antibody titers and shedding of organism and presence or severity of disease. It is unknown if exposed rabbits eventually become seronegative. Available tests include ELISA, indirect IFA, and carbon immunoassay.
• Serology for *Pasteurella*—usefulness is severely limited and generally not helpful in the diagnosis of pasteurellosis in pet rabbits. An ELISA is available and results are reported as negative, low positive, or high positive. Positive results, even when high, only indicate prior exposure to *Pasteurella* and the development of antibodies and do not confirm active infection. Low-positive results may occur due to cross-reaction with other, nonpathogenic bacteria (false positive). False-negative results are common with immunosuppression or early infection. No evidence exists to support correlation of titers to the presence or absence of disease.
• Serologic testing for toxoplasmosis—anecdotal reports of using serum antibody titers available for testing in dogs and cats to diagnose infection in rabbits exist.

### IMAGING
• Tympanic bullae and skull radiography—may help rule out otitis interna/media; however, normal radiographs do not rule out bulla disease.
• CT and MRI—valuable for confirming bulla lesions and CNS extension of otitis interna/media or to identify localized tumor, granuloma, and extent of inflammation

### PATHOLOGIC FINDINGS
May be local to extensive necrosis, malacia, vascular rupture and hemorrhage, vascular emboli, granulomatous proliferation, or obstructive hydrocephalus

## TREATMENT
None effective

## MEDICATIONS

### DRUG(S) OF CHOICE
Oxibendazole (60 mg/kg PO q24h) anecdotally slowed progression of clinical signs in mildly affected rabbits.

### CONTRAINDICATIONS/INTERACTIONS
Topical and systemic corticosteroids—rabbits are very sensitive to the immunosuppressive effects of corticosteroids; use may exacerbate subclinical bacterial or *E. cuniculi* infection.

## FOLLOW-UP

### PATIENT MONITORING
N/A

### PREVENTION/AVOIDANCE
Avoid grazing in areas where raccoons are present.

### POSSIBLE COMPLICATIONS
N/A

### EXPECTED COURSE AND PROGNOSIS
Usually progressive after acute or insidious onset; euthanasia often warranted

## MISCELLANEOUS

### ZOONOTIC POTENTIAL
Potential risks to humans, especially the immunosuppressed

### SEE ALSO
• Ataxia
• Encephalitis and meningoencephalitis
• Encephalitozoonosis
• Head Tilt
• Paresis and Paralysis

### ABBREVIATIONS
• CNS = central nervous system
• CT = computed tomography
• ELISA = enzyme-linked immunosorbent assay
• IFA = immunofluorescent assay
• MRI = magnetic resonance imaging

*Suggested Reading*

Cox JC. Altered immune responsiveness associated with *Encephalitozoon cuniculi* in rabbits. Lab Anim 2000;34:281–289.

Deeb BJ, Carpenter JW. Neurologic and musculoskeletal diseases. In: Quesenberry KE, Carpenter JW, eds. Ferrets, Rabbits and Rodents: Clinical Medicine and Surgery. 2nd Ed. Philadelphia: WB Saunders, 2004:203–210.

Harcourt-Brown F. Neurological and locomotor diseases. In: Harcourt-Brown F, ed. Textbook of Rabbit Medicine. Oxford: Butterworth-Heinemann, 2002:307–323.

Paul-Murphy J, Ramer JC. Urgent care of the pet rabbits. Vet Clin North Am Exotic Anim Pract 1998;1(1):127–152.

Rosenthal KR. Torticollis in rabbits. Proc North Am Vet Conf 2005;1378–1379.

*Portions Adapted From*

Lin-Baker CB. Encephalitis Secondary to Parasitic Migration. In: Tilley LP, Smith FWK, Jr., eds. The 5-Minute Veterinary Consult: Canine and Feline, 3rd Ed. Baltimore: Lippincott Williams & Wilkins, 2004.

# BASICS

## DEFINITION
Abnormal overflow of the aqueous portion of the precorneal tear film

## PATHOPHYSIOLOGY
• Caused by blockage of the nasolacrimal drainage system, overproduction of the aqueous portion of tears (usually in response to ocular irritation), or poor eyelid function secondary to malformation or deformity
• In rabbits, epiphora is most often caused by dental disease, resulting in blockage of the nasolacrimal duct, or irritation to the globe from tooth root elongation or abscess.
• Rabbits have only one nasolacrimal punctum, with a nasolacrimal duct that runs in close association with the roots of the cheek teeth (premolars and molars) and upper incisors. Elongation of the tooth roots is an extremely common disorder in pet rabbits. Root elongation and tooth root abscesses can impinge on or erode into the nasolacrimal duct, resulting in blockage and/or dacryocystitis. In most cases, the blocked duct fills with inflammatory cells, oil and debris; however, secondary bacterial infections can occur.
• Also commonly caused by blockage of the nasolacrimal duct with inspissated exudate or scarring secondary to chronic upper respiratory infections

## SYSTEMS AFFECTED
Ophthalmic

## SIGNALMENT
• Acquired cheek tooth elongation causing blockage of nasolacrimal duct or intrusion into the retrobulbar space—usually seen in middle-aged rabbits
• Young animals—congenital tooth malocclusion, congenital eyelid deformities
• Dwarf and lop breeds—congenital tooth malocclusion
• Dwarf and Himalayan breeds—glaucoma more common
• Rex and New Zealand White breeds—entropion and trichiasis more common

## SIGNS

### Historical Signs
• History of previous treatment for dental disease
• History of incisor overgrowth. In rabbits with dental disease, owners generally notice incisor overgrowth first, as these teeth are readily visible. In nearly all cases, incisor overgrowth is only a symptom of cheek teeth elongation and generalized dental disease.
• Inability to prehend food, dropping food out of the mouth
• History of nasal discharge or previous upper respiratory infection
• Facial asymmetry, masses, or exophthalmos in rabbits with tooth root abscesses
• Signs of pain—reluctance to move, depression, lethargy, hiding, hunched posture in rabbits with underlying dental disease
• Unilateral or bilateral alopecia, crusts, and matted fur in periocular area, cheeks, and/or nasal rostrum
• History of red or painful eyes in rabbits with primary ocular disease

### Physical Examination Findings
• Facial pyoderma—alopecia, erythema, and matted fur, in periocular area, cheeks, and/or nasal rostrum; due to constant moisture from epiphora
• Thick, white exudate accumulation in medial canthus in rabbits with dacryocystitis
• Corneal ulcers associated with dacryocystitis are usually superficial and ventrally located; ulcers secondary to exposure keratitis are usually central and may be superficial or deep.
• Depending on the underlying cause, may see blepharospasm, conjunctival hyperemia, exophthalmia, entropion, or corneal disease. Perform a complete ocular examination including pupillary light reflex, Schirmer tear test, tonometry; examination of the orbit, cornea, anterior chamber, iris, fundus, conjunctiva, nictitating membrane, and eyelids

### Oral Examination
• A thorough examination of the oral cavity is indicated in every rabbit with epiphora. A thorough examination includes the incisors, molars, and buccal and lingual mucosa to rule out dental disease. Use of an otoscope or speculum may be useful in identifying severe abnormalities; however, many problems will be missed by using this method alone. Complete examination requires heavy sedation or general anesthesia and specialized equipment.
• A focused, directed light source and magnification (or a rigid endoscope) will provide optimal visualization.
• Use a rodent mouth gag and cheek dilators (Jorgensen Laboratories, Inc., Loveland, CO) to open the mouth and pull buccal tissues away from teeth surfaces to allow adequate exposure. Use a cotton swab or tongue depressor to retract the tongue from lingual surfaces.
• Identify cheek teeth elongation, irregular crown height, spikes, curved teeth, tooth discoloration, tooth mobility, missing teeth, purulent exudate, oral ulceration, or abscesses.
• Significant tooth root abnormalities may be present despite normal-appearing crowns. Skull films are required to identify apical disorders.
• Incisors—may see overgrowth, horizontal ridges or grooves, malformation, discoloration, fractures, or increased or decreased curvature

## CAUSES AND RISK FACTORS

### Obstruction of the Nasolacrimal Drainage System—Most Common Cause
*Congenital*
Imperforate nasolacrimal puncta, ectopic nasolacrimal openings, and nasolacrimal atresia—not yet documented in rabbits
*Acquired*
• Dacryocystitis—inflammation of the canaliculi, lacrimal sac, or nasolacrimal ducts. Often sterile and secondary to blockage from dental disease—inflammatory cells, oil, and debris present. Can also be infectious, extending from primary rhinitis or conjunctivitis. If bacterial infection is present (primary or secondary), *Staphylococcus* spp., *Pseudomonas* spp., *Moraxella* spp., *Pasteurella multocida*, *Neisseria* spp., and *Bordetella* spp. are frequently cultured.
• Cheek tooth or incisor elongation—extremely common cause; the nasolacrimal duct is normally very closely associated with the roots of the cheek teeth; elongation or abscessation of the tooth roots (most commonly the second upper premolar) impinges or invades into the nasolacrimal duct.
• Rhinitis or sinusitis—causes swelling adjacent to the nasolacrimal duct
• Trauma or fractures of the lacrimal or maxillary bones
• Neoplasia—conjunctiva, medial eyelids, nasal cavity, maxillary bone, or periocular sinuses

### Overproduction of Tears Secondary to Ocular Irritants
*Congenital*
• Distichiasis or trichiasis
• Entropion
*Acquired*
• Corneal or conjunctival foreign bodies (especially hay, litter, or bedding)
• Corneal stromal abscess
• Conjunctivitis—often associated with upper respiratory infections, environmental irritants, or, rarely, blepharoconjunctivitis due to myxomatosis
• Ulcerative keratitis—trauma most common; exposure to keratitis following anesthesia, facial nerve paralysis; corneal abrasion in rabbits with torticollis
• Anterior uveitis—most commonly bacterial or *Encephalitozoon cuniculi*
• Glaucoma
• Eyelid neoplasms
• Blepharitis

# EPIPHORA

### Eyelid Abnormalities or Poor Eyelid Function

Tears never reach the nasolacrimal puncta but instead spill over the eyelid margin.
*Congenital*
Entropion
*Acquired*
• Posttraumatic eyelid scarring
• Facial nerve paralysis

## DIAGNOSIS

### DIFFERENTIAL DIAGNOSIS
• Other ocular discharges (e.g., mucous or purulent)—epiphora is a watery, serous discharge.
• Eye—often red when caused by overproduction of tears; quiet when secondary to impaired outflow. However, chronic blockage of the nasolacrimal duct and dacryocystitis can lead to corneal ulceration or secondary conjunctivitis so that eyes eventually appear red.
• Unilateral condition with ocular pain (blepharospasm)—usually indicates a tooth root disorder, foreign body, or corneal injury
• Chronic, bilateral condition—usually due to chronic upper respiratory tract infection (scarring, inflammation of duct); can indicate a congenital problem; bilateral tooth root disorders also seen
• Acute, bilateral condition with severe eyelid edema—consider myxomatosis.
• Facial pain, swelling, nasal discharge, or sneezing—seen with tooth root elongation or abscess; may indicate nasal or sinus infection; may indicate obstruction from neoplasm
• White discharge confined to the medial canthus—usually indicates dacryocystitis

### CBC/BIOCHEMISTRY/URINALYSIS
N/A

### OTHER LABORATORY TESTS
N/A

### IMAGING
• Skull radiographs are mandatory to identify dental disease, nasal, sinus, or maxillary bone lesions; and, if present, to plan treatment strategies and to monitor progression of treatment.
• Perform under general anesthesia
• Five views are recommend for thorough assessment: ventral–dorsal, lateral, two lateral obliques, and rostral–caudal.
• CT—superior to radiographs to localize obstruction and characterize associated lesions
• Dacryocystorhinography—radiopaque contrast material to help localize obstruction

### DIAGNOSTIC PROCEDURES
• Bacterial culture and sensitivity testing and cytologic examination of the material—

with purulent material at the medial canthus (e.g., dacryocystitis); performed before instilling any substance into the eye. Often, only normal organisms are isolated (*Bacillus subtilis, Staphylococcus aureus, Bordetella* sp.)
• Topical fluorescein dye application to the eye—most physiologic test for nasolacrimal function; should be performed first; dye flows through the nasolacrimal system and reaches the external nares in approximately 10 seconds in normal rabbits.
• Rhinoscopy—with or without biopsy or bacterial culture; may be indicated if previous tests suggest a nasal or sinus lesion

### Nasolacrimal Flush
• Confirms obstruction
• May dislodge foreign material
• Topical administration of an ophthalmic anesthetic is generally sufficient for this procedure; nervous rabbits may require mild sedation.
• Rabbits have only a single nasolacrimal punctum located in the ventral eyelid at the medial canthus. A 23-gauge lacrimal cannula or a 24-gauge Teflon intravenous catheter can be used to flush the duct. Irrigation will generally produce a thick, white exudate from the nasal meatus.

## TREATMENT

• Remove cause of ocular irritation—removal of a conjunctival or corneal foreign body; treatment of the primary ocular disease (e.g., conjunctivitis, ulcerative keratitis, and uveitis), correction of entropion
• Treat primary obstructing lesion (e.g., dental disease, nasal or sinus mass, and infection)—can be frustrating with advanced underlying dental disease
• Nasolacrimal duct irrigation—as described above
• Irrigation of the duct often needs to be repeated, either daily for 2–3 consecutive days or once every 3–4 days until irrigation produces a clear fluid.
• Instill an ophthalmic antibiotic solution such as ciprofloxacin or chloramphenicol 4–6 times a day for 14–21 days.
• Keep fur around face clean and dry.

### CLIENT EDUCATION
• Warn client that recurrence is common in patients with nasolacrimal obstruction.
• Inform client that early detection and intervention provide a better long-term prognosis.
• The nasolacrimal duct may become completely obliterated in rabbits with severe tooth root disease (abscesses, elongation, neoplasia). Epiphora may be lifelong. Home management, including keeping the face clean and dry, is crucial to prevent sec-

ondary pyoderma. In many cases, acquisition of a second rabbit can be beneficial if the second rabbit grooms discharges from the face.
• Rabbits with cheek tooth root elongation—by the time clinical signs are noted, disease is usually advanced. Lifelong treatment, consisting of periodic coronal reduction (teeth trimming), is required, usually every 1–3 months.
• Severe dental disease, especially those with tooth root abscesses and severe bony destruction, carry a guarded to poor prognosis for complete resolution. Most will require extensive surgery, sometimes multiple surgeries and multiple follow-up visits. Recurrences in the same or other locations are common. Clients must be aware of the monetary and time investment.

### SURGICAL CONSIDERATIONS
• Trimming of cheek teeth (coronal reduction)—may control progression of root elongation
• Tooth extraction—because rabbits have very long, deeply embedded and curved tooth roots, extraction per os can be extremely time consuming and labor intensive as compared to dogs and cats. If the germinal bud is not completely removed, the teeth may regrow or a new abscess may form. If not experienced with tooth extraction in rabbits, the author recommends referral to a veterinarian with special expertise whenever feasible.
• In rabbits with extensive tooth root abscesses, aggressive debridement is indicated, and special expertise may be required. Maxillary and retrobulbar abscesses can be particularly challenging. If not experienced with facial abscesses in rabbits, the author recommends referral to a veterinarian with special expertise whenever feasible.

## MEDICATIONS

### DRUG(S) OF CHOICE
• Topical broad-spectrum antibiotic ophthalmic solutions—while awaiting results of diagnostic tests (e.g., bacterial culture and sensitivity testing; diagnostic radiographs), q4–6h may try triple antibiotic solution, ciprofloxacin, gentocin, or ophthalmic chloramphenicol solution
• Dacryocystitis—based on bacterial culture and sensitivity test results; continued for at least 21 days
• Systemic antibiotics—indicated in rabbits with tooth root abscess as cause of conjunctivitis
• Topical NSAIDs—0.03% flurbiprofen or 1% diclofenac may help reduce inflammation and irritation associated with flushes
• Sedation for nasolacrimal duct flushing or

oral examination—light sedation with midazolam (0.5–2 mg/kg IM) or diazepam (1–2 mg/kg IM); oral examinations or longer procedures require deeper sedation: the author prefers ketamine (15–20 mg/kg IM) plus midazolam (0.5–1.0 mg/kg IM); many other sedation protocols exist. Alternatively, administer general anesthesia with isoflurane.
• Long-term pain management—indicated in rabbits with tooth root elongation. NSAIDs have been used for short- or long-term therapy to reduce pain and inflammation: meloxicam (0.2–0.5 mg/kg PO q24h) or carprofen (2.2 mg/kg PO q12–24h)

## CONTRAINDICATIONS
• Topical corticosteroids or antibiotic–corticosteroid combinations—avoid; associated with gastrointestinal ulceration and hemorrhage, delayed wound healing, and heightened susceptibility to infection; rabbits are very sensitive to the immunosuppressive effects of both topic and systemic corticosteroids; use may exacerbate subclinical bacterial infection.
• Topical corticosteroids—never use if the cornea retains fluorescein stain.

## PRECAUTIONS
Aggressive flushing of the nasolacrimal duct may cause temporary swelling of the periocular tissues. Swelling using resolves within 12–48 hours.

## POSSIBLE INTERACTIONS
N/A

## ALTERNATIVE DRUGS
N/A

## FOLLOW-UP

### PATIENT MONITORING

*Dacryocystitis*
• Reevaluate every 3–4 days until the condition is resolved.
• Problem persists more than 7–10 days with treatment or recurs soon after cessation of treatment—indicates a foreign body or nidus of persistent infection or obstruction; requires further diagnostics (e.g., skull films, dacryostorhinography)

## POSSIBLE COMPLICATIONS
• Recurrence—most common complication; caused by nonresolution of underlying dental disease, recurrence of ocular irritation (e.g., corneal ulceration, distichiasis, entropion)
• In rabbits with chronic dental disease, lifelong treatment is required.
• Permanent blockage of the nasolacrimal duct may occur due to scarring from chronic URI, abscess, or neoplasia

## MISCELLANEOUS

### ASSOCIATED CONDITIONS
• Immunosuppression
• Recurrent eye "infections"
• Moist dermatitis ventral to the medial canthus
• Nasal discharge

### AGE-RELATED FACTORS
N/A

### ZOONOTIC POTENTIAL
N/A

### PREGNANCY
N/A

### SEE ALSO
• Cheek tooth malocclusion and elongation
• Conjunctivitis
• Incisor malocclusion and overgrowth
• Pyoderma
• Tooth root abscesses

## ABBREVIATIONS
• CT = computed tomography
• NSAIDs = nonsteroidal antiinflammatory drugs
• URI = upper respiratory infection

*Suggested Reading*
Andrew SE. Corneal disease of rabbits. Vet Clin Noth Am Exotic Anim Pract 2002;5(2):341–356.
Crossley DA. Oral biology and disorders of lagomorphs. Vet Clin Noth Am Exotic Anim Pract 2003;6(3):629–659.
Crossley DA, Aiken S. Small mammal dentistry. In: Quesenberry KE, Carpenter JW, eds. Ferrets, Rabbits and Rodents: Clinical Medicine and Surgery. 2nd Ed. Philadelphia: WB Saunders, 2004:370–382.
Van der Woerdt A. Ophthalmologic disease in small pet animals. In: Quesenberry KE, Carpenter JW, eds. Ferrets, Rabbits and Rodents: Clinical Medicine and Surgery. 2nd Ed. Philadelphia: WB Saunders, 2004:421–428.
Williams DL. Laboratory animal ophthalmology. In: Gelatt KN, ed. Veterinary Ophthalmology. 3rd Ed. Philadelphia: Lippincott Williams & Wilkins, 1999:151–181.

*Portions Adapted From*
Gilger BC. Epiphora. In: Tilley LP, Smith FWK, Jr., eds. The 5-Minute Veterinary Consult: Canine and Feline, 3rd Ed. Baltimore: Lippincott Williams & Wilkins, 2004.

# EPISTAXIS

## BASICS

### DEFINITION
Bleeding from the nose

### PATHOPHYSIOLOGY
Results from one of three abnormalities—coagulopathy, space-occupying lesion, or vascular or systemic disease

### SYSTEMS AFFECTED
- Respiratory—hemorrhage; sneezing
- Hemic/lymphatic/immune—anemia
- Gastrointestinal—melena

### SIGNALMENT
Depends on underlying cause

### SIGNS

#### Historical Findings
- Nasal hemorrhage
- Sneezing, nasal discharge, staining of the front paws
- Ptyalism, anorexia with dental disease
- Epiphora, ocular discharge with nasolacrimal duct obstruction
- With coagulopathy—hematochezia, melena, hematuria, or hemorrhage from other areas of the body—rare in rabbits
- Melena—may be from swallowing blood

#### Physical Examination Findings
- Nasal discharge—with rhinitis or sinusitis; unilateral suggests foreign body, tooth root abscess, or neoplasm; secretions or dried discharges are found on the hair around the nose and front limbs; facial alopecia and pyoderma seen secondary to chronic discharge
- Ocular discharge—serous with nasolacrimal obstruction; purulent with extension of bacterial infection to conjunctiva; exophthalmos with retrobulbar abscess
- Concurrent dental disease, especially tooth root impaction, malocclusion, and incisor overgrowth; findings may include ptyalism, anorexia, nasal discharge, ocular discharge, exophthalmia. Always perform a thorough oral examination.
- Frontal and facial bone deformity—abscess or neoplastic disease
- Nasal hemorrhage
- With coagulopathy—possibly petechia, ecchymosis, hematomas, hematochezia, melena, and hematuria

### CAUSES

#### Space-Occupying Lesion
- Infection—most common cause bacterial (*Pasteurella multocida, Staphylococcus aureus, Bordetella bronchiseptica, Moraxella catarrhalis, Pseudomonas aeruginosa, Mycobacterium* spp., and various anaerobes have also been implicated); fungal (*Aspergillus* spp., *Cryptococcus* spp.)—rare in rabbits; usually blood-tinged mucopurulent exudate rather than frank hemorrhage

- Tooth root abscess—common cause; generally anaerobes
- Foreign body—mostly inhaled vegetable matter (e.g., grass and seeds)
- Trauma; chewing on electric cords
- Neoplasia—squamous cell carcinoma, osteosarcoma, chondrosarcoma, and fibrosarcoma
- Coagulopathy—not well described in rabbits; may be seen secondary to anticoagulant rodenticide intoxication or severe hepatopathy

### RISK FACTORS
- Immunosuppression—caused by stress, concurrent disease, or corticosteroid use most important risk factor in developing pasteurellosis
- Poor husbandry—dirty, molding bedding; dusty cat litter; diets too low in fiber content may predispose to dental disease.

## DIAGNOSIS

### DIFFERENTIAL DIAGNOSIS
See causes.

### CBC/BIOCHEMISTRY/URINALYSIS
- Anemia—if enough hemorrhage has occurred
- Thrombocytopenia—possible
- TWBC elevations are usually not seen with bacterial diseases. A relative heterophilia and/or lymphopenia are more common.
- Pancytopenia—may suggest bone marrow disease
- Hypoproteinemia—if enough hemorrhage has occurred
- High ALT, AST, and total bilirubin—severe hepatic disease with coagulopathy possible; high BUN due to ingested blood

### OTHER LABORATORY TESTS
Coagulation profile—not well described in rabbits. May simultaneously obtain a coagulation profile from a normal rabbit to use as control. One study reported PT range of 7.5 +/− 1.5 seconds to 14.6 +/− 4.3 seconds (n = 12). APTT values were 32.8 +/− 4.5 seconds (n = 6).

### IMAGING
- Skull series radiology—must be taken under general anesthesia: patients with nasal discharge (e.g., hemorrhagic, mucous, or serous) have fluid density that obscures nasal detail; bony lysis or proliferation of the turbinate and facial bones important radiographic finding, consistent with chronic bacterial (especially tooth root abscess) and neoplastic invasion. Always assess the apical roots of the incisors; elongation of the roots of the cheek teeth may penetrate the sinuses and be visible radiographically.

- Thoracic radiographs are indicated in rabbits with bacterial rhinitis. Subclinical pneumonia is common; often detected only radiographically; screen for metastasis with suspected neoplasia.
- CT scans or MRI—more accurate in delineating nasal or sinus disease; may not be widely available

### DIAGNOSTIC PROCEDURES
- Rhinoscopy, nasal lavage, nasal biopsy (via rhinoscopy)—indicated for suspected space-occupying disease; aimed at removing foreign bodies and evaluating and sampling nasal tissue for a causal diagnosis (e.g., neoplasia and infection)
- Cytologic and histopathologic examination and bacterial and fungal culture and sensitivity testing—nasal tissue sample
- Bone marrow aspiration biopsy—with pancytopenia

## TREATMENT
- Coagulopathy—usually inpatient
- Space-occupying lesion or vascular or systemic disease—outpatient or inpatient, depending on the disease and its severity
- Minimize activity or stimuli that precipitate hemorrhage episodes.
- Treatment must be directed toward the underlying disease.
- Anticoagulant rodenticide intoxication—plasma or whole blood transfusion for acute bleeding; perform in-house crossmatch prior to administration; blood types not described for rabbits
- Liver disease—treat and support the underlying cause; plasma may be beneficial.
- Discontinue all NSAIDs
- Rhinoscopy—to remove nasal foreign bodies
- Radiotherapy—nasal tumors, various response rates, depending on tumor type
- Surgery—foreign body unremovable by rhinoscopy; neoplasia; dental abscesses

## MEDICATIONS

### DRUG(S) OF CHOICE
- Anticoagulant rodenticide intoxication—plasma or whole blood transfusion for acute bleeding. Perform in-house crossmatch prior to administration; blood types not described for rabbits. Vitamin K1—2.5 mg/kg PO q24h for 10–30 days (depending on the specific product); the injectable form may be administered orally; bioavailability enhanced by the concurrent feeding of a small amount of fat; has also been administered IM (2–10 mg/kg PRN); however, anaphylactic reactions have been reported anecdo-

tally with IV or SC administration. Administer for 1 (warfarin) to 4 (longer-acting formulations) weeks. Apply Elizabethan collar for several days to prevent coprophagy.
• Serious hemorrhage—control with cage rest; intranasal instillation of Neo-Synephrine or dilute epinephrine may help (promotes vasoconstriction).
• Bacterial infection—antibiotics; based on culture and sensitivity testing whenever possible. When antibiotics are indicated, always use broad-spectrum antibiotics such as enrofloxacin (5–20 mg/kg PO, IM, SC q12–24h) or trimethoprim sulfa (30 mg/kg PO q12h). Anaerobic bacteria are usually causative agents of tooth root abscess; use antibiotics effective against anaerobes such as azithromycin (30 mg/kg PO q24h); can be used alone or combined with metronidazole (20 mg/kg PO q12h). Alternatively, use penicillin g (40,000–60,000 IU/kg SC q2–7d) or chloramphenicol (50 mg/kg PO q8h). Combine with topical treatment.

## CONTRAINDICATIONS
• Oral administration of antibiotics that select against Gram-positive bacteria (penicillins, macrolides, lincosamides, and cephalosporins) can cause fatal enteric dysbiosis and enterotoxemia.
• The use of corticosteroids (systemic or topical in otic preparations) can severely exacerbate bacterial infection.
• Avoid drugs that may predispose patient to hemorrhage—NSAIDs, heparin, phenothiazine tranquilizers
• Topical nasal decongestants containing phenylephrine can exacerbate nasal inflammation and cause nasal ulceration and purulent rhinitis.

## PRECAUTIONS
N/A

## POSSIBLE INTERACTIONS
N/A

## ALTERNATIVE DRUGS
N/A

# FOLLOW-UP

## PATIENT MONITORING
• Coagulation profile
• Monitor clinical signs.

## POSSIBLE COMPLICATIONS
Anemia and collapse rare

# MISCELLANEOUS

## ASSOCIATED CONDITIONS
N/A

## AGE-RELATED FACTORS
N/A

## ZOONOTIC POTENTIAL
N/A

## PREGNANCY
N/A

## SEE ALSO
See causes.

## ABBREVIATIONS
• ALT = alanine transferase
• AST = aspartate aminotransferase
• APTT = activated partial thromboplastin time
• BUN = blood urea nitrogen
• CT = computed tomography
• MRI = magnetic resonance imaging
• NSAIDs = nonsteroidal antiinflammatory drugs
• PT = prothrombin time

## Suggested Reading
Bennet RA. Treatment of abscesses in the head of rabbits. Proc North Am Vet Conf 1999;821–823.
Crossley DA. Oral biology and disorders of lagomorphs. Vet Clin North Am Exotic Anim Pract 2003;6(3):629–660.

Crossley DA, Aiken S. Small mammal dentistry. In: Quesenberry KE, Carpenter JW, eds. Ferrets, Rabbits and Rodents: Clinical Medicine and Surgery. 2nd Ed. Philadelphia: WB Saunders, 2004:370–382.
Deeb BJ. Respiratory disease and pasteurellosis. In: Quesenberry KE, Carpenter JW, eds. Ferrets, Rabbits and Rodents: Clinical Medicine and Surgery. 2nd Ed. Philadelphia: WB Saunders, 2004:172–182.
Deeb BJ, DiGiacomo RF. Respiratory diseases of rabbits. Vet Clin North Am Exotic Anim Pract 2000;3(2):465–480.
Dodds WJ. Rabbit and ferret hemostasis. In: Fudge AM, ed. Laboratory Medicine, Avian and Exotic Pets. Philadelphia: WB Saunders, 2000.
Harcourt-Brown F. Dental disease. In: Harcourt-Brown F, ed. Textbook of Rabbit Medicine. Oxford: Butterworth-Heinemann, 2002:165–205.
Hendricks JC. Respiratory condition in critical patients. Critical care. Vet Clin North Am Small Anim Pract 1989;19:1167–1188.
Paul-Murphy J, Ramer JC. Urgent care of the pet rabbits. Vet Clin North Am Exotic Anim Pract 1998;1(1):127–152.
Tyrell KC, Citron DM, Jenkins JR, et al. Periodontal bacteria in rabbit mandibular and maxillary abscesses. J Clin Microbiol 2002;40(3):1044–1047.

*Portions Adapted From*
Crystal MA. Epistaxis. In: Tilley LP, Smith FWK, Jr., eds. The 5-Minute Veterinary Consult: Canine and Feline, 3rd Ed. Baltimore: Lippincott Williams & Wilkins, 2004.

# EXOPHTHALMOS AND ORBITAL DISEASES

 **BASICS**

## DEFINITION
• Abnormal position of the eye
• Exophthalmos—anterior displacement of the globe; common presenting complaint in pet rabbits; usually associated with acquired cheek tooth elongation and tooth root abscesses; less often retrobulbar fat pads or neoplasia
• Enophthalmos—posterior displacement of the globe; unusual finding in rabbits
• Strabismus—deviation of the globe from the correct position of fixation, which the patient cannot correct

## PATHOPHYSIOLOGY
• Exophthalmos—caused by space-occupying lesions posterior to the equator of the globe; retrobulbar abscess is the most common cause of exophthalmia in the rabbit
• Retrobulbar abscesses are almost always caused by extension of tooth root abscesses; occasionally may be secondary to upper respiratory infections or trauma
• Unlike cats and dogs, abscesses in rabbits do not rupture and drain. Rabbit abscesses are filled with a thick, caseous exudate, surrounded by a fibrous capsule.
• Most tooth root abscesses are secondary to acquired cheek tooth elongation. All rabbit teeth are open-rooted and grow continuously at a rate of approximately 3 mm per week, with growth originating from the germinal bud located at the apex of the tooth.
• The rate of normal wear should equal the rate of eruption. Normal wear requires proper occlusion with the opposing set of teeth and a highly abrasive diet to grind coronal surfaces.
• The cause of acquired cheek teeth elongation is likely multifactorial and not completely known. The most significant contributing or exacerbating factor is feeding diets that contain inadequate amounts of the coarse roughage material required to properly grind coronal surfaces. Inherited or congenital malocclusion may also be a significant factor.
• Pulpitis, pulp necrosis, and apical abscess formation are common sequelae to tooth root elongation; abscesses may also be caused by trauma or penetration into sinus cavities and subsequent bacterial invasion or feed impaction in interdental spaces created by abnormal tooth growth.
• Malpositioned eye—caused by changes in volume (loss or gain) of the orbital contents or abnormal extraocular muscle function
• Enophthalmos—caused by loss of orbital volume or space-occupying lesions anterior to the equator of the globe

• Strabismus—usually caused by an imbalance of extraocular muscle tone or lesions that restrict extraocular muscle mobility

## SYSTEMS AFFECTED
• Ophthalmic
• Oral cavity—exophthalmia commonly associated with dental disease
• Respiratory—because of the close proximity, the nasal cavity and frontal and maxillary sinuses are often involved.

## SIGNALMENT
• Acquired cheek tooth elongation or tooth root abscess causing intrusion into the retrobulbar space—usually seen in middle-aged rabbits
• Young animals—congenital tooth malocclusion, congenital eyelid deformities
• Dwarf and lop breeds—congenital tooth malocclusion
• Orbital neoplasia—more common in middle-aged to old rabbits

## SIGNS

### Historical Signs
• History of previous treatment for dental disease
• History of incisor overgrowth. In rabbits with dental disease, owners generally notice incisor overgrowth first, as these teeth are readily visible. In nearly all cases, incisor overgrowth is only a symptom of cheek teeth elongation and generalized dental disease.
• Inability to prehend food, dropping food out of the mouth
• Preference for soft foods, change in eating or drinking behaviors
• Ptyalism, bruxism
• History of nasal discharge or previous upper respiratory infection
• Facial asymmetry, masses in rabbits with tooth root abscesses
• Signs of pain—reluctance to move, depression, lethargy, hiding, hunched posture in rabbits with underlying dental disease

### Physical Examination Findings
*Exophthalmos*
• Secondary signs of space-occupying orbital disease
• Difficulty in retropulsing the globe
• Serous to mucopurulent ocular discharge
• Chemosis
• Eyelid swelling
• Lagophthalmos—inability to close the eyelids over the cornea adequately during blinking
• Exposure keratitis—with or without ulceration
• Third eyelid protrusion
• Visual impairment caused by optic neuropathy
• Fundic abnormalities
• Signs of dental disease: ptyalism, facial asymmetry, pain, nasal discharge

*Enophthalmos*
• Ptosis
• Third eyelid protrusion
• Extraocular muscle atrophy
• Entropion—with severe disease
*Strabismus*
• Deviation of one or both eyes from the normal position
• May note exophthalmos or enophthalmos

### Oral Examination
• A thorough examination of the oral cavity is indicated in every rabbit with epiphora. Complete examination requires heavy sedation or general anesthesia and specialized equipment. Use of an otoscope or speculum may be useful in identifying severe abnormalities; however, many problems will be missed by using this method alone.
• A focused, directed light source and magnification will provide optimal visualization.
• Use a rodent mouth gag and cheek dilators (Jorgensen Laboratories, Inc., Loveland, CO) to open the mouth and pull buccal tissues away from teeth surfaces to allow adequate exposure. Use a cotton swab or tongue depressor to retract the tongue and examine lingual surfaces.
• Identify cheek teeth elongation, irregular crown height, spikes, curved teeth, oral ulceration, abscesses, loose or discolored teeth, halitosis, or purulent discharge.
• Significant tooth root abnormalities may be present despite normal-appearing crowns. Skull films are required to identify apical disorders.
• Incisors—may see overgrowth, horizontal ridges or grooves, malformation, discoloration, fractures, increased or decreased curvature, or malocclusion

## CAUSES

### Exophthalmos
• Tooth root elongation and tooth root abscess—extremely common cause; *Pasteurella* usually not cultured; common isolates from these sites include *Streptococcus* spp; anaerobic bacteria such as *Fusobacterium nucleatum*, *Prevotella* spp., *Peptostreptococcus micros*, *Actinomyces israelii*, and *Arcanobacterium haemolyticum*. Less commonly may culture *Pasteurella multocida*, *Staphylococcus aureus*, *Pseudomonas* spp., *Escherichia coli*, b-hemolytic *Streptococcus* spp., *Proteus* spp., and *Bacteroides* spp.
• Retrobulbar neoplasm—primary or secondary; lymphoma most common
• Excessive orbital fat deposits—obese rabbits
• Myositis—muscles of mastication or extraocular muscles
• Orbital hemorrhage secondary to trauma
• Thymoma—increased venous pressure from space-occupying effects

*Enophthalmos*
• Ocular pain
• Collapsed globe
• Horner's syndrome
• Loss of orbital fat or muscle

*Strabismus*
• Abnormal innervation of extraocular muscle
• Restriction of extraocular muscle motility by scar tissue from previous trauma or inflammation
• Destruction of extraocular muscle attachments after proptosis

## RISK FACTORS

For retrobulbar abscess—chronic respiratory infection; poor diet; immunosuppression

## DIAGNOSIS

### DIFFERENTIAL DIAGNOSIS

• Buphthalmic globe—may simulate a space-occupying mass and cause the eye to be displaced anteriorly owing to its size in relationship to the orbital volume; IOP usually high; corneal diameter is greater than normal; affected eye is usually blind
• Thymoma—eyes can be retropulsed; no pain present
• Bilateral exophthalmos—retroorbital fat pads, bilateral tooth root abscesses, increased venous pressure (thymoma most common)
• Unilateral exophthalmos—tooth root abscess, neoplasia

### CBC/BIOCHEMISTRY/URINALYSIS
Usually normal

### OTHER LABORATORY TESTS
Serology for *Pasteurella*—usefulness is severely limited and generally not helpful in the diagnosis of pasteurellosis in pet rabbits. An ELISA is available and results are reported as negative, low positive, or high positive. Positive results, even when high, only indicate prior exposure to *Pasteurella* and the development of antibodies and do not confirm active infection. Low-positive results may occur due to cross-reaction with other, nonpathogenic bacteria (false positive). False-negative results are common with immunosuppression or early infection. No evidence exists to support correlation of titers to the presence or absence of disease.

### IMAGING

#### Skull Radiographs
• Mandatory to identify retrobulbar lesions and type and extent of dental disease, to plan treatment strategies, and to monitor progression of treatment.
• Perform under general anesthesia
• Five views are recommended for thorough assessment of the teeth and skull:

ventral–dorsal, lateral, two lateral obliques, and rostral–caudal.
• Orbital ultrasonography—helpful in defining the extent of the lesion
• Thoracic radiographs—may help identify metastatic disease
• CT—superior to radiographs to evaluate retrobulbar pathology and dental disease

### DIAGNOSTIC PROCEDURES
• Lack of globe retropulsion—confirms a space-occupying mass
• Oral examination, skull radiographs, and fine needle aspiration of the orbit—may be completed after anesthetizing the patient
• Fine needle aspiration (18–20-gauge)—if the retrobulbar mass is accessible; submit samples for aerobic, anaerobic, and fungal cultures; Gram's staining; and cytologic examination
• Cytology—often diagnostic for abscess and neoplasia
• Biopsy—indicated if needle aspiration is nondiagnostic and mass lesion is accessible

## TREATMENT

### DIFFERENTIAL DIAGNOSIS

#### General Comments
• For orbital neoplasms or thymoma—consultation with an oncologist is recommended once the diagnosis is made.
• For retrobulbar fat pads—weight reduction
• For retrobulbar abscess—aggressive surgical debridement, followed by long-term local and systemic antibiotic therapy; limited (palliative) response to antibiotic treatment alone

### NURSING CARE
• Keep fur around face clean and dry.
• Supportive care in debilitated or anorectic patients; assisted feeding; subcutaneous or intravenous fluid therapy

### ACTIVITY
N/A

### DIET
• It is absolutely imperative that the rabbit continue to eat during and following treatment. Many rabbits with dental disease or retrobulbar masses will become anorectic. Rabbits may be unable to eat solid food following radical coronal reduction, extractions, or surgical treatment of abscesses. Anorexia will cause or exacerbate gastrointestinal hypomotility, derangement of the gastrointestinal microflora, and overgrowth of intestinal bacterial pathogens.
• Syringe feed a gruel such as Critical Care for Herbivores (Oxbow Pet Products, Murdock, NE) 10–15 mL/kg PO q6–8h. Larger volumes and more frequent feedings are often accepted; feed as much as the rabbit will

readily accept. Alternatively, pellets can be ground and mixed with fresh greens, vegetable baby foods, water, or juice to form a gruel.
• Most rabbits will require assisted feeding for 36–48 hours postoperatively following radical abscess debridement; assisted feeding may be needed for several weeks.
• High-carbohydrate, high-fat nutritional supplements are contraindicated.
• Return the rabbit to a solid-food diet as soon as possible to encourage normal occlusion and wear. Increase the amount of tough, fibrous foods and foods containing abrasive silicates such as hay and wild grasses; avoid pelleted food and soft fruits or vegetables.
• Encourage oral fluid intake by offering fresh water or wetting leafy vegetables.

### CLIENT EDUCATION
• Most rabbits with apical abscesses have generalized dental disease. Diet change and lifelong treatment, consisting of periodic coronal reduction (teeth trimming), is required, usually every 1–3 months.
• Most retrobulbar tooth root abscesses carry a fair to poor prognosis for complete resolution. Most will require extensive surgical debridement, including enucleation and multiple follow-up visits. Recurrences in the same or other locations are common. Clients must be aware of the monetary and time investment.
• With severe disease causing intractable pain and anorexia, euthanasia may be the most humane option. However, many rabbits will continue to eat well and appear comfortable with assisted feeding and analgesics for many months.

### SURGICAL CONSIDERATIONS

#### Retrobulbar Tooth Root Abscesses
• In rabbits with extensive tooth abscesses, aggressive debridement is indicated, and special expertise may be required. Maxillary and retrobulbar abscesses can be particularly challenging. If not experienced with facial abscesses in rabbits, the author recommends referral to a veterinarian with special expertise whenever feasible.
• Enucleation and/or exenteration are usually required. All material within the abscess should be removed with the capsule intact until maxillary bone is reached. All teeth associated with the abscess must be removed. All bone involved in the abscess must be thoroughly debrided.
• The defect should be filled with antibiotic-impregnated polymethyl methacrylate (AIPMMA) beads.
• AIPMMA beads release a high concentration of antibiotic into local tissues for several months. Selection of antibiotic is limited to those known to elute appropriately from bead to tissues and should be

# EXOPHTHALMOS AND ORBITAL DISEASES

based on culture and susceptibility testing. AIPMMA beads are not commercially available but can be made using PMMA by Surgical Simplex Bone Cement (Howmedica, Rutherford, NJ) or Bone Cement (Zimmer, Charlotte, NC). Antibiotics successfully used include cephalothin, cefazolin, or ceftiofur (2 g/20 g PMMA); gentamicin or tobramycin (1 g/2 g PMMA); or amikacin (1.25 g/2 g PMMA). Antibiotic is added to the copolymer powder before adding the liquid and formed into small, spherical beads. Beads must be manufactured and inserted aseptically, and unused beads should be gas sterilized prior to future use. Beads should be left in the incision site for at least 2 months, but can be left in indefinitely.
• Samples for aerobic and anaerobic bacterial culture and cytologic examination should be obtained from the abscess wall.
• Place on long-term antibiotic therapy; appropriate pain management

### Orbital Neoplasms
• Early exenteration or orbital exploratory surgery and debulking of the mass via a lateral approach to the orbit to save the globe are rational therapeutic choices.
• Adjunctive chemotherapy or radiotherapy—depending on neoplasm type and extent of the lesion.

## MEDICATIONS

### DRUG(S) OF CHOICE
• Exophthalmos (all patients)—lubricate cornea (e.g., artificial tear ointment q6h) to prevent desiccation and ulceration.
• Ulceration—topical antibiotic (e.g., bacitracin–neomycin–polymyxin, ciprofloxacin, gentamicin, or ophthalmic chloramphenicol solution, q8h); 1% atropine q12–24h may help reduce ciliary spasm; however, some rabbits produce atropinase; application may not be effective.

### Orbital Abscess or Cellulitis
*Antibiotics*
• Choice of antibiotic is ideally based on results of culture and susceptibility testing. Depending on the severity of infection, long-term antibiotic therapy is required (3 months minimum to several months or years). Most tooth root abscesses are caused by anaerobic bacteria; use antibiotics effective against anaerobes such as azithromycin (30 mg/kg PO q24h); metronidazole (20 mg/kg PO q12h); azithromycin and metronidazole can be used alone or in combination. Alternatively, use penicillin g (40,000–60,000 IU/kg SC q2–7d) or chloramphenicol (50 mg/kg PO q8h). Combine with topical treatment (surgical debridement, AIPPMA beads). If aerobic bacteria are isolated, use broad-spectrum antibiotics such as enrofloxacin (5–20 mg/kg PO, SC, IM q12–24h) or trimethoprimsulfa (30 mg/kg PO q12h).
• Long-term parenteral penicillin has been used with limited success as palliative treatment if surgery is not an option.
*Acute Pain Management*
• Buprenorphine (0.01–0.05 mg/kg SC, IM, IV q8–12h)—use preoperatively for surgical abscess treatment.
• Butorphanol (0.1–1.0 mg/kg SC, IM, IV q4–6h)—may cause profound sedation; short-acting
• Morphine (2–5 mg/kg SC, IM q2–4h) or oxymorphone (0.05–0.2 mg/kg SC, IM q8–12h)—use with caution; more than one to two doses may cause gastrointestinal stasis.
• Meloxicam (0.2 mg/kg SC, IM q24h)
• Carprofen (1–4 mg/kg SC q12h)
*Long-Term Pain Management*
• NSAIDs have been used for short- or long-term therapy to reduce pain and inflammation: meloxicam (0.2–0.5 mg/kg PO q24h) or carprofen (2.2 mg/kg PO q12–24h)
• Sedation for oral examination—ketamine (15–20 mg/kg IM) plus midazolam (0.5–1.0 mg/kg IM); many other sedation protocols exist. Alternatively, administer general anesthesia with isoflurane.

### CONTRAINDICATIONS
• Oral administration of most antibiotics effective against anaerobes will cause a fatal gastrointestinal dysbiosis in rabbits. Do not administer penicillins, macrolides, lincosamides, and cephalosporins by oral administration.
• Corticosteroids—associated with gastrointestinal ulceration and hemorrhage, delayed wound healing, and heightened susceptibility to infection; rabbits are very sensitive to the immunosuppressive effects of both topical and systemic corticosteroids; use may exacerbate subclinical bacterial infection.

### PRECAUTIONS
• Chloramphenicol—avoid human contact with chloramphenicol due to potential blood dyscrasia. Advise owners of potential risks.
• Meloxicam—use with caution in rabbits with compromised renal function.

### POSSIBLE INTERACTIONS
N/A

### ALTERNATIVE DRUGS
If AIPPMA beads are not available, packing the postdebridement deficit with antibiotic-laden gauze, 50% dextrose solution, or honey has been used as an alternative. Effectiveness varies, depending on the severity of disease and owner compliance.

## FOLLOW-UP

### PATIENT MONITORING
• Reevaluate 7–10 days postoperatively, then as needed every 1–3 months for patients in which regular teeth trimming is indicated.
• Evaluate the entire oral cavity and the skull with each recheck and repeat skull radiographs at least every 3–6 months to monitor for possible recurrence at the surgical site or other locations.

### POSSIBLE COMPLICATIONS
• Recurrence, chronic pain, or extensive tissue destruction warranting euthanasia due to poor quality of life
• Loss of the eye

### EXPECTED COURSE AND PROGNOSIS
• Orbital neoplasms—fair to poor depending on the tumor type and size
• Thymoma—generally poor
• Retrobulbar tooth root abscess—depends on severity of bone involvement, underlying disease, condition of the cheek teeth, and presence of other abscesses. Fair to guarded prognosis with single, small retrobulbar abscesses, adequate surgical debridement, and medical treatment. Rabbits with abscesses in the nasal passages or with multiple or severe maxillary abscesses have a guarded to poor prognosis. Euthanasia may be warranted; however, some rabbits can live for weeks to months comfortably with antibiotic treatment, assisted feeding, and analgesics.
• If surgical debridement of retrobulbar abscess is not possible, treatment with long-term antibiotic and pain medication may be palliative.

## MISCELLANEOUS

### ASSOCIATED CONDITIONS
N/A

### AGE-RELATED FACTORS
N/A

### ZOONOTIC POTENTIAL
N/A

### PREGNANCY
NA

### SEE ALSO
• Abscesses
• Cheek tooth malocclusion and elongation
• Conjunctivitis
• Incisor malocclusion and overgrowth
• Red eye

# EXOPHTHALMOS AND ORBITAL DISEASES

## ABBREVIATIONS
- CT = computed tomography
- ELISA = enzyme-linked immunosorbent assay
- IOP = intraocular pressure
- NSAIDs = nonsteroidal antiinflammatory drugs

### Suggested Reading

Crossley DA. Oral biology and disorders of lagomorphs. Vet Clin Noth Am Exotic Anim Pract 2003;6(3):629–659.

Crossley DA, Aiken S. Small mammal dentistry. In: Quesenberry KE, Carpenter JW, eds. Ferrets, Rabbits and Rodents: Clinical Medicine and Surgery. 2nd Ed. Philadelphia: WB Saunders, 2004:370–382.

Harcourt-Brown F. Dental disease. In: Harcourt-Brown F, ed. Textbook of Rabbit Medicine. Oxford: Butterworth-Heinemann, 2002:165–205.

Lukehart SA, Fohn MJ, Baker-Zander SA. Efficacy of azithromycin for therapy of active syphilis in the rabbit model. J Antimicrob Chemother 1990;25 Suppl A:91–99.

Tyrell KC, Citron DM, Jenkins JR, et al. Periodontal bacteria in rabbit mandibular and maxillary abscesses. J Clin Microbiol 2002;;40(3):1044–1047.

Van der Woerdt A. Ophthalmologic disease in small pet animals. In: Quesenberry KE, Carpenter JW, eds. Ferrets, Rabbits and Rodents: Clinical Medicine and Surgery. 2nd Ed. Philadelphia: WB Saunders, 2004:421–428.

Williams DL. Laboratory animal ophthalmology. In: Gelatt KN, ed. Veterinary Ophthalmology. 3rd Ed. Philadelphia: Lippincott Williams & Wilkins, 1999:151–181.

### Portions Adapted From

Colitz CMH. Orbital Diseases (Exophthalmos, Enophthalmus, Strabismus). In: Tilley LP, Smith FWK, Jr., eds. The 5-Minute Veterinary Consult: Canine and Feline, 3rd Ed. Baltimore: Lippincott Williams & Wilkins, 2004.

# FACIAL NERVE PARESIS/PARALYSIS

## BASICS

### DEFINITION
Dysfunction of the facial nerve (seventh cranial nerve), causing paralysis or weakness of the muscles of the ears, eyelids, lips, and nostrils

### PATHOPHYSIOLOGY
Weakness or paralysis caused by impairment of the facial nerve or the neuromuscular junction peripherally or the facial nucleus in the brainstem

### SYSTEMS AFFECTED
• Nervous—facial nerve peripherally or its nucleus in the brainstem
• Ophthalmic—if parasympathetic preganglionic neurons that supply the lacrimal glands and course with the facial nerve are involved, keratoconjunctivitis sicca develops because of lack of tear secretion.

### GENETICS
N/A

### INCIDENCE/PREVALENCE
Common sequela to otic and dental disease in rabbits

### GEOGRAPHIC DISTRIBUTION
N/A

### SIGNALMENT
• Lop-eared rabbits may be more likely to develop otitis externa, dental disease, and subsequent facial nerve paralysis.
• Dwarf breeds are more likely to have dental disease and subsequent facial nerve paralysis.
• No age or sex predilection

### SIGNS

#### General Comments
• Assess strength of the palpebral closure; there should be full eyelid closure when a finger is gently passed over both eyelids simultaneously.
• Bilateral nerve involvement is rare in rabbits—consider systemic disease or bilateral otitis.
• Unilateral paresis or paralysis—may accompany other clinical signs; may indicate focal or systemic disease

#### Historical Findings
• History of otitis externa, interna, or media
• History of vestibular disease
• Head tilt
• Holding one ear down
• Excessive drooling
• Facial asymmetry
• Eye—inability to close, rubbing, discharge, cloudy cornea, redness

### Physical Examination Findings
Findings associated with facial nerve disorder:
• Ipsilateral ear and lip drooping
• Excessive drooling
• Food falling from the side of mouth
• Collapse of the nostril
• Inability to close the eyelids
• Wide palpebral fissure
• Palpebral reflex decreased or absent
• Chronic—patient may have deviation of the face toward the affected side.
• Nasal discharge, facial abscesses
Findings associated with ear disease:
• Evidence of aural erythema, white creamy discharge, and thick and stenotic canals support otitis externa.
• White, dull, opaque, and bulging tympanic membrane on otoscopic examination sometimes visible when middle ear exudate is present
• Abscess at the base of the ear common finding
• Pain—upon opening the mouth or bulla palpation may be detected.
Other findings:
• Mucopurulent discharge from the affected eye and exposure conjunctivitis or keratitis—may be noted
• When secondary to brainstem disease—altered mentation (e.g., depression or stupor); other cranial nerve and gait abnormalities may be noted.

### CAUSES

#### Unilateral Peripheral
• Inflammatory—otitis media or interna
• Trauma—fracture of the petrous temporal bone; injury to the facial nerve or secondary to surgical ablation of external ear canal
• Neoplasia
• Idiopathic and metabolic causes not reported in rabbits

#### Bilateral Peripheral
• Bilateral ear disease
• Idiopathic, metabolic, inflammatory, and immune-mediated—not reported in rabbits
• Toxic—botulism

#### CNS
• Most unilateral
• Inflammatory—infectious (bacterial abscess as extension from ear or dental disease), protozoal (*Encephalitozoon cuniculi*), fungal (not well described in rabbits), and noninfectious (granulomatous meningoencephalomyelitis)
• Neoplastic—primary brain tumor, metastatic tumor

### RISK FACTORS
Chronic ear disease

## DIAGNOSIS

### DIFFERENTIAL DIAGNOSIS
• Differentiate unilateral from bilateral.
• Look for other neurologic deficits.
• Be sure that abnormal head posture is not due to holding one ear down due to pain, as may occur in otitis externa alone, and not associated with neurologic pathology.
• *E. cuniculi*—this is a diagnosis of exclusion. Every attempt should be made to rule out otic disease prior to assuming *E. cuniculi* infection. Antemortem diagnosis of *E. cuniculi* is usually presumed based on clinical signs, exclusion of other diagnoses, positive antibody titers and, sometimes, response to treatment. Definitive antemortem diagnosis is problematic, since a positive antibody titer indicates exposure only, some rabbits respond minimally or not at all to anthelmintic treatment, and many rabbits will improve spontaneously with supportive care alone. Definitive diagnosis requires identification of organisms and characteristic inflammation in tissues anatomically correlated with clinical signs, generally acquired at postmortem examination.
• Central vestibular diseases—difficult to differentiate in rabbits; may see lethargy, somnolence, stupor, and other brainstem signs
• Neoplasia—uncommon causes of refractory and relapsing otitis media and interna; diagnosed by imaging of the head
• Trauma—history and physical evidence of injury
• Idiopathic—rare, consider if patient has no historical or physical signs of ear disease and no other neurologic deficits

### CBC/BIOCHEMISTRY/URINALYSIS
Usually normal

### OTHER LABORATORY TESTS
• Serologic testing for *E. cuniculi*—many tests are available, but usefulness is extremely limited since a positive titer indicates only exposure and does not confirm *E. cuniculi* as the cause of neurologic signs. *E. cuniculi* can only be definitively diagnosed by finding organisms and resultant lesions on histopathologic examination in areas that anatomically correlate with observed clinical signs. Antibody titers usually become positive by 2 weeks postinfection but generally do not continue to rise with active infection or decline with treatment. No correlation exists between antibody titers and shedding of organism and presence or severity of disease. It is unknown if exposed rabbits eventually become seronegative. Available tests include ELISA, indirect IFA, and carbon immunoassay.

• Serology for *Pasteurella*—has been used to attempt to rule out pasteurellosis as a cause of underlying disease. However, the usefulness of antibody titers is severely limited and generally not helpful in the diagnosis of pasteurellosis in pet rabbits. An ELISA is available and results are reported as negative, low positive, or high positive. Positive results, even when high, only indicate prior exposure to *Pasteurella* and the development of antibodies and do not confirm active infection. Low-positive results may occur due to cross-reaction with other, nonpathogenic bacteria (false positive). False-negative results are common with immunosuppression or early infection. No evidence exists to support correlation of titers to the presence or absence of disease. May be useful in the establishment of SPF colonies

### IMAGING
• Bullae radiographs—tympanic bullae may appear cloudy if exudate is present; may see thickening of the bullae and petrous temporal bone with chronic disease; may see lysis of the bone with severe cases of osteomyelitis; may be normal in some rabbits, even with severe otitis interna and/or bullae disease; normal-appearing radiographs do not rule out bullae disease.
• CT—superior to radiographs to diagnose bullae disease. Detailed evidence of fluid and soft tissue density within the middle ear and the extent of involvement of the adjacent structures; defines brainstem disease

### DIAGNOSTIC PROCEDURES
• Schirmer tear test—evaluate tear production. Average values reported as 5 mm/min; however, even lower values can be seen in normal rabbits.
• CSF examination—may be helpful in detecting brainstem disease
• Bacterial culture and sensitivity testing—sample from myringotomy or surgical removal of exudate from the tympanic bulla is most accurate.

## TREATMENT

### APPROPRIATE HEALTH CARE
• Outpatient—otherwise healthy rabbits
• Inpatient—initial medical workup and management of systemic or CNS disease

### NURSING CARE
• Concurrent otitis externa—culture and clean the ear; use warm normal saline if the tympanum is ruptured; if a cleaning solution is used, follow with a thorough flush with normal saline; dry the ear canal with a cotton swab and low vacuum suction; sedation or general anesthesia may be necessary in rabbits with painful ears.

• Keep fur around face clean and dry.
• Instill artificial tears if indicated.

### ACTIVITY
N/A

### DIET
• It is absolutely imperative that the rabbit continue to eat during and following treatment. Many rabbits with vestibular signs or pain from otic or dental disease will become anorectic. Anorexia will often cause gastrointestinal hypomotility, derangement of the gastrointestinal microflora, and overgrowth of intestinal bacterial pathogens.
• Offer a large selection of fresh, moistened greens such as cilantro, romaine lettuce, parsley, carrot tops, dandelion greens, spinach, collard greens, etc., and good-quality grass hay. Many rabbits will begin to eat these foods, even if they were previously anorectic. Bring food to recumbent animals or hand feed.
• If the patient refuses these foods, syringe feed a gruel such as Critical Care for Herbivores (Oxbow Pet Products, Murdock, NE) 10–15 mL/kg PO q6–8h. Many rabbits will eat larger volumes at more frequent intervals; feed amounts that the rabbit will readily accept. Alternatively, pellets can be ground and mixed with fresh greens, vegetable baby foods, water, or juice to form a gruel.
• High-carbohydrate, high-fat nutritional supplements are contraindicated.
• Encourage oral fluid intake by offering fresh water and wetting leafy vegetables. CAUTION: Be aware of aspiration secondary to abnormal body posture in patients with severe head tilt and vestibular disequilibrium or brainstem dysfunction.

### CLIENT EDUCATION
• Advise client that the clinical signs are usually permanent, but as muscle fibrosis develops, a natural "tuck up" may occur that reduces asymmetry.
• Inform client that the other side can become affected.
• Discuss eye care: the cornea on the affected side may need lubrication; must regularly check for corneal ulcers
• Inform client that most animals tolerate this nerve deficit well.

### SURGICAL CONSIDERATIONS
Bulla osteotomy—may be useful in patients with disorders of the middle ear

## MEDICATIONS

### DRUG(S) OF CHOICE
• Treat specific disease if possible.
• Tear replacement—if Schirmer tear test value low; with ectropion or exophthalmic globes

### CONTRAINDICATIONS
• Corticosteroids—no evidence of improvement with use; will exacerbate infectious disease
• Oral administration of antibiotics that select against Gram-positive bacteria (penicillins, macrolides, lincosamides, and cephalosporins) can cause fatal enteric dysbiosis and enterotoxemia.

### PRECAUTIONS
N/A

### POSSIBLE INTERACTIONS
N/A

### ALTERNATIVE DRUGS
N/A

## FOLLOW-UP

### PATIENT MONITORING
• Reevaluate early for evidence of corneal ulcers.
• Assess monthly for palpebral reflexes and lip and ear movements to evaluate return of function and condition of affected eye, although damage is often permanent.

### PREVENTION AVOIDANCE
Treating otitis or upper respiratory infections in early stages may prevent otitis media/interna and/or brain abscesses.

### POSSIBLE COMPLICATIONS
• Keratoconjunctivitis sicca
• Corneal ulcers
• Severe contracture on side of lesion
• Progression of underlying disease

### EXPECTED COURSE AND PROGNOSIS
• Depend on cause
• Improvement may take weeks or months or may never occur.
• Lip contracture sometimes develops.

## MISCELLANEOUS

### ASSOCIATED CONDITIONS
N/A

### AGE-RELATED FACTORS
N/A

### ZOONOTIC POTENTIAL
N/A

### PREGNANCY
N/A

### SYNONYMS
Idiopathic facial paresis and paralysis

### SEE ALSO
• Conjunctivitis
• *Encephalitozoon cuniculi*
• Head tilt
• Otitis media and interna

# FACIAL NERVE PARESIS/PARALYSIS

## ABBREVIATIONS
- CNS = central nervous system
- CSF = cerebrospinal fluid
- CT = computed tomography
- ELISA = enzyme-linked immunosorbent assay
- IFA = immunofluorescence assay
- SPF = specific pathogen free

## Suggested Reading
Deeb BJ, Carpenter JW. Neurologic and musculoskeletal diseases. In: Quesenberry KE, Carpenter JW, eds. Ferrets, Rabbits and Rodents: Clinical Medicine and Surgery. 2nd Ed. Philadelphia: WB Saunders, 2004:203–210.

de Lahunta A. Veterinary neuroanatomy and clinical neurology. 2nd Ed. Philadelphia: Saunders, 1983.

Harcourt-Brown F. Neurological and locomotor diseases. In Harcourt-Brown F, ed. Textbook of Rabbit Medicine. Oxford: Butterworth-Heinemann, 2002:307–323.

Oliver JE, Lorenz MD. Handbook of veterinary neurologic diagnosis. 2nd Ed. Philadelphia: Saunders, 1993.

Paul-Murphy J, Ramer JC. Urgent care of the pet rabbits. Vet Clin North Am Exotic Anim Pract 1998;1(1):127–152.

Rosenthal KR. Torticollis in rabbits. Proc North Am Vet Conf 2005;1378–1379.

## Portions Adapted From
Neer TM. Facial Nerve Paresis and Paralysis. In: Tilley LP, Smith FWK, Jr., eds. The 5-Minute Veterinary Consult: Canine and Feline, 3rd Ed. Baltimore: Lippincott Williams & Wilkins, 2004.

## BASICS

### OVERVIEW
• Flea infestation—the presence of fleas and flea dirt; *Ctenocephalides canis* or *C. felis* most commonly found on rabbits
• Heavy infestations may cause anemia, especially in young rabbits.
• Fleabite hypersensitivity has not been documented in rabbits; however, some rabbits appear to be significantly more pruritic than others, suggesting that a hypersensitivity reaction may exist in these animals.

### SIGNALMENT
• Incidence varies with climatic conditions and flea population.
• No age or sex predilection
• Clinical signs vary with individual animals.
• Young animals more likely to develop anemia

### SIGNS

#### Historical Findings
• History of flea infestation in other pets, including dogs and cats
• Some animals asymptomatic
• Biting, chewing, scratching, or excessive licking
• Signs of fleas and flea dirt

#### Physical Examination Findings
• Depends on the severity of the reaction and the degree of exposure to fleas (i.e., seasonal vs. year-round)
• Finding fleas and flea dirt
• Papules, alopecia, excoriations, and scaling may appear anywhere on the body.
• Secondary bacterial infections sometimes seen
• Pale mucous membranes, tachycardia in anemic animals

### CAUSES AND RISK FACTORS
Exposure to other flea-infested animals within the household; keeping animals outdoors in hutches

## DIAGNOSIS

### DIFFERENTIAL DIAGNOSIS
• Fur mites—*Cheyletiella* spp. or, less commonly, *Leporacarus gibbus*. May be concurrent with flea infestation. Fur mite lesions are usually located in the intrascapular or tail base region and associated with copious amounts of large, white scale. Mites are readily identified in skin scrapes or acetate tape preparations under low magnification.
• Ear mites (*Psoroptes cuniculi*)—usually intensely pruritic; lesions typically localized to areas inside of pinnae, surrounding ears, face, and neck. Skin thickening and exuda-

tive crusts form with chronic infestation. Mites can be seen with unaided eye or with microscopic examination under low power.
• Other ectoparasites—*Sarcoptes scabiei* and *Notoedres cati* rarely infest rabbits. Lesions are located around the head and neck and are intensely pruritic.
• Contact dermatitis—usually ventral distribution of lesions; acute onset
• Sebaceous adenitis—often profuse amounts of white scale and flakes, alopecia; diagnose by skin biopsy.
• Barbering—by cage mates or self-inflicted—causes hair loss alone without pruritus, scale, or skin lesions
• Lack of grooming due to obesity or underlying dental or musculoskeletal disease may cause an accumulation of scale.
• Injection site reactions, especially with irritating substances such as enrofloxacin, may cause alopecia and crusting.

### CBC/BIOCHEMISTRY/URINALYSIS
Usually normal; hypereosinophilia inconsistently detected and not well documented

### OTHER LABORATORY TESTS
• Skin scrapings—negative
• Flea combings—fleas or flea dirt usually found in affected rabbits
• Cytology of ear exudate—no mites seen

### IMAGING
N/A

### DIAGNOSTIC PROCEDURES
• Diagnosis usually based on historical information and ruling out other causes of dermatitis
• Fleas or flea dirt is supportive but may be difficult to find.
• The most accurate test may be response to appropriate treatment.

### PATHOLOGIC FINDINGS
• Superficial dermatitis
• Histopathologic lesions not well described

## TREATMENT

### CLIENT EDUCATION
• Inform owners that controlling exposure to fleas is currently the only means of therapy.
• Treat all animals in the household.

## MEDICATIONS

### DRUG(S) OF CHOICE
• Imidacloprid (Advantage, Bayer)—monthly spot treatment for cats and dogs; one dose for cats <9 lbs., divided onto two to three spots topically q30d anecdotal dosage, appears to be safe and effective in rabbits.

• Selamectin (Revolution, Pfizer)—monthly spot treatment for cats and dogs; appears to be safe and effective at 6–12 mg/kg applied topically q30d
• Fipronil (Frontline, Rhone Merieux)—not recommended, toxicity reported in rabbits
• Systemic treatments—limited benefit because they require a flea bite to be effective; may help animals with flea infestation; primarily licensed for use in only dogs; lufenuron (Program, CIBA Animal Health), a chitin inhibitor available as an oral formulation for cats and dogs, has been used anecdotally in rabbits at 30 mg/kg PO q30d.
• Sprays and powders—usually contain pyrethrins and pyrethroids (synthetic pyrethrins) or carbaryl with an insect growth regulator or synergist; products labeled for use in kittens and puppies are anecdotally considered safe and generally effective, advantages are low toxicity and repellent activity; disadvantages are frequent applications and expense.
• Indoor treatment—fogs and premises sprays; usually contain organophosphates, pyrethrins, and/or insect growth regulators; apply according to manufacturer's directions; treat all areas of the house; can be applied by the owner; advantages are weak chemicals and generally inexpensive; disadvantage is labor intensity; premises sprays concentrate the chemicals in areas that most need treatment. Safety of product usage in a rabbit's environment is unknown.
• Professional exterminators—advantages are less labor intensive, relatively few applications, sometimes guaranteed; disadvantages are strength of chemicals and cost; specific recommendations and guidelines must be followed. Safety of product usage in a rabbit's environment is unknown.
• Inert substances—boric acid, diatomaceous earth, and silica aerogel; treat every 6–12 months; follow manufacturer's recommendations; very safe and effective if applied properly
• Outdoor treatment—concentrated in shaded areas; sprays usually contain pyrethroids or organophosphates and an insect growth regulator; powders are usually organophosphates; product containing nematodes (*Steinerma carpocapsae*) is safe and chemical free.
• Antibiotics—may be necessary to treat secondary pyoderma, if severe

### CONTRAINDICATIONS
• Oral administration of antibiotics that select against Gram-positive bacteria (penicillins, macrolides, lincosamides, and cephalosporins) can cause fatal enteric dysbiosis and enterotoxemia.
• Do not use corticosteroids (systemic or topical) to treat pruritic dermatitis in rabbits with fleas. Corticosteroid use is associ-

# FLEAS AND FLEA INFESTATON

ated with gastrointestinal ulceration and hemorrhage, delayed wound healing, and hepatopathy, hepatic abscess formation, and heightened susceptibility to infection.
• Do not use fipronil on rabbits.
• Do not use flea collars on rabbits.
• Do not use organophosphate-containing products on rabbits.
• Do not use straight permethrin sprays or permethrin spot-ons on rabbits.

### PRECAUTIONS
• Use extreme caution when dipping or bathing rabbits due to the high risk of skeletal fractures and excessive chilling with inexperienced owners.
• Most flea control products discussed above are off-label use. Safety and efficacy has not been evaluated in rabbits. Use with caution, especially in young or debilitated animals.
• Prevent rabbits or their cage mates from licking topical spot-on products before they are dry.
• Pyrethrin/pyrethroid-type flea products—adverse reactions include depression, hypersalivation, muscle tremors, vomiting, ataxia, dyspnea, and anorexia.
• Toxicity—if any signs are noted, the animal should be bathed thoroughly to remove any remaining chemicals and treated appropriately.
• Rodents and fish are very sensitive to pyrethrins.

### POSSIBLE INTERACTIONS
With the exception of lufenuron used concurrently with imidacloprid, do not use more than one flea treatment at a time.

### ALTERNATIVE DRUGS
N/A

## FOLLOW-UP

### PATIENT MONITORING
• Pruritus and alopecia—should decrease with effective flea control; if signs persist evaluate for other causes.

• Fleas and flea dirt—should decrease with effective flea control; however, absence is not always a reliable indicator of successful treatment in very sensitive animals.

### PREVENTION/AVOIDANCE
• Flea control for all other pets in the household, especially dogs and cats
• See medications
• Year-round warm climates—may require year-round flea control
• Seasonally warm climates—usually begin flea control in May or June

### POSSIBLE COMPLICATIONS
• Secondary bacterial infections
• Adverse reaction to flea-control products
• Anemia

### EXPECTED COURSE AND PROGNOSIS
Prognosis is good if strict flea control is instituted.

## MISCELLANEOUS

### ASSOCIATED CONDITIONS
N/A

### AGE-RELATED FACTORS
Use caution with flea-control products in young animals; remove fleas with a flea comb instead and treat other pets in the household.

### ZOONOTIC POTENTIAL
In areas of moderate to severe flea infestation, people can be bitten by fleas; usually papular lesions are located on the wrists and ankles.

### PREGNANCY
Carefully follow the label directions of each individual product to estimate its safety; however, bear in mind that these products have not been used extensively in pregnant rabbits, and safety is unknown.

### SYNONYMS
N/A

### ABBREVIATIONS
N/A

### SEE ALSO
• Cheyletiellosis
• Dermatophytosis
• Ear mites

*Suggested Reading*
Clyde VL. Practical treatment and control of common ectoparasites in exotic pets. Vet Med 1996;91(7):632–637.
Harcourt-Brown, F. Skin diseases. In: Harcourt-Brown F, ed. Textbook of Rabbit Medicine. Oxford: Butterworth-Heinemann, 2002:224–248.
Hess L. Dermatologic diseases. In: Quesenberry KE, Carpenter JW, eds. Ferrets, Rabbits and Rodents: Clinical Medicine and Surgery. 2nd Ed. Philadelphia: WB Saunders, 2004:194–202.
Jenkins, JR. Skin disorders of the rabbit. Vet Clin North Am Exotic Anim Pract 2001;4(2):543–563.
McTier TL, Hair A, Walstrom DJ, et al. Efficacy and safety of topical administration of selamectin for treatment of ear mite infestation in rabbits. J Am Vet Med Assoc 2003;223(3):322–324.

*Portions Adapted From*
Kuhl KA, Greek JS. Fleas and Flea Control. In: Tilley LP, Smith FWK, Jr., eds. The 5-Minute Veterinary Consult: Canine and Feline, 2nd Ed. Baltimore: Lippincott Williams & Wilkins, 2000.

# BASICS

## OVERVIEW
• A syndrome of rabbits in which the stomach fills with gas and fluid, which results in complex local and systemic pathologic and physiologic changes
• Fluid or ingesta accumulates in the stomach in conjunction with a mechanical or functional obstruction of the pyloric orifice.
• In most cases dilation is due to foreign body obstruction of the pylorus or duodenum; in rare instances, the stomach dilates in the absence of a foreign body;, the cause of this is unknown.
• Dilation of the stomach may progress, adding to functional obstruction.
• Twisting of the stomach rarely occurs but has been anecdotally reported.
• Direct gastric damage and multiple systemic abnormalities can occur secondary to ischemia from rising intragastric pressures.
• These changes may account for the acute clinical signs, which can include severe abdominal pain, hypovolemic shock, and cardiovascular failure.

## SIGNALMENT
• Can occur in any-aged rabbit, but gastrointestinal foreign bodies are more commonly seen in older rabbits on low-fiber diets
• No breed or sex predilections

## SIGNS

### Historical Findings
• May have history of anorexia of short duration
• Weakness or collapse most common historical finding
• Progressive abdominal distension
• Depression

### Physical Examination Findings
• Tympanic cranial abdomen
• Tachycardia initially; bradycardia if shocky
• Tachypnea
• Signs of hypovolemic shock (e.g., pale mucous membranes, decreased capillary refill time, weak pulses, hypothermic)
• Severe abdominal pain on palpation

## CAUSES AND RISK FACTORS
• Most acute pyloric or duodenal obstructions are caused by ingested hair mats, cloth, or other fibers; less commonly by small pieces of rubber or plastic objects.
• Craving for fiber may occur in rabbits fed diets deficient in coarse, long-stemmed hay and may contribute to excessive chewing on household items (cloth, cords, towels, etc.) or barbering. Ingestion of these objects can result in acute obstruction.

• Peritoneal adhesions, fibrosis, or intraabdominal abscesses occasionally cause pyloric outflow obstruction; presentation is usually more chronic (preceded by signs of gastrointestinal hypomotility), but acute obstruction resulting in gastric dilation occasionally is seen.
• Intestinal intussusception is a rare cause of gastric dilation.
• Occasionally, the stomach dilates and fills with fluid and gas in the absence of an obstructing foreign body. The cause of this is unknown; functional pyloric outflow obstruction, gastric myoelectric abnormalities, dynamic movement of the stomach following ingestion of food or water, aerophagia, and severe ileus or stress may play a role.

# DIAGNOSIS

## DIFFERENTIAL DIAGNOSIS
• Gastrointestinal hypomotility—usually present for anorexia, lack of fecal production; patients generally bright and alert or only mild to moderately depressed; abdominal palpation reveals a large, doughy or firm mass within the stomach (vs. air- or fluid-filled stomach with gastric dilation); radiographics demonstrate stomach full of ingesta; sometimes surrounded by air; air is often also visible in the remainder of the intestinal tract as well.
• Overgrowth of gas-producing *Clostridia* spp.—similar presentation, as patients also are often in shock on presentation. With clostridial overgrowth, gas is usually palpable and visible radiographically throughout the entire intestinal tract; there is a history of inappropriate antibiotic use, gastric stasis, or feeding of foods high in simple carbohydrates. Overgrowth may occur simultaneously with mechanical causes of gastric dilation.
• Aerophagia—rabbits with severe dyspnea; history of respiratory tract disease; can be due to upper respiratory tract disorders alone as rabbits are obligate nasal breathers.
• Differentiate nongastric dilation conditions via examination and imaging; rabbits with gastric dilation are in extreme pain; often present in shock or moribund; tympanic, gas- or fluid-filled stomach is palpable; borborygmus is often increased on abdominal auscultation; radiographs demonstrate dilated, gas- and/or fluid-filled stomach.

## CBC/BIOCHEMISTRY/URINALYSIS
• Expect hemogram abnormalities consistent with hemoconcentration/shock.
• Electrolyte abnormalities and acid-base alterations may be seen.

## OTHER LABORATORY TESTS
N/A

## IMAGING
• Abdominal radiography—severe distention of the stomach with fluid and/or gas; remainder of intestines usually appear normal.
• Stabilization may be necessary prior to imaging procedures.
• Abdominal ultrasound—helpful to identify intestinal foreign material, extraluminal intestinal obstruction, or intussusception

## DIAGNOSTIC PROCEDURES
N/A

# TREATMENT

## APPROPRIATE HEALTH CARE
• Emergency inpatient medical management
• Patients require immediate medical therapy with special attention to establishing improved cardiovascular function and then gastric decompression.
• Fluid therapy for hypovolemic shock—LRS or other crystalloid (60–90 mg/kg/hr IV, IO over 20–60 minutes, followed by maintenance rate) or crystalloid bolus (30 mL/kg) plus hetastarch bolus (5 mL/kg initially) followed by crystalloids at a maintenance rate and hetastarch at 20mL/kg divided over 24 hours.
• Supportive fluids on the basis of hydration status are recommended for animals not in shock.
• Perform gastric decompression by orogastric intubation; light sedation may facilitate this process. Make sure the rabbit is securely restrained in a towel; a large-diameter otoscope is useful as a mouth gag through which a well-lubricated, open-ended, flexible rubber tube is passed into the stomach.
• Decompression by other techniques such as trocarization and in-dwelling catheters have not been described in rabbits; leakage of gastric contents into the peritoneum potentially a life-threatening consequence.
• Surgery is indicated in most cases to remove outflow obstruction, though the time interval from presentation to surgery may vary depending on response or lack of response to treatment.
• Most obstructions occur in the proximal duodenum where a sharp turn occurs near the ileocecal junction.

## NURSING CARE
• Maintain blood pressure with ample fluid support following volume replacement/shock therapy.
• Monitor patients closely for reoccurrence of dilation or cardiorespiratory decompensation.

## GASTRIC DILATION

### ACTIVITY
Surgical patients may resume normal activity after the foreign body is removed.

### DIET
• Patients should be NPO until obstruction is relieved; then resume normal feeding if rabbit is willing to eat. If rabbit refuses food, assist-feed gruel such as Critical Care for Herbivores (Oxbow Pet Products, Murdock, NE) 10–15 mL/kg PO q6–8h. Larger volumes and more frequent feedings are often accepted; feed as much as the rabbit will readily accept. Alternatively, pellets can be ground and mixed with fresh greens, vegetable baby foods, water, or juice to form a gruel. If sufficient volumes of food are not accepted in this manner, nasogastric intubation is indicated.
• High-carbohydrate, high-fat nutritional supplements are contraindicated.

### CLIENT EDUCATION
• Most rabbits with gastric dilation present in critical condition. Prognosis is guarded, even with immediate decompression and treatment for shock.
• Discuss potential risks of surgery, especially when patients are critical.
• Explain signs of recurrence of gastric dilation, so the client may detect the condition early.

### SURGICAL CONSIDERATIONS
• Indicated in patients with intestinal foreign body, extraluminal obstruction, or intussusception—exploratory celiotomy
• Timing of surgery—based on the patient's cardiovascular condition, gastric decompression, and other physical parameters
• Prolonged delay may result in death of the patient.
• Surgical exploration should be thorough and yet efficient to minimize surgical time.
• Occasionally, no obstruction is visible on preoperative imaging or at surgery and patients recover uneventfully, although bloat may recur; the cause of gastric dilation is unknown in these cases.

## MEDICATIONS

### DRUG(S) OF CHOICE
• Antibiotics are indicated because of the potential for endotoxemia associated with shock, gastric compromise, and potential abdominal contamination at the time of surgery.
• Effective antibiotic choices include trimethoprim sulfa (30 mg/kg PO q12h) or enrofloxacin (5–20 mg/kg PO, SC, IM q12–24h).

• For sedation—light sedation with midazolam (0.5–1 mg/kg IM) or diazepam (1–2 mg/kg IM); many other sedation protocols exist.
• H$_2$-receptor antagonists may ameliorate or prevent gastric ulceration—cimetidine (5–10 mg/kg PO, SC, IM, IV q6–12h) or ranitidine (2 mg/kg IV q24h or 2–5 mg/kg PO q12h)

#### Acute Pain Management
• Buprenorphine (0.01–0.05 mg/kg SC, IM, IV q8–12h)—use preoperatively and for postoperative pain management as needed.
• Butorphanol (0.1–1.0 mg/kg SC, IM, IV q4–6h)—may cause profound sedation; short-acting
• Morphine (2–5 mg/kg SC, IM q2–4h) or oxymorphone (0.05–0.2 mg/kg SC, IM q8–12h)—use with caution; more than one to two doses may cause gastrointestinal stasis.
• Meloxicam (0.2 mg/kg SC, IM q24h)
• Carprofen (1–4 mg/kg SC q12h)

#### Postoperative Pain Management
• Meloxicam (0.2–0.5 mg/kg PO q24h); carprofen (2.2 mg/kg PO q12–24h)

### CONTRAINDICATIONS AND PRECAUTIONS
• The use of antibiotics that are primarily Gram positive in spectrum is contraindicated in rabbits. Use of these antibiotics will suppress the growth of commensal flora, allowing overgrowth of enteric pathogens. Do not orally administer lincomycin, clindamycin, erythromycin, ampicillin, amoxicillin cephalosporins, or penicillins.
• Prior to surgical removal, the use of gastrointestinal motility enhancers is contraindicated in rabbits with complete gastrointestinal tract obstruction due to the possibility of intestinal rupture.
• Avoid drugs that may lead to renal compromise until shock and hypovolemia are corrected (e.g., aminoglycosides, NSAIDs)
• Corticosteroids—avoid; associated with gastrointestinal ulceration and hemorrhage, delayed wound healing, and heightened susceptibility to infection; rabbits are very sensitive to the immunosuppressive effects of both topic and systemic corticosteroids; use may exacerbate subclinical bacterial infection.
• Corticosteroids—do not use with NSAIDs because of combined negative effects on the gastrointestinal tract.

### POSSIBLE INTERACTIONS
N/A

### ALTERNATIVE DRUGS
N/A

## FOLLOW-UP

### PATIENT MONITORING
• Cardiorespiratory function for at least 24 hours after surgery; blood pressure and perfusion
• Monitor for recurrence of gastric dilation.
• Monitor the appetite and production of fecal pellets. Anesthetic agents used during surgical removal of foreign bodies contribute to gastrointestinal hypomotility and subsequent overgrowth of toxin-forming bacteria. Rabbits with postoperative gastrointestinal stasis are anorectic and produce little to no feces.
• With successful treatment, see return of appetite, normal feces produced

### PREVENTION/AVOIDANCE
• Strict feeding of diets containing adequate indigestible fiber and low-carbohydrate content along with access to fresh water will usually prevent the formation of gastric trichobezoars or retention of small foreign bodies.
• The rabbit should be closely supervised during times when access to potential foreign bodies is likely.
• Regularly brush rabbits to remove shed hair and prevent ingestion of hair mats.

### POSSIBLE COMPLICATIONS
• Death due to gastric rupture
• Postoperative gastrointestinal stasis and subsequent overgrowth of bacterial pathogens
• Stricture formation at the site of removal
• Gastric dilation may recur.

### EXPECTED COURSE AND PROGNOSIS
• Most rabbits with gastric dilation present in critical condition. Prognosis is guarded, even with immediate decompression and treatment for shock.
• Prognosis based on surgical assessment and postoperative recovery, but generally guarded
• Patients recovering well after 7 days appear to have a good prognosis for complete recovery.

## MISCELLANEOUS

### ASSOCIATED CONDITIONS
• Gastrointestinal hypomotility
• Clostridial enterotoxicosis

### AGE-RELATED FACTORS
N/A

**ZOONOTIC POTENTIAL**
N/A

**PREGNANCY**
N/A

**SYNONYMS**
Bloat

**SEE ALSO**
• Gastrointestinal foreign body
• Gastrointestinal hypomotility and gastrointestinal statis

**ABBREVIATIONS**
• LRS = lactated Ringer's solution
• NPO = nothing by mouth

• NSAIDs = nonsteroidal antiinflammatory drugs

*Suggested Reading*

Brown SA, Rosenthal KL. The anorexic rabbit. Proc North Am Vet Conf, 1997:788.
Jenkins JR. Feeding recommendations for the house rabbit. Vet Clin Noth Am Exotic Anim Pract 1999;2(1):143–151.
Jenkins JR. Gastrointestinal diseases. In: Quesenberry KE, Carpenter JW, eds. Ferrets, Rabbits and Rodents: Clinical Medicine and Surgery. 2nd Ed. Philadelphia: WB Saunders, 2004:161–171.
Paul-Murphy JA, Ramer JC. Urgent care of the pet rabbits. Vet Clin North Am Exotic Anim Pract 1998;1(1):127–152.
Rees Davies R, Rees Davies JAE. Rabbit gastrointestinal physiology. Vet Clin North Am Exotic Anim Pract 2003;6(1): 139–153.

*Portions Adapted From*

Waschak MJ. Gastric Dilation and Volvulus Syndrome. In: Tilley LP, Smith FWK, Jr., eds. The 5-Minute Veterinary Consult: Canine and Feline, 3rd Ed. Baltimore: Lippincott Williams & Wilkins, 2004.

# GASTROINTESTINAL FOREIGN BODIES

 **BASICS**

## DEFINITION
A nonfood item located in the esophagus, stomach, or intestines

## PATHOPHYSIOLOGY
- Proper gastrointestinal tract motility and hind-gut fermentation are dependent on the ingestion of large amounts of roughage and long-stemmed hay. Diets that contain inadequate amounts of long-stemmed, coarse fiber (such as the feeding of only commercial pelleted food without hay or grasses) cause gastrointestinal tract hypomotility.
- The presence of "hairballs" or trichobezoars in the stomach is not a disease, but a symptom or consequence of gastrointestinal hypomotility or stasis. Rabbits normally ingest hair during grooming. Healthy rabbits will always have some amount of hair and ingesta in the stomach. These stomach contents are both palpable and visible radiographically in the normal, healthy rabbit.
- With proper nutrition and gastrointestinal tract motility, fur ingested as a result of normal grooming behavior and some small or easily deformed foreign bodies will pass through the gastrointestinal tract with the ingesta uneventfully.
- When gastrointestinal motility slows or stops, ingesta, including fur and other material, accumulates in the stomach. Rabbits cannot vomit to expel nonfood contents from the stomach.
- Dehydration of stomach contents often occurs, making the contents more difficult to pass. With medical treatment of gastrointestinal hypomotility, motility usually returns, stomach contents soften, and hair and other ingesta will usually pass. Without treatment, rentention of inspissated gastric contents and subsequent metabolic derangements combined with shifts in intestinal microbial flora can be fatal.
- Large, nondeformable, or severely inspissated ingested material may cause a partial or complete outflow obstruction, most commonly in the pylorus or small intestine.
- Rabbits are extremely fond of chewing, especially on cloth, bedding, or fur. When fed diets containing insufficient coarse fiber, chewing behavior is often exacerbated, perhaps due to a craving for fiber. The combination of excessive chewing and gastrointestinal tract hypomotility predisposes rabbits to retention of gastric foreign material.
- Anorexia due to infectious or metabolic disease or pain may cause or exacerbate gastrointestinal hypomotility.
- Ingestion of toxic foreign bodies, such as heavy metals, may cause a functional ileus, thereby contributing to foreign body retention.
- Retained objects of insufficient size to cause an outflow obstruction may cause a mechanical irritation to the gastric mucosa.
- Chronic ingestion of cat litter, especially scoopable litter, often accumulates in the cecum and can cause severe cecal impaction.
- Acute, complete obstruction of the gastrointestinal tract occasionally occurs and is usually due to the presence of a hair mat combined with other ingested foreign material (chewed pieces of cloth, towels, carpet, cords, etc.) in the intestines, especially the duodenum. These may be related to gastrointestinal hypomotility or ingestion of a hair mat too large to pass through the intestine, or may be the result of local intestinal inflammation or neoplasia.
- Complete gastrointestinal tract obstruction is an acute, life-threatening emergency.

## SYSTEMS AFFECTED
- Gastrointestinal—if an obstruction has occurred, the patient may refuse food or water and become dehydrated. If a perforation has occurred, mediastinitis or peritonitis may develop.
- Musculoskeletal—loss of muscle mass may occur due to inappetence.
- Cardiovascular—shock with acute gastrointestinal tract obstruction

## INCIDENCE/PREVALENCE
- Gastrointestinal hypomotility resulting in anorexia, abdominal pain, ill-thrift, scant or lack of feces, or chronic intermittent diarrhea is one of the most common clinical problems seen in the rabbit.
- Acute obstruction of the gastrointestinal tract is uncommon.

## SIGNALMENT
- More commonly seen in older rabbits on inappropriate diets, but can occur in any-aged rabbit
- No breed or gender predilections

## SIGNS

### Historical Findings
*Esophageal Foreign Body*
- Esophageal foreign bodies are extremely rare in rabbits.
- Ptyalism, anorexia, and persistent attempts at swallowing may be seen.

*Chronic Gastric Foreign Body—Accumulation of Hair and Other Ingesta Secondary to Gastrointestinal Hypomotility*
- Rabbits often initially stop eating pellets but continue to eat treats, followed by complete anorexia.
- Fecal pellets become scant and small in size.
- Patients are usually bright and alert.
- Signs of pain, such as teeth grinding, a hunched posture, and reluctance to move
- History of inappropriate diet (e.g., cereals, grains, commercial pellets only, sweets, large quantities of fruits, lack of feeding long-stemmed hay)
- Recent history of illness or stressful event

*Acute Pyloric or Intestinal Obstruction*
- May have history of anorexia of short duration
- Weakness or collapse most common historical finding
- Progressive abdominal distension
- Often quickly progresses to lateral recumbency and signs of shock
- Diarrhea may also occur.

### Physical Examination Findings
*Gastrointestinal Hypomotility, Accumulation of Stomach Contents*
- Palpation of the stomach is an extremely valuable tool in the diagnosis of abnormal retention of stomach contents. Ingesta normally should be palpable in the stomach of a healthy rabbit. The normal stomach should be easily deformable, feel soft and pliable, and not remain pitted on compression. Rabbits with early gastrointestinal hypomotility will have a firm, often enlarged stomach that remains pitted when compressed. With complete gastrointestinal stasis, severe dehydration, or prolonged hypomotility, the stomach may be severely distended, hard, and nondeformable.
- The presence of firm ingesta in the stomach of a rabbit that has been anorectic for 1–3 days is compatible with the diagnosis of gastrointestinal hypomotility.
- Small, hard fecal pellets or absence of fecal pellets palpable in the colon
- Fluid or gas may be palpable within the cecum.
- Emaciation may be seen in chronic cases.
- Little to no borborygmus on abdominal auscultation

*Acute Pyloric or Intestinal Obstruction*
- Tachycardia initially; bradycardia if shocky
- Tachypnea
- Signs of hypovolemic shock (e.g., pale mucous membranes, decreased capillary refill time, weak pulses, hypothermic)
- Severe abdominal pain on palpation
- Stomach filled with fluid and/or gas palpable; stomach usually extremely distended and tympanic
- These rabbits are usually in shock and require emergency decompression.
- Often increased borborygmus on abdominal auscultation

## CAUSES
- In most cases ingesta, including hair and foreign material, are retained in the gastrointestinal tract due to a lack of normal gastrointestinal motility. Gastrointestinal

# GASTROINTESTINAL FOREIGN BODIES

hypomotility is often the result of feeding diets with insufficient long-stem hair or coarse fiber content. Gastrointestinal hypomotility may also be caused by anorexia. Common causes of anorexia include dental disease (malocclusion, molar impaction, tooth root abscesses), metabolic disease (renal disease, liver disease), pain (oral, trauma, postoperative pain, adhesions), neoplasia (gastrointestinal, uterine), and toxins.
• Anesthetic agents may cause or exacerbate gastrointestinal hypomotility.
• Some retained foreign bodies are simply too large to pass through the intestinal tract. This is an unusual condition and occurs when rabbits ingest large mats of hair, chewed bedding or fabric, or other materials that pass through the stomach but cannot pass through the intestines.
• Focal intestinal inflammation, neoplasia, or stricture may trap foreign body

## RISK FACTORS
• Diets with inadequate indigestible coarse fiber content
• Inactivity due to pain, obesity, cage confinement
• Anesthesia and surgical procedures
• Unsupervised chewing behavior
• Underlying dental, gastrointestinal tract, or metabolic disease

## DIAGNOSIS

### DIFFERENTIAL DIAGNOSIS
• For palpable mass in the cranial abdomen—neoplasia, abscess, normal gastric contents
• For anorexia—dental disease, gastrointestinal stasis, metabolic disease, pain, neoplasia, cardiac disease, toxin
• For decreased fecal output—anorexia, gastrointestinal stasis, intussusception, intestinal neoplasia

### CBC/BIOCHEMISTRY/URINALYSIS
• These tests are often normal.
• May be used to identify underlying causes of gastrointestinal hypomotility
• If the intestinal tract has been perforated, an inflammatory leukogram may be seen.
• PCV and TS elevation in dehydrated patients
• Serum ALT elevation in rabbits with liver disease, especially hepatic lipidosis in anorectic rabbits
• Anemia from gastric bleeding is rare.

### OTHER LABORATORY TESTS
N/A

### IMAGING
• Radiographs are valuable to delineate the type and location of some radiopaque foreign bodies; however, most retained foreign material in the rabbit intestinal tract is the

same density as normal ingesta.
• Rabbits should not be fasted prior to taking radiographs.
• Gastric contents (primarily food and hair) are normally present and visible radiographically, even if the rabbit has been inappetent. The presence of ingesta (including hair) in the stomach is a normal finding.
• Moderate to severe distension of the stomach with ingesta is usually visible with gastrointestinal hypomotility. In some rabbits with gastrointestinal stasis, a halo of gas can be observed around the inspissated stomach contents. Gas distension is also common throughout the intestinal tract, including the cecum in rabbits with gastrointestinal hypomotility or stasis.
• Cecal distention with ingesta and/or gas may be seen.
• Severe distension of the stomach with fluid and/or gas is usually seen with acute small intestinal obstructions.
• Contrast studies are generally not useful in the detection of intestinal foreign bodies.
• Localized free gas in the peritoneal cavity is seen with peritonitis resulting from gastrointestinal perforation.
• Abdominal ultrasound can be useful for documenting an intestinal foreign body; may be difficult to interpret when large amounts of gas are present within the intestinal tract; may help define extraluminal mass

### OTHER DIAGNOSTIC PROCEDURES
Upper gastrointestinal endoscopy may be used to diagnose esophageal and gastric foreign bodies. In addition, this allows assessment of the extent of mucosal injury. However, the presence of large amounts of gastric ingesta, the small size of the patient and subsequent limitations on instrument size often limit the use of endoscopy.

### PATHOLOGIC FINDINGS
N/A

## TREATMENT

### APPROPRIATE HEALTH CARE
• Esophageal foreign bodies are considered an emergency since the incidence of complications increases with the length of time the foreign body is present.
• Severe gastric distention with fluid or gas (bloat) is a life-threatening emergency.
• Most gastric foreign bodies, including retention of gastric contents secondary to gastrointestinal hypomotility, are considered an urgency rather than an emergency, unless the patient has evidence of complete obstruction, gastric erosion, or signs of toxicosis.
• Intestinal foreign bodies are an emergency since the incidence of complications increases with the length of time the foreign body is present.

• Cecal foreign material or impaction is generally considered an urgency rather than emergency, unless the patient has signs of severe metabolic derangements or toxicosis.

### NURSING CARE
#### Fluid Therapy
• Fluid therapy is an essential component of the medical management of patients with retained and inspissated stomach contents secondary to gastrointestinal hypomotility. Administer both oral and parenteral fluids. Oral fluid administration will aid in the rehydration of inspissated gastric contents. Mildly affected rabbits will usually respond well to oral and subcutaneous fluid administration, dietary modification described below, and, in some cases, treatment with intestinal motility modifiers and analgesics.
• Intravenous or intraosseous fluids are required in patients that are severely dehydrated or depressed. Maintenance fluid requirements are estimated at 100 mL/kg/day. Rehydration is essential to treatment success in severely ill rabbits. Initially, a balanced fluid (e.g., lactated Ringer's solution) may be used.
• Fluid therapy for rabbits with acute pyloric or small intestinal obstruction that are often presented in shock—LRS or other crystalloid (60–90 mg/kg/hr IV, IO over 20–60 minutes, followed by maintenance rate) or crystalloid bolus (30 mL/kg) plus hetastarch bolus (5 mL/kg initially) followed by crystalloids at a maintenance rate and hetastarch at 20 mL/kg divided over 24 hours.
• A warm, quiet environment should be provided.

#### Gastric Decompression
• Patients with an extremely dilated gas- and/or fluid-filled stomach (secondary to acute obstruction) require immediate medical therapy with special attention to establishing improved cardiovascular function and gastric decompression.
• Administer fluid therapy as described above for critical patients; supportive fluids on the basis of hydration status are recommended for animals not in shock.
• Perform gastric decompression by orogastric intubation using a well-lubricated, open-ended red rubber catheter. A large-diameter otoscope cone can be used as a mouth gag. Make sure the rabbit is securely restrained in a towel. Sedation is generally required, unless the patient is extremely depressed.
• Surgery is indicated following decompression in most cases to remove outflow obstruction, though the time interval from presentation to surgery may vary depending on response or lack of response to treatment.

# GASTROINTESTINAL FOREIGN BODIES

## ACTIVITY
• If patient is not debilitated, encourage exercise (hopping) for at least 10–15 minutes every 6–8 hours because activity promotes gastric motility; provide supervised freedom from the cage or access to a safe grazing area.
• Surgical patients may resume normal activity after the foreign body is removed.

## DIET
• Critical patients with acute small intestinal or pyloric obstruction should be NPO until obstruction is relieved; then resume normal feeding if rabbit is willing to eat.
• It is absolutely imperative that the rabbit continue to eat during and following medical treatment, and within 12 hours of surgical treatment. Continued anorexia will exacerbate gastrointestinal hypomotility and cause further derangement of the gastrointestinal microflora and overgrowth of intestinal bacterial pathogens.
• Offer a large selection of fresh, moistened greens such as cilantro, romaine lettuce, parsley, carrot tops, dandelion greens, spinach, collard greens, etc., and good-quality grass hay. Many rabbits will begin to eat these foods, even if they were previously anorectic. Also offer the rabbit's usual pelleted diet, as the initial goal is to get the rabbit to eat.
• If the patient refuses these foods, syringe feed a gruel such as Critical Care for Herbivores (Oxbow Pet Products, Murdock, NE) 10–15 mL/kg PO q6–8h. Larger volumes and more frequent feedings are often accepted; feed as much as the rabbit will readily accept. Alternatively, pellets can be ground and mixed with fresh greens, vegetable baby foods, water, or juice to form a gruel. If sufficient volumes of food are not accepted in this manner, nasogastric intubation is indicated.
• High-carbohydrate, high-fat nutritional supplements are contraindicated.
• The diet should be permanently modified to include sufficient amounts of indigestible, coarse fiber. Offer long-stemmed grass or timothy hay (commercially available hay cubes are not sufficient) and an assortment of washed, fresh leafy greens. These foods should always constitute the bulk of the diet. Pellets should be limited (if offered at all) and foods high in simple carbohydrates prohibited or limited to the occasional treat.

## CLIENT EDUCATION
• Discuss possible complications prior to treatment, especially if surgery is required.
• Discuss the importance of dietary modification.
• Limit unsupervised access to objects commonly ingested from the environment, especially bedding and cloth.

## SURGICAL CONSIDERATIONS
• Gastrointestinal hypomotility—accumulation of inspissated gastric contents (including ingested hair) will usually pass with medical treatment alone; surgery is generally contraindicated in rabbits with gastrointestinal hypomotility. Surgical manipulation of the intestinal tract, hypothermia, anesthetic agents, and pain all exacerbate gastrointestinal hypomotility; gastrointestinal stasis is often worse postoperatively. The combination of these factors results in a significantly worsened prognosis with surgical treatment.
• Ingested foreign material—surgery may be indicated to remove foreign material such as cloth from the stomach; in extremely rare cases, inspissated ingesta forms a concretion in the stomach that does not respond to medical treatment.
• Acute gastric dilation due to small intestinal or pyloric foreign body—is a surgical emergency; patients usually present in shock and require decompression prior to surgery.
• If surgery is performed, the entire gastrointestinal tract and liver should be assessed, and biopsy specimens collected when indicated.

### Endoscopy
Objects in the stomach are rarely amenable to removal by flexible endoscopy. Endoscopy is less traumatic than surgery; however, object retrieval is usually impaired due to the presence of gastric ingesta, the small size of the patient, and subsequent limitations on instrument size.

# MEDICATIONS
Use parenteral medications in animals with severely compromised intestinal motility; oral medications may not be properly absorbed; begin oral medication when intestinal motility begins to return (fecal production, return of appetite, radiographic evidence)

## DRUG(S) OF CHOICE
• Motility modifiers may be helpful in rabbits with gastrointestinal hypomotility. Cisapride (0.5 mg/kg PO q8–12h) enhances gastric emptying and is available through many compounding pharmacies.
• Analgesics such as meloxicam (0.2 mg/kg SC, IM q24h or 0.2–0.5 mg/kg PO q24h), buprenorphine (0.01–0.05 mg/kg SC, IM, IV q8–12h), or flunixin meglumine (1.1 mg/kg SC, IM q12h for no more than 3 days) are essential to treatment of most rabbits with gastrointestinal hypomotility. Intestinal pain, either postoperative or from gas distention and ileus, impairs mobility and decreases appetite, and may severely inhibit recovery.

• Antibiotic therapy indicated in patients with acute gastric dilation; also indicated in patients with bacterial overgrowth that sometimes occurs secondary to gastrointestinal hypomotility (more common in patients that have been anorectic for several days) indicated in patients with diarrhea, abnormal fecal cytology, and disruption of the intestinal mucosa (evidenced by blood in the feces)
• When antibiotics are indicated, always use broad-spectrum antibiotics such as trimethoprim sulfa (30 mg/kg PO q12h) or enrofloxacin (5–20 mg/kg PO, SC, IM q12–24h).
• If secondary overgrowth of *Clostridium* spp. is evident, use metronidazole (20 mg/kg PO q12h).
• Simethicone 65–130 mg/rabbit q1h for two to three treatments may be helpful in alleviating painful intestinal gas.
• For sedation—light sedation with midazolam (0.5–2 mg/kg IM) or diazepam (1–2 mg/kg IM) many other sedation protocols exist.
• $H_2$-receptor antagonists may ameliorate or prevent gastric ulceration—cimetidine (5–10 mg/kg PO, SC, IM, IV q6–12h) or ranitidine (2 mg/kg IV q24h or 2–5 mg/kg PO q12h)

## CONTRAINDICATIONS
• The use of antibiotics that are primarily Gram positive in spectrum is contraindicated in rabbits. Use of these antibiotics will suppress the growth of commensal flora, allowing overgrowth of enteric pathogens. Do not orally administer lincomycin, clindamycin, erythromycin, ampicillin, amoxicillin cephalosporins, or penicillins.
• Prior to surgical removal, the use of gastrointestinal motility enhancers is contraindicated in rabbits with complete gastrointestinal tract obstruction due to the possibility of intestinal rupture.
• Corticosteroids—avoid; associated with gastrointestinal ulceration and hemorrhage, delayed wound healing, and heightened susceptibility to infection; rabbits are very sensitive to the immunosuppressive effects of both topic and systemic corticosteroids; use may exacerbate subclinical bacterial infection.

## PRECAUTIONS
• NSAIDs—use with caution in rabbits with compromised renal function; avoid until shock and hypovolemia are corrected; do not use if gastric ulceration is present.
• Oral administration of any antibiotic may potentially cause enteric dysbiosis; discontinue use if diarrhea or anorexia occurs.

## POSSIBLE INTERACTIONS
N/A

# GASTROINTESTINAL FOREIGN BODIES

## ALTERNATIVE DRUGS

• Metoclopramide (0.2–0.05 mg/kg PO, SC q6–8h)—has also been used as a gastrointestinal promotility agent; efficacy is questionable.

• Enzymatic digestion of small trichobezoars with fresh pineapple juice, papaya extract, or pancreatic enzymes has been advocated. However, these substances should be used with caution (or preferably, not at all), as they may exacerbate gastric mucosal ulceration/erosions and may contribute to gastric rupture. Additionally, these substances do nothing to treat the underlying cause of trichobezoars, gastrointestinal hypomotility.

• Intestinal lubricants such as cat laxatives are unlikely to aid in the passage of trichobezoars as they simply lubricate the intestinal contents and do nothing to treat the underlying motility disorder.

• The addition of psyllium-based food supplements is not an adequate substitution for long-stemmed hay in the diet.

## FOLLOW-UP

### PATIENT MONITORING

• Monitor all patients for return of appetite and production of fecal pellets, indicating successful treatment.

• Surgical patients—after the foreign body has been removed, assess the mucosa for damage. Mucosal ulceration may occur due to mucosal injury. Usually, the degree of mucosal injury is proportional to the length of time the object is within the gastrointestinal tract and the texture of the object.

• Anesthetic agents used during surgical removal of foreign bodies contribute to gastrointestinal hypomotility and subsequent overgrowth of toxin-forming bacteria. Rabbits with postoperative gastrointestinal stasis are anorectic and produce little to no feces. Be certain that postoperative patients are eating and passing feces prior to release.

• Monitor the patient for at least 2 months after the foreign body removal for evidence of stricture formation at the site of the foreign body or intraabdominal adhesions.

### PREVENTION/AVOIDANCE

• Strict feeding of diets containing adequate amounts of indigestible coarse fiber (long-stemmed hay) and low simple carbohydrate content along with access to fresh water will often prevent episodes.

• The rabbit should be closely supervised during times when access to potential foreign bodies is likely.

• Regularly brush rabbits to remove shed hair and prevent ingestion.

### POSSIBLE COMPLICATIONS

• Persistent ileus and death

• Postoperative gastrointestinal stasis and subsequent overgrowth of bacterial pathogens

• Stricture formation at the site of removal; intraabdominal adhesions postoperatively

• Death due to gastric rupture

### EXPECTED COURSE AND PROGNOSIS

• The prognosis is dependent upon the chronicity of obstruction, the extent of gastrointestinal mucosal damage, and the degree of disruption of enteric commensal flora.

• Early medical management of animals with gastrointestinal hypomotility usually carries a good to excellent prognosis.

• The prognosis following surgical removal of foreign material or acute small intestinal obstructions is guarded to poor. Patients recovering well after 7 days appear to have a good prognosis for complete recovery.

## MISCELLANEOUS

### ASSOCIATED CONDITIONS

• Bacterial dysbiosis
• Bacterial endotoxemia
• Hepatic lipidosis
• Dental disease
• Hypercalciuria

### AGE-RELATED FACTORS

Middle-aged to older rabbits are more likely to develop gastrointestinal hypomotility or ingest foreign material (carpet, cloth).

### ZOONOTIC POTENTIAL

N/A

### PREGNANCY

N/A

### SYNONYMS

Wool block

### SEE ALSO

• Clostridial enterotoxemia
• Gastric dilation
• Gastrointestinal hypomotility

### ABBREVIATIONS

• ALT = alanine aminotransferase
• LRS = lactated Ringer's solution
• NSAIDs = nonsteroidal antiinflammatory drugs
• NPO = nothing by mouth
• PCV = packed cell volume
• TS = total solids

*Suggested Reading*

Brown SA, Rosenthal KL. The anorexic rabbit. Proc North Am Vet Conf, 1997:788.

Cheeke PR. Rabbit Feeding and Nutrition. Orlando, FL: Academic Press, 1987.

Donoghue S. Nutrition and pet rabbits. In: Rosenthal KL, ed. Practical Exotic Animal Medicine: The Compendium Collection. Trenton, NJ: Veterinary Learning Systems, 1997:107.

Jenkins JR. Feeding recommendations for the house rabbit. Vet Clin Noth Am Exotic Anim Pract 1999;2(1):143–151.

Jenkins JR. Gastrointestinal diseases. In: Quesenberry KE, Carpenter JW, eds. Ferrets, Rabbits and Rodents: Clinical Medicine and Surgery. 2nd Ed. Philadelphia: WB Saunders, 2004:161–171.

Paul-Murphy JA, Ramer JC. Urgent care of the pet rabbits. Vet Clin North Am Exotic Anim Pract 1998;1(1):127–152.

Rees Davies R, Rees Davies JAE. Rabbit gastrointestinal physiology. Vet Clin North Am Exotic Anim Pract 2003;6(1):139–153.

# GASTROINTESTINAL HYPOMOTILITY AND GASTROINTESTINAL STASIS

 BASICS

## DEFINITION
• Gastrointestinal hypomotility—increased gastrointestinal transit time characterized by decreased frequency of cecocolonic segmental contractions
• Gastrointestinal stasis—severe ileus with little to no caudal movement of ingesta

## PATHOPHYSIOLOGY
• Rabbits are hind-gut fermenters and are extremely sensitive to alterations in diet.
• Proper hind-gut fermentation and gastrointestinal tract motility are dependent on the ingestion of large amounts of roughage and long-stemmed hay. Diets that contain inadequate amounts of long-stemmed, coarse fiber (such as the feeding of only commercial pelleted food without hay or grasses) cause gastrointestinal tract hypomotility.
• The presence of "hairballs" or trichobezoars in the stomach is not a disease, but a symptom or consequence of gastrointestinal hypomotility or stasis. Rabbits normally ingest hair during grooming. Healthy rabbits will always have some amount of hair and ingesta in the stomach. These stomach contents are both palpable and visible radiographically in the normal, healthy rabbit.
• With proper nutrition and gastrointestinal tract motility, fur ingested as a result of normal grooming behavior and some small or easily deformed foreign bodies will pass through the gastrointestinal tract with the ingesta uneventfully.
• When gastrointestinal motility slows or stops, ingesta, including fur and other material, accumulates in the stomach. Rabbits cannot vomit to expel nonfood contents from the stomach.
• Dehydration of stomach contents often occurs, making the contents more difficult to pass. With medical treatment of gastrointestinal hypomotility, motility usually returns, stomach contents soften, and hair and other ingesta will usually pass. Without treatment, rentention of inspissated gastric contents and subsequent metabolic derangements combined with shifts in intestinal microbial flora can be fatal.
• Affected rabbits suddenly or gradually refuse food; as motility slows, ingesta accumulates proximal to the colon (stomach, cecum); fecal pellets become small and scant; water is removed from fecal pellets in the colon, making the fecal pellets drier than normal.
• Cecocolonic hypomotility also causes alterations in cecal fermentation, pH, and substrate production resulting in alteration of enteric microflora populations. Diets low in coarse fiber typically contain high simple carbohydrate concentrations, which provide a ready source of fermentable products and promote the growth of bacterial pathogens such as *Escherichia coli* and *Clostridium* spp. Bacterial dysbiosis can cause acute diarrhea, enterotoxemia, ileus, or chronic intermittent diarrhea.
• Anorexia due to infectious or metabolic disease, pain, stress, or starvation may cause or exacerbate gastrointestinal hypomotility.
• The process is often self-perpetuating; gastrointestinal hypomotility and dehydration promote anorexia and exacerbation of stasis.

## SYSTEMS AFFECTED
• Gastrointestinal
• Musculoskeletal—loss of muscle mass may occur due to inappetence.

## INCIDENCE/PREVALENCE
Gastrointestinal hypomotility resulting in scant or lack of feces, chronic intermittent diarrhea, abdominal pain, and ill-thrift is one of the most common clinical problems seen in the rabbit.

## SIGNALMENT
• More commonly seen in middle-aged to older rabbits on inappropriate diets, but can occur in any-aged rabbit
• No breed or gender predilections

## SIGNS
### Historical Findings
• History of inappropriate diet (e.g., cereals, grains, commercial pellets only, sweets, large quantities of fruits, lack of feeding long-stemmed hay)
• Recent history of illness or stressful event
• History of decreased activity—cage confinement, orthopedic or neuromuscular disease
• Weight loss in rabbits with underlying or chronic disease
• Obesity in rabbits on diets consisting of mainly commercial pellets
• Patients are usually bright and alert, except for those with enterotoxemia or acute small intestinal obstruction (gastric dilation), which are depressed, lethargic, or shocky.
• Inappetence or anorexia is the most common sign. Rabbits often initially stop eating pellets but continue to eat treats, followed by complete anorexia.
• Fecal pellets often become scant and small in size; no fecal pellets produced with complete gastrointestinal stasis
• Signs of pain, such as teeth grinding, a hunched posture, and reluctance to move, are common.
• Chronic, intermittent diarrhea characterized by soft, sticky stools

### Physical Examination Findings
• Small, hard fecal pellets or absence of fecal pellets palpable in the colon; examine feces in cage or carrier—appear small, firm, and scant with gastrointestinal hypomotility
• Cecum may be filled with gas, fluid, or firm, dry contents, depending on the underlying cause.
• Palpation of the stomach is an extremely valuable tool in the diagnosis of abnormal retention of stomach contents. Ingesta normally should be palpable in the stomach of a healthy rabbit. The normal stomach should be easily deformable, feel soft and pliable, and not remain pitted on compression. Rabbits with early gastrointestinal hypomotility will have a firm, often enlarged stomach that remains pitted when compressed. With complete gastrointestinal stasis, severe dehydration, or prolonged hypomotility, the stomach may be severely distended, hard, and nondeformable.
• The presence of firm ingesta in the stomach of a rabbit that has been anorectic for 1–3 days is compatible with the diagnosis of gastrointestinal hypomotility.
• Little or no borborygmus is heard on abdominal auscultation in rabbits with gastrointestinal hypomotility.
• Other physical examination findings depend on the underlying cause; perform a complete physical examination, including a thorough oral examination.

## CAUSES AND RISK FACTORS
### Dietary and Environmental Causes
• In the majority of cases, gastrointestinal hypomotility is caused by feeding diets with insufficient roughage such as grasses and long-stemmed hay and/or excessive simple carbohydrate content. Examples of improper diets include a diet consisting primarily of commercial pellets, especially those containing seeds, oats, or other high-carbohydrate treats; feeding of cereal products (bread, crackers, breakfast cereals); and feeding large amounts of fruits containing simple carbohydrates. Proper hind-gut fermentation and gastrointestinal motility rely on large quantities of indigestible coarse fiber, as found in long-stemmed hay and grasses. Most commercial pelleted diets contain inadequate roughage, coarse fiber, and excessive calories. This high caloric content often contributes to obesity and hepatic lipidosis, both of which may exacerbate intestinal disease.
• Hair—excessive consumption (barbering) may contribute; a craving for fiber due to a fiber-deficient diet may contribute to barbering. However, ingestion of hair is normal in rabbits and, if the gastrointestinal tract is functioning normally, hair will pass uneventfully. Consumption of a whole, large hair mat may act as a small intestinal foreign body.

# GASTROINTESTINAL HYPOMOTILITY AND GASTROINTESTINAL STASIS

• Foreign material—ingestion of cloth (towels, carpeting, etc.) may cause gastrointestinal tract obstruction; scoopable cat litters can cause severe cecal impaction.

• Change of environment—hospitalization, boarding; can cause significant stress and contribute to gastrointestinal hypomotility

• New animals in the household, social stress, fighting

• Lack of exercise (cage confinement, obesity)—often a significant contributing factor

## Drugs

• Anesthetic agents may cause or exacerbate gastrointestinal hypomotility.

• Anticholinergics

• Opioids

## Anorexia or Inappetence

Conditions that result in inappetence or anorexia may also cause gastrointestinal hypomotility. Common causes of anorexia include dental disease (malocclusion, molar elongation, tooth root abscesses), metabolic disease (renal disease, liver disease), pain (oral, trauma, postoperative pain, adhesions), neoplasia (gastrointestinal, uterine), toxins, changes in the environment, or accidental starvation.

# DIAGNOSIS

## DIFFERENTIAL DIAGNOSIS

• It is important to differentiate acute pyloric or small intestinal obstruction from gastrointestinal hypomotility, as acute intestinal obstruction is usually a life-threatening emergency. With acute gastrointestinal obstruction—acute-onset of anorexia, abdominal pain, reluctance to move, often progresses to lateral recumbency and signs of hypovolemic shock (e.g., pale mucous membranes, decreased capillary refill time, weak pulses, hypothermic). Stomach is severely distended, tympanic, and full of gas and/or fluid. Patients are often in shock and require emergency decompression. Monitor rectal temperature; rabbits that become hypothermic are critically ill.

• For palpable mass in the cranial abdomen—neoplasia, abscess, hepatomegaly, normal gastric contents

• For anorexia—dental disease, metabolic disease, pain, neoplasia, cardiac disease, toxin

• For decreased fecal output—anorexia, intestinal foreign body, intussusception, intestinal neoplasia

• For chronic, intermittent diarrhea—cecotrophs, bacterial or parasitic infections, alterations in gastrointestinal tract flora due to antibiotic use or stress, partial obstruction by gastrointestinal foreign body or neoplasia, infiltrative bowel disease

## CBC/BIOCHEMISTRY/URINALYSIS

• These tests are often normal.

• May be used to identify underlying causes of gastrointestinal hypomotility or anorexia

• PCV and TS elevation in dehydrated patients

• Serum ALT elevation in rabbits with liver disease, especially lipidosis

• If the intestinal tract has been perforated, an inflammatory leukogram may be seen.

## OTHER LABORATORY TESTS
N/A

## IMAGING

### Radiography

• Rabbits should not be fasted prior to taking radiographs.

• Gastric contents (primarily food and hair) are normally present and visible radiographically, even if the rabbit has been inappetent. The presence of ingesta (including hair) in the stomach is a normal finding.

• Moderate to severe distension of the stomach with ingesta is usually visible with gastrointestinal hypomotility. In some rabbits with gastrointestinal stasis, a halo of gas can be observed around the inspissated stomach contents. Gas distension is also common throughout the intestinal tract, including the cecum in rabbits with gastrointestinal hypomotility or stasis.

• Small fecal balls or the absence of fecal balls in the colon is highly suggestive.

• Severe distention of the stomach with fluid and/or gas is usually seen with acute small intestinal obstructions and usually constitutes an emergency.

## OTHER DIAGNOSTIC PROCEDURES
N/A

## PATHOLOGIC FINDINGS
N/A

# TREATMENT

## APPROPRIATE HEALTH CARE

• Rabbits that have been anorectic for 1–3 days should be evaluated and treated as soon as possible.

• Rabbits that have been anorectic for >3 days should be seen on an emergency basis.

## NURSING CARE

### Fluid Therapy

• Fluid therapy is an essential component of the medical management of all patients with gastrointestinal hypomotility. Administer both oral and parenteral fluids. Oral fluid administration will aid in the rehydration of inspissated gastric contents. Mildly affected rabbits will usually respond well to oral and subcutaneous fluid administration, treatment with intestinal motility modifiers,

analgesics, and dietary modification described below.

• Intravenous or intraosseous fluids are required in patients that are severely dehydrated or depressed and to replace fluid losses from acute diarrhea. Maintenance fluid requirements are estimated at 100 mL/kg/day.

• Rehydration is essential to treatment success in severely ill rabbits. Initially, a balanced fluid (e.g., lactated Ringer's solution) may be used.

• A warm, quiet environment should be provided.

## ACTIVITY

If patient is not debilitated, encourage exercise (hopping) for at least 10–15 minutes every 6–8 hours since activity promotes gastric motility; provide supervised freedom from the cage or access to a safe grazing area.

## DIET

• It is absolutely imperative that the rabbit continue to eat during and following treatment. Continued anorexia will exacerbate gastrointestinal hypomotility and cause further derangement of the gastrointestinal microflora and overgrowth of intestinal bacterial pathogens.

• Offer a large selection of fresh, moistened greens such as cilantro, romaine lettuce, parsley, carrot tops, dandelion greens, spinach, collard greens, etc., and good-quality grass hay. Many rabbits will begin to eat these foods, even if they were previously anorectic. Also offer the rabbit's usual, pelleted diet, as the initial goal is to get the rabbit to eat.

• If the patient refuses these foods, syringe feed a gruel such as Critical Care for Herbivores (Oxbow Pet Products, Murdock, NE) 10–15 mL/kg PO q6–8h. Larger volumes and more frequent feedings are often accepted; feed as much as the rabbit will readily accept. Alternatively, pellets can be ground and mixed with fresh greens, vegetable baby foods, water, or juice to form a gruel. If sufficient volumes of food are not accepted in this manner, nasogastric intubation is indicated.

• High-carbohydrate, high-fat nutritional supplements are contraindicated.

• Encourage oral fluid intake by offering fresh water, wetting leafy vegetables, or flavoring water with vegetable juices.

• The diet should be permanently modified to include sufficient amounts of indigestible, coarse fiber. Offer long-stemmed grass or timothy hay (commercially available hay cubes are not sufficient) and an assortment of washed, fresh leafy greens. These foods should always constitute the bulk of the diet. Pellets should be limited (if

# GASTROINTESTINAL HYPOMOTILITY AND GASTROINTESTINAL STASIS

offered at all) and foods high in simple carbohydrates prohibited or limited to the occasional treat.

## CLIENT EDUCATION

• Discuss the importance of dietary modification and increasing activity level.
• Advise owners to regularly monitor food consumption and fecal output; seek veterinary attention with a noticeable decrease in either.

## SURGICAL CONSIDERATIONS

• Gastrointestinal hypomotility—accumulation of inspissated gastric contents (including ingested hair) will usually pass with medical treatment alone; surgery is generally contraindicated in rabbits with gastrointestinal hypomotility. Surgical manipulation of the intestinal tract, hypothermia, anesthetic agents, and pain all exacerbate gastrointestinal hypomotility; gastrointestinal stasis is often worse postoperatively. The combination of these factors results in a significantly worsened prognosis with surgical treatment.
• Ingested foreign material—surgery may be indicated to remove foreign material such as cloth from the stomach; in extremely rare cases, inspissated ingesta forms a concretion in the stomach that does not respond to medical treatment alone.
• Acute gastric dilation due to small intestinal or pyloric foreign body—is a surgical emergency; patients usually present in shock and require decompression prior to surgery.

## MEDICATIONS

Use parenteral medications in animals with severely compromised intestinal motility; oral medications may not be properly absorbed; begin oral medication when intestinal motility begins to return (fecal production, return of appetite, radiographic evidence).

## DRUG(S) OF CHOICE

• Motility modifiers may be helpful in rabbits with gastrointestinal hypomotility. Cisapride (0.5 mg/kg PO q8–12h) enhances gastric emptying and is available through many compounding pharmacies.
• Analgesics such as meloxicam (0.2 mg/kg SC, IM q24h or 0.2–0.5 mg/kg PO q24h), or buprenorphine (0.01–0.05 mg/kg SC, IM, IV q8–12h) are essential for treatment of most rabbits with gastrointestinal hypomotility. Intestinal pain, either postoperative or from gas distention and ileus, impairs mobility and decreases appetite, and may severely inhibit recovery.
• Antibiotic therapy—indicated in patients with bacterial overgrowth that sometimes occurs secondary to gastrointestinal hypo-

motility; more common in patients that have been anorectic for several days. Indicated in patients with diarrhea, abnormal fecal cytology, and disruption of the intestinal mucosa (evidenced by blood in the feces)
• When antibiotics are indicated, always use broad-spectrum antibiotics such as trimethoprim sulfa (30 mg/kg PO q12h) or enrofloxacin (5–20 mg/kg PO, SC, IM q12–24h)
• If secondary overgrowth of *Clostridium* spp. is evident, use metronidazole (20 mg/kg PO q12h).

### Other Treatment

• $H_2$-receptor antagonists may ameliorate or prevent gastric ulceration: cimetidine (5–10 mg/kg PO, SC, IM, IV q6–12h) and ranitidine (2 mg/kg IV q24h or 2–5 mg/kg PO q12h)
• Simethicone 65–130 mg/rabbit q1h for two to three treatments may be helpful in alleviating painful intestinal gas.

## CONTRAINDICATIONS

• The use of antibiotics that are primarily Gram positive in spectrum is contraindicated in rabbits. Use of these antibiotics will suppress the growth of commensal flora, allowing overgrowth of enteric pathogens. Do not orally administer lincomycin, clindamycin, erythromycin, ampicillin, amoxicillin cephalosporins, or penicillins.
• The use of gastrointestinal motility enhancers is contraindicated in rabbits with complete gastrointestinal tract obstruction due to the possibility of intestinal rupture.

## PRECAUTIONS

• NSAIDs—use with caution in rabbits with compromised renal function or if gastric ulceration is suspected.
• Oral administration of any antibiotic may potentially cause enteric dysbiosis; discontinue use if diarrhea or anorexia occurs.

## POSSIBLE INTERACTIONS

N/A

## ALTERNATIVE DRUGS

• Metoclopramide (0.2–0.05 mg/kg PO, SC q6–8h) has also been used as a gastrointestinal promotility agent; efficacy is questionable.
• Enzymatic digestion of small trichobezoars with fresh pineapple juice, papaya extract, or pancreatic enzymes has been advocated. However, these substances should be used with caution (or preferably, not at all), as they may exacerbate gastric mucosal ulceration/erosions and may contribute to gastric rupture. Additionally, these substances do nothing to treat the underlying cause of trichobezoars, gastrointestinal hypomotility.
• Intestinal lubricants such as cat laxatives are unlikely to aid in the passage of tri-

chobezoars as they simply lubricate the intestinal contents and do nothing to treat the underlying motility disorder.
• The addition of psyllium-based food supplements is not an adequate substitution for long-stemmed hay in the diet.

## FOLLOW-UP

### PATIENT MONITORING

Monitor hydration, appetite, and production of fecal pellets. Rabbits that are successfully treated will regain a normal appetite and begin to produce normal volumes of feces. Initially, the fecal pellets are sometimes expelled bound together with hair.

### PREVENTION/AVOIDANCE

• Strict feeding of diets containing adequate amounts of indigestible coarse fiber (long-stemmed hay) and low simple carbohydrate content along with access to fresh water will often prevent episodes.
• Allow sufficient daily exercise.
• Prevent obesity.
• Be certain that all postoperative patients are eating and passing feces prior to release.

### POSSIBLE COMPLICATIONS

• Continued ileus leading to metabolic derangements and death
• Death due to gastric rupture
• Overgrowth of bacterial pathogens; clostridial enterotoxicosis

### EXPECTED COURSE AND PROGNOSIS

• Depends on the underlying cause
• Chronic intermittent diarrhea—excellent to good prognosis with proper dietary modification
• Early medical management of animals with gastrointestinal hypomotility carries a good to excellent prognosis.
• The prognosis following gastrotomy or enterotomy is guarded to poor. Most patients will survive the surgery, but gastrointestinal tract motility may never return to normal.

## MISCELLANEOUS

### ASSOCIATED CONDITIONS

• Dental disease
• Hypercalciuria
• Hepatic lipidosis
• Bacterial dysbiosis
• Bacterial endotoxemia

### AGE-RELATED FACTORS

Middle-aged to older rabbits on a poor diet are more likely to develop gastrointestinal hypomotility.

### ZOONOTIC POTENTIAL

N/A

# GASTROINTESTINAL HYPOMOTILITY AND GASTROINTESTINAL STASIS

**PREGNANCY**
N/A

**SYNONYMS**
Wool block

**SEE ALSO**
• Anorexia
• Clostridial enterotoxicosis
• Diarrhea, chronic

**ABBREVIATIONS**
• ALT = alanine aminotransferase
• NSAIDs = nonsteroidal antiinflammatory drugs
• PCV = packed cell volume
• TS = total solids

*Suggested Reading*

Brown, SA, Rosenthal KL. The anorexic rabbit. Proc North Am Vet Conf, 1997:788.

Cheeke PR. Rabbit Feeding and Nutrition. Orlando, FL: Academic Press, 1987.

Donoghue S. Nutrition and pet rabbits. In: Rosenthal KL, ed. Practical Exotic Animal Medicine: The Compendium Collection. Trenton, NJ: Veterinary Learning Systems, 1997:107.

Jenkins JR. Feeding recommendations for the house rabbit. Vet Clin North Am Exotic Anim Pract 1999;2(1):143–151.

Jenkins JR. Gastrointestinal diseases. In: Quesenberry KE, Carpenter JW, eds. Ferrets, Rabbits and Rodents: Clinical Medicine and Surgery. 2nd Ed. Philadelphia: WB Saunders, 2004:161–171.

Paul-Murphy JA, Ramer JC. Urgent care of the pet rabbits. Vet Clin North Am Exotic Anim Pract 1998;1(1):127–152.

Rees Davies R, Rees Davies JAE. Rabbit gastrointestinal physiology. Vet Clin North Am Exotic Anim Pract 2003;6(1):139–153.

# HEAD TILT (VESTIBULAR DISEASE)

 **BASICS**

## DEFINITION
Tilting of the head away from its normal orientation with the trunk and limbs; associated with disorders of the vestibular system

## PATHOPHYSIOLOGY
• Vestibular system—coordinates position and movement of the head with that of the eyes, trunk, and limbs by detecting linear acceleration and rotational movements of the head; includes vestibular nuclei in the rostral medulla of the brainstem, vestibular portion of the vestibulocochlear nerve (cranial nerve VIII), and receptors in the semicircular canals of the inner ear
• Head tilt—most consistent sign of diseases affecting the vestibular system and its projections to the cerebellum, spinal cord, cerebral cortex, reticular formation, and extraocular eye muscles
• In rabbits, vestibular disease is most commonly caused by bacterial otitis interna/media, brain abscess, *Encephalitozoon cuniculi* infection, or trauma.

## SYSTEMS AFFECTED
• Nervous—peripheral or CNS
• Gastrointestinal—associated nausea, inappetence

## SIGNALMENT
• Lop-eared rabbits may be more likely to show signs of otitis externa.
• Dwarf breeds and older and immunosuppressed rabbits may be more predisposed to signs due to infection with *E. cuniculi.*

## SIGNS
• Often acute presentation regardless of the cause
• Often severe initially—see rolling, torticollis, lateral recumbency, unable or unwilling to lift head from the ground
• Head tilt usually accompanied by other vestibular signs; abnormal nystagmus (resting, positional); mild ventral deviation of the eye (vestibular strabismus); ataxia and disequilibrium with a tendency to fall, lean, or roll toward the side of the tilt; often acute in onset
• Peripheral deficits—horizontal or rotatory nystagmus with fast phase in the direction opposite the head tilt; patient may have concomitant ipsilateral facial nerve paresis or paralysis.
• Central deficits—vertical, horizontal, or rotatory nystagmus that can change with the position of the head; altered mentation possible; ipsilateral paresis or proprioceptive deficits possible; other signs related to the cerebellum such as intention tremors possible
• Rolling common with both peripheral and central disease

• Anorexia, inappetence due to nausea
• Nasal/ocular discharge—historical or present on physical examination; spread of upper respiratory infection to inner/middle ear common
• In rabbits with otitis externa, thick, white, creamy exudate may be found in the horizontal and/or vertical canals.
• In rabbits with otitis media only, the external canal may have a normal appearance on otoscopic examination, but the tympanum bulges out into the external canal and a white, creamy exudate can sometimes be seen behind the tympanum.
• Some rabbits with otitis internal media have no visible otoscopic lesions.

## CAUSES
### Peripheral Disease
• Inflammatory—otitis media and interna most common cause; primarily bacterial but occasionally related to parasitic (e.g., *Psoroptes cuniculi*) and fungal origins. *Pasteurella multocida, Staphylococcus aureus, Pseudomonas aeruginosa, Escherichia coli* and *Listeria monocytogenes* most often cultured in otitis media/interna; foreign body (rare)
• Idiopathic—not well described in rabbits; however, a definitive diagnosis is often not found, and many rabbits improve with supportive care.
• Traumatic—tympanic bulla or petrosal bone fracture; aggressive ear flush
• Neoplastic—neoplasia of the bone and surrounding tissue (rare)
• Toxic—lead; aminoglycosides
• Metabolic and immune mediated—not described in rabbits

### Central Disease
*Inflammatory, Infectious*
• Bacterial—most common cause; central erosion caused by otitis media and interna; encephalitis due to *Pasteurella* spp. or other bacteria
• Protozoal—*E. cuniculi* infections are believed to be a very common cause of vestibular disease in rabbits; however, the prevalence of *E. cuniculi* as a cause of CNS disease is controversial since definitive antemortem diagnosis is not possible and postmortem lesions do not always correlate well with clinical disease; toxoplasmosis (rare)
• Aberrant larval migrans—*Baylisascaris* sp. (raccoon roundworm)
• Viral—rabies very rarely reported, but should be considered in any rabbit with neurologic disease; herpesvirus also described
• Fungal (e.g., cryptococcosis, blastomycosis, histoplasmosis)—not yet described in rabbits
*Inflammatory, Noninfectious*
Granulomatous meningoencephalomyelitis—common postmortem finding in rabbits both with and without ante-

mortem signs of vestibular disease; has been attributed to *E. cuniculi* infection, but organisms not always found
*Degenerative*
Demyelinating disease; vascular event; incidence unknown
*Trauma*
Bone fracture with brainstem injury
*Neoplastic*
Nervous system neoplasia rarely reported in rabbits; skull tumor (e.g., osteosarcoma); metastasis (e.g., hemangiosarcoma and melanoma)
*Nutritional*
Hypovitaminosis A (rare)
*Toxic*
Lead; metronidazole (rare)

## RISK FACTORS
• Immunosuppression, especially for *E. cuniculi* or bacterial infection—predisposes to clinical disease: stress, poor diet, concurrent disease, and glucocorticoid or antitumor chemotherapy
• For otitis interna/media—abnormal or breed-related conformation of the external canal (e.g., stenosis, lop-eared breeds); excessive moisture (e.g., from frequent cleanings with improper solutions) can lead to infection.

 **DIAGNOSIS**

## DIFFERENTIAL DIAGNOSIS
### General Comments
Every attempt should be made to rule out otic disease prior to assuming *E. cuniculi* infection. Antemortem diagnosis of *E. cuniculi* is presumed based on clinical signs, exclusion of other diagnoses, positive antibody titers, and, sometimes, response to treatment. Definitive antemortem diagnosis is problematic, since a positive antibody titer indicates exposure only, some rabbits respond minimally or not at all to anthelmintic treatment, and many rabbits will improve spontaneously with supportive care alone. Definitive diagnosis requires identification of organisms and characteristic inflammation in affected tissues that anatomically correlate with clinical signs; generally acquired at postmortem examination

### Nonvestibular Head Tilt and Head Posture
• Be sure that abnormal head posture is not due to holding one ear down due to pain, as may occur in otitis externa/media alone, and is not associated with vestibular pathology.
• Rabbits with vestibular dysfunction demonstrate nystagmus, torticollis, ataxia, and/or tremors in addition to head tilt.

## CBC/BIOCHEMISTRY/URINALYSIS
• Usually normal
• May reflect underlying disorder in stressed immunosuppressed rabbits

## OTHER LABORATORY TESTS
• Serologic testing for *E. cuniculi*—many tests are available, but usefulness is extremely limited since a positive titer indicates only exposure and does not confirm *E. cuniculi* as the cause of neurologic signs. *E. cuniculi* can only be definitively diagnosed by finding organisms and resultant lesions on histopathologic examination in areas that anatomically correlate with observed clinical signs. Antibody titers usually become positive by 2 weeks postinfection, but generally do not continue to rise with active infection or decline with treatment. No correlation exists between antibody titers and shedding of organism and presence or severity of disease. It is unknown if exposed rabbits eventually become seronegative. Available tests include ELISA, indirect IFA, and carbon immunoassay.
• Serology for *Pasteurella*—usefulness is severely limited and generally not helpful in the diagnosis of pasteurellosis in pet rabbits. An ELISA is available and results are reported as negative, low positive, or high positive. Positive results, even when high, only indicate prior exposure to *Pasteurella* and the development of antibodies and do not confirm active infection. Low-positive results may occur due to cross-reaction with other, nonpathogenic bacteria (false positive). False-negative results are common with immunosuppression or early infection. No evidence exists to support correlation of titers to the presence or absence of disease.
• Bacterial culture and sensitivity testing—sample from myringotomy or surgical drainage of tympanic bulla if otitis media or interna is suspected.
• Microscopic examination of ear swab

## IMAGING
• Tympanic bullae and skull radiography—may help rule out otitis interna/media; however, normal radiographs do not rule out bulla disease.
• CT and MRI—valuable for confirming bulla lesions and CNS extension from otitis or to document localized tumor, granuloma, and extent of inflammation

## DIAGNOSTIC PROCEDURES
• Otoscopic examination—in rabbits with otitis externa, thick, white, creamy exudate may be found in the horizontal and/or vertical canals. Otitis interna/media may occur in the absence of otitis externa via extension through the eustachian tube; may see bulging tympanum. Some rabbits with otitis interna have no visible otoscopic abnormalities.

• CSF analysis—sample from the cerebellomedullary cistern; may be valuable for evaluating central vestibular disease; detects inflammatory process; sample collection may put the patient at risk for herniation if there is a mass or high intracranial pressure.
• Biopsy—when a tumor or osteomyelitis is suspected

## TREATMENT

### APPROPRIATE HEALTH CARE
Inpatient vs. outpatient—depends on severity of the signs (especially vestibular ataxia and need for supportive care)

### NURSING CARE
• Supportive fluids—replacement or maintenance fluids (depend on clinical state); may be required in the acute phase when disorientation and nausea preclude oral intake
• Drug affecting vestibular function—discontinue offending agent; signs are usually, but not always, reversible.
• Trauma—supportive care (e.g., antiinflammatory drugs, antibiotics, intravenous fluid administration); specific fracture repair or hematoma removal is difficult, considering the location.

### ACTIVITY
Restrict (e.g., avoid stairs and slippery surfaces) according to the degree of disequilibrium; encourage return to activity as soon as safely possible; activity may enhance recovery of vestibular function.

### DIET
• It is absolutely imperative that the rabbit continue to eat during and following treatment. Anorexia will often cause gastrointestinal hypomotility, derangement of the gastrointestinal microflora, and overgrowth of intestinal bacterial pathogens.
• Offer a large selection of fresh, moistened greens such as cilantro, romaine lettuce, parsley, carrot tops, dandelion greens, spinach, collard greens, etc., and good-quality grass hay. Many rabbits will begin to eat these foods, even if they were previously anorectic. Also, try offering the rabbit's usual pelleted diet, as the initial goal is to get the rabbit to eat. Bring the food to the rabbit if nonambulatory, or offer food by hand.
• If the patient refuses these foods, syringe feed a gruel such as Critical Care for Herbivores (Oxbow Pet Products, Murdock, NE) 10–15 mL/kg PO q6–8h. Larger volumes and more frequent feedings are often accepted; feed as much as the rabbit will readily accept. Alternatively, pellets can be ground and mixed with fresh greens, vegetable baby foods, water, or juice to form a gruel.

• High-carbohydrate, high-fat nutritional supplements are contraindicated.
• Encourage oral fluid intake by offering fresh water, wetting leafy vegetables, or flavoring water with vegetable juices.
CAUTION: Be aware of aspiration secondary to abnormal body posture in patients with severe head tilt and vestibular disequilibrium or brainstem dysfunction.

### CLIENT EDUCATION
• Advise client that the prognosis for central vestibular disorders is usually poorer than that for peripheral disorders.

### SURGICAL CONSIDERATIONS
Total ear canal ablation and/or bullae osteotomy may be required to treat bulla disease and otitis media or interna; surgical resection of abscess or tumor may be indicated, if accessible; vestibular signs may persist following surgery.

## MEDICATIONS

### DRUG(S) OF CHOICE
• Otitis media or interna, bacterial encephalitis—antibiotics; choice is ideally based on results of culture and susceptibility testing, if possible. Depending on the severity of infection, long-term antibiotic therapy is required (4–6 weeks minimum to several months). Use broad-spectrum antibiotics such as enrofloxacin (5–20 mg/kg PO, SC, IM q12–24h) or trimethoprim sulfa (30 mg/kg PO q12h); if anaerobic infections are suspected, use chloramphenicol (50 mg/kg PO q8h) or azithromycin (30 mg/kg PO q24h); can be used alone or combined with metronidazole (20 mg/kg PO q24h). Alternatively, use penicillin g (40,000–60,000 IU/kg SC q2–7d).
• *E. cuniculi*—benzimidazole anthelmintics are effective against *E cuniculi* in vitro and have been shown to prevent experimental infection in rabbits. However, efficacy in rabbits with clinical signs is unknown. Anecdotal reports suggest a response to treatment; however, many rabbits with neurologic signs improve with or without treatment. Published treatments include oxibendazole (20 mg/kg PO q24h × 7–14 days, then reduce to 15 mg/kg q24h × 30–60 days), albendazole (20–30 mg/kg q24h × 30 days, then 15 mg/kg PO q24h × 30 days), and fenbendazole (20 mg/kg q24h × 5–28 days).
• Severe vestibular signs (continuous rolling, torticollis) or seizures—diazepam 1–2 mg/kg IM or midazolam 1–2 mg/kg IM
• Meclizine (2–12 mg/kg PO q8–12h) may reduce clinical signs, control nausea, and induce mild sedation.

# HEAD TILT (VESTIBULAR DISEASE)

## CONTRAINDICATIONS
• Oral administration of antibiotics that select against Gram-positive bacteria (penicillins, macrolides, lincosamides, and cephalosporins) can cause fatal enteric dysbiosis and enterotoxemia.
• Drugs potentially toxic to the vestibular system—aminoglycoside antibiotics; prolonged high-dose metronidazole

## PRECAUTIONS
• Topical and systemic corticosteroids—rabbits are very sensitive to the immunosuppressive effects of corticosteroids; use may exacerbate subclinical bacterial infection. The use of corticosteroids (systemic or topical in otic preparations) can severely exacerbate otitis.
• Albendazole has been associated with bone marrow toxicity in dogs and cats; toxicity in rabbits is unknown; however, anecdotal reports of pancytopenia leading to death in rabbits exist.
• Avoid topical otic preparations if the tympanic membrane is ruptured.

## POSSIBLE INTERACTIONS
Several topical otic medications may induce contact irritation or allergic response; reevaluate all worsening cases.

## ALTERNATIVE DRUGS
Systemic corticosteroids have been advocated by practitioners for treatment of *E. cuniculi*–induced CNS granulomatous inflammation. Use of corticosteroids is controversial. Although clinical improvement has been anecdotally reported, rabbits are very sensitive to the immunosuppressive effects of corticosteroids; immunosuppression may exacerbate subclinical bacterial or *E. cuniculi* infection.

# FOLLOW-UP

## PATIENT MONITORING
• Monitor for corneal ulceration—secondary to facial nerve paralysis or abrasion during vestibular episodes

• Repeat the neurologic examination at a frequency dictated by the underlying cause
• Head tilt may persist.

## POSSIBLE COMPLICATIONS
• Progression of disease with deterioration of mental status
• Corneal ulceration

## EXPECTED COURSE AND PROGNOSIS
• Following acute episode, head tilt often persists. Most rabbits adapt well to this, will ambulate, eat well, and appear to live comfortable lives. Recurrence of acute episodes may occur.
• Prognosis—guarded depending on underlying cause; varied response to drug treatment; many rabbits improve with antibiotic therapy and/or supportive care alone.
• Residual deficits (especially neurologic) cannot be predicted until after a course of therapy; long-term quality of life is good for the majority of rabbits with mild to moderate residual head tilt or facial nerve paralysis.

# MISCELLANEOUS

## ASSOCIATED CONDITIONS
• Dental disease
• Facial abscesses
• Upper respiratory infections
• Gastrointestinal hypomotility

## AGE-RELATED FACTORS
*E. cuniculi* and bacterial otitis interna/media may be more common in older, especially immunosuppressed, animals.

## ZOONOTIC POTENTIAL
• Rabies—consider in endemic areas if the patient is an outdoor animal that has rapidly progressive encephalitis.
• *E. cuniculi*—unlikely, but possible in immunosuppressed humans. Mode of transmission and susceptibility in humans are unclear.

## PREGNANCY
N/A

## SYNONYMS
Wry neck

## SEE ALSO
• *E. cuniculi*
• Otitis media and interna
• Pasteurellosis

## ABBREVIATIONS
• CNS = central nervous system
• CSF = cerebrospinal fluid
• CT = computed tomography
• ELISA = enzyme-linked immunosorbent assay
• IFA = immunofluorescence assay
• MRI = magnetic resonance imaging

## Suggested Reading
Deeb BJ, Carpenter JW. Neurologic and musculoskeletal diseases. In: Quesenberry KE, Carpenter JW, eds. Ferrets, Rabbits and Rodents: Clinical Medicine and Surgery. 2nd Ed. Philadelphia: WB Saunders, 2004:203–210.

de Lahunta A. Veterinary Neuroanatomy and Clinical Neurology. 2nd Ed. Philadelphia: Saunders, 1983.

Harcourt-Brown F. Neurological and locomotor diseases. In: Harcourt-Brown F, ed. Textbook of Rabbit Medicine. Oxford: Butterworth-Heinemann, 2002:307–323.

Oliver JE, Lorenz MD. Handbook of Veterinary Neurologic Diagnosis. 2nd ed. Philadelphia: Saunders, 1993.

Paul-Murphy J, Ramer JC. Urgent care of the pet rabbits. Vet Clin North Am Exotic Anim Pract 1998;1(1):127–152.

Rosenthal KR. Torticollis in rabbits. Proc North Am Vet Conf 2005;1378–1379.

## Portions Adapted From
Cochrane SM. Head Tilt. In: Tilley LP, Smith FWK, Jr., eds. The 5-Minute Veterinary Consult: Canine and Feline, 3rd Ed. Baltimore: Lippincott Williams & Wilkins, 2004.

# HEAT STROKE AND HEAT STRESS

## BASICS

### DEFINITION
• Heat stroke—a form of nonpyrogenic hyperthermia that occurs when heat-dissipating mechanisms of the body cannot accommodate excessive heat; can lead to multisystemic organ dysfunction
• Rabbits are very sensitive to heat stroke and heat stress.
• Temperatures of 105°F or above without signs of inflammation suggest nonpyrogenic hyperthermia.
• Other possible causes of nonpyrogenic hyperthermia include excessive exercise, thyrotoxicosis, and hypothalamic lesions, but these have not been described in rabbits.

### PATHOPHYSIOLOGY
The primary pathophysiologic processes of heat stroke are related to thermal damage that can lead to cellular necrosis, hypoxemia, and protein denaturalization.

### SYSTEMS AFFECTED
• Nervous—neuronal damage, parenchymal hemorrhage, and cerebral edema
• Cardiovascular—hypovolemia, cardiac arrhythmias, myocardial ischemia, and necrosis
• Gastrointestinal—mucosal ischemia and ulceration, bacterial translocation, and endotoxemia
• Hepatobiliary—hepatocellular necrosis
• Renal/urologic—acute renal failure
• Hemic/lymph/immune—hemoconcentration, thrombocytopenia, disseminated intravascular coagulopathy
• Musculoskeletal—rhabdomyolysis

### GENETICS
N/A

### GEOGRAPHIC DISTRIBUTION
May be seen in any climate but more common in warm and or humid environments

### SIGNALMENT
No breed, age, or sex predilection

### SIGNS

#### Historical Findings
• Identifiable underlying cause—hot day, outdoor rabbits in the sun, ambient temperature >85°F, lack of shade, lack of ventilation, lack of drinking water, excessive exercise
• Predisposing underlying disease—cardiovascular disease, neuromuscular disease, obesity, previous history of heat-related disease

#### Physical Examination Findings
• Weakness, depression, ataxia early findings
• Panting
• Seizures
• Coma

• Hyperthermia
• Hyperemic mucous membranes
• Tachycardia
• Cardiac arrhythmias
• Respiratory distress
• Muscle tremors
• Hematochezia
• Melena
• Petechiation
• Shock
• Oliguria/anuria
• Respiratory arrest
• Cardiopulmonary arrest

### CAUSES AND RISK FACTORS
• Excessive environmental heat and humidity—may be due to weather conditions or accidents such as enclosed in unventilated room or car or housed outdoors with a lack of shade and ventilation
• Exercise
• Toxicosis—strychnine and metaldehyde cause hyperthermia secondary to seizure activity.
• Previous history of heat-related disease
• Age extremes
• Heat intolerance due to poor acclimatization
• Obesity
• Poor cardiopulmonary conditioning
• Underlying cardiopulmonary disease
• Thick hair coat
• Dehydration

## DIAGNOSIS

### DIFFERENTIAL DIAGNOSIS
• If temperatures exceed 105°F without evidence of inflammation, consider heat stroke.
• Early clinical signs are nonspecific (lethargy, ataxia) and may resemble many other diseases. History is the most helpful factor in differentiating cause. However, many owners do not realize that the environment may have been too warm or ventilation inadequate for a pet rabbit. Always carefully question owners if heat stress is suspected.

### CBC/BIOCHEMISTRY/URINALYSIS
• May help identify underlying disease process
• May help identify sequelae to hyperthermia
• CBC abnormalities may include anemia, thrombocytopenia, or hemoconcentration.
• Biochemistry profile may show azotemia, hyperalbuminemia, high ALT, high AST, high CK, and electrolyte abnormalities.

### OTHER LABORATORY TESTS
N/A

### IMAGING
Thoracic and abdominal radiographs may help identify underlying cardiopulmonary disease or predisposing factors.

### DIAGNOSTIC PROCEDURES
Frequent body temperature monitoring

## TREATMENT

### APPROPRIATE HEALTH CARE
• Hospitalize patient until temperature is stabilized.
• Most patients need intensive care for several days; however, many rabbits do not survive.

### NURSING CARE
• Immediate correction of hyperthermia—wet rabbit by spraying with water or soaking with cool, wet cloths before transporting to veterinary facility, if possible. Wet rabbit in veterinary hospital by above means, or immersing body in cool water; convection cool with fans; evaporative cool (e.g., alcohol on foot pads, axilla, and groin).
• Stop cooling procedures when temperature reaches 103°F to avoid hypothermia.
• Supplement oxygen via oxygen cage, mask, or nasal catheter.
• Give ventilatory support if required.
• Give fluid support with shock doses of crystalloids.
• Treat complications such as renal failure and cerebral edema.
• Treat underlying disease or correct predisposing factors.

### ACTIVITY
Restricted

### DIET
Nothing per OS until animal is stable. Then, be certain the rabbit continues to eat throughout treatment to prevent gastrointestinal hypomotility.

### CLIENT EDUCATION
• Be aware of clinical signs.
• Know how to cool animals.
• An episode of heat stroke may predispose pets to additional episodes.

### SURGICAL CONSIDERATIONS
N/A

## MEDICATIONS

### DRUG(S) OF CHOICE
• No specific drugs are required for hyperthermia or heat stroke; therapy depends on clinical presentation.

# HEAT STROKE AND HEAT STRESS

• Fluid therapy for hypovolemic shock—LRS or other crystalloid (60–90 mg/kg/hr IV, IO over 20–60 minutes, followed by maintenance rate) or crystalloid bolus (30 mL/kg) plus hetastarch bolus (5 mL/kg initially) followed by crystalloids at a maintenance rate and hetastarch at 20 mL/kg divided over 24 hours.
• Cerebral edema—mannitol using canine/feline protocols
• Ventricular arrhythmia—lidocaine bolus (1–2 mg/kg IV or 2–4 mg/kg IT) followed by continuous-rate intravenous infusion using feline dosage if necessary
• Metabolic acidosis—sodium bicarbonate (2 mEq/kg IV)
• Hemorrhagic diarrhea—broad-spectrum antibiotics
• Seizures—diazepam (1–2 mg/kg IV to effect)

## CONTRAINDICATIONS
• Oral administration of antibiotics that select against Gram-positive bacteria (penicillins, macrolides, lincosamides, and cephalosporins) can cause fatal enteric dysbiosis and enterotoxemia.
• NSAIDs—not indicated in nonpyrogenic hyperthermia because the hypothalamic set point is not altered
• Corticosteroids—not demonstrated to be of benefit. Rabbits are extremely sensitive to the immunosuppressive effects and gastrointestinal ulceration subsequent to systemic or topical administration of corticosteroids.
• Cooling with ice—may lead to peripheral vasoconstriction and poor heat dissipation

## PRECAUTIONS
N/A

## POSSIBLE INTERACTIONS
N/A

## ALTERNATIVE DRUGS
N/A

## FOLLOW-UP

### PATIENT MONITORING
Monitor closely during cooling-down period and for a minimum of 24 hours postepisode; most need several days of treatment, depending on clinical presentation and sequelae. Perform a thorough physical examination daily; also consider monitoring:
• Body temperature
• Body weight
• Blood pressure
• ECG
• Thoracic auscultation
• Urinalysis and urine output
• PCV, TP
• CBC, biochemical profile

### PREVENTION/AVOIDANCE
Avoid risk factors.

### POSSIBLE COMPLICATIONS
• Cardiac arrhythmias
• Hemorrhagic diarrhea
• Organ failure
• Coma
• Seizures
• Acute renal failure
• Pulmonary edema—acute respiratory distress
• Hepatocellular necrosis
• Disseminated intravascular coagulation
• Respiratory arrest
• Cardiopulmonary arrest

### EXPECTED COURSE AND PROGNOSIS
• Guarded—depending on complications and duration of episode
• May predispose to further episodes due to damage to thermoregulatory center

## MISCELLANEOUS

### ASSOCIATED CONDITIONS
N/A

### AGE-RELATED FACTORS
N/A

### ZOONOTIC POTENTIAL
N/A

### PREGNANCY
N/A

### SYNONYMS
• Heat exhaustion
• Heat prostration
• Heat-related disease

### ABBREVIATIONS
• ALT = alanine aminotransferase
• AST = aspartate aminotransferase
• CBC = complete blood count
• CK = creatine kinase
• ECG = electrocardiogram
• LRS = lactated Ringer's solution
• NSAIDs = nonsteroidal antiinflammatory drugs
• PCV = packed cell volume
• TS = total solids

*Suggested Reading*

Deeb BJ, Carpenter JW. Neurologic and musculoskeletal diseases. In: Quesenberry KE, Carpenter JW, eds. Ferrets, Rabbits and Rodents: Clinical Medicine and Surgery. 2nd Ed. Philadelphia: WB Saunders, 2004:203–210.

Haskins SC. Thermoregulation, hypothermia, hyperthermia. In: Ettinger SJ, Feldman EC, eds. Textbook of Veterinary Internal Medicine. Philadelphia: Saunders, 1995:26–30.

Lee-Parritz DE, Pavletic MM. Physical and chemical injuries: heatstroke, hypothermia, burns, and frostbite. In: Murtaugh RJ, Kaplan PM, eds. Veterinary Emergency and Critical Care Medicine. St. Louis: Mosby Year Book, 1992:194–196.

Paul-Murphy J, Ramer JC. Urgent care of the pet rabbits. Vet Clin North Am Exotic Anim Pract 1998;1(1):127–152.

*Portions Adapted From*

Marks SL. Heat Stroke and Hyperthermia. In: Tilley LP, Smith FWK, Jr., eds. The 5-Minute Veterinary Consult: Canine and Feline, 2nd Ed. Baltimore: Lippincott Williams & Wilkins, 2000.

# BASICS

## DEFINITION
The presence of blood in the urine. It is important to differentiate true hematuria from red or red-brown–colored urine caused by the excretion of dietary pigments in urine or from blood originating from the reproductive tract in females

## PATHOPHYSIOLOGY
• Secondary to loss of endothelial integrity in the urinary tract
• Clotting factor deficiency or thrombocytopenia possible, but not commonly reported
• Must distinguish from blood originating from the reproductive tract in female rabbits. Blood expressed from the uterus or vaginal vault during micturition is a much more common cause of perceived "hematuria" than actual urinary tract bleeding.

## SYSTEMS AFFECTED
• Renal/urologic
• Reproductive

## SIGNALMENT
N/A

## SIGNS

### Historical Findings
• Red-tinged urine with or without pollakiuria
• Blood clots expelled during micturition

### Physical Examination Findings
• May be normal
• Palpable mass in patients with neoplasia
• Turgid, sometimes painful bladder on abdominal palpation in rabbits with hypercalciuria or cystitis
• Detect urocystoliths by abdominal palpation; failure to palpate uroliths does not exclude them from consideration. Often, one single, large calculus is palpated.
• In rabbits with crystalluria, the bladder palpates as a soft, doughy mass.
• With chronic disease, the bladder may markedly increase in size and may even fill most of the abdomen.
• Petechia or ecchymoses in patients with coagulopathies

## CAUSES

### Lower Urinary Tract—Most Common
• Hypercalciuria, urolithiasis
• Infectious—bacterial cystitis
• Neoplasia
• Trauma

### Upper Urinary Tract
• Nephrolithiasis
• Neoplasia
• Infectious—bacterial
• Inflammatory—glomerulonephritis
• Trauma

### Genitalia
• Most common cause of hematuria in intact females
• Uterine neoplasia, endometrial hyperplasia, or endometrial venous aneurysm—female rabbits with uterine disease often expel blood when urinating. Blood may mix with urine and be mistaken for hematuria.
• Pyometra
• Trauma

### Systemic
• Coagulopathy (anticoagulant rodenticides)
• Thrombocytopenia

## RISK FACTORS
• Sedentary, obese rabbits on diets consisting mainly of commercial pellets or high alfalfa hay content are at high risk for hypercalciuria, urolithiasis, and nephrolithiasis.
• Middle-aged to older intact females at risk for uterine neoplasia or pyometra

# DIAGNOSIS

## DIFFERENTIAL DIAGNOSIS
• Rule out physiologic red-brown–colored urine—may be mistaken for hematuria; normal rabbits may have brown- to red-colored urine. This color change may be intermittent and is caused by the excretion of plant pigments. Differentiate blood from pigment excretion by cytologic examination; pigments may also fluoresce using an ultraviolet light (black light) or Wood's lamp.
• Rule out blood originating from uterus in intact females—perform urinalysis, collect sample via ultrasound-guided cystocentesis to differentiate true hematuria from uterine bleeding
• Rule out other causes of discolored urine (myoglobinuria, hemoglobinuria).

## LABORATORY FINDINGS

### Drugs That May Alter Laboratory Results
High doses of vitamin C (ascorbic acid) may cause false-negative reagent test strip results; newer generations of reagent strips are more resistant to interference by reducing substances such as ascorbic acid.

### Disorders That May Alter Laboratory Results
• Common urine reagent strip tests for blood are designed to detect RBCs, hemoglobin, or myoglobin.
• Low specific urine gravity may lyse RBCs.
• Bacteriuria (bacterial peroxidase) may cause false-positive test strip results.

### CBC/BIOCHEMISTRY/URINALYSIS
• Elevated serum calcium concentration (normal range 12–16 mg/dL) in rabbits with hypercalciuria; the significance of this

is unclear since many normal rabbits have high serum calcium concentration and never develop hypercalciuria.
• With urinary tract infection, leukocytosis may be seen, but this finding is rare.
• Azotemia in some patients with bilateral renal disease or urinary tract obstruction
• Thrombocytopenia, anemia with bleeding disorders
• Mild anemia with uterine adenocarcinoma
• Urinary sediment evaluation usually reveals calcium oxalate or calcium carbonate crystals; however, this is a normal finding in rabbits and the presence of large amounts of crystals in the urine does not necessarily indicate disease. Disease occurs only when the concentration of crystals is excessive, forming thick, white to brown, sandlike urine and subsequent inflammatory cystitis or partial to complete blockage of the urethra.
• Pyuria (normal value 0–1 WBC/hpf), hematuria (normal value 0–1 RBC/hpf), and proteinuria (normal value 0–33 mg/dL) indicate urinary tract inflammation, but these are nonspecific findings that may result from infectious and noninfectious causes of lower urinary tract disease.
• Identification of neoplastic cells in urine sediment indicates urinary tract neoplasia.

## OTHER LABORATORY TESTS
Bacterial culture of urine to identify urinary tract infection

## IMAGING
Ultrasonography, radiography, and possibly contract radiographs may be useful in obtaining a diagnosis.

## DIAGNOSTIC PROCEDURES
• Cystoscopy
• Biopsy of mass lesions

# TREATMENT
• Hematuria may indicate a serious disease process.
• Hypercalciuria requires diet and husbandry modification. Diuresis and mechanical removal of urine "sludge" are often necessary.
• Uroliths require surgical removal.
• Uterine disease requires surgical intervention.

# MEDICATIONS

## DRUG(S) OF CHOICE
• Blood transfusion may be necessary if patient is severely anemic.
• Fluids to treat dehydration
• Symptomatic rabbits with hypercalciuria or urinary calculi are sometimes in pain and

## HEMATURIA

therefore reluctant to urinate. Pain management may aid in urination and promote appetite and water consumption. NSAIDs (meloxicam, carprofen) reduce pain and may decrease inflammation in the bladder.

### CONTRAINDICATIONS

• Glucocorticoids or other immunosuppressive agents
• Oral administration of antibiotics that select against Gram-positive bacteria (penicillins, macrolides, lincosamides, and cephalosporins) can cause fatal enteric dysbiosis and enterotoxemia.

### PRECAUTIONS
N/A

### ALTERNATIVE DRUGS
N/A

 FOLLOW-UP

### PATIENT MONITORING

• Response to treatment by clinical signs, serial physical examinations, laboratory testing, and radiographic and ultrasonic evaluations appropriate for each specific cause
• Refer to specific chapters describing diseases listed in section on causes.

### POSSIBLE COMPLICATIONS

• Anemia
• Urinary tract obstruction with urolithiasis or hypercalciuria
• Renal failure with urolithiasis or hypercalciuria
• Metastases with uterine adenocarcinoma

 MISCELLANEOUS

### ASSOCIATED CONDITIONS

• Obesity
• Gastrointestinal hypomotility
• Musculoskeletal disorders

### AGE-RELATED FACTORS

• Neoplasia tends to occur in middle-aged to older rabbits.
• Hypercalciuria tends to occur in middle-aged to older rabbits.

### ZOONOTIC POTENTIAL
N/A

### PREGNANCY
N/A

### SYNONYMS
N/A

### SEE ALSO

• Hypercalciuria and urolithiasis
• Lower urinary tract infections
• Pyometra and nonneoplastic endometrial disorders
• Uterine adenocarcinoma
• Vaginal discharge

### ABBREVIATIONS

• NSAIDs = nonsteroidal antiinflammatory drugs
• RBC = red blood cell
• WBC = white blood cell

*Suggested Reading*

Brown SA. Rabbit urinary tract disease. Proc North Am Vet Conf 1997;785–787.
Cheeke PR, Amberg JW. Comparative calcium excretion by rats and rabbits. J Anim Sci 1973;37:450–454.
Donoghue S. Nutrition and pet rabbits. In: Rosenthal KL, ed. Practical Exotic Animal Medicine: The Compendium Collection. Trenton, NJ: Veterinary Learning Systems, 1997:107.
Harkness JE, Wagner JE. The Biology and Medicine of Rabbits and Rodents. 3rd Ed. Baltimore: Williams & Wilkins, 1989.
Harcourt-Brown F. Urogenital disease. In: Harcourt-Brown F, ed. Textbook of Rabbit Medicine. Oxford: Butterworth-Heinemann, 2002:335–351.
Pare JA, Paul-Murphy J. Disorders of the reproductive and urinary systems. In: Quesenberry KE, Carpenter JW, eds. Ferrets, Rabbits and Rodents: Clinical Medicine and Surgery. 2nd Ed. Philadelphia:WB Saunders, 2004:183–193.
Paul-Murphy J, Ramer JC. Urgent care of the pet rabbits. Vet Clin North Am Exotic Anim Pract 1998;1(1):127–152.
Redrobe S. Calcium metabolism in rabbits. Semin Avian Exotic Pet Med 2002;11(2):94–101.

*Portions Adapted From*

Bartges JW. Hematuria. In: Tilley LP, Smith FWK, Jr., eds. The 5-Minute Veterinary Consult: Canine and Feline, 2nd Ed. Baltimore: Lippincott Williams & Wilkins, 2000.

# BASICS

## DEFINITION
Formation of crystals or uroliths composed of calcium salts (usually calcium oxalate and calcium carbonate) within the urinary tract and associated clinical conditions. Excessive crystal formation and retention in the bladder result in thick, sand- or pastelike urine ("sludge") and inflammation of the bladder wall. Crystals can condense to form uroliths in the bladder, urethra, ureters, or renal pelvis.

## PATHOPHYSIOLOGY
• In rabbits, intestinal calcium absorption is not dependent on vitamin D, and nearly all calcium in the diet is absorbed. Calcium excretion occurs primarily through the kidneys (vs. the gallbladder in other mammals); the fractional urinary excretion is 45–60% in rabbits compared to less than 2% in other mammals.
• Rabbits normally eat a diet high in calcium; however, not all rabbits develop hypercalciuria.
• The factors leading to hypercalciuria and urolith formation in rabbits is unclear; however, the disease is seen more commonly in obese, sedentary rabbits fed a diet composed primarily of commercial alfalfa-based pellets. Most commercial diets contain excessive amounts of calcium. The dietary requirement of calcium for rabbits is only 0.22 g of calcium/100 g food, but most commercial diets contain up to 0.9–1.6 g of calcium/100 g of food. It is unlikely that high dietary calcium content alone is the cause of hypercalciuria, but it may exacerbate urinary sludge formation when combined with other factors leading to urine retention.
• Inadequate water intake leading to a more concentrated urine and factors that impair complete evacuation of the bladder, such as lack of exercise, obesity, cystitis, neoplasia, or neuromuscular disease, may also contribute. Without frequent urination and dilute urine, calcium crystals may precipitate out of solution within the bladder. Precipitated crystals form a thick sand or sludge within the bladder that does not mix normally with urine and is not eliminated during voiding.

## SYSTEMS AFFECTED
• Renal/urologic
• Skin—urine scald, perineal and ventral dermatitis

## GENETICS
Unknown, but may play a role in determining which rabbits develop hypercalciuria

## INCIDENCE/PREVALENCE
Clinical conditions related to hypercalciuria and urolith formation are extremely common in pet rabbits.

## GEOGRAPHIC DISTRIBUTION
Ubiquitous

## SIGNALMENT
### Breed Predilections
All breeds are equally affected.

### Mean Age and Range
Seen most commonly in middle-aged rabbits 3–5 years old

### Predominant Sex
N/A

## SIGNS
### General Comments
• Some animals remain asymptomatic, despite large amounts of calcium sludge accumulation in the bladder.
• Depend on location, size, and amount of material in the bladder

### Historical Findings
• Pollakiuria, dysuria, hematuria, and urine staining in the perineum in rabbits with urocystoliths, ureteroliths, or large amounts of crystalline sludge in the bladder
• Owners may report thick, pasty, beige- to brown-colored urine; sometimes this urine is so thick that it is mistaken for diarrhea.
• Abnormal-appearing urine is not always reported. Some rabbits void clear urine while sludge remains in the bladder; sometimes cloudy urine is reported.
• Hunched posture, ataxia, or difficulty ambulating in rabbits with neurologic or orthopedic disorders leading to urine retention
• Anorexia, weight loss, lethargy, tooth grinding, tenesmus, and a hunched posture in rabbits with large urocystoliths, large amounts of sludge in the bladder, or complete or partial obstruction of the ureters or urethra

### Physical Examination Findings
• Detect urocystoliths by abdominal palpation; failure to palpate uroliths does not exclude them from consideration. Most often, one single large calculus is palpated. In rabbits with crystalluria (urine "sludge"), the bladder palpates as a soft, doughy mass.
• With chronic disease, the bladder loses tone, may markedly increase in size, and may even fill most of the abdomen.
• A large urinary bladder may also be palpable in patients with partial or complete urethral obstruction.
• Manual expression of the bladder may reveal thick, beige- to brown-colored urine. Manual expression of the bladder may expel thick, brown urine even in rabbits that have normal-appearing voided urine.

• A large kidney may be palpated in rabbits with ureteroliths and subsequent hydronephrosis (rare).

## CAUSES
See pathophysiology.

## RISK FACTORS
• Inadequate water intake (dirty water bowls, unpalatable water, changing water sources, inadequate water provision)
• Urine retention (underlying bladder pathology, neuromuscular disease)
• Inadequate cleaning of litter box or cage may cause some rabbits to avoid urinating for abnormally long periods.
• Obesity
• Pain and a reluctance to ambulate
• Lack of exercise; cage confinement
• Feeding of exclusively commercial pelleted diets
• Renal disease
• Calcium or vitamin/mineral supplements added to the diet

# DIAGNOSIS

## DIFFERENTIAL DIAGNOSIS
• Other, less common causes of hematuria, dysuria, and pollakiuria, with or without urethral obstruction, include urinary tract infection and lower urinary tract neoplasia.
• Female rabbits with pyometra or uterine neoplasia may expel blood or a thick, often blood-tinged vaginal discharge when urinating. This discharge may mix with urine and mimic hypercalciuria.
• Uroliths composed of magnesium ammonium phosphate are also radiopaque, but these are extremely rare in the rabbit.

## CBC/BIOCHEMISTRY/URINALYSIS
• Most affected rabbits are hypercalcemic (normal range 12–16 mg/dL); however, the significance of this is unclear since many normal rabbits have high serum calcium concentration and never develop hypercalciuria.
• With urinary tract infection, leukocytosis may be seen, but this finding is rare.
• Complete urinary outflow obstruction can cause postrenal azotemia (e.g., high BUN, creatinine).
• Urinary sediment evaluation reveals calcium oxalate or calcium carbonate crystals; however, this is a normal finding in rabbits, and the presence of large amounts of crystals in the urine does not necessarily indicate disease. Disease occurs only when the concentration of crystals is excessive, forming thick, white to brown, sandlike urine and subsequent inflammatory cystitis or partial to complete blockage of the urethra.

# HYPERCALCIURIA AND UROLITHIASIS

• Pyuria (normal value 0–1 WBC/hpf), hematuria (normal value 0–1 RBC/hpf), and proteinuria (normal value 0–33 mg/dL) indicate urinary tract inflammation, but these are nonspecific findings that may result from infectious and noninfectious causes of lower urinary tract disease.

### OTHER LABORATORY TESTS
Quantitative mineral analysis of uroliths retrieved during cystotomy.

### IMAGING
• Calcium oxalate uroliths are radiopaque and may be detected by survey radiography. Uroliths must be differentiated from calcium "sand" or "sludge" in the bladder, which resembles a bladder full of contrast material. Ultrasonic examination of the bladder and palpation can be helpful to distinguish solitary calculi from amorphous "sand."
• A small amount of "sand" or "sludge" in the bladder is frequently discovered serendipitously in rabbits undergoing radiographs for other causes
• Nephroliths and/or ureteroliths may also been seen. Renal calcification can resemble renoliths on abdominal radiographs. Renal calcification can be differentiated from renoliths on ultrasound.
• Occasionally, relatively large uroliths can be found in the urethra, sometimes causing only partial obstruction.

### DIAGNOSTIC PROCEDURES
Perform a urine culture—many rabbits with hypercalciuria have concurrent bacterial cystitis.

### PATHOLOGIC FINDINGS
N/A

# TREATMENT

### APPROPRIATE HEALTH CARE
• Look for and treat any underlying medical problem that may cause a reluctance or inability to urinate.
• Retrograde urohydropropulsion to flush urethral stones back into the urinary bladder or voiding urohydropropulsion to eliminate bladder "sand" can be performed on an outpatient basis. Voiding urohydropropulsion is contraindicated in patients with urethral obstruction.
• Surgery requires a short period of hospitalization.

### NURSING CARE
• Asymptomatic rabbits diagnosed with hypercalciuria based on incidental radiographic evidence may respond to diuresis via subcutaneous fluid administration, increasing water consumption, dietary modification, weight loss, and increase in exercise alone.

• Symptomatic rabbits with large amounts of calcium precipitate ("sand" or "sludge") in the urinary bladder may respond to medical treatment with fluid therapy and voiding urohydropropulsion. Manually express the bladder to remove as much precipitated calcium sand as possible. Gentle ballottement or agitation of the bladder may help to mobilize sludge. Administer fluid therapy, either IV or SC, daily for 2–4 days to increase the amount of urine in the bladder. If precipitated calcium sand is detected in the bladder (via palpation or imaging) after this time, continue fluid therapy and manually express the bladder once daily for 3–4 days, gently forcing the nonvoided "sludge" out the urethra. This may be a painful procedure; anesthesia with isoflurane during manual expression and administration of butorphanol (0.1–0.5 mg/kg SC, IM, IV q4h) or meloxicam (0.2–0.5 mg/kg PO q24h) for pain management are necessary. Administration of diazepam (1–5 mg/kg IM) prior to manual expression of the bladder may aid in smooth muscle relaxation and subsequent dilation of the urethra.
• If large amounts of precipitate are present and manual expression does not remove sufficient amounts of precipitate, flushing the bladder via urethral catheterization may be effective. Begin fluid diuresis as described above. Administer diazepam and induce general anesthesia, catheterize the urethra, flush with warm saline, and aspirate the contents of the bladder. Continue to flush and aspirate until most of the sand is removed. Administer butorphanol, buprenorphine, or meloxicam for pain relief.
• Fortunately, ureteroliths are relatively rare. However, when present they can be surprisingly large and may only cause partial obstruction. Retrograde urohydropropulsion can sometimes be used to push small stones back into the bladder, which can then be removed via cystotomy. Catheterization should be attempted under isoflurane anesthesia. Attempt to dislodge the calculus using a 5.t–5 Fr. rubber catheter. Administration of 1–2 mg/kg diazepam IM and infusing 0.02–0.3 mL of 1% or 2% lidocaine locally into the urethra may aid in urethral dilation and passage of the catheter. Flush with saline as the catheter is advanced. Advance the catheter slowly and carefully, since the urethra is fragile and may easily tear. Large urethral calculi may require surgical removal.
• If the bladder does not empty completely during micturition, some owners can be taught to manually express the bladder several times daily to prevent buildup of sludge.
• Treat associated urine scald with gentle cleaning; keep the area clean and dry; apply zinc oxide plus menthol powder (Gold

Bond, Martin Himmel, Inc.) to clean skin q24h.

### ACTIVITY
• Increase activity level by providing large exercise areas to encourage voiding and prevent recurrence—important part of treatment and prevention
• Reduce during the period of tissue repair after surgery.

### DIET
• It is absolutely imperative that the rabbit continue to eat during and following treatment. Many urinary tract disorders are painful and may lead to a decreased appetite. Anorexia may cause or exacerbate gastrointestinal hypomotility and cause derangement of the gastrointestinal microflora and overgrowth of intestinal bacterial pathogens.
• Offer a large selection of fresh, moistened greens such as cilantro, romaine lettuce, parsley, carrot tops, dandelion greens, spinach, or collard greens and good-quality grass hay. Many rabbits will begin to eat these foods, even if they were previously anorectic.
• If the patient refuses these foods, syringe feed a gruel such as Critical Care for Herbivores (Oxbow Pet Products, Murdock, NE) 10–15 mL/kg PO q6–8h. Larger volumes and more frequent feedings are often accepted; feed as much as the rabbit will readily accept. Alternatively, pellets can be ground and mixed with fresh greens, vegetable baby foods, water, or juice to form a gruel. The addition of canned pumpkin to this gruel is a palatable source of fiber and calories. If sufficient volumes of food are not accepted in this manner, nasogastric intubation is indicated.
• High-carbohydrate, high-fat nutritional supplements are contraindicated.
• Increasing water consumption is essential to the prevention and treatment of hypercalciuria. Provide multiple sources of fresh water. Automatic, continuously pouring water fountains available for cats entice some rabbits to drink. Flavoring the water with fruit or vegetable juices (with no added sugars) may be helpful. Provide a variety of clean, fresh, leafy vegetables sprayed or soaked with water.
• No reports of dissolution of calcium oxalate uroliths with special diets
• Following treatment, reduction in the amount of calcium in the diet may help to prevent or delay recurrence. Eliminate feeding of alfalfa pellets and switch to a high-fiber timothy-based pellet (Oxbow Pet Products, Murdock, NE). The form of calcium found in alfalfa-based commercial pellets and alfalfa hay is calcium carbonate, which is 50% more bioavailable than the calcium oxalate found in most green, leafy

vegetables. Feed timothy and grass hay instead of alfalfa hay and offer large volumes of fresh, green, leafy vegetables.

## CLIENT EDUCATION
Urolith removal or removal of calcium "sand" does not alter the factors responsible for their formation; eliminating risk factors such as obesity, sedentary life, and poor diet combined with increasing water consumption is necessary to minimize or delay recurrence. Even with these changes, however, recurrence is likely.

## SURGICAL CONSIDERATIONS
• Uroliths within the bladder, ureters, or renal pelvis must be removed surgically. The procedures are similar to those performed on dogs or cats.
• Calcium "sludge" in the bladder that does not respond to medical therapy may require cystotomy for removal.

## MEDICATIONS

### DRUG(S) OF CHOICE
• No available drugs effectively dissolve calcium oxalate uroliths.
• Many rabbits with large amounts of calcium precipitate or uroliths have an underlying chronic bacterial cystitis. Treat with antibiotics, based on culture and susceptibility testing when possible for 3–4 weeks following surgery or urohydropropulsion; may also be indicated in the treatment of severe urine scald
• Pain management is essential during and following surgery, urohydropropulsion, and urinary catheterization, or if pain is causing reduced frequency of voiding. Perioperative choices include butorphanol (0.1–1.0 mg/kg SC, IM, IV q4–6h) or buprenorphine (0.01–0.05 mg/kg SC, IM, IV q6–12h). Meloxicam (0.2–0.5 mg/k PO q24h) and carprofen (1–2.2 mg/kg PO q12h) have been used for long-term pain management.
• If the bladder is chronically distended and will not empty completely during micturition, bethanechol chloride has been anecdotally used at feline dosages (2.5–5 mg/kg q 8–12h).

### CONTRAINDICATIONS
Oral administration of antibiotics that select against Gram-positive bacteria (penicillins, macrolides, lincosamides, and

cephalosporins) can cause fatal enteric dysbiosis and enterotoxemia.

### PRECAUTIONS
Steroids and furosemide promote calciuria.

### POSSIBLE INTERACTIONS
N/A

### ALTERNATIVE DRUGS
N/A

## FOLLOW-UP

### PATIENT MONITORING
• Following general anesthesia, monitor for postoperative ileus. Be certain the rabbit is eating and defecating normally prior to release from the hospital.
• Radiographs are essential following surgery or urohydropropulsion to verify complete removal.

### PREVENTION/AVOIDANCE
• Increase water consumption for the remainder of the rabbit's life.
• Place patients on a lowered calcium diet (described above).
• Increase exercise.

### POSSIBLE COMPLICATIONS
• Rabbits undergoing general anesthesia are at high risk for developing life-threatening postoperative ileus. This is especially common with obese rabbits fed a poor-quality diet, as many rabbits with hypercalciuria are.
• Renal failure, urinary tract obstruction, hydronephrosis, bladder atony
• Urine scald

### EXPECTED COURSE AND PROGNOSIS
The prognosis following surgical removal of uroliths or urohydropropulsion for the removal of calcium "sand" is fair to good. Although husbandry changes and dietary management may decrease the likelihood of recurrence, many rabbits will develop clinical disease again within 1–2 years.

## MISCELLANEOUS

### ASSOCIATED CONDITIONS
• Gastrointestinal hypomotility
• Dental disease
• Lower urinary tract infection

### AGE-RELATED FACTORS
Rare in young animals

### ZOONOTIC POTENTIAL
None

### PREGNANCY
N/A

### SYNONYMS
Calcium oxalate urolithiasis

### SEE ALSO
• Dysuria and pollakiuria
• Lower urinary tract infection
• Nephrolithiasis and urolithiasis
• Urinary tract obstruction

### ABBREVIATIONS
• BUN = blood urea nitrogen
• RBC = red blood cell
• WBC = white blood cell

*Suggested Reading*

Brown SA. Rabbit urinary tract disease. Proc North Am Vet Conf 1997;785–787.

Cheeke PR, Amberg JW. Comparative calcium excretion by rats and rabbits. J Anim Sci 1973;37:450–454

Donoghue S. Nutrition and pet rabbits. In: Rosenthal KL, ed. Practical Exotic Animal Medicine: The Compendium Collection. Trenton, NJ: Veterinary Learning Systems, 1997:107.

Garibaldi BA, Pecquet-Goad ME. Hypercalcemia with secondary nephrolithiasis in a rabbit. Lab Anim Sci 1988;38:331–333.

Harkness JE, Wagner JE. The Biology and Medicine of Rabbits and Rodents. 3rd Ed. Baltimore: Williams & Wilkins, 1989.

Harcourt-Brown F. Urogenital disease. In: Harcourt-Brown F, ed. Textbook of Rabbit Medicine. Oxford: Butterworth-Heinemann, 2002:335–351.

Kampheus J. Calcium metabolism of rabbits as an etiological factor for urolithiasis. J Nutr 1991;121:595–596.

Pare JA, Paul-Murphy J. Disorders of the reproductive and urinary systems. In: Quesenberry KE, Carpenter JW, eds. Ferrets, Rabbits and Rodents: Clinical Medicine and Surgery. 2nd Ed. Philadelphia: WB Saunders, 2004:183–193.

Paul-Murphy J, Ramer JC. Urgent care of the pet rabbits. Vet Clin North Am Exotic Anim Pract 1998;1(1):127–152.

Redrobe S. Calcium metabolism in rabbits. Semin Avian Exotic Pet Med 2002;11(2):94–101.

# INCISOR MALOCCLUSION AND OVERGROWTH

 BASICS

## DEFINITION
• Incisor overgrowth—occurs when normal occlusion does not occur. Rabbit teeth are open-rooted and grow continuously throughout life. Normal rabbit incisors are very long and curved and rely on proper contact of the upper incisors with the lower incisors during chewing to create a chisel shape.
• Malocclusion of the incisors—can occasionally be caused by congenital skeletal malocclusion or by trauma, but is usually the result of pathologic elongation of the cheek teeth.

## PATHOPHYSIOLOGY
• Normal dentition—total of six incisors, including two sets (lower and upper) of large incisor teeth and two small peg teeth located lingual to the large, upper incisors. No canine teeth, but instead a large diastema followed by the cheek teeth. The premolars and molars are aligned as one functional unit and are therefore referred to as cheek teeth. Cheek teeth consist of three upper premolars, three upper molars, two lower premolars, and three lower molars on each side.
• All teeth are open-rooted and grow continuously at a rate of approximately 3 mm per week, with growth originating from the germinal bud located at the apex of the tooth.
• The rate of normal wear should equal the rate of eruption, approximately 3 mm per week. Normal wear requires proper occlusion with the opposing set of teeth and a highly abrasive diet to stimulate chewing and grind coronal surfaces.
• Most incisor overgrowth and malocclusion is caused by overgrown cheek teeth. Elongation of the cheek teeth prohibits complete closure of the mouth, preventing the upper incisors from contacting the lower incisors, which allows unopposed growth of the incisors.
• Incisor growth—can be as much as 1 mm/day if unopposed
• The cause of cheek teeth overgrowth is likely multifactorial and not completely known. The most significant contributing or exacerbating factor is feeding diets that contain inadequate amounts of the coarse roughage material required to properly grind coronal surfaces. Congenital or inherited malocclusion may also play a role.
• Incisors may grow into or damage adjacent soft tissues; secondary bacterial infections may occur.

## SYSTEMS AFFECTED
• Oral cavity
• Ocular—nasolacrimal duct obstruction, retroorbital invasion of tooth roots
• Respiratory—apical (tooth root) invasion of the sinuses
• Musculoskeletal—weight loss, muscle wasting

## GENETICS
Unknown

## INCIDENCE/PREVALENCE
One of the most common presenting complaints in pet rabbits

## GEOGRAPHIC DISTRIBUTION
N/A

## SIGNALMENT
• Usually seen in middle-aged rabbits—incisor overgrowth secondary to cheek tooth elongation
• Young animals—congenital malocclusion
• Dwarf and lop breeds—congenital malocclusion
• No breed or gender predilection for incisor overgrowth secondary to cheek tooth elongation

## SIGNS

### General Comments
• Owners generally notice incisor overgrowth first, as these teeth are readily visible. In nearly all cases, incisor overgrowth is a symptom of generalized dental disease.
• Always perform a thorough oral examination under sedation or general anesthesia to examine the cheek teeth. Rabbits have a long, narrow mouth; use of a directed light source (or endoscope), a nasal speculum, cheek dilators, mouth gag are needed to thoroughly examine the teeth.
• Significant cheek teeth apical abnormalities may be present despite normal-appearing crowns. Skull films are required to identify apical (root) disorders.

### Historical Findings
• Inability to prehend food, dropping food out of the mouth, preference for softer foods
• Weight loss
• Anorexia or decreased appetite
• Preference for a water bowl over a sipper bottle
• Excessive drooling and moist dermatitis on the chin and dewlap
• Nasal discharge
• Tooth grinding
• Excessive tear production
• Facial asymmetry or exophthalmos in rabbits with tooth root abscesses
• Signs of pain—reluctance to move, depression, lethargy, hiding, hunched posture
• Unkempt haircoat, lack of grooming

### Physical Examination Findings
Incisors—overgrown, horizontal ridges or grooves, malformation, discoloration, fractures, increased or decreased curvature, loose teeth; malocclusion—bite appears level or the mandibular incisors are rostral to maxillary incisors

### Oral Examination
• A thorough examination of the cheek teeth requires heavy sedation or general anesthesia and specialized equipment. A cursory examination using an otoscope for illumination and visualization is insufficient for rabbits with dental disease.
• A focused, directed light source and magnification will provide optimal visualization.
• Use a rodent mouth gag and cheek dilators (Jorgensen Laboratories, Inc., Loveland, CO) to open the mouth and pull buccal tissues away from teeth surfaces to allow adequate exposure. Use a cotton swab or tongue depressor to retract the tongue from lingual surfaces.
• Normal cheek teeth—do not have a flat surface, but small vertical cusps; normal crown length for maxillary cheek teeth: approximately 1 mm (maximum 2 mm); normal crown length for mandibular cheek teeth: approximately 3 mm (maximum 5 mm)
• Identify cheek teeth abnormalities—elongation, irregular crown height, spikes, curved teeth, discolored teeth, missing teeth, purulent exudate, odor, impacted food, oral ulceration, or abscesses
• Buccal or lingual mucosa and lip margins—ulceration, abrasions, secondary bacterial infection, or abscess formation if incisors or cheek teeth spikes have damaged soft tissues

### Other Findings
• Ptyalism, secondary moist pyoderma around the mouth, neck, and dewlap areas
• A scalloped edge or single bony protrusion may be palpable on the ventral rim of the mandible in some rabbits with apical cheek teeth disorders
• Soft tissue swelling, abscess most commonly located on the mandible or below the eye
• Exophthalmus in rabbits with retrobulbar abscesses from periapical cheek tooth abscesses
• Weight loss, emaciation
• Nasal discharge
• Ocular discharge—blocked nasolacrimal duct; pressure on the eye from retrobulbar abscess or overgrown tooth roots
• Signs of gastrointestinal hypomotility—scant feces, intestinal pain, diarrhea

## CAUSES
• Congenital skeletal malocclusion—unusual cause; most likely in young, dwarf, or lop-eared breeds
• Trauma—traumatic fracture of the incisors; iatrogenic damage from inappropriate incisor clipping
• Elongated cheek teeth—likely multiple etiologies; inadequate hay or tough foods to properly grind teeth so that coronal surfaces cannot wear normally

## RISK FACTORS
• Feeding pelleted diets (without supplementing long-stemmed hay and grasses)—these diets lack sufficient abrasive material to properly wear teeth; pellets are small and calorically dense, requiring less chewing.
• Breeding rabbits with congenital malocclusion
• Broken incisors—improper restraint or inappropriate clipping of the incisors

## DIAGNOSIS

### DIFFERENTIAL DIAGNOSIS
• Overgrowth due to trauma—may have history of trauma (jumping, falling, being dropped) or history of having the teeth "clipped." May see fractured incisors and discoloration secondary to pulpitis. Rule out cheek teeth elongation by performing thorough oral examination under anesthesia and skull radiographs.
• Congenital malocclusion—seen in young animals. Diagnosis of exclusion if cheek teeth elongation has been ruled out by performing thorough oral examination under anesthesia and mandatory skull radiographs

### CBC/BIOCHEMISTRY/URINALYSIS
Usually normal; may see abnormalities in liver enzymes in rabbits with hepatic lipidosis secondary to anorexia

### OTHER LABORATORY TESTS
N/A

### IMAGING
*Skull Radiographs*
• Mandatory to identify type and extent of dental disease, to plan treatment strategies, and to monitor progression of treatment
• Perform under general anesthesia.
• Five views are recommend for thorough assessment—ventral–dorsal, lateral, two lateral obliques, and rostral–caudal.
• Common incisor abnormalities—lower incisors no longer occlude with the peg teeth; with unopposed growth, they will often lose their normal curvature and protrude rostrally from the mandible; the apex of the mandibular incisors may invade into the roots of the premolars; increased curvature of the upper incisors is usually seen.

• With early disease—elongation of the crowns and roots, loss of normal coronal occlusal pattern, mild radiolucency around tooth roots, enlargement of germinal bud, lysis of bone
• Moderate to severe disease—crooked teeth, reduction in the diameter or obliteration of the pulp cavity, widening of the interdental space, apical radiolucency and bony lysis, penetration of the tooth roots into surrounding cortical bone
• Periapical abscess—severe lysis of cortical bone, bony proliferation
• CT—superior to radiographs to evaluate the extent of dental disease and bony destruction

### DIAGNOSTIC PROCEDURES
• Fine needle aspiration of facial swelling—may be helpful to identify abscess
• Bacterial culture of affected tissue and/or exudate—aerobic and anaerobic bacteria; growth more likely if wall or capsule is sampled; bacteria deep within exudate are often nonviable.
• Bacterial susceptibility testing to direct antibiotic therapy

## TREATMENT

### APPROPRIATE HEALTH CARE
• Outpatient—patients with mild to moderate dental disease requiring coronal reduction
• Inpatient—patients with periapical or facial abscess, patients requiring extraction, or debilitated patients

### NURSING CARE
Keep fur around face clean and dry.

### ACTIVITY
N/A

### DIET
• It is absolutely imperative that the rabbit continue to eat during and following treatment. Many rabbits with dental disease will become anorectic. Rabbits may be unable to eat solid food following radical coronal reduction, extractions, or surgical treatment of abscesses. Anorexia will cause or exacerbate gastrointestinal hypomotility, derangement of the gastrointestinal microflora, and overgrowth of intestinal bacterial pathogens.
• Syringe feed a gruel such as Critical Care for Herbivores (Oxbow Pet Products, Murdock, NE) 10–15 mL/kg PO q6–8h. Larger volumes and more frequent feedings are often accepted; feed as much as the rabbit will readily accept. Alternatively, pellets can be ground and mixed with fresh greens, vegetable baby foods, water, or juice to form a gruel.

• Most rabbits will require assisted feeding for 36–48 hours postoperatively; following coronal reduction assisted feeding may be needed for several weeks.
• High-carbohydrate, high-fat nutritional supplements are contraindicated.
• Return the rabbit to a solid-food diet as soon as possible to encourage normal occlusion and wear. Increase the amount of tough, fibrous foods such as hay and wild grasses; avoid pelleted food and soft fruits or vegetables.
• Encourage oral fluid intake by offering fresh water or wetting leafy vegetables.

### CLIENT EDUCATION
• Unless incisor malocclusion is temporary due to trauma, it can only be managed, not cured.
• Most incisor malocclusions are acquired secondary to cheek teeth elongation. By the time clinical signs are noted, disease is usually advanced. Lifelong treatment, consisting of periodic coronal reduction (teeth trimming), is required, usually every 1–3 months.
• Severe dental disease, especially those with tooth root abscesses and severe bony destruction, carries a guarded to poor prognosis for complete resolution. Most will require extensive surgery, sometimes multiple surgeries and multiple follow-up visits. Recurrences in the same or other locations are common. Clients must be aware of the monetary and time investment.
• Teach owners how to recognize signs of oral pain.

### SURGICAL CONSIDERATIONS
*Trimming of Incisors (Coronal Reduction)*
• Trimming of incisors alone will be of little to no benefit for most rabbits, since in most cases malocclusion is acquired secondary to cheek teeth elongation.
• Treat all predisposing or coexisting dental disease, cheek teeth elongation, and tooth root abscesses in addition to trimming the incisors.
• Most rabbits require sedation or general anesthesia to trim the incisors, although some will tolerate it with restraint only. The decision is based on the rabbit's temperament and the practitioner's level of proficiency. Err on the side of caution; rabbits may unexpectedly jump, resulting in significant soft tissue or spinal trauma.
• If performed under general anesthesia—premedicate with buprenorphine (add ketamine and midazolam in nervous patients), induce with isoflurane via mask, move the mask over nose to maintain anesthesia (rabbits are obligate nasal breathers), or intubate.

# INCISOR MALOCCLUSION AND OVERGROWTH

• Do not clip the teeth with nail trimmers, rongeurs, or any other clipping device—clipping may cause longitudinal fractures of the teeth, leading to pulpitis and subsequent periapical abscessation, or damage periapical tissues.

• Trim incisors with Dremel tool using a diamond cutting blade or using a high- or low-speed thin cutting dental bur.

• Protect soft tissues from the cutting blade.

• Avoid cutting through the pulp—the pulp grows beyond the level of gingiva with overgrown teeth and is visible as a pink coloration. Cutting the pulp is painful and may cause pulpitis, pulp necrosis, and periapical abscess formation.

• If the pulp is accidentally cut, indicated by bleeding at the cut surface of the tooth, perform a partial pulpectomy and cap the pulp with calcium hydroxide cement. Do not use conventional filling materials as these prevent normal tooth wear.

## Incisor Extraction

• May be a preferred option, since teeth will need to be trimmed every 4–8 weeks, often for life. Each trimming can be stressful to the rabbit and expensive and time consuming for the client, and carries the risk of pulp exposure or trauma to teeth during trimming.

• Incisor extraction will not limit food prehension.

• Regular examination of the cheek teeth to monitor for overgrowth is still required.

• Indicated in rabbits with loose incisors or periapical abscesses

• Because rabbits have very long, deeply embedded, and curved incisor roots, incisor extraction can be extremely time consuming and labor intensive as compared to for dogs and cats. If the germinal bud is not completely removed, an abscess may form. If not experienced with tooth extraction in rabbits, the author recommends referral to a veterinarian with special expertise whenever feasible.

# MEDICATIONS

## DRUG(S) OF CHOICE

### Antibiotics

Indicated in rabbits with periapical abscesses. Choice of antibiotic is ideally based on results of culture and susceptibility testing. Depending on the severity of infection, long-term antibiotic therapy is required (4–6 weeks minimum to several months or years). Most facial or dental abscesses are caused by anaerobic bacteria; use antibiotics effective against anaerobes such as azithromycin (30 mg/kg PO q24h); can be used alone or combined with metronidazole (20 mg/kg PO q12h). Alternatively, use penicillin g (40,000–60,000 IU/kg SC q2–7d), chloramphenicol (50 mg/kg PO q8h) or metronidazole alone. Combine with topical treatment (surgical debridement, AIPPMA beads). If aerobic bacteria are isolated, use broad-spectrum antibiotics such as enrofloxacin (5–20 mg/kg PO, SC, IM q12–24h) or trimethoprim sulfa (30 mg/kg PO q12h).

### Acute Pain Management

Buprenorphine (0.01–0.05 mg/kg SC, IM, IV q8–12h)—use preoperatively for extractions, coronal reduction, or surgical abscess treatment.

### Long-Term Pain Management

NSAIDs have been used for short- or long-term therapy to reduce pain and inflammation—meloxicam (0.2–0.5 mg/kg PO q24h) or carprofen (2.2 mg/kg PO q12–24h)

### Heavy Sedation for Oral Examination or Trimming of Incisors

Ketamine (15–20 mg/kg IM) plus midazolam (0.5–1.0 mg/kg IM); many other sedation protocols exist; alternatively, administer general anesthesia with isoflurane.

## CONTRAINDICATIONS

• Oral administration of most antibiotics effective against anaerobes will cause a fatal gastrointestinal dysbiosis in rabbits. Do not administer penicillins, macrolides, lincosamides, and cephalosporins by oral administration.

• Corticosteroids—associated with gastrointestinal ulceration and hemorrhage, delayed wound healing, and heightened susceptibility to infection; rabbits are very sensitive to the immunosuppressive effects of both topical and systemic corticosteroids; use may exacerbate subclinical bacterial infection.

## PRECAUTIONS

• Chloramphenicol—avoid human contact with chloramphenicol due to potential blood dyscrasia. Advise owners of potential risks.

• Meloxicam—use with caution in rabbits with compromised renal function.

## POSSIBLE INTERACTIONS
N/A

## ALTERNATIVE DRUGS
N/A

# FOLLOW-UP

## PATIENT MONITORING

• Reevaluate, and trim as needed, every 4–8 weeks. Evaluate the entire oral cavity with each recheck.

• Monitor for signs of apical abscess or invasion of the tooth roots into surrounding bone or sinuses (epiphora, nasal discharge, facial swelling).

## PREVENTION/AVOIDANCE

• In rabbits with acquired dental disease, prevention is not possible once clinical signs of malocclusion are present. With periodic coronal reduction and appropriate diet, progression of disease may be arrested, but treatment is lifelong.

• Provide adequate tough, fibrous foods such as hay and grasses to encourage normal wear of teeth.

## POSSIBLE COMPLICATIONS

• Periapical abscesses, recurrence, chronic pain, or extensive tissue destruction may warrant euthanasia due to poor quality of life

• Hepatic lipidosis with prolonged anorexia

• Chronic epiphora with nasolacrimal duct occlusion

## EXPECTED COURSE AND PROGNOSIS

• Incisor overgrowth only (congential malocclusion or trauma)—good to fair prognosis; lifelong incisor trimming may be required.

• Incisor overgrowth due to cheek teeth elongation—fair to poor prognosis, depending on severity of disease; lifelong treatment is required.

• Periapical or facial abscesses, osteomyelitis—depend on severity of bone involvement and location. Rabbits with abscesses in the nasal passages or with exophthalmos or multiple or severe maxillary abscesses have a guarded to poor prognosis. Multiple surgeries and follow-up treatments are usually required; recurrence rates are high. Euthanasia may be warranted with severe or advanced disease, especially in rabbits that are in pain or cannot eat.

• Severity of physical examination and radiographic findings do not always correlate well with the degree of apparent discomfort. Some rabbits appear to remain comfortable for extended periods with long-term administration of antibiotics and analgesics.

# MISCELLANEOUS

## ASSOCIATED CONDITIONS
N/A

## AGE-RELATED FACTORS
N/A

## ZOONOTIC POTENTIAL
N/A

## PREGNANCY
N/A

# INCISOR MALOCCLUSION AND OVERGROWTH

**SYNONYMS**
N/A

**SEE ALSO**
- Abscessation
- Epiphora
- Cheek teeth malocclusion and elongation

**ABBREVIATIONS**
- AIPPMA = antibiotic-impregnated polymethyl methacrylate
- NSAIDs = nonsteroidal antiinflammatory drugs

*Suggested Reading*
Crossley DA. Oral biology and disorders of lagomorphs. Vet Clin North Am Exotic Anim Pract 2003;6(3):629–659.
Crossley DA, Aiken S. Small mammal dentistry. In: Quesenberry KE, Carpenter JW, eds. Ferrets, Rabbits and Rodents: Clinical Medicine and Surgery. 2nd Ed. Philadelphia: WB Saunders, 2004:370–382.
Harcourt-Brown F. Dental disease. In: Harcourt-Brown F, ed. Textbook of Rabbit Medicine. Oxford: Butterworth-Heinemann, 2002:165–205.
Lukehart SA, Fohn MJ, Baker-Zander SA. Efficacy of azithromycin for therapy of active syphilis in the rabbit model. J Antimicrob Chemother 1990;25 Suppl A:91–99.
Tyrell KC, Citron DM, Jenkins JR, et al. Periodontal bacteria in rabbit mandibular and maxillary abscesses. J Clin Microbiol 2002;40(3):1044–1047.

# INCONTINENCE, URINARY

 BASICS

## DEFINITION
Loss of voluntary control of micturition, usually observed as involuntary urine leakage

## PATHOPHYSIOLOGY
Usually a disorder of the storage phase of micturition. Urine storage failure is caused by failure of urinary bladder accommodation, failure of urethral continence mechanisms, or anatomic bypass of urinary storage structures. Partial outlet obstruction and other causes of urinary bladder overdistension may result in paradoxical, or overflow, urinary incontinence.

## SYSTEMS AFFECTED
- Renal/urologic
- Nervous
- Skin—urine scald, perineal and ventral dermatitis

## SIGNALMENT
Most common in middle-aged rabbits 3–5 years old

## SIGNS

### Historical Findings
- Owners often observe urine scald or report dribbling of urine when the rabbit is picked up.
- Trauma, rear limb paresis, or paralysis in rabbits with spinal disease
- Other CNS signs in rabbits with CNS abscess or *Encephalitozoon cuniculi*
- Cloudy or thick, beige- to brown-colored urine in rabbits with hypercalciuria
- May be only historical finding in rabbits with hypercalciuria or urinary calculi

### Physical Examination Findings
- Rear limb paresis or paralysis
- Urine scald in perineal region
- Detect urocystoliths by abdominal palpation; failure to palpate uroliths does not exclude them from consideration.
- In rabbits with crystalluria, the bladder palpates as a soft, doughy mass.
- With chronic disease, the bladder may markedly increase in size and may even fill most of the abdomen.
- Manual expression of the bladder may reveal thick, beige- to brown-colored urine in rabbits with hypercalciuria. Manual expression of the bladder may expel thick, brown urine even in rabbits that have normal-appearing voided urine.

## CAUSES

### Neurologic
- Disruption of local neuroreceptors, peripheral nerves, spinal pathways, or higher centers involved in the control of micturition can disrupt urine storage.
- Lesion of the sacral spinal cord, such as traumatic fractures or dislocation (very common), disk disease, or spinal neoplasia can result in a flaccid, overdistended urinary bladder with weak outlet resistance. Urine retention and overflow incontinence develop.
- Lesions of the cerebellum or cerebral micturition center (most commonly abscess or *E. cuniculi*) affect inhibition and voluntary control of voiding.

### Urinary Bladder Storage Dysfunction
Hypercalciuria/urinary calculi, urinary tract infection, infiltrative neoplastic lesion, external compression, and chronic partial outlet obstruction

### Urethral Disorders
- Acquired urethral incompetence—estrogen-responsive urinary incontinence in ovariohysterectomized females has been reported.
- Urinary tract infection or inflammation from hypercalciuria

### Anatomic
- Developmental or acquired anatomic abnormalities that divert urine from normal storage mechanisms or interfere with urinary bladder or urethral function
- Ectopic ureters—the only congenital abnormality reported in the literature

## RISK FACTORS
- For hypercalciuria/urinary calculi—inadequate water intake (dirty water bowls, unpalatable water, changing water sources, inadequate water provision); inadequate cleaning of litter box or cage may cause some rabbits to avoid urinating for abnormally long periods; obesity, lack of exercise, feeding of exclusively alfalfa-based pelleted diets, renal disease, and adding calcium or vitamin/mineral supplements to the diet
- For neurologic causes—improper restraint (fracture/luxation); debility, stress, or immunosuppression (bacterial infection and *E. cuniculi*)
- For estrogen-responsive incontinence—ovariohysterectomy

 DIAGNOSIS

## DIFFERENTIAL DIAGNOSIS

### Differentiating Similar Signs
- Voluntary but inappropriate urination
- Inability to maintain proper stance for micturition due to musculoskeletal disease or obesity—rabbits normally lift their hindquarters and spray urine caudally; an inability to maintain this posture causes urine to soak the perineal region and ventrum and may mimic incontinence.
- Urine spraying—territorial marking in intact animals

### Differentiating Causes
- Polyuria—may precipitate or exacerbate urinary incontinence or lead to nocturia and inappropriate urination
- Hypercalciuria—urinary incontinence occasionally the only clinical sign; urine scald in perineum or ventrum; doughy consistency to bladder on palpation; manual expression of the bladder may reveal thick, beige- to brown-colored urine in rabbits with hypercalciuria.
- Other neurologic signs are usually present in rabbits with CNS disease or spinal disorders.
- A large, distended urinary bladder may be seen in rabbits with neurologic causes of incontinence or chronic, severe hypercalciuria.

## CBC/BIOCHEMISTRY/URINALYSIS
- Hematologic and biochemical analyses may be helpful in identifying causes or polyuric disorders.
- Hypercalciuria—urinary sediment evaluation reveals calcium oxalate or calcium carbonate crystals; however, this is a normal finding in rabbits, and the presence of large amounts of crystals in the urine does not necessarily indicate disease. Disease occurs only when the concentration of crystals is excessive, forming thick, white to brown, paste- or sandlike urine and subsequent inflammatory cystitis or partial to complete blockage of the urethra.
- Pyuria (normal value 0–1 WBC/hpf), hematuria (normal value 0–1 RBC/hpf), and proteinuria (normal value 0–33 mg/dL) indicate urinary tract inflammation, but these are nonspecific findings that may result from infectious and noninfectious causes of lower urinary tract disease.

## OTHER LABORATORY TESTS
Serologic testing for *E. cuniculi*—many tests are available, but usefulness is extremely limited since a positive titer indicates only exposure and does not confirm *E. cuniculi* as the cause of neurologic signs. *E. cuniculi* can only be definitively diagnosed by finding organisms and resultant lesions on histopathologic examination in areas that anatomically correlate with observed clinical signs. Antibody titers usually become positive by 2 weeks postinfection, but generally do not continue to rise with active infection or decline with treatment. No correlation exists between antibody titers and shedding of organism and presence or severity of disease. It is unknown if exposed rabbits eventually become seronegative. Available tests include ELISA, indirect IFA, and carbon immunoassay.

## IMAGING

### Radiographic finding
- Calcium oxalate uroliths and sand are radiopaque and may be detected by survey radiography. Uroliths must be differentiated

from calcium "sand" or "sludge" in the bladder, which resembles a bladder full of contrast material. With chronic disease, the bladder may enlarge significantly.

• Skull films may demonstrate otitis media; increased soft tissue density in the bullae, bony lysis, or periosteal proliferation in rabbits with bacterial otitis interna/media or brain abscesses. CT scans or MRI is much more accurate.

• Radiographs may demonstrate spinal fractures, luxations, or other orthopedic abnormalities that prohibit normal posture during micturition.

### Ultrasonographic Findings
Can evaluate the kidneys and urinary bladder to identify uroliths, hypercalciuria, masses, hydroureter, or evidence of pyelonephritis.

### DIAGNOSTIC PROCEDURES
• Neurologic examination—examination of anal tone, tail tone, and perineal sensation provides a brief assessment of caudal spinal and peripheral nerve function.
• Urethral catheterization may be required to assess patency of the urethra if urine retention is observed.

# TREATMENT
• Usually outpatient
• Address primary neurologic disorders specifically, if possible.
• Identify urinary tract infection and treat appropriately.
• Ectopic ureters and urolithiasis may be surgically corrected.
• Symptomatic rabbits with calcium precipitate ("sand" or "sludge") in the urinary bladder often respond to medical treatment with fluid therapy and voiding urohydropropulsion.
• Treat secondary urine scald; keep area clean and dry.

# MEDICATIONS

### DRUG(S) OF CHOICE
• Urethral incompetence in ovariohysterectomized rabbits may respond to 0.5 mg of diethylstilbestrol PO one to two times per week.

• Some rabbits with large amounts of calcium precipitate or uroliths have an underlying chronic bacterial cystitis. Treat with antibiotics, based on culture and susceptibility testing when possible, for 3–4 weeks.

### CONTRAINDICATIONS
Oral administration of antibiotics that select against Gram-positive bacteria (penicillins, macrolides, lincosamides, and cephalasporins) cause fatal enteric dysbiosis and enterotoxemia.

### PRECAUTIONS
Estrogen compounds (rarely) cause signs of estrus or bone marrow suppression.

### POSSIBLE INTERACTIONS
N/A

### ALTERNATIVE DRUGS
N/A

# FOLLOW-UP

### PATIENT MONITORING
• Radiographs are essential following treatment of hypercalciuria to verify complete removal of calcium precipitate or uroliths.
• Periodic urinalysis
• Periodic hemogram in patients receiving estrogens
• Rabbits with incontinence caused by neurologic disease carry a poor prognosis.

### POSSIBLE COMPLICATIONS
• Recurrent and ascending urinary tract infection
• Urine scald with perineal and ventral dermatitis, myiasis, pododermatitis
• Refractory and unmanageable incontinence

# MISCELLANEOUS

### ASSOCIATED CONDITIONS
• Gastrointestinal hypomotility
• Pyoderma

### AGE-RELATED FACTORS
N/A

### ZOONOTIC POTENTIAL
Possible with *E. cuniculi*

### PREGNANCY
N/A

### SEE ALSO
• Encephalitis and meningioencephalitis
• Hypercalciuria and urolithiasis
• Polydipsia and polyuria

### ABBREVIATIONS
• CNS = central nervous system
• CT = computed tomography
• ELISA = enzyme-linked immunosorbent assay
• IFA = immunofluorescence assay
• MRI = magnetic resonance imaging
• RBC = red blood cell
• WBC = white blood cell

### Suggested Reading
Brown SA. Rabbit urinary tract disease. Proc North Am Vet Conf 1997;785–787.
Donoghue S. Nutrition and pet rabbits. In: Rosenthal KL, ed. Practical Exotic Animal Medicine: The Compendium Collection. Trenton, NJ: Veterinary Learning Systems, 1997:107.
Harkness JE, Wagner JE. The Biology and Medicine of Rabbits and Rodents. 3rd Ed. Baltimore: Williams & Wilkins, 1989.
Harcourt-Brown F. Urogenital disease. In: Harcourt-Brown F, ed. Textbook of Rabbit Medicine. Oxford: Butterworth-Heinemann, 2002:335–351.
Pare JA, Paul-Murphy J. Disorders of the reproductive and urinary systems. In: Quesenberry KE, Carpenter JW, eds. Ferrets, Rabbits and Rodents: Clinical Medicine and Surgery. 2nd Ed. Philadelphia: WB Saunders, 2004:183–193.
Paul-Murphy J, Ramer JC. Urgent care of the pet rabbits. Vet Clin North Am: Exotic Anim Pract 1998;1(1):127–152.
Redrobe S. Calcium metabolism in rabbits. Semin Avian Exotic Pet Med 2002;11(2):94–101.

### Portions Adapted From
Lane IF. Incontinence, Urinary. In: Tilley LP, Smith FWK, Jr., eds. The 5-Minute Veterinary Consult: Canine and Feline, 3rd Ed. Baltimore: Lippincott Williams & Wilkins, 2004.

# LAMENESS

## BASICS

### DEFINITION
A disturbance in gait and locomotion in response to pain or injury

### PATHOPHYSIOLOGY
• Severe, sharp pain—when moving, patient carries or puts no weight on the affected limb.
• Milder, dull, or aching pain—when moving, patient limps or bears little weight on the affected limb; at rest, the patient bears less weight on the affected limb.
• If the rear limbs are affected, the rabbit may appear to walk rather than hop.
• Many rabbits are reluctant to move at all with mild to moderate limb pain.
• Pain produced only during certain phases of movement—patient adjusts its motion and gait to minimize discomfort.

### SYSTEMS AFFECTED
• Musculoskeletal
• Nervous
• Dermatologic—secondary disorders (urine scald, dermatitis)

### SIGNALMENT
Age, breed, and sex predilection—depend on specific disease

### SIGNS

#### General Comments
Always assess the patient's neurologic status, especially with a suspected proximal lesion.

#### Historical Findings
• Complete history—mandatory; signalment; identification of affected limb(s); known trauma; changes with exercise or rest; responsiveness to previous treatments
• Determine onset of lameness—acute or chronic
• Determine progression—static, slow, rapid
• Signs of pain—depression, lethargy, hunched posture while sitting, reluctance to move, hiding, teeth grinding, grunting or crying with movement, decreased appetite or water intake, lack of grooming

#### Physical Examination Findings
• Use secure restraint when examining rabbits in pain.
• Perform a complete routine examination.
• Observe gait—hopping, climbing
• Palpate—asymmetry of muscle mass, bony prominences, swelling over joints
• Manipulate bones and joints, beginning distally and working proximally.
• Assess—instability, luxation or subluxation, pain, abnormal range of motion, abnormal sounds
• Examine suspected area of involvement last—by starting with normal limbs, patient may relax, allowing assessment of normal reaction to maneuvers.

• Urine scald in the perineal region, dermatitis or alopecia due to inappropriate grooming, pododermatitis

### CAUSES

#### General Comments
The causes listed below are the most common causes of lameness in rabbits, with most common listed first. Also consider other causes common to dogs and cats; these may also occur in rabbits, but have not been well documented.

#### Forelimb
• Infection—abscess, septic arthritis, pododermatitis
• Degenerative joint disease
• Shoulder luxation or subluxation
• Elbow luxation or subluxation
• Trauma—soft tissue, bone, joint
• Congenital anomalies
• Soft tissue or bone neoplasia—primary, metastatic

#### Hindlimb
• Infection—ulcerative pododermatitis (sore hocks), abscess, septic arthritis
• Trauma—soft tissue, bone, joint
• Hip luxation or subluxation
• Degenerative joint disease
• Cruciate ligament disease
• Patella luxation
• Congenital anomalies
• Hip dysplasia
• Soft tissue or bone neoplasia—primary, metastatic

#### Spinal Disease
• Fractures, luxation
• Spondylosis
• Intervertebral disc disease

### RISK FACTORS
• Trauma, dislocations—improper restraint, trauma in caged rabbits suddenly startled, possibly disuse atrophy from confinement
• Ulcerative pododermatitis (sore hocks)—excoriation, friction, or constant moisture on the skin and soft tissues of the plantar aspect of the hock; caused by lack of protective fur covering and/or feces and urine coating the feet
• Abscesses, infection—immunosuppression (stress, corticosteroid use, concurrent disease); poor husbandry
• Obesity, lack of exercise

## DIAGNOSIS

### DIFFERENTIAL DIAGNOSIS
• Must differentiate musculoskeletal from neurogenic causes
• Lameness affecting one limb—fracture, soft tissue injury, abscess, ulcerative pododermatitis, neoplasia

• Lameness affecting multiple limbs—spinal trauma, spondylosis, disc disease, septic arthritis

### CBC/BIOCHEMISTRY/URINALYSIS
Usually normal; relative heterophilia and/or lymphopenia sometimes seen with bacterial diseases

### OTHER LABORATORY TESTS
Depend on suspected cause

### IMAGING
• Radiographs—recommended for all suspected musculoskeletal causes
• CT, MRI—help identify and delineate causative lesions

### DIAGNOSTIC PROCEDURES
• Cytologic examination of joint fluid—identify and differentiate intraarticular disease.
• EMG—differentiate neuromuscular from musculoskeletal disease.
• Muscle and/or nerve biopsy—reveal and identify neuromuscular disease.

## TREATMENT
Depends on underlying cause

### NURSING CARE
• Depends on severity of disease
• Bandage or splint care
• Anorectic rabbits may require forced alimentation.
• Soft bedding; daily bedding changes
• Remove soiled bedding; keep fur clean and dry.

### ACTIVITY
Restricted until resolution of symptoms

### DIET
• It is absolutely imperative that the rabbit continue to eat during and following treatment. Disorders causing lameness are often painful, resulting in anorexia. Anorexia will often cause gastrointestinal hypomotility, derangement of the gastrointestinal microflora, and overgrowth of intestinal bacterial pathogens.
• Offer a large selection of fresh, moistened greens such as cilantro, romaine lettuce, parsley, carrot tops, dandelion greens, spinach, collard greens, etc., and good-quality grass hay. Many rabbits will begin to eat these foods, even if they were previously anorectic.
• If the patient refuses these foods, syringe feed a gruel such as Critical Care for Herbivores (Oxbow Pet Products) 10–15 mL/kg PO q6–8h. Larger volumes and more frequent feedings are often accepted; feed as much as the rabbit will readily accept. Alternatively, pellets can be ground and mixed

with fresh greens, vegetable baby foods, water, or juice to form a gruel. If sufficient volumes of food are not accepted in this manner, nasogastric intubation is indicated.
• High-carbohydrate, high-fat nutritional supplements are contraindicated.
• Encourage oral fluid intake by offering fresh water and wetting leafy vegetables.

### SURGICAL CONSIDERATIONS
• Most abscesses, osteomyelitis, and septic joints require aggressive surgical management.
• Simple, closed fractures may respond to external coaptation; most other fractures require open reduction.
• Joint injuries—closed reduction of coxofemoral luxation is difficult due to powerful hindlimb musculature; most require open reduction, FHO with chronic luxation, or severe DJD; most elbow luxations require internal fixation as the shoulder is difficult to incorporate in a bandage; cruciate tears often heal with cage rest.

## MEDICATIONS
### DRUG(S) OF CHOICE
*Acute Pain Management*
• Butorphanol (0.1–1.0 mg/kg SC, IM, IV q4–6h)—may cause profound sedation; short-acting
• Buprenorphine (0.01–0.05 mg/kg SC, IM, IV q8–12h)—less sedating, longer-acting than butorphanol
• Morphine (2–5 mg/kg SC, IM q2–4h) or oxymorphone (0.05–0.2 mg/kg SC, IM q8–12h)—use with caution; more than one to two doses may cause gastrointestinal stasis.
• Meloxicam (0.2 mg/kg SC, IM q24h)
• Carprofen (1–4 mg/kg SC q12h)

*Long-Term Pain Management*
NSAIDs—have been used for short- or long-term therapy to reduce pain and inflammation in rabbits with spinal cord disease: meloxicam (0.2–0.5 mg/kg PO q24h) or carprofen (2.2 mg/kg PO q12–24h)

*Bacterial Infection*
Use antimicrobial drugs effective against the infectious agent; gain access to site of infection. Choice of antibiotic is based on results of culture and susceptibility testing. Use

broad-spectrum antibiotics such as enrofloxacin (5–20 mg/kg PO, SC, IM q12–24h) or trimethoprim sulfa (30 mg/kg PO q12h); if anaerobic infections are suspected, use metronidazole (20 mg/kg PO q12h) or parenteral penicillin g (40,000–60,000 IU/kg SC q2–7d).

### CONTRAINDICATIONS
• Oral administration of antibiotics that select against Gram-positive bacteria (penicillins, macrolides, lincosamides, and cephalosporins) cause fatal enteric dysbiosis and enterotoxemia.
• Corticosteroids—associated with gastrointestinal ulceration and hemorrhage, delayed wound healing, and heightened susceptibility to infection; rabbits are very sensitive to the immunosuppressive effects of both topical and systemic corticosteroids; use may exacerbate subclinical bacterial infection.

### PRECAUTIONS
Meloxicam—use with caution in rabbits with compromised renal function.

### POSSIBLE INTERACTIONS
N/A

### ALTERNATIVE DRUGS
• Chondroprotective agents, nutraceuticals (oral glycosaminoglycans, cosequin)—use not well described in rabbits; have been anecdotally used at feline dosages in addition to analgesics
• Acupuncture may be effective for rabbits with chronic pain.

## FOLLOW-UP
### PATIENT MONITORING
• Depends on underlying cause
• Monitor for complications arising secondary to chronic pain and immobility such as urine scald, hypercalciuria, obesity, sore hocks, and gastrointestinal hypomotility.

### POSSIBLE COMPLICATIONS
Secondary to chronic pain and immobility—urine scald, hypercalciuria, obesity, sore hocks, gastrointestinal hypomotility; ankylosis common with severe joint disorders

## MISCELLANEOUS
### ASSOCIATED CONDITIONS
N/A

### AGE-RELATED FACTORS
N/A

### ZOONOTIC POTENTIAL
N/A

### PREGNANCY
N/A

### SEE ALSO
• Abscessation
• Pododermatitis
• Vertebral fracture and luxation

### ABBREVIATIONS
• CT = computed tomography
• DJD = degenerative joint disease
• EMG = electromyogram
• FHO = femoral head osteotomy
• MRI = magnetic resonance imaging

*Suggested Reading*

Deeb BJ, Carpenter JW. Neurologic and musculoskeletal diseases. In: Quesenberry KE, Carpenter JW, eds. Ferrets, Rabbits and Rodents: Clinical Medicine and Surgery. 2nd Ed. Philadelphia: WB Saunders, 2004:194–210.

Greenaway JB, Partlow GD, Gonsholt NL, et al. Anatomy of the lumbosacral spinal cord in rabbits. J Am Anim Hosp Assoc 2001;37(1):27–34.

Harcourt-Brown F. Neurological and locomotor diseases. In: Harcourt-Brown F, ed. Textbook of Rabbit Medicine. Oxford: Oxford: Butterworth-Heinemann, 2002:307–323.

Kapatkin A. Orthopedics in small mammals. Quesenberry KE, Carpenter JW, eds. Ferrets, Rabbits and Rodents: Clinical Medicine and Surgery. 2nd Ed. Philadelphia: WB Saunders, 2004:383–391.

Paul-Murphy J, Ramer JC. Urgent care of the pet rabbits. Vet Clin North Am Exotic Anim Pract 1998;1(1):127–152.

*Portions Adapted From*

Schwarz PD. Lameness. In: Tilley LP, Smith FWK, Jr., eds. The 5-Minute Veterinary Consult: Canine and Feline, 3rd Ed. Baltimore: Lippincott Williams & Wilkins, 2004.

# LEAD TOXICITY

 BASICS

## OVERVIEW
- Intoxication (blood lead concentrations >10 µg/dL) owing to acute or chronic exposure to some form of lead
- Many rabbits chew or lick lead-containing household substances, especially painted surfaces, occasionally metallic objects
- Lead—interferes with numerous enzymes, including those involved in heme synthesis; causes fragility and decreased survival of RBCs
- Damage to CNS capillaries—may account for brain lesions

## SYSTEMS AFFECTED
- Hemic/lymph/immune—interference with hemoglobin synthesis
- Gastrointestinal—unknown mechanism
- Nervous—capillary damage; possible direct toxic affect
- Renal/urologic—damage to proximal tubule cells

## SIGNALMENT
- Incidence unknown; more common in rabbits living in older homes and rabbits that roam free in the house
- No age, breed, or gender predisposition

## SIGNS
- Nonspecific signs such as weight loss, anorexia, depression, and lethargy predominate.
- Gastrointestinal—decreased appetite, anorexia, gastrointestinal hypomotility or stasis; rarely diarrhea
- CNS—blindness, weakness, lethargy, ataxia, seizures

## CAUSES
- Ingestion of some form of lead—paint and paint residues or dust from sanding; linoleum; solder; plumbing materials and supplies; lubricating compounds; putty; tar paper; lead foil; lead objects
- Use of improperly glazed ceramic food or water bowl
- Lead paint or solder on cages

## RISK FACTORS
- Living in economically depressed areas or old housing that is being renovated
- Unsupervised chewing
- Lead-containing cages or cage contents

 DIAGNOSIS

## DIFFERENTIAL DIAGNOSIS
For CNS signs:
- Other, more common causes of encephalopathy—infectious diseases most common, especially bacterial (brain abscess, extension from otitis interna/media, menin-

goencephalitis) or protozoal (encephalitozoonosis); parasitic migration (*Baylisascaris*—raccoon roundworm), viral, fungal rare in rabbits; brain tumor; hepatic or ischemic encephalopathy also rare
- Heat stroke—acute onset, supportive history
- Physical examination findings helpful in diagnosing more common problems: nasal/ocular discharge—either historical or currently present, common finding with spread of upper respiratory infection to inner/middle ear; otitis externa—thick, white, creamy exudate may be found in the horizontal and/or vertical canals; otitis interna/media—may occur in the absence of otitis externa via extension through the eustachian tube, may see bulging tympanum. Some rabbits with otitis interna have no visible otoscopic abnormalities.
For anorexia, depression, and weight loss:
- Almost any systemic disease process
- Gastrointestinal disease is one of the most common causes—especially problems related to gastrointestinal hypomotility or stasis
- Pain
- Dental disease

## CBC/BIOCHEMISTRY/URINALYSIS
- Anemia common finding; may be only abnormality found in rabbit that is otherwise clinically normal or exhibiting vague, nonspecific signs
- Nucleated erythrocytes, hypochromasia, poikilocytosis, and cytoplasmic basophilic stippling of RBCs sometimes seen

## OTHER LABORATORY TESTS
### Lead Concentration
- Submit whole, unclotted blood; lithium heparin tube or check with diagnostic laboratory for anticoagulant preference
- Toxic—antemortem whole blood lead concentrations >10 µg/dL
- Lower values—must be interpreted in conjunction with history and clinical signs
- Blood levels—may not correlate with occurrence or severity of clinical signs

## IMAGING
May note radiopaque material in gastrointestinal tract; not diagnostic. Radiopaque densities often not present with ingestion of paint

## DIAGNOSTIC PROCEDURES
N/A

 TREATMENT

## APPROPRIATE HEALTH CARE
- Inpatient—first course of chelation, depending on severity of clinical signs; for rabbits that are actively seizing, debilitated, or anorectic and require supportive care

- Outpatient—rabbits that are stable and eating; if owner can administer injections

## NURSING CARE
Balanced electrolyte fluids—replacement of hydration deficit

## ACTIVITY
N/A

## DIET
- It is absolutely imperative that the rabbit continue to eat during and following treatment. Anorexia will often cause gastrointestinal hypomotility, derangement of the gastrointestinal microflora, and overgrowth of intestinal bacterial pathogens.
- Offer a large selection of fresh, moistened greens such as cilantro, romaine lettuce, parsley, carrot tops, dandelion greens, spinach, collard greens, etc., and good-quality grass hay. Many rabbits will begin to eat these foods, even if they were previously anorectic.
- If the patient refuses these foods, syringe feed a gruel such as Critical Care for Herbivores (Oxbow Pet Products, Murdock, NE) 10–15 mL/kg PO q6–8h. Larger volumes and more frequent feedings are often accepted; feed as much as the rabbit will readily accept. Alternatively, pellets can be ground and mixed with fresh greens, vegetable baby foods, water, or juice to form a gruel.
- High-carbohydrate, high-fat nutritional supplements are contraindicated.
- Encourage oral fluid intake by offering fresh water, wetting leafy vegetables, or flavoring water with vegetable juices.

## CLIENT EDUCATION
- Inform client of the potential of adverse human health effects of lead.
- Notify public health officials.
- Determine the source of the lead.

## SURGICAL CONSIDERATIONS
Removal of lead objects from the gastrointestinal tract may be indicated.

 MEDICATIONS

## DRUG(S) OF CHOICE
- Control of seizures—diazepam (1–5 mg/kg IV, IM; begin with 0.5–1.0 mg/kg IV bolus); may repeat if gross seizure activity has not stopped within 5 minutes; can be administered rectally if IV access cannot be obtained; may diminish or stop the gross motor seizure activity to allow IV catheter placement
- Reduction of lead body burden—CaEDTA (25 mg/kg SC q6h for 5 days); dilute to 1% solution with D5W before administration; may need multiple treatments; allow a 5-day rest period between treatments.

• For gastrointestinal hypomotility—cisapride (0.5–1.0 mg/kg PO q8–12h) is usually helpful in regaining normal motility; cisapride is available through many compounding pharmacies.

## CONTRAINDICATIONS
CaEDTA—do not administer to patients with renal impairment or anuria; establish urine flow before administration.

## PRECAUTIONS
CaEDTA—safety in pregnancy not established

## POSSIBLE INTERACTIONS
N/A

## ALTERNATIVE DRUGS
Alternatives to CaEDTA—D-penicillamine or succimer—use not reported in rabbits

## FOLLOW-UP

### PATIENT MONITORING
Blood lead—assess 10–14 days after cessation of chelation therapy and again 2–3 months later.

### PREVENTION/AVOIDANCE
Determine source of lead and remove it from the patient's environment.

### POSSIBLE COMPLICATIONS
• Permanent neurologic signs (e.g., blindness) occasionally

• Derangement of the gastrointestinal microflora and overgrowth of intestinal bacterial pathogens secondary to gastrointestinal hypomotility or stasis

## EXPECTED COURSE AND PROGNOSIS
• Signs should dramatically improve within 24–48 hours after initiating chelation therapy.
• Prognosis—favorable with treatment
• Uncontrolled seizures—guarded prognosis

## MISCELLANEOUS

### ASSOCIATED CONDITIONS
N/A

### AGE-RELATED FACTORS
N/A

### ZOONOTIC POTENTIAL
None; however, humans in the same environment may be at risk for exposure.

### PREGNANCY
• Transplacental passage—may cause neonatal poisoning
• Lactation—lead mobilized from bones unlikely to poison nursing animals

### SYNONYMS
Plumbism

### SEE ALSO
• Gastrointestinal hypomotility
• Seizures

### ABBREVIATIONS
• CNS = central nervous system
• RBC = red blood cell

*Suggested Reading*

Bailey EM, Garland T. Toxicologic emergencies. In: Murtaugh RJ, Kaplan PM, eds. Veterinary Emergency and Critical Care Medicine. St. Louis: Mosby Year Book, 1992:427–452.

Deeb BJ, Carpenter JW. Neurologic and musculoskeletal diseases. In: Quesenberry KE, Carpenter JW, eds. Ferrets, Rabbits and Rodents: Clinical Medicine and Surgery. 2nd Ed. Philadelphia: WB Saunders, 2004:203–210.

Harcourt-Brown F. Neurological and locomotor diseases. In: Harcourt-Brown F, ed. Textbook of Rabbit Medicine. Oxford: Butterworth-Heinemann, 2002:307–323.

Paul-Murphy J, Ramer JC. Urgent care of the pet rabbits. Vet Clin North Am Exotic Anim Pract 1998;1:127–152.

Swartout MS, Gerken DF. Lead-induced toxicosis in two domestic rabbits. J Am Vet Med Assoc 1987;191:717–719.

*Portions Adapted From*

Popenga RH. Lead Poisoning. In: Tilley LP, Smith FWK, Jr., eds. The 5-Minute Veterinary Consult: Canine and Feline, 2nd Ed. Baltimore: Lippincott Williams & Wilkins, 2000.

# LOWER URINARY TRACT INFECTION

## BASICS

### OVERVIEW
• Result of microbial colonization of the urinary bladder and/or proximal portion of the urethra
• Microbes, usually aerobic bacteria, ascend the urinary tract under conditions that permit them to persist in the urine or adhere to the epithelium and subsequently multiply. Urinary tract colonization requires at least transient impairment of the mechanisms that normally defend against infection. In rabbits, the most common cause of impairment is hypercalciuria. Inflammation of infected tissues results in the clinical signs and laboratory test abnormalities exhibited by patients.

### SYSTEMS AFFECTED
Renal/urologic—lower urinary tract

### INCIDENCE/PREVALENCE
Hypercalciuria is one of the most common problems seen in rabbits housed indoors. Secondary bacterial cystitis is seen in many of these rabbits.

### SIGNALMENT
• Seen most commonly in middle-aged rabbits 3–5 years old
• Seen most often in obese rabbits with a sedentary lifestyle and poor nutrition

### SIGNS

#### Historical Findings
• None in some patients
• Pollakiuria—frequent voiding of small volumes
• Beige to brown thick urine—may be mistaken for diarrhea by some owners
• Urinating in places that are not customary
• Hematuria
• Urine scald

#### Physical Examination Findings
• Detect urocystoliths by abdominal palpation; failure to palpate uroliths does not exclude them from consideration. Usually, one single, large calculus is palpated. In rabbits with crystalluria, the bladder palpates as a soft, doughy mass.
• With chronic hypercalciuria, the bladder may markedly increase in size, and may even fill most of the abdominal cavity.
• With hypercalciuria, manual expression of the bladder may reveal thick, beige- to brown-colored urine. Manual expression of the bladder may expel thick, brown urine even in rabbits that have normal-appearing voided urine.
• No abnormalities in some animals

### CAUSES AND RISK FACTORS
• *Escherichia coli* and *Pseudomonas* sp. are common causes of bacterial cystitis.

• Conditions that cause urine stasis or incomplete emptying of the bladder predispose to lower urinary tract infection. Common causes include inadequate exercise, cage confinement, or painful conditions (reluctance to move).
• Inadequate water intake (dirty water bowls, unpalatable water, changing water sources, inadequate water provision)
• Urine retention (underlying bladder pathology, neuromuscular disease)
• Inadequate cleaning of litter box or cage may cause some rabbits to avoid urinating for abnormally long periods.
• Obesity
• Lack of exercise
• Feeding of exclusively alfalfa-based pelleted diets
• Calcium or vitamin/mineral supplements added to the diet

## DIAGNOSIS

### DIFFERENTIAL DIAGNOSIS
• Female rabbits with pyometra or uterine neoplasia may expel blood or a thick, often blood-tinged vaginal discharge when urinating. This discharge may mix with urine and mimic lower urinary tract infection or hypercalciuria
• Female rabbits with uterine disorders may expel a bright red fluid while urinating that may be confused with hematuria—obtain a urine sample via cystocentesis to differentiate.
• Urolithiasis or hypercalciuria without secondary bacterial cystitis
• Lower urinary tract neoplasia
• Differentiate from other causes by urinalysis, urine culture, radiography, and ultrasonography.

### CBC/BIOCHEMISTRY/URINALYSIS
• Most rabbits with hypercalciuria are hypercalcemic (normal range 12–16 mg/dL); however, the significance of this is unclear since many normal rabbits have high serum calcium concentration and never develop hypercalciuria or lower urinary tract infection.
• With urinary tract infection, leukocytosis may be seen, but this finding is rare.
• Complete urinary outflow obstruction can cause postrenal azotemia (e.g., high BUN, creatinine, and phosphorus).
• Urinary sediment evaluation reveals calcium oxalate or calcium carbonate crystals; however, this is a normal finding in rabbits, and the presence of large amounts of crystals in the urine does not necessarily indicate disease. Disease occurs only when the concentration of crystals is excessive, forming thick, white to brown, sandlike

urine and subsequent inflammatory cystitis or partial to complete blockage of the urethra.
• Pyuria (normal value 0–1 WBC/hpf), hematuria (normal value 0–1 RBC/hpf), and proteinuria (normal value 0–33 mg/dL) indicate urinary tract inflammation, but these are nonspecific findings that may result from infectious and noninfectious causes of lower urinary tract disease.
• Bacteria are rarely observed on urinalysis, even in rabbits with significant lower urinary tract infection.

### OTHER LABORATORY TESTS

#### Urine Culture and Sensitivity Testing
• Urine culture is necessary for definitive diagnosis.
• Correct interpretation of urine culture results requires obtaining the specimen in a manner that minimizes contamination, handling and storing the specimen so that numbers of viable bacteria do not change in vitro, and using a quantitative culture method. Keep the specimen in a sealed sterile container; if the culture is not started right away, the urine can be refrigerated for up to 8 hours without important changes in the results.
• Cystocentesis is the preferred technique for obtaining urine for culture.
• Culture biopsy samples collected from bladder wall if cystotomy is performed.

### IMAGING
• Survey and contrast radiographic studies as well as ultrasound of the bladder or urethra may detect an underlying urinary tract lesion.
• Calcium oxalate uroliths and sand are common in rabbits with lower urinary tract infection. Uroliths are radiopaque and may be detected by survey radiography. Uroliths must be differentiated from calcium "sand" or "sludge" in the bladder, which resembles a bladder full of contrast material. Since rabbits tend to form a single large calculus in the urinary bladder, differentiating the two can be difficult. Ultrasonic examination of the bladder and palpation can be helpful to distinguish solitary calculi from amorphous "sand."
• A small amount of "sand" or "sludge" in the bladder is often found serendipitously in rabbits that are radiographed for other reasons.
• Radiographs and ultrasonic examination are used to differentiate a fluid-filled uterus from bladder in females with pyometra, uterine neoplasia, or hyperplasia.

### DIAGNOSTIC PROCEDURES
N/A

### PATHOLOGIC FINDINGS
N/A

## TREATMENT

### APPROPRIATE HEALTH CARE
Treat as outpatient unless another urinary abnormality (e.g., obstruction) requires inpatient treatment.

### NURSING CARE
• Asymptomatic rabbits diagnosed with hypercalciuria and lower urinary tract infection based on incidental radiographic evidence and urinalysis/urine culture may respond to antibiotic therapy, increasing water consumption, dietary modification, weight loss, and increase in exercise alone.
• Symptomatic rabbits with large amounts of calcium precipitate ("sand" or "sludge") in the urinary bladder may require medical treatment with fluid therapy and voiding urohydropropulsion. Manually express the bladder to remove as much precipitated calcium sand as possible. Gentle ballottement or agitation of the bladder may help to mobilize sludge. Administer fluid therapy, either IV or SC, daily for 3–4 days to increase the amount of urine in the bladder. If precipitated calcium sand is detected in the bladder (via palpation or imaging) after this time, continue fluid therapy and manually express the bladder once daily for 3–4 days, gently forcing the nonvoided "sludge" out the urethra. This may be a painful procedure; anesthesia with isoflurane during manual expression and administration of butorphanol (0.1–0.5 mg/kg SC, IM, IV q4h) or meloxicam (0.2–0.5 mg/kg PO q24h) for pain management is necessary. Administration of diazepam (1–5 mg/kg IM) prior to manual expression of the bladder may aid in smooth muscle relaxation and subsequent dilation of the urethra.
• If large amounts of precipitate are present and manual expression does not remove sufficient amounts of precipitate, flushing the bladder via urethral catheterization may be effective. Begin fluid diuresis as described above. Administer diazepam and induce general anesthesia, catheterize the urethra, flush with warm saline, and aspirate the contents of the bladder. Continue to flush and aspirate until most of the sand is removed. Administer butorphanol, buprenorphine, or meloxicam for pain relief.
• Treat associated urine scald with gentle cleaning; keep the area clean and dry; apply zinc oxide plus menthol powder (Gold Bond, Martin Himmel, Inc) to clean skin q24h.

### ACTIVITY
Increase activity level by providing large exercise areas to encourage voiding and prevent recurrence.

### DIET
• Increasing water consumption is essential to prevention and treatment of hypercalciuria. Provide multiple sources of fresh water. Flavoring the water with fruit juices (with no added sugars) is usually helpful. Provide a variety of clean, fresh, leafy vegetables sprayed or soaked with water.
• No reports of dissolution of calcium oxalate uroliths with special diets
• Following treatment, reduction in the amount of calcium in the diet may help to prevent or delay recurrence. Eliminate feeding of alfalfa pellets or alfalfa hay and switch to a high-fiber timothy-based pellet (Oxbow Pet Products, Murdock, NE). The form of calcium found in alfalfa-based commercial pellets is calcium carbonate, which is 50% more bioavailable than the calcium oxalate found in most green, leafy vegetables. Feed timothy and grass hay instead of alfalfa hay, and offer large volumes of fresh, green, leafy vegetables.

### CLIENT EDUCATION
Urolith removal or removal of calcium "sand" does not alter the factors responsible for their formation; eliminating risk factors such as obesity, sedentary life, and poor diet combined with increasing water consumption is necessary to minimize recurrence. Even with these changes, however, recurrence is likely.

### SURGICAL CONSIDERATIONS
• Except when a concomitant disorder requires surgical intervention, management does not involve surgery.
• Uroliths within the bladder, urethra, ureters, or renal pelvis must be removed surgically. The procedures are similar to those performed on dogs or cats.

## MEDICATIONS

### DRUG(S) OF CHOICE
• Base choice of drug on results of sensitivity test.
• Antibiotics that concentrate in the urine are most appropriate. Initial choices include enrofloxacin (5–20 mg/kg PO, SC, IM q12–24h) and trimethoprim sulfa (30 mg/kg PO q12h).
• For acute, uncomplicated infection, treat with antimicrobial drugs for at least 2 weeks. Appropriate duration of treatment for complicated lower urinary tract infection depends on the underlying problem.

### CONTRAINDICATIONS
Oral administration of antibiotics that select against Gram-positive bacteria (penicillins, macrolides, lincosamides, and cephalosporins) can cause fatal enteric dysbiosis and enterotoxemia.

## FOLLOW-UP

### PATIENT MONITORING
• When antibacterial drug efficacy is in doubt, culture the urine 2–3 days after starting treatment. If the drug is effective, the culture will be negative.
• Rapid recrudescence of signs when treatment is stopped generally indicates either a concurrent urinary tract abnormality or that the infection extends into some deep-seated site (e.g., renal parenchyma).
• Successful cure of an episode of urinary tract infection is best demonstrated by performing a urine culture 7–10 days after completing antimicrobial therapy.

### PREVENTION/AVOIDANCE
• Treat underlying hypercalciuria when present.
• Increase water consumption for the remainder of the rabbit's life.
• Place patients on a lowered calcium diet (described above).
• Increase exercise.

### POSSIBLE COMPLICATIONS
• Urine scald; myiasis; pododermatitis
• Failure to detect or treat effectively may lead to pyelonephritis.

### EXPECTED COURSE AND PROGNOSIS
• If not treated, expect infection to persist indefinitely.
• Generally, the prognosis for animals with uncomplicated lower urinary tract infection is good to excellent. The prognosis for animals with complicated infection is determined by the prognosis for the other urinary abnormality.
• The prognosis following surgical removal of uroliths or urohydropropulsion for the removal of calcium "sand" is fair to good. Although dietary management may decrease the likelihood of recurrence, many rabbits will develop clinical disease again within 1–2 years.

## MISCELLANEOUS

### ASSOCIATED CONDITIONS
• Hypercalciuria
• Gastrointestinal hypomotility

### AGE-RELATED FACTORS
Complicated infection is more common in middle-aged to old than in young animals.

### SYNONYMS
Bacterial cystitis

### SEE ALSO
• Hypercalciuria and urolithiasis
• Nephrolithiasis and ureterolithiasis

# LOWER URINARY TRACT INFECTION

## ABBREVIATIONS
- BUN = blood urea nitrogen
- RBC = red blood cell
- WBC = white blood cell

*Suggested Reading*

Brown SA. Rabbit urinary tract disease. Proc North Am Vet Conf 1997;785–787.

Donoghue S. Nutrition and pet rabbits. In: Rosenthal KL, ed. Practical Exotic Animal Medicine: The Compendium Collection. Trenton, NJ: Veterinary Learning Systems, 1997:107.

Harkness JE, Wagner JE. The Biology and Medicine of Rabbits and Rodents. 3rd Ed. Baltimore: Williams & Wilkins, 1989.

Harcourt-Brown F. Urogenital disease. In: Harcourt-Brown F, ed. Textbook of Rabbit Medicine. Oxford: Butterworth-Heinemann, 2002:335–351.

Pare JA, Paul-Murphy J. Disorders of the reproductive and urinary systems. In: Quesenberry KE, Carpenter JW, eds. Ferrets, Rabbits and Rodents: Clinical Medicine and Surgery. 2nd Ed. Philadelphia: WB Saunders, 2004:183–193.

Paul-Murphy J, Ramer JC. Urgent care of the pet rabbits. Vet Clin North Am Exotic Anim Pract 1998;1(1):127–152.

Redrobe S. Calcium metabolism in rabbits. Semin Avian Exotic Pet Med 2002;11(2):94–101.

*Portions Adapted From*

Lees GE. Lower Urinary Tract Infection. In: Tilley LP, Smith FWK, Jr., eds. The 5-Minute Veterinary Consult: Canine and Feline, 3rd Ed. Baltimore: Lippincott Williams & Wilkins, 2004.

## BASICS

### OVERVIEW

#### Septic Mastitis
• Bacterial infection of one or more lactating glands; result of ascending infection, trauma to the gland, or hematogenous spread
• Potentially life-threatening infection; may lead to septic shock
• Mammary gland abscesses—may occur in nonlactating does due to trauma or hematogenous spread

#### Cystic Mastitis
• Sterile, fluid-filled cysts arising from mammary papillary ducts; usually single, but may be multiple, coalesce and involve several glands
• Associated with endometrial cystic hyperplasia or uterine adenocarcinoma; hormonally mediated; resolves with ovariohysterectomy.
• May progress to mammary adenocarcinoma if untreated

### SIGNALMENT
• Septic mastitis—postpartum lactating does or pseudopregnant does; no age predilection
• Cystic mastitis—highest incidence in does >3–4 years old, as this is the age range in which associated endometrial disorders occur; all breeds at risk; occurrence rate independent of breeding status

### SIGNS

#### Historical Findings
*Septic Mastitis*
• Anorexia, lethargy, depression
• Polydipsia/polyuria
• May have had signs of pseudopregnancy—pulling hair, nest building
• Illness or death in suckling young
*Cystic Mastitis*
• Patients usually bright, alert, not in pain
• May have history of hematuria—due to associated endometrial disorder; not true hematuria, since blood originates from the uterus, but is expelled during micturition. Hematuria is often reported as intermittent or cyclic; usually occurs at the end of micturition

#### Physical Examination Findings
*Septic Mastitis*
• Firm, swollen, warm, erythematous (possibly deep-purple to cyanotic), and painful mammary gland(s) from which purulent or hemorrhagic fluid can be expressed
• May involve single or multiple glands
• Fever, dehydration—with systemic involvement

• Abscessation of gland(s)
*Cystic Mastitis*
• Swelling around nipple(s) or within mammary gland; filled with clear or serosanguinous fluid; no signs of inflammation (heat, pain, induration)
• May see signs of associated uterine disorder—palpably enlarged uterus; fresh blood or serosanguinous vaginal discharge; usually expelled during urination, but can appear independent of micturition; may see discharge adhered to fur

### CAUSES AND RISK FACTORS

#### Septic Mastitis
• Trauma
• Poor hygiene
• Systemic infection originating elsewhere (e.g., metritis)
• *Staphylococcus aureus*, *Streptococcus* sp., and *Pasteurella* sp. most common isolates

#### Cystic Mastitis
• Intact reproductive status
• Endometrial disorders—endometrial hyperplasia, endometriosis, endometritis, pyometra
• Uterine adenocarcinoma

## DIAGNOSIS

### DIFFERENTIAL DIAGNOSIS
• Mammary gland hyperplasia—has been reported secondary to pituitary tumors
• Inflammatory mammary adenocarcinoma—differentiated by biopsy; may have simultaneous mammary abscess
• Subcutaneous abscess—may or may not involve mammary gland

### CBC/BIOCHEMISTRY/URINALYSIS
• CBC—usually normal or lymphopenia; neutrophilia and left shift not common
• Azotemia, increases in ALT, electrolyte disturbances—all can be abnormal in rabbits with septicemia or severe dehydration, depending on clinical course
• Urinalysis—in rabbits with associated vaginal bleeding; sample collected by ultrasound-guided cystocentesis to differentiate true hematuria from uterine bleeding

### IMAGING
• Abdominal radiography—in rabbits with cystic mastitis—may detect a large uterus with uterine adenocarcinoma or other endometrial disorder
• Thoracic radiographs—if mammary or uterine neoplasia is suspected; assess for metastasis.
• Ultrasonography—assess size of uterus and nature of uterine contents.

### OTHER LABORATORY TESTS
• Fine needle aspirate of firm masses—may be helpful in differentiating mammary neoplasia from abscess; can be misleading if necrotic, septic foci are present within tumor
• Fine needle aspirate of fluid—usually serosanguineous fluid with atypical epithelial cells in does with cystic mastitis
• Fine needle aspirate of regional lymph node—to identify metastases if adenocarcinoma is suspected
• Excisional biopsy—may be required to identify adenocarcinoma
• Bacterial culture and susceptibility testing—from wall of abscess or expressed fluid/milk
• Serology for *Pasteurella* in rabbits with septic mastitis or abscesses—usefulness is severely limited and generally not helpful in the diagnosis of pasteurellosis in pet rabbits. An ELISA is available and results are reported as negative, low positive, or high positive. Positive results, even when high, only indicate prior exposure to *Pasteurella* and the development of antibodies and do not confirm active infection. Low-positive results may occur due to cross-reaction with other, nonpathogenic bacteria (false positive). False-negative results are common with immunosuppression or early infection. No evidence exists to support correlation of titers to the presence or absence of disease.

### DIAGNOSTIC PROCEDURES
Express milk or fluid from teats—if septic may see degenerative neutrophils with intracellular bacteria or macrophages; obtain bacterial culture to identify the organism; expressed fluid is serosanguineous with atypical epithelial cells in rabbits with cystic mastitis

## TREATMENT

### SEPTIC MASTITIS
• Inpatient until stable
• Neonates—do not foster to surrogate doe as may transmit infection to surrogate
• Dehydration or sepsis—intravenous fluid therapy
• Apply warm compress and milk out affected gland(s) several times daily.
• Abscessed or necrotic glands—require surgical debridement
• Assist-feed any rabbit that is anorectic or inappetent to avoid secondary gastrointestinal disorders.
• Clean and disinfect the environment.

### CYSTIC MASTITIS
Usually resolves with ovariohysterectomy; no other treatment indicated

## MASTITIS, CYSTIC AND SEPTIC

### MAMMARY NEOPLASIA
Mastectomy and ovariohysterectomy; insufficient data on prognosis exist.

## MEDICATIONS

### DRUG(S) OF CHOICE

*Septic Mastitis*
- Antibiotics—choice is ideally based on results of culture and susceptibility testing. Use broad-spectrum antibiotics such as enrofloxacin (5–20 mg/kg PO, SC, IM q12–24h), trimethoprim sulfa (30 mg/kg PO q12h), or chloramphenicol (50 mg/kg PO q8h). Alternatively, use parenteral penicillin g (40,000–60,000 IU/kg SC q2–7d) if *Pasteurella* or streptococcus is isolated (not usually effective for staphylococcus).
- Pain management—NSAIDs to reduce pain and inflammation: meloxicam (0.2–0.5 mg/kg PO q24h) or carprofen (2.2 mg/kg PO q12–24h)

### CONTRAINDICATIONS
- Oral administration of most antibiotics effective against anaerobes will cause a fatal gastrointestinal dysbiosis in rabbits. Do not administer penicillins, macrolides, lincosamides, and cephalosporins by oral administration.
- Corticosteroids—associated with gastrointestinal ulceration and hemorrhage, delayed wound healing, and heightened susceptibility to infection; rabbits are very sensitive to the immunosuppressive effects of both topical and systemic corticosteroids; use may exacerbate subclinical bacterial infection.

### PRECAUTIONS
- Chloramphenicol—avoid human contact with chloramphenicol due to potential blood dyscrasia. Advise owners of potential risks.
- Meloxicam—use with caution in rabbits with compromised renal function.

## FOLLOW-UP

### PATIENT MONITORING
Physical examination; monitor for development of neoplasia in intact females.

### PREVENTION/AVOIDANCE
- Septic mastitis—clean environment.
- Cystic mastitis—ovariohysterectomy for all nonbreeding rabbits; usually performed between 6 months and 2 years of age. Breeding rabbits—recommend stop breeding and spay after 4 years of age, as this is when most endometrial disorders (including adenocarcinoma) occur.

### POSSIBLE COMPLICATIONS
- Abscessation may cause loss of gland(s), septicemia, death, death of suckling neonates
- Cystic mastitis—progression to mammary adenocarcinoma with metastasis to lymph nodes and lungs if owner elects not to spay; hemorrhage, possible death in rabbits with associated bleeding uterine disorders

### EXPECTED COURSE AND PROGNOSIS
- Septic mastitis—fair to guarded with treatment, depending on severity
- Cystic mastitis—good if ovariohysterectomy is performed; affected glands usually return to normal within 3–4 weeks.
- Mammary neoplasia—frequently metastasizes to regional lymph nodes and lungs; survival times not reported

## MISCELLANEOUS

### ASSOCIATED CONDITIONS
- Mammary neoplasia
- Endometrial disorders
- Uterine adenocarcinoma
- Ovarian neoplasia
- Ovarian abscess

### AGE-RELATED FACTORS
Uterine neoplasia—rare in rabbits under 2 years of age; risk increases with age; seen in up to 60% of does over 3 years old

### SEE ALSO
- Pyometra and nonneoplastic endometrial disorders
- Uterine adenocarcinoma

### ABBREVIATIONS
- ALT = alanine aminotransferase
- CBC = complete blood count
- ELISA = enzyme-linked immunosorbent assay

*Suggested Reading*

Baba N, von Haam E. Animal model for human disease: spontaneous adenocarcinoma in aged rabbits. Am J Pathol 1972;68:653–656.

Jenkins JR. Surgical sterilization in small mammals: spay and castration. Vet Clin North Am Exotic Anim Pract 2000;3(3):617–627.

Lewis, B. Uterine adenocarcinoma in a rabbit. Exotic DVM 2003;5(1):11.

Saito K, Nakanishi M, Hasegawa A. Uterine disorders diagnosed by ventrotomy in 47 rabbits. J Vet Med Sci 2002;64(6):495–497.

Pare JA, Paul-Murphy J. Disorders of the reproductive and urinary systems. In: Quesenberry KE, Carpenter JW, eds. Ferrets, Rabbits and Rodents: Clinical Medicine and Surgery. 2nd Ed. Philadelphia: WB Saunders, 2004:183–193.

*Portions Adapted From*

Freshman JL. Mastitis. In: Tilley LP, Smith FWK, Jr., eds. The 5-Minute Veterinary Consult: Canine and Feline, 3rd Ed. Baltimore: Lippincott Williams & Wilkins, 2004.

BASICS

## DEFINITION
Presence of digested blood in the feces; appears as green–black, tarry stool. Melena is an unusual finding in pet rabbits.

## PATHOPHYSIOLOGY
Usually the result of upper gastrointestinal bleeding. However, melena can also be associated with ingested blood from the oral cavity or upper respiratory tract.

## SYSTEMS AFFECTED
• Gastrointestinal
• Hematopoietic
• Respiratory

## SIGNALMENT
No breed or gender predilections

## SIGNS

### Historical Findings
• Melena may be accompanied by anorexia, weight loss, or bruxism.
• Feces may be formed or diarrheic.
• Question owner about the rabbit's chewing habits, such as barbering and possible ingestion of foreign bodies (especially carpeting, cloth, or bedding material) or anticoagulant rodenticides.
• Gastric ulceration may be more common in stressed rabbits; history of recent illness, surgery, hospitalization, or environmental changes

### Physical Examination Findings
• Pallor of the mucous membranes
• Weight loss—indicates chronic disease
• Poor haircoat or alopecia due to barbering
• Dehydration
• Fecal staining of the perineum
• Abdominal distention may be due to gastric distention, cecal distention, thickened or fluid-filled intestinal loops, masses, or organomegaly.

## CAUSES
• Gastric ulceration—associated with recent stress (disease, surgery, hospitalization, environmental changes), corticosteroid administration, NSAIDs, gastrointestinal hypomotility
• Bacterial infection/enterotoxemia—*Escherichia coli*, *Clostridium spiroforme*, *Salmonella* spp., *Pseudomonas* spp.
• Gastric neoplasia—adenocarcinoma, leiomyosarcoma, leiomyoma, papilloma
• Gastrointestinal obstruction—neoplasia, foreign body, intussusception
• Drugs and toxins—anticoagulant rodenticides, plant toxins, heavy metals, antibiotics, NSAIDs, corticosteroids
• Metabolic disorders—liver disease, renal disease

• Ingestion of blood—oropharyngeal, nasal, or sinus lesions (abscess, trauma, neoplasia, aspergillosis)
• Coagulopathy
• Septicemia

## RISK FACTORS
• Unsupervised chewing
• Recent stress
• Diets high in simple carbohydrates, low in coarse fiber content

 DIAGNOSIS

## DIFFERENTIAL DIAGNOSIS

### Differentiating Similar Signs
Melenic feces should be differentiated from cecotrophs (or night feces). Cecotrophs are formed in the cecum, are rich in nutrients, and are usually eliminated during the early morning hours. Normally, cecotrophs are not observed because rabbits will ingest them directly from the anus. Occasionally rabbits are unable to consume the cecotroph, which may be mistaken for melenic feces due to the dark color. Cecotrophs have a soft consistency, tend to clump together, are usually covered with mucous, and may be differentiated from melenic feces by performing a fecal occult blood test.

## CBC/BIOCHEMISTRY
• Regenerative anemia may be seen with chronic gastrointestinal bleeding.
• Serum albumin concentration seen with dehydration
• TWBC elevation may be seen with bacterial enteritis; however, a relative neutrophilia and lymphopenia are more common.
• Serum biochemistry abnormalities may suggest renal or hepatic disease.
• Serum glucose concentration may be elevated due to stress.

## OTHER LABORATORY TESTS
N/A

## IMAGING

### Radiographic Findings
• Survey abdominal radiography may indicate intestinal obstruction, cecal impaction, organomegaly, mass, foreign body, or intraperitoneal fluid.
• Gastric contents (primarily food and hair) are normally present and visible radiographically, even if the rabbit has been inappetent. The presence of ingesta (including hair) in the stomach is a normal finding.
• Moderate to severe distension of the stomach with ingesta is usually visible in rabbits with gastrointestinal hypomotility. In some rabbits with gastrointestinal stasis, a halo of gas can be observed around the inspissated stomach contents. Gas distension is also common throughout the intestinal tract, in-

cluding the cecum in rabbits with gastrointestinal hypomotility or stasis
• Contrast radiography is usually not helpful in demonstrating gastric ulceration in rabbits
• Abdominal ultrasonography may demonstrate intestinal wall thickening, gastrointestinal mass, foreign body, or ileus.

### Fecal Examination
• Fecal Gram's stain—may demonstrate spore-forming bacteria consistent with *Clostridia* spp. or excessive numbers of Gram-negative bacteria
• Fecal cytology—may reveal RBC or fecal leukocytes, which are associated with inflammatory disease or invasive bacterial strains
• Fecal culture may be difficult to interpret since *E. coli* and *Clostridia sp.* may be present in small numbers in normal rabbits. A heavy growth of these bacteria is considered significant. Fecal culture should be performed if other bacterial infections, such salmonellosis, is suspected.
• Fecal occult blood testing—in patients with dark brown–black stool to confirm melena

### Surgical Considerations
Exploratory laparotomy and surgical biopsy should be pursued if there is evidence of obstruction or intestinal mass.

### Endoscopy
Upper gastrointestinal endoscopy—generally not useful to diagnose gastric foreign bodies or ulceration. The small size of the patient and subsequent limitations on instrument size often limit the use of endoscopy. The stomach is usually full of ingesta, precluding visibility.

 TREATMENT

• Treatment must be specific to the underlying cause to be successful.
• Patients with melena usually require hospitalization and 24-hour care for parenteral medication and fluid therapy.
• Fluid therapy and correction of electrolyte imbalances are important parts of treatment; maintenance fluid requirements are estimated at 100 mL/kg/day.
• Exploratory laparotomy to remove foreign bodies or tumors

## DIET
• It is imperative that the rabbit continue to eat during and following treatment. Continued anorexia will exacerbate gastrointestinal motility disorders and cause further derangement of the gastrointestinal microflora and overgrowth of intestinal bacterial pathogens.
• Offer a good-quality grass hay and a large selection of fresh, moistened greens such as

## MELENA

cilantro, romaine lettuce, parsley, carrot tops, dandelion greens, spinach, collard greens, etc. Many rabbits will begin to eat these foods, even if they were previously anorectic.
• In some rabbits, addition of leafy greens may exacerbate diarrhea. For these patients, offer good-quality grass hay alone.
• If the patient refuses these foods, syringe feed a gruel such as Critical Care for Herbivores (Oxbow Pet Products, Murdock, NE) 10–15 mL/kg PO q6–8h. Alternatively, pellets can be ground and mixed with fresh greens, vegetable baby foods, water, or juice to form a gruel. If sufficient volumes of food are not accepted in this manner, nasogastric intubation is indicated.
• High-carbohydrate, high-fat nutritional supplements are contraindicated.
• The diet should be permanently modified to include sufficient amounts of indigestible fiber. Initially, feed only grass or timothy hay and washed fresh greens. These foods should always constitute the bulk of the diet.

## MEDICATIONS

### DRUG(S) OF CHOICE
• Antibiotic therapy—indicated in patients with melena due to disruption of the intestinal mucosa. Selection should be based on results of culture and susceptibility testing when possible.
• If antibiotics are indicated, always use broad-spectrum antibiotics such as trimethoprim sulfa (30 mg/kg PO q12h) or enrofloxacin (5–20 mg/kg PO, SC, IM q12–24h).
• *Clostridium* spp.—metronidazole (20 mg/kg PO q12h)
• Antisecretory agents—cimetidine (5–10 mg/kg PO, SC q8–12h) or ranitidine (2 mg/kg IV q24h or 2–5 mg/kg PO q12h)
• Sucralfate—25 mg/kg PO q8–12h

### CONTRAINDICATIONS
• The use of antibiotics that are primarily Gram positive in spectrum is contraindicated in rabbits. Use of these antibiotics will suppress the growth of commensal flora, allowing overgrowth of enteric pathogens.
• Corticosteroids—rabbits are extremely sensitive to the immunosuppressive effects and gastrointestinal ulceration subsequent to systemic or topical administration of corticosteroids.

### POSSIBLE INTERACTIONS
N/A

### ALTERNATE DRUGS
N/A

## FOLLOW-UP

### PATIENT MONITORING
• PCV daily until anemia is stabilized, then weekly
• Fecal volume and character, appetite, attitude, and body weight
• If melena does not resolve, consider reevaluation of the diagnosis.

### POSSIBLE COMPLICATIONS
• Septicemia due to bacterial invasion of enteric mucosal
• Dehydration due to fluid loss
• Gastrointestinal perforation with gastrointestinal ulceration

## MISCELLANEOUS

### ASSOCIATED CONDITIONS
• Septicemia
• Gastrointestinal hypomotility

### AGE-RELATED FACTORS
*E. coli, Clostridia* sp., or related diarrhea more severe in neonates. Gastrointestinal hypomotility more common in middle-aged to older rabbits.

### ZOONOTIC POTENTIAL
N/A

### PREGNANCY
N/A

### SEE ALSO
• Anticoagulant rodenticide toxicosis
• Clostridial enterotoxemia
• Gastrointestinal hypomotility

### ABBREVIATIONS
• NSAIDs = nonsteroidal antiinflammatory drugs
• PCV = packed cell volume
• RBC = red blood cell
• TWBC = total white blood cell

### Suggested Reading
Brown SA, Rosenthal KL. The anorexic rabbit. Proc North Am Vet Conf, 1997:788.
Dodds WJ. Rabbit and ferret hemostasis. In: Fudge AM, ed. Laboratory Medicine, Avian and Exotic Pets. Philadelphia: WB Saunders, 2000.
Donoghue S. Nutrition and pet rabbits. In: Rosenthal KL, ed. Practical Exotic Animal Medicine: The Compendium Collection. Trenton, NJ: Veterinary Learning Systems, 1997:107.
Jenkins JR. Gastrointestinal diseases. In: Quesenberry KE, Carpenter JW, eds. Ferrets, Rabbits and Rodents: Clinical Medicine and Surgery. 2nd Ed. Philadelphia: WB Saunders, 2004:161–171.
Murphy M, Gerken D. The anticoagulant rodenticides. In: Kirk RW, Bonagura J, eds. Current Veterinary Therapy X. Philadelphia: Saunders, 1989:143–146.
Paul-Murphy JA, Ramer JC. Urgent care of the pet rabbit. Vet Clin North Am Exot Anim Pract 1998;1(1):127–152.

# BASICS

## OVERVIEW
• A systemic, usually fatal disease in domestic and wild, old-world rabbits caused by a myxoma virus in the poxvirus family
• Disease in wild rabbits is less severe due to the development of genetic resistance to the virus.
• The virus was originally intentionally introduced into Australia and Europe in an effort to control wild rabbit populations; resistance has since developed.
• Several strains of myxoma viruses exist, and pathogenicity varies with strain and host immunity.
• Virus is spread primarily through insect bites (mosquitos, flies, fur mites, fleas), but can also be transmitted by mechanical vectors (nonbiting insects, thorns, bedding, food).
• Wild rabbits often only show mild disease, with the development of firm cutaneous nodules at the site of transmitting bites.
• Clinical signs in pet rabbit depend on how long the rabbit survives; most pet rabbits will die within 2 weeks.

## GEOGRAPHIC DISTRIBUTION
• Europe, South America, North America, and Australia
• In the United States, seen primarily in California. The California strain is extremely virulent, with mortality rates exceeding 99%.

## SIGNALMENT
• Domestic, pet rabbits (*Oryctolagus cuniculus*) more susceptible to disease than wild cotton-tail rabbits (*Sylviagus* spp.) and other North American species of rabbits
• Outdoor rabbits may be at greater risk due to mode of viral transmission
• At the time of writing, seen primarily in rabbits living in California; ease of transportation of pet rabbits raises concern over spread to other parts of the country.

## SIGNS

### California Strain in Pet (Domestic) Rabbits
• Incubation period is usually 1–3 days.
• Peracute—death with few premonitory signs, lethargy, eyelid edema, pyrexia, death within 7 days
• Acute form—eyelid edema usually develops first; perioral and perineal swelling and edema; cutaneous hemorrhage; lethargy; anorexia; dyspnea; seizures or other CNS signs (excitement, opisthotonus); death within 1–2 weeks

• Chronic form—few rabbits live long enough to develop this form; see blepharo-conjunctivitis; swelling; edema around base of ears; generalized cutaneous tumors; lethargy; anorexia; dyspnea; high fever; death within 2 weeks

### Wild Rabbits
• Cutaneous nodules at the site of transmission (insect bite, scratch)—firm fibromalike swellings may be only clinical signs.
• Young wild or feral rabbits may develop disease similar to pet rabbits.

## CAUSES AND RISK FACTORS
• Myxoma virus, a strain of Leporipoxvirus
• Outbreaks may be more likely when mosquitos are numerous (summer, fall).

# DIAGNOSIS

## DIFFERENTIAL DIAGNOSIS
• For periocular, perioral, and perineal rash—*Treponema cuniculi* (rabbit syphilis); usually not associated with edema or fever; usually otherwise healthy
• For neurologic signs—meningitis, otitis interna/media, rabies; usually not associated with dermatologic signs

## CBC/BIOCHEMISTRY/URINALYSIS
N/A

## OTHER LABORATORY TESTS
Serologic testing—various serologic tests are available for research purposes; may not be commercially available in North America

## IMAGING
N/A

## DIAGNOSTIC PROCEDURES
Virus isolation

## PATHOLOGIC FINDINGS

### Gross
• Cutaneous nodules—characteristic lesions are fibrous nodules with mucinous material in the center.
• Hepatic necrosis, splenomegaly, infarcts, or hemorrhage in lungs, trachea, and thymus
• Subcutaneous ecchymoses; ecchymoses in serosal surfaces of the gastrointestinal tract
• May be no gross lesions in peracute cases

### Histopathologic
• Undifferentiated mesenchymal cells, inflammatory cells, mucin, and edema
• Necrotizing lesions—may be seen in fetal placentas

# TREATMENT
• None effective
• Supportive care—generally unsuccessful

# MEDICATIONS

## DRUG(S) OF CHOICE
N/A

## CONTRADINDICATIONS/POSSIBLE INTERACTIONS
N/A

# FOLLOW-UP

## PREVENTION/AVOIDANCE
• Control of vectors—screening to keep out insects; flea control; keep indoors
• Disinfection—10% bleach, 10% NaOH, 1–1.4% formalin
• Quarantine new rabbits; do not house wild rabbits with domestic pet rabbits.
• Vaccination with an attenuated myxoma virus vaccine may provide temporary protection; not available in the United States; vaccination may cause atypical myomatosis.

# MISCELLANEOUS

## ZOONOTIC POTENTIAL
None

## ABBREVIATION
CNS = central nervous system

*Suggested Reading*

Harcourt-Brown F. Infectious diseases of domestic rabbits. In: Harcourt-Brown F. Textbook of Rabbit Medicine. Oxford: Butterworth-Heinemann, 2002:361–385.

Hess L. Dermatologic diseases. In: Quesenberry KE, Carpenter JW, eds. Ferrets, Rabbits and Rodents: Clinical Medicine and Surgery. 2nd Ed. Philadelphia: WB Saunders, 2004:194–202.

Langan GP, Schaeffer DO. Rabbit microbiology and virology. In: Fudge AM, ed. Laboratory Medicine Avian and Exotic Pets. Philadelphia: WB Saunders, 2000:325–333.

Murray MJ. Myxomatosis. North Am Vet Conf 2005;1349–1350.

# NASAL DISCHARGE AND SNEEZING

## BASICS

### DEFINITION
• Nasal discharges may be serous, mucoid, mucopurulent, purulent, blood tinged, or frank blood (epistaxis).
• Sneezing is the reflexive expulsion of air through the nasal cavity and is commonly associated with nasal discharge.

### PATHOPHYSIOLOGY
• Secretions are produced by mucous cells of the epithelium and glands. Irritation of the nasal mucosa (by mechanical, chemical, or inflammatory stimulation) increases nasal secretion production.
• Mucosal irritation and accumulated secretions are a potent stimulus of the sneeze reflex; sneezing may be the first sign of nasal discharge. Sneezing frequency often decreases with chronic disease.
• The most common cause of nasal discharge and sneezing in rabbits is bacterial infection. Infection usually begins in the nasal cavity and may spread via the eustachian tubes to the inner or middle ears into the sinuses and bones of the face, via the nasolacrimal duct to the eye, via the trachea to the lower respiratory tract, and hematogenously to joints, bones, and other organ systems.
• Recurrent or refractory infections are common due to foci of infection in inaccessible regions (deep within the sinuses, bone, etc.) and destruction of turbinates.

### Types of Nasal Discharge and Common Associations
• Serous—mild irritation, allergies, acute phase of inflammation, early bacterial infection
• Mucoid—allergies or contact irritation, acute inflammation or infection, early neoplastic conditions
• Purulent (or mucopurulent)—bacterial infections, nasal foreign bodies, rarely mycotic in rabbits
• Serosanguineous—destructive processes (bacterial pathogens, primary nasal tumors), associated with coagulopathies

### SYSTEMS AFFECTED
• Respiratory—mucosa of the upper respiratory tract, including the nasal cavities, sinuses, and nasopharynx
• Ophthalmic—extension to the eyes via nasolacrimal duct
• Musculoskeletal—extension of infection into bones of the skull
• Neurologic—extension of infection via eustachian tube causing vestibular signs from otitis interna/media
• Hemic/lymphatic/immune—systemic diseases may cause blood-tinged nasal discharge or epistaxis due to hemostasis disorders.

### SIGNALMENT
• Young animals—bacterial infections
• Middle-aged to older animals—nasal tumors, dental disease, bacterial infections

### SIGNS

#### Historical Findings
• Nasal discharge and sneezing may be reported as concurrent problems. Information concerning both the initial and present character of the discharge and whether it was originally unilateral or bilateral are important historical findings.
• The response to previous antibiotic therapy may be helpful in determining secondary bacterial involvement. Bacterial infections, dental disease, or foreign bodies will often respond initially to antibiotic therapy but commonly relapse after treatment. Nasal tumors typically show little response.
• History of ocular discharge; ptyalism with tooth involvement; head tilt; vestibular signs; scratching at ears with extension into the ears
• History of feeding diets consisting of commercial pelleted foods without the addition of long-stemmed hay or grasses common in rabbits with dental disease

#### Physical Examination Findings
• Secretions or dried discharges on the hair around the nose and front limbs
• Concurrent dental disease, especially tooth root impaction, malocclusion, and incisor overgrowth. Findings may include ptyalism, anorexia, nasal discharge, ocular discharge, and exophthalmia. Always perform a thorough oral examination.
• Ocular discharge—may be serous with nasolacrimal duct occlusion or mucopurulent with conjunctivitis secondary to nasolacrimal duct obstruction or extension of upper respiratory infection; exophthalmos with retrobulbar abscess
• Bony involvement (tooth root abscess, tumor, pasteurellosis or other bacteria) may cause facial swelling or pain.
• Lethargy, anorexia, or depression with pain, extension to lower respiratory tract, or hematogenous spread
• Dyspnea, stridor—especially with exertion if extension to lower respiratory tract or complete nasal occlusion has occured (rabbits are obligate nasal breathers)

### CAUSES
• Pyogenic bacteria—*Pasteurella multocida, Staphylococcus aureus, Bordetella bronchiseptica, Moraxella catarrhalis, Pseudomonas aeruginosa, Mycobacterium* sp., and various anaerobes have also been implicated.
• Odontogenic abscesses—*Pasteurella* usually not causative; common isolates from these sites include anaerobic bacteria such as *Fusobacterium nucleatum, Prevotella* spp., *Peptostreptococcus micros, Actinomyces israelii,* and *Arcanobacterium haemolyticum.* Aerobic bacteria—*Streptococcus* sp. most common isolate

• Dental disease—periapical or tooth root abscesses, elongated maxillary tooth roots penetrating into nasal passages
• Foreign objects, especially hay, straw, or other bedding material
• Allergies or irritants—dust, cat litter, bedding, plant material
• Neoplasia
• Unilateral discharge often is associated with nonsystemic processes—dental-related disease, nasal tumors, or foreign bodies
• Discharge may be unilateral or bilateral with bacterial respiratory tract infections, allergies, nasal tumors, dental disease, or foreign bodies

### RISK FACTORS
• Dental disease
• Immunosuppression
• Stress
• Corticosteroid use
• Poor husbandry—inappropriate diet; urine-soaked bedding

## DIAGNOSIS

### DIFFERENTIAL DIAGNOSIS
Allergic, irritant, neoplastic, infectious, inflammatory, and traumatic disorders

### CBC/BIOCHEMISTRY
• TWBC elevations are usually not seen with bacterial diseases. A relative neutrophilia and/or lymphopenia are more common.
• Although not specific for any particular cause of nasal discharge, a chemistry profile may be valuable for detecting concurrent problems and as part of a thorough evaluation prior to any procedure requiring anesthesia.

### OTHER LABORATORY TESTS
Serology for *Pasteurella*—usefulness is severely limited and generally not helpful in the diagnosis of pasteurellosis in pet rabbits. An ELISA is available and results are reported as negative, low positive, or high positive. Positive results, even when high, only indicate prior exposure to *Pasteurella* and the development of antibodies, but do not confirm active infection. Low-positive results may occur due to cross-reaction with other, nonpathogenic bacteria (false positive). False-negative results are common with immunosuppression or early infection. No evidence exists to support correlation of titers to the presence or absence of disease.

### IMAGING

#### Radiographic Findings
• Radiography of the nasal cavities can be helpful in cases of chronic nasal discharge, especially to rule out bacterial rhinitis/sinusitis, neoplasia, foreign body, or associated dental disease. Because of difficulties

with overlying structures, the patient should be anesthetized and carefully positioned.
• The lateral view is useful in detecting any periosteal reaction over the nasal bones, for detecting gross changes in the maxillary teeth, nasal cavity, and frontal sinus, and for evaluating the air column of the nasopharynx.
• The ventrodorsal view is useful for evaluating the nasal cavities and turbinates; disease may be localized to the affected side.
• The lateral oblique views are best for detecting maxillary teeth abnormalities.
• The rostrocaudal view is used to evaluate each frontal sinus (e.g., periosteal reaction, filling).
• CT scans or MRI is extremely helpful in detecting the extent of bony changes associated with pasteurellosis and nasal tumors.

## OTHER DIAGNOSTIC PROCEDURES
• Cultures—may be difficult to interpret, since commonly isolated bacteria (e.g., *Pasteurella* sp., *Bordetella* sp.) often represent only commensal organisms or opportunistic pathogens. A heavy growth of a single organism is usually significant. Deep cultures obtained by inserting a mini-tipped culturette 2–4 cm into each nostril are sometimes reliable. However, samples taken from the nares should not be overinterpreted, since the causative agent may be located only deep within the sinuses and not be present at the rostral portion of the nostrils, where samples are readily accessible.
• A lack of growth does not rule out bacterial disease, since the infection may be in an inaccessible, deep area of the nasal cavity or sinuses, and many organisms (especially anaerobes and *Pasteurella* sp.) can be difficult to grow on culture.
• PCR assay for pasteurellosis may also be performed on samples taken from deep nasal swabs. Positive results should not be overinterpreted. *Pasteurella* is often a co-pathogen with other bacteria; presence of organism alone does not confirm *Pasteurella* as the sole causative agent.
• Nasal cytology—nonspecific inflammation is most commonly found.
• Biopsy of the nasal cavity is indicated in any animal with chronic nasal discharge in which neoplasia is suspected. Specimens may be obtained by direct endoscopic biopsy or rhinotomy. Multiple samples may be necessary to ensure adequate representation of the disease process.
• Rhinoscopy can be extremely valuable to visualize nasal abnormalities, retrieve foreign bodies, or obtain biopsy samples; sometimes the only method of identifying foreign bodies

## TREATMENT
• Outpatient treatment is acceptable unless surgery is required or the patient is exhibiting signs of systemic illness in addition to nasal discharge.
• Symptomatic treatment and nursing care are important in the treatment of rabbits with sneezing and nasal discharge. Patient hydration, nutrition, warmth, and hygiene (keeping nares clean) are important.
• Surgery may be necessary to remove foreign bodies, to obtain samples for biopsy, or to debulk abscesses, tumors, or granulomas.
• Treat associated dental disease—extractions, complete debridement of abscesses
• If epiphora or ocular discharge is present, always flush the nasolacrimal duct.
• Remove environmental allergens/irritants (dusty litters, moldy hay or bedding); provide clean airspace.

### DIET
• Rabbits with nasal discharge are often inappetent. It is absolutely imperative that the rabbit continue to eat during and following treatment. Anorexia will often cause gastrointestinal hypomotility, derangement of the gastrointestinal microflora, and overgrowth of intestinal bacterial pathogens.
• Offer a large selection of fresh, moistened greens such as cilantro, romaine lettuce, parsley, carrot tops, dandelion greens, spinach, collard greens, etc., and good-quality grass hay. Many rabbits will begin to eat these foods, even if they were previously anorectic.
• If the patient refuses these foods, syringe feed a gruel such as Critical Care for Herbivores (Oxbow Pet Products, Murdock, NE) 10–15 mL/kg PO q6–8h. Alternatively, pellets can be ground and mixed with fresh greens, vegetable baby foods, water, or juice to form a gruel.
• High-carbohydrate, high-fat nutritional supplements are contraindicated.
• Encourage oral fluid intake by offering fresh water, wetting leafy vegetables, or flavoring water with vegetable juices.

### CLIENT EDUCATION
• Discuss need to correct or prevent risk factors.
• Warn clients that signs may recur following discontinuation of antibiotic therapy. Rabbits with chronic nasal discharge and turbinate destruction are unlikely to be cured; the goal of medication is to control more severe signs, and lifelong therapy may be required.

## MEDICATIONS
### DRUG(S) OF CHOICE
• Nasal secretions clear more easily if the patient is well hydrated; fluid therapy should be considered if hydration is marginal.
• Antimicrobial drugs effective against the infectious agent; gain access to site of infection. Choice of antibiotic is ideally based on results of culture and susceptibility testing. Depending on the severity of infection, long-term antibiotic therapy is required (2 weeks minimum to several months or even years in cases of chronic, recurrent bacterial rhinitis/sinusitis). Use broad-spectrum antibiotics such as enrofloxacin (5–20 mg/kg PO, IM, SC q12–24h) or trimethoprim sulfa (30 mg/kg PO q12h). Anaerobic bacteria are usually causative agents of tooth root abscess; use antibiotics effective against anaerobes such as azithromycin (30 mg/kg PO q24h); can be used alone or combined with metronidazole (20 mg/kg PO q12h). Alternatively, use penicillin g (40,000–60,000 IU/kg SC q2–7d), chloramphenicol (50 mg/kg PO q8h) or metronidazole alone. Combine with topical treatment.
• Antihistamines have been used in rabbits with allergic rhinitis and symptomatically in rabbits with infectious rhinitis. Use is anecdotal and dosages have been extrapolated from feline dosages: hydroxyzine (2 mg/kg PO q8–12h) or diphenhydramine (2 mg/kg PO, SC q8–12h)
• Nebulization with saline may be beneficial.
• Topical ophthalmic preparations, such as those containing quinolones, to treat associated conjunctivitis

### CONTRAINDICATIONS
• Topical nasal decongestants containing phenylephrine can exacerbate nasal inflammation and cause nasal ulceration and purulent rhinitis.
• Oral administration of antibiotics that select against Gram-positive bacteria (penicillins, macrolides, lincosamides, and cephalosporins) can cause fatal enteric dysbiosis and enterotoxemia.
• The use of corticosteriods (systemic or topical in ophthalmic preparations) can severely exacerbate bacterial infection.

### PRECAUTIONS
N/A

### POSSIBLE INTERACTIONS
N/A

### ALTERNATIVE DRUGS
Topical (intranasal) administration of ciprofloxacin ophthalmic drops in nares may be used in conjunction with systemic antibiotic therapy. Use with caution and with adequate restraint. Rabbits strongly object to

## NASAL DISCHARGE AND SNEEZING

any nasal stimulation. Jumping or kicking may result in serious musculoskeletal injury.

## FOLLOW-UP

### PATIENT MONITORING
Clinical assessment and monitoring for relapse of clinical signs

### POSSIBLE COMPLICATIONS
• Loss of appetite
• Extension of primary disease into mouth, eyes, ears, lungs, or brain
• Dyspnea as a result of nasal obstruction

## MISCELLANEOUS

### ASSOCIATED CONDITIONS
• Cheek teeth malocclusion and elongation
• Gastrointestinal hypomotility
• Abscessation

### AGE-RELATED FACTORS
N/A

### ZOONOTIC POTENTIAL
N/A

### PREGNANCY
N/A

### SYNONYMS
Snuffles

### SEE ALSO
• Abscessation
• Cheek teeth malocclusion and elongation
• Pasteurellosis
• Rhinitis and sinusitis

### ABBREVIATIONS
• CT = computed tomography
• ELISA = enzyme-linked immunosorbent assay
• MRI = magnetic resonance imaging
• PCR = polymerase chain reaction
• TWBC = total white blood cell

*Suggested Reading:*
Crossley DA. Oral biology and disorders of lagomorphs. Vet Clin North Am Exotic Anim Pract 2003;6(3):629–659.
Deeb BL. Respiratory disease and the pasteurella complex. In: Hillyer EV, Quesenberry K, eds. Ferrets, Rabbits and Rodents: Clinical Medicine and Surgery. Philadelphia: WB Saunders 1997:189–201.
Deeb BL, DiGiacomo RF. Respiratory diseases of rabbits. Vet Clin North Am Exotic Anim Pract 2000;3(2):465–480.
DeLong D, Manning PJ. Bacterial diseases. In: Manning P, Ringler DH, Newcomer CE, eds. The Biology of the Laboratory Rabbit. Orlando, FL: Academic Press, 1994:129–170.
Harcourt-Brown F. Cardiorespiratory diseases. In: Harcourt-Brown F, ed. Textbook of Rabbit Medicine. Oxford: Butterworth-Heinemann, 2002:324–335.
Langan GP, Schaeffer DO. Rabbit microbiology and virology. In: Fudge AM, ed. Laboratory Medicine Avian and Exotic Pets. Philadelphia: WB Saunders, 2000:325–333.

*Portions Adapted From*
McKiernan BC. Nasal Discharge (Sneezing, Reverse Sneezing). In: Tilley LP, Smith FWK, Jr., eds. The 5-Minute Veterinary Consult: Canine and Feline, 3rd Ed. Baltimore: Lippincott Williams & Wilkins, 2004.

# BASICS

## DEFINITION
Discomfort along the spinal column

## PATHOPHYSIOLOGY
Pain may originate in the epaxial muscles, vertebrae and associated structures, spinal nerves, nerve roots or dorsal root ganglia, and meninges.

## SYSTEMS AFFECTED
• Nervous
• Musculoskeletal

## SIGNALMENT
No age, breed, or sex predilection

## SIGNS

### Historical Findings
• Owner may describe an abnormal gait; the rabbit may be unable to hop; be reluctant to jump or climb; have difficulty getting in and out of litter box, climbing stairs, and hopping onto furniture; and may drag the affected limbs or be unable get up.
• Sudden onset of paresis/paralysis is common with traumatic vertebral fractures or luxation.
• History of improper restraint—inexperienced handlers or owners; restraint for mask induction of anesthesia; very nervous animals escaping from appropriate restraint
• Trauma may not have been witnessed. Many rabbits fracture or luxate vertebrae by suddenly jumping while in their cages. History may include startling event such as a loud thunderstorm, fireworks, or unfamiliar people or pets in the house.
• Ataxia, rear limb weakness
• Perineal dermatitis, urine scald
• Flaking, alopecia in intrascapular region or tail head due to inability to groom
• Feces or cecotrophs pasted to perineum
• Teeth grinding or reluctance to move due to pain

### Physical Examination Findings
• Pain on epaxial palpation
• Neurologic deficits referable to the spinal cord or nerve root compression
• Ataxia, rear limb weakness
• Perineal dermatitis—matted fur, urine-soaked perineum or ventrum, feces pasted to perineum, alopecia, erythema, ulceration, myiasis; seen secondary to inability to groom and in rabbits with fecal or urinary incontinence
• Pododermatitis (sore hocks) due to inactivity or inability to groom
• Alopecia, flaking, *Cheyletiella* sp. mites in intrascapular or tail head region due to inadequate grooming
• Accumulation of wax in ear canals from inadequate grooming
• Hypercalciuria secondary to insufficient voiding in chronically painful rabbits or rabbits with loss of bladder control
• Obesity

## CAUSES

### Epaxial Muscles
• Traumatic myositis
• Abscess, cellulitis

### Vertebrae and Associated Structures
• Fracture
• Luxation and subluxation
• Disk disease
• Spondylosis
• Vertebral osteomyelitis
• Vertebral neoplasia
• Malformation and malarticulation
• Diskospondylitis

### Spinal Nerves
• Entrapment by disk herniation
• Neoplasia—primary or metastatic
• Traumatic entrapment, tearing, or laceration
• Compression or inflammation of dorsal root ganglion
• Meningitis—bacterial, protozoal

## RISK FACTORS
• Trauma
• Spinal fractures, luxations, or intervertebral disk disease—improper restraint, trauma in caged rabbits suddenly startled, possibly disuse atrophy from confinement

# DIAGNOSIS

## DIFFERENTIAL DIAGNOSIS
• Diseases involving thoracic structures—pleura, cardiovascular system, and lungs
• Diseases involving abdominal structures—uterine neoplasia, hypercalciuria or urolithiasis, abdominal abscesses
• Rule out limb musculoskeletal pain, especially coxofemoral DJD
• *Encephalitozoon cuniculi*—nonpainful disease of the spinal cord

## CBC/BIOCHEMISTRY/URINALYSIS
• Creatine kinase—can be high with any diseases affecting the muscle
• CBC—TWBC elevations are usually not seen with bacterial diseases. A relative heterophilia and/or lymphopenia are more common.

## OTHER LABORATORY TESTS
N/A

## IMAGING
• Survey radiographs—identify DJD, hypercalciuria, or other causes of pain and reluctance to move.
• Spinal radiographs—lesion localized to the spinal cord; may reveal fracture or luxation, narrowed disc spaces, disc herniation, spondylosis, diskospondylitis, bony tumor, congenital vertebral malformation
• Thoracic radiography—detect metastasis
• Myelography—if survey radiography is not diagnostic and when considering surgery
• CT or MRI—evaluate potential brain disease; CT is of limited value for evaluation of spine in rabbits; MRI more accurate, but not widely available and technically difficult to perform
• Abdominal ultrasonography—if underlying metabolic disease is suspected

## DIAGNOSTIC PROCEDURES

### Epaxial Muscle
• Muscle biopsy—may reveal neoplastic or inflammatory cells
• EMG—may identify an irritating or denervating process affecting the muscles
• Bone biopsy—helps confirm vertebral neoplasia and infection
• Cytology and culture—from the affected intervertebral space; may help identify cause
• CSF analysis—sample from the cerebellomedullary cistern; may be valuable for evaluating central disease; detect inflammatory process; sample collection may put the patient at risk for herniation if there is a mass or high intracranial pressure.

# TREATMENT
• Varies widely according to the nature and extent of the tissues involved
• Caution: symptomatic treatment without first establishing a diagnosis can be dangerous.
• Inpatient vs. outpatient—depends on severity of disease

## NURSING CARE
• Keep perineum clean, dry, and free of fecal matter.
• Use soft bedding; keep bedding clean and dry to prevent dermatitis or bed sores.
• Manual expression of the bladder if unable to urinate
• Comb frequently to remove matted hair and scale from areas in which the rabbit cannot groom.

## ACTIVITY
Restrict until spinal trauma and disk herniation can be ruled out.

## DIET
• It is absolutely imperative that the rabbit continue to eat during and following treatment. Animals in pain are often anorectic. Anorexia will often cause gastrointestinal hypomotility, derangement of the gastrointestinal microflora, and overgrowth of intestinal bacterial pathogens.

# NECK AND BACK PAIN

• Offer a large selection of fresh, moistened greens such as cilantro, romaine lettuce, parsley, carrot tops, dandelion greens, spinach, collard greens, etc., and good-quality grass hay. Many rabbits will begin to eat these foods, even if they were previously anorectic.
• If the patient refuses these foods, syringe feed a gruel such as Critical Care for Herbivores (Oxbow Pet Products, Murdock, NE) 10–15 mL/kg PO q6–8h. Alternatively, pellets can be ground and mixed with fresh greens, vegetable baby foods, water, or juice to form a gruel.
• Encourage oral fluid intake by offering fresh water, wetting leafy vegetables, or flavoring water with vegetable juices.

## MEDICATIONS

### DRUG(S) OF CHOICE
• NSAIDs—have been used for short- or long-term therapy to reduce pain and inflammation in rabbits with musculoskeletal disease: meloxicam (0.2–0.5 mg/kg PO q12–24h) or carprofen (2.2 mg/kg PO q12–24); use only when the patient is exhibiting signs.
• Glucocorticosteroids—contraindicated in most rabbits with neck or back pain; indicated only in rabbits with acute spinal trauma; establish a diagnosis before initiating.
• Antimicrobial therapy—for infection; depends on the causative agent
• Chemotherapy and radiotherapy—depends on tumor type

### CONTRAINDICATIONS
• Oral administration of antibiotics that select against Gram-positive bacteria (penicillins, macrolides, lincosamides, and cephalosporins) can cause fatal enteric dysbiosis and enterotoxemia.
• Corticosteroids—do not use with diskospondylitis or other infectious diseases; do not use for routine treatment of inflammatory or painful musculoskeletal disorders; associated with gastrointestinal ulceration and hemorrhage, delayed wound healing, and heightened susceptibility to infection; rabbits are very sensitive to the immunosuppressive effects of both topic and systemic corticosteroids; use may exacerbate subclinical bacterial infection.

### PRECAUTIONS
• Corticosteroids—use with caution, only in acute spinal trauma; associated with gastrointestinal ulceration and hemorrhage, delayed wound healing, and heightened susceptibility to infection; rabbits are very sensitive to the immunosuppressive effects of both topic and systemic corticosteroids; use may exacerbate subclinical bacterial infection.
• Meloxicam—use with caution in rabbits with compromised renal function.
• Steroids and NSAIDs—do not use in combination; life-threatening gastroenteritis may result.

### POSSIBLE INTERACTIONS
N/A

### ALTERNATIVE DRUGS
• Chondroitin sulfate (Cosequin, Nutramax) has been used anecdotally using feline dosage protocols; polysulfate glycosaminoglycan (Adequan, Luitpold) 2.2 mg/kg SC, IM q3d × 21–28 days, then q14d.
• Acupuncture may be effective for rabbits with chronic pain.

## FOLLOW-UP

### PATIENT MONITORING
• Monitor response to treatment closely and make adjustments as necessary.
• Instruct client to watch for signs of gastrointestinal hypomotility, pyoderma, and urinary tract disease.

### POSSIBLE COMPLICATIONS
• Fibrous replacement of muscle fibers, causing chronic pain and immobility
• Permanent paralysis or dysfunction
• Urinary tract infection, bladder atony, urine scalding and pyoderma, fecal incontinence, decubital ulcer formation, myiasis
• Exacerbation of bacterial infections (possibly life-threatening), gastric ulceration with corticosteroid usage
• Chronic pain

## MISCELLANEOUS

### ASSOCIATED CONDITIONS
• Gastrointestinal hypomotility
• Hypercalciuria
• Ulcerative pododermatitis (sore hocks)

### AGE-RELATED FACTORS
• Anomalous conditions—usually seen in younger animals
• Neoplastic conditions—more often seen in middle-aged to old animals

### ZOONOTIC POTENTIAL
N/A

### PREGNANCY
Use of corticosteroids is contraindicated.

### SEE ALSO
See causes.

### ABBREVIATIONS
• CBC = complete blood count
• CSF = cerebrospinal fluid
• CT = computed tomography
• EMG = electromyelogram
• DJD = degenerative joint disease
• MRI = magnetic resonance imaging
• NSAIDs = nonsteroidal antiinflammatory drugs
• TWBC = total white blood cell

*Suggested Reading*

Deeb BJ, Carpenter JW. Neurologic and musculoskeletal diseases. In: Quesenberry KE, Carpenter JW, eds. Ferrets, Rabbits and Rodents: Clinical Medicine and Surgery. 2nd Ed. Philadelphia: WB Saunders, 2004:203–210.

Greenaway JB, Partlow GD, Gonsholt NL, et al. Anatomy of the lumbosacral spinal cord in rabbits. J Am Anim Hosp Assoc 2001;37(1):27–34.

Harcourt-Brown F. Neurological and locomotor diseases. In: Harcourt-Brown F, ed. Textbook of Rabbit Medicine. Oxford: Butterworth-Heinemann, 2002:307–323.

Kapatkin A. Orthopedics in small mammals. In: Quesenberry KE, Carpenter JW, eds. Ferrets, Rabbits and Rodents: Clinical Medicine and Surgery. 2nd Ed. Philadelphia: WB Saunders, 2004:383–391.

Oliver JE, Lorenz MD, Kornegay JN. Pain. In: Handbook of Veterinary Neurology. Philadelphia: Saunders, 1997:333–340.

Paul-Murphy J, Ramer JC. Urgent care of the pet rabbits. Vet Clin North Am Exotic Anim Pract 1998;1(1):127–152.

*Portions Adapted From*

Luttgen PJ. Neck and Back Pain. In: Tilley LP, Smith FWK, Jr., eds. The 5-Minute Veterinary Consult: Canine and Feline, 3rd Ed. Baltimore: Lippincott Williams & Wilkins, 2004.

## BASICS

### DEFINITION
• Nephroliths—uroliths (i.e., polycrystalline concretions or calculi) located in the renal pelvis or collecting diverticula of the kidney
• Ureteroliths—uroliths located within a ureter; many originate within the renal pelvis and so are associated with nephrolithiasis.
• Nephroliths or nephrolith fragments may pass into the ureters (ureteroliths).
• Nephroliths that are not infected, not causing obstruction or clinical signs, and not progressively enlarging are termed inactive. Inactive nephroliths are unusual in rabbits; most will progressively enlarge, eventually causing obstruction.

### PATHOPHYSIOLOGY
• Nephroliths and ureteroliths can cause partial or complete obstruction of the renal pelvis or ureter, predispose to pyelonephritis, and result in compressive injury of the renal parenchyma, leading to renal failure.
• Most uroliths are composed of calcium salts (calcium oxalate and calcium carbonate). Excessive crystal formation and retention in the bladder initially results in thick, sandlike urine ("sludge") and inflammation of the bladder wall. Crystals can condense to form uroliths in the bladder, urethra, ureters, or renal pelvis.
• In rabbits, intestinal calcium absorption is not dependent on vitamin D, and nearly all calcium in the diet is absorbed. Calcium excretion occurs primarily through the kidneys (vs. the gallbladder in other mammals); the fractional urinary excretion is 45–60% in rabbits compared to less than 2% in other mammals.
• Rabbits normally eat a diet high in calcium; however, not all rabbits develop hypercalciuria.
• The factors leading to hypercalciuria and urolith formation in rabbits is unclear; however, the disease is seen more commonly in obese, sedentary rabbits fed a diet composed primarily of alfalfa-based commercial pellets and alfalfa hay. Most commercial diets contain excessive amounts of calcium. The dietary requirement of calcium for rabbits is only 0.22 g of calcium/100 g food, but most commercial diets contain up to 0.9–1.6 g of calcium/100 g of food. It is unlikely that high dietary calcium content alone is the cause of hypercalciuria, but it may exacerbate urinary sludge formation when combined with other factors leading to urine retention.
• Inadequate water intake leading to a more concentrated urine and factors that impair complete evacuation of the bladder, such as lack of exercise, obesity, cystitis, neoplasia or neuromuscular disease, may also contribute. Without frequent urination and dilute urine, calcium crystals may precipitate out of solution. Precipitated crystals form a thick sand or sludge.

### SYSTEMS AFFECTED
Renal/urologic—affects the urinary tract, with potential for obstruction, recurrent urinary tract infections, or renal failure

### GENETICS
Unknown

### INCIDENCE/PREVALENCE
Clinical conditions related to hypercalciuria and urolith formation are extremely common in pet rabbits.

### GEOGRAPHIC DISTRIBUTION
Ubiquitous

### SIGNALMENT
*Breed Predilections*
All breeds are equally affected.

*Mean Age and Range*
Seen most commonly in middle-aged rabbits 3–5 years old

*Predominant Sex*
N/A

### SIGNS
*General Comments*
Many patients are asymptomatic despite large amounts of calcium sludge accumulation in the bladder and/or the presence of nephroliths or ureteroliths; diagnosis is made during workup of other problems.

*Historical Findings*
• Pollakiuria, dysuria, hematuria, and urine staining in the perineum in rabbits with associated urolithiasis or large amounts of crystalline sludge in the bladder (generally precedes or accompanies nephroliths/ureteroliths)
• Anorexia, weight loss, lethargy, tooth grinding, tenesmus, and a hunched posture in rabbits with large urocystoliths, large amounts of sludge in the bladder, or complete or partial obstruction of the ureters or urethra
• Signs attributable to uremia in animals with bilateral obstruction or renal failure
• Pain (renal colic) with acute abdominal/lumbar pain

*Physical Examination Findings*
• Abdominal or lumbar pain upon palpation sometimes present
• Renomegaly if ureteral obstruction leads to hydronephrosis
• Unilateral ureteral obstruction results in azotemia and uremic clinical signs only when the function of the contralateral kidney is compromised.

• Detect urocystoliths by abdominal palpation; failure to palpate uroliths does not exclude them from consideration. Often, one single, large calculus is palpated. In rabbits with crystalluria, the bladder palpates as a soft, doughy mass.
• Renoliths/ureteroliths are often preceded by or accompanied with calcium precipitates ("sludge") in the bladder. Manual expression of the bladder may reveal thick, beige- to brown-colored urine. Manual expression of the bladder may expel thick, brown urine even in rabbits that have normal-appearing voided urine.

### CAUSES
See pathophysiology.

### RISK FACTORS
• Inadequate water intake (dirty water bowls, unpalatable water, changing water sources, inadequate water provision)
• Urine retention—underlying bladder pathology, neuromuscular disease, painful conditions causing a reluctance to ambulate (musculoskeletal disease, dental disease, abscess)
• Inadequate cleaning of litter box or cage may cause some rabbits to avoid urinating for abnormally long periods.
• Obesity
• Lack of exercise
• Feeding of exclusively alfalfa-based commercial pelleted diets
• Renal disease
• Calcium or vitamin/mineral supplements added to the diet
• Lower urinary tract infection—ascending infection and pyelonephritis

## DIAGNOSIS

### DIFFERENTIAL DIAGNOSIS
• Consider in all cases of renal failure, unilateral or bilateral renomegaly, abdominal pain, or fluid accumulation in the retroperitoneal space.
• Renal calcification can resemble renoliths on abdominal radiographs. Renal calcification can be differentiated from renoliths on ultrasound.
• Radiopacities on abdominal radiographs that may be confused with ureteroliths, including particulate fecal material in the colon, mammary gland nipples, and mineralization of the renal pelvis
• Other causes of ureteral obstruction include intraluminal tumors, ureteral strictures (following surgery or trauma), and extraluminal compression. Hydroureter and hydronephrosis may occur because of ureteral ectopia, pyelonephritis, and obstruction of the ureteral opening at the trigone; none of these conditions is common in rabbits.

# NEPHROLITHIASIS AND URETEROLITHIASIS

## CBC/BIOCHEMISTRY/URINALYSIS

These tests evaluate renal function and screen for concurrent disease before the treatment of ureterolithiasis. They do not directly contribute to the diagnosis of nephrolithiasis/ureterolithiasis.

- CBC results—usually normal unless the patient has pyelonephritis (rare)
- Serum biochemistry analysis—most affected rabbits are hypercalcemic (normal range 12–16 mg/dL); however, the significance of this is unclear since many normal rabbits have high serum calcium concentration and never develop hypercalciuria.
- Remainder of the serum biochemistry is usually normal unless bilateral obstruction, pyelonephritis, or compressive renal injury leads to renal failure.
- Urinary sediment evaluation reveals calcium oxalate or calcium carbonate crystals; however, this is a normal finding in rabbits, and the presence of large amounts of crystals in the urine does not necessarily indicate disease. Disease occurs only when the concentration of crystals is excessive, forming thick, white to brown, sandlike urine and subsequent inflammatory cystitis or partial to complete blockage of the urethra, ureters, or renal pelvis
- Pyuria (normal value 0–1 WBC/hpf), hematuria (normal value 0–1 RBC/hpf), and proteinuria (normal value 0–33 mg/dL) indicate urinary tract inflammation, but these are nonspecific findings that may result from infectious and noninfectious causes of lower urinary tract disease.

## OTHER LABORATORY TESTS

- Submit retrieved uroliths for quantitative analysis.
- Results of bacterial culture of urine may confirm urinary tract infection in animals with concurrent pyelonephritis.

## IMAGING

- Calcium oxalate uroliths are radiopaque and may be detected by survey radiography. If obstruction and hydronephrosis have occurred, renomegaly may be apparent. If ureteral rupture occurs, contrast in the retroperitoneal space may be lost.
- Renal calcification can resemble renoliths on abdominal radiographs. Renal calcification can be differentiated from renoliths on ultrasound.
- Most rabbits with ureteroliths/nephroliths also have urocystoliths or "sand" or "sludge" in the bladder.
- May use ultrasonography or excretory urography to confirm the presence, size, and number of nephroliths or ureteroliths; changes suggesting pyelonephritis may also be observed by ultrasound.

## DIAGNOSTIC PROCEDURES

Perform excretory urography to confirm function in the remaining kidney prior to nephrectomy.

## PATHOLOGIC FINDINGS

Histopathology required only to confirm the presence of secondary renal lesions

# TREATMENT

## APPROPRIATE HEALTH CARE

Manage patients with inactive nephroliths as outpatients. Surgical patients require hospitalization.

## NURSING CARE

- Patients in ARF or uremic crisis—correct estimated fluid deficits with normal (0.9%) saline or balanced polyionic solution within 4–6 hours to prevent additional renal injury from ischemia; once the patient is hydrated, ongoing fluid requirements are provided in balanced electrolyte solution (approximately 100 mL/kg/day).
- Use caution when hydrating extremely stressed rabbits. Severe stress may cause a decrease in GFR and subsequent overhydration. Be sure that the volume of urine excreted is appropriate to the amount of fluids received.
- Hypervolemia—stop fluid administration and eliminate excess fluid by diuretic administration.
- Patients in CRF—subcutaneous fluid therapy (daily or every other day) may benefit patients with moderate to severe CRF.

## ACTIVITY

- Reduce during the period of tissue repair after surgery.
- Long term—increase activity level by providing large exercise areas to encourage voiding and prevent recurrence.

## DIET

- It is absolutely imperative that the rabbit continue to eat during and following treatment. Many rabbits with urinary tract disease have a decreased appetite. Anorexia may cause or exacerbate gastrointestinal hypomotility, derangement of the gastrointestinal microflora, and overgrowth of intestinal bacterial pathogens.
- Offer a large selection of fresh, moistened greens such as cilantro, romaine lettuce, parsley, carrot tops, dandelion greens, spinach, or collard greens and good-quality grass hay. Many rabbits will begin to eat these foods, even if they were previously anorectic.
- If the patient refuses these foods, syringe feed a gruel such as Critical Care for Herbivores (Oxbow Pet Products, Murdock, NE) 10–15 mL/kg PO q6–8h. Larger volumes and more frequent feedings are often

accepted; feed as much as the rabbit will readily accept. Alternatively, pellets can be ground and mixed with fresh greens, vegetable baby foods, water, or juice to form a gruel. The addition of canned pumpkin to this gruel is a palatable source of fiber and calories. If sufficient volumes of food are not accepted in this manner, nasogastric intubation is indicated.

- High-carbohydrate, high-fat nutritional supplements are contraindicated.
- Increasing water consumption is essential to prevention and treatment of hypercalciuria. Provide multiple sources of fresh water. Automatic, continuously pouring water fountains available for cats entice some rabbits to drink. Flavoring the water with fruit or vegetable juices (with no added sugars) may be helpful. Provide a variety of clean, fresh, leafy vegetables sprayed or soaked with water.
- No reports of dissolution of calcium oxalate uroliths with special diets
- Following treatment, reduction in the amount of calcium in the diet may help to prevent or delay recurrence. Eliminate feeding of alfalfa pellets and switch to a high-fiber timothy-based pellet (Oxbow Pet Products, Murdock, NE). The form of calcium found in alfalfa-based commercial pellets and alfalfa hay is calcium carbonate, which is 50% more bioavailable than the calcium oxalate found in most green, leafy vegetables. Feed timothy and grass hay instead of alfalfa hay and offer large volumes of fresh, green, leafy vegetables.

## CLIENT EDUCATION

- Inactive nephroliths/ureteroliths—may not require removal but should be monitored periodically; most nephroliths will continue to increase in size and can potentially cause obstruction at any time. Resulting hydronephrosis or renal parenchymal injury may initially be asymptomatic, so conservative management and monitoring carries a slight risk of undetected and potentially irreversible renal damage, which must be weighed against the potential renal damage from nephrotomy.
- Urolith removal does not alter the factors responsible for their formation; eliminating risk factors such as obesity, sedentary life, and poor diet combined with increasing water consumption may help to minimize or delay recurrence. Even with these changes, however, recurrence is highly likely.

## SURGICAL CONSIDERATIONS

- Indications for removal of nephroliths/ureteroliths—obstruction, recurrent infection, symptomatic nephroliths, progressive nephrolith enlargement, and a nonfunctional contralateral kidney
- Surgical techniques recommended for removal of ureteroliths vary, depending on the

site of obstruction, the presence or absence of infection, and the degree of function of the associated kidney. Performance of a ureterotomy or ureteroneocystotomy requires experience in microsurgical techniques.
• When the contralateral kidney functions normally or when severe hydronephrosis or pyelonephritis is present in the affected kidney, ureteronephrectomy may be appropriate.

## MEDICATIONS

### DRUG(S) OF CHOICE
• Medical dissolution is ineffective.
• Dietary therapy aimed at prevention of recurrent disease (See diet, above) is imperative following relief of obstruction.
• Pain management is essential during and following surgery or if pain is causing reduced frequency of voiding. Perioperative choices include butorphanol (0.1–1.0 mg/kg SC, IM, IV q4–6h) or buprenorphine (0.01–0.05 mg/kg SC, IM, IV q6–12h). Meloxicam (0.2–0.5 mg/k PO q24h) and carprofen (1–2.2 mg/kg PO q12h) have been used for long-term pain management.

### CONTRAINDICATIONS
N/A

### PRECAUTIONS
• Steroids and furosemide promote calciuria.
• NSAIDs—use with caution in patients with renal disease.

### POSSIBLE INTERACTIONS
N/A

### ALTERNATIVE DRUGS
N/A

## FOLLOW-UP

### PATIENT MONITORING
• Following general anesthesia, monitor for postoperative ileus. Be certain the rabbit is eating and defecating normally prior to release from the hospital.

• Following successful removal of uroliths, recheck every 3–6 months for recurrence of uroliths and to ensure owner compliance with preventive measures; urinalysis, radiographs (or ultrasound), and a urine culture are usually appropriate.

### PREVENTION/AVOIDANCE
• Increase water consumption for the remainder of the rabbit's life.
• Place patients on a lowered calcium diet (described above).
• Increase exercise.

### POSSIBLE COMPLICATIONS
• Rabbits undergoing general anesthesia are at high risk for developing life-threatening postoperative ileus. This is especially common with obese rabbits fed a poor-quality diet, as many rabbits with hypercalciuria are.
• Hydronephrosis, renal failure, recurrent urinary tract infection, pyelonephritis, sepsis, ureteral rupture

### EXPECTED COURSE AND PROGNOSIS
• Highly variable; depend on urolith location, size, and the presence of secondary complications (e.g., obstruction, infection, renal failure)
• Most nephroliths continue to increase in size.
• Although dietary management may decrease the likelihood of recurrence, many rabbits will develop clinical disease again within 1–2 years.

## MISCELLANEOUS

### ASSOCIATED CONDITIONS
• Commonly associated with uroliths in the bladder
• Gastrointestinal hypomotility

### AGE-RELATED FACTORS
Rare in young animals

### PREGNANCY
N/A

### SEE ALSO
• Gastrointestinal hypomotility
• Hypercalciuria
• Renal failure
• Urinary tract obstruction

### ABBREVIATIONS
• ARF = acute renal failure
• CBC = complete blood count
• CRF = chronic renal failure
• GFR = glomerular filtration rate
• NSAIDs = nonsteroidal antiinflammatory drugs
• RBC = red blood cell
• WBC = white blood cell

*Suggested Reading*

Brown SA. Rabbit urinary tract disease. Proc North Am Vet Conf 1997;785–787.

Cheeke PR, Amberg JW. Comparative calcium excretion by rats and rabbits. J Anim Sci 1973;37:450–454.

Donoghue S. Nutrition and pet rabbits. In: Rosenthal KL, ed. Practical Exotic Animal Medicine: The Compendium Collection. Trenton, NJ: Veterinary Learning Systems, 1997:107.

Garibaldi BA, Pecquet-Goad ME. Hypercalcemia with secondary nephrolithiasis in a rabbit. Lab Anim Sci 1988;38:331–333.

Harkness JE, Wagner JE. The Biology and Medicine of Rabbits and Rodents. 3rd Ed. Baltimore: Williams & Wilkins, 1989.

Harcourt-Brown F. Urogenital disease. In: Harcourt-Brown F, ed. Textbook of Rabbit Medicine. Oxford: Butterworth-Heinemann, 2002:335–351.

Kampheus J. Calcium metabolism of rabbits as an etiological factor for urolithiasis. J Nutr 1991;121:595–596.

Pare JA, Paul-Murphy J. Disorders of the reproductive and urinary systems. In: Quesenberry KE, Carpenter JW, eds. Ferrets, Rabbits and Rodents: Clinical Medicine and Surgery 2nd Ed. Philadelphia:WB Saunders, 2004:183–193.

Paul-Murphy J, Ramer JC. Urgent care of the pet rabbits. Vet Clin North Am Exotic Anim Pract 1998;1(1):127–152.

Redrobe S. Calcium metabolism in rabbits. Semin Avian Exotic Pet Med 2002;11(2):94–101.

*Portions Adapted From*

Adams LG. Nephrolithiasis. In: Tilley LP, Smith FWK, Jr., eds. The 5-Minute Veterinary Consult: Canine and Feline, 3rd Ed. Baltimore: Lippincott Williams & Wilkins, 2004.

# OBESITY

## BASICS

### DEFINITION
The presence of body fat in sufficient excess to compromise normal physiologic function or predispose the animal to metabolic, surgical, and/or mechanical problems. Obesity has become an extremely common, and often debilitating, problem in pet rabbits.

### PATHOPHYSIOLOGY
• Caging—inactivity is an important risk factor since many pet rabbits are kept in small cages for long periods of time. Most cages sold commercially are inadequate in size. Access to exercise areas is often limited.
• Dietary factors—most commercial pelleted diets are alfalfa based and very nutrient dense. Free-choice feeding of pellets is one of the primary causes of obesity in rabbits. Most pelleted diets are low in fiber and high in protein, calories, and carbohydrates. The feeding of commercially marketed rabbit "treats" such as honey sticks, yogurt drops, and pellets containing seed or grains contribute to obesity. Additionally, the high simple carbohydrate content of these treats can cause or exacerbate serious disorders such as gastrointestinal hypomotility and dysbiosis.
• Feeding management—some rabbits will overeat and become obese if pelleted food is left in the cage all day, due to boredom and lack of exercise.
• Animal factors—some rabbits refuse to eat hay or other foods high in coarse, indigestible fiber (this behavior not only contributes to obesity, but also to dental disease and gastrointestinal hypomotility). Rabbits with orthopedic, musculoskeletal, or painful disorders may be unwilling or unable to ambulate; inactivity contributes to obesity. Increasing age may also contribute to it.
• Owner factors—rabbits tend to prefer sweet-tasting treats; overfeeding of these treats contributes to obesity in pet rabbits. Rabbits are often treated as family members and owners have difficulty denying these treats.

### SYSTEMS AFFECTED
• Musculoskeletal—articular and locomotor problems
• Hepatobiliary—hepatic lipidosis
• Cardiovascular
• Gastrointestinal—gastrointestinal hypomotility and stasis; dysbiosis associated with inappropriate diets
• Urogenital—hypercalciuria common in obese, sedentary rabbits
• Dermatologic—poor grooming, fecal pasting of perineum, moist dermatitis, pododermatitis, myiasis

### SIGNALMENT
• Caged, inactive, middle-aged animals of either gender are at increased risk.
• Dwarf and lop breeds may be predisposed to obesity.

### SIGNS
• Excess amounts of body fat for body size are often measured as body condition score of 4 on a 1–5 scale in which 1 is cachectic (>20% underweight), 2 is lean (10–20% underweight), 3 is moderate, 4 is stout (20–40% overweight), and 5 is obese (>40% overweight).
• Sites of adipose tissue to evaluate during physical examination include the ribcage, abdomen, axilla, and dewlap.
• In some overweight rabbits, fat accumulation in the axillary region is multilobulated and may resemble neoplasia.
• In a normal, nonobese rabbit, the ribs should be palpable without an overlying layer of fat; no rolls of fat should extend over the rear limbs or hindquarters.
• Lethargy, weakness
• Perineal pyoderma, feces, or cecotrophs pasted to perineal region due to inability to groom or consume cecotrophs
• Flaky dermatitis in intrascapular region due to inability to groom
• Moist dermatitis of dewlap in females

### CAUSES
Most commonly, excessive access to pelleted diets and treats, often combined with insufficient activity

### RISK FACTORS
• Owner lifestyle
• Diet palatability and energy density
• Cage confinement

## DIAGNOSIS

### DIFFERENTIAL DIAGNOSIS
• Pregnancy
• Increased muscle mass
• Intraabdominal neoplasia or organomegaly
• Similar problems/diseases should be differentiated via history, physical examination, laboratory evaluation, and imaging.

### CBC/BIOCHEMISTRY/URINALYSIS
Normal

### OTHER LABORATORY TESTS
Normal

### IMAGING
Demonstrates excess body fat

### DIAGNOSTIC PROCEDURES
N/A

## TREATMENT
Success is lifelong amelioration of the problem.

### NURSING CARE
• Keep perineum clean, dry, and free of fecal matter.
• Remove matted hair. Be extremely cautious when clipping hair or pulling on mats since rabbit skin is extremely fragile and will easily tear. Sedation may be required.
• Treat secondary dermatitis.
• Provide soft, clean flooring to help prevent secondary pododermatitis.

### ACTIVITY
Increase activity level by providing access to exercise areas.

### DIET
• Either eliminate or reduce the volume of pelleted foods. A maximum volume of one-quarter cup pellets per 5 lb. body weight has been recommended. Switch to a high-fiber, timothy-based pelleted diet (Oxbow Pet Products, Murdock, NE).
• Do not feed alfalfa-based pelleted foods or pellet mixes containing seeds and/or dried fruits and vegetables.
• Do not feed commercial rabbit treats or dried fruits, because these are more calorie dense.
• Offer a large selection of fresh, moistened greens such as cilantro, romaine lettuce, parsley, carrot tops, dandelion greens, collard greens, broccoli leaves and tops, endive, basil, escarole, kale, swiss chard, chicory, or mustard greens.
• Feed high-quality timothy or grass hay ad lib in addition to fresh greens daily.
• Limit fresh fruits and nonleafy vegetable treats to 2–3 tsp per 5 lb. of body weight daily.
• Strictly prohibit simple sugars (such as yogurt drops, candies, or cookies), high-starch foods (such as bread products, grains, nuts, cereals, oats, corn, and peas), and legumes.

### CLIENT EDUCATION
• It is the most important part of obesity therapy; it must be tailored to each particular circumstance
• In addition to obesity, advise clients that feeding high-calorie, high-carbohydrate, low-fiber diets can lead to gastrointestinal hypomotility, chronic soft stools, hypercalciuria, dental disease, and hepatic lipidosis, all of which can be life threatening.
• Therapeutic suggestions include reasonable, functional weight loss goals, rather than recommending achieving a poorly

defined "optimal adult weight" for aesthetic reasons. Keeping a food record that identifies all food sources may help some clients appreciate how much the pet consumes. Suggest that "snacks" replace regular food rather than supplement it and that the snacks consist of a portion of the regularly allotted food.

• The amount fed should be tailored to the specific needs of individual pets. Caloric requirements reported for rabbits are 150–175 kcal/kg for growing, pregnant, lactating small breed rabbits, and 40–50 kcal/kg for adult large breed maintenance.

## MEDICATIONS

### DRUG(S) OF CHOICE
N/A

### CONTRAINDICATIONS
N/A

### PRECAUTIONS
N/A

### POSSIBLE INTERACTIONS
N/A

### ALTERNATIVE DRUGS
N/A

## FOLLOW-UP

### PATIENT MONITORING
• Lifelong follow-up and support are essential to maintain the reduced weight.

• At the initial visit instruct clients to recognize a moderate body condition score and to feed the quantity of food necessary to maintain this condition during the changing physiologic and environmental conditions of the pet's life; remind them at checkups.

### POSSIBLE COMPLICATIONS
• Do not fast rabbits or make sudden, drastic reductions in available food; this may predispose them to hepatic lipidosis or gastrointestinal hypomotility.
• Increased anesthetic risk
• Cardiovascular disease
• Orthopedic disease
• Hepatic lipidosis
• Moist dermatitis, pododermatitis; myiasis

## MISCELLANEOUS

### ASSOCIATED CONDITIONS
• Orthopedic problems
• Skin problems
• Respiratory problems
• Hepatic lipidosis

### AGE-RELATED FACTORS
N/A

### ZOONOTIC POTENTIAL
N/A

### PREGNANCY
Obesity may increase risk of dystocia, but because of potential risk to fetus, do not treat pregnant animals.

### SYNONYMS
N/A

### SEE ALSO
• Gastrointestinal hypomotility
• Hypercalciuria and urolithiasis
• Pyoderma

### ABBREVIATIONS
N/A

*Suggested Reading*

Cheeke PR. Rabbit Feeding and Nutrition. Orlando, FL: Academic Press, 1987.

Donoghue S. Nutrition and pet rabbits. In: Rosenthal KL, ed. Practical Exotic Animal Medicine: The Compendium Collection. Trenton, NJ: Veterinary Learning Systems, 1997:107.

Jenkins JR. Gastrointestinal diseases. In: Quesenberry KE, Carpenter JW, eds. Ferrets, Rabbits and Rodents: Clinical Medicine and Surgery. 2nd Ed. Philadelphia: WB Saunders, 2004:161–171.

Jenkins JR. Feeding recommendations for the house rabbit. Vet Clin Noth Am Exotic Anim Pract

*Portions Adapted From*

Crandell J. Obesity. In: Tilley LP, Smith FWK, Jr., eds. The 5-Minute Veterinary Consult: Canine and Feline, 3rd Ed. Baltimore: Lippincott Williams & Wilkins, 2004.

# OTITIS EXTERNA AND MEDIA

 BASICS

## OVERVIEW
• Inflammation of the external ear canal—not a diagnosis but a description of clinical signs
• Otitis media often results as an extension of otitis externa through a ruptured tympanum.
• Otitis media may occur as an extension of upper respiratory infection (rhinitis, sinusitis) via the eustachian tube. In this case, the tympanum may be intact.
• A thorough otic examination, including visualization of the tympanum, should be part of routine physical examination. The normal rabbit ear has a small amount of yellow/beige wax, which may need to be removed with a small curette to visualize the tympanum. Dwarf, lop-eared breeds tend to form more wax than other breeds.
• Rabbits with otitis externa/media have thick, white exudate in the horizontal or vertical canal. Often, this exudate is located deep within the horizontal canal, near the tympanum, and may not be associated with signs of inflammation. A thorough otic examination is required to detect this exudate.
• Some rabbits are asymptomatic—otitis is detected on otic examination.
• Exudate is generally extremely caseous, does not drain, and is difficult to flush. Successful removal of all exudate from the horizontal canal can be challenging and requires consistent owner compliance and, frequently, multiple office visits.

## SIGNALMENT
• Lop-eared rabbits may be more likely to show signs of otitis externa.
• No age or sex predilection

## SIGNS

### Historical Findings
• Pain—may be manifested by anorexia, holding the ear down, depression, or repeated digging at the floor.
• Head shaking
• Scratching at the pinnae
• Malodorous ears (uncommon)

### Physical Examination Findings
• Thick, white, creamy exudate in the horizontal and/or vertical canals
• In rabbits with otitis media only, the external canal may have a normal appearance on otoscopic examination; the tympanum may bulge out into the external canal, and a white, creamy exudate may be seen behind the tympanum.
• In some cases, the otic examination appears normal, despite significant otitis media.
• Redness and swelling of the external canal, leading to stenosis

• Exudate caused by ear mites often forms distinctive, large, tan foliated crusts that may entirely fill the pinna.
• Excessive wax production
• Scaling and exudation—may result in canal obstruction
• Holding the pinna down or tilting the head due to pain
• Alopecia, excoriations at the base of the ear
• Vestibular signs (with head tilt, nystagmus, anorexia, ataxia, and rolling) indicate development of otitis interna/media.

## CAUSES
• Parasitic—*Psoroptes cuniculi* (ear mites)
• Bacterial infections—common; *Pasteurella multocida* and *Staphylococcus aureus* are most often cultured from the horizontal canal in otitis externa; *P. multocida, S. aureus, Pseudomonas aeruginosa, Escherichia coli,* and *Listeria monocytogenes* are most often cultured in otitis interna/media.
• Yeast infections—bacterial infections can be mixed with, or entirely the result of, *Malassezia* sp. or other yeast species.
• Hypersensitivities—rabbits often develop hypersensitivity reactions to many of the topical ear cleaning solutions or medications commonly used in other mammalian species.
• Obstruction—neoplasia, excessive cerumen production, foreign bodies
• Progressive changes—canal hypertrophy, fibrosis, cartilage calcification
• Otitis media—can produce symptoms on its own; can act as a reservoir for organisms, causing recurrent condition

## RISK FACTORS
• Abnormal or breed-related conformation of the external canal (e.g., stenosis, pendulous pinnae) restricts proper air flow into the canal.
• Excessive moisture (e.g., from frequent cleanings with improper solutions) can lead to infection.
• Topical drug reaction and irritation and trauma from abrasive cleaning techniques

 DIAGNOSIS

## DIFFERENTIAL DIAGNOSIS

### Exudate in the Ear Canal
• Normal wax—most rabbits normally have a light yellow/beige, waxy exudate in the ear canal. Exudate from bacterial otitis is typically creamy white to beige in color. However, white exudate may turn yellow/brown on the surface after drying out and be mistaken for wax. To differentiate, remove a small amount of dried exudate to reveal white, creamy exudate below.
• Ear mites—intense pruritus primarily located around the ears, head, and neck is occasionally generalized. Thick, brown,

beige crusty exudate is in the ear canal and extending onto the pinna. With severe infestations, crust layer may be very thick.

### Head Tilt
• Rabbits with otitis externa/media may hold the ear down or tilt the head due to pain. This must be differentiated from a head tilt caused by lesions affecting the vestibular apparatus. Rabbits with vestibular dysfunction demonstrate nystagmus, torticollis, ataxia, and/or tremors in addition to head tilt.
• Progression of otitis interna/media may lead to lesions of the vestibular apparatus, so that clinical signs of both may be seen concurrently.

## CBC/BIOCHEMISTRY/URINALYSIS
May indicate a primary underlying disease

## OTHER LABORATORY TESTS
Serology for *Pasteurella*—usefulness is severely limited and generally not helpful in the diagnosis of pasteurellosis in pet rabbits. An ELISA is available and results are reported as negative, low positive, or high positive. Positive results, even when high, may only indicate prior exposure to *Pasteurella* and the development of antibodies and do not confirm active infection. Low-positive results may occur due to cross-reaction with other, nonpathogenic bacteria (false positive). False-negative results are common with immunosuppression or early infection. No evidence exists to support correlation of titers to the presence or absence of disease.

## IMAGING
Bullae radiographs—may demonstrate otitis media; increased soft tissue density in the bullae, bony lysis, or periosteal proliferation. Normal appearance of bullae radiographs does not rule out otitis media. Occasionally, rabbits with severely affected bullae have normal-appearing radiographs. The bullae are best evaluated using CT scans or MRI when available; in many cases, severe abnormalities are found on CT scans even when bullae radiographs appeared normal.

## DIAGNOSTIC PROCEDURES
• Gross appearance of the exudate—bacterial infections commonly produce a thick, creamy white exudate; yeast infections commonly produce a yellow–tan thick exudate; however, appearance does not allow an accurate diagnosis of the type of infection; microscopic examination is necessary. Ear mites produce a characteristic profuse, tan foliated crusting on the pinnae.
• Microscopic examination of aural exudate—extremely important diagnostic tool. Make preparations from both canals (the contents of the canals may not be the same); spread samples thinly on a glass microscope

slide; findings: type(s) of bacteria or yeast assist in the choice of therapy; WBCs within the exudate indicate active infection.
• Culture of exudate—perform both aerobic and anaerobic culture to identify bacterial pathogens and base antibiotic selection.
• Culture of the nasal cavity—to direct antibiotic therapy in rabbits with intact tympanum and evidence of concurrent respiratory infection. In these rabbits, otitis media is assumed to be the result of extension of upper respiratory infections. To obtain a sample, a mini-tip culturette (#4 Calgiswab) is inserted 1–4 cm inside the nares near the nasal septum. Sedation and appropriate restraint are required to obtain a deep, meaningful sample. The nasal cavity is extremely sensitive, and rabbits that appear sedated may jump or kick when the nasal mucosa is touched. Inadequate sedation or restraint may result in serious spinal or other musculoskeletal injury.
• Skin scrapings from the pinnae—parasites
• Skin biopsy—neoplasia

## PATHOLOGIC FINDINGS
N/A

## TREATMENT

### APPROPRIATE HEALTH CARE
#### General Comments
• Many rabbits have thick, white exudate in the horizontal canal, preventing visualization of the tympanum. Frequently, no signs of inflammation of the ear canal are present. Many of these rabbits are asymptomatic and may remain so lifelong. One study demonstrated that 32% of asymptomatic rabbits had exudate in the horizontal canal and/or otitis media on necropsy. The decision as to how aggressively one should treat asymptomatic rabbits, or whether to treat at all, is multifactorial; age of the animal, concurrent diseases, owner compliance, and financial issues should be considered. Exudate is generally extremely caseous, does not drain, and can be difficult to flush. Successful removal of all exudate from the horizontal canal can be challenging and requires consistent owner compliance and, frequently, multiple office visits for cleaning under anesthesia. Occasionally, aggressive cleaning and medication of the ear canal will irritate the lining of the ear canal and/or may cause rupture of the tympanum, resulting in clinical signs of otitis externa and/or interna in a previously asymptomatic rabbit. However, when possible, treatment of asymptomatic animals is recommended, since many of these rabbits are in pain (even if that pain is not recognized by the owner) and the ear may serve as a nidus for infection. Early intervention in asymptomatic rabbits may

prevent severe disease, such as otitis interna or brain abscess, from occurring.
• Treatment is indicated in all rabbits showing clinical signs of otitis externa/media.
• Outpatient, unless severe vestibular signs are noted

### NURSING CARE
• Ear cleaning under sedation may be helpful in rabbits with large amounts of exudate in the horizontal canal or otitis media. Warmed, physiologic saline is recommended, especially if the tympanum is not intact. Even if the tympanum is intact, use caution with commercial otic cleaning solutions. Rabbits often develop hypersensitivity reactions to many of the topical ear cleaning solutions or medications commonly used in other mammalian species.
• Rabbits with ear mites—do not attempt to clean the ears; it is not necessary since crusts will fall off following treatment with ivermectin; cleaning can cause painful ulceration and worsening of otitis.

### ACTIVITY
No restrictions

### DIET
• It is absolutely imperative that the rabbit continue to eat during and following treatment. Anorexia will often cause gastrointestinal hypomotility, derangement of the gastrointestinal microflora, and overgrowth of intestinal bacterial pathogens.
• Offer a large selection of fresh, moistened greens such as cilantro, romaine lettuce, parsley, carrot tops, dandelion greens, spinach, collard greens, etc., and good-quality grass hay. Many rabbits will begin to eat these foods, even if they were previously anorectic.
• If the patient refuses these foods, syringe feed a gruel such as Critical Care for Herbivores (Oxbow Pet Products, Murdock, NE) 10–15 mL/kg PO q6–8h. Alternatively, pellets can be ground and mixed with fresh greens, vegetable baby foods, water, or juice to form a gruel. If sufficient volumes of food are not accepted in this manner, nasogastric intubation is indicated.
• High-carbohydrate, high-fat nutritional supplements are contraindicated.
• Encourage oral fluid intake by offering fresh water, wetting leafy vegetables, or flavoring water with vegetable juices.

### CLIENT EDUCATION
• Chronic otitis can be extremely frustrating to treat, especially once otitis media develops. Successful outcome requires long-term therapy, consistent client compliance, and, possibly, surgical intervention.
• Teach clients, by demonstration, the proper method for medicating ears. Proper restraint is critical—severe injury to the back may occur if proper restraint is not employed.

### SURGICAL CONSIDERATIONS
• Indicated when the canal is severely stenotic, when medical treatment fails, or when neoplasia is diagnosed
• Medical treatment failure is common. A total ear canal ablation is indicated with severe or long-standing disease, especially when aural pain diminishes the quality of life. In most rabbits with disease severe enough to warrant surgery, otitis media is often present, requiring concurrent bullae osteotomy. The two procedures are similar to those performed in dogs and cats. However, careful pain management and the use of antibiotic-impregnated polymethyl methacrylate (AIPMMA) beads are necessary for a successful outcome. Complete excision of all abnormal tissue, followed by filling the defect with AIPMMA beads, will usually prevent postsurgical abscess formation. Unlike dogs and cats, bullae and ear canals in affected rabbits are filled with a thick, caseous exudate, surrounded by a fibrous capsule, and often extend aggressively into surrounding soft tissue and bone.
• Without as complete an excision as possible of all abnormal tissue followed by filling the defect with AIPMMA beads, recurrence rates are extremely high. Given the expense and pain involved in these procedures, the author recommends referral to a specialist if surgical expertise or AIPMMA beads are not available.
• AIPMMA beads release a high concentration of antibiotic into local tissues for several months. Selection of antibiotic is limited to those known to elute appropriately from bead to tissues and should be based on culture and susceptibility testing. AIPMMA beads are not commercially available, but can be made using PMMA by Surgical Simplex Bone Cement (Howmedica, Rutherford, NJ) or Bone Cement (Zimmer, Charlotte, NC). Antibiotics successfully used include cephalothin, cefazolin, or ceftiofur (2 g/20 g PMMA); gentamicin or tobramycin (1 g/2 g PMMA); or amikacin (1.25 g/2 g PMMA). Antibiotic is added to the copolymer powder before adding the liquid and formed into small, spherical beads. Beads must be inserted aseptically, and unused beads should be gas sterilized prior to future use. Beads should be left in the incision site for at least 2 months, but can be left in indefinitely.
• Lateral ear canal resection is generally an ineffective procedure in rabbits. Ceruminous gland hyperplasia, as seen in canine patients, does not occur in rabbits. Most rabbits with chronic otitis have middle ear involvement or exudate deep within the horizontal canal. Exudates are extremely caseated and do not drain well. Complete excision of all affected soft tissue, cartilage, and bone, often coupled with the use of AIPMMA beads, is usually necessary for a successful outcome.

## OTITIS EXTERNA AND MEDIA

## MEDICATIONS

### DRUG(S) OF CHOICE

#### Systemic
• Antibiotics—necessary in most cases of bacterial otitis externa; mandatory when the tympanum has ruptured. Choice of antibiotic is ideally based on results of culture and susceptibility testing. Depending on the severity of infection, long-term antibiotic therapy is required (4–6 weeks minimum to several months). Use broad-spectrum antibiotics such as enrofloxacin (5–20 mg/kg PO, SC, IM q12–24h) or trimethoprim-sulfa (30 mg/kg PO q12h); if anaerobic infections are suspected, use chloramphenicol (50 mg/kg PO q8h) or azithromycin (30 mg/kg PO q24h) (can be used alone or combined with metronidazole [20 g/kg PO q12h]). Alternatively, use penicillin g (40,000–60,000 IU/kg SC q2–7d). Combine with topical or surgical treatment.
• For ear mites—1% ivermectin (0.4 mg/kg SC q10–14d for two to three doses) or selamectin (Revolution, Pfizer) (6–12 mg/kg applied topically q30d). It is not necessary and may be detrimental to clean the ears thoroughly to remove debris during this treatment period.
• For pain management—meloxicam (0.2–0.5 mg/kg PO q24h) or carprofen (2.2 mg/kg PO q12h)
• For sedation—light sedation with midazolam (0.5–2 mg/kg IM) or diazepam (1–2 mg/kg IM); for deeper sedation and longer procedures, the author prefers ketamine (15–20 mg/kg IM) plus midazolam (0.5 mg/kg IM); many other sedation protocols exist.

#### Topical
• Topical therapy is paramount for resolution and control of otitis externa.
• First, clean the external ear canal as completely as possible; complete flushing under sedation or general anesthesia for severe cases, including otitis media. Do not clean the ear canals when treating for ear mites.
• Apply appropriate topical medications frequently and in sufficient quantity to completely treat the entire canal.
• Not recommended—combination and steroid-containing ointments (e.g., Otomax, Panalog, Liquachlor), which often accumulate and perpetuate the condition
• Recommended—antibacterial (e.g., enrofloxacin, gentocin) or antiyeast drops (miconazole) without corticosteroids; treatment duration is generally longer than in cats and dogs.
• Commercial ear cleansers with cerumenolytics, antiseptics, and astringents available for dogs and cats should be used with caution as some rabbits will develop contact irritation or an allergic response. Routine use of these products at home is not recommended; liquids tend to accumulate in rabbit's deep ear canals.

### CONTRAINDICATIONS
• Oral administration of antibiotics that select against Gram-positive bacteria (penicillins, macrolides, lincosamides, and cephalosporins) can cause fatal enteric dysbiosis and enterotoxemia.
• Ruptured tympanum—use caution with topical cleansers and medications other than sterile saline or dilute acetic acid; potential for ototoxicity is a concern; and controversial.
• The use of corticosteroids (systemic or topical in otic preparations) can severely exacerbate otitis.

### PRECAUTIONS
• Proper restraint is critical when examining, cleaning, or medicating the ears—severe injury to the spine may occur if proper restraint is not employed.
• Use extreme caution when cleaning the external ear canals of all animals with severe and chronic otitis externa, because the tympanum can easily be ruptured.
• Postflushing vestibular complications are common, sometimes temporary, but can be permanent if otitis media is present; warn clients of possible complications and residual effects.

### POSSIBLE INTERACTIONS
Several topical medications may induce contact irritation or allergic response; reevaluate all worsening cases.

### ALTERNATIVE DRUGS
N/A

## FOLLOW-UP

### PATIENT MONITORING
Repeat exudate examinations can assist in monitoring infection.

### PREVENTION/AVOIDANCE
Control of underlying diseases

### POSSIBLE COMPLICATIONS
• Uncontrolled otitis externa can lead to otitis media, deafness, vestibular disease, cellulitis, facial nerve paralysis, progression to otitis interna, and rarely meningoencephalitis.
• Pain may contribute to gastrointestinal hypomotility or stasis.

### EXPECTED COURSE AND PROGNOSIS
• Otitis externa—very mild cases, with proper therapy, usually resolve in 3–4 weeks; failure to correct underlying primary cause results in recurrence.
• Otitis media—may take months of systemic antibiotic therapy; most will improve, but some are nonresponsive to medical treatment; guarded to good prognosis with proper surgical treatment

## MISCELLANEOUS

### ASSOCIATED CONDITIONS
• Upper respiratory infections
• Dental disease
• Abscesses
• Epiphora

### AGE-RELATED FACTORS
N/A

### ZOONOTIC POTENTIAL
N/A

### PREGNANCY
N/A

### SYNONYMS
N/A

### SEE ALSO
Causes

### ABBREVIATIONS
• CT = computed tomography
• ELISA = enzyme-linked immunosorbent assay
• MRI = magnetic resonance imaging
• WBC = white blood cell

#### Suggested Reading
Bennet RA. Treatment of abscesses in the head of rabbits. Proc North Am Vet Conf 1999;821–823.

Ethell MT, Bennett RA, Brown MP, et al. In vitro elution of gentamicin, amikacin, and ceftiofur from polymethylmethacrylate and hydroxyapatite cement. Vet Surg 2000;29:375–382.

Hess L. Dermatologic diseases. In: Quesenberry KE, Carpenter JW, eds. Ferrets, Rabbits and Rodents: Clinical Medicine and Surgery. 2nd Ed. Philadelphia: WB Saunders, 2004:194–202.

Jenkins, JR. Skin disorders of the rabbit. Vet Clin North Am Exotic Anim Pract 2001;4(2):543–563.

Langan GP, Schaeffer DO. Rabbit microbiology and virology. In: Fudge AM, ed. Laboratory Medicine: Avian and Exotic Pets. Philadelphia: WB Saunders, 2000:325–333.

McTier TL, Hair A, Walstrom DJ, et al. Efficacy and safety of topical administration of selamectin for treatment of ear mite infestation in rabbits. J Am Vet Med Assoc 2003;223(3):322–324.

Rosenthal KR. Torticollis in rabbits. Proc North Am Vet Conf 2005;1378–1379.

## OTITIS MEDIA AND INTERNA

# BASICS

## DEFINITION
Inflammation of the middle (otitis media) and inner (otitis interna) ears most commonly caused by bacterial infection

## PATHOPHYSIOLOGY
• May arise from extension of infection of the external ear through the tympanic membrane or extension from the oral and nasopharyngeal cavities via the eustachian tube
• Interna—may also result from hematogenous spread of a systemic infection

## SYSTEMS AFFECTED
• Nervous—vestibulocochlear receptors in the inner ear and the facial nerve in the middle ear (peripheral) with possible extension of infection intracranially (central)
• Ophthalmic—cornea and conjunctiva; from exposure and/or lack of tear production after nerve damage
• Gastrointestinal—hypomotility secondary to anorexia from nausea in the acute phase

## INCIDENCE/PREVALENCE
One of the most common disorders seen in pet rabbits

## GEOGRAPHIC DISTRIBUTION
N/A

## SIGNALMENT
• Lop-eared rabbits may be more likely to show signs of otitis externa.
• No age or sex predilection

## SIGNS

### General Comments
Related to the severity and extent of the infection; may range from none to those related to bulla discomfort and nervous system involvement

### Historical Findings
• Most commonly an acute onset of vestibular signs; often severe initially
• Torticollis can be severe; affected rabbit is often unwilling or unable to lift its head off the ground
• Head tilt
• Patient may lean, veer, or roll toward the side affected with peripheral vestibulitis.
• Owners often mistake severe episodes of rolling for seizures.
• Anorexia or bruxism due to nausea—may occur during the acute phase; rabbits cannot vomit.
• Pain manifested as reluctance to chew, shaking the head, pawing at the affected ear, holding the affected ear down, inappetence, reluctance to move, and digging at the cage floor.
• Facial nerve damage—facial asymmetry, an inability to blink, ocular discharge

### Physical Examination Findings
*Neurologic Examination Findings*
• Damage to the associated neurologic structures depends on the severity and location.
• Vestibular portion of cranial nerve VIII—when vestibular portion is affected, there is an ipsilateral head tilt.
• Nystagmus—resting or positional (more common); rotatory or horizontal may be seen; does not appear to aid in differentiating central from peripheral
• Vestibular strabismus—ipsilateral ventral deviation of eyeball with neck extension may be noted.
• Ipsilateral leaning, veering, falling, or rolling
• Facial nerve damage—ipsilateral paresis/paralysis of the ear, eyelids, lips, and nares; there may be reduced tear production; with chronic facial nerve paralysis, contracture of the affected side of the face caused by fibrosis of the denervated muscles; deficits can be bilateral.
*Other Findings*
• Evidence of aural erythema, white creamy discharge, and thick and stenotic canals support otitis externa (not always present; extension from eustachian tube more common source of infection).
• White, dull, opaque, and bulging tympanic membrane on otoscopic examination indicates a middle ear exudate.
• In some cases, the otic examination appears normal, despite significant otitis media/interna.
• Nasal discharge, facial abscesses—may be associated
• Abscess at the base of the ear is a common finding.
• Pain—upon opening the mouth or bulla palpation may be detected.
• Corneal ulcer—may be caused by inability to blink or a dry eye

## CAUSES
• Bacteria—most common; primary agents include *Pasteurella multocida, Staphylococcus aureus, Pseudomonas aeruginosa, Escherichia coli, Listeria monocytogenes,* and various anaerobes.
• Yeast (*Malassezia* sp., *Candida* sp.)—agents to consider
• Mites—*Psoroptes cuniculi* infestation infrequently leads to secondary bacterial infections.
• Unilateral disease—usually bacterial; look for foreign bodies, trauma, and tumor.

## RISK FACTORS
• Immunosuppression (stress, corticosteroid use, concurrent disease, debility) increases susceptibility to and extension of bacterial infections, especially pasteurellosis.
• Abnormal or breed-related conformation of the external canal (e.g., stenosis,

pendulous pinnae) restricts proper air flow into the canal.
• Vigorous ear flush
• Ear cleaning solutions—may be irritating to the middle and inner ear; avoid if the tympanum is ruptured.

# DIAGNOSIS

## DIFFERENTIAL DIAGNOSIS
• Be sure that abnormal head posture is not due to holding one ear down due to pain, as it may occur in otitis externa alone, and not associated with vestibular pathology; rabbits with vestibular dysfunction demonstrate nystagmus, torticollis, ataxia, and/or tremors in addition to head tilt.
• *Encephalitozoon cuniculi*—this is a diagnosis of exclusion. Every attempt should be made to rule out otic disease prior to assuming *E. cuniculi* infection in rabbits with vestibular signs. Antemortem diagnosis of *E. cuniculi* is usually presumed based on clinical signs, exclusion of other diagnoses, and, possibly, response to treatment. Definitive antemortem diagnosis is problematic, since a positive antibody titer indicates exposure only, some rabbits respond minimally or not at all to anthelmintic treatment, and many rabbits will improve spontaneously with supportive care alone. Definitive diagnosis requires identification of organisms and characteristic inflammation in tissues that correspond anatomically to observed clinical signs, generally acquired at postmortem examination.
• Central vestibular diseases—abscess most common; difficult to differentiate in rabbits; may see lethargy, somnolence, stupor, and other brainstem signs
• Neoplasia—uncommon causes of refractory and relapsing otitis media and interna; diagnosed by imaging of the head
• Trauma—history and physical evidence of injury

## CBC/BIOCHEMISTRY/URINALYSIS
• Usually normal; abnormalities may suggest concurrent disease causing immunosuppression.
• Hemogram—TWBC elevations are usually not seen with bacterial diseases. A relative heterophilia and/or lymphopenia are more common.

## OTHER LABORATORY TESTS
• Serologic testing for *E. cuniculi*—many tests are available, but usefulness is extremely limited since a positive titer indicates only exposure and does not confirm *E. cuniculi* as the cause of neurologic signs. *E. cuniculi* can only be definitively diagnosed by finding organisms and resultant lesions on histopathologic examination in areas that anatomically correlate with observed

clinical signs. Antibody titers usually become positive by 2 weeks postinfection but generally do not continue to rise with active infection or decline with treatment. No correlation exists between antibody titers and shedding of organisms and presence or severity of disease. It is unknown if exposed rabbits eventually become seronegative. Available tests include ELISA, indirect IFA, and carbon immunoassay.
• Serology for *Pasteurella*—usefulness is severely limited and generally not helpful in the diagnosis of pasteurellosis in pet rabbits. An ELISA is available and results are reported as negative, low positive, or high positive. Positive results, even when high, only indicate prior exposure to *Pasteurella* and the development of antibodies and do not confirm active infection. Low-positive results may occur due to cross-reaction with other, nonpathogenic bacteria (false positive). False-negative results are common with immunosuppression or early infection. No evidence exists to support correlation of titers to the presence or absence of disease.

### IMAGING
• Bullae radiographs—tympanic bullae may appear cloudy if exudate is present; may see thickening of the bullae and petrous temporal bone with chronic disease; may see lysis of the bone with severe cases of osteomyelitis; may be normal in some rabbits, even with severe otitis interna and/or bullae disease; normal-appearing radiographs do not rule out bullae disease.
• CT—superior to radiographs to diagnose bullae disease. Detailed evidence of fluid and soft tissue density within the middle ear and the extent of involvement of the adjacent structures; CT better at revealing associated bony changes

### DIAGNOSTIC PROCEDURES
• Bacterial culture and sensitivity testing—sample from myringotomy or surgical debridement of tympanic bulla is most accurate.
• Culture of the nasal cavity—to direct antibiotic therapy in rabbits with intact tympanum and evidence of concurrent respiratory infection. In these rabbits, otitis media is assumed to be the result of extension of upper respiratory infections. To obtain a sample, a mini-tip culturette (#4 Calgiswab) is inserted 1–4 cm inside the nares near the nasal septum. Sedation and appropriate restraint are required to obtain a deep, meaningful sample. The nasal cavity is extremely sensitive, and rabbits that appear sedated may jump or kick when the nasal mucosa is touched. Inadequate sedation or restraint may result in serious spinal or other musculoskeletal injury.
• Microscopic examination of ear swab if otitis externa is also present

• Biopsy—when a tumor or osteomyelitis is suspected

### PATHOLOGIC FINDINGS
Purulent exudate within the middle ear cavity surrounded by a thickened bullae and microscopic evidence of degenerative neutrophils with intracellular bacteria; variable degree of osteomyelitis

# TREATMENT

### APPROPRIATE HEALTH CARE
• Inpatient—severe debilitating infection; neurologic signs
• Discharge stable patients, pending further diagnostics and surgery, if indicated.

### NURSING CARE
• Fluid therapy—if unable to eat or drink owing to nausea and disorientation
• Concurrent otitis externa—culture and clean the ear; use warm normal saline if the tympanum is ruptured; if a cleaning solution is used, follow with a thorough flush with normal saline; dry the ear canal with a cotton swab and low vacuum suction; sedation or general anesthesia necessary in rabbits with painful ears

### ACTIVITY
Restrict with substantial vestibular signs to avoid injury; encourage return to activity as soon as safely possible; activity may enhance recovery of vestibular function.

### DIET
• It is absolutely imperative that the rabbit continue to eat during and following treatment. Many rabbits with vestibular signs will become anorectic. Anorexia will often cause gastrointestinal hypomotility, derangement of the gastrointestinal microflora, and overgrowth of intestinal bacterial pathogens.
• Offer a large selection of fresh, moistened greens such as cilantro, romaine lettuce, parsley, carrot tops, dandelion greens, spinach, collard greens, etc., and good-quality grass hay. Many rabbits will begin to eat these foods, even if they were previously anorectic. Bring food to recumbent animals or hand feed.
• If the patient refuses these foods, syringe feed a gruel such as Critical Care for Herbivores (Oxbow Pet Products, Murdock, NE) 10–15 mL/kg PO q6–8h. Some rabbits will accept greater volumes more frequently; feed as much as the rabbit will readily accept. Alternatively, pellets can be ground and mixed with fresh greens, vegetable baby foods, water, or juice to form a gruel.
• High-carbohydrate, high-fat nutritional supplements are contraindicated.
• Encourage oral fluid intake by offering fresh water and wetting leafy vegetables.

CAUTION: Be aware of aspiration secondary to abnormal body posture in patients with severe head tilt and vestibular disequilibrium or brainstem dysfunction.

### CLIENT EDUCATION
• Inform client that otitis media/interna can be extremely frustrating to treat, especially in chronic cases. Successful outcome requires long-term therapy, consistent client compliance, and, frequently, surgical intervention.
• Warn client that neurologic signs, especially head tilt and facial nerve paralysis, may persist. Although most rabbits improve and seem to maintain a good quality of life despite residual neurologic deficits, some rabbits improve minimally or not at all, even with aggressive therapy.

### SURGICAL CONSIDERATIONS
• Indicated when the canal is severely stenotic, when evidence of middle ear exudate or osteomyelitis is present and refractory to medical management, or when neoplasia is diagnosed
• Total ear canal ablation—indicated when otitis media is associated with recurrent otitis externa or neoplasia, especially when aural pain diminishes the quality of life
• Bullae osteotomy and total ear canal ablation—procedures are similar to those performed in dogs and cats. However, careful pain management and the use of antibiotic-impregnated polymethyl methacrylate (AIPMMA) beads are necessary for a successful outcome. Complete excision of all abnormal tissue, followed by filling the defect with AIPMMA beads, will usually prevent postsurgical abscess formation. Unlike dogs and cats, bullae in affected rabbits are filled with a thick, caseous exudate; infection often extends aggressively into surrounding soft tissue and bone. Without the use of AIPMMA beads, an abscess is likely to form at the surgical site, resulting in treatment failure. Given the expense and pain involved in these procedures, the author recommends referral to a specialist if surgical expertise or AIPMMA beads are not available.
• AIPMMA beads release a high concentration of antibiotic into local tissues for several months. Selection of antibiotic is limited to those known to elute appropriately from bead to tissues and should be based on culture and susceptibility testing. AIPMMA beads are not commercially available, but can be made using PMMA by Surgical Simplex Bone Cement (Howmedica, Rutherford, NJ) or Bone Cement (Zimmer, Charlotte, NC). Antibiotics successfully used include cephalothin, cefazolin, or ceftiofur (2 g/20 g PMMA); gentamicin or tobramycin (1 g/2 g PMMA); or amikacin (1.25 g/2 g PMMA).

Antibiotic is added to the copolymer powder before adding the liquid and formed into small, spherical beads. Beads must be inserted aseptically, and unused beads should be gas sterilized prior to future use. Beads should be left in the incision site for at least 2 months, but can be left in indefinitely.
• Cytologic examination, both aerobic and anaerobic culture/susceptibility testing of middle ear exudate and histopathologic evaluation of samples of abnormal tissue—perform at the time of surgery.

## MEDICATIONS

### DRUG(S) OF CHOICE
• Systemic antibiotics—choice is ideally based on results of culture and susceptibility testing. Depending on the severity of infection, long-term antibiotic therapy is required (4–6 weeks minimum to several months or lifelong treatment in some cases). Use broad-spectrum antibiotics such as enrofloxacin (5–20 mg/kg PO, SC, IM q12–24h) or trimethoprim sulfa (30 mg/kg PO q12h); if anaerobic infections are suspected, use chloramphenicol (50 mg/kg PO q8h) or azithromycin (30 mg/kg PO q24h) (can be used alone or combined with metronidazole [20 mg/kg PO q12h]). Alternatively, use penicillin g (40,000–60,000 IU/kg SC q2–7d).
• Topical antibiotics—for treatment of concurrent otitis externa, use antibacterial (e.g., enrofloxacin, gentamicin) or antiyeast drops (miconazole) without corticosteroids.
• For pain management—meloxicam (0.2–0.5 mg/kg PO q24h) or carprofen (2.2 mg/kg PO q12h); imperative in postoperative period
• Severe vestibular signs (continuous rolling, torticollis) or seizures—diazepam (1–2 mg/kg IM) or midazolam (1–2 mg/kg IM) during acute phase
• Meclizine (2–12 mg/kg PO q24h) may reduce clinical signs, control nausea, and induce mild sedation.

### CONTRAINDICATIONS
• Oral administration of antibiotics that select against Gram-positive bacteria (penicillins, macrolides, lincosamides, and cephalosporins) can cause fatal enteric dysbiosis and enterotoxemia.
• Topical and systemic corticosteroids—rabbits are very sensitive to the immunosuppressive effects of corticosteroids; use will exacerbate otitis.
• Ruptured tympanum or associated neurologic deficits—avoid oil-based or irritating external ear preparations (e.g., chlorhexidine) and aminoglycosides, which are toxic to inner ear structures.

### PRECAUTIONS
Avoid rigorously flushing the external ear; it may result in or exacerbate signs of otitis media or interna

### POSSIBLE INTERACTIONS
Several topical otic medications may induce contact irritation or allergic response; reevaluate all worsening cases.

### ALTERNATIVE DRUGS
N/A

## FOLLOW-UP

### PATIENT MONITORING
• Monitor for corneal ulceration—secondary to facial nerve paralysis or abrasion during vestibular episodes
• Evaluate for resolution of signs after 10–14 days or sooner if the patient is deteriorating.

### PREVENTION/AVOIDANCE
Treating otitis or upper respiratory infections in early stages may prevent otitis media/interna and/or brain abscesses.

### POSSIBLE COMPLICATIONS
• Corneal ulcers
• Signs associated with vestibular and facial nerve damage may persist.
• Severe infections—may spread to the brainstem
• Osteomyelitis of the petrous temporal bone and middle ear cavity effusion—common sequela to severe, chronic infections
• Bulla osteotomy—postoperative complications include facial paralysis, postoperative abscess formation, and onset or exacerbation of vestibular dysfunction.

### EXPECTED COURSE AND PROGNOSIS
• Otitis media and interna—may take months of systemic antibiotic therapy; most will improve, but some are nonresponsive to medical treatment.
• When medical management is ineffective, a surgical evaluation should be explored.
• Vestibular signs often improve after surgery; however, recurrence is common.
• Residual deficits (especially neurologic) cannot be predicted until after a course of therapy; long-term quality of life is good for the majority of rabbits with mild to moderate residual head tilt or facial nerve paralysis.

## MISCELLANEOUS

### ASSOCIATED CONDITIONS
• Upper respiratory infection
• Facial abscesses
• Dental disease

### AGE-RELATED FACTORS
N/A

### ZOONOTIC POTENTIAL
N/A

### PREGNANCY
N/A

### SYNONYMS
Middle and inner ear infections

### SEE ALSO
• *Encephalitozoon cuniculi*
• Head tilt (vestibular disease)
• Otitis externa and media

### ABBREVIATIONS
• CT = computed tomography
• ELISA = enzyme-linked immunosorbent assay
• IFA = immunofluorescent assay
• TWBC = total white blood cell

*Suggested Reading*
Deeb BJ, Carpenter JW. Neurologic and musculoskeletal diseases. In: Quesenberry KE, Carpenter JW, eds. Ferrets, Rabbits and Rodents: Clinical Medicine and Surgery. 2nd Ed. Philadelphia: WB Saunders, 2004:194–210.
Greenaway JB, Partlow GD, Gonsholt NL, et al. Anatomy of the lumbosacral spinal cord in rabbits. J Am Anim Hosp Assoc 2001;37(1):27–34.
Harcourt-Brown F. Neurological and locomotor diseases. In: Harcourt-Brown F, ed. Textbook of Rabbit Medicine. Oxford: Butterworth-Heinemann, 2002:307–323.
Lukehart SA, Fohn MJ, Baker-Zander SA. Efficacy of azithromycin for therapy of active syphilis in the rabbit model. J Antimicrob Chemother 1990;25 Suppl A:91–99.
Paul-Murphy J, Ramer JC. Urgent care of the pet rabbits. Vet Clin North Am Exotic Anim Pract 1998;1(1):127–152.
Rosenthal KR. Torticollis in rabbits. Proc North Am Vet Conf 2005;1378–1379.
Tyrell KC, Citron DM, Jenkins JR, et al. Periodontal bacteria in rabbit mandibular and maxillary abscesses. J Clin Microbiol 2002;40(3):1044–1047.

*Portions Adapted From*
Joseph RJ. Otitis Media and Interna. In: Tilley LP, Smith FWK, Jr., eds. The 5-Minute Veterinary Consult: Canine and Feline, 3rd Ed. Baltimore: Lippincott Williams & Wilkins, 2004.

# PARESIS AND PARALYSIS

 BASICS

## DEFINITION
- Paresis—weakness of voluntary movement
- Paralysis—lack of voluntary movement
- Quadriparesis (tetraparesis)—weakness of voluntary movements in all limbs
- Quadriplegia (tetraplegia)—absence of all voluntary limb movement
- Paraparesis—weakness of voluntary movements in pelvic limbs
- Paraplegia—absence of all voluntary pelvic limb movement

## PATHOPHYSIOLOGY
- Weakness—may be caused by lesions in the upper or lower motor neuron system. In rabbits, weakness, especially paraparesis, can be due to the effects of systemic or metabolic disease, obesity, or due to structural damage to the CNS or PNS.
- Evaluation of limb reflexes—determine which system (upper or lower motor neuron) is involved.
- Upper motor neurons and their axons—inhibitory influence on the large motor neurons of the lower motor neuron system; maintain normal muscle tone and normal spinal reflexes; if injured, spinal reflexes are no longer inhibited or controlled and reflexes become exaggerated or hyperreflexic.
- In lower motor neurons or their processes (peripheral nerves)—if injured, spinal reflexes cannot be elicited (areflexic) or are reduced (hyporeflexic).

## SYSTEMS AFFECTED
Nervous

## SIGNALMENT
No specific age, breed, or gender predisposition

## SIGNS

### General Comments
Limb weakness—may be acute or gradual onset; most present acutely.

### Historical Findings
- Owner may describe an abnormal gait; the rabbit may be unable to hop, may walk only, may drag the affected limbs, or may be unable to get up.
- Sudden onset of paresis/paralysis is common with traumatic vertebral fractures or luxation and has been described in rabbits with encephalitozoonosis.
- Trauma may not have been witnessed. Many rabbits fracture or luxate vertebrae by suddenly jumping while in their cages. History may include a startling event such as a loud thunderstorm or fireworks or unfamiliar people or pets in the house.
- Focal compressive spinal cord diseases often begin with ataxia and progress to weakness and finally to paralysis.

- Urinary incontinence or urine scalding in the perineal region is common in rabbits with paraparesis. Rabbits must be able to assume a normal stance during micturition. Rear limb paresis, paralysis, or pain prevents normal stance, resulting in urine soaking of the perineum and ventrum.
- Alopecia, flaking over the shoulders and tail head—due to inability to properly groom
- Severe obesity may cause locomotor difficulty.

### Physical Examination Findings
- Patient is usually alert.
- If in pain, patient may resent handling and manipulation during the examination.
- Urine scald in the perineal region; dermatitis or alopecia due to inappropriate grooming
- Ulcerative pododermatitis—alopecia, erythema, scabs, or abscesses on the plantar aspect of the feet may occur with chronic rear limb weakness.
- With systemic or metabolic disease—weight loss, splenomegaly, depression, or dehydration may be seen.

### Neurologic Examination Findings
- Confirm that the problem is weakness or paralysis.
- Localize problem to either lower or upper motor neuron system.
- Paraplegia—bladder may also be paralyzed in rabbits with spinal cord damage, negating voluntary urination.

## CAUSES

### Generalized Quadriplegia
Cervical spinal cord or multifocal cord diseases—trauma, disk herniation, *Encephalitozoon cuniculi,* neoplasia, malformations, spondylosis, and discospondylitis

### Paraplegia
*Front Limb Paresis With Normal Rear Limbs*
- Trauma—bilateral brachial plexus or nerve root injury
- Cord lesion (vascular, *E cuniculi,* neoplasia, abscess) at C6–T2 affecting gray matter only
*Rear Limb Paresis*
- Trauma (lumbosacral fracture or luxation at L6–L7 most common), disk herniation, *E. cuniculi,* spondylosis, discospondylitis, degenerative myelopathy (anecdotally reported in rabbits)
- Weakness due to systemic or metabolic disease, dental disease, severe obesity

### Generalized Quadriplegia With Cranial Nerve Deficits, Seizures, or Stupor
Diseases of the brain—encephalitis (bacteria, *E. cuniculi,* toxoplasmosis, rabies), neoplasia, trauma, vascular accidents, congenital or inherited disorders

## RISK FACTORS
- Spinal fractures, luxations, or intervertebral disk disease—improper restraint, trauma in caged rabbits suddenly startled, possibly disuse atrophy from confinement
- *E. cuniculi*—immunosuppression (stress, corticosteroid use, concurrent disease)
- Spondylosis—unknown, possibly related to small caging, lack of exercise

 DIAGNOSIS

## DIFFERENTIAL DIAGNOSIS

### Weak Pelvic Limbs
- Pain or hyperesthesia elicited at site of spinal cord damage usually seen with trauma, IVD disease, discospondilitis, and, rarely, bone tumors
- Lack of pain along spinal column—consider *E. cuniculi,* CNS lesions, systemic or metabolic disease, vascular disease (rare), degenerative myelopathy, neoplasia
- Acute onset—most common with spinal cord trauma, but has been anecdotally reported with *E. cuniculi*
- Gradual onset or intermittent weakness—usually systemic or metabolic disease, spondylosis, occasionally seen with IVD extrusion, if extrusion is gradual.
- Other clinical signs—lethargy, weight loss, signs referable to a specific system seen in rabbits with metabolic disease causing weakness; severe obesity
- Spinal reflexes—localize weakness to the cervical, thoracolumbar, or lower lumbar cord segments.
- Musculoskeletal disorders—typically produce lameness and a reluctance to move
- Urolithiasis—affected rabbits are in pain; postural changes may mimic weakness.

## CBC/BIOCHEMISTRY/URINALYSIS
Usually normal, unless systemic or metabolic diseases involved (e.g., electrolyte imbalance and anemia)

## OTHER LABORATORY TESTS
Electrolyte imbalance—correct the problem; see if paresis resolves.

## IMAGING
- Spinal radiographs—lesion localized to the spinal cord; may reveal fracture or luxation, calcified disc, narrowed disc spaces, spondylosis, discospondylitis, bony tumor, congenital vertebral malformation
- Skull films—identify dental disease (cause of weakness, chronic debility); severe bullae disease with extension into brain
- Whole body radiographs—identify heart disease, neoplasia, urolithiasis, orthopedic disorders
- Myelography—if survey radiography is not diagnostic and when considering surgery

• CT or MRI—evaluate potential brain disease; CT is of limited value for evaluation of spine in rabbits; MRI more accurate, but not widely available and technically difficult to perform
• Abdominal ultrasonography—if underlying metabolic disease (renal, hepatic) is suspected

### DIAGNOSTIC PROCEDURES
• CSF analysis—sample from the cerebellomedullary cistern; it may be valuable for evaluating CNS disease; detect inflammatory process; sample collection may put the patient at risk for herniation if there is a mass or high intracranial pressure.
• Muscle and nerve biopsy—to evaluate patients with generalized lower motor neuron weakness

## TREATMENT
• Inpatient—with severe weakness/paralysis or until bladder function can be ascertained
• Bedding—move paralyzed, paretic, or painful rabbits away from soiled bedding; check and clean frequently to prevent urine scalding and moist pyoderma; use padded bedding to help prevent decubital ulcer formation.
• Keep fur clean and dry.
• Turning—turn recumbent patients from side to side four to eight times daily; prevent hypostatic lung congestion and decubital ulcer formation.
• Manual expression of the bladder if unable to urinate
• Carts available for small breed dogs can sometimes be fitted for larger rabbits, and may be tolerated for limited periods.

### ACTIVITY
Restrict until spinal trauma and disk herniation can be ruled out.

### DIET
• It is absolutely imperative that the rabbit continue to eat during and following treatment. Painful rabbits may become anorectic. Anorexia will often cause gastrointestinal hypomotility, derangement of the gastrointestinal microflora, and overgrowth of intestinal bacterial pathogens.
• Offer a large selection of fresh, moistened greens such as cilantro, romaine lettuce, parsley, carrot tops, dandelion greens, spinach, collard greens, etc., and good-quality grass hay. Place the food in front of recumbent rabbits or feed by hand.
• If the patient refuses these foods, syringe feed a gruel such as Critical Care for Herbivores (Oxbow Pet Products, Murdock, NE) 10–15 mL/kg PO q6–8h. Alternatively, pellets can be ground and mixed with fresh greens, vegetable baby foods, water, or juice to form a gruel.

• High-carbohydrate, high-fat nutritional supplements are contraindicated.
• Encourage oral fluid intake by offering fresh water and by wetting leafy vegetables. Place water bottles or dishes within reach of recumbent rabbits.

## MEDICATIONS

### DRUG(S) OF CHOICE
• Not recommended until the source or cause of the problem is identified
• NSAIDs—have been used for short- or long-term therapy to reduce pain and inflammation in rabbits with musculoskeletal disease: meloxicam (0.2–0.5 mg/kg PO q24h; 0.2 mg/kg SC, IM q24h) or carprofen (2.2 mg/kg PO q12–24h)
• Corticosteroids have been used in rabbits with disc extrusion or spinal cord trauma with some success. Although clinical improvement has been anecdotally reported, rabbits are very sensitive to the immunosuppressive and gastrointestinal side effects of corticosteroids; immunosuppression may exacerbate subclinical bacterial infections or *E. cuniculi.*
• With acute spinal trauma (fracture/luxation) or disk herniation only—methylprednisolone sodium succinate administered IV may be of benefit. Reported canine dose—30 mg/kg IV followed by 15 mg/kg 2 and 6 hours later; doses for rabbits not reported.
• Administer with gastrointestinal protectant to reduce risk of ulceration: cimetidine (5–10 mg/kg PO, SC, IM, IV q8–12h) or ranitidine (2 mg/kg IV q24h or 2–5 mg/kg PO q12h).

### CONTRAINDICATIONS
• Oral administration of antibiotics that select against Gram-positive bacteria (penicillins, macrolides, lincosamides, and cephalosporins) can cause fatal enteric dysbiosis and enterotoxemia.
• Corticosteroids—do not use with discospondylitis or other infectious diseases.

### PRECAUTIONS
Corticosteroids—use with caution, only in acute spinal trauma; associated with gastrointestinal ulceration and hemorrhage, delayed wound healing, and heightened susceptibility to infection; rabbits are very sensitive to the immunosuppressive effects of both topical and systemic corticosteroids; use may exacerbate subclinical bacterial infection.

### POSSIBLE INTERACTIONS
N/A

### ALTERNATIVE DRUGS
For acute spinal trauma—prednisolone (0.25 mg/kg q12h × 5 days); dexamethasone (0.5–2 mg/kg IV, IM); use with caution.

## FOLLOW-UP

### PATIENT MONITORING
• Neurologic examinations—perform daily to monitor status.
• Bladder—evacuate (via manual expression or catheterization) three to four times a day to prevent overdistension and subsequent bladder atony; once bladder function has returned, patient can be managed at home.
• Monitor for uremia secondary to urine retention.

### POSSIBLE COMPLICATIONS
• Urinary tract infection, bladder atony, urine scalding and pyoderma, constipation, decubital ulcer formation, myiasis
• Exacerbation of bacterial infections (possibly life threatening), hepatic abscesses, and gastric ulceration with corticosteroid usage
• Myelomalacia—with severe spinal cord trauma or disk herniations
• Permanent paralysis

### EXPECTED COURSE AND PROGNOSIS
• Depend on the cause
• Insufficient information exists on the prognosis following surgery for intervertebral disc disease in rabbits.
• Rabbits with rear limb paresis or paralysis due to mild to moderate spinal disease may regain partial or full function with exercise restriction, supportive care, and long-term administration of NSAIDs, depending on the cause.
• Most paralyzed rabbits with severe spinal trauma (fracture, luxation) do not regain mobility; euthanasia may be warranted; rate of complicating conditions (bladder, cutaneous) is very high; quality of life is often poor.
• Wheeled carts manufactured for small dogs have been used successfully in a limited number of rabbits.

## MISCELLANEOUS

### ASSOCIATED CONDITIONS
Gastrointestinal hypomotility

### AGE-RELATED FACTORS
N/A

### ZOONOTIC POTENTIAL
*E. cuniculi*—unlikely, but possible in immunosuppressed humans. Mode of transmission and susceptibility in humans are unclear.

### PREGNANCY
N/A

## PARESIS AND PARALYSIS

**ABBREVIATIONS**
- CNS = central nervous system
- CSF = cerebrospinal fluid
- CT = computed tomography
- IVD = intervertebral disc disease
- MRI = magnetic resonance imaging
- NSAIDs = nonsteroidal antiinflammatory drugs
- PNS = peripheral nervous system

*Suggested Reading*

Deeb BJ, Carpenter JW. Neurologic and musculoskeletal diseases. In: Quesenberry KE, Carpenter JW, eds. Ferrets, Rabbits and Rodents: Clinical Medicine and Surgery. 2nd Ed. Philadelphia: WB Saunders, 2004:194–210.

Harcourt-Brown F. Neurological and loco-motor diseases. In Harcourt-Brown F, ed. Textbook of Rabbit Medicine. Oxford: Butterworth-Heinemann, 2002:307–323.

Felchle LM, Sigler RL. Phacoemulsification for the management of *Encephalitozoon cuniculi*-induced phacoclastic uveitis in a rabbit. Vet Ophthalmol 2002;5(3):211–215.

Paul-Murphy J, Ramer JC. Urgent care of the pet rabbits. Vet Clin North Am Exotic Anim Pract 1998;1(1):127–152.

*Portions Adapted From*

Shell LG. Paralysis. In: Tilley LP, Smith FWK, Jr., eds. The 5-Minute Veterinary Consult: Canine and Feline, 3rd Ed. Baltimore: Lippincott Williams & Wilkins, 2004.

# BASICS

## DEFINITION
• A bacterial disease that can be a cause of rhinitis, sinusitis, otitis, conjunctivitis, dacryocystitis, pleuropneumonia, bacteremia, and abscesses in subcutaneous tissues, bone, joints, or internal organs in rabbits; caused by many different serotypes of *Pasteurella*
• Often a copathogen with other, more common bacterial causes of rhinitis or sinusitis

## PATHOPHYSIOLOGY
• *Pasteurella multocida*—a Gram-negative, nonmotile coccobacillus; aerobic and facultatively anaerobic
• Transmission may be by direct contact, aerosol, or fomites; most rabbits are infected at birth from does with vaginal infection, or shortly after birth.
• Colonizes the nasal cavity and upper respiratory tract; usually remains subclinical or eliminated if host's defenses are intact
• May cause rhinitis initially; may spread into the sinuses and bones of the face and/or spread via the eustachian tubes to the ears, via the nasolacrimal duct to the eye, via the trachea to the lower respiratory tract, and hematogenously to joints, bones, and other organ systems
• Not all infected rabbits become clinically ill. Outcome of infection depends on virulence of serotype and host's defenses. More virulent serotypes produce toxins that may cause nasal turbinate atrophy; purified toxin may produce pleuritis, pneumonia, and osteoclastic bone resorption; endotoxin in plasma may cause fever, depression, and shock.
• Often a coinfection with other bacteria—*Staphylococcus aureus, Bordetella bronchiseptica, Moraxella catarrhalis, Pseudomonas aeruginosa, Mycobacterium* spp., and various anaerobes are all as common or more common causes of rhinitis/sinusitis and facial abscesses.
• Several outcomes are possible, including (1) elimination of infection, (2) chronic subclinical infection, (3) development of clinical signs that improve with antibiotic therapy and recur following discontinuation of therapy, and (4) chronic, progressive disease.

## SYSTEMS AFFECTED
• Respiratory—mucosa of the upper respiratory tract, including the nasal cavities, sinuses, and nasopharynx
• Ophthalmic—extension to the eyes via nasolacrimal duct
• Musculoskeletal—extension of infection into bones of the skull

• Neurologic—extension of infection through eustachian tube causing vestibular signs from otitis interna/media; extension into CNS; extension into joints/bones
• Potential cause of abscess formation in any organ system via hematogenous spread

## GENETICS
Genetic susceptibility not well known

## INCIDENCE/PREVALENCE
• True incidence in pet population is unknown
• Many infections are subclinical.

## GEOGRAPHIC DISTRIBUTION
Worldwide

## SIGNALMENT
No breed, age, or gender predilection

## SIGNS

### General Comments
Disease severity has a wide range—subclinical to mild, moderate, and severe clinical disease, especially in stressed rabbits

### Historical Findings
• Usually begins with rhinitis—sneezing, nasal discharge, staining of the front paws
• Ptyalism, facial swelling, anorexia with sinusitis or head abscess
• Epiphora; ocular discharge with extension into the eyes via nasolacrimal duct or blockage of the nasolacrimal duct
• Head tilt; scratching at ears with extension into the ears via eustachian tubes or CNS
• Dyspnea with severe rhinitis (rabbits are obligate nasal breathers), pneumonia, or large intrathoracic abscesses
• Anorexia, depression, pain from skeletal abscesses; often only clinical sign is intrathoracic or hepatic abscess until abscess is large enough to cause space-occupying effects.
• Lameness; reluctance to move with plantar or digital abscesses
• Subcutaneous swelling with subcutaneous mammary abscess

### Physical Examination Findings
• No clinical signs in rabbits with subclinical disease
• Depend on area of body involved
• Sneezing
• Serous to purulent nasal discharge
• Epiphora, purulent ocular discharge, exophthalmia, intraocular abscess
• Facial swelling, ptyalism
• Fever, malaise, depression, anorexia
• Head tilt, torticollis, nystagmus, scratching at ears
• Dyspnea, tachypnea—auscultation may be helpful to differentiate between upper airway obstruction and lung disease; however, referred upper respiratory tract noise hinders thoracic auscultation, especially in dyspneic rabbits.

• Lameness, reluctance to move, single to multiple swellings with limb abscesses

## CAUSES
Any one of many serotypes of *Pasteurella*

## RISK FACTORS

### Disease Agent
*Pasteurella* serotype—virulence factors, infectious dose

### Host Factors That Increase Susceptibility
• Age—neonatal/young rabbits; immature immune system
• Overall health status—debilitated animals: other concurrent disease (especially other respiratory bacterial pathogens)
• Stress is an important determining factor in outcome of disease.
• Corticosteroid use can severely exacerbate disease and cause activation of subclinical infection; hepatic abscesses is common.

### Environmental Factors
• Poor husbandry—dirty, molding bedding and poor nutrition contribute to stress.
• Grooming habits may result in contaminated hair coat, environment, feed, and water dishes.

# DIAGNOSIS

## DIFFERENTIAL DIAGNOSIS
• Head or facial abscesses—dental disease; tooth root abscesses are nearly always caused by anaerobic bacterial and/or *Streptococcus* sp.; *Pasteurella* usually not a contributing pathogen
• Nasal discharge—other bacterial infection (*Staphylococcus aureus, Bordetella bronchiseptica, Moraxella catarrhalis, Pseudomonas aeruginosa, Mycobacterium* spp., and various anaerobes all are common causes of URI (may be copathogen with *Pasteurella*); dental disease; periapical or tooth root abscesses; elongated maxillary tooth roots penetrating into nasal passages with secondary bacterial infection; foreign body (mostly inhaled grass and seeds); allergen or irritant (inhaled pollen, moldy bedding, dusty litter, bleach, or cigarette smoke); mycotic infection (rare)
• Dyspnea—laryngeal swelling from traumatic intubation, other upper airway obstruction, thoracic neoplasia, cardiovascular disease
• Facial swelling—primary dental disease, abscess from other bacteria, neoplasia, mycoses (rare)
• Epiphora—incisor root impaction or abscess blocking the nasolacrimal duct, primary conjunctivitis, irritation
• Head tilt, vestibular signs—other causes of otitis interna/media; neoplasia, *Encephalitozoon cuniculi*

# PASTEURELLOSIS

• Lameness, reluctance to move—orthopedic injury, spinal cord disease, pain

## CBC/BIOCHEMISTRY/URINALYSIS

Hemogram—TWBC elevations are usually not seen with bacterial diseases. A relative neutrophilia and/or lymphopenia are more common.

## OTHER LABORATORY TESTS

Serology for *Pasteurella*—usefulness is severely limited and generally not helpful in the diagnosis of pasteurellosis in pet rabbits. An ELISA is available and results are reported as negative, low positive, or high positive. Positive results, even when high, only indicate prior exposure to *Pasteurella* and the development of antibodies and do not confirm active infection. Low-positive results may occur due to cross-reaction with other, nonpathogenic bacteria (false positive). False-negative results are common with immunosuppression or early infection. No evidence exists to support correlation of titers to the presence or absence of disease. Test may be useful to monitor SPF colonies.

## IMAGING

• Thoracic radiographs are indicated in rabbits with bacterial rhinitis. Subclinical pneumonia is common; often detected only radiographically
• Skull series radiology—must be taken under general anesthesia; necessary to rule out dental disease
• Patients with nasal discharge (e.g., hemorrhagic, mucous, or serous) have fluid density that obscures nasal detail.
• Bony lysis or proliferation of the turbinate and facial bones important radiographic finding; consistent with chronic bacterial or neoplastic invasion
• Assess the apical roots of the incisors.
• CT scans or MRI is extremely helpful in detecting the extent of bony changes associated with pasteurellosis and nasal tumors.
• Ultrasonography—determine organ system affected; extent of disease

## DIAGNOSTIC PROCEDURES

• Cytology—nasal swab or flush rarely yields diagnostic sample; nonspecific inflammation is most commonly found.
• Cultures—may be difficult to interpret, since commonly isolated bacteria (e.g., *Bordetella*) often represent only commensal organisms or opportunistic pathogens. Deep cultures obtained by inserting a mini-tipped culturette 2–4 cm into each nostril are sometimes reliable. However, samples taken from the nares should not be overinterpreted, since the causative agent may be located only deep within the sinuses and may not be present at the rostral portion of the nostrils, where samples are readily accessible.

• A lack of growth does not rule out *Pasteurella*, since the infection may be in an inaccessible, deep area of the nasal cavity or sinuses, and *Pasteurella* is sometimes difficult to grow on culture.
• *Pasteurella* PCR assay may also be performed on samples taken from deep nasal swabs. PCR may be more sensitive in detecting the presence of *Pasteurella*; however, it should be combined with anaerobic and aerobic culture to identify other bacterial primary or copathogens.
• NOTE: use of antimicrobials in a patient before sampling may produce false-negative cultures.

## PATHOLOGIC FINDINGS

Nasal turbinate atrophy, bony lysis, abscess formation

# TREATMENT

## APPROPRIATE HEALTH CARE

Outpatient treatment is acceptable unless surgery is required or the patient is exhibiting signs of systemic illness in addition to nasal discharge.

## NURSING CARE

• Varies according to severity and location of disease
• Symptomatic treatment and nursing care are important in the treatment of rabbits with sneezing and nasal discharge. Patient hydration, nutrition, warmth, and hygiene (keeping nares clean) are important.
• Humidification of environment often helps mobilize nasal discharge; enhances patient comfort
• Saline nebulization may be helpful to humidify airways in rabbits with chronic rhinitis or sinusitis.
• Oxygen supplementation, low stress environment important in rabbits with dyspnea
• If epiphora or ocular discharge is present, always cannulate and flush the nasolacrimal duct. Topical administration of an ophthalmic anesthetic is generally sufficient for this procedure; nervous rabbits may require sedation with midazolam (1–2 mg/kg IM). Rabbits have only a single nasolacrimal punctum located in the ventral eyelid at the medial canthus. A 23-gauge lacrimal cannula or a 24-gauge Teflon intravenous catheter can be used to flush the duct. Irrigation will generally produce a thick, white exudate from the nasal meatus. Irrigation of the duct often needs to be repeated, either daily for 2–3 consecutive days, or once every 3–4 days until irrigation produces a clear fluid. Instill an ophthalmic antibiotic solution such as ciprofloxacin or chloramphenicol four to six times a day for 14–21 days.

• Postoperative wound care, bandaging necessary in rabbits treated for abscesses

## ACTIVITY

Restrict in dyspneic and postsurgical patients.

## DIET

• It is absolutely imperative that the rabbit continue to eat during and following treatment. Anorexia will often cause gastrointestinal hypomotility, derangement of the gastrointestinal microflora, and overgrowth of intestinal bacterial pathogens.
• Offer a large selection of fresh, moistened greens such as cilantro, romaine lettuce, parsley, carrot tops, dandelion greens, spinach, collard greens, etc., and good-quality grass hay. Many rabbits will begin to eat these foods, even if they were previously anorectic.
• If the patient refuses these foods, syringe feed a gruel such as Critical Care for Herbivores (Oxbow Pet Products, Murdock, NE), giving approximately 10–15 mL/kg PO q6–8h. Alternatively, pellets can be ground and mixed with fresh greens, vegetable baby foods, water, or juice to form a gruel.
• High-carbohydrate, high-fat nutritional supplements are contraindicated.
• Encourage oral fluid intake by offering fresh water, wetting leafy vegetables. or flavoring water with vegetable juices.

## CLIENT EDUCATION

• If underlying disease (dental disease, severe tissue destruction) is not correctable, warn client that a cure is unlikely with chronic sinusitis. The goal of treatment is to control the more severe clinical signs with medication; inform client that treatment may be lifelong.
• Abscesses of the head and those involving bone have a guarded to poor prognosis for complete resolution. Most will require extensive surgery, sometimes multiple surgeries and multiple follow-up visits. Recurrences in the same or other locations are common. Clients must be aware of the monetary and time investment.

## SURGICAL CONSIDERATIONS

• Unlike cats and dogs, abscesses in rabbits do not often rupture and drain. Rabbit abscesses are filled with a thick, caseous exudate, surrounded by a fibrous capsule, and often extend aggressively into surrounding soft tissue and bone. Abscesses with bony involvement (facial, plantar, joints) can be extremely difficult to treat, often requiring surgical intervention and prolonged medical care.
• Abscesses—do an en bloc excision of entire abscess, leaving wide margins; exercise care not to rupture capsule.
• If entire abscess cannot be removed, lance, remove exterior wall, curette all exudates,

and leave wound to heal via second intention; remove, in entirety, all teeth involved in the abscess; remove abscess at the level of the bone, curette/debride all grossly abnormal bone and soft tissue.
• In most cases of head abscesses, the use of antibiotic-impregnated polymethyl methacrylate (AIPMMA) beads will ensure the best outcome. Given the expense and pain involved in these procedures, the author recommends referral to a specialist if surgical expertise or AIPMMA beads are not available.
• AIPMMA beads release a high concentration of antibiotic into local tissues for several months. Selection of antibiotic is limited to those known to elute appropriately from bead to tissues and should be based on culture and susceptibility testing. AIPMMA beads are not commercially available, but can be made using PMMA by Surgical Simplex Bone Cement (Howmedica, Rutherford, NJ) or Bone Cement (Zimmer, Charlotte, NC). Antibiotics successfully used include cephalothin, cefazolin, or ceftiofur (2 g/20 g PMMA); gentamicin or tobramycin (1 g/2 g PMMA); or amikacin (1.25 g/2 g PMMA). Antibiotic is added to the copolymer powder before adding the liquid and formed into small, spherical beads. Beads must be inserted aseptically, and unused beads should be gas sterilized prior to future use. Beads should be left in the incision site for at least 2 months, but can be left in indefinitely.
• Place on long-term antibiotic therapy; appropriate pain management

## MEDICATIONS

### DRUG(S) OF CHOICE
• Choice of antibiotic is ideally based on results of culture and susceptibility testing. Depending on the severity of infection, long-term antibiotic therapy is required (4–6 weeks minimum to several months or even lifelong in some cases).
• Antimicrobial drugs generally effective against *Pasteurella* include enrofloxacin (5–20 mg/kg PO, SC, IM q12–24h), trimethoprim sulfa (30 mg/kg PO q12h), chloramphenicol (50 mg/kg PO q8h), azithromycin (30 mg/kg PO q24h), or parenteral penicillin g benzathine/penicillin g procaine (40,000 IU/kg SC q24h × 2 weeks, then q48h × 2 or more weeks).
• For pain management—meloxicam (0.2–0.5 mg/kg PO q24h) or carprofen (2.2 mg/kg PO q12h)

• For sedation—light sedation with midazolam (0.5–2 mg/kg IM) or diazepam (1–2 mg/kg IM); for deeper sedation and longer procedures, the author prefers ketamine (15–20 mg/kg IM) plus midazolam (0.5 mg/kg IM); many other sedation protocols exist.

### CONTRAINDICATIONS
• Oral administration of antibiotics that select against Gram-positive bacteria (penicillins, macrolides, lincosamides, and cephalosporins) can cause fatal enteric dysbiosis and enterotoxemia.
• The use of corticosteroids (systemic or topical in otic preparations) can severely exacerbate bacterial infection.
• Topical nasal decongestants containing phenylephrine can exacerbate nasal inflammation and cause nasal ulceration and purulent rhinitis.

### PRECAUTIONS
N/A

### POSSIBLE INTERACTIONS
N/A

### ALTERNATIVE DRUGS
N/A

## FOLLOW-UP

### PATIENT MONITORING
Clinical assessment and monitoring for relapse of clinical signs

### PREVENTION/AVOIDANCE
Avoid stressful conditions and corticosteroid use; provide excellent diet and husbandry.

### POSSIBLE COMPLICATIONS
• Extension of infection into the brain, mouth, eyes, ears, or lungs
• Loss of appetite
• Dyspnea as a result of nasal obstruction

### EXPECTED COURSE AND PROGNOSIS
• Prognosis depends on chronicity, strain of bacteria, and host factors.
• Chronic infection prognosis guarded to poor for complete resolution of clinical signs, depending on invasiveness (e.g., poor with extensive turbinate destruction, CNS signs). Many will remain comfortable on lifelong antibiotic therapy.
• Thoracic abscess—usually not amenable to surgical treatment; treat with supportive care, long-term antibiotics; fair to grave prognosis depending on location
• Recovered animals may shed *Pasteurella* intermittently.

## MISCELLANEOUS

### ASSOCIATED CONDITIONS
N/A

### AGE-RELATED FACTORS
N/A

### ZOONOTIC POTENTIAL
N/A

### PREGNANCY
• May complicate disease
• Abortion may be a sequela to infection.

### SYNONYMS
Snuffles

### ABBREVIATIONS
• CNS = central nervous system
• CT = computed tomography
• ELISA = enzyme-linked immunosorbent assay
• MRI = magnetic resonance imaging
• PCR = polymerase chain reaction
• SPF = specific pathogen free
• TWBC = total white blood cell
• URI = upper respiratory infection

*Suggested Reading*
Bennet RA. Treatment of abscesses in the head of rabbits. Proc North Am Vet Conf 1999;821–823.
Deeb BJ. Respiratory disease and pasteurellosis. In: Quesenberry KE, Carpenter JW, eds. Ferrets, Rabbits and Rodents: Clinical Medicine and Surgery. 2nd Ed. Philadelphia: WB Saunders, 2004:172–182.
Deeb BL, DiGiacomo RF. Respiratory diseases of rabbits. Vet Clin N Am Exotic Anim Pract 2000;3(2);465–480.
DeLong D, Manning PJ. Bacterial diseases. In: Manning P, Ringler DH, Newcomer CE, eds. The Biology of the Laboratory Rabbit. Orlando, FL: Academic Press, 1994:129–170.
Harcourt-Brown F. Cardiorespiratory diseases. In: Harcourt-Brown F, ed. Textbook of Rabbit Medicine. Oxford: Butterworth-Heinemann, 2002:324–335.
Kapatkin A. Orthopedics in small mammals. Quesenberry KE, Carpenter JW, eds. Ferrets, Rabbits and Rodents: Clinical Medicine and Surgery. 2nd Ed. Philadelphia: WB Saunders, 2004:383–391.
Langan GP, Schaeffer DO. Rabbit microbiology and virology. In: Fudge AM, ed. Laboratory Medicine: Avian and Exotic Pets. Philadelphia: WB Saunders, 2000:325–333.
Rosenthal KR. Torticollis in rabbits. Proc North Am Vet Conf 2005;1378–1379.

# PINWORMS (OXYURIDS)

 **BASICS**

## OVERVIEW
• Pinworms in rabbits—caused by the oxyurid *Passalurus ambiguus*.
• These small worms can inhabit the cecum, small intestine, and colon.
• Pinworms are generally considered to be nonpathogenic, rarely cause clinical signs, and may be an incidental finding at necropsy.
• Transmission is fecal–oral; eggs are passed in the feces and ingested by the same or other rabbits in the environment.
• The rabbit pinworm is host specific.

## SIGNALMENT
No age, gender, or breed predilection

## SIGNS
### Historical Findings
• Usually asymptomatic
• May cause moderate to severe perineal pruritus
• Ill thrift
• Poor reproductive performance in breeding colonies

### Physical Examination Findings
• Perineal dermatitis possible
• Poor haircoat, weight loss, or rectal prolapse possible (rare) with heavy infestation
• May be an incidental finding during abdominal surgery or necropsy

## CAUSES AND RISK FACTORS
• *Passalurus ambiguus*
• Infected rabbits in the environment
• Food or environment contaminated with feces

 **DIAGNOSIS**

## DIFFERENTIAL DIAGNOSIS
For perineal pruritus/dermatitis—urine scald, fleas, contact dermatitis; all are more common causes.

## CBC/BIOCHEMISTRY/URINALYSIS
Usually normal

## OTHER LABORATORY TESTS
N/A

## IMAGING
N/A

## DIAGNOSTIC PROCEDURES
• Ova or adult worms can be identified in fecal float or fecal direct smear (not usually found on fur around anus).
• Adult worms are seen around anus or incidentally found in cecum or colon during abdominal surgery or necropsy.
• Worms are sexually dimorphic; male pinworms are 300 μm in diameter, 4.1 mm long, and have a single curved spicule; females are slightly longer (6.6 mm) and have a long tail.

 **TREATMENT**

• Usually asymptomatic—no treatment indicated if found incidentally (e.g., at surgery)
• Treat if symptomatic or if owners see worms around anus.
• Clean adult pinworms from perineal area.
• Treat secondary perineal pyoderma, if present.
• Recurrence is common, even in rabbits housed alone, since rabbits ingest their own feces and continue to reinfect themselves.

 **MEDICATIONS**

## DRUG(S) OF CHOICE
### Adulticide/Larvicide Anthelmintics
• Fenbendazole (10–20 mg/kg once, repeat in 10–14 days)
• Thiabendazole (50 mg/kg PO once, repeat in 10–14 days)
• Piperazine (200 mg/kg PO, repeat in 14 days)
• Retreatment may be required.
• Treat all rabbits in the environment.

## CONTRAINDICATIONS/POSSIBLE INTERACTIONS
Ivermectin is not effective.

 **FOLLOW-UP**

Monitor fecal egg counts posttreatment.

 **MISCELLANEOUS**

## ZOONOTIC POTENTIAL
Host-specific parasite; not transmissible to humans

### Suggested Reading
Hess L. Dermatologic diseases. In: Quesenberry KE, Carpenter JW, eds. Ferrets, Rabbits and Rodents: Clinical Medicine and Surgery. 2nd Ed. Philadelphia, WB Saunders:194–202.
Jenkins JR. Gastrointestinal diseases. In: Quesenberry KE, Carpenter JW, eds. Ferrets, Rabbits and Rodents: Clinical Medicine and Surgery. 2nd Ed. Philadelphia: WB Saunders, 2004: 161–171.

# BASICS

## DEFINITION
The fully developed inflammatory response to virulent bacteria, deep mycoses, or inhaled foreign material in lung parenchyma with subsequent pulmonary dysfunction

## PATHOPHYSISOLOGY
• Bacteria, the most common cause, enter the lower respiratory tract primarily by inhalation, aspiration, or hematogenous routes; infections incite an overt inflammatory reaction.
• Tracheobronchial tree and lungs—normally not continuously sterile
• Oropharyngeal bacteria—frequently aspirated; may be present for an unknown interval in the normal tracheobronchial tree and lung; have the potential to cause or complicate respiratory infection
• Respiratory infection—development depends on the complex interplay of many factors: size, inoculation site, number of organisms and their virulence, and resistance of the host.
• Leukocytes infiltrate the airways and alveoli and cause consolidation, ischemia, tissue necrosis, and atelectasis owing to bronchial occlusion, obstructive bronchiolitis, and impaired collateral ventilation.
• Abscess formation in lung parenchyma and/or pleural space is extremely common; rabbit's abscesses are filled with a thick, caseous exudate, surrounded by a fibrous capsule. They can be either slow-growing or become large very quickly, and often extend aggressively into surrounding soft tissue and bone.
• Mortality—associated with severe hypoxemia (low arterial oxygen concentration) and sepsis

## SYSTEMS AFFECTED
Respiratory—primary or secondary infection

## GENETICS
N/A

## INCIDENCE/PREVALENCE
N/A

## GEOGRAPHIC DISTRIBUTION
Widespread

## SIGNALMENT
No breed, age, or gender predilection

## SIGNS

### Historical Findings
• Anorexia, weight loss, and/or lethargy often only complaint
• Fever
• Exercise intolerance—difficult to recognize in caged rabbits

• Signs of previous upper respiratory disease—nasal discharge, ocular discharge, sneezing, facial abscess, dental disease, ptyalism
• Labored breathing—usually late in the course of disease
• Coughing not seen in rabbits

### Physical Examination Findings
• Lethargy
• Weight loss
• Fever
• Dehydration
• Dyspnea
• Abnormal breath sounds on auscultation—increased intensity or bronchial breath sounds, crackles, and wheezes; decreased or absent breath sounds with pulmonary abscesses. In rabbits with concurrent upper respiratory disease, referred sounds can make thoracic auscultation difficult; obtain thoracic radiographs if pneumonia is suspected.
• Serous or mucopurulent nasal discharge, ocular discharge, facial abscess, dental disease, ptyalism
• Anorectic rabbits—may show signs of gastrointestinal hypomotility; scant, dry feces, dehydration, firm stomach or cecal contents, gas-filled intestinal loops

## CAUSES
• Bacterial—*Staphylococcus aureus, Bordetella bronchiseptica, Moraxella catarrhalis, Pseudomonas aeruginosa, Mycobacterium* sp., *Pasteurella multocida,* and various anaerobes have been implicated.
• Mycotic—*Aspergillus* sp. and *Cryptococcus* sp. have been anecdotally reported; they appear to be very rare, but should be considered.
• Aspiration pneumonia—in general, rabbits do not vomit so aspiration pneumonia is rare; it may be seen as a result of dysphagia or following administration of oral medications, forced feeding, or tube feeding.

## RISK FACTORS

### Disease Agent
Bacterial serotype, virulence factors, infectious dose

### Host Factors That Increase Susceptibility
• Age—neonatal/young rabbits; immature immune system
• Overall health status—debilitated animals: other concurrent disease, stress, corticosteroid use
• Dental disease—periapical or tooth root abscesses, fractured teeth; malocclusions causing sharp points on crowns to penetrate oral mucosa; provides entry route for bacteria; cause general debility
• Dysphagia, aspiration
• Reduced level of consciousness—stupor, coma, and anesthesia

### Environmental Factors
• Grooming habits may result in bacteria-contaminated haircoat, which contaminates environment, feed, and water dishes.
• Close contact may spread bacterial infection.
• Poor husbandry—dirty, molding bedding; poor nutrition
• Inhaled irritants—ammonia buildup from urine-soaked bedding, bleach or other disinfectants, smoke

# DIAGNOSIS

## DIFFERENTIAL DIAGNOSIS
• Bacterial rhinitis or foreign body—rabbits are obligate nasal breathers and may become dyspneic with severe upper respiratory disease.
• Chronic sinusitis
• Pulmonary abscess
• Pleural infection—pyothorax
• Bronchial foreign body
• Congestive heart failure
• Dyspnea from abdominal distension
• Tachypnea from pain, fear, heat stroke, or metabolic disease

## CBC/BIOCHEMISTRY/URINALYSIS
Hemogram—TWBC elevations are usually not seen with bacterial diseases. A relative neutrophilia and/or lymphopenia are more common.

## OTHER LABORATORY TESTS
Serology for *Pasteurella*—usefulness is severely limited and generally not helpful in the diagnosis of pasteurellosis in pet rabbits. An ELISA is available and results are reported as negative, low positive, or high positive. Positive results, even when high, only indicate prior exposure to *Pasteurella* and the development of antibodies and do not confirm active infection. Low-positive results may occur due to cross-reaction with other, nonpathogenic bacteria (false positive). False-negative results are common with immunosuppression or early infection. No evidence exists to support correlation of titers to the presence or absence of disease. Test may be useful to monitor SPF colonies.

## IMAGING

### Thoracic Radiography
• Alveolar pattern characterized by increased pulmonary densities (margins indistinct; air bronchograms or lobar consolidation)
• Obese rabbits often have intrathoracic fat that should not be misinterpreted as pulmonary abscess or pneumonia.

## DIAGNOSTIC PROCEDURES
• Microbiologic and cytologic examinations—aspirates or washings; definitive diagnosis

## PNEUMONIA

• Samples—transtracheal washing and bronchoalveolar lavage are difficult procedures in rabbits due to the location of glottis; fine needle lung aspiration can be performed under ultrasound guidance.

### PATHOLOGIC FINDINGS

*Gross*
• Irregular consolidation of lung parenchyma
• Multifocal white nodules of caseous exudates of varying size within lung parenchyma
• Palpable firmness of the tissue

## TREATMENT

### APPROPRIATE HEALTH CARE
Inpatient—recommended with multisystemic signs (e.g., anorexia, fever, weight loss, and lethargy)

### NURSING CARE
• Maintain normal systemic hydration—important to aid mucociliary clearance and secretion mobilization; use a balanced multielectrolyte solution.
• Nebulization with bland aerosols—may contribute to a more rapid resolution if used in conjunction with antibacterials
• Oxygen therapy—for respiratory distress

### ACTIVITY
Restrict during treatment (inpatient or outpatient)

### DIET
• It is absolutely imperative that the rabbit continue to eat during and following treatment. Anorexia will often cause gastrointestinal hypomotility, derangement of the gastrointestinal microflora, and overgrowth of intestinal bacterial pathogens.
• Offer a large selection of fresh, moistened greens such as cilantro, romaine lettuce, parsley, carrot tops, dandelion greens, spinach, collard greens, etc., and good-quality grass hay. Many rabbits will begin to eat these foods, even if they were previously anorectic.
• If the patient refuses these foods, syringe feed a gruel such as Critical Care for Herbivores (Oxbow Pet Products, Murdock, NE) 10–15 mL/kg PO q6–8h. Alternatively, pellets can be ground and mixed with fresh greens, vegetable baby foods, water, or juice to form a gruel.
• High-carbohydrate, high-fat nutritional supplements are contraindicated.
• Encourage oral fluid intake by offering fresh water, wetting leafy vegetables, or flavoring water with vegetable juices.

### CLIENT EDUCATION
Warn client that morbidity and mortality are associated with severe hypoxemia, thoracic abscesses, and sepsis.

### SURGICAL CONSIDERATIONS
Surgery (lung lobectomy)—may be indicated with pulmonary abscessation or bronchopulmonary foreign body with secondary pneumonia; may be indicated if unresponsive to conventional treatment and disease is limited to one or two lobes.

## MEDICATIONS

### DRUG(S) OF CHOICE
• Antimicrobial drugs are effective against the infectious agent; gain access to site of infection. Choice of antibiotic is ideally based on results of culture and susceptibility testing. Depending on the severity of infection, long-term antibiotic therapy is required (4–6 weeks minimum to several months or years). Use broad-spectrum antibiotics such as enrofloxacin (5–20 mg/kg PO, SC, IM q12–24h) or trimethoprim sulfa (30 mg/kg PO q12h); if anaerobic infections are suspected, use chloramphenicol (50 mg/kg PO q8h), metronidazole (20 mg/kg PO q12h), azithromycin (30 mg/kg PO q24h) (can be used alone or combined with metronidazole), or parenteral penicillin g (40,000–60,000 IU/kg SC q2–7d).
• For sedation—light sedation with midazolam (0.5–2 mg/kg IM) or diazepam (1–2 mg/kg IM); for deeper sedation and longer procedures, the author prefers ketamine (15–20 mg/kg IM) plus midazolam (0.5–1.0 mg/kg IM); many other sedation protocols exist.

### CONTRAINDICATIONS
• Oral administration of antibiotics that select against Gram-positive bacteria (penicillins, macrolides, lincosamides, and cephalosporins) can cause fatal enteric dysbiosis and enterotoxemia.
• The use of corticosteroids (systemic or topical preparations) can severely exacerbate bacterial infection.
• Anticholinergics and antihistamines—may thicken secretions and inhibit mucokinesis and exudate removal from airways

### PRECAUTIONS
N/A

### POSSIBLE INTERACTIONS
N/A

### ALTERNATIVE DRUGS
N/A

## FOLLOW-UP

### PATIENT MONITORING
• Clinical assessment and monitoring for relapse of clinical signs
• Thoracic radiographs—improve more slowly than the clinical appearance

### PREVENTION/AVOIDANCE
• Avoid stressful conditions, corticosteroid use; provide excellent diet and husbandry.
• Treating upper respiratory infections in early stages may prevent spread to the lungs.
• Prevent progressive dental disease by selecting pets without congenital predisposition (when possible), providing high-fiber foods, good-quality hay, and periodic trimming of overgrown crowns.

### POSSIBLE COMPLICATIONS
N/A

### EXPECTED COURSE AND PROGNOSIS
• Prognosis depends on chronicity and severity.
• Early, mild disease—prognosis is good with aggressive antibacterial and supportive therapy; more guarded in young animals and patients that are debilitated, immunocompromised, or have severe underlying disease
• Chronic infection with widespread lung involvement—prognosis guarded to grave
• Thoracic abscess—usually not amenable to surgical treatment; treat with supportive care, long-term antibiotics; fair to grave prognosis depending on location

## MISCELLANEOUS

### ASSOCIATED CONDITIONS
• Dental disease
• Gastrointestinal hypomotility

### AGE-RELATED FACTORS
Young rabbits may have a poorer prognosis.

### ZOONOTIC POTENTIAL
N/A

### PREGNANCY
Rabbits infected with *Pasteurella*—may transmit infection to neonates

### SEE ALSO
• Cheek tooth malocclusion and elongation
• Pasteurellosis
• Rhinitis/sinusitis

### ABBREVIATIONS
• SPF = specific pathogen free
• TWBC = total white blood cell

*Suggested Reading*

Deeb BJ. Respiratory disease and pasteurellosis. In: Quesenberry KE, Carpenter JW, eds. Ferrets, Rabbits and Rodents: Clinical Medicine and Surgery. 2nd Ed. Philadelphia: WB Saunders, 2004:172–182.

Deeb BL, DiGiacomo RF. Respiratory diseases of rabbits. Vet Clin N Am Exotic Anim Pract 2000;3(2):465–480.

DeLong D, Manning PJ. Bacterial diseases. In: Manning P, Ringler DH, Newcomer CE, eds. The Biology of the Laboratory Rabbit. Orlando, FL: Academic Press, 1994:129–170.

Harcourt-Brown F. Cardiorespiratory diseases. In Harcourt-Brown F, ed. Textbook of Rabbit Medicine. Oxford: Butterworth-Heinemann, 2002:324–335.

Langan GP, Schaeffer DO. Rabbit microbiology and virology. In: Fudge AM, ed. Laboratory Medicine: Avian and Exotic Pets. Philadelphia: WB Saunders, 2000: 325–333.

*Portions Adapted From*

Roudebush P. Pneumonia, Bacterial. In: Tilley LP, Smith FWK, Jr., eds. The 5-Minute Veterinary Consult: Canine and Feline, 3rd Ed. Baltimore: Lippincott Williams & Wilkins, 2004.

# POISONING (INTOXICATION)

 **BASICS**

## OVERVIEW
- Rabbits frequently ingest poisonous plants, rodent poisons, and lead.
- Many antibiotics commonly administered to other mammals can be fatal to rabbits.
- Rabbits frequently have severe adverse reactions to many topical products (cosmetic soaps, shampoos, sprays) that are safe for use in other mammals.
- Acutely ill patients are often diagnosed as poisoned when no other diagnosis is obvious.
- Make the diagnosis after determining pre-existing conditions and initially controlling clinical signs.
- Goals of treatment—providing emergency intervention, preventing further exposure, preventing further absorption, applying specific antidotes, hastening elimination, providing supportive measures, and offering client education
- Suspected intoxication—suspected toxic materials and specimens may be valuable from a medicolegal aspect; maintain a proper chain of physical evidence; keep good medical records.

## CAUSES AND RISK FACTORS
### Ingested Toxins
- Poisonous plants—especially rabbits grazing outdoors; some indoor houseplants
- Lead—chewing or licking lead-containing household substances, especially painted surfaces; occasionally metallic objects
- Anticoagulant rodenticides

### Oral Drug Administration/Overdosage
- Antibiotics that select against Gram-positive bacteria (penicillins, macrolides, lincosamides, and cephalosporins) cause fatal enteric dysbiosis and enterotoxemia.
- NSAIDs

### Topically Applied Products
- Fipronil
- Flea collars
- Organophosphate-containing products
- Permethrin sprays or permethrin spot-on products—when applied in high concentrations
- D-Limonene
- Environmental insecticides/herbicides—many lawn care products; avoid contact for 3–7 days following application; consult manufacturer for specific recommendations.
- Some heavily scented shampoos and soaps manufactured for human use have anecdotally caused depression, lethargy, and anorexia when used on rabbits.

 **DIAGNOSIS**

- Usually presumed, based on history of exposure, clinical signs, and exclusion of other diagnoses
- Resources for emergencies—National Poison Control Center; state diagnostic laboratories; local poison control centers are great value for cases of suspected intoxication, especially when labels or containers are available. PDR often has LD50 for rabbits used in pharmacologic research.
- Confirmation of diagnosis—by chemical analysis (may occur after the fact); accurate diagnosis and detailed records may help with future patients affected by the same intoxicant and are invaluable in medicolegal proceedings.

 **TREATMENT**

## SUPPORTIVE
- Control of body temperature—normal rabbit rectal temperature is 101.3°F–104.0°F. Warm chilled rabbits using a circulating hot water blanket, hot water bottles, or a circulating hot air blanket or by placing in a warmed incubator. Gradually warm over a 20- to 30-minute period. Cool overheated rabbits by spraying with water or soaking with cool, wet cloths; convection cool with fans or evaporative cool (e.g., alcohol on foot pads, axilla, and groin). Stop cooling procedures when temperature reaches 103°F to avoid hypothermia.
- Supplement oxygen if necessary via oxygen cage, mask, or nasal catheter.
- Control seizures.
- Encourage food intake once rabbit is completely stabilized. Offer a good-quality grass hay and a large selection of fresh, moistened greens. If the patient refuses these foods, syringe feed a gruel such as Critical Care for Herbivores (Oxbow Pet Products, Murdock, NE). Alternatively, pellets can be ground and mixed with fresh greens, vegetable baby foods, water, or juice to form a gruel. Fiber in the diet will promote gastrointestinal motility and elimination of ingested toxins.

## EMERGENCY
- Establishment of a patent airway—intubate using a 2.0-mm endotracheal tube in small rabbits, 2.5- to 3.5-mm in large rabbits. Rabbits may be difficult to intubate; the glottis often cannot be directly visualized due to an elongated, curved oral cavity and small mouth opening. Place rabbit in sternal recumbency, extending head and neck forward and slightly upward. Use a laryngoscope to depress the tongue, and apply pressure to the base of the tongue to expose the epiglottis; apply a topical anesthetic to the larynx to prevent laryngospasm prior to introducing the endotracheal tube. When available, a rigid endoscope can be used to visualize the trachea to guide intubation. If intubation is not readily accomplished, administer oxygen via a face mask securely fitted over the mouth and nose while rocking the rabbit's body. The rocking motion causes diaphragmatic excursion and may be adequate to successfully ventilate some rabbits.
- Artificial respiration
- Cardiac massage—external or internal
- Correct any cardiac abnormalities
- After stabilization—may proceed with more specific therapeutic measures

## PREVENT ABSORPTION
- Major treatment factor
- Available measures—washing, gastric lavage techniques, use of adsorbents and cathartics

### Washing Skin
- Rid skin of external toxicants.
- Bathe with a mild liquid detergent or shampoo to remove the noxious agent. Use extreme caution when bathing rabbits due to the high risk of stress, skeletal fractures, and excessive chilling. Dry the rabbit immediately, monitor body temperature, and house in a warm, quiet cage to decrease stress.
- Avoid contamination of the people handling the patient.

### Emetics
Cannot be used in rabbits

### Activated Charcoal
- Does not detoxify but prevents absorption if properly used
- Highly absorptive of many toxicants—organic poisons, bacterial toxins, organophosphate insecticides, other insecticides, rodenticides, mercuric chloride, strychnine, other alkaloids (e.g., morphine and atropine), barbiturates, ethylene glycol
- Ineffective against cyanide, heavy metals, arsenic, or caustic materials
- Dosage—1–3 g/kg body weight in a concentration of 1 g charcoal/5–10 mL water. Dosage may need to be repeated.
- Administer via syringe (when possible) or via orogastric tube.
- Monitor rabbit for signs of gastrointestinal hypomotility and treat accordingly for several days after treatment.
- Cathartic—the use of sodium sulfate or sorbitol has not been described in rabbits. Use with caution if at all.

### Gastric Lavage
- An effective means of emptying the stomach; use only if a potentially lethal substance has been ingested. Do not perform if petroleum distillate products or caustic agents have been ingested.
- Always anesthetize and intubate with a cuffed endotracheal tube to prevent aspiration prior to gastric lavage.
- Stomach tube size—use the largest possible; a good rule: use the same size as the cuffed endotracheal tube (1 mm = 3 Fr).
- Volume of water or lavage solution for each washing—5–10 mL/kg body weight
- Infusion and aspiration cycle—10–15 repetitions recommended for small animals
- Activated charcoal in the solution enhances the effectiveness.
- Precautions—(1) use low pressure to prevent forcing the toxicant into the duodenum; (2) reduce the infused volume or do not lavage rabbits with obviously weakened stomachs (e.g., in a patient that has ingested a caustic or corrosive toxicant); (3) do not force the stomach tube through either the esophagus or the stomach wall.
- It carries risk of gastric rupture.

### ENHANCED ELIMINATION
- Absorbed toxicants—generally excreted by the kidneys; may be excreted by other routes (e.g., bile, feces, lungs, and other body secretions)
- Apply an Elizabethan collar to prevent coprophagy and reingestion of ingested toxins.
- Renal and urinary excretion—may be enhanced by the use of diuretics; requires maintenance of adequate renal function
- Diuresis is also beneficial in rabbits with exposure to potential nephrotoxins (e.g., NSAIDs overdose).
- Fluid diuresis—0.9% NaCl, LRS, or other balanced crystalloid solution. Maintenance is 50–100 mL/kg/day. Attempt diuresis by IV administration of two to three times hourly maintenance volumes. Carefully monitor patients undergoing fluid diuresis for overhydration by monitoring urine output, weight, thoracic auscultation, and electrolytes.
- For additional diuresis—furosemide (1–4 mg/kg IV, SC, IM q4–6h)

## MEDICATIONS
### DRUG(S) OF CHOICE
- Specific antidotes or procedures may be available for the more common toxicants. Contact national or local poison control;

information may need to be extrapolated from canine/feline treatments when specific treatment for rabbits is lacking.
- Control of seizures—diazepam (1–5 mg/kg IV, IM; begin with 0.5–1.0 mg/kg IV bolus); may repeat if gross seizure activity has not stopped within 5 minutes; can be administered rectally if IV access cannot be obtained
- Anticoagulant rodenticide intoxication—plasma or whole blood transfusion for acute bleeding. Perform in-house crossmatch prior to administration; blood types not described for rabbits. Vitamin K1 (2.5 mg/kg PO q24h for 10–30 days) (depending on the specific product); the injectable form may be administered orally; bioavailability enhanced by the concurrent feeding of a small amount of fat has also been administered IM (2–10 mg/kg PRN); however, anaphylactic reactions have been reported anecdotally with IV or SC administration. Administer for 1 (warfarin) to 4 (longer-acting formulations) weeks.
- For antibiotic induced enteric dysbiosis—metronidazole (20 mg/kg PO, IV q12h); cholestyramine (Questran, Bristol Laboratories) is an ion-exchange resin that binds clostridial iota toxins. A dose of 2 g in 20 mL of water administered by gavage has been reported to be effective in preventing death in rabbits with acute clostridial enterotoxemia.
- For lead intoxication—CaEDTA (25 mg/kg SC q6h for 5 days); dilute to 1% solution with D5W before administration; may need multiple treatments; allow a 5-day rest period between treatments.
- Hemorrhagic diarrhea—broad-spectrum antibiotics such as enrofloxacin (5–15mg/kg PO, IM, SC q12h) or trimethoprim sulfa (30 mg/kg PO q12h)
- Gastric irritation/ulceration following NSAID intoxication—cimetidine (10 mg/kg PO, SC, IV, IM q8–12h) or sucralfate (25 mg/kg PO q8–12h)
- For gastrointestinal hypomotility—metoclopramide (0.2–1.0 mg/kg PO, SC q6–8h) or cisapride (0.5–1.0 mg/kg PO q8–12h) is usually helpful in regaining normal motility; cisapride is available through many compounding pharmacies.
- Analgesics such as buprenorphine (0.01–0.05 mg/kg SC, IM q6–12h) or meloxicam (0.2–0.5 mg/kg PO q24h) may be beneficial for rabbits with intestinal pain. Intestinal pain from gas distention and ileus impairs mobility and decreases appetite and may severely inhibit recovery.

- Glycopyrrolate and 2-PAM have been anecdotally used at feline dosages to treat organophosphate toxicosis.

### CONTRAINDICATIONS
Do not administer lincomycin, clindamycin, erythromycin, ampicillin, amoxicillin cephalosporins, or penicillins orally to rabbits.

## FOLLOW-UP
- Specific monitoring depends on the toxicant, clinical signs, and laboratory abnormalities.
- Observe for improvement in the rabbit's general demeanor.
- Regularly assess the cardiopulmonary status.
- Carefully monitor for signs of overhydration in rabbits undergoing fluid diuresis.
- Observe for and treat signs of gastrointestinal hypomotility following successful treatment of any type of poisoning in rabbits.

## MISCELLANEOUS
### ABBREVIATIONS
- CaEDTA = calcium ethylenediaminetetra acetate
- LRS = lactated Ringer's solution
- NSAIDs = nonsteroidal antiinflammatory drugs
- PDR = physician's desk reference

### Suggested Reading
Bailey EM, Garland T. Toxicologic emergencies. In: Murtaugh RJ, Kaplan PM, eds. Veterinary Emergency and Critical Care Medicine. St. Louis: Mosby Year Book, 1992:427–452.
Ofoefule SI, Onuoha LC, Okonta MJ, et al. Effect of activated charcoal on isoniazid absorption in rabbits. Bull Chim Farm 2001;140:183–186.
Paul-Murphy J, Ramer JC. Urgent care of the pet rabbits. Vet Clin North Am Exotic Anim Pract 1998;1(1):127–152.
Swartout MS, Gerken DF. Lead-induced toxicosis in two domestic rabbits. J Am Vet Med Assoc 1987;191:717–719.

### Portions Adapted From
Bailey EM, Garland T. Poisoning. In: Tilley LP, Smith FWK, Jr., eds. The 5-Minute Veterinary Consult: Canine and Feline, 3rd Ed. Baltimore: Lippincott Williams & Wilkins, 2004.

# POLYURIA AND POLYDIPSIA

 BASICS

## DEFINITION
Polyuria is defined as greater than normal urine production, and polydipsia as greater than normal water consumption. Average normal water intake may vary from 50–150 mL/kg body weight daily. Rabbits fed large amounts of water-containing foods, such as leafy vegetables, will drink less water than those on a dry diet of hay and pellets. Urine production has been reported as between 120–130 mL/kg body weight per day.

## PATHOPHYSIOLOGY
• Urine production and water consumption (thirst) are controlled by interactions between the kidneys, pituitary gland, and hypothalamus.
• Usually, polydipsia occurs as a compensatory response to polyuria to maintain hydration. The patient's plasma becomes relatively hypertonic and activates thirst mechanisms. Occasionally, polydipsia may be the primary process and polyuria is the compensatory response. Then, the patient's plasma becomes relatively hypotonic because of excessive water intake, and ADH secretion is reduced, resulting in polyuria.

## SYSTEMS AFFECTED
• Renal/urologic—kidneys
• Cardiovascular—alterations in "effective" circulating volume

## SIGNALMENT
• More likely to be seen in middle-aged to older rabbits
• No sex predilection

## SIGNS
N/A

## CAUSES
• Primary polyuria due to impaired renal response to ADH—renal failure, pyelonephritis, pyometra, hepatic failure, hypokalemia, drugs
• Primary polyuria caused by osmotic diuresis—diabetes mellitus, postobstructive diuresis, some diuretics (e.g., mannitol and furosemide), ingestion or administration of large quantities of solute (e.g., sodium chloride or glucose)
• Primary polyuria due to ADH deficiency (not reported in rabbits, but should be considered)—traumatic, neoplastic; some drugs (e.g., alcohol and phenytoin)
• Primary polydipsia—behavioral problems (especially boredom), pyrexia, or pain. Organic disease of the anterior hypothalamic thirst center of neoplastic, traumatic, or inflammatory origin have not been reported in rabbits but should be considered.

## RISK FACTORS
• Renal disease or liver disease
• Selected electrolyte disorders
• Administration of diuretics and anticonvulsants

 DIAGNOSIS

## DIFFERENTIAL DIAGNOSIS
### Differentiating Similar Signs
• Differentiate polyuria from an abnormal increase in the frequency of urination (pollakiuria). Pollakiuria is often associated with dysuria, stranguria, or hematuria. Patients with polyuria void large quantities of urine; patients with pollakiuria typically void small quantities of urine.
• Measuring urinary-specific gravity may provide evidence of adequate urine-concentrating ability (1.020).

### Differentiating Causes
• If associated with progressive weight loss—consider renal failure, hepatic failure, pyometra, neoplasia, pyelonephritis, and possibly diabetes mellitus.
• If associated with hypercalciuria—consider renal failure and nephrolithiasis.
• If associated with polyphagia—consider diabetes mellitus (rare).
• If associated with recent estrus in an intact female—consider pyometra.
• If associated with abdominal distention—consider hepatic failure and neoplasia.

## CBC/BIOCHEMISTRY/URINALYSIS
• Relative hypernatremia or high serum osmolarity suggests primary polyuria.
• Hyponatremia or low serum osmolarity suggests primary polydipsia.
• BUN elevation (normal 9.1–22.7 mg/dL); creatinine elevation (normal 0.5–2.0 mg/dL) is consistent with renal causes for polyuria/polydipsia but may also indicate dehydration resulting from inadequate compensatory polydipsia.
• High hepatic enzyme activities are consistent with hepatic disease.
• Hypercalcemia—rabbits have a high normal serum calcium concentration (12–15 mg/dL) that varies with dietary intake. Hypercalcemia can be a potential cause of renal failure, rather than the result of renal failure in the rabbit.
• Hypoalbuminemia supports renal or hepatic causes of polyuria/polydipsia.
• Neutrophilia may suggest infectious or inflammatory disease.
• White blood cell casts and/or bacteriuria should prompt consideration of pyelonephritis.
• Urinary sediment evaluation often reveals calcium oxalate or calcium carbonate crystals; however, this is a normal finding in rabbits, and the presence of large amounts of crystals in the urine does not necessarily indicate disease. Disease occurs only when the concentration of crystals is excessive, forming thick, white to brown, sandlike urine and subsequent inflammatory cystitis or partial to complete blockage of the urethra.
• Pyuria (normal value 0–1 WBC/hpf), hematuria (normal value 0–1 RBC/hpf), and proteinuria (normal value 0–33 mg/dL) indicate urinary tract inflammation, but these are nonspecific findings that may result from infectious and noninfectious causes of lower urinary tract disease.

## OTHER LABORATORY TESTS
Urine culture—chronic pyelonephritis cannot be conclusively ruled out by absence of pyuria or bacteriuria.

## IMAGING
Abdominal survey radiography and ultrasonography may provide additional evidence of renal (e.g., primary renal diseases and hypercalciuria), hepatic (e.g., microhepatica, hepatic infiltrate), or uterine (e.g., pyometra) disorders that can contribute to polyuria/polydipsia.

## DIAGNOSTIC PROCEDURES
N/A

 TREATMENT

• Serious medical consequence for the patient is rare if patient has free access to water and is willing and able to drink. Until the mechanism of polyuria is understood, discourage owners from limiting access to water. Direct treatment at the underlying cause.
• Provide polyuric patients with free access to water. Also provide fluids parenterally when other conditions limit oral intake or dehydration persists despite polydipsia.
• Base fluid selection on knowledge of the underlying cause for fluid loss. In most patients, lactated Ringer's solution is an acceptable replacement fluid.

## DIET
• Many rabbits with polyuria/polydipsia develop inappetence. Be certain that the rabbit continues to eat to prevent the development of, or exacerbation of, gastrointestinal hypomotility.
• Increasing water consumption is essential to prevention and treatment of hypercalciuria. Provide multiple sources of fresh water. Flavoring the water with fruit juices (with no added sugars) is usually helpful. Provide a variety of clean, fresh, leafy vegetables sprayed or soaked with water.

• No reports of dissolution of calcium oxalate uroliths with special diets
• Following treatment, reduction in the amount of calcium in the diet may help to prevent or delay recurrence of hypercalciuria. Eliminate feeding of alfalfa pellets and switch to a high-fiber timothy-based pellet (Oxbow Pet Products, Murdock, NE). The form of calcium found in alfalfa-based commercial pellets and alfalfa hay is calcium carbonate, which is 50% more bioavailable than the calcium oxalate found in most green, leafy vegetables. Feed timothy and grass hay instead of alfalfa hay, and offer large volumes of fresh, green, leafy vegetables.

 MEDICATIONS

### DRUG(S) OF CHOICE
Vary with underlying cause

### CONTRAINDICATIONS
N/A

### PRECAUTIONS
Until renal and hepatic failure have been excluded as potential causes for polyuria/polydipsia, use caution in administering any drug eliminated via these pathways.

### POSSIBLE INTERACTIONS
N/A

### ALTERNATIVE DRUGS
N/A

 FOLLOW-UP

### PATIENT MONITORING
• Hydration status by clinical assessment of hydration and serial evaluation of body weight
• Fluid intake and urine output—provide a useful baseline for assessing adequacy of hydration therapy

### POSSIBLE COMPLICATIONS
• Gastrointestinal hypomotility
• Dehydration
• Urine scald, pododermatitis, myiasis

 MISCELLANEOUS

### ASSOCIATED CONDITIONS
• Bacterial urinary tract infection
• Hypercalciuria

### AGE-RELATED FACTORS
N/A

### ZOONOTIC POTENTIAL
N/A

### PREGNANCY
N/A

### SYNONYMS
N/A

### SEE ALSO
• Dysuria and pollakiuria
• Gastrointestinal hypomotility and gastrointestinal stasis
• Hematuria
• Hypercalciuria
• Pyometra
• Renal failure

### ABBREVIATIONS
• ADH = antidiuretic hormone
• BUN = blood urea nitrogen
• RBC = red blood cell
• WBC = white blood cell

*Suggested Reading*

Brown SA. Rabbit urinary tract disease. Proc North Am Vet Conf 1997;785–787.
Donoghue S. Nutrition and pet rabbits. In: Rosenthal KL, ed. Practical Exotic Animal Medicine: The Compendium Collection. Trenton, NJ: Veterinary Learning Systems, 1997:107.
Harcourt-Brown F. Urogenital disease. In: Harcourt-Brown F, ed. Textbook of Rabbit Medicine. Oxford: Butterworth-Heinemann, 2002:335–351.
Harkness JE, Wagner JE. The Biology and Medicine of Rabbits and Rodents. 3rd Ed. Baltimore: Williams & Wilkins, 1989.
Pare JA, Paul-Murphy J. Disorders of the reproductive and urinary systems. In: Quesenberry KE, Carpenter JW, eds. Ferrets, Rabbits and Rodents: Clinical Medicine and Surgery. 2nd Ed. Philadelphia: WB Saunders, 2004:183–193.
Paul-Murphy J, Ramer JC. Urgent care of the pet rabbits. Vet Clin North Am Exotic Anim Pract 1998;1(1):127–152.
Redrobe S. Calcium metabolism in rabbits. Semin Avian Exotic Pet Med 2002;11(2): 94–101.

*Portions Adapted From*

Polzin DJ. Polyuria and Polydipsia. In: Tilley LP, Smith FWK, Jr., eds. The 5-Minute Veterinary Consult: Canine and Feline, 3rd Ed. Baltimore: Lippincott Williams & Wilkins, 2004.

## PRURITUS

## BASICS

### DEFINITION
The sensation that provokes the desire to scratch, rub, chew, or lick; often an indicator of inflamed skin. Pruritus, or itching, is a primary cutaneous sensation that may be elicited from the epidermis, dermis, or mucous membranes.

### SYSTEMS AFFECTED
Skin/exocrine

### SIGNALMENT
Variable; depends on the underlying cause

### SIGNS
• The act of scratching, licking, biting, or chewing
• Evidence of self-trauma and cutaneous inflammation is often present.
• Alopecia may be seen.

### CAUSES
• Parasitic—*Psoroptes cuniculi* (ear mites) extremely pruritic; fleas—usually pruritic; cheyletiellosis (fur mites)—can be severely pruritic; *Passalurus ambiguus* (rabbit pinworm)—severe perineal pruritus sometimes seen; *Sarcoptes scabiei* and *Notoedres cati*—rarely infest rabbits, but can be intensely pruritic; *Haemodipsus ventricosus* (rabbit louse)—very rare in pet house rabbits, may be pruritic
• Neoplastic—cutaneous lymphosarcoma; other primary or metastatic neoplasia
• Bacterial/fungal—pyoderma, moist dermatitis, dermatomycosis
• Immunologic—contact dermatitis has been anecdotally reported in rabbits. Cutaneous lesions resembling urticaria or histologic lesions characteristic of allergic reactions in other species have also been anecdotally reported; however, there are no confirmed cases of atopy, food allergy, or other allergic dermatitis in rabbits.
• Injection reactions
• Irritants—soaps, shampoos, bedding, or harsh cleaning solutions

### RISK FACTORS
N/A

## DIAGNOSIS

### DIFFERENTIAL DIAGNOSIS
• Alopecia—focal: in most cases, a clear history of pruritus is noted; some animals may excessively lick themselves without the owner's knowledge; ear mites, fleas, *Cheyletiella*, dermatomycosis, bacterial pyoderma, and some cutaneous neoplasms may all cause alopecia with varying degrees of inflammation and pruritus.

• Alopecia—barbering; often associated with craving for fiber in rabbits fed diets deficient in coarse fiber such as long-stemmed hay; may mimic pruritus

### Distribution of Lesions
• *Cheyletiella* (or less commonly, *Leporacarus gibbus*)—lesions are usually located in the intrascapular or tail base region and associated with copious amounts of large, white scale. Mites are readily identified in skin scrapes or acetate tape preparations under low magnification.
• Ear mites—alopecia around ear base, pinna; may extend to face, neck, abdomen, perineal region; intense pruritus; brown, beige crusty exudate in the ear canal and pinna
• Fleas—patchy alopecia and pruritus; finding flea dirt will help to differentiate them secondary pyoderma sometimes seen
• Other ectoparasites – *Sarcoptes scabiei* and *Notoedres cati* rarely infest rabbits. Lesions are located around the head and neck and are intensely pruritic.
• Pinworms—heavy infections of intestinal pinworms sometimes causes intense perineal dermatitis and self-mutilation. Ova or adult worms can be identified in fecal float or fecal direct smear.
• Injection reactions—alopecia, scabs, scale, erythema; usually in the intrascapular region as this is a common site of subcutaneous injections
• Contact dermatitis—alopecia with or without erythema; scale on ventral abdomen or other contact areas
• Moist dermatitis—alopecia, with or without erythema, scale, or ulceration. Facial—associated with epiphora or ptyalism; perineal/ventral—associated with urinary disease, diarrhea, or uneaten cecotrophs
• Dermatophytosis—partial to complete alopecia with scaling; with or without erythema; not always ringlike; may begin as small papules; no specific distribution
• Sebaceous adenitis—excessive scale, alopecia; usually not pruritic

### CBC/BIOCHEMISTRY/URINALYSIS
To identify underlying disease, especially in rabbits with perineal dermatitis or urine scald

### OTHER LABORATORY TESTS
N/A

### IMAGING
Radiographs—skull/dental to identify underlying dental disease in rabbits with moist dermatitis secondary to chronic epiphora or ptyalism; whole body radiographs may be helpful in identifying hypercalciuria, spinal, orthopedic, renal, or gastrointestinal diseases contributing to perineal or ventral moist dermatitis.

### DIAGNOSTIC PROCEDURES
• Skin scrapes, acetate tape preparations, epidermal cytology, and dermatophyte cultures (with microscopic identification)—identify primary or coexisting diseases caused by parasites or other microorganisms.
• Microscopic examination of ear crust placed in mineral oil—usually a very effective means of identifying ear mites; mites may also be visualized with an otoscope.
• Wood's lamp—do not use as the sole means of diagnosing or excluding dermatomycosis, owing to false negatives and misinterpretations of fluorescence.
• Skin biopsy or fine needle aspirate—useful to diagnose cutaneous neoplasms

## TREATMENT
• More than one disease may be contributing to the itching; if treatment for an identified condition does not result in improvement, consider other causes.
• Moist dermatitis—identify and correct underlying cause (dental disease in facial dermatitis; urinary, gastrointestinal, musculoskeletal disease in perineal/ventral dermatitis); keep the area clean and dry; apply zinc oxide plus menthol powder (Gold Bond, Martin Himmel, Inc) to clean skin q24h.

## MEDICATIONS

### DRUG(S) OF CHOICE

#### Symptomatic Therapy
• Antihistamines—use is anecdotal and dosages have been extrapolated from feline dosages: hydroxyzine (2 mg/kg PO q8–12h) or diphenhydramine (2 mg/kg PO, SC q8–12h)
• Topical sprays, lotions, creams, and shampoos used in dogs and cats have not been evaluated in rabbits. Use with caution as rabbits are fastidious groomers and may ingest topical medications.

#### Systemic/Topical Therapy
Varies with specific cause
• Ear mites—1% ivermectin (0.4 mg/kg SC q10–14d for two to three doses) or selamectin (Revolution, Pfizer) (6–12 mg/kg applied topically q30d); treat all in contact animals
• *Cheyletiella*—1% ivermectin (0.4 mg/kg SC q10–14d for two to three doses) or selamectin (Revolution, Pfizer) (6–12 mg/kg applied topically q30d); treat all in contact animals
• Fleas—imidacloprid (Advantage, Bayer)—one cat dose divided onto two to three spots topically q30d (anecdotal dosage) or

selamectin (Revolution, Pfizer)—6–12 mg/kg applied topically q30d; treat all in contact animals
• Sarcoptic mange—ivermectin (0.2–0.4 mg/kg SC q14d for three to four doses); treat all in contact animals
• Bacterial folliculitis—shampoos and antibiotic therapy, preferably based on culture and susceptibility testing; good initial choices include enrofloxacin (5–20 mg/kg PO q12–24h) and trimethoprim sulfa (30 mg/kg PO q12h).
• Dermatomycosis—lime sulfur dip q7d has been used successfully; lime sulfur is oderiferous and can stain; dipping is often difficult to perform on rabbits; clotrimazole cream (Lotrimin Cream 1%, Schering-Plough Corp.) for focal lesions; itraconazole (5 mg/kg PO q24h × 4–6 weeks) or griseofulvin (25 mg/kg PO q24h × 4–6 weeks) for refractory cases
• Intestinal pinworms—thiabendazole (50 mg/kg PO) or fenbendazole (10–20 mg/kg PO) q10–14d for two treatments; treat all in contact animals

### CONTRAINDICATIONS
• Corticosteroids, topical or systemic—associated with gastrointestinal ulceration and hemorrhage, delayed wound healing, and heightened susceptibility to infection; rabbits are very sensitive to the immunosuppressive effects of both topical and systemic corticosteroids; use may exacerbate subclinical bacterial infection.
• Oral administration of antibiotics that select against Gram-positive bacteria (penicillins, macrolides, lincosamides, and cephalosporins) can cause fatal enteric dysbiosis and enterotoxemia.
• Do not use fipronil on rabbits.
• Do not use flea collars on rabbits.
• Do not use organophosphate-containing products on rabbits.
• Do not use straight permethrin sprays or permethrin spot-ons on rabbits.

### PRECAUTIONS
• Use extreme caution when recommending dipping or bathing rabbits due to the high risk of stress, skeletal fractures, and excessive chilling with inexperienced owners.
• All flea control products discussed above are off-label use. Safety and efficacy have not been evaluated in rabbits. Use with caution, especially in young or debilitated animals.
• Prevent rabbits or their cage mates from licking topical spot-on products before they are dry.
• Toxicity—if any signs are noted, the animal should be bathed thoroughly to remove any remaining chemicals and treated appropriately.
• Topical flea preparation for use in dogs and cats, such as permethrins and pyrethrins, are less effective and may be toxic to rabbits.
• Griseofulvin—bone marrow suppression reported in dogs/cats as an idiosyncratic reaction or with prolonged therapy; it is not yet reported in rabbits but may occur; weekly or biweekly CBC is recommended. Neurologic side effects reported in dogs and cats—monitor for this possibility in rabbits; do not use during the first two trimesters of pregnancy; it is teratogenic.
• Sometimes the application of anything topically, including water, soap products, and products containing alcohol, iodine, and benzoyl peroxide, can exacerbate itching; cool water may be soothing.

### POSSIBLE INTERACTIONS
N/A

### ALTERNATIVE DRUGS
N/A

 **FOLLOW-UP**

### PATIENT MONITORING
Monitor for alleviation of itching and hair regrowth.

### POSSIBLE COMPLICATIONS
Secondary pyoderma

 **MISCELLANEOUS**

### ASSOCIATED CONDITIONS
• Dental disease
• Musculoskeletal disease
• Obesity

### AGE-RELATED FACTORS
N/A

### ZOONOTIC POTENTIAL
Dermatophytosis and *Cheyletiella* can cause skin lesions in people.

### PREGNANCY
Avoid griseofulvin and ivermectin in pregnant animals.

### SEE ALSO
• Cheyletiellosis
• Dermatophytosis
• Ear mites
• Fleas and flea infestations

### ABBREVIATION
CBC = complete blood count

*Suggested Reading*

Harcourt-Brown, F. Skin diseases. In: Harcourt-Brown F, ed. Textbook of Rabbit Medicine. Oxford: Butterworth-Heinemann, 2002:224–248.
Hess L. Dermatologic diseases. In: Quesenberry KE, Carpenter JW, eds. Ferrets, Rabbits and Rodents: Clinical Medicine and Surgery. 2nd Ed. Philadelphia: WB Saunders, 2004: 194–202.
Jenkins, JR. Skin disorders of the rabbit. Vet Clin North Am Exotic Anim Pract 2001;4(2):543–563.
McTier TL, Hair A, Walstrom DJ, et al. Efficacy and safety of topical administration of selamectin for treatment of ear mite infestation in rabbits. J Am Vet Med Assoc 2003;223(3):322–324.

*Portions Adapted From*

Gram WD, Williamson N. Pruritus. In: Tilley LP, Smith FWK, Jr., eds. The 5-Minute Veterinary Consult: Canine and Feline, 3rd Ed. Baltimore: Lippincott Williams & Wilkins, 2004.

# PTYALISM (SLOBBERS)

 **BASICS**

## DEFINITION
• Excessive production of saliva
• Pseudoptyalism is the excessive release of saliva that has accumulated in the oral cavity.
• "Slobbers" is the layman's term for moist pyoderma around the face or dewlap, usually secondary to ptyalism and dental disease.

## PATHOPHYSIOLOGY
• Saliva is constantly produced and secreted into the oral cavity from the salivary glands (parotid, sublingual, mandibular, zygomatic, buccal).
• Normal saliva production may appear excessive in patients with an anatomic abnormality that allows saliva to dribble out of the mouth or a condition that affects swallowing.
• Salivation increases because of excitation of the salivary nuclei in the brainstem.
• Stimuli that lead to this are taste and tactile sensations involving the mouth and tongue.
• Higher centers in the CNS can also excite or inhibit the salivary nuclei.
• Lesions involving either the CNS or the oral cavity can cause excessive salivation.

## SYSTEMS AFFECTED
N/A

## SIGNALMENT
• Underlying dental disease—usually seen in middle-aged to older rabbits
• Dwarf and lop breeds—congenital malocclusion of teeth
• No gender predilection

## SIGNS

### Historical Findings
• Anorexia—seen most often in patients with oral lesions, gastrointestinal disease, and systemic disease
• History of incisor overgrowth. In rabbits with dental disease, owners generally notice incisor overgrowth first, as these teeth are readily visible. In nearly all cases, incisor overgrowth is only a symptom of cheek teeth elongation and generalized dental disease.
• Inability to prehend food, dropping food out of the mouth, preference for soft foods
• Weight loss
• Nasal discharge
• Tooth grinding
• Excessive tear production
• Facial asymmetry or exophthalmos in rabbits with tooth root abscesses
• Signs of pain—reluctance to move, depression, lethargy, hiding, hunched posture
• Unkempt haircoat, lack of grooming
• Neurologic signs—patients that have been exposed to causative drugs or toxins

### Physical Examination Findings
• Dewlap pyoderma—alopecia, erythema, matted fur, enlarged, thickened skin folds, variable crusts. Due to constant moisture from ptyalism; usually is a symptom of dental disease. Always perform a thorough oral examination.
• Complete oral cavity examination requires heavy sedation or general anesthesia and specialized equipment. Use of an otoscope or speculum may be useful in identifying severe abnormalities; however, many problems will be missed by using this method alone.
• A focused, directed light source and magnification will provide optimal visualization.
• Use a rodent mouth gag and cheek dilators (Jorgensen Laboratories, Inc., Loveland, CO) to open the mouth and pull buccal tissues away from teeth surfaces to allow adequate exposure. Use a cotton swab or tongue depressor to retract the tongue and examine lingual surfaces.
• Identify cheek teeth elongation, irregular crown height, spikes, curved teeth, oral ulceration, abscesses, loose or discolored teeth, halitosis, or purulent discharge.
• Significant tooth root abnormalities may be present despite normal-appearing crowns. Skull films are required to identify apical disorders.
• Incisors—practitioners may see overgrowth, horizontal ridges or grooves, malformation, discoloration, fractures, increased or decreased curvature, or malocclusion.
• Stomatitis—ulceration and inflammation of many different causes is associated with ptyalism.
• Mass in the oral cavity
• Lesions of the tongue—inflammation, ulceration, mass, and foreign body
• Blood in the saliva—suggests bleeding from the oral cavity, pharynx, or esophagus
• Halitosis—usually caused by oral cavity disease
• Facial pain—caused by dental disease
• Cranial nerve deficits—trigeminal nerve (CN V) lesions can cause drooling due to inability to close the mouth; facial nerve palsy (CN VII) can cause drooling from the affected side; glossopharyngeal (CN IX), vagus (CN X), and hypoglossal (CN XII) nerve lesions can cause a loss of the gag reflex or inability to swallow.

## CAUSES

### Oral Disease
• Cheek teeth elongation caused by improper wear or congenital malocclusion—most common cause; from oral pain; spikes on occlusal surfaces may cause inflammation, laceration, or ulceration of soft tissues; secondary bacterial infections may occur.
• Tooth root abscesses
• Gingivitis or stomatitis—may also be secondary to ingestion of a caustic agent, poisonous plant, burns (e.g., those from biting on an electrical cord), or uremia
• Foreign body
• Neoplasm
• Metabolic, esophageal, and gastrointestinal disorders, or nausea—usually do not cause ptyalism in rabbits

### Neurologic Disorders
• Rabies
• Tetanus
• Disorders that cause dysphagia
• Disorders that cause facial nerve palsy—especially otitis interna and media
• Disorders that cause seizures—during a seizure, ptyalism may occur because of autonomic discharge or reduced swallowing of saliva and may be exacerbated by chomping of the jaws.

### Drugs and Toxins
• Those that are caustic (e.g., household cleaning products and some common house plants)
• Those with a disagreeable taste—many antibiotics and anthelminthics
• Those that induce hypersalivation, including organophosphate compounds, cholinergic drugs, insecticides containing boric acid, pyrethrin and pyrethroid insecticides, and illicit drugs such as amphetamines, cocaine, and opiates
• Animal venom (e.g., black widow spiders, Gila monsters, and North American scorpions)

## RISK FACTORS
• Cheek teeth elongation—likely multiple etiologies; feeding pelleted foods containing inadequate fibrous, tough foods needed for normal wear of occlusal surfaces; elongation in geriatric rabbits
• Tooth root abscess—usually secondary to acquired or congenital malocclusion, trauma to the pulp
• Unsupervised roaming in the house—increased risk for electric cord shock, ingestion of caustic agents

 **DIAGNOSIS**

## DIFFERENTIAL DIAGNOSIS
• Differentiate from moist dewlap pyoderma caused by sloppy drinking from a water bowl; change rabbit to sipper bottle.
• Differentiating causes of ptyalism requires a thorough history, including current medications and possible toxin exposure.
• Complete physical examination (with special attention to the oral cavity) and neurologic examination are critical; wear examination gloves when rabies exposure is possible.

## CBC/BIOCHEMISTRY/URINALYSIS
• CBC—often normal
• Biochemical analysis—usually normal except in patients with renal disease or hepatic lipidosis secondary to anorexia

## OTHER LABORATORY TESTS
Postmortem fluorescent antibody testing of the brain if rabies is suspected

## IMAGING
• Skull radiographs are mandatory to identify dental disease and, if present, to plan treatment strategies and to monitor progression of treatment.
• Perform under general anesthesia
• Five views are recommend for thorough assessment—ventral–dorsal, lateral, two lateral obliques, and rostral–caudal.
• CT—superior to radiographs to evaluate the extent of dental disease and bony destruction
• Ultrasonography—may be useful in the diagnosis of underlying urinary or gastrointestinal disorders

## DIAGNOSTIC PROCEDURES
• Cytologic examination of oral lesions or fine needle aspiration of oral mass
• Biopsy and histopathology of oral lesion or mass if dental disease has been ruled out

# TREATMENT
Treat the underlying cause.

## NURSING CARE
• Keep fur around face clean and dry.
• Supportive care in debilitated or anorectic patients; assisted feeding, subcutaneous or intravenous fluid therapy
• Symptomatic treatment to reduce the flow of saliva—generally unnecessary, may be of little value to the patient and may mask other signs of the underlying cause

## ACTIVITY
N/A

## DIET
• It is absolutely imperative that the rabbit continue to eat during and following treatment. Many rabbits with dental disease will become anorectic.
• If anorectic syringe feed a gruel such as Critical Care for Herbivores (Oxbow Pet Products, Murdock, NE) 10–15 mL/kg PO q6–8h. Larger volumes and more frequent feedings are often accepted; feed as much as the rabbit will readily accept. Alternatively, pellets can be ground and mixed with fresh greens, vegetable baby foods, water, or juice to form a gruel.
• Tooth extraction or abscess debridement—most rabbits will require assisted feeding for 36–48 hours postoperatively;

following radical abscess debridement, assisted feeding may be needed for several weeks.
• High-carbohydrate, high-fat nutritional supplements are contraindicated.
• Following treatment, return the rabbit to a solid-food diet as soon as possible to encourage normal occlusion and wear. Increase the amount of tough, fibrous foods and foods containing abrasive silicates such as hay and wild grasses; avoid pelleted food and soft fruits or vegetables.
• Encourage oral fluid intake by offering fresh water or wetting leafy vegetables.

## CLIENT EDUCATION
• Inform owner that resolution requires correction of underlying cause. The most common cause, chronic dental disease, requires a long-term time and financial commitment. Diet change and lifelong treatment, consisting of periodic coronal reduction (teeth trimming), is required, usually every 1–3 months.
• Discuss need to correct or prevent risk factors.

## SURGICAL CONSIDERATIONS
• Trimming of cheek teeth (coronal reduction)—trimming of spurs and sharp points alone will be of little benefit for most rabbits; in most cases all the crowns of the cheek teeth are elongated and maloccluded and will need to be reduced.
• Tooth extraction—because rabbits have very long, deeply embedded and curved tooth roots, extraction per os can be extremely time consuming and labor intensive as compared to with dogs and cats. If the germinal bud is not completely removed, the teeth may regrow or a new abscess may form. If not experienced with tooth extraction in rabbits, the author recommends referral to a veterinarian with special expertise whenever feasible.
• In rabbits with extensive tooth root abscesses, aggressive debridement is indicated, and special expertise may be required. Maxillary and retrobulbar abscesses can be particularly challenging. If not experienced with facial abscesses in rabbits, the author recommends referral to a veterinarian with special expertise whenever feasible.

# MEDICATIONS

## DRUG(S) OF CHOICE

### Antibiotics
• Moist pyoderma—initially may be treated empirically with broad-spectrum antibiotics such as enrofloxacin (5–20 mg/kg PO, SC, IM q12–24h) or trimethoprim sulfa (30

mg/kg PO q12h); for recurrent, resistant, or deep pyoderma, base antibiotic therapy on culture and sensitivity testing.
• Superficial, moist dermatitis—apply zinc oxide plus menthol powder (Gold Bond, Martin Himmel, Inc.) to clean, clipped skin q24h.
• Tooth root abscess—choice of antibiotic is ideally based on results of culture and susceptibility testing. Depending on the severity of infection, long-term antibiotic therapy is required (4–6 weeks minimum to several months or years). Most tooth root abscesses are caused by anaerobic bacteria; use antibiotics effective against anaerobes such as azithromycin (30 mg/kg PO q24h); can be used alone or combined with metronidazole (20 mg/kg PO q12h). Alternatively use penicillin g (40,000–60,000 IU/kg SC q2–7d) or chloramphenicol (50 mg/kg PO q8h); usually only effective when combined with topical treatment (surgical debridement, antibiotic-impregnated acrylic beads)

### Long-Term Pain Management
Most rabbits with dental disease are in pain. NSAIDs have been used for short- or long-term therapy to reduce pain and inflammation: meloxicam (0.2–0.5 mg/kg PO q24h) or carprofen (2.2 mg/kg PO q12–24h)

### Sedation for Oral Examination
Ketamine (15–20 mg/kg IM) plus midazolam (0.5–1.0 mg/kg IM); many other sedation protocols exist. Alternatively, administer general anesthesia with isoflurane.

## CONTRAINDICATIONS
• Oral administration of antibiotics that select against Gram-positive bacteria (penicillins, macrolides, lincosamides, and cephalosporins) can cause fatal enteric dysbiosis and enterotoxemia.
• Corticosteroids—associated with gastrointestinal ulceration and hemorrhage, delayed wound healing, and heightened susceptibility to infection; rabbits are very sensitive to the immunosuppressive effects of both topical and systemic corticosteroids; use may exacerbate subclinical bacterial infection.

## PRECAUTIONS
• Chloramphenicol—avoid human contact with chloramphenicol due to potential blood dyscrasia. Advise owners of potential risks.
• Meloxicam—use with caution in rabbits with compromised renal function.

## POSSIBLE INTERACTIONS
N/A

## ALTERNATIVE DRUGS
N/A

## PTYALISM (SLOBBERS)

 **FOLLOW-UP**

### PATIENT MONITORING
• Depends on the underlying cause (see Causes)
• Continually monitor hydration and nutritional status in anorectic animals.

### PREVENTION AVOIDANCE
• Do not use clippers to trim incisors.
• Prevent progressive dental disease by selecting pets without congenital predisposition (when possible), providing high-fiber foods and good-quality hay, discontinuing or limiting the feeding of pellets and soft fruits or vegetables, and periodically trimming overgrown crowns.
• Do not allow unsupervised roaming or chewing; remove all potential risks from the rabbit's environment.

### POSSIBLE COMPLICATIONS
• Moist pyoderma; myiasis
• Bacteremia and septicemia
• Hepatic lipidosis with prolonged anorexia
• With underlying dental disease—recurrence, chronic pain, or extensive tissue destruction

### EXPECTED COURSE AND PROGNOSIS
• Depend on the underlying cause
• In rabbits with chronic dental disease, lifelong treatment is required.

 **MISCELLANEOUS**

### ASSOCIATED CONDITIONS
• Immunosuppression
• Gastrointestinal hypomotility

### AGE-RELATED FACTORS
• Congenital malocclusion in young rabbits
• Acquired tooth elongation in middle-aged to older rabbits

### ZOONOTIC POTENTIAL
Rabies

### PREGNANCY
N/A

### SYNONYMS
• Hypersalivation
• Drooling
• Sialorrhea

### SEE ALSO
• Abscessation
• Cheek tooth malocclusion and elongation
• Incisor malocclusion and overgrowth
• Pyoderma

### ABBREVIATIONS
• CBC = complete blood count
• CN = cranial nerve
• CNS = central nervous system
• CT = computed tomography
• NSAIDS = nonsteroidal antiinflammatory drugs

*Suggested Reading*

Bennet RA. Treatment of abscesses in the head of rabbits. Proc North Am Vet Conf 1999;821–823.

Crossley DA. Oral biology and disorders of lagomorphs. Vet Clin North Am Exotic Anim Pract 2003;6(3):629–659.

Crossley DA, Aiken S. Small mammal dentistry. In: Quesenberry KE, Carpenter JW, eds. Ferrets, Rabbits and Rodents: Clinical Medicine and Surgery. 2nd Ed. Philadelphia: WB Saunders, 2004: 370–382.

Harcourt-Brown F. Dental disease. In: Harcourt-Brown F, ed. Textbook of Rabbit Medicine. Oxford: Butterworth-Heinemann, 2002:165–205.

Tyrell KC, Citron DM, Jenkins JR, et al. Periodontal bacteria in rabbit mandibular and maxillary abscesses. J Clin Microbiol 2002;40(3):1044–1047.

*Portions Adapted From*

Crandell J. Ptyalism. In: Tilley LP, Smith FWK, Jr., eds. The 5-Minute Veterinary Consult: Canine and Feline, 3rd Ed. Baltimore: Lippincott Williams & Wilkins, 2004.

# BASICS

## DEFINITION
Bacterial infection of the skin

## PATHOPHYSIOLOGY
• Skin infections occur when the surface integrity of the skin has been broken, the skin has become macerated by chronic exposure to moisture, normal bacterial flora have been altered, circulation has been impaired, or immunocompetency has been compromised.
• Pyoderma in rabbits is secondary to an underlying condition that prevents normal grooming or causes chronic exposure to moisture and/or contact with excrement. Identification and correction of the underlying cause(s) are essential for successful treatment.

## SYSTEMS AFFECTED
Skin/exocrine

## GENETICS
N/A

## INCIDENCE/PREVALENCE
Pyoderma is an extremely common problem in pet rabbits.

## GEOGRAPHIC DISTRIBUTION
N/A

## SIGNALMENT

### Breed Predilections
• Breeds with dense fur or long coats such as dwarf or miniature lops and angoras are more prone to perineal dermatitis.
• Any breed with underlying dental, musculoskeletal, gastrointestinal, or urinary disease may develop secondary pyoderma.

### Mean Age and Range
Age of onset usually related to underlying cause

### Predominant Sex
Female rabbits are somewhat more prone to perineal and dewlap pyodermas.

## SIGNS

### General Comments
• Determined by underlying cause. The location of pyoderma is important for establishing a differential diagnosis and determining the underlying cause. Three locations are most common: facial, dewlap, and perineal. Pododermatitis is also a common problem; this topic is discussed in another section. Ulcerative Pododermatitis (Sore Hocks)
• Multifocal pyoderma or pyoderma localized to regions other than the face, dewlap, or perineal region is less common and most frequently secondary to ectoparasites or trauma.

### Historical Findings
• Facial pyoderma—history of dental disease, epiphora, nasal or ocular discharge, exophthalmia
• Dewlap dermatitis (chin, neck)—history of dental disease, ptyalism, anorexia, nasal or ocular discharge
• Perineal dermatitis—history of polydipsia/polyuria, lower urinary tract disease, obesity, intermittent diarrhea, uneaten cecotrophs, lameness, reluctance to move, poor sanitation
• Multifocal or focal pyoderma—history of trauma or ectoparasites

### Physical Examination Findings
Determined by the underlying disease or area affected
• Facial pyoderma—unilateral or bilateral alopecia, crusts, matted fur in periocular area, cheeks, and/or nasal rostrum. Pyoderma is secondary to chronic ocular discharge or epiphora. Most common cause of ocular discharge/epiphora is blockage of the nasolacrimal duct, usually by the elongated tooth roots or chronic upper respiratory infection. Findings may include ptyalism, anorexia, nasal discharge, ocular discharge, and exophthalmia. Always perform a thorough oral examination.
• Dewlap pyoderma—alopecia; erythema; matted fur; enlarged, thickened skin folds; variable crusts. Most commonly caused by constant moisture from ptyalism as a symptom of dental disease. May see fractured teeth, food lodged between teeth and/or gingival mucosal; malocclusion causing sharp points on crowns, which penetrate oral mucosa. Always perform a thorough oral examination.
• Perineal dermatitis—alopecia or matted fur may extend from perineal region to inner thighs and abdomen; fur may be urine soaked or matted with feces/cecotrophs; underlying skin may appear ulcerated, erythremic; purulent exudate and necrotic debris may be present, especially in animals with deep perineal skin folds; may lead to myiasis (fly strike). Depending on the underlying cause, may find palpable sand within the urinary bladder, cystic calculi, obesity, and musculoskeletal pain.

## CAUSES
• *Staphylococcus aureus, Pseudomonas aeruginosa,* or *Pasteurella multocida* most frequent
• Chronic exposure to moisture—from epiphora (facial) or ptyalism (dewlap); both are most commonly caused by dental disease or chronic upper respiratory tract infection. From urine (perineal, ventral)—due to underlying urinary tract disease, polyuria, or conditions that do not allow the rabbit to maintain a normal posture while urinating (musculoskeletal disease, obesity). Rabbits normally lift their hindquarters and spray urine caudally; an inability to maintain this posture causes urine to soak the perineal region and ventrum. Urine may also collect in perineal skin folds in rabbits with excessive folds. From feces (perineal, ventral)—uneaten cecotrophs, chronic diarrhea. From the environment—water bowls (dewlap), urine-soaked bedding (perineal, ventral)
• Matting of fur—from an inability to properly groom. Matted fur traps moisture, feces, and bacteria near the skin. Inability to groom may be due to dental disease, musculoskeletal disease, obesity, or pain with severe pyoderma.

## RISK FACTORS
• Dental disease—periapical or tooth root abscesses, tooth root impaction, fractured teeth, food lodged between teeth and/or gingival mucosa; malocclusion causing sharp points on crowns, which penetrate oral mucosa. May cause ptyalism or blockage of nasolacrimal duct leading to epiphora. May inhibit grooming
• Chronic upper respiratory tract infection—may cause obstruction of the nasolacrimal duct leading to epiphora
• Obesity—interferes with normal grooming; prevents normal posture while urinating; excessive skin folds retain moisture.
• Musculoskeletal disease—arthritis, spondylosis, spinal injury, fractures, pododermatitis: interferes with normal grooming and/or prevents normal posture while urinating; may prevent ingestion of cecotrophs
• Excessive skin folds—in dewlap or perineal region: traps moisture, debris, and bacteria
• Husbandry—urine- or water-soaked bedding; water bowls may cause chronic soaking of the chin and dewlap in rabbits with large dewlaps.
• Parasites—fleas, *Cheyletiella*
• Contact irritants
• Fungal infection—dermatophyte
• Immune incompetency—glucocorticoids; young animals
• Trauma pressure points, scratching, bite wounds, injection site reaction

# DIAGNOSIS

## DIFFERENTIAL DIAGNOSIS
• Barbering—hair loss along the flanks, body wall. Close examination reveals broken hairs. Dominant cage mate pulls/chews hairs on submissive rabbit; owners may not observe this behavior. Self-barbering is usually due to a craving for fiber seen in rabbits fed diets deficient in coarse fibers such as long-stemmed hay.
• *Cheyletiella* (or less commonly, *Leporacarus gibbus*)—lesions are usually located in the intrascapular or tail base region and

associated with copious amounts of large, white scale. Mites are readily identified in skin scrapes or acetate tape preparations under low magnification.
• Ear mites—alopecia around ear base, pinna; may extend to face, neck, abdomen, perineal region; intense pruritus; brown, beige crusty exudate in the ear canal and pinna
• Fleas—patchy alopecia; finding flea dirt will help make diagnosis; secondary pyoderma sometimes seen
• Injection reactions—alopecia, scabs, scale, erythema, usually in the intrascapular region as this is a common site of subcutaneous injections
• Lack of grooming—may cause alopecia and an accumulation of scale in intrascapular or tail base regions
• Dermatophytosis—partial to complete alopecia with scaling; with or without erythema; not always ringlike; may begin as small papules
• *Treponema cuniculi* (rabbit syphilis)—alopecia, crusts at mucocutaneous junctions, especially nose, lips, and genitalia
• Neoplasia—basal cell tumors, cutaneous lymphoma, cutaneous epitheliotropic lymphoma (mycoses fungoides), or mast cell tumors: rare in rabbits; focal or diffuse truncal alopecia; scaling and erythema; may see plaque formation
• Sebaceous adenitis—large amounts of white scale; alopecia; usually begins around the head and neck. Differentiate by skin biopsy and histologic examination.

### CBC/BIOCHEMISTRY/URINALYSIS
• May reflect the underlying cause (e.g., causes of polydipsia/polyuria, diarrhea, urinary tract infection)
• CBC changes due to pyoderma alone are usually not present.

### OTHER LABORATORY TESTS
N/A

### IMAGING
• Dental or skull radiographs—to identify type and extent of dental disease in rabbits with facial or dewlap pyoderma; perform under general anesthesia.
• Radiographs are generally very useful in identifying the underlying cause of perineal pyoderma (e.g., spinal lesions, osteoarthritis, urinary tract disease).
• Ultrasonography—may be useful in the diagnosis of underlying urinary or gastrointestinal disorders

### DIAGNOSTIC PROCEDURES
• Skin scrapings, dermatophyte culture—identify the underlying cause
• Skin biopsy—to rule out neoplasia, if suspected
• Culture—usually positive for *S. aureus*; other organisms may be identified; may be useful to direct antibiotic therapy

### PATHOLOGIC FINDINGS
• Folliculitis
• Furunculosis
• Inflammatory reaction—suppurative or pyogranulomatous
• Special stains—identify Gram-negative bacteria or treponema

 TREATMENT

### APPROPRIATE HEALTH CARE
Usually outpatient, unless treatment of underlying cause requires hospitalization

### NURSING CARE
• Matted hair must be removed for treatment to be effective. Be extremely cautious when clipping hair or pulling on mats since rabbit skin is extremely fragile and will easily tear. Electric clippers are often ineffective in removing thick mats. Curved scissors work best. Work slowly and carefully so as not to damage the skin. Rabbits with large matted areas will require sedation.
• Bathing should not be performed until all mats are removed. Wet hair mats readily retain moisture and may exacerbate pyoderma. After removing matted hair, or on alopecic areas, gentle cleaning with chlorhexidine shampoos will remove surface debris.
• Use extreme caution when dipping or bathing rabbits due to the high risk of skeletal fractures, excessive chilling, and severe stress.
• Thoroughly dry the rabbit after bathing.

### ACTIVITY
No restriction

### DIET
No restrictions

### CLIENT EDUCATION
• Stress the importance of good hygiene—clean wet, soiled bedding.
• Inform owner that resolution of dermatitis requires correction of underlying cause. Some conditions, such as chronic dental disease and orthopedic disorders, require a long-term time and financial commitment.

### SURGICAL CONSIDERATIONS
Fold pyodermas may require surgical correction to prevent recurrence.

 MEDICATIONS

### DRUG(S) OF CHOICE
• Superficial—initially may be treated empirically with broad-spectrum antibiotics such as enrofloxacin (5–20 mg/kg PO, SC, IM q12–24h) or trimethoprim sulfa (30 mg/kg PO q12h)

• Recurrent, resistant, or deep—base antibiotic therapy on culture and sensitivity testing.
• Superficial, moist dermatitis—apply zinc oxide plus menthol powder (Gold Bond, Martin Himmel, Inc.) to clean, clipped skin q24h.
• Perineal dermatitis can be extremely painful—administer meloxicam (0.2–0.5 mg/kg PO q24h) or carprofen (2.2 mg/kg PO q12h).
• For sedation—light sedation with midazolam (0.5–2 mg/kg IM) or diazepam (1–2 mg/kg IM); for deeper sedation and longer procedures, the author prefers ketamine (15–20 mg/kg IM) plus midazolam (0.5 mg/kg IM); many other sedation protocols exist.

### CONTRAINDICATIONS
• Oral administration of antibiotics that select against Gram-positive bacteria (penicillins, macrolides, lincosamides, and cephalosporins) can cause fatal enteric dysbiosis and enterotoxemia.
• Steroids, topical or systemic—will encourage resistance and recurrence even when used concurrently with antibiotics

### PRECAUTIONS
Use extreme caution when dipping or bathing rabbits due to the high risk of skeletal fractures and excessive chilling especially when performed by inexperienced owners; sudden death has been reported following bathing.

### POSSIBLE INTERACTIONS
N/A

### ALTERNATIVE DRUGS
N/A

 FOLLOW-UP

### PATIENT MONITORING
Administer antibiotics for a minimum of 2 weeks beyond clinical cure.

### PREVENTION/AVOIDANCE
• Prevent progressive dental disease by selecting pets without congenital predisposition (when possible), providing high-fiber foods and good-quality hay, discontinuing or limiting the feeding of pellets and soft fruits or vegetables, and periodically trimming overgrown crowns.
• Prevent obesity.
• Provide clean, appropriate surface substrates.

### POSSIBLE COMPLICATIONS
• Myiasis
• Pododermatitis
• Bacteremia and septicemia

**EXPECTED COURSE AND PROGNOSIS**
Likely to be recurrent or nonresponsive if underlying cause is not identified and effectively managed

 **MISCELLANEOUS**

**ASSOCIATED CONDITIONS**
Gastrointestinal hypomotility

**AGE-RELATED FACTORS**
N/A

**ZOONOTIC POTENTIAL**
N/A

**PREGNANCY**
N/A

**SEE ALSO**
• Hypercalciuria and urolithiasis
• Obesity
• Ptyalism

**ABBREVIATION**
CBC = complete blood count

*Suggested Reading*
Clyde VL. Practical treatment and control of common ectoparasites in exotic pets. Vet Med 1996;91(7):632–637.
Harcourt-Brown, F. Skin diseases. In: Harcourt-Brown F, ed. Textbook of Rabbit Medicine. Oxford: Butterworth-Heinemann, 2002:224–248.

Hess L. Dermatologic diseases. In: Quesenberry KE, Carpenter JW, eds. Ferrets, Rabbits and Rodents: Clinical Medicine and Surgery. 2nd Ed. Philadelphia: WB Saunders, 2004:194–202.
Jenkins JR. Skin disorders of the rabbit. Vet Clin North Am Exotic Anim Pract 2001; 4(2):543–563.

*Portions Adapted From*
Codner EC, Rhodes KH. Phyoderma. In: Tilley LP, Smith FWK, Jr., eds. The 5-Minute Veterinary Consult: Canine and Feline, 3rd Ed. Baltimore: Lippincott Williams & Wilkins, 2004.

# PYOMETRA AND NONNEOPLASTIC ENDOMETRIAL DISORDERS

## BASICS

### OVERVIEW
• Pyometra—develops when bacterial invasion of abnormal endometrium leads to intraluminal accumulation of purulent exudate. Occurs less commonly than other endometrial disorders, including adenocarcinoma
• Endometrial disorders—common endometrial disorders of rabbits include endometrial hyperplasia (most common), endometrial venous aneurysms, endometriosis, and endometritis. Less common disorders include hydrometra and mucometra.
• Most endometrial disorders can result in significant uterine hemorrhage.
• Frequently practitioners see more than one disorder in the same rabbit, especially in rabbits with uterine adenocarcinoma. For instance, many rabbits with uterine neoplasia also have areas of cystic endometrial hyperplasia.
• May be difficult clinically to differentiate nonneoplastic endometrial disorders from uterine adenocarcinoma prior to ovariohysterectomy
• Normal cycling rabbit (female rabbit is called a doe)—induced ovulators with silent estrus; estrous cycles last 7–14 days; most does are receptive to males approximately 14 of every 16 days.
• Pseudopregnancy—can occur even in solitary does; lasts 16–17 days (normal gestation 30–33 days); commonly followed by hydrometra, pyometra, or endometrial hyperplasia
• Bacteria—endometrial secretions provide excellent media for growth; ascend from the vagina through the partially open cervix during proestrus and estrus; may be transmitted from male during copulation; hematogenous spread also reported
• The cause of endometrial venous aneurysm is unknown; it often multiple aneurysms are present; rupture results in significant, possibly life-threatening hemorrhage.

### SIGNALMENT
• Intact females
• Highest incidence in does >3–4 years old
• All breeds at risk

### SIGNS
#### Historical Findings
• Hematuria—most common presenting complaint. Not true hematuria, since blood originates from the uterus, but is released during micturition. Hematuria is often reported as intermittent or cyclic; usually occurs at the end of micturition
• Does with mild or early endometrial disease may have no clinical signs.
• Serosanguineous to purulent, blood-tinged vaginal discharge
• Increased aggressiveness
• May have had signs of pseudopregnancy—pulling hair, nest building
• Closed cervix pyometra—signs of systemic illness, may progress to signs of septicemia and shock
• Breeding does—small litter size; increased number of stillborn or resorbed fetuses; infertility; dystocia; abandonment of litters
• Polydipsia and polyuria may be seen with pyometra.

#### Physical Examination Findings
• Uterus—often palpably large; careful palpation may allow determination of size; overly aggressive palpation may induce rupture in rabbits with pyometra, as the uterus can be extremely friable.
• Serosanguineous to purulent, blood-tinged vaginal discharge
• Blood-stained perineum
• Enlarged mammary gland—one or multiple; may be firm and multilobulated (mammary tumors) or fluid filled (cystic); septic mastitis may also occur.
• Pale mucous membranes, tachycardia in rabbits that have had significant uterine hemorrhage
• Depression, lethargy, and anorexia in rabbits with pyometra or uterine hemorrhage

### CAUSES AND RISK FACTORS
• Intact sexual status
• Risk increases with age—seen more often in rabbits >3 years of age
• Risk may increase with sterile mating or when does mount each other.
• Common bacterial pathogens in pyometra—*Pasteurella multocida* and *Staphylococcus aureus* most common; others include *Chlamydia*, *Listeria monocytogenes*, *Moraxella bovis*, *Actinomyces pyogenes*, *Brucella melitensis*, and *Salmonella* sp.

## DIAGNOSIS

### DIFFERENTIAL DIAGNOSIS
• Pregnancy
• Uterine adenocarcinoma—more common uterine disorder
• Other uterine neoplasia (leiomyoma)

### CBC/BIOCHEMISTRY/URINALYSIS
• Often unremarkable
• Neutrophilia—sometimes seen in rabbits with pyometra; most often with relative lymphopenia; TWBC elevations usually not seen
• Regenerative (and occasionally nonregenerative) anemia possible in rabbits with uterine hemorrhage
• Azotemia, increases in ALT, electrolyte disturbances—all can be abnormal in rabbits with pyometra, septicemia, or severe dehydration, depending on clinical course.
• Urinalysis—sample collected by ultrasound-guided cystocentesis to differentiate hematuria from uterine bleeding

### OTHER LABORATORY TESTS
• Cytologic examination of vaginal discharge—polymorphonuclear cells and bacteria
• Bacterial culture and sensitivity test of uterine contents—obtained during ovariohysterectomy to direct antibiotic therapy; vaginal culture not helpful in confirming diagnosis (bacteria cultured are usually normal vaginal flora)
• Histopathologic examination of uterus following ovariohysterectomy—necessary for definitive diagnosis

### IMAGING
#### Radiography
• Detect a large uterus.
• Rule out pregnancy—average gestation lasts 30–33 days; calcification of skeletons occurs in last trimester.
• Pyometra—uterus may appear as a distended, tubular structure in the caudal ventral abdomen.

#### Ultrasonography
• Assess size of uterus and nature of uterine contents.
• Rule out pregnancy.

### DIAGNOSTIC PROCEDURES
N/A

## TREATMENT

### APPROPRIATE HEALTH CARE
Inpatient in does with pyometra or uterine hemorrhage; can be life threatening

### NURSING CARE
• Supportive care—immediate intravenous fluid administration and antibiotics in does with pyometra
• Blood transfusion may be required in does with significant uterine hemorrhage.

### ACTIVITY
N/A

### DIET
• It is absolutely imperative that the rabbit continue to eat during and following treatment. Anorexia will often cause gastrointestinal hypomotility, derangement of the gastrointestinal microflora, and overgrowth of intestinal bacterial pathogens.
• Offer a large selection of fresh, moistened greens such as cilantro, romaine lettuce, parsley, carrot tops, dandelion greens, spinach, collard greens, etc., and good-quality grass hay. Many rabbits will begin to eat these foods, even if they were previously anorectic.

# PYOMETRA AND NONNEOPLASTIC ENDOMETRIAL DISORDERS

• If the patient refuses these foods, syringe feed a gruel such as Critical Care for Herbivores (Oxbow Pet Products, Murdock, NE) 10–15 mL/kg PO q6–8h. Alternatively, pellets can be ground and mixed with fresh greens, vegetable baby foods, water, or juice to form a gruel. If sufficient volumes of food are not accepted in this manner, nasogastric intubation is indicated.
• High-carbohydrate, high-fat nutritional supplements are contraindicated.
• Encourage oral fluid intake by offering fresh water and wetting leafy vegetables.

## CLIENT EDUCATION
• Inform client that ovariohysterectomy is indicated with any uterine disorder.
• Medical treatment is not recommended—uterus contains thick exudate that does not drain in does with endometritis or pyometra.
• Most other uterine disorders carry risk of hemorrhage in the uterus; can become life threatening; can progress; all are at risk for developing uterine adenocarcinoma; reproductive performance is reduced in does with endometrial disorders.
• Inform client that medical treatment does not cure underlying endometrial disease; progression of disease can be life threatening.

## SURGICAL CONSIDERATIONS
• Ovariohysterectomy preferred treatment for all uterine disorders
• Premedicate with buprenorphine (plus ketamine and diazepam in nervous patients); chamber or mask induction; intubate when possible.
• Proceed cautiously; enlarged uterus may be friable; adhesions and ovarian abscesses may accompany pyometra.
• Ligate caudal to the cervix in the proximal vagina, so that the bicornate cervix (double cervix) is also removed.
• Handle tissues minimally and keep tissues moist intraoperatively to help prevent postoperative adhesion formation.
• Avoid reactive suture materials (especially catgut); use hemoclips or nonreactive suture to prevent postoperative adhesion formation.
• Uterine rupture or leakage of purulent material from the uterine stump—repeated lavage of the peritoneal cavity with sterile saline

# MEDICATIONS
## DRUG(S) OF CHOICE
### Antibiotics
• Empirical, pending results of bacterial culture and sensitivity test
• For all patients with pyometra on endometritis

• Use broad-spectrum antibiotics such as enrofloxacin (5–20 mg/kg PO, SC, IM q12–24h), trimethoprim sulfa (30 mg/kg PO q12h), or chloramphenicol (50 mg/kg PO q8h).

### Acute Pain Management
• Buprenorphine (0.01–0.05 mg/kg SC, IM, IV q8–12h); use preoperatively
• Butorphanol (0.1–1.0 mg/kg SC, IM, IV q4–6h); may cause profound sedation; short-acting
• Morphine (2–5 mg/kg SC, IM q2–4h) or oxymorphone (0.05–0.2 mg/kg SC, IM q8–12h); use with caution; more than one to two doses may cause gastrointestinal stasis.
• Meloxicam (0.2 mg/kg SC, IM q24h)
• Carprofen (1–4 mg/kg SC q12h)

### Postoperative Pain Management
• NSAIDs have been used for short- or long-term therapy to reduce pain and inflammation: meloxicam (0.2–0.5 mg/kg PO q24h) or carprofen (2.2 mg/kg PO q12–24h)
• Sedation—ketamine (15–20 mg/kg IM) plus midazolam (0.5–1.0 mg/kg IM); many other sedation protocols exist.

## CONTRAINDICATIONS
• Oral administration of most antibiotics effective against anaerobes will cause a fatal gastrointestinal dysbiosis in rabbits. Do not administer penicillins, macrolides, lincosamides, and cephalosporins by oral administration.
• Corticosteroids—associated with gastrointestinal ulceration and hemorrhage, delayed wound healing, and heightened susceptibility to infection; rabbits are very sensitive to the immunosuppressive effects of both topical and systemic corticosteroids; use may exacerbate subclinical bacterial infection.

## PRECAUTIONS
• Chloramphenicol—avoid human contact with chloramphenicol due to potential blood dyscrasia. Advise owners of potential risks.
• Meloxicam—use with caution in rabbits with compromised renal function.

## POSSIBLE INTERACTIONS
N/A

## ALTERNATIVE DRUGS
Prostaglandins—PGF2α has not been used successfully in rabbits.

# FOLLOW-UP
## PATIENT MONITORING
• Monitor carefully for signs of pain (reluctance to move, teeth grinding) postoperatively.
• Make certain the doe continues to eat postoperatively.

• If owners elect not to perform surgery—monitor carefully for signs of uterine hemorrhage (blood passed during micturition) or sepsis in rabbits with endometritis or mastitis.

## PREVENTION/AVOIDANCE
• Ovariohysterectomy for all nonbreeding rabbits; usually performed between 6 months and 2 years of age.
• For breeding rabbits—recommend the client stop breeding and spay after 4 years of age, as this is when most endometrial disorders (including adenocarcinoma) occur.

## POSSIBLE COMPLICATIONS
• Peritonitis, sepsis in does with endometritis or pyometra
• Postoperative intraabdominal adhesions—may contribute to chronic pain and gastrointestinal motility disorders
• Uterine adenocarcinoma in does >3 years of age
• Hemorrhage and possible death in rabbits with bleeding uterine disorders

## EXPECTED COURSE AND PROGNOSIS
• Good prognosis with timely ovariohysterectomy for most uterine disorders, including adenocarcinoma that has not metastasized
• Guarded prognosis in does presented with vigorous vaginal hemorrhage; emergency stabilization and hysterectomy are indicated to control hemorrhage.
• Guarded to poor in does with pyometra that is not treated early; sepsis or peritonitis may follow.

# MISCELLANEOUS
## ASSOCIATED CONDITIONS
• Mammary neoplasia
• Mastitis
• Ovarian neoplasia
• Ovarian abscess
• Pyometra of the uterine stump in spayed animals—may develop any time after ovariohysterectomy

## AGE-RELATED FACTORS
Risk increases with age.

## ZOONOTIC POTENTIAL
N/A

## PREGNANCY
N/A

## SEE ALSO
• Mastitis, septic and cystic
• Uterine adenocarcinoma

## ABBREVIATIONS
• ALT = alanine transferase
• PGF2α = prostaglandin F2-alpha
• TWBC = total white blood cell

## PYOMETRA AND NONNEOPLASTIC ENDOMETRIAL DISORDERS

*Suggested Reading*

Baba N, von Haam E. Animal model for human disease: spontaneous adenocarcinoma in aged rabbits. Am J Pathol 1972;68:653–656.

Jenkins JR. Surgical sterilization in small mammals: spay and castration. Vet Clin North Am Exotic Anim Pract 2000;3(3):617–627.

Lewis B. Uterine adenocarcinoma in a rabbit. Exotic DVM 2003;5(1):11.

Pare JA, Paul-Murphy J. Disorders of the reproductive and urinary systems. In: Quesenberry KE, Carpenter JW, eds. Ferrets, Rabbits and Rodents: Clinical Medicine and Surgery. 2nd Ed. Philadelphia: WB Saunders, 2004:183–193.

Saito K, Nakanishi M, Hasegawa A. Uterine disorders diagnosed by ventrotomy in 47 rabbits. J Vet Med Sci 2002;64(6): 495–497.

*Portions Adapted From*

Rootkustritz MV. Pyometra and Cystic Endometrial Hyperplasia. In: Tilley LP, Smith FWK, Jr., eds. The 5-Minute Veterinary Consult: Canine and Feline, 3rd Ed. Baltimore: Lippincott Williams & Wilkins, 2004.

# BASICS

## DEFINITION
A severe, invariably fatal, viral polioencephalitis of warm-blooded animals, including humans

## PATHOPHYSIOLOGY
Virus—enters body through a wound (usually from a bite of rabid animal) or via mucous membranes; replicates in myocytes; spreads to the neuromuscular junction and neurotendinal spindles; travels to the CNS via intraaxonal fluid within peripheral nerves; spreads throughout the CNS; finally spreads centrifugally within peripheral, sensory, and motor neurons

## SYSTEMS AFFECTED
• Nervous—clinical encephalitis, either paralytic or furious
• Salivary glands—contain large quantities of infectious virus particles that are shed in saliva

## GENETICS
None

## INCIDENCE/PREVALENCE
• Incidence of disease within infected rabbits not reported
• Prevalence—overall low; 30 cases reported in the United States between 1971 and 1997

## GEOGRAPHIC DISTRIBUTION
Worldwide

## SIGNALMENT

### Species
All warm-blooded animals, including dogs, cats, and humans

### Breed, Age, and Sex Predilections
None

## SIGNS

### General Comments
• In one documented case of rabies in a rabbit, neurologic signs (blindness, forelimb paresis) did not develop until 1 month postexposure.
• The clinical signs of rabies in rabbits are usually nonspecific and include fever, anorexia, lethargy, fever, and posterior paresis. These signs are very similar to many common diseases in rabbits. The furious form of rabies seen in other mammals is unusual in rabbits. However, consider rabies as a differential diagnosis in any rabbit displaying neurologic signs.

### Historical Findings
History of signs similar to those seen in other mammals with rabies warrants consideration of rabies as a diagnosis in the rabbit. Consider rabies in rabbits with a history of:

• Being housed outdoors, even if confined to a hutch
• Contact or bites from wild or possibly infected animals
• Change in attitude—apprehension, nervousness, anxiety, unusual shyness or aggressiveness
• Erratic behavior—biting; biting at cage; wandering and roaming; excitability; irritability; viciousness
• Disorientation
• Muscular function—incoordination, seizures, paralysis
• Blindness
• Excess salivation or frothing

### Physical Examination Findings
• All or some of the historical findings
• Mandibular and laryngeal paralysis, with dropped jaw
• Inability to swallow
• Hypersalivation
• Fever

## CAUSES
Rabies virus—a single-stranded RNA virus; genus Lyssavirus; family Rhabdoviridae

## RISK FACTORS
• Exposure to wildlife, especially skunks, raccoons, bats, and foxes
• Lack of vaccination against rabies for rabbits
• Bite or other skin-penetrating wounds from unvaccinated dogs, cats, or wildlife
• Exposure to aerosols in bat caves
• Use of modified live virus rabies vaccine

# DIAGNOSIS

## DIFFERENTIAL DIAGNOSIS
• Seriously consider rabies for any rabbit showing unusual mood or behavior changes or exhibiting any unaccountable neurologic signs. Caution: Handle with considerable care to prevent possible transmission of the virus to individuals caring for or treating the animal.
• Any neurologic disease—otitis interna/media; brain tumor; brain abscess; encephalitis, lead poisoning; aberrant parasite migration
• Head wound—identify lesions from wound
• Choking
• Tetanus
• Lead poisoning

## CBC/BIOCHEMISTRY/URINALYSIS
No characteristic hematologic or biochemical changes

## OTHER LABORATORY TESTS
N/A

## IMAGING
N/A

## DIAGNOSTIC PROCEDURES
DFA test of nervous tissue—rapid and sensitive test; collect brain, head, or entire body of a small rabbit that has died or has been euthanatized; chill sample immediately; submit to a state-approved laboratory for rabies diagnosis. Caution: Use extreme care when collecting, handling, and shipping these specimens.

## PATHOLOGIC FINDINGS
• Gross changes—generally absent, despite dramatic neurologic disease
• Histopathologic changes—acute to chronic polioencephalitis; gradual increase in the severity of the nonsuppurative inflammatory process in the CNS as disease progresses; large neurons within the brain may contain the classic intracytoplasmic inclusions (Negri bodies).

# TREATMENT

## APPROPRIATE HEALTH CARE
Strictly inpatient

## NURSING CARE
Administer with extreme caution.

## ACTIVITY
• Confine to secured quarantine area with clearly posted signs indicating suspected rabies.
• Cages should be locked; only designated people should have access.
• Feed and water without opening the cage door.

## DIET
N/A

## CLIENT EDUCATION
• Thoroughly inform client of the seriousness of rabies to the animal and the zoonotic potential.
• Ask client about any human exposure (e.g., contact, bite) and strongly urge client to see a physician immediately.
• Local public health official must be notified.

## SURGICAL CONSIDERATIONS
N/A

# MEDICATIONS

## DRUG(S) OF CHOICE
• No treatment
• Once the diagnosis is certain, euthanasia is indicated.

## CONTRAINDICATIONS
None

## PRECAUTIONS
N/A

## RABIES

### POSSIBLE INTERACTIONS
N/A

### ALTERNATIVE DRUGS
N/A

## FOLLOW-UP

### PATIENT MONITORING
• All suspected rabies patients should be securely isolated and monitored for any development of mood change, attitude change, or clinical signs that might suggest the diagnosis.
• An apparently healthy rabbit that bites a person should be confined and monitored; contact local public health regulatory agency for instructions on quarantining rabbits inflicting bite wounds.
• If the rabbit dies during quarantine, the head should be submitted for testing as outlined above.
• A rabbit that is bitten by or exposed to a known rabid animal must be euthanized or quarantined for up to 6 months or according to local or state regulations.

### PREVENTION/AVOIDANCE
• Vaccines—no vaccine is currently approved for use in rabbits in the United States. However, in areas where rabies is endemic, some practitioners have vaccinated rabbits according to standard recommendations and state and local requirements for cats and dogs using a killed vaccine.

• Prevent contact with wildlife—especially rabbits housed outdoors.
• Disinfection—any contaminated area, cage, food dish, or instrument must be thoroughly disinfected; use a 1:32 dilution (4 ounces per gallon) of household bleach to quickly inactivate the virus.

### POSSIBLE COMPLICATIONS
Paralysis or attitude changes

### EXPECTED COURSE AND PROGNOSIS
Prognosis—grave; invariably fatal; euthanasia is indicated to confirm diagnosis.

## MISCELLANEOUS

### ASSOCIATED CONDITIONS
None

### AGE-RELATED FACTORS
None

### ZOONOTIC POTENTIAL
• Extreme
• Humans must avoid being bitten by or having contact with saliva from a rabid animal or an asymptomatic animal that is incubating the disease.
• Suspected rabies cases must be strictly quarantined and confined to prevent exposure to humans and other animals.
• Local and state regulations must be adhered to carefully and completely.

### PREGNANCY
Infection during pregnancy will be fatal.

### SYNONYMS
Rage, hydrophobia

### ABBREVIATIONS
• CNS = central nervous system
• DFA = direct immunofluorescent antibody

### Suggested Reading
Eng TR, Fishbein DB. National Study Group on Rabies. Epidemiologic factors, clinical findings, and vaccination status of rabies in cats and dogs in the United States in 1988. J Am Vet Med Assoc 1990;197:201–209.
Greene CE, Dreesen DW. Rabies. In: Greene CE, ed. Infectious Diseases of the Dog and Cat. 2nd Ed. Philadelphia: Saunders, 1998:114–126.
Jenkins SR, Auslander M, Conti L, et al. Compendium of Animal Rabies Control, 2002. J Am Vet Med Assoc 2002;221:44–48.

### Portions Adapted From
Scott FW. Rabies. In: Tilley LP, Smith FWK, Jr., eds. The 5-Minute Veterinary Consult: Canine and Feline, 3rd Ed. Baltimore: Lippincott Williams & Wilkins, 2004.

# BASICS

## DEFINITION
Hyperemia of the eyelids, conjunctiva, ocular vasculature, or hemorrhage within the eye

## PATHOPHYSIOLOGY
• Active dilation of ocular vessels—in response to extraocular or intraocular inflammation or passive congestion
• Hemorrhage from existing or newly formed blood vessels
• Many rabbits with ocular disease have underlying chronic respiratory or dental disease.
• Most dental disease is secondary to tooth root elongation.

## SYSTEMS AFFECTED
• Ophthalmic—eye and/or ocular adnexa
• Oral cavity—related dental disease
• Respiratory—related respiratory infections and apical (tooth root) invasion of the sinuses

## SIGNALMENT
• Middle-aged to older rabbits—acquired cheek tooth elongation causing blockage of nasolacrimal duct or intrusion into the retrobulbar space
• Young animals—congenital tooth malocclusion, congenital eyelid deformities
• Dwarf and lop breeds—congenital tooth malocclusion
• Dwarf and Himalayan breeds—glaucoma more common
• Rex and New Zealand White breeds—entropion and trichiasis more common
• Other ocular diseases—no breed, age, or sex predilection

## SIGNS

### Historical Findings
• Depend on cause
• History of previous treatment for dental disease
• History of nasal discharge or previous upper respiratory infection
• Facial asymmetry, masses, or exophthalmos in rabbits with tooth root abscesses
• Signs of pain—reluctance to move, depression, lethargy, hiding, and hunched posture in rabbits with painful ocular conditions or underlying dental disease
• Unilateral or bilateral alopecia, crusts, and matted fur in periocular area, cheeks, and/or nasal rostrum

### Physical Examination Findings
• Depend on cause
• Blepharospasm
• Ocular discharge—serous, mucoid, or mucopurulent

• Thick, white exudate accumulation in medial canthus in rabbits with dacryocystitis
• Corneal ulcers associated with dacryocystitis are usually superficial and ventrally located; ulcers secondary to exposure keratitis are usually central and may be superficial or deep.
• Chemosis
• Excessive conjunctival tissue—may partially or completely occlude the cornea
• Facial pyoderma—alopecia, erythema, and matted fur in periocular area, cheeks, and/or nasal rostrum; due to constant moisture in rabbits with epiphora

### Oral Examination
• A thorough examination of the oral cavity is indicated in every rabbit with ocular discharge. A thorough examination includes the incisors, molars, and buccal and lingual mucosa to rule out dental disease. Use of an otoscope or speculum may be useful in identifying severe abnormalities; however, many problems will be missed by using this method alone. Complete examination requires heavy sedation or general anesthesia and specialized equipment.
• A focused, directed light source and magnification (or a rigid endoscope) will provide optimal visualization.
• Use a rodent mouth gag and cheek dilators (Jorgensen Laboratories, Inc., Loveland, CO) to open the mouth and pull buccal tissues away from teeth surfaces to allow adequate exposure. Use a cotton swab or tongue depressor to retract tongue from lingual surfaces.
• Identify cheek teeth elongation, irregular crown height, spikes, curved teeth, tooth discoloration, tooth mobility, missing teeth, purulent exudate, oral ulceration, or abscesses.
• Significant tooth root abnormalities may be present despite normal-appearing crowns. Skull films are required to identify apical disorders.
• Incisors—you may see overgrowth, horizontal ridges or grooves, malformation, discoloration, fractures, increased or decreased curvature.

## CAUSES
Virtually every case fits into one or more of the following categories:
• Blepharitis—bacterial, *Treponema cuniculi* (rabbits syphilis), or myxomatosis
• Conjunctivitis—primary (rare), secondary to eyelid or lash disorders, foreign bodies, environmental irritants, dacryocystitis, or upper respiratory tract disease
• Aberrant conjunctival overgrowth—unknown cause; conjunctiva grows from the limbus, is nonadherent to the cornea, and may completely cover the cornea; does not appear to be painful or associated with significant inflammation

• Keratitis—traumatic most common; exposure to keratitis following anesthesia, facial nerve paralysis; corneal abrasion in rabbits with torticollis; secondary to eyelash or eyelid disorder, keratoconjunctivitis sicca
• Anterior uveitis—most commonly bacterial or *Encephalitozoon cuniculi*
• Episcleritis or scleritis
• Glaucoma
• Hyphema—trauma, iridal abscess, or *E. cuniculi* most common cause
• Orbital disease—usually the orbital abnormality is more prominent.
• Dacryocystitis—inflammation of the canaliculi, lacrimal sac, or nasolacrimal ducts. Usually sterile and secondary to blockage from dental disease—inflammatory cells, oil, and debris present. If secondary bacterial infection, *Staphylococcus* spp., *Pseudomonas* spp., *Moraxella* spp., *Pasteurella multocida, Neisseria* spp., and *Bordetella* spp. frequently cultured. Cheek tooth or incisor elongation—most common cause; the nasolacrimal duct is normally very closely associated with the roots of the cheek teeth; elongation or abscessation of the tooth roots (most commonly the second upper premolar) impinges or invades into the nasolacrimal duct. Chronic upper respiratory infection is also a common cause of nasolacrimal duct obstruction (thick or dried exudates, abscess, stricture).

## RISK FACTORS
• Systemic infectious or inflammatory diseases
• Immunocompromise
• Coagulopathies
• Topical ophthalmic medications—aminoglycosides, pilocarpine, epinephrine
• Neoplasia
• Trauma
• Malocclusion and tooth root elongation

# DIAGNOSIS

## DIFFERENTIAL DIAGNOSIS
More than one cause may occur simultaneously.

### Similar Signs
• Rule out normal variations.
• Palpebral conjunctiva—normally redder than bulbar conjunctiva
• One or two large episcleral vessels—may be normal if the eye is otherwise quiet
• Transient mild hyperemia—with excitement, exercise, and straining; transient prolapse of the tear gland/nictitans may occur.
• Horner's syndrome—may cause mild conjunctival vascular dilation; differentiated by other signs and pharmacologic testing

# RED EYE

## DIFFERENTIATING CAUSES

• Superficial (conjunctival) vessels—originate near the fornix; move with the conjunctiva; branch repeatedly; blanch quickly with topical 2.5% phenylephrine or 1:100,000 epinephrine; suggests ocular surface disorders (e.g., conjunctivitis, superficial keratitis, blepharitis)
• Deep (episcleral) vessels—originate near the limbus; branch infrequently; do not move with the conjunctiva; blanch slowly or incompletely with topical sympathomimetics; suggest episcleritis or intraocular disease (e.g., anterior uveitis or glaucoma)
• Discharge—mucopurulent to purulent: typical of ocular surface disorders and blepharitis; serous or none: typical of intraocular disorders or blockage of the nasolacrimal duct
• Unilateral condition with ocular pain (blepharospasm)—usually indicates a tooth root disorder, keratitis, or foreign body. Can be seen with anterior uveitis secondary to *E. cuniculi* or iridal or corneal stromal abscess
• Chronic, bilateral condition—can indicate a congenital problem or chronic upper respiratory tract infection; bilateral tooth root disorders also seen
• Acute, bilateral condition with severe eyelid edema—consider myxomatosis
• Bilateral blepharitis—rule out *Treponema cuniculi* (rabbit syphilis); most have perineal and perioral dermatitis.
• Facial pain, swelling, nasal discharge, or sneezing—seen with tooth root elongation or abscess; may indicate nasal or sinus infection; may indicate obstruction from neoplasm
• White discharge confined to the medial canthus—usually indicates dacryocystitis
• Corneal opacification, neovascularization, or fluorescein stain retention—suggests keratitis
• Aqueous flare or cell (increased protein or cells in the anterior chamber)—confirms diagnosis of anterior uveitis
• Pupil—miotic: common with anterior uveitis; dilated: common with glaucoma; normal: with blepharitis and conjunctivitis
• Abnormally shaped or colored irides—suggest anterior uveitis, iridal abscess, *E. cuniculi*
• Luxated or cataractous lenses—suggest glaucoma or anterior uveitis
• IOP—high: diagnostic for glaucoma; low: suggests anterior uveitis
• Loss of vision—suggests glaucoma, anterior uveitis, or severe keratitis. Vision can be difficult to assess in rabbits; rabbits typically do not menace; pupillary light response may not correlate well with vision; rabbits often refuse to negotiate obstacles and may not respond to objects such as cotton balls tossed near face.

• Glaucoma and anterior uveitis—may complicate hyphema

## CBC/BIOCHEMISTRY/URINALYSIS

Usually normal, except with underlying systemic disease

## OTHER LABORATORY TESTS

Serologic testing for *E. cuniculi* in rabbits with cataracts or phacoclastic uveitis—many tests are available, but usefulness is extremely limited since a positive titer indicates only exposure and does not confirm *E. cuniculi* as the cause of uveitis. *E. cuniculi* can only be definitively diagnosed by finding organisms and resultant lesions on ocular histopathology or by positive DNA probe on removed lens material. Antibody titers usually become positive by 2 weeks postinfection but generally do not continue to rise with active infection or decline with treatment. No correlation exists between antibody titers and shedding of organism and presence or severity of disease. It is unknown if exposed rabbits eventually become seronegative. Available tests include ELISA, indirect IFA, and carbon immunoassay.

## IMAGING

• Skull radiographs are mandatory to identify dental disease and nasal, sinus, or maxillary bone lesions, and, if present, to plan treatment strategies and to monitor progression of treatment.
• Perform under general anesthesia.
• Five views are recommend for thorough assessment—ventral–dorsal, lateral, two lateral obliques, and rostral–caudal.
• CT—superior to radiographs to localize obstruction and characterize associated lesions
• Dacryocystorhinography—radiopaque contrast material to help localize nasolacrimal duct obstruction
• Chest radiographs—consider with anterior uveitis or if intraocular neoplasia is a possibility.
• Abdominal radiography or ultrasonography—may help rule out infectious or neoplastic causes
• Ocular ultrasonography—if the ocular media are opaque; may define the extent and nature of intraocular disease or identify an intraocular tumor

## DIAGNOSTIC PROCEDURES

• Tonometry—must perform in every patient with an unexplained red eye. Normal intraocular pressure reported as 10–20 mm Hg when measured by applanation tonometry.
• Schirmer tear test—average values reported as 5 mm/min; however, even lower values can be seen in normal rabbits.
• Cytologic examination of affected tissue—lid, conjunctiva, cornea

• Fluorescein stain—rule out ulcerative keratitis; test for nasolacrimal function; dye flows through the nasolacrimal system and reaches the external nares in approximately 10 seconds in normal rabbits.
• Conjunctival biopsies—with chronic conjunctivitis or with a mass lesion
• Perform a nasolacrimal flush—rule out nasolacrimal disease; may dislodge foreign material. Topical administration of an ophthalmic anesthetic is generally sufficient for this procedure; nervous rabbits may require mild sedation. Rabbits have only a single nasolacrimal punctum located in the ventral eyelid at the medial canthus. A 23-gauge lacrimal cannula or a 24-gauge Teflon intravenous catheter can be used to flush the duct. Irrigation will generally produce a thick, white exudate from the nasal meatus.
• Aerobic bacterial culture and sensitivity—consider with mucopurulent discharge; ideally specimens taken before anything is placed in the eye (e.g., topical anesthetic, fluorescein, and flush) to prevent inhibition or dilution of bacterial growth; not routinely indicated for KCS and a mucopurulent discharge (secondary bacterial overgrowth almost certain). Often, only normal organisms are isolated (*Bacillus subtilis, Staphylococcus aureus, Bordetella* spp.).

 **TREATMENT**

• Usually outpatient
• Elizabethan collar—consider to prevent self-trauma
• Avoid dirty environments or those that may lead to ocular trauma.
• Because there is a narrow margin for error, consider referral if you cannot attribute the condition to one of the listed causes, if you cannot rule out glaucoma on the initial visit, or if the diagnosis is so uncertain that administration of a topical antibiotic alone or a topical corticosteroid alone would be questionable.
• Underlying tooth root disorders—trimming of cheek teeth (coronal deduction) may correct or control progression of root elongation. If tooth extraction is required or tooth root abscess is diagnosed it may require referral to a veterinarian with special expertise, if feasible. Because rabbits have very long, deeply embedded tooth roots, extraction per os can be extremely time consuming and labor intensive as compared to with dogs and cats. In rabbits with extensive tooth root abscesses, aggressive debridement is indicated. Maxillary and retrobulbar abscesses can be particularly challenging.
• Aberrant conjunctival overgrowth—surgical excision of the excessive conjunctiva; often only palliative and may re-form.

• Few causes are fatal; however, a workup may be indicated (especially with anterior uveitis and hyphema) to rule out potentially fatal systemic diseases.
• Deep corneal ulcers and glaucoma—may be best treated surgically

## MEDICATIONS

### DRUG(S) OF CHOICE
• Depends on specific cause
• Generally, controls ocular pain, inflammation, infection, and IOP
• Topical broad-spectrum antibiotic ophthalmic solutions—for keratitis, conjunctivitis, dacryocystitis; while waiting for results of diagnostic tests; may try triple antibiotic solution, ciprofloxacin, gentamicin, or ophthalmic chloramphenicol solution q4–6h
• 1% atropine q12–24h may help reduce ciliary spasm in patients with corneal ulcer or anterior uveitis; however, some rabbits produce atropinase; application may not be effective.
• Dacryocystitis—antibiotic choice based on bacterial culture and sensitivity test results; continue for at least 21 days
• Systemic antibiotics—indicated in rabbits with tooth root abscess or upper respiratory tract infection causing dacryocystitis or conjunctivitis
• Topical NSAIDs—0.03% flurbiprofen or 1% diclofenac may help reduce inflammation and irritation associated with flushes.
• Sedation for nasolacrimal duct flushing or oral examination—light sedation with midazolam (0.5–2 mg/kg IM) or diazepam (1–2 mg/kg IM); oral examinations or longer procedures require deeper sedation; the author prefers ketamine (15–20 mg/kg IM) plus midazolam (0.5–1.0 mg/kg IM); many other sedation protocols exist. Alternatively, administer general anesthesia with isoflurane.
• Long-term pain management—indicated in rabbits with tooth root elongation. NSAIDs have been used for short or long term therapy to reduce pain and inflammation: meloxicam (0.2–0.5 mg/kg PO q24h) or carprofen (2.2 mg/kg PO q12–24h).

### CONTRAINDICATIONS
• Topical corticosteroids—never use if the cornea retains fluorescein stain.

• Oral administration of most antibiotics effective against anaerobes will cause a fatal gastrointestinal dysbiosis in rabbits. Do not administer penicillins, macrolides, lincosamides, and cephalosporins by oral administration.

### PRECAUTIONS
• Topical corticosteroids or antibiotic–corticosteroid combinations—avoid; associated with gastrointestinal ulceration and hemorrhage, delayed wound healing, and heightened susceptibility to infection; rabbits are very sensitive to the immunosuppressive effects of both topical and systemic corticosteroids; use may exacerbate subclinical bacterial infection.
• Topical aminoglycosides—may be irritating; may impede reepithelization if used frequently or at high concentrations
• Topical solutions—may be preferable to ointments if corneal perforation is possible
• Atropine—may exacerbate KCS and glaucoma
• NSAIDs—use with caution in hyphema

### POSSIBLE INTERACTIONS
N/A

### ALTERNATIVE DRUGS
N/A

## FOLLOW-UP

### PATIENT MONITORING
• Depends on cause
• Repeat ophthalmic examinations—as required to ensure that IOP, ocular pain, and inflammation are well controlled
• The greater the risk of loss of vision, the more closely the patient needs to be followed; may require daily or more frequent examination

### POSSIBLE COMPLICATIONS
• Chronic epiphora
• Loss of the eye or permanent vision loss
• Chronic ocular inflammation and pain

## MISCELLANEOUS

### ASSOCIATED CONDITIONS
• Dental disease
• Gastrointestinal hypomotility

### AGE-RELATED FACTORS
N/A

### ZOONOTIC POTENTIAL
N/A

### PREGNANCY
N/A

### SEE ALSO
• Anterior uveitis
• Conjunctivitis
• Epiphora
• Myxomatosis

### ABBREVIATIONS
• CT = computed tomography
• IFA = immunofluorescence assay
• ELISA = enzyme-linked immunosorbent assay
• IOP = intraocular pressure
• KCS = keratoconjunctivitis sicca
• NSAIDs = nonsteroidal antiinflammatory drugs

*Suggested Reading*
Andrew SE. Corneal disease of rabbits. Vet Clin Noth Am Exotic Anim Pract 2002;5(2):341–356.
Crossley DA. Oral biology and disorders of lagomorphs. Vet Clin Noth Am Exotic Anim Pract 2003;6(3):629–659.
Crossley DA, Aiken S. Small mammal dentistry. In: Quesenberry KE, Carpenter JW, eds. Ferrets, Rabbits and Rodents: Clinical Medicine and Surgery. 2nd Ed. Philadelphia: WB Saunders, 2004:370–382.
Van der Woerdt A. Ophthalmologic disease in small pet animals. In: Quesenberry KE, Carpenter JW, eds. Ferrets, Rabbits and Rodents: Clinical Medicine and Surgery. 2nd Ed. Philadelphia: WB Saunders, 2004:421–428.
Williams DL. Laboratory Animal Ophthalmology. In: Gelatt KN, ed. Veterinary ophthalmology. 3rd Ed. Philadelphia: Lippincott Williams & Wilkins, 1999:151–181.

*Portions Adapted From*
Miller PE. Red Eye. In: Tilley LP, Smith FWK, Jr., eds. The 5-Minute Veterinary Consult: Canine and Feline, 3rd Ed. Baltimore: Lippincott Williams & Wilkins, 2004.

# RENAL FAILURE

 **BASICS**

## DEFINITION
• Azotemia and an inability to concentrate urine, or in the absence of dehydration
• Acute renal failure (ARF) is a syndrome characterized by sudden onset of filtration failure by the kidneys, accumulation of uremic toxins, and dysfunction of fluid, electrolyte, and acid–base balance.
• Chronic renal failure (CRF) results from primary renal disease that has persisted for months to years; characterized by irreversible renal dysfunction that tends to deteriorate progressively.

## PATHOPHYSIOLOGY
• Reduction in functional renal mass results in impaired urine-concentrating ability (leading to polyuria and polydipsia [PU/PD]) and retention of nitrogenous waste products of protein catabolism (leading to azotemia).
• Adrenaline release in response to pain or stress can cause significant reduction in renal plasma flow and glomerular filtration rate, predisposing stressed rabbits to ARF.
• In rabbits, intestinal calcium absorption is not dependent on vitamin D, and nearly all calcium in the diet is absorbed. Calcium excretion occurs primarily through the kidneys; the fractional urinary excretion is 45–60% in rabbits compared to less than 2% in most other mammals. This predisposes rabbits to urinary and renal calculi and may cause renal failure.
• Ascending lower urinary tract infection may cause pyelonephritis and subsequent renal failure.
• With chronicity, decreased erythropoietin and calcitriol production by the kidneys can result in hypoproliferative anemia.

## SYSTEMS AFFECTED
• Renal/urologic—impaired renal function leading to PU/PD and signs of uremia
• Nervous, gastrointestinal, musculoskeletal, and other body systems—secondarily affected by uremia
• Hemic/lymph/immune—anemia

## GENETICS
N/A

## INCIDENCE/PREVALENCE
Not well documented; however, renal failure is a common sequela to many conditions affecting rabbits

## SIGNALMENT
Animals of any age can be affected, but prevalence increases with increasing age.

### Predominant Sex
None

## SIGNS
### General Comments
Clinical signs are related to the severity of renal dysfunction and presence or absence of complications.

### Historical Findings
• ARF—sudden onset of anorexia, listlessness, diarrhea or lack of stool production (ileus), ataxia, seizures, known toxin exposure, recent medical or surgical conditions, and oliguria/anuria or polyuria
• CRF—PU/PD, anorexia, diarrhea or lack of stool production (ileus), weight loss, lethargy, poor haircoat; ataxia, seizures or coma are seen in late stages. Asymptomatic animals with stable CRF may decompensate, resulting in a uremic crisis.

### Physical Examination Findings
• ARF—depression, dehydration (sometimes overhydration), hypothermia, fever, tachypnea, bradycardia, nonpalpable urinary bladder if oliguric, kidneys may be painful on palpation
• CRF—small, irregular kidneys sometimes palpable, dehydration, cachexia, mucous membrane pallor; evidence of gastrointestinal hypomotility (stomach full of desiccated ingesta, gas or fluid in cecum) is common.

## CAUSES
• Shock, severe stress, prolonged anesthesia, heat stroke, heart failure, or septicemia can cause ARF.
• ARF or CRF—nephroliths, glomerulonephritis, pyelonephritis, chronic urinary obstruction, drugs (e.g., aminoglycoside, sulfonamides, chemotherapeutic agents), heavy metals, lymphoma or other neoplasia, *Encephalitozoon cuniculi*, amyloidosis

## RISK FACTORS
• ARF—preexisting renal disease, dehydration, hypovolemia, severe stress, hypotension, advanced age, concurrent disease, prolonged anesthesia or surgery, and administration of nephrotoxic drugs
• CRF—aging, nephroliths, urinary tract infection, diabetes mellitus

 **DIAGNOSIS**

## DIFFERENTIAL DIAGNOSIS
• For PU/PD—hypercalciuria, pyometra, hepatic failure, diabetes mellitus, postobstructive diuresis, behavioral disorders
• For renomegaly—renal neoplasia (lymphoma), hydronephrosis, renal abscess, cystic kidneys (rare)
• Prerenal azotemia (decreased renal perfusion)—characterized by azotemia with concentrated urine (specific gravity >1.020); correctable with fluid repletion; seen commonly in stressed rabbits

• Postrenal azotemia—characterized by azotemia with obstruction or rupture of the excretory system

## CBC/BIOCHEMISTRY/URINALYSIS
• Nonregenerative anemia with CRF; normal or high PCV with ARF
• BUN elevation (normal 9.1–22.7 mg/dL); creatinine elevation (normal 0.5–2.0 mg/dL)
• Normal serum calcium concentration in rabbits is high (12–16 mg/dL) and corresponds directly with dietary calcium intake. In some cases of renal failure, calcium absorption from the intestines continues, while renal elimination is impaired, and may result in increases in serum calcium concentration; however, this is not a consistent finding.
• Hyperphosphatemia is seen with decreased GFR, and elevations may be prerenal, renal, or postrenal. Hyperphosphatemia is more commonly observed in rabbits with CRF.
• Hyperkalemia is occasionally seen with ARF or postrenal obstruction.
• Inability to concentrate urine, mild to moderate proteinuria, glucosuria; WBCs, RBCs, and variable bacteriuria may be seen depending on the underlying cause.
• WBC casts should prompt consideration of pyelonephritis.
• Urinary sediment evaluation often reveals calcium oxalate or calcium carbonate crystals; however, this is a normal finding in rabbits, and the presence of large amounts of crystals in the urine does not necessarily indicate disease. Disease occurs only when the concentration of crystals is excessive, forming thick, white to brown, sandlike urine and subsequent inflammatory cystitis, partial to complete blockage of the urethra or nephrolithiasis.

## OTHER LABORATORY TESTS
• Serum lead or zinc concentration
• *E. cuniculi* titers—many tests are available, but usefulness is limited since a positive titer indicates only exposure and does not confirm *E. cuniculi* as the cause of clinical signs. *E. cuniculi* is not a common cause of renal failure.

## IMAGING
• Abdominal radiographs may reveal calcium oxalate "sand" or uroliths in rabbits with hypercalciuria. Uroliths must be differentiated from calcium "sand" or "sludge" in the bladder, which resembles a bladder full of contrast material. Since rabbits tend to form a single large calculus in the urinary bladder, differentiating the two can be difficult. Ultrasonic examination of the bladder with simultaneous palpation can be helpful to distinguish solitary calculi from amorphous "sand." It may be an incidental finding or cause of CRF.

• Calculi may also form in the renal pelvis and/or ureters. The presence of renal calculi alone does not imply renal failure; excretory urography is necessary to determine if the affected kidney is patent.

• Abdominal radiographs may demonstrate small kidneys (or large kidneys secondary to hydronephrosis, renal cysts, renal abscess, or neoplasia) in animals with CRF.

• Rabbits with ARF often have normal-sized to large kidneys.

• Metastatic calcification of soft tissues, including kidneys and aorta, or hyperostosis is sometimes seen in rabbits with CRF. Absorption of calcium from the gastrointestinal tract is not dependent on vitamin D and continues normally in rabbits with renal failure. However, in some cases, renal excretion of calcium is impaired, leading to excessive mineralization of bone and soft tissues.

• Ultrasonography may be useful in identifying pyelonephritis, renal cysts, renal abscess, degeneration, or neoplasia.

### DIAGNOSTIC PROCEDURES

• Evaluation of ultrasound-guided fine needle aspirates of the kidney may be helpful in the diagnosis of renal neoplasia, abscesses, or cysts.

• Although not indicated in most rabbits, renal biopsy may be helpful in selected patients to document underlying cause.

### PATHOLOGIC FINDINGS

• Gross findings—small kidneys with a lumpy or granular surface may be seen with CRF. Rabbits with previous *E. cuniculi* infections often have focal, irregular areas of pitting on the surface of the kidney. This is usually an incidental finding. Large, irregular kidneys with neoplasia or abscess are commonly found.

• Histopathologic findings—frequently nonspecific; chronic generalized nephropathy or end-stage kidneys; findings are specific for diseases causing CRF in some patients. Rabbits with previous *E. cuniculi* infectious have focal interstitial fibrosis, usually an incidental finding without clinical significance. Nephrosis or nephritis may be seen in rabbits with ARF.

## TREATMENT

### APPROPRIATE HEALTH CARE

Patients with compensated CRF may be managed as outpatients; patients in ARF or uremic crisis should be managed as inpatients.

### NURSING CARE

• Patients in ARF or uremic crisis—correct estimated fluid deficits with normal (0.9%) saline or balanced polyionic solution within 4–6 hours to prevent additional renal injury

from ischemia; once the patient is hydrated, ongoing fluid requirements are provided as a balanced electrolyte solution (approximately 100 mL/kg/day). Use caution when hydrating extremely stressed rabbits. Severe stress may cause a decrease in GFR and subsequent overhydration. Be sure that the volume of urine excreted is appropriate to the amount of fluids received.

• Hypervolemia—stop fluid administration and eliminate excess fluid by diuretic administration.

• Patients in CRF—subcutaneous fluid therapy (daily or every other day) may benefit patients with moderate to severe CRF.

### ACTIVITY

Unrestricted

### DIET

• Increase water consumption. Provide multiple sources of fresh water. Flavoring the water with fruit or vegetable juices (with no added sugars) may be helpful. Provide a variety of clean, fresh, leafy vegetables sprayed or soaked with water.

• It is absolutely imperative that the rabbit continue to eat during and following treatment. Many rabbits with renal failure have a decreased appetite. Anorexia may cause or exacerbate gastrointestinal hypomotility and cause derangement of the gastrointestinal microflora and overgrowth of intestinal bacterial pathogens.

• Offer a large selection of fresh, moistened greens such as cilantro, romaine lettuce, parsley, carrot tops, dandelion greens, spinach, collard greens, etc., and good-quality grass hay. Many rabbits will begin to eat these foods, even if they were previously anorectic.

• If the patient refuses these foods, syringe feed a gruel such as Critical Care for Herbivores (Oxbow Pet Products, Murdock, NE). Alternatively, pellets can be ground and mixed with fresh greens, vegetable baby foods, water, or juice to form a gruel. The addition of canned pumpkin to this gruel is a palatable source of fiber and calories. If sufficient volumes of food are not accepted in this manner, nasogastric intubation is indicated.

• High-carbohydrate, high-fat nutritional supplements are contraindicated.

• Further protein restriction is not indicated; the normal recommended diet for rabbits is already protein restricted.

• No reports of dissolution of calcium oxalate uroliths with special diets

• Reduction in the amount of calcium in the diet may help to prevent or delay recurrence of hypercalciuria, and prevent metastatic tissue calcification with CRF. Eliminate feeding of alfalfa pellets and switch to a high-fiber timothy-based pellet (Oxbow Pet Products, Murdock, NE). The

form of calcium found in alfalfa-based commercial pellets and alfalfa hay is calcium carbonate, which is 50% more bioavailable than the calcium oxalate found in most green, leafy vegetables. Feed timothy and grass hay instead of alfalfa hay and offer large volumes of fresh, green, leafy vegetables.

### CLIENT EDUCATION

• CRF—tends to progress over months, possibly to years

• ARF—inform of the poor prognosis for complete recovery, potential for morbid complications of treatment (e.g., fluid overload, sepsis, and multiple organ failure), and expense of prolonged hospitalization.

### SURGICAL CONSIDERATIONS

Avoid hypotension during anesthesia to prevent additional renal injury.

## MEDICATIONS

### DRUG(S) OF CHOICE

• Inadequate urine production (anuric or oliguric renal failure)—ensure patient is fluid volume replete; provide additional isonatric fluid to achieve mild (3–5%) volume expansion; failure to induce diuresis by fluid replacement indicates severe parenchymal damage or underestimation of fluid deficit; if fluid replete, administration of diuretics (furosemide [1–4 mg/kg IV] or mannitol at feline dosages) to induce diuresis may be successful; reduce stress. If these treatments fail to induce diuresis within 4–6 hours, the prognosis is grave.

• Anorexia, inappetence—reduce gastric acid production: cimetidine (5–10 mg/kg PO, SC, q 8–12h) or ranitidine (2 mg/kg IV q24h or 2.5 mg/kg PO q12h)

• Severe chronic anemia—erythropoietin (50–150 IU/kg SC q2–3d until PCV normalizes, then q7d × 4 weeks)

### CONTRAINDICATIONS

Avoid nephrotoxic agents (NSAIDs, aminoglycosides).

### PRECAUTIONS

Modify dosages of all drugs that require renal metabolism or elimination.

### POSSIBLE INTERACTIONS

N/A

### ALTERNATIVE DRUGS

N/A

### PATIENT MONITORING

• ARF—monitor urinalysis, PCV, BUN, creatinine and electrolytes, body weight, urine output, and clinical status daily

• CRF—monitor at 1–3 month intervals, depending on therapy and severity of disease.

## RENAL FAILURE

### POSSIBLE COMPLICATIONS
• ARF—seizures, gastrointestinal bleeding, cardiac arrhythmias, congestive heart failure, pulmonary edema, hypovolemic shock, coma, cardiopulmonary arrest, and death
• CRF—gastroenteritis, anemia, death

### PREVENTION/AVOIDANCE
Anticipate the potential for ARF in patients that are hemodynamically unstable, receiving nephrotoxic drugs, have multiple organ failure, or are undergoing prolonged anesthesia and surgery; maintenance of hydration and/or mild saline volume expansion may be preventive.

### EXPECTED COURSE AND PROGNOSIS
• Nonoliguric ARF—milder than oliguric; recovery may occur, but the prognosis remains guarded to unfavorable.
• Oliguric ARF—extensive renal injury is difficult to manage, and has a poor prognosis for recovery.
• Anuric ARF—generally fatal
• CRF—short-term prognosis depends on severity; long-term prognosis guarded to poor because CRF tends to be progressive

 **MISCELLANEOUS**

### ASSOCIATED CONDITIONS
• Hypercalciuria
• Urolithiasis
• Gastrointestinal hypomotility

### AGE-RELATED FACTORS
Increased incidence in older animals; normal renal function decreases with aging.

### ZOONOTIC POTENTIAL
*E. cuniculi* is common in rabbits and may have zoonotic potential.

### PREGNANCY
ARF is a rare complication of pregnancy in animals; promoted by acute metritis, pyometra, and postpartum sepsis or hemorrhage

### SYNONYMS
Kidney failure

### SEE ALSO
• Hypercalciuria
• Nephrolithiasis and ureterolithiasis
• PU/PD
• Urinary tract obstruction

### ABBREVIATIONS
• BUN = blood urea nitrogen
• GFR = glomerular filtration rate
• NSAIDs = nonsteroidal antiinflammatory drugs
• PCV = packed cell volume

### Suggested Reading
Brown SA. Rabbit urinary tract disease. Proc North Am Vet Conf 1997;785–787.
Cheeke PR, Amberg JW. Comparative calcium excretion by rats and rabbits. J Anim Sci 1973;37:450–454.
Donoghue S. Nutrition and pet rabbits. In: Rosenthal KL, ed. Practical Exotic Animal Medicine: The Compendium Collection. Trenton, NJ: Veterinary Learning Systems, 1997:107.
Garibaldi BA, Pecquet-Goad ME: Hypercalcemia with secondary nephrolithiasis in a rabbit. Lab Anim Sci 1988;38:331–333.
Harcourt-Brown F. Urogenital disease. In: Harcourt-Brown F. Textbook of Rabbit Medicine. Oxford: Butterworth-Heinemann, 2002:335–351.
Harkness JE, Wagner JE. The Biology and Medicine of Rabbits and Rodents. 3rd Ed. Baltimore: Williams & Wilkins, 1989.
Kampheus J. Calcium metabolism of rabbits as an etiological factor for urolithiasis. J Nutr 1991;121:595–596.
Pare JA, Paul-Murphy J. Disorders of the reproductive and urinary systems. In: Quesenberry KE, Carpenter JW, eds. Ferrets, Rabbits and Rodents: Clinical Medicine and Surgery. 2nd Ed. Philadelphia: WB Saunders, 2004:183–193.
Paul-Murphy J, Ramer JC. Urgent care of the pet rabbits. Vet Clin North Am Exotic Anim Pract 1998;1(1):127–152.
Redrobe S. Calcium metabolism in rabbits. Semin Avian Exotic Pet Med 2002;11(2):94–101.

### Portions Adapted From
Cowgill LP. Renal Failure, Acute. Adams LG. Renal Failure, Chronic. In: Tilley LP, Smith FWK, Jr., eds. The 5-Minute Veterinary Consult: Canine and Feline, 3rd Ed. Baltimore: Lippincott Williams & Wilkins, 2004.

# RHINITIS AND SINUSITIS

## BASICS

### DEFINITION
• Rhinitis—inflammation of the mucous membrane of the nose
• Sinusitis—inflammation of the associated paranasal sinuses
• Rhinosinusitis is a coined term, because one rarely occurs without the other.

### PATHOPHYSIOLOGY
• May be acute or chronic, noninfectious or infectious
• All causes are often complicated by opportunistic secondary microbial invasion.
• Associated mucosal vascular congestion and friability, excessive mucous gland secretion, neutrophil chemotaxis, and nasolacrimal duct obstruction—lead to congestion, obstructed airflow, sneezing, epistaxis, nasal discharge (mucopurulent), and epiphora
• In rabbits, the most common cause is bacterial infection. Infection usually begins in the nasal cavity and may spread via the eustachian tubes to the ears, into the sinuses and bones of the face, via the nasolacrimal duct to the eye, via the trachea to the lower respiratory tract, and hematogenously to joints, bones, and other organ systems.
• Recurrent or refractory bacterial infections are common due to foci in inaccessible regions (deep within the sinuses, bone, etc.) and destruction of turbinates.
• Turbinate and facial bone destruction commonly occurs secondary to dental disease and tooth root abscesses.
• Turbinate and facial bone destruction may also develop with neoplastic or fungal disease (less common).

### SYSTEMS AFFECTED
• Respiratory—mucosa of the upper respiratory tract, including the nasal cavities, sinuses, and nasopharynx
• Ophthalmic—extension to the eyes via nasolacrimal duct
• Musculoskeletal—extension of infection into bones of the skull
• Neurologic—extension of infection through eustachian tube causing vestibular signs from otitis interna/media
• Oral cavity—dental disease, tooth root abscess

### GENETICS
Unknown

### INCIDENCE/PREVALENCE
• Bacterial respiratory infection—one of the most common diseases encountered in clinical practice
• Tooth roots extending into sinuses also common cause

• Nasal tumors and foreign bodies seen occasionally

### GEOGRAPHIC DISTRIBUTION
N/A

### SIGNALMENT
No breed or sex predilection

#### Mean Age and Range
• Infectious and congenital disease—younger animals
• Tumor, infectious disease, and dental disease—middle-aged to old animals

### SIGNS

#### Historical Findings
• Sneezing, nasal discharge, staining of the front paws, epistaxis
• Ptyalism, anorexia, preference for soft foods with dental disease
• Epiphora, ocular discharge with extension into the eyes via nasolacrimal duct or with nasolacrimal duct obstruction (dried exudates, strictures)
• Head tilt, scratching at ears with extension into the ears via eustachian tubes

#### Physical Examination Findings
• Nasal discharge—bilateral with bacterial; unilateral suggests foreign body, tooth root abscess, or neoplasm; secretions or dried discharges on the hair around the nose and front limbs, facial alopecia and pyoderma
• Epistaxis—suggests neoplastic disease, tooth root abscesses, invasive bacterial infection and foreign body; erosion may bleed; violent sneezing may cause traumatic epistaxis.
• Diminished nasal airflow—unilateral or bilateral
• Ocular discharge—serous or purulent with nasolacrimal obstruction; purulent with extension of bacterial infection to conjunctiva; exophthalmos with retrobulbar abscess
• Concurrent dental disease, especially tooth root impaction or abscess, malocclusion and incisor overgrowth; findings may include ptyalism, anorexia, nasal discharge, ocular discharge, exophthalmia. Always perform a thorough oral examination.
• Frontal and facial bone deformity—bacterial or neoplastic disease

### CAUSES

#### Infectious
• *Staphylococcus aureus, Bordetella bronchiseptica, Moraxella catarrhalis, Pseudomonas aeruginosa, Mycobacterium* spp., *Pasteurella multocida,* and various anaerobes have been implicated.
• Odontogenic abscesses—*Pasteurella* usually not present; common isolates from these sites include *Streptococcus* spp.; anaerobic bacteria cultured include *Fusobacterium nucleatum, Prevotella* spp., *Peptostreptococcus micros, Actinomyces israelii,* and *Arcanobacterium haemolyticum.*

#### Noninfectious
• Dental disease—periapical or tooth root abscesses, elongated maxillary tooth roots penetrating into nasal passages with secondary bacterial infection
• Facial trauma
• Foreign body—mostly inhaled vegetable matter (e.g., grass and seeds)
• Allergic or irritant—inhaled pollen, moldy bedding, dusty litter, or cigarette smoke
• Neoplasia—squamous cell carcinoma, osteosarcoma, chondrosarcoma, and fibrosarcoma

### RISK FACTORS
• Immunosuppression—caused by stress, concurrent disease, or corticosteroid use most important risk factor in developing pasteurellosis
• Poor husbandry—dirty, molding bedding; ammonia buildup from urine-soaked bedding, dusty cat litter, cleaning agents. Dietary—diets too low in coarse fiber content (long-stemmed hay) predispose to dental disease.

## DIAGNOSIS

### DIFFERENTIAL DIAGNOSIS
• Epistaxis—coagulopathy or hypertension
• Facial swelling—abscess, neoplasia, primary dental disease
• Epiphora—incisor root impaction, abscess or dried exudate blocking the nasolacrimal duct, primary conjunctivitis, irritation

### CBC/BIOCHEMISTRY/URINALYSIS
Hemogram—TWBC elevations are usually not seen with bacterial diseases. A relative neutrophilia and/or lymphopenia are more common.

### OTHER LABORATORY TESTS
Serology for *Pasteurella*—usefulness is severely limited and generally not helpful in the diagnosis of pasteurellosis in pet rabbits. An ELISA is available and results are reported as negative, low positive, or high positive. Positive results, even when high, only indicate prior exposure to *Pasteurella* and the development of antibodies and do not confirm active infection. Low-positive results may occur due to cross-reaction with other, nonpathogenic bacteria (false positive). False-negative results are common with immunosuppression or early infection. No evidence exists to support correlation of titers to the presence or absence of disease.

### IMAGING
• Thoracic radiographs are indicated in rabbits with bacterial rhinitis. Subclinical pneumonia is common; often detected only radiographically

## RHINITIS AND SINUSITIS

• Skull series radiology—must be taken under general anesthesia; especially indicated with suspected dental disease
• Patients with nasal discharge (e.g., hemorrhagic, mucous, or serous) have fluid density that obscures nasal detail.
• Bony lysis or proliferation of the turbinate and facial bones are important radiographic finding, consistent with chronic bacterial and neoplastic invasion.
• Assess the apical roots of the incisors; elongation of the roots of the cheek teeth may penetrate the sinuses and be visible radiographically.
• CT scans or MRI is extremely helpful in detecting the extent of bony changes associated with bacterial rhinitis/sinusitis and delineating dental disease and nasal tumors.

### DIAGNOSTIC PROCEDURES
• Cytology—nasal swab or flush rarely yields diagnostic sample; nonspecific inflammation is most commonly found.
• Cultures—may be difficult to interpret, since commonly isolated bacteria (e.g., *Bordetella* sp.) often represent only commensal organisms or opportunistic pathogens. A heavy growth of a single organism is usually significant. Deep cultures obtained by inserting a mini-tipped culturette 2–4 cm into each nostril are sometimes reliable. However, samples taken from the nares should not be overinterpreted, since the causative agent may be located only deep within the sinuses and not present at the rostral portion of the nostrils, where samples are readily accessible.
• A lack of growth does not rule out bacterial disease, since the infection may be in an inaccessible, deep area of the nasal cavity or sinuses and many organisms (especially anaerobes and *Pasteurella* sp.) can be difficult to grow on culture.
• PCR assay for pasteurellosis may also be performed on samples taken from deep nasal swabs. Positive results should not be overinterpreted. *Pasteurella* is often a co-pathogen with other bacteria; presence of organism alone does not confirm *Pasteurella* as the sole causative agent.
• Biopsy of the nasal cavity is indicated in any animal with chronic nasal discharge in which neoplasia is suspected. Specimens may be obtained by direct endoscopic biopsy or rhinotomy. Multiple samples may be necessary to ensure adequate representation of the disease process.
• Rhinoscopy can be extremely valuable to visualize nasal abnormalities, retrieve foreign bodies, or obtain biopsy samples; sometimes it is the only method of identifying foreign bodies.

 TREATMENT

### APPROPRIATE HEALTH CARE
Depends on underlying cause

### NURSING CARE
• Provide oxygen supplementation if patient appears to be dyspneic; rabbits are obligate nasal breathers; nasal discharge can cause severe dyspnea.
• Symptomatic treatment and nursing care are important in the treatment of rabbits with nasal discharge. Patient hydration, nutrition, warmth, and hygiene (keeping nares clean) are important.
• Humidification of environment often helps mobilize nasal discharge and enhances patient comfort.
• Nebulization with normal saline may be useful to humidify airways.
• If epiphora or ocular discharge is present and the patient is not dyspneic, cannulate and flush the nasolacrimal duct. Topical administration of an ophthalmic anesthetic is generally sufficient for this procedure; nervous rabbits may require sedation with midazolam (1–2 mg/kg IM). Rabbits have only a single nasolacrimal punctum located in the ventral eyelid at the medial canthus. A 23-gauge lacrimal cannula or a 24-gauge Teflon intravenous catheter can be use to flush the duct. Irrigation will generally produce a thick, white exudate from the nasal meatus. Irrigation of the duct often needs to be repeated, either daily for 2–3 consecutive days, or once every 3–4 days until irrigation produces a clear fluid. Instill an ophthalmic antibiotic solution such as ciprofloxacin or chloramphenicol four to six times a day for 14–21 days.
• Remove environmental allergens/irritants (dusty litters, moldy hay or bedding); provide clean bedding and airspace.

### ACTIVITY
No change

### DIET
• It is absolutely imperative that the rabbit continue to eat during and following treatment. Anorexia will often cause gastrointestinal hypomotility, derangement of the gastrointestinal microflora, and overgrowth of intestinal bacterial pathogens.
• Offer a large selection of fresh, moistened greens such as cilantro, romaine lettuce, parsley, carrot tops, dandelion greens, spinach, collard greens, etc., and good-quality grass hay. Many rabbits will begin to eat these foods, even if they were previously anorectic.

• If the patient refuses these foods, syringe feed a gruel such as Critical Care for Herbivores (Oxbow Pet Products, Murdock, NE), giving approximately 10–15 mL/kg PO q6–8h. Alternatively, pellets can be ground and mixed with fresh greens, vegetable baby foods, water, or juice to form a gruel.
• High-carbohydrate, high-fat nutritional supplements are contraindicated.
• Encourage oral fluid intake by offering fresh water, wetting leafy vegetables, or flavoring water with vegetable juices.

### CLIENT EDUCATION
If underlying disease (dental disease, severe tissue destruction, chronic bacterial disease) is not correctable, warn client that a cure is unlikely in rabbits with chronic bacterial sinusitis. The goal of treatment is to control the more severe clinical signs with medication. Also warn the client that treatment may be lifelong.

### SURGICAL CONSIDERATIONS
Treat associated dental disease—extractions; debride abscesses.

 MEDICATIONS

### DRUG(S) OF CHOICE
*Antibiotics*
• Improvement noted in most patients, irrespective of the underlying cause
• Secondary bacterial infection may cause many clinical signs.
• Relapse common with cessation of treatment
• Systemic therapy—at least 4–6 weeks often is indicated to help prevent deep colonization by the resident flora; lifelong treatment may be indicated in some cases.
• Low-dose, once-daily treatment may be continued indefinitely to maintain remission in some patients; never a substitute for a thorough diagnostic evaluation
• Selection based on results of nasal culture or empirically
• Use broad-spectrum antibiotics such as enrofloxacin (5–20 mg/kg PO, IM, SC q12–24h) or trimethoprim sulfa (30 mg/kg PO q12h). Anaerobic bacteria are usually causative agents of tooth root abscess; use of antibiotics is effective against anaerobes such as azithromycin (30 mg/kg PO q24h); it can be used alone or combined with metronidazole (20 mg/kg PO q12h). Alternatively, use penicillin g (40,000–60,000 IU/kg SC q2–7d) or chloramphenicol (50 mg/kg PO q8h).

## CONTRAINDICATIONS

• Topical nasal decongestants containing phenylephrine can exacerbate nasal inflammation and cause nasal ulceration and purulent rhinitis.
• Oral administration of antibiotics that select against Gram-positive bacteria (penicillins, macrolides, lincosamides, and cephalosporins) can cause fatal enteric dysbiosis and enterotoxemia.
• The use of corticosteroids (systemic or topical in otic preparations) can severely exacerbate bacterial infection.

## PRECAUTIONS
N/A

## POSSIBLE INTERACTIONS
N/A

## ALTERNATIVE DRUGS

• Antihistamines have been used in rabbits with suspected allergic rhinitis and symptomatically in rabbits with infectious rhinitis. Use is anecdotal and dosages have been extrapolated from feline dosages: hydroxyzine (2 mg/kg PO q8–12h); diphenhydramine (2 mg/kg PO, SC q8–12h).
• Topical (intranasal) administration of ciprofloxacin ophthalmic drops in nares may be used in conjunction with systemic antibiotic therapy.
• Nebulization with saline may be beneficial.

 FOLLOW-UP

## PATIENT MONITORING
Clinical assessment and monitoring for relapse of clinical signs

## PREVENTION/AVOIDANCE
Avoid stressful conditions, corticosteroid use; provide excellent diet and husbandry.

## POSSIBLE COMPLICATIONS
• Extension of infection into the brain, mouth, eyes, ears, or lungs

• Loss of appetite
• Dyspnea as a result of nasal obstruction

## EXPECTED COURSE AND PROGNOSIS
• Prognosis depends on cause and chronicity
• Chronic infection—prognosis guarded to poor for complete resolution of clinical signs, depending on invasiveness (e.g., poor with extensive turbinate destruction, CNS signs)
• Neoplasms—prognosis grave to poor

 MISCELLANEOUS

## ASSOCIATED CONDITIONS
• Dental disease
• Gastrointestinal hypomotility
• Abscessation

## AGE-RELATED FACTORS
• Most of the infectious causes are found in young animals.
• Neoplasms—more common in old animals

## ZOONOTIC POTENTIAL
N/A

## PREGNANCY
N/A

## SEE ALSO
• Abscessation
• Cheek tooth malocclusion and elongation
• Dyspnea and tachypnea
• Pasteurellosis

## ABBREVIATIONS
• CNS = central nervous system
• CT = computed tomography
• ELISA = enzyme-linked immunosorbent assay
• MRI = magnetic resonance imaging
• PCR = polymerase chain reaction
• TWBC = total white blood cell

*Suggested Reading*

Bennet RA. Treatment of abscesses in the head of rabbits. Proc North Am Vet Conf 1999;821–823.

Crossley DA. Oral biology and disorders of lagomorphs. Vet Clin North Am Exotic Anim Pract 2003;6(3):629–659.

Crossley DA, Aiken S. Small mammal dentistry. In: Quesenberry KE, Carpenter JW, eds. Ferrets, Rabbits and Rodents: Clinical Medicine and Surgery. 2nd Ed. Philadelphia: WB Saunders, 2004:370–382.

Deeb BJ. Respiratory disease and pasteurellosis. In: Quesenberry KE, Carpenter JW, eds. Ferrets, Rabbits and Rodents: Clinical Medicine and Surgery. 2nd Ed. Philadelphia: WB Saunders, 2004:172–182

Deeb BL, DiGiacomo RF. Respiratory diseases of rabbits. Vet Clin North Am Exotic Anim Pract 2000;2(2):465–480.

DeLong D, Manning PJ. Bacterial diseases. In: Manning P, Ringler DH, Newcomer CE, eds. The Biology of the Laboratory Rabbit. Orlando, FL: Academic Press, 1994:129–170.

Harcourt-Brown F. Cardiorespiratory diseases. In Harcourt-Brown F, ed. Textbook of Rabbit Medicine. Oxford: Butterworth-Heinemann, 2002:324–335.

Langan GP, Schaeffer DO. Rabbit microbiology and virology. In: Fudge AM, ed. Laboratory Medicine: Avian and Exotic Pets. Philadelphia: WB Saunders, 2000:325–333.

*Portions Adapted From*

Mason RA. Rhinitis and Sinusitis. In: Tilley LP, Smith FWK, Jr., eds. The 5-Minute Veterinary Consult: Canine and Feline, 2nd Ed. Baltimore: Lippincott Williams & Wilkins, 2000.

**BASICS**

## DEFINITION
• Clinical manifestation of excessive discharges of hyperexcitable cerebrocortical neurons
• Clinical signs vary depending on the area of the cortex involved.

## PATHOPHYSIOLOGY
• Intracranial and extracranial—result in focal or diffuse hyperexcitability of cerebrocortical neurons
• High-frequency and sustained activity may recruit other parts of the brain into the epileptic discharge and cause neuronal damage, leading to more frequent and refractory seizures (in both acute and chronic disorders).

## SYSTEMS AFFECTED
Nervous

## SIGNALMENT
• White, blue-eyed rabbits may be more likely to have idiopathic epilepsy.
• Dwarf breeds and older and immunosuppressed rabbits may be more predisposed to infection with *Encephalitozoon cuniculi*.
• Lop-eared rabbits may be predisposed to otitis interna/media with subsequent brain involvement.

## SIGNS
### General Comments
• Usually sudden onset; short duration (<2 minutes); abrupt termination; often followed by postictal disturbances (e.g., mental confusion, apparent blindness)
• May occur as isolated events, cluster seizures (more than two within 24 hours), or status epilepticus
• Generalized more common than partial

### Historical Findings
• Seizure history (e.g., age at first seizure; type; initial and subsequent frequency)—may reveal clues about the underlying cause
• History of upper respiratory infection, dental disease, otitis externa/interna in rabbits with bacterial encephalitis or brain abscesses
• History of grazing outdoors consistent with parasitic encephalitis (*Baylisascaris*, toxoplasmosis)
• History of head trauma

### Physical Examination Findings
• Physical abnormalities—may be related to the seizures, indicating multisystemic disease (e.g., infectious, metabolic)
• Head tilt accompanied by other vestibular signs often seen in rabbits with brain abscess, encephalitozoonosis

• In rabbits with otitis, thick, white, creamy exudate may be found in the horizontal and/or vertical canals.
• Some rabbits with otitis interna have no visible otoscopic lesions. Infection is due to extention via eustacian tube.

## CAUSES
### Extracranial Causes
• Metabolic—severe hypoglycemia and hypocalcemia; advanced hepatic encephalopathy
• Toxicities—heavy metal; many other intoxications in their advanced stages
• Hypoxic—cardiovascular diseases

### Intracranial Causes (Most Common)
• Functional (idiopathic and genetic) epilepsy—poorly documented
• Structural brain lesions—infectious encephalitides (bacterial infections, encephalitozoonosis, toxoplasmosis, and *Baylisascaris*) most common; less frequent: ischemic encephalopathy and brain tumors

## RISK FACTORS
Any brain lesion involving the forebrain

 **DIAGNOSIS**

## DIFFERENTIAL DIAGNOSIS
### Similar Signs
• Severe vestibular disease—continuous rolling, distress, and paddling may mimic seizures or accompany seizures; differentiated by history and physical examination (torticollis, abnormal nystagmus)
• Syncope—rare in rabbits; sudden loss of consciousness and muscle tone resulting in flaccid recumbency and followed by complete recovery within seconds; differentiated by history and physical examination (e.g., episodes induced by stress or exercise, cardiovascular abnormalities such as heart murmur and arrhythmias)

### Differentiating Causes
• Metabolic and hypoxic disorders—other historical, clinical, and laboratory signs
• Toxins—history of exposure to lead: may have intermittent seizures; other toxins: a progression from shaking to trembling and finally to sustained status epilepticus until treatment or death
• Structural brain lesions—other forebrain signs; acute onset of high-frequency seizures with no sign of extracranial causes

## CBC/BIOCHEMISTRY/URINALYSIS
Usually normal unless multisystemic disease exists

## OTHER LABORATORY TESTS
• Serologic testing for *E. cuniculi*—many tests are available, but usefulness is extremely limited since a positive titer indicates only exposure and does not confirm

*E. cuniculi* as the cause of neurologic signs. *E. cuniculi* can only be definitively diagnosed by finding organisms and resultant lesions on histopathologic examination in areas that anatomically correlate with observed clinical signs. Antibody titers usually become positive by 2 weeks postinfection, but generally do not continue to rise with active infection or decline with treatment. No correlation exists between antibody titers and shedding of organism and presence or severity of disease. It is unknown if exposed rabbits eventually become seronegative. Available tests include ELISA, indirect IFA, and carbon immunoassay.
• Serology for *Pasteurella*—suspected brain abscess, encephalitis; usefulness is severely limited and generally not helpful in the diagnosis of pasteurellosis in pet rabbits. An ELISA is available and results are reported as negative, low positive, or high positive. Positive results, even when high, only indicate prior exposure to *Pasteurella* and the development of antibodies and do not confirm active infection. Low-positive results may occur due to cross-reaction with other, nonpathogenic bacteria (false positive). False-negative results are common with immunosuppression or early infection. No evidence exists to support correlation of titers to the presence or absence of disease.

## IMAGING
• Tympanic bullae—may help rule out otitis interna/media; however, normal radiographs do not rule out bulla disease.
• Skull radiography—usually unrewarding; calcified meningiomas or associated calvarial hyperostosis reported in other species, but not in rabbits
• CT and MRI—extremely valuable for confirming bulla lesions and CNS extension from peripheral locations; document or localize tumor, granuloma, and extent of inflammation.

## DIAGNOSTIC PROCEDURES
CSF analysis—may be helpful to detect active brain diseases; findings often nonspecific

 **TREATMENT**
• Known cause—treat, if possible.
• Outpatient—isolated seizures
• Inpatient—cluster seizures; status epilepticus; treat rapidly and aggressively.

## NURSING AND SUPPORTIVE CARE
• Constantly supervise hospitalized patient.
• Cool down if hyperthermic.
• Install IV line for drug and fluid administration.
• Use 0.9% sodium chloride over 5% glucose to avoid drug precipitation.

## CLIENT EDUCATION
- Emphasize the importance of the diagnostic workup.
- Inform client that antiepileptic treatment is only symptomatic and may not consistently help unless a primary cause can be identified and treated.
- Instruct the client to keep a seizure calendar.

## MEDICATIONS

### DRUG(S) OF CHOICE

*Severe Cluster Seizures and Status Epilepticus*
- Diazepam—1–5 mg/kg IV; begin with 0.5–1.0 mg/kg IV bolus; may repeat if gross seizure activity has not stopped within 5 minutes; can be administered rectally if IV access cannot be obtained; may diminish or stop the gross motor seizure activity to allow IV catheter placement
- Constant rate infusion protocols used in dogs and cats have been anecdotally used.
- Administer 50% dextrose, 0.25–2.0 ml IV slow bolus (1–3 minutes) to effect in hypoglycemic animals.

*Chronically Recurrent Seizures*
Phenobarbital—has been anecdotally used at dosages used in dogs and cats: 1–2.5 mg/kg PO q12h

*For Bacterial Meningoencephalitis and Abscess*
Antibiotics—choice is ideally based on results of culture and susceptibility testing when possible (otitis, extension from sinuses). Long-term antibiotic therapy is generally required (4–6 weeks minimum to several months). Use broad-spectrum antibiotics such as enrofloxacin (10–20 mg/kg PO q12–24h) or trimethoprim sulfa (30 mg/kg PO q12h); if anaerobic infections are suspected use chloramphenicol (50 mg/kg PO q8h), metronidazole (20 mg/kg PO q12h), azithromycin (30 mg/kg PO q24h) (can be used alone or combined with metronidazole), or parenteral penicillin g (40,000–60,000 IU/kg SC q2–7d).

*For Encephalitozoonosis*
Benzimidazole anthelmintics are effective against *E. cuniculi* in vitro and have been shown to prevent experimental infection in rabbits. However, efficacy in rabbits with clinical signs is unknown. Anecdotal reports suggest a response to treatment; however, many rabbits with neurologic signs improve with or without treatment. Published treatments include oxibendazole (20–30 mg/kg PO q24h × 7–14 days, then reduce to 15 mg/kg q24h × 30–60 days), albendazole (20–30 mg/kg q24h × 30 days, then 15 mg/kg PO q24h × 30 days), and fenbendazole (20 mg/kg q24h × 5–28 days).

*For Toxoplasmosis*
Trimethoprim sulfa (15–30 mg/kg PO q12h); sulfadiazine in combination with pyrimethamine for 2 weeks has also been recommended.

### CONTRAINDICATIONS
- Dexamethasone—contraindicated in patients with infectious diseases, but may help decrease brain edema when impending brain herniation or life-threatening edema is suspected
- Oral administration of antibiotics that select against Gram-positive bacteria (penicillins, macrolides, lincosamides, and cephalosporins) can cause fatal enteric dysbiosis and enterotoxemia.
- Acepromazine, ketamine, xylazine, bronchodilators (e.g., aminophylline, terbutaline, theophylline), and estrogens—do not administer to any patient with documented or potential seizures; lower seizure threshold.

### PRECAUTIONS
- Intensive parenteral antiepileptic drug therapy—requires constant monitoring and care; hypothermia common; persistent subtle seizure activity difficult to recognize; potential cardiovascular and respiratory depression with overdosage
- Albendazole has been associated with bone marrow toxicity in dogs and cats; toxicity in rabbits is unknown; however, anecdotal reports of pancytopenia leading to death in rabbits exist.
- Never leave a patient with historical, actual, or potential seizures hospitalized without constant supervision; if monitoring cannot be provided on a 24-hour basis, send the patient home or refer it to an emergency clinic.

### POSSIBLE INTERACTIONS
Cimetidine, ranitidine, and chloramphenicol—may decrease the metabolism of phenobarbital

### ALTERNATIVE DRUGS
Phenobarbital, propofol for status epilepticus; potassium bromide—anecdotally used following canine and feline protocols

## FOLLOW-UP

### PATIENT MONITORING
- CBC, biochemistry, and urinalysis—evaluate before initiation of maintenance oral antiepileptic drug therapy; then monitor every 6–12 months.
- Have owners keep a diary of seizure activity—adjust medications based on clinical response.
- Measurement of serum phenobarbital concentration after treatment initiation—optimal concentration unknown in rabbits; anecdotally lower than expected; may not correlate well with clinical control of seizures

- Epilepsy secondary to treated primary disease—slowly and gradually wean patient off the antiepileptic drug after 6 months without seizures; if seizures recur, reinstate the drug.

### POSSIBLE COMPLICATIONS
- Phenobarbital—hepatotoxicity possible with chronic use; although not reported in rabbits, thrombocytopenia, neutropenia, pruritus, and swelling of the feet may occur in other mammals.
- Diazepam—acute hepatic necrosis reported in other species
- Seizures may continue despite adequate antiepileptic therapy; refractoriness to diazepam may develop.
- Hypoglycemia and hyperthermia with prolonged seizures
- Status epilepticus, leading to death
- Permanent neurologic deficits may follow severe status epilepticus regardless of the cause.
- Progression of disease with deterioration of mental status

### EXPECTED COURSE AND PROGNOSIS
Prognosis—guarded depending on underlying cause; varied response to drug treatment

## MISCELLANEOUS

### ASSOCIATED CONDITIONS
- Dental disease
- Upper respiratory infections
- Facial abscesses
- Gastrointestinal hypomotility

### AGE-RELATED FACTORS
Encephalitozoonosis and bacterial disease may be more common in older, especially immunosuppressed animals.

### ZOONOTIC POTENTIAL
Encephalitozoonosis—unlikely, but possible in immunosuppressed humans. Mode of transmission and susceptibility in humans are unclear.

### PREGNANCY
N/A

### SEE ALSO
- Ataxia
- Encephalitis and meningioencephalitis
- Poisoning (Intoxication)

### ABBREVIATIONS
- CBC = complete blood count
- CNS = central nervous system
- CSF = cerebrospinal fluid
- CT = computed tomography
- IFA = immunofluorescence assay
- ELISA = enzyme-linked immunosorbent assay
- MRI = magnetic resonance imaging

## SEIZURES

*Suggested Reading*

de Lahunta A. Veterinary Neuroanatomy and Clinical Neurology. 2nd Ed. Philadelphia: Saunders, 1983.

Deeb BJ, Carpenter JW. Neurologic and musculoskeletal diseases. In: Quesenberry KE, Carpenter JW, eds. Ferrets, Rabbits and Rodents: Clinical Medicine and Surgery. 2nd Ed. Philadelphia: WB Saunders, 2004:203–210.

Harcourt-Brown F. Neurological and locomotor diseases. In: Harcourt-Brown F, ed. Textbook of Rabbit Medicine. Oxford: Butterworth-Heinemann, 2002:307–323.

Oliver JE, Lorenz MD. Handbook of Veterinary Neurologic Diagnosis. 2nd Ed. Philadelphia: Saunders, 1993.

Paul-Murphy J, Ramer JC. Urgent care of the pet rabbits. Vet Clin North Am Exotic Anim Pract 1998;1(1):127–152.

Rosenthal KR. Torticollis in rabbits. Proc North Am Vet Conf 2005;1378–1379.

*Portions Adapted From*

Quesnel AD. Seizures (Convulsions, Status Epilepticus)—Cats. In: Tilley LP, Smith FWK, Jr., eds. The 5-Minute Veterinary Consult: Canine and Feline, 3rd Ed. Baltimore: Lippincott Williams & Wilkins, 2004.

## BASICS

### OVERVIEW
• A sporadic cutaneous viral disease of pet rabbits caused by a virus in the Papovaviridae family
• Virus is oncogenic; characteristic cutaneous lesions can progress to malignant squamous cell carcinoma; metastasis may occur.
• It is seen in domestic and wild rabbits.
• Virus is spread via biting arthropods, primarily mosquitos and ticks.
• Clinical signs in pet rabbit consist of characteristic skin lesions.

### SIGNALMENT
• Pet rabbits (*Oryctolagus cuniculus*) and wild cottontail rabbits (*Sylvilagus* spp.)
• Outdoor rabbits may be at greater risk due to mode of viral transmission.
• Highest incidence in rabbits living in California; occurs sporadically all over North America

### SIGNS
• Raised, red, well-demarcated, rough, usually circular cutaneous lesions; often 1 cm or more in diameter
• Lesions are often friable; bleed readily with trauma
• Cutaneous nodules occur most commonly on the eyelids, ears, and feet in domestic (pet) rabbits.
• Nodules occur around the neck and shoulder areas most commonly in wild rabbits.
• Lesions sometimes spontaneously regress.

### CAUSES AND RISK FACTORS
• Oncogenic, DNA virus in the Papovaviridae family
• Outbreaks may be more likely when mosquitos are numerous (summer, fall).

## DIAGNOSIS

### CBC/BIOCHEMISTRY/URINALYSIS
N/A

### OTHER LABORATORY TESTS
Virus isolation

### IMAGING
N/A

### DIAGNOSTIC PROCEDURES
Histologic examination of excised nodules to confirm diagnosis

### PATHOLOGIC FINDINGS
Cutaneous nodules—raised, round, red, keratinized epithelial nodules

*Histopathology*
Hyperkeratosis; may contain characteristic inclusions bodies

## TREATMENT

• Surgical excision of nodules is indicated. Nodules are frequently friable and bleed easily; may transform into malignant squamous cell carcinoma
• Nodules sometimes regress spontaneously.

## MEDICATIONS

### DRUG(S) OF CHOICE
N/A

### CONTRADINDICATIONS/POSSIBLE INTERACTIONS
N/A

## FOLLOW-UP

### PREVENTION/AVOIDANCE
Control of vectors—screening to keep out insects; flea control; keep indoors.

## MISCELLANEOUS

### ZOONOTIC POTENTIAL
None

*Suggested Reading*

Harcourt-Brown F. Infectious diseases of domestic rabbits. In: Harcourt-Brown F, ed. Textbook of Rabbit Medicine. Oxford: Butterworth-Heinemann, 2002:361–385.

Hess L. Dermatologic diseases. In: Quesenberry KE, Carpenter JW, eds. Ferrets, Rabbits and Rodents: Clinical Medicine and Surgery. 2nd Ed. Philadelphia: WB Saunders, 2004:194–202.

Jenkins JR. Skin disorders of the rabbit. Vet Clin North Am Exotic Anim Pract 2001;4(2):543–563.

Langan GP, Schaeffer DO. Rabbit microbiology and virology. In: Fudge AM, ed. Laboratory Medicine: Avian and Exotic Pets. Philadelphia: WB Saunders, 2000:325–333.

# SPONDYLOSIS DEFORMANS

## BASICS

### OVERVIEW
• Degenerative, noninflammatory condition of the vertebral column characterized by the production of osteophytes along the ventral, lateral, and dorsolateral aspects of the vertebral endplates
• Lumbar spine is most commonly affected.
• Most rabbits are asymptomatic, and radiographic evidence of spondylosis often does not correlate well with clinical signs. Pain from any source will often make a rabbit reluctant to move or groom. A thorough history and physical examination should be performed to rule out other, more common causes of pain before attributing radiographic lesions of spondylosis to clinical signs.

### SIGNALMENT
• Seen more often in medium to large breeds
• Occurrence increases with age; most often in rabbits >3 years old

### SIGNS

#### General Comments
• Many rabbits are asymptomatic. Clinical signs often do not correlate well with radiographic findings.
• Always rule out other, more common causes of pain and reluctance to ambulate (degenerative joint disease, septic arthritis, intervertebral disc disease, spinal trauma, dental disease, urolithiasis).
• If signs are present, they are most often referable to an inability to properly groom or attain a normal stance while urinating due to stiffness or pain. Affected rabbits may be unable to groom the intrascapular, perineal, or tail head region, or may be unable to consume cecotrophs from the rectum. If unable to attain a normal stance while urinating, urine may soak the ventrum, resulting in urine scald.
• Gait abnormalities, reluctance to jump anecdotally reported as second most common clinical sign

#### Physical Examination Findings
• Neurologic deficits referable to the spinal cord or nerve root compression
• Ataxia, rear limb weakness
• Ulcerative pododermatitis
• Perineal dermatitis—matted fur, urine-soaked perineum or ventrum, feces pasted to perineum, alopecia, erythema, ulceration, myiasis
• Alopecia, flaking, *Cheyletiella* mites in intrascapular or tail head region due to inadequate grooming

• Accumulation of wax in ear canals from inadequate grooming
• Hypercalciuria secondary to insufficient voiding
• Obesity

### CAUSES AND RISK FACTORS
• Repeated microtrauma
• Major trauma
• Inherited predisposition possible
• May be related to small cage size, lack of exercise
• Obesity may predispose

## DIAGNOSIS

### DIFFERENTIAL DIAGNOSIS
• Pain from nonorthopedic disorders—rabbits may be reluctant to ambulate or groom when in pain, regardless of the source of pain.
• Discospondylitis—differentiated by radiographic evidence of end-plate lysis
• Spinal osteoarthritis—degeneration of the articular facet joints
• Degenerative joint disease
• Intervertebral disc disease

### CBC/BIOCHEMISTRY/URINALYSIS
• CBC/biochemistry profile usually normal
• Urinalysis may reflect hypercalciuria or urinary tract infection; may be secondary to insufficient voiding or primary cause of pain and reluctance to ambulate

### OTHER LABORATORY TESTS
N/A

### IMAGING
• Spinal radiography—initially shows osteophytes as projecting from the edge of the vertebral body; with progression, they appear to bridge the intervertebral space. Signs do not always correlate well with clinical signs. Many rabbits with significant radiographic abnormalities remain pain free.
• Skull radiographs—to rule out dental disease as a cause of pain and reluctance to groom or ambulate
• Whole body radiographs—to rule out other, more common causes of pain and reluctance to groom or ambulate (arthritis, urolithiasis, etc.)

### DIAGNOSTIC PROCEDURES
Myelography and CT or MRI—to rule out intervertebral disc disease or other spinal disorders; unusual cases of spondylosis may demonstrate an atypical dorsal osteophyte compressing the spinal cord or nerve roots or encroaching on critical soft tissue structures.

## TREATMENT

### APPROPRIATE HEALTH CARE
• Treat as outpatient with limited exercise and analgesic administration.
• Obesity—recommend a weight-reduction program.

### NURSING CARE
For all rabbits that do not groom or are nonambulatory:
• Keep perineum clean, dry, and free of fecal matter.
• Remove matted hair. Be extremely cautious when clipping hair or pulling on mats since rabbit skin is extremely fragile and will easily tear. Sedation may be required.
• Use soft bedding; keep bedding clean and dry to prevent dermatitis or bed sores.

## MEDICATIONS

### DRUG(S) OF CHOICE
• NSAIDs—have been used for short- or long-term therapy to reduce pain and inflammation in rabbits with musculoskeletal disease: meloxicam (0.2–0.5 mg/kg PO q12–24h) or carprofen (2.2 mg/kg PO q12–24h); use only when the patient is exhibiting signs.
• Dermatitis—initially may be treated empirically with broad-spectrum antibiotics such as enrofloxacin (5–20 mg/kg PO, SC, IM q12–24h) or trimethoprim sulfa (30 mg/kg PO q12h)
• Superficial, moist dermatitis—apply zinc oxide plus menthol powder (Gold Bond, Martin Himmel, Inc.) to clean, clipped skin q24h

### CONTRAINDICATIONS
• Oral administration of antibiotics that select against Gram-positive bacteria (penicillins, macrolides, lincosamides, and cephalosporins) can cause fatal enteric dysbiosis and enterotoxemia.
• Corticosteroids—associated with gastrointestinal ulceration and hemorrhage, delayed wound healing, and heightened susceptibility to infection; rabbits are very sensitive to the immunosuppressive effects of both topical and systemic corticosteroids; use may exacerbate subclinical bacterial infection.

### PRECAUTIONS
Meloxicam—use with caution in rabbits with compromised renal function.

### ALTERNATIVE DRUGS
• Chondroitin sulfate (Cosequin, Nutramax) has been used anecdotally using feline dosage protocols; polysulfate glycosaminoglycan (Adequan, Luitpold) 2.2 mg/kg SC, IM q3d × 21–28 days, then q14d.
• Acupuncture may be effective for rabbits with chronic pain.

### FOLLOW-UP
• Gradually return the animal to normal activity after signs have subsided for several weeks.
• Relapse can occur with strenuous activity.

### PREVENTION/AVOIDANCE
• Prevent obesity.
• Encourage regular exercise throughout life.

### POSSIBLE COMPLICATIONS
• Dermatitis, urine scald, ulcerative pododermatitis (sore hocks), myiasis
• Hypercalciuria

### EXPECTED COURSE AND PROGNOSIS
Unknown; if clinical signs are present, they are likely to recur; likely to be progressive with age

### MISCELLANEOUS

### ABBREVIATIONS
• CBC = complete blood count
• CT = computed tomography
• MRI = magnetic resonance imaging
• NSAIDs = nonsteroidal antiinflammatory drugs

*Suggested Reading*

Deeb BJ, Carpenter JW. Neurologic and musculoskeletal diseases. In: Quesenberry KE, Carpenter JW, eds. Ferrets, Rabbits and Rodents: Clinical Medicine and Surgery. 2nd Ed. Philadelphia: WB Saunders, 2004:203–210.

Harcourt-Brown F. Neurological and locomotor diseases. In: Harcourt-Brown F, ed. Textbook of Rabbit Medicine. Oxford: Butterworth-Heinemann, 2002:307–323.

Kapatkin A. Orthopedics in small mammals. In: Quesenberry KE, Carpenter JW, eds. Ferrets, Rabbits and Rodents: Clinical Medicine and Surgery. 2nd Ed. Philadelphia: WB Saunders, 2004:383–391.

*Portions Adapted From*

Gram WD. Spondylosis Deformans. In: Tilley LP, Smith FWK, Jr., eds. The 5-Minute Veterinary Consult: Canine and Feline, 3rd Ed. Baltimore: Lippincott Williams & Wilkins, 2004.

# STERTOR AND STRIDOR

## BASICS

### DEFINITION
• Abnormally loud sounds that result from air passing through an abnormally narrowed upper airway and meeting resistance because of partial obstruction of these regions. In rabbits, nasal obstruction is the most common source.
• Stertor—low-pitched snoring sound that usually arises from the vibration of flaccid tissue or fluid; can arise from pharyngeal, nasal, laryngeal, or tracheal obstruction
• Stridor—higher-pitched sounds that result when relatively rigid tissues are vibrated by the passage of air; result of nasal, laryngeal, pharyngeal, or tracheal obstruction

### PATHOPHYSIOLOGY
• Rabbits are obligate nasal breathers. The rim of the epiglottis is normally situated dorsal to the elongated soft palate to allow air passage from the nose to the trachea during normal respiration. Obstruction of nasal passages, larynx, or pharynx may cause stertor or stridor.
• Airway obstruction causes turbulence as air passes through a narrowed passage; with worsening obstruction or increasing air velocity, the amplitude of the sound increases as the tissue, secretion, or foreign body composing the obstruction is vibrated.
• Obstruction sufficient enough to increase the work of breathing—respiratory muscles increase their effort and the turbulence is exacerbated; inflammation and edema of the tissues in the region of the obstruction may develop, further reducing the airway lumen and further increasing the work of breathing, creating a vicious circle. Discomfort and poor gas exchanged can produce considerable anxiety in rabbits, further worsening dyspnea.

### SYSTEMS AFFECTED
Respiratory

### SIGNALMENT
• Tumor—usually old animal
• No breed or sex predilection for other causes

### SIGNS

#### Historical Findings
• Varies with underlying cause
• Sneezing, nasal discharge, staining of the front paws, epistaxis with sinusitis/rhinitis
• Ptyalism, anorexia, bruxism, and preference for soft foods with dental disease
• History of recent intubation or attempts at intubation
• Epiphora, ocular discharge with secondary nasolacrimal duct obstruction

#### Physical Examination Findings
• Nasal discharge—bilateral with bacterial; unilateral suggests nasal foreign body, tooth root abscess, or neoplasm; secretions or dried discharges on the hair around the nose and front limbs, facial alopecia and pyoderma
• Epistaxis—suggests neoplastic disease, tooth root abscesses, invasive bacterial infection, and foreign body; erosion may bleed; violent sneezing may cause traumatic epistaxis.
• Ocular discharge—serous or purulent with secondary nasolacrimal obstruction; purulent with extension of bacterial infection to conjunctiva; exophthalmos with retrobulbar abscess
• Concurrent dental disease, especially tooth root abscess or impaction, malocclusion, and incisor overgrowth; findings may include ptyalism, anorexia, nasal discharge, ocular discharge, exophthalmia. Always perform a thorough oral examination.
• Frontal and facial bone deformity—abscess or neoplastic disease
• Partial obstruction—produces an increase in airway sounds before producing an obvious change in respiratory pattern and before producing a change in the respiratory function of gas exchange; increased sound may precede any obvious change in behavior.
• Breath sounds audible from a distance without a stethoscope—suspect narrowing of the upper airway.
• You may note increased respiratory effort and paradoxical respiratory movements (chest wall collapses inward during inspiration and springs outward during expiration) when the effort is extreme; they are often accompanied by obvious postural changes (e.g., abducted forelimbs, extended head and neck, and open-mouth breathing).

### CAUSES
• Sinusitis/rhinitis—*Staphylococcus aureus, Bordetella bronchiseptica, Moraxella catarrhalis, Pseudomonas aeruginosa, Mycobacterium* spp., *Pasteurella multocida,* and various anaerobes have been implicated.
• Dental disease—periapical or tooth root abscesses, elongated maxillary tooth roots penetrating into nasal passages with secondary bacterial infection
• Facial, nasal, or neck trauma (bite wounds, crushing injuries)
• Foreign body—mostly inhaled vegetable matter (e.g., grass and seeds)
• Allergy or irritant—inhaled pollen, moldy bedding, dusty litter, chemical irritants, or smoke
• Airway tumors
• Neuromuscular dysfunction—brainstem disease, polyneuropathy, polymyopathy, hypothyroidism
• Edema or inflammation of the palate, pharynx, and larynx—secondary to turbulent airflow, upper respiratory infection, and hemorrhage
• Edema of the epiglottis from intubation or multiple attempts at intubation
• Physiologic causes—mild to moderate upper airway noise may be heard with dyspnea of any cause, including anxiety, lower respiratory tract, and nonrespiratory causes of dyspnea.

### RISK FACTORS
• Immunosuppression—caused by stress, concurrent disease, or corticosteroid use (most important risk factor in developing bacterial rhinitis/sinusitis)
• Traumatic intubation or multiple attempts at intubation—causes severe laryngeal swelling
• Poor husbandry—dirty, molding bedding; high ammonia concentration from urine-soaked bedding, dusty cat litter
• Diet—feeding diets with insufficient coarse fiber (such as long-stemmed hay) predisposes to dental disease.
• Anxiety
• Any respiratory or cardiovascular disease that increases ventilation
• Turbulence caused by the increased airflow may lead to swelling and worsen the airway obstruction.

## DIAGNOSIS

### DIFFERENTIAL DIAGNOSIS
• Must differentiate sounds from nasal, pharyngeal and laryngeal narrowing from sounds arising elsewhere in the respiratory system
• Systematically auscultate over the nose, pharynx, larynx, and trachea to attempt to identify the point of maximal intensity of any abnormal sound and to identify the phase of respiration when it is most obvious.
• Identify the anatomic location from which the abnormal sound arises and seek exacerbating causes.

### CBC/BIOCHEMISTRY/URINALYSIS
Hemogram—TWBC elevations are usually not seen with bacterial diseases. A relative neutrophilia and/or lymphopenia are more common.

### OTHER LABORATORY TESTS
Serology for *Pasteurella*—if suspected cause of respiratory signs; usefulness is severely limited and generally not helpful in the diagnosis of pasteurellosis in pet rabbits. An ELISA is available and results are reported as negative, low positive, or high positive. Positive results, even when high, only indicate prior exposure to *Pasteurella* and the development of antibodies and do not confirm active infection. Low-positive results may occur due to cross-reaction with other,

nonpathogenic bacteria (false positive). False-negative results are common with immunosuppression or early infection. No evidence exists to support correlation of titers to the presence or absence of disease.

### IMAGING
• Skull series radiology—must be taken under general anesthesia—patients with nasal discharge (e.g., hemorrhagic, mucous, or serous) have fluid density that obscures nasal detail; bony lysis or proliferation of the turbinate and facial bones are important radiographic finding, consistent with chronic bacterial (especially tooth root abscess) and neoplastic invasion. Always assess the apical roots of the incisors; elongation of the roots of the cheek teeth may penetrate the sinuses and be visible radiographically.
• Lateral radiographs of the head and neck—may help identify abnormal soft tissues of the airway; limited use for identifying laryngeal disease; may allow further evaluation of external masses compressing the upper airway
• Thoracic radiographs are indicated in rabbits with bacterial rhinitis. Subclinical pneumonia is common; often detected only radiographically
• CT scans or MRI—more accurate in delineating nasal, sinus, or dental disease; may not be widely available

### DIAGNOSTIC PROCEDURES
• Cytology—nasal swab or flush rarely yields diagnostic sample; nonspecific inflammation is most commonly found.
• Cultures—may be difficult to interpret, since commonly isolated bacteria (e.g., *Bordetella* sp.) often represent only commensal organisms or opportunistic pathogens. A heavy growth of a single organism is usually significant. Deep cultures obtained by inserting a mini-tipped culturette 2–4 cm into each nostril are sometimes reliable. However, samples taken from the nares should not be overinterpreted, since the causative agent may be located only deep within the sinuses and not present at the rostral portion of the nostrils, where samples are readily accessible.
• A lack of growth does not rule out bacterial disease, since the infection may be in an inaccessible, deep area of the nasal cavity or sinuses and many organisms (especially anaerobes and *Pasteurella* sp.) can be difficult to grow on culture.
• Biopsy of the nasal cavity is indicated in any animal with chronic nasal discharge in which neoplasia is suspected. Specimens may be obtained by direct endoscopic biopsy or rhinotomy.

• Pharyngoscopy and laryngoscopy—using an otoendoscope or 2.7-mm rigid endoscope; allows direct visualization of pharyngeal or laryngeal disease. Requires general anesthesia; must consider risk to patient. Remember that the patient's ability to use muscles to open the airway is compromised by anesthesia. Normal palate—very long compared to dogs and cats; completely entraps the rim of the epiglottis to accommodate normal obligate nasal breathing
• Patient should be as stable as possible before undergoing general anesthesia, but do not unduly delay procedure; appropriate surgical treatment is usually the only means of reducing the airway obstruction.

## TREATMENT
• Hypoxia and hypoventilation—occur only after prolonged severe obstruction; supplemental oxygen not always critical for sustaining patients with partial airway obstruction
• Keep patient cool, quiet, and calm—anxiety, exertion, and pain lead to increased oxygen demands and increased ventilation, potentially worsening the obstruction.
• All sedatives—may relax the upper airway muscles and worsen the obstruction; closely monitor effects of sedatives; be prepared with emergency means for securing the airway if complete obstruction occurs.
• Keep nares clear of nasal discharges in rabbits with URT disease
• Extreme airway obstruction—attempt an emergency intubation; if obstruction prevents intubation, emergency tracheostomy or passage of a tracheal catheter to administer oxygen may be the only available means for sustaining life; a tracheal catheter can only briefly sustain oxygenation while a more permanent solution is sought.

### DIET
• Provide adequate nutrition.
• It is imperative that the rabbit continue to eat during and following treatment. Anorexia will often cause gastrointestinal hypomotility, derangement of the gastrointestinal microflora, and overgrowth of intestinal bacterial pathogens.
• If the patient refuses these foods, syringe feed a gruel such as Critical Care for Herbivores (Oxbow Pet Products, Murdock, NE), giving approximately 10–15 mL/kg PO q6–8h.
• Alternatively, pellets can be ground and mixed with fresh greens, vegetable baby foods, water, or juice to form a gruel.
• Encourage oral fluid intake by offering fresh water, wetting leafy vegetables, or flavoring water with vegetable juices.

## MEDICATIONS
### DRUG(S) OF CHOICE
• Antibiotics—improvement noted in most patients with primary or secondary bacterial sinusitis or rhinitis. Systemic therapy for 4–6 weeks is usually indicated. Selection is based on results of nasal culture or empirically. Use broad-spectrum antibiotics such as enrofloxacin (5–20mg/kg PO, IM, SC q12–24h) or trimethoprim sulfa (30 mg/kg PO q12h). Anaerobic bacteria are usually causative agents of tooth root abscess; use antibiotics effective against anaerobes such as azithromycin (30 mg/kg PO q24h); can be used alone or combined with metronidazole (20mg/kg PO q12h). Alternatively, use penicillin g (40,000–60,000 IU/kg SC q2–7d) or chloramphenicol (50 mg/kg PO q8h). Combine with topical treatment.
• Terbutaline has been used at feline doses to treat intubation-induced bronchoconstriction.
• Steroids—may be indicated if laryngeal edema or inflammation (posttraumatic or multiple intubation attempts)

### CONTRAINDICATIONS
• Oral administration of antibiotics that select against Gram-positive bacteria (penicillins, macrolides, lincosamides, and cephalosporins) can cause fatal enteric dysbiosis and enterotoxemia.
• Topical nasal decongestants containing phenylephrine can exacerbate nasal inflammation and cause nasal ulceration and purulent rhinitis.

### PRECAUTIONS
• The use of corticosteroids (systemic or topical in otic preparations) can severely exacerbate bacterial infection. Use only if absolutely necessary to reduce known laryngeal edema. Do not use for stertor of unknown cause or if infectious causes of respiratory tract disease are present.
• Sedatives and anesthetics

### POSSIBLE INTERACTIONS
N/A

### ALTERNATIVE DRUGS
Diuretics—may be administered; efficacy doubtful

## FOLLOW-UP
### PATIENT MONITORING
Clinical assessment and monitoring for relapse of clinical signs

## STERTOR AND STRIDOR

### POSSIBLE COMPLICATIONS
• Serious complications—may occur and persist despite efforts to relieve the obstruction; include airway edema, pulmonary edema (may progress to life-threatening acute lung injury), and hypoventilation; may require tracheostomy and/or artificial ventilation
• Take particular care when inducing general anesthesia or when using sedatives in any patient with upper airway obstruction.
• When owner chooses to take an apparently stable patient home, or if continual observation is not feasible, inform client that complete obstruction could occur.

 **MISCELLANEOUS**

### ASSOCIATED CONDITIONS
• Dental disease
• Gastrointestinal hypomotility
• Abscessation

### AGE-RELATED FACTORS
N/A

### ZOONOTIC POTENTIAL
N/A

### PREGNANCY
N/A

### SYNONYM
N/A

### SEE ALSO
• Cheek tooth malocclusion and elongation
• Rhinitis/sinusitis
• Tooth root abscesses (apical abscesses)

### ABBREVIATIONS
• CT = computed tomography
• ELISA = enzyme-linked immunosorbent assay
• MRI = magnetic resonance imaging
• URT = upper respiratory tract

*Suggested Reading*
Bennet RA. Treatment of abscesses in the head of rabbits. Proc North Am Vet Conf 1999;821–823.
Crossley DA. Oral biology and disorders of lagomorphs. Vet Clin North Am Exotic Anim Pract 2003;6(3):629–659.
Crossley DA, Aiken S. Small mammal dentistry. In: Quesenberry KE, Carpenter JW, eds. Ferrets, Rabbits and Rodents: Clinical Medicine and Surgery. 2nd Ed. Philadelphia: WB Saunders, 2004:370–382.
Deeb BJ. Respiratory disease and pasteurellosis. In: Quesenberry KE, Carpenter JW, eds. Ferrets, Rabbits and Rodents: Clinical Medicine and Surgery. 2nd Ed. Philadelphia: WB Saunders, 2004:172–182.
Deeb BJ, DiGiacomo RF. Respiratory diseases of rabbits. Vet Clin North Am Exotic Anim Pract 2000;3(2):465–480.
Ethell MT, Bennett RA, Brown MP, et al. In vitro elution of gentamicin, amikacin, and ceftiofur from polymethylmethacrylate and hydroxyapatite cement. Vet Surg 2000;29:375–382.
Harcourt-Brown F. Dental disease. In: Harcourt-Brown F, ed. Textbook of Rabbit Medicine. Oxford: Butterworth-Heinemann, 2002:165–205.
Hendricks JC. Respiratory condition in critical patients. Critical care. Vet Clin North Am Small Anim Pract 1989;19:1167–1188.
Tyrell KC, Citron DM, Jenkins JR, et al. Periodontal bacteria in rabbit mandibular and maxillary abscesses. J Clin Microbiol 2002;40(3):1044–1047.

*Portions Adapted From*
Prueter JC. Stertor and Stridor. In: Tilley LP, Smith FWK, Jr., eds. The 5-Minute Veterinary Consult: Canine and Feline, 3rd Ed. Baltimore: Lippincott Williams & Wilkins, 2004.

# BASICS

## OVERVIEW
• Neoplasia originating from thymic epithelium
• Infiltrated with lymphocytes and reticular epithelial cells
• Can occur alone or with multiorgan systemic lymphoma

## SIGNALMENT
• Anecdotally, the most common cause of mediastinal mass in rabbits
• Insufficient information exists to assess the true incidence, age, gender, or breed predilection.

## SIGNS
• Exophthalmus, third eyelid protrusion—bilateral, due to increased venous pressure from space-occupying effects of the tumor (cranial caval syndrome)
• Swelling of the head, neck, or forelimbs—cranial caval syndrome
• Tachypnea
• Dyspnea
• Muscle weakness and megaesophagus—not reported in rabbits

## CAUSES AND RISK FACTORS
N/A

# DIAGNOSIS

## DIFFERENTIAL DIAGNOSIS
• Lymphoma
• Normal thymus (does not completely regress with age in rabbits)
• Thyroid carcinoma
• Other mediastinal masses not reported in rabbits, but should be considered
• For radiographically evident soft tissue density in mediastinum—abscess, consolidated lung lobe, thymic remnant, intrathoracic fat pad

• For bilateral exophthalmos—tooth root abscess, retrobulbar neoplasia: usually painful; eyes cannot be retropulsed; with thymoma, eyes can be retropulsed and no pain is present.

## CBC/BIOCHEMISTRY/URINALYSIS
Lymphocytosis—occasionally

## OTHER LABORATORY TESTS
N/A

## IMAGING
Thoracic radiographs—may reveal a cranial mediastinal mass and/or pleural effusion

## DIAGNOSTIC PROCEDURES
Fine needle aspirate—cytologic examination shows lymphocytes (mature or pleomorphic reported) and thymic epithelial cells.

# TREATMENT
• Inpatient
• Surgical excision—may be treatment of choice; limited number of case reports available
• Radiotherapy—potentially beneficial by reducing the lymphoid component of the mass

# MEDICATIONS

## DRUG(S) OF CHOICE
• Chemotherapy—little information available; consult with oncologist.
• Prednisone—used in a very limited number of patients; may see partial remission

## CONTRAINDICATIONS/POSSIBLE INTERACTIONS
Immunosuppressive drugs—use with extreme caution; only with definitive diagnosis; immunosuppression may exacerbate subclinical *Encephalitozoon cuniculi* or bacterial infections, the result of which could be fatal.

# FOLLOW-UP
• Thoracic radiography—every 3 months recommended in other species; monitor for recurrence
• Cure—may be possible if tumor is surgically resectable
• Prognosis—poor with nonresectable tumor

# MISCELLANEOUS

## ASSOCIATED CONDITIONS
• Multiorgan system lymphoma

## SEE ALSO
• Dyspnea and tachypnea
• Exophthalmus

## Suggested Reading
Clippinger TL, Bennett RA, Alleman AR, et al. Removal of a thymoma via median sternotomy in a rabbit with recurrent appendicular neurofibrosarcoma. J Am Vet Med Assoc 1998;213:1131, 1140–1143.
Huston SM, Quesenberry KE. Cardiovascular and lymphoproliferative diseases. In: Quesenberry KE, Carpenter JW, eds. Ferrets, Rabbits and Rodents: Clinical Medicine and Surgery. 2nd Ed. Philadelphia: WB Saunders, 2004:211–220.
Vernau KM, Grahm BH, Clarke-Scott HA, et al. Thymoma in a geriatric rabbit with hypercalcemia and periodic exophthalmus. J Am Vet Med Assoc 1995;206:820–822.

# TOOTH ROOT ABSCESSES (APICAL ABSCESSES)

## BASICS

### DEFINITION
- An abscess is a localized collection of purulent exudate contained within a fibrous capsule formed by the disintegration of tissues.
- Accumulation of inflammatory cells at the apex of a nonvital tooth—periapical abscess
- Systemic spread of bacteria (bacteremia and pyemia) can affect other organ systems.
- Tooth root abscesses are one of the most common problems seen in rabbits.

### PATHOPHYSIOLOGY
- An abscess spreads along the pathway of least resistance from the tooth apex, resulting in osteomyelitis and, if perforated through the cortex forms a subcutaneous abscess that can burst through the skin to create a cutaneous sinus.
- Unlike cats and dogs, abscesses in rabbits do not often rupture and drain. Rabbit abscesses are filled with a thick, caseous exudate, surrounded by a fibrous capsule. Abscesses that perforate through bone can be extremely difficult to treat, requiring aggressive surgical intervention and prolonged medical care. Prognosis is fair to poor depending on the severity and location.
- Abscesses on the face (especially the mandible, retrobulbar and periorbital lobes) are almost always caused by extension of tooth root abscesses; occasionally they may be secondary to upper respiratory infections, otitis, or trauma.
- Most tooth root abscesses are secondary to acquired cheek tooth elongation. All rabbit teeth are open-rooted and grow continuously at a rate of approximately 3 mm per week, with growth originating from the germinal bud located at the apex of the tooth.
- The rate of normal wear should equal the rate of eruption, approximately 3 mm per week. Normal wear requires proper occlusion with the opposing set of teeth and a highly abrasive diet to grind coronal surfaces.
- The cause of acquired cheek teeth elongation is likely multifactorial and not completely known. The most significant contributing or exacerbating factor is feeding diets that contain inadequate amounts of the coarse roughage material required to properly grind coronal surfaces. Malocclusion may also be an inherited or congenital defect.
- Cheek teeth are naturally curved. When erupted crowns are a normal length, they will contact the apposing set of cheek teeth at an angle such that the teeth will occlude with a flat grinding surface. If normal wear does not occur and teeth overgrow, the exposed coronal surfaces will curve away from the apposing set of teeth, contact at an abnormal angle, and cause the formation of sharp spikes.
- Spikes on the cheek teeth can become very long and either erode into adjacent soft tissues or, in some cases, entrap the tongue. Secondary bacterial infections are common.
- Cheek teeth that no longer can occlude normally will continue to elongate into the oral cavity, until normal jaw tone arrests upward growth. At this point, pressure from the apposing set of cheek teeth will cause the teeth to grow in an apical direction (ventrally into the mandible or upward into the maxilla) such that the apices intrude into cortical bone.
- Pulpitis, pulp necrosis, and apical abscess formation are common sequela that may also be caused by trauma, food lodged between abnormal teeth, penetration into sinus cavities, and subsequent bacterial invasion.

### SYSTEMS AFFECTED
- Oral cavity
- Ocular—nasolacrimal duct obstruction, retroorbital invasion of tooth roots
- Respiratory—apical (tooth root) invasion of the sinuses
- Musculoskeletal—weight loss, muscle wasting

### GENETICS
Unknown

### INCIDENCE/PREVALENCE
One of the most common presenting complaints in pet rabbits

### GEOGRAPHIC DISTRIBUTION
N/A

### SIGNALMENT
- Usually seen in middle-aged rabbits—acquired cheek tooth elongation
- Young animals—congenital malocclusion
- Dwarf and lop breeds—congenital malocclusion
- No breed or gender predilection for acquired cheek tooth elongation

### SIGNS

#### Historical Findings
- History of incisor overgrowth—owners generally notice incisor overgrowth first, as these teeth are readily visible. In nearly all cases, incisor overgrowth is a symptom of cheek teeth elongation and generalized dental disease.
- Inability to prehend food, dropping food out of the mouth, preference for soft foods
- Weight loss
- Anorexia with an interest in food but inability to eat, or decreased appetite due to pain
- Preference for a water bowl over a sipper bottle
- Excessive drooling
- Nasal discharge
- Tooth grinding
- Excessive tear production
- Facial asymmetry or exophthalmos in rabbits with large tooth root abscesses
- Signs of pain—reluctance to move, depression, lethargy, hiding, hunched posture
- Unkempt haircoat, lack of grooming

#### Physical Examination Findings
- Soft tissue swelling; abscesses most commonly located along the mandible or below the eye
- Cutaneous sinus exuding pus

#### Oral Examination
- A thorough examination of the cheek teeth requires heavy sedation or general anesthesia and specialized equipment. A cursory examination using an otoscope for illumination and visualization is insufficient for rabbits with dental disease.
- A focused, directed light source and magnification will provide optimal visualization.
- Use a rodent mouth gag and cheek dilators (Jorgensen Laboratories, Inc., Loveland, CO) to open the mouth and pull buccal tissues away from teeth surfaces to allow adequate exposure. Use a cotton swab or tongue depressor to retract the tongue from lingual surfaces.
- Normal cheek teeth—do not have a flat surface, but small vertical cusps; normal crown length for maxillary cheek teeth: approximately 1 mm (maximum 2 mm); normal crown length for mandibular cheek teeth: approximately 3 mm (maximum 5 mm)
- Identify cheek teeth abnormalities—elongation, irregular crown height, spikes, curved teeth, discolored teeth, missing teeth, purulent exudate, odor, impacted food, oral ulceration, or abscesses
- Affected tooth may be loose and painful on palpation.
- Buccal or lingual mucosa and lip margins—ulceration, abrasions, secondary bacterial infection, or abscess formation if incisors or cheek teeth spikes have damaged soft tissues
- Significant tooth root abnormalities may be present despite normal-appearing crowns. Skull films are required to identify apical disorders.
- Incisors—may see overgrowth, horizontal ridges or grooves, malformation, discoloration, fractures, increased or decreased curvature. Malocclusion—bite appears level or the mandibular incisors occlude rostral to maxillary incisors.

#### Other Findings
- Ptyalism, secondary moist pyoderma around the mouth, neck, and dewlap areas
- Halitosis
- A scalloped edge or single bony protrusion may be palpable on the ventral rim of the

# TOOTH ROOT ABSCESSES (APICAL ABSCESSES)

mandible in rabbits into which the cheek teeth have intruded and distorted surrounding bone.
• Tartar accumulation, periodontal disease, and caries are rare in rabbits.
• Exophthalmus in rabbits with retrobulbar abscesses arising from periapical cheek tooth abscesses
• Weight loss, emaciation
• Nasal discharge—tooth root invasion into the sinuses; tooth root abscesses
• Ocular discharge—blocked nasolacrimal duct from diseased tooth roots (usually the second upper premolar); pressure on the eye from retrobulbar abscess or overgrown molar roots
• Signs of gastrointestinal hypomotility—scant feces, intestinal pain, diarrhea

## CAUSES AND RISK FACTORS
• Pyogenic bacteria—*Pasteurella* usually not present; common isolates from these sites include *Streptococcus* spp.; anaerobic bacteria cultured include *Fusobacterium nucleatum*, *Prevotella* spp., *Peptostreptococcus micros*, *Actinomyces israelii*, and *Arcanobacterium haemolyticum*. Occasionally may culture *Staphylococcus aureus*, *Pseudomonas* spp., *Escherichia coli*, b-hemolytic *Streptococcus* spp., *Proteus* spp., and *Bacteroides* spp.
• Any pulpal trauma—especially inappropriate clipping of the teeth; cutting through the pulp during teeth trimming; creates portal of entry for bacteria
• Direct blow causing fracture of the crown, severe pulpitis, and pulpal necrosis
• Malocclusive trauma in rabbits with cheek tooth elongation—most common cause
• Acquired cheek teeth elongation—likely multiple etiologies; feeding pelleted foods containing inadequate fibrous, tough foods needed for normal wear of occlusal surfaces
• Immunosuppression—systemic or topical corticosteroid use, immunosuppressive chemotherapy, underlying predisposing disease (e.g., liver disease, chronic renal failure)

## DIAGNOSIS

### DIFFERENTIAL DIAGNOSIS
• Subcutaneous abscess—from trauma, puncture wound, or hematogenous spread; abscess is freely moveable on palpation; does not adhere to or appear contiguous with bone
• Neoplasia—differentiate by radiography, CT scan, and cytologic or histologic examination.

### CBC/BIOCHEMISTRY/URINALYSIS
• CBC—normal or lymphopenia; neutrophilia and left shift not usually seen in rabbits with abscesses

• May see abnormalities in liver enzymes in rabbits with hepatic lipidosis secondary to anorexia

### OTHER LABORATORY TESTS
N/A

### IMAGING

#### Skull Radiographs
• Mandatory to identify type and extent of dental disease, to plan treatment strategies, and to monitor progression of treatment
• Perform under general anesthesia.
• Five views are recommend for thorough assessment—ventral–dorsal, lateral, two lateral obliques, and rostral–caudal.
• With early disease—elongation of the crowns and roots, loss of normal coronal occlusal pattern, mild radiolucency around tooth roots, enlargement of germinal bud, lysis of bone
• Moderate to severe disease—crooked teeth, reduction in the diameter or obliteration of the pulp cavity; widening of the interdental space, apical radiolucency and bony lysis, penetration of the tooth roots into surrounding cortical bone
• Periapical abscess—severe lysis of cortical bone, bony proliferation
• CT—superior to radiographs to evaluate the extent of dental disease and bony destruction

### DIAGNOSTIC PROCEDURES
• Fine needle aspiration of facial swelling—may be helpful to identify abscess
• Bacterial culture of affected tissue and/or exudate—aerobic and anaerobic bacteria; growth more likely if wall or capsule is sampled; bacteria deep within exudate are often nonviable
• Bacterial susceptibility testing to direct antibiotic therapy

## TREATMENT

### APPROPRIATE HEALTH CARE
• Outpatient—patients with small periapical abscess that can be treated by extraction per os
• Inpatient—patients with large, palpable periapical or facial abscess requiring extensive debridement; debilitated patients

### NURSING CARE
• Keep fur around face clean and dry.
• Supportive care in debilitated or anorectic patients, assisted feeding, subcutaneous or intravenous fluid therapy

### ACTIVITY
N/A

### DIET
• It is absolutely imperative that the rabbit continue to eat during and following treat-

ment. Many rabbits with dental disease will become anorectic. Rabbits may be unable to eat solid food following radical coronal reduction, extractions, or surgical treatment of abscesses. Anorexia will cause or exacerbate gastrointestinal hypomotility, derangement of the gastrointestinal microflora, and overgrowth of intestinal bacterial pathogens.
• Syringe feed a gruel such as Critical Care for Herbivores (Oxbow Pet Products, Murdock, NE) 10–15 mL/kg PO q6–8h. Alternatively, pellets can be ground and mixed with fresh greens, vegetable baby foods, water, or juice to form a gruel.
• Most rabbits will require assisted feeding for 36–48 hours postoperatively; following radical abscess debridement, assisted feeding may be needed for several weeks.
• High-carbohydrate, high-fat nutritional supplements are contraindicated.
• Return the rabbit to a solid-food diet as soon as possible to encourage normal occlusion and wear. Increase the amount of tough, fibrous foods and foods containing abrasive silicates such as hay and wild grasses; avoid pelleted food and soft fruits or vegetables.
• Encourage oral fluid intake by offering fresh water or wetting leafy vegetables.

### CLIENT EDUCATION
• Discuss need to correct or prevent risk factors.
• Most rabbits with apical abscesses have generalized dental disease. Diet change and lifelong treatment, consisting of periodic coronal reduction (teeth trimming), are required, usually every 1–3 months.
• Large tooth root abscesses with severe bony destruction carry a fair to poor prognosis for complete resolution. Most will require extensive surgery, sometimes multiple surgeries and multiple follow-up visits. Recurrences in the same or other locations are common. Clients must be aware of the monetary and time investment.
• With severe disease, euthanasia may be the most humane option, especially in rabbits with intractable pain or those that cannot eat.

### SURGICAL CONSIDERATIONS

#### Small Apical Abscess
• Without significant osteomyelitis; has not perforated through cortex; has not caused cellulitis or perforated into subcutaneous spaces
• Can usually be treated by tooth extraction per os
• Because rabbits have very long, deeply embedded and curved tooth roots, extraction per os can be extremely time consuming and labor intensive as compared to with dogs and cats. If the germinal bud is not completely removed, the teeth may regrow or a new abscess may form. If not experi-

# TOOTH ROOT ABSCESSES (APICAL ABSCESSES)

enced with tooth extraction in rabbits, the author recommends referral to a veterinarian with special expertise whenever feasible.
• Anesthetic considerations—premedicate with buprenorphine, induce with isoflurane via mask, move the mask over nose to maintain anesthesia (rabbits are obligate nasal breathers), or intubate.
• Use a focused, directed light source and magnification (e.g., lighted magnification loops).
• Adequate exposure of the teeth and protection of soft tissues are crucial. Use a rodent mouth gag and cheek dilators (Jorgensen Laboratories, Inc., Loveland, CO) to open the mouth and pull buccal tissues away from teeth surfaces.
• Specialized root elevators developed for curved rabbit teeth (Crossley Rabbit Incisor or Molar Luxator, Jorgensen Laboratories Inc., Loveland, CO) should be used.
• Curette and flush all visible exudate; fill the pocket with Doxirobe Gel (Pfizer AH, Kalamazoo, MI) or antibiotic-impregnated polymethyl methacrylate (AIPMMA) beads.
• Place on long-term antibiotic therapy; appropriate pain management
• Extraction of multiple cheek teeth in a single procedure can be extremely traumatic; some rabbits may not recover.

### Large Tooth Root Abscesses
• In rabbits with extensive tooth abscesses, aggressive debridement is indicated, and special expertise may be required. Maxillary and retrobulbar abscesses can be particularly challenging. If not experienced with facial abscesses in rabbits, the author recommends referral to a veterinarian with special expertise whenever feasible.
• Abscess causing extensive osteomyelitis, penetration through the cortex, and subcutaneous swelling should be removed via a cutaneous approach. All material within the abscess should be removed with the capsule intact until bone is reached. All teeth associated with the abscess must be removed. All bone and soft tissues involved in abscess must be thoroughly debrided.
• Fill the defect with AIPMMA beads.
• AIPMMA beads release a high concentration of antibiotic into local tissues for several months. Selection of antibiotic is limited to those known to elute appropriately from bead to tissues and should be based on culture and susceptibility testing. AIPMMA beads are not commercially available, but can be made using PMMA by Surgical Simplex Bone Cement (Howmedica, Rutherford, NJ) or Bone Cement (Zimmer, Charlotte, NC). Antibiotics successfully used include cephalothin, cefazolin, or ceftiofur (2 g/20 g PMMA); gentamicin or tobramycin (1 g/2 g PMMA); or amikacin (1.25 g/2 g PMMA). Antibiotic is added to

the copolymer powder before adding the liquid and formed into small, spherical beads. Beads must be manufactured and inserted aseptically, and unused beads should be gas sterilized prior to future use. Beads should be left in the incision site for at least 2 months, but can be left in indefinitely.
• Place on long-term antibiotic therapy with appropriate pain management.

## MEDICATIONS

### DRUG(S) OF CHOICE

*Antibiotics*
Choice of antibiotic is ideally based on results of culture and susceptibility testing. Depending on the severity of infection, long-term antibiotic therapy is required (4–6 weeks minimum to several months or years). Most tooth root abscesses are caused by anaerobic bacteria; use antibiotics effective against anaerobes such as azithromycin (30 mg/kg PO q24h); can be used alone or combined with metronidazole (20 mg/kg PO q12h). Alternatively, use penicillin g (40,000–60,000 IU/kg SC q2–7d) or chloramphenicol (50 mg/kg PO q8h). Combine with topical treatment (surgical debridement, AIPMMA beads). If aerobic bacteria are isolated, use broad-spectrum antibiotics such as enrofloxacin (5–20 mg/kg PO, SC, IM q12–24h) or trimethoprim sulfa (30 mg/kg PO q12h).

*Acute Pain Management*
• Buprenorphine (0.01–0.05 mg/kg SC, IM, IV q8-12h)—use preoperatively for extractions, coronal reduction, or surgical abscess treatment.
• Butorphanol (0.1–1.0 mg/kg SC, IM, IV q4–6h)—may cause profound sedation; short-acting
• Morphine (2–5 mg/kg SC, IM q2–4h) or oxymorphone (0.05–0.2 mg/kg SC, IM q8–12h)—use with caution; more than one to two doses may cause gastrointestinal stasis.
• Meloxicam (0.2 mg/kg SC, IM q24h)
• Carprofen (1–4 mg/kg SC q12h)

*Long-Term Pain Management*
• NSAIDs have been used for short- or long-term therapy to reduce pain and inflammation: meloxicam (0.2–0.5 mg/kg PO q24h) or carprofen (2.2 mg/kg PO q12–24h)
• Sedation for oral examination—ketamine (15–20 mg/kg IM) plus midazolam (0.5–1.0 mg/kg IM); many other sedation protocols exist. Alternatively, administer general anesthesia with isoflurane.

### CONTRAINDICATIONS
• Oral administration of most antibiotics effective against anaerobes will cause a fatal gastrointestinal dysbiosis in rabbits. Do not

administer penicillins, macrolides, lincosamides, and cephalosporins by oral administration.
• Corticosteroids—associated with gastrointestinal ulceration and hemorrhage, delayed wound healing, and heightened susceptibility to infection; rabbits are very sensitive to the immunosuppressive effects of both topical and systemic corticosteroids; use may exacerbate subclinical bacterial infection.
• Placement of Penrose or similar drains—these do not provide drainage and can serve as a route for continued contamination.
• The placement of calcium hydroxide paste in the defect following debridement is contraindicated, as extensive tissue necrosis may occur.

### PRECAUTIONS
• Chloramphenicol—avoid human contact with chloramphenicol due to potential blood dyscrasia. Advise owners of potential risks.
• Meloxicam—use with caution in rabbits with compromised renal function.

### POSSIBLE INTERACTIONS
N/A

### ALTERNATIVE DRUGS
• If AIPMMA beads are not available, packing the postdebridement deficit with antibiotic-laden gauze has been used as an alternative. The choice of antibiotic is based on culture and susceptibility testing. Antibiotics used include penicillin (80,000 IU/kg), ampicillin (20 mg/kg), cefazolin (25 mg/kg), and metronidazole (50 mg/kg). Oral antibiotic therapy is used simultaneously during the entire treatment period. The wounds are evaluated and the gauze removed and repacked every 7 days under general anesthesia, until complete resolution occurs. Effectiveness varies, depending on severity of disease and owner compliance.
• 50% dextrose-soaked gauze has been anecdotally used with success as a topical abscess treatment following surgical debridement. Dextrose has bactericidal properties and promotes granulation bed formation. The abscess cavity is filled with dextrose-laden gauze and replaced daily until a healthy granulation bed appears. Honey has been used in a similar manner. Effectiveness varies, depending on the severity of disease and owner compliance.

## FOLLOW-UP

### PATIENT MONITORING
• Make sure the patient is eating, passing stools, and maintaining normal hydration.
• Reevaluate 7–10 days postoperatively, then as needed every 1–3 months if regular teeth trimming is indicated.

# TOOTH ROOT ABSCESSES (APICAL ABSCESSES)

• Evaluate the entire oral cavity and radiograph the skull with each recheck to monitor for possible recurrence at extraction site or other abnormal teeth.

## PREVENTION/AVOIDANCE
• Do not use clippers to trim incisors or cheek teeth.
• Discontinue or limit the feeding of pellets and soft fruits or vegetables; provide adequate tough, fibrous foods such as hay and grasses to encourage normal wear of teeth.
• Do not breed rabbits with congenital malocclusion.

## POSSIBLE COMPLICATIONS
• Recurrence, chronic pain, or extensive tissue destruction warranting euthanasia due to poor quality of life
• Hepatic lipidosis with prolonged anorexia
• Chronic epiphora with nasolacrimal duct occlusion

## EXPECTED COURSE AND PROGNOSIS
• Small periapical abscesses with limited bone destruction—good to fair prognosis with extraction and topical and long-term systemic antibiotic treatment
• Severe osteomyelitis, multiple tooth involvement—depend on severity of bone involvement and location. Rabbits with abscesses in the nasal passages, or exophthalmos, or multiple or severe maxillary abscesses have a guarded to poor prognosis. Euthanasia may be warranted if pain is intractable.

• If surgical debridement of tooth root abscess is not possible, treatment with long-term antibiotic and pain medication may be palliative; many tooth root abscesses are slow growing and patients can live for months in comfort, even with relatively large abscesses.

 MISCELLANEOUS

## ASSOCIATED CONDITIONS
Gastrointestinal hypomotility

## AGE-RELATED FACTORS
• Congenital malocclusion in young rabbits
• Acquired tooth elongation in middle-aged to older rabbits

## ZOONOTIC POTENTIAL
N/A

## PREGNANCY
N/A

## SYNONYMS
N/A

## SEE ALSO
• Abscessation
• Epiphora
• Incisor malocclusion and overgrowth

## ABBREVIATIONS
• CBC = complete blood count
• CT = computed tomography
• NSAIDs = nonsteroidal antiinflammatory drugs

*Suggested Reading*

Bennet RA. Treatment of abscesses in the head of rabbits. Proc North Am Vet Conf 1999;821–823.

Crossley DA. Oral biology and disorders of lagomorphs. Vet Clin North Am Exotic Anim Pract 2003;6(3):629–659.

Crossley DA, Aiken S. Small mammal dentistry. In: Quesenberry KE, Carpenter JW, eds. Ferrets, Rabbits and Rodents: Clinical Medicine and Surgery. 2nd Ed. Philadelphia: WB Saunders, 2004:370–382.

Ethell MT, Bennett RA, Brown MP, et al. In vitro elution of gentamicin, amikacin, and ceftiofur from polymethylmethacrylate and hydroxyapatite cement. Vet Surg 2000;29:375–382.

Harcourt-Brown F. Dental disease. In: Harcourt-Brown F, ed. Textbook of Rabbit Medicine. Oxford: Butterworth-Heinemann, 2002:165–205.

Lukehart SA, Fohn MJ, Baker-Zander SA. Efficacy of azithromycin for therapy of active syphilis in the rabbit model. J Antimicrob Chemother 1990;25 Suppl A:91–9.

Tyrell KC, Citron DM, Jenkins JR, et al. Periodontal bacteria in rabbit mandibular and maxillary abscesses. J Clin Microbiol 2002;40(3):1044–1047.

# TOXOPLASMOSIS

## BASICS

### OVERVIEW
• *Toxoplasma gondii*—an obligate intracellular coccidian protozoan parasite that infects nearly all mammals; Felidae the definitive hosts; all other warm-blooded animals are intermediate hosts. Uncommon cause of neurologic disease in rabbits
• Severity and manifestation—depend on location and degree of tissue injury caused by tissue cysts
• Infection—acquired by ingestion of tissue cysts or oocysts; organisms spread to extraintestinal organs via blood or lymph; results in focal necrosis to many organs (heart, eye, CNS)
• Chronic disease—tissue cysts form; low-grade disease; in other mammals, usually not clinically apparent unless immunosuppression or concomitant illness allows organism to proliferate, causing an acute inflammatory response; assumed to be true in rabbits also

### SIGNALMENT
Rare cause of neurologic disease in rabbits

### SIGNS
• Neurologic—reflect diffuse neurologic inflammation, seizures, tremors, torticollis, ataxia, paresis, paralysis, muscle weakness, and tetraparesis
• Other signs (cardiac, gastrointestinal, ocular)—not well described in rabbits

### CAUSES AND RISK FACTORS
• Exposure to vegetation contaminated by cat feces
• Immunosuppression—may predispose to infection or reactivation

## DIAGNOSIS

### DIFFERENTIAL DIAGNOSIS
• Other, more common causes of (focal) encephalopathy—infectious diseases most common, especially bacterial (brain abscess, extension from otitis interna/media, meningoencephalitis) or encephalitozoonosis; viral, fungal diseases rare in rabbits; brain tumor; ischemic encephalopathy also rare
• Physical examination findings helpful in diagnosing more common problems: nasal/ocular discharge—historical or current, common with spread of upper respiratory infection to inner/middle ear; otitis—thick, white, creamy exudate may be found in the horizontal and/or vertical canals.

### CBC/BIOCHEMISTRY/URINALYSIS
Normal unless the parasite also affects non-neural tissues

### OTHER LABORATORY TESTS
• Serologic testing for *Encephalitozoon cuniculi*—may be helpful in ruling out encephalitozoonosis; however, usefulness is limited since a positive titer indicates only exposure and does not confirm *E. cuniculi* as the cause of clinical signs.
• Serologic testing for *Pasteurella*—may be helpful in ruling out pasteurellosis; a paired, rising titer indicates active infection; single titers only indicate exposure to *Pasteurella* spp. and are of limited usefulness since most rabbits in North America have been exposed.
• Serologic testing for toxoplasmosis—anecdotal reports of using serum antibody titers available for testing in dogs and cats to support diagnosis in rabbits exist; however, no data exist to direct proper interpretation of results.

### IMAGING
• Tympanic bullae and skull radiography—may help rule out otitis interna/media; however, normal radiographs do not rule out bulla disease.
• CT and MRI—valuable for confirming bulla lesions and CNS extension from peripheral regions, localized tumor, granuloma, and extent of inflammation

### PATHOLOGIC FINDINGS
Brain—focal areas of necrosis; nonsuppurative meningoencephalitis; organisms can be differentiated from *E. cuniculi* by their strong uptake of hematoxylin stain; incidental finding in heart and skeletal muscle

## TREATMENT
• Inpatient vs. outpatient—depends on severity of the signs and need for supportive care
• Intravenous or subcutaneous fluids may be required when disorientation and nausea preclude oral intake.

### ACTIVITY
Restrict (e.g., avoid stairs and slippery surfaces) according to the degree of disequilibrium; encourage return to activity as soon as safely possible; activity may enhance recovery of vestibular function.

### DIET
• It is absolutely imperative that the rabbit continue to eat during and following treatment. Anorexia will often cause gastrointestinal hypomotility, derangement of the gastrointestinal microflora, and overgrowth of intestinal bacterial pathogens.

• Offer a large selection of fresh, moistened greens such as cilantro, romaine lettuce, parsley, carrot tops, dandelion greens, spinach, collard greens, etc., and good-quality grass hay. Many rabbits will begin to eat these foods, even if they were previously anorectic.
• If the patient refuses these foods, syringe feed gruel such as Critical Care for Herbivores (Oxbow Pet Products, Murdock, NE). Alternatively, pellets can be ground and mixed with fresh greens, vegetable baby foods, water, or juice to form a gruel.
• High-carbohydrate, high-fat nutritional supplements are contraindicated.
• Encourage oral fluid intake by offering fresh water, wetting leafy vegetables, or flavoring water with vegetable juices.
CAUTION: Be aware of aspiration secondary to abnormal body posture in patients with severe head tilt and vestibular disequilibrium or brainstem dysfunction.

## MEDICATIONS

### DRUG(S) OF CHOICE
Trimethoprim sulfa (15–30 mg/kg PO q12h); sulfadiazine in combination with pyrimethamine for 2 weeks used at feline doses has also been recommended.

### CONTRAINDICATIONS
Oral administration of clindamycin should not be used to treat toxoplasmosis in rabbits. This antibiotic and other antibiotics that select against Gram-positive bacteria (penicillins, macrolides, lincosamides, and cephalosporins) can cause fatal enteric dysbiosis and enterotoxemia.

### PRECAUTIONS
Sulfadiazine/pyrimethamine combination—causes depression, anemia, leukopenia, and thrombocytopenia in cats; toxicity in rabbits not described

### POSSIBLE INTERACTIONS
N/A

### ALTERNATIVE DRUGS
Doxycycline (2.5 mg/kg PO q12h) has also been used to treat toxoplasmosis in rabbits; efficacy uncertain

## FOLLOW-UP

### PATIENT MONITORING
Periodic examination to assess neuromuscular deficits; progression of disease warrants further evaluation for other causes of neuromuscular disease.

### PREVENTION/AVOIDANCE
Prevent ingestion of bedding, feed, or outdoor grazing of vegetation contaminated with cat feces.

### POSSIBLE COMPLICATIONS
N/A

### EXPECTED COURSE AND PROGNOSIS
• Prognosis—guarded; varied response to drug treatment
• Residual deficits (especially neurologic) likely; however, severity cannot be predicted until after a course of therapy.

## MISCELLANEOUS

### ASSOCIATED CONDITIONS
• Pasteurellosis
• Gastrointestinal hypomotility
• Dental disease
• Upper respiratory infections

### AGE-RELATED FACTORS
N/A

### ZOONOTIC POTENTIAL
Rabbits are intermediate hosts and do not shed organism; possible human transmission occurs by eating undercooked rabbit meat.

### PREGNANCY
Parasitemia during pregnancy—spread of organism to fetus possible

### ABBREVIATIONS
• CNS = central nervous system
• CT = computed tomography
• MRI = magnetic resonance imaging

*Suggested Readings*

Deeb BJ, Carpenter JW. Neurologic and musculoskeletal diseases. In: Quesenberry KE, Carpenter JE, eds. Ferrets, Rabbits and Rodents: Clinical Medicine and Surgery. 2nd Ed. Philadelphia: WB Saunders, 2004:203–210.

Harcourt-Brown F. Neurologic and locomotor diseases. In: Harcourt-Brown F, ed. Textbook of Rabbit Medicine. Oxford: Butterworth-Heinemann, 2002:307–323.

*Portions Adapted From*

Barr SC. Toxoplasmosis. In: Tilley LP, Smith FWK, Jr., eds. The 5-Minute Veterinary Consult: Canine and Feline, 3rd Ed. Baltimore: Lippincott Williams & Wilkins, 2004.

# TREPONEMATOSIS (RABBIT SYPHILIS)

 BASICS

## OVERVIEW
• A sexually transmitted bacterial infection caused by the spirochete *Treponema cuniculi*
• Transmission occurs via sexual contact or other direct contact with lesions or from does to offspring during passage through the vagina at birth.
• Incubation period can be prolonged, as long as 3–12 weeks.
• Lesions are confined to mucocutaneous junctions; beginning in the prepuce or vulva, may progress to the anus and perianal region and spread to the lips, nose, and eyelids during grooming

## SIGNALMENT
• Clinical signs are uncommon in pet rabbits; serologic findings suggest approximately 25% of asymptomatic rabbits may have been infected.
• Clinical signs most commonly seen in young rabbits

## SIGNS
### Historical Findings
• History of recent breeding in adult rabbits or contact with infected animals
• Seen in young rabbits with no breeding history if transmitted from doe at birth
• History of erythema and swelling around the vulva or prepuce, anus, lips, and nose followed by papules and crusts
• Occasionally, a history of abortion or neonatal death in breeding does
• Signs may wax and wane, spontaneously resolve, and reappear following stress.

### Physical Examination Findings
• Initially erythema, swelling at mucocutaneous junction surrounding the external genitalia, spreading to anus and then mouth, nose, and sometimes periocular region with grooming
• Lesions sometimes found on the face only, in the absence of genital lesions (contact by sniffing affected rabbits)
• Lesions progress to papules, vesicles that ulcerate and form crusts.
• Lesions may be painful.

## CAUSES AND RISK FACTORS
• *T. cuniculi*, a spirochete antigenically similar to *Treponema pallidum*, the causative agent of human syphilis
• Rabbit to human transmission does not occur
• Risk factor—sexual or direct contact with affected rabbits; transmission by asymptomatic animals possible

 DIAGNOSIS

### General Comments
Diagnosis is often presumptive, based on history, characteristic clinical signs, and response to treatment.

## DIFFERENTIAL DIAGNOSIS
• Ear mites—although lesions may be seen around the face, neck, abdomen, and perineal region, the majority of lesions are around ear base and pinna; intense pruritus
• Contact hypersensitivity—may see lesions around face or perineal region; does not progress to papules, ulceration, or crusts
• Pyoderma—moist pyoderma in perineal region or face extremely common, secondary to chronic exposure to moisture; larger area usually affected than with *T. cuniculi*; dry crusts usually not present with pyoderma; underlying cause usually identifiable
• Autoimmune dermatoses—not reported in rabbits

## CBC/BIOCHEMISTRY/URINALYSIS
N/A

## OTHER LABORATORY TESTS
Serologic testing—demonstrates exposure to *T. cuniculi*; titers may take 12 weeks to develop following exposure; lesions may be present before titers become positive; titers eventually decline over several months with treatment, but usually remain elevated following spontaneous resolution of clinical signs. May be important to identify asymptomatic carriers

## IMAGING
N/A

## DIAGNOSTIC PROCEDURES
• History, physical examination findings, and response to treatment are usually sufficient for diagnosis.
• Skin biopsy and histologic examination—identify organisms with silver staining. Lesions consist of ulcers, necrotic crusts surrounded by inflammatory cells.

 TREATMENT

• Outpatient treatment
• Treat all rabbits in contact with affected rabbit.
• Topical treatment, other than keeping the lesions clean and dry, is generally not needed.

 MEDICATIONS

Penicillin g, benzathine (42,000–84,000 IU/kg SC q7d) for three treatments; lesions often diminish significantly after only one or two injections.

## CONTRAINDICATIONS/POSSIBLE INTERACTIONS
Do not administer any penicillin by an oral route—can cause fatal dysbiosis

 FOLLOW-UP

## PATIENT MONITORING
• Treat other rabbits in contact with affected rabbits; monitor for resolution of lesions.
• Monitor for signs of dysbiosis (diarrhea, anorexia) in treated rabbits; dysbiosis is unlikely but possible with high doses of parenteral penicillin.

## PREVENTION/AVOIDANCE
Avoid contact with clinically affected or seropositive rabbits.

## EXPECTED COURSE AND PROGNOSIS
Prognosis is excellent with treatment; treatment is considered to be curative and lesions typically resolve in 1–3 weeks; treat all in-contact rabbits to prevent reinfection.

 MISCELLANEOUS

## ZOONOTIC POTENTIAL
*T. cuniculi* is not transmissible to humans.

### Suggested Readings
Harcourt-Brown, F. Skin diseases. In: Harcourt-Brown F, ed. Textbook of Rabbit Medicine. Oxford: Butterworth-Heinemann, 2002:224–248.
Hess L. Dermatologic diseases. In: Quesenberry KE, Carpenter JW, eds. Ferrets, Rabbits and Rodents: Clinical Medicine and Surgery. 2nd Ed. Philadelphia: WB Saunders, 2004:194–202.
Jenkins JR. Skin disorders of the rabbit. Vet Clin North Am Exotic Anim Pract 2001;4(2):543–563.
Pare JA, Paul-Murphy J. Disorders of the reproductive and urinary systems. In: Quesenberry KE, Carpenter JW, eds. Ferrets, Rabbits and Rodents: Clinical Medicine and Surgery. 2nd Ed. Philadelphia: WB Saunders, 2004:183–193.

# BASICS

## DEFINITIION
- A mat of ingested hair, often combined with inspissated food, located in the stomach or intestines
- Hair in the stomach is a normal finding in all healthy rabbits. The finding of hair in the stomach is not a disease or symptom of disease in normal, healthy rabbits.
- Inspissated stomach contents, often including hair secondary to gastrointestinal hypomotility, stasis, or outflow obstruction is an abnormal finding. Diagnostic and treatment efforts are directed toward the cause of accumulated and inspissated stomach contents, not at removal of the hair.

## PATHOPHYSIOLOGY
- Rabbits are hind-gut fermenters and are extremely sensitive to alterations in diet.
- Proper hind-gut fermentation and gastrointestinal tract motility are dependent on the ingestion of large amounts of roughage and long-stemmed hay. Diets that contain inadequate amounts of long-stemmed, coarse fiber (such as the feeding of only commercial pelleted food without hay or grasses) cause gastrointestinal tract hypomotility.
- The presence of "hairballs" or trichobezoars in the stomach is not a disease, but a symptom or consequence of gastrointestinal hypomotility or stasis. Rabbits normally ingest hair during grooming. Healthy rabbits will always have some amount of hair and ingesta in the stomach. These stomach contents are both palpable and visible radiographically in the normal, healthy rabbit.
- With proper nutrition and gastrointestinal tract motility, fur ingested as a result of normal grooming behavior will pass through the gastrointestinal tract with the ingesta uneventfully.
- When gastrointestinal motility slows or stops, ingesta, including fur and other material, accumulates in the stomach. Rabbits cannot vomit to expel nonfood contents from the stomach.
- Dehydration of stomach contents often occurs, making the contents more difficult to pass. With medical treatment of gastrointestinal hypomotility, motility usually returns, stomach contents soften, and hair and other ingesta will usually pass. Without treatment, rentention of inspissated gastric contents and subsequent metabolic derangements combined with shifts in intestinal microbial flora can be fatal.
- Cecocolonic hypomotility also causes alterations in cecal fermentation, pH, and substrate production, resulting in alteration of enteric microflora populations. Diets low in coarse fiber typically contain high simple carbohydrate concentrations, which provide

a ready source of fermentable products and promote the growth of bacterial pathogens such as *Escherichia coli* and *Clostridium* spp. Bacterial dysbiosis can cause acute diarrhea, enterotoxemia, ileus, or chronic intermittent diarrhea.
- In some rabbits, other foreign materials such as cloth or carpet may become incorporated into the compacted stomach contents. Rabbits are fond of chewing, and when fed diets containing insufficient coarse fiber, chewing behavior is often exacerbated.
- Anorexia due to infectious or metabolic disease, pain, stress, or starvation may cause or exacerbate gastrointestinal hypomotility.
- The process is often self-perpetuating; gastrointestinal hypomotility and dehydration promote anorexia and exacerbation of stasis.
- Trichobezoars occasionally occur in the intestines, especially in the duodenum, causing an acute intestinal blockage. These may be related to gastrointestinal hypomotility or ingestion of a hair mat too large to pass through the intestine, or may be the result of local intestinal inflammation or neoplasia. Complete gastrointestinal tract obstruction is a life-threatening emergency.

## SYSTEMS AFFECTED
- Gastrointestinal
- Musculoskeletal—loss of muscle mass may occur due to inappetence.

## INCIDENCE/PREVALENCE
- Gastrointestinal hypomotility resulting in retention of stomach contents, scant or lack of feces, chronic intermittent diarrhea, abdominal pain, and ill-thrift is one of the most common clinical problems seen in the rabbit.
- Acute small intestinal obstruction by hair or foreign material is a less common, acute, life-threatening condition.

## SIGNALMENT
- More commonly seen in middle-aged to older rabbits on inappropriate diets, but can occur in any aged rabbit.
- No breed or gender predilection

## SIGNS

### Historical Findings
*Gastrointestinal Hypomotility, Accumulation of Stomach Contents*
- History of inappropriate diet (e.g., cereals, grains, commercial pellets only, sweets, large quantities of fruits, lack of feeding long-stemmed hay)
- Recent history of illness or stressful event
- History of decreased activity—cage confinement, orthopedic or neuromuscular disease
- Weight loss in rabbits with underlying or chronic disease
- Obesity in rabbits on diets consisting of mainly commercial pellets
- Chronic, intermittent diarrhea

- Patients are usually bright and alert, except those with enterotoxemia or acute small intestinal obstruction (gastric dilation), which are depressed, lethargic, or shocky.
- Inappetence or anorexia is the most common sign. Rabbits often initially stop eating pellets but continue to eat treats, followed by complete anorexia.
- Fecal pellets often become scant and small in size; no fecal pellets are produced with complete gastrointestinal stasis.
- Signs of pain, such as teeth grinding, a hunched posture and reluctance to move, are common.
*Acute Small Intestinal or Pyloric Obstruction*
- May have history of anorexia of short duration
- Weakness or collapse most common historical finding
- Progressive abdominal distension
- Often quickly progresses to lateral recumbency and signs of shock
- Diarrhea may also occur.

### Physical Examination Findings
*Gastrointestinal Hypomotility, Accumulation of Stomach Contents*
- Small, hard fecal pellets or absence of fecal pellets palpable in the colon; examine feces in cage or carrier—appear small, firm, and scant with gastrointestinal hypomotility
- Palpation of the stomach is an extremely valuable tool in the diagnosis of abnormal retention of stomach contents. Ingesta normally should be palpable in the stomach of a healthy rabbit. The normal stomach should be easily deformable, feel soft and pliable, and not remain pitted on compression. Rabbits with early gastrointestinal hypomotility will have a firm, often enlarged stomach that remains pitted when compressed. With complete gastrointestinal stasis, severe dehydration, or prolonged hypomotility, the stomach may be severely distended, hard, and nondeformable.
- The presence of firm ingesta in the stomach of a rabbit that has been anorectic for 1–3 days is compatible with the diagnosis of gastrointestinal hypomotility.
- Little or no borborygmus is heard on abdominal auscultation in rabbits with gastrointestinal hypomotility.
- Other physical examination findings depend on the underlying cause; perform a complete physical examination, including a thorough oral examination.
*Acute, Small Intestinal or Pyloric Obstruction*
- Tachycardia initially; bradycardia if shocky
- Tachypnea
- Signs of hypovolemic shock (e.g., pale mucous membranes, decreased capillary refill time, weak pulses, hypothermia)
- Severe abdominal pain on palpation
- Stomach filled with fluid and/or gas palpable; stomach usually extremely distended and tympanic

# TRICHOBEZOARS

• These rabbits are usually in shock and require emergency decompression.
• Often increased borborygmus on abdominal auscultation

## CAUSES
• In most cases ingesta, including hair and foreign material, are retained in the gastrointestinal tract due to a lack of normal gastrointestinal motility. Gastrointestinal hypomotility is often caused by feeding diets with insufficient long-stemmed hay or coarse fiber content. Gastrointestinal hypomotility may also be caused by anorexia. Common causes of anorexia include dental disease (malocclusion, molar impaction, tooth root abscesses), metabolic disease (renal disease, liver disease), pain (oral, trauma, postoperative pain, adhesions), neoplasia (gastrointestinal, uterine), and toxins.
• Anesthetic agents may cause or exacerbate gastrointestinal hypomotility.
• Some ingested foreign material is simply too large to pass through the intestinal tract. This is an unusual condition and occurs when rabbits ingest large mats of hair, chewed bedding or fabric, or other materials that pass through the stomach but cannot pass through the intestines.
• Focal intestinal inflammation, neoplasia, or stricture may contribute to outflow obstruction.

## RISK FACTORS
• Diets with inadequate indigestible coarse fiber content
• Inactivity due to pain, obesity, cage confinement
• Anesthesia and surgical procedures
• Unsupervised chewing behavior
• Long-haired breeds, excessive grooming or barbering
• Underlying dental, gastrointestinal tract, or metabolic disease

# DIAGNOSIS

## DIFFERENTIAL DIAGNOSIS
• Normal stomach contents—hair and other ingesta are often palpable and visible radiographically in normal, healthy rabbits. Treatment is warranted in rabbits displaying clinical signs of gastrointestinal hypomotility or stasis, described above.
• It is important to differentiate acute pyloric or small intestinal obstruction from gastrointestinal hypomotility, as acute intestinal obstruction is usually a life-threatening emergency. With acute gastrointestinal obstruction—sudden onset of anorexia, abdominal pain, reluctance to move often progresses to lateral recumbency and signs of hypovolemic shock (e.g., pale mucous membranes, decreased capillary refill time, weak pulses, hypothermia). Stom-

ach is severely distended, tympanic, and full of gas and/or fluid. Patients are often critical and require emergency decompression. Monitor rectal temperature; rabbits that become hypothermic are critically ill.
• For palpable mass in the cranial abdomen—neoplasia, abscess, hepatomegaly, normal gastric contents
• For anorexia—dental disease, metabolic disease, pain, neoplasia, cardiac disease, toxin
• For decreased fecal output—anorexia, intestinal foreign body, intussusception, intestinal neoplasia
• For chronic, intermittent diarrhea—cecotrophs, bacterial or parasitic infections, alterations in gastrointestinal tract flora due to antibiotic use or stress, partial obstruction by gastrointestinal foreign body or neoplasia, infiltrative bowel disease

## CBC/BIOCHEMISTRY/URINALYSIS
• These tests are often normal.
• May be used to identify underlying causes of gastrointestinal hypomotility
• PCV and TS elevation in dehydrated patients
• Serum ALT elevation in rabbits with liver disease, especially lipidosis
• If the intestinal tract has been perforated, an inflammatory leukogram may be useful.
• Anemia from gastric bleeding is rare.

## OTHER LABORATORY TESTS
N/A

## IMAGING
### Radiography
• Gastric contents (primarily food and hair) are normally present and visible radiographically, even if the rabbit has been inappetent. The presence of ingesta (including hair) in the stomach is a normal finding.
• Moderate to severe distension of the stomach with ingesta is usually visible with gastrointestinal hypomotility. In some rabbits with gastrointestinal stasis, a halo of gas can be observed around the inspissated stomach contents. Gas distension is also common throughout the intestinal tract, including the cecum in rabbits with gastrointestinal hypomotility or stasis.
• Cecal distention with ingesta and/or gas may be seen.
• Severe distention of the stomach with fluid and/or gas is usually seen with acute small intestinal obstructions.

### Ultrasound
Abdominal ultrasound can be useful for documenting an intestinal foreign body; may be difficult to interpret when large amounts of gas are present within the intestinal tract; may help define extraluminal mass

## OTHER DIAGNOSTIC PROCEDURES
N/A

## PATHOLOGIC FINDINGS
N/A

# TREATMENT

## APPROPRIATE HEALTH CARE
• Severe gastric distention with fluid or gas (bloat) is a life-threatening emergency.
• Rabbits that have been anorectic for 1–3 days should be evaluated and treated as soon as possible.
• Rabbits that have been anorectic for >3 days should be seen on an emergency basis.

## NURSING CARE
• Fluid therapy is an essential component of the medical management of patients with retained and inspissated stomach contents secondary to gastrointestinal hypomotility. Administer both oral and parenteral fluids. Oral fluid administration will aid in the rehydration of inspissated gastric contents. Mildly affected rabbits will usually respond well to oral and subcutaneous fluid administration, dietary modification described below, and in some cases, treatment with intestinal motility modifiers and analgesics.
• Intravenous or intraosseous fluids are required in patients that are severely dehydrated or depressed. Maintenance fluid requirements are estimated at 100 mL/kg/day. Rehydration is essential to treatment success in severely ill rabbits. Initially, a balanced fluid (e.g., lactated Ringer's solution) may be used.
• Fluid therapy for rabbits with acute pyloric or small intestinal obstruction (are often presented in shock)—LRS or other crystalloid (60–90 mg/kg/hr IV, IO over 20–60 minutes, followed by maintenance rate) or crystalloid bolus (30 mL/kg) plus hetastarch bolus (5 mL/kg initially), followed by crystalloids at a maintenance rate and hetastarch at 20 mL/kg divided over 24 hours.
• A warm, quiet environment should be provided.
• Gentle massage of the stomach may help to soften and loosen compacted stomach contents. Do not perform if acute obstruction is suspected.

### Gastric Decompression
• Patients with acute intestinal obstruction and an extremely dilated, gas- and/or fluid-filled stomach require immediate medical therapy with special attention to establishing improved cardiovascular function and gastric decompression.
• Administer fluid therapy as described above for critical patients; supportive fluids on the basis of hydration status are recommended for animals not in shock.

• Perform gastric decompression by orogastric intubation using a well-lubricated, open-ended red rubber catheter. A large-diameter otoscope cone can be used as a mouth gag. Make sure the rabbit is securely restrained in a towel. Sedation is generally required, unless the patient is extremely depressed.

## ACTIVITY

If patient is not debilitated, encourage exercise (hopping) for at least 10–15 minutes every 6–8 hours because activity promotes gastric motility; provide supervised freedom from the cage or access to a safe grazing area.

## DIET

• Critical patients with acute small intestinal or pyloric obstruction should be NPO until obstruction is relieved; then resume normal feeding if rabbit is willing to eat.
• It is absolutely imperative that the rabbit continue to eat during and following medical treatment, and within 12 hours of surgical treatment. Continued anorexia will exacerbate gastrointestinal hypomotility and cause further derangement of the gastrointestinal microflora and overgrowth of intestinal bacterial pathogens.
• Offer a large selection of fresh, moistened greens such as cilantro, romaine lettuce, parsley, carrot tops, dandelion greens, spinach, collard greens, etc., and good-quality grass hay. Many rabbits will begin to eat these foods, even if they were previously anorectic. Also offer the rabbit's usual pelleted diet, as the initial goal is to get the rabbit to eat.
• If the patient refuses these foods, syringe feed a gruel such as Critical Care for Herbivores (Oxbow Pet Products, Murdock, NE) 10–15 mL/kg PO q6–8h. Alternatively, pellets can be ground and mixed with fresh greens, vegetable baby foods, water, or juice to form a gruel. If sufficient volumes of food are not accepted in this manner, nasogastric intubation is indicated.
• High-carbohydrate, high-fat nutritional supplements are contraindicated.
• The diet should be permanently modified to include sufficient amounts of indigestible, coarse fiber. Offer long-stemmed grass or timothy hay (commercially available hay cubes are not sufficient) and an assortment of washed, fresh leafy greens. These foods should always constitute the bulk of the diet. Pellets should be limited (if offered at all) and foods high in simple carbohydrates prohibited or limited to the occasional treat.

## CLIENT EDUCATION

• Discuss possible complications prior to treatment, especially if surgery is required.
• Discuss the importance of dietary modification.

• Limit unsupervised access to objects commonly ingested from the environment, especially bedding and cloth.

## SURGICAL CONSIDERATIONS

• Gastrointestinal hypomotility—accumulation of inspissated gastric contents (including ingested hair) will usually pass with medical treatment alone; surgery is generally contraindicated in rabbits with gastrointestinal hypomotility. Surgical manipulation of the intestinal tract, hypothermia, anesthetic agents, and pain all exacerbate gastrointestinal hypomotility; gastrointestinal stasis is often worse postoperatively. The combination of these factors results in a significantly worsened prognosis with surgical treatment.
• Ingested foreign material—surgery may be indicated to remove foreign material such as cloth from the stomach; in extremely rare cases, inspissated ingesta form a concretion in the stomach that does not respond to medical treatment alone.
• Gastric dilation due to small intestinal or pyloric foreign body—is a surgical emergency; patients usually present in shock and require decompression prior to surgery.

## MEDICATIONS

Use parenteral medications in animals with severely compromised intestinal motility; oral medications may not be properly absorbed; begin oral medication when intestinal motility begins to return (fecal production, return of appetite, radiographic evidence).

## DRUG(S) OF CHOICE

• Motility modifiers may be helpful in rabbits with gastrointestinal hypomotility. Cisapride (0.5 mg/kg PO q8–12h) enhances gastric emptying and is available through many compounding pharmacies.
• Analgesics such as meloxicam (0.2 mg/kg SC, IM q24h or 0.2–0.5 mg/kg PO q24h) or buprenorphine (0.01–0.05 mg/kg SC, IM, IV q8–12h) are essential to treatment of most rabbits with gastrointestinal hypomotility. Intestinal pain, either postoperative or from gas distention and ileus, impairs mobility and decreases appetite and may severely inhibit recovery.
• Antibiotic therapy—indicated in patients with bacterial overgrowth that sometimes occurs secondary to gastrointestinal hypomotility; more common in patients that have been anorectic for several days; indicated in patients with diarrhea, abnormal fecal cytology, and disruption of the intestinal mucosa (evidenced by blood in the feces)
• When antibiotics are indicated, always use broad-spectrum antibiotics such as trimethoprim sulfa (30 mg/kg PO q12h) or enrofloxacin (5–20 mg/kg PO, SC, IM q12–24h).

• If secondary overgrowth of *Clostridium* spp. is evident, use metronidazole (20 mg/kg PO q12h).
• Simethicone (65–130 mg/rabbit q1h for two to three treatments) may be helpful in alleviating painful intestinal gas.
• For sedation—light sedation with midazolam (0.5–2 mg/kg IM) or diazepam (1–2 mg/kg IM); for deeper sedation and longer procedures, the author prefers ketamine (15–20 mg/kg IM) plus midazolam (0.5–1.0 mg/kg IM); many other sedation protocols exist.
• $H_2$-receptor antagonists may ameliorate or prevent gastric ulceration: cimetidine (5–10 mg/kg PO, SC, IM, IV q6–12h) or ranitidine (2 mg/kg IV q24h or 2–5 mg/kg PO q12h).

## CONTRAINDICATIONS

• The use of antibiotics that are primarily Gram positive in spectrum is contraindicated in rabbits. Use of these antibiotics will suppress the growth of commensal flora, allowing overgrowth of enteric pathogens. Do not orally administer lincomycin, clindamycin, erythromycin, ampicillin, amoxicillin cephalosporins, or penicillins.
• Prior to surgical removal, the use of gastrointestinal motility enhancers is contraindicated in rabbits with complete gastrointestinal tract obstruction due to the possibility of intestinal rupture.
• Corticosteroids—avoid; associated with gastrointestinal ulceration and hemorrhage, delayed wound healing, and heightened susceptibility to infection; rabbits are very sensitive to the immunosuppressive effects of both topic and systemic corticosteroids; use may exacerbate subclinical bacterial infection.

## PRECAUTIONS

• NSAIDs—use with caution in rabbits with compromised renal function; avoid until shock and hypovolemia are corrected; do not use if gastric ulceration is present.
• Oral administration of any antibiotic may potentially cause enteric dysbiosis; discontinue use if diarrhea or anorexia occurs.

## POSSIBLE INTERATIONS
N/A

## ALTERNATIVE DRUGS

• Metoclopramide (0.2–0.05 mg/kg PO, SC q6–8h) has also been used as a gastrointestinal promotility agent; efficacy is questionable.
• Enzymatic digestion of small trichobezoars with fresh pineapple juice, papaya extract, or pancreatic enzymes have been advocated. However, these substances should be used with caution (or preferably, not at all), as they may exacerbate gastric mucosal ulceration/erosions and may contribute to gastric rupture. Additionally, these substances do nothing to treat the underlying

## TRICHOBEZOARS

cause of trichobezoars, gastrointestinal hypomotility.
• Intestinal lubricants such as cat laxatives are unlikely to aid in the passage of trichobezoars as they simply lubricate the intestinal contents and do nothing to treat the underlying motility disorder.
• The addition of psyllium-based food supplements is not an adequate substitution for long-stemmed hay in the diet.

 FOLLOW-UP

### PATIENT MONITORING
• Monitor all patients for return of appetite and production of fecal pellets, indicating successful treatment.
• Surgical patients—anesthetic agents used during surgical removal of intestinal foreign material contribute to gastrointestinal hypomotility and subsequent overgrowth of toxin-forming bacteria. Rabbits with postoperative gastrointestinal stasis are anorectic and produce little to no feces. Be certain that postoperative patients are eating and passing feces prior to release.
• Monitor the patient for at least 2 months after surgery for evidence of stricture formation at the site of the foreign body or intraabdominal adhesions.

### PREVENTION/AVOIDANCE
• Strict feeding of diets containing adequate amounts of indigestible coarse fiber (long-stemmed hay) and low simple carbohydrate content along with access to fresh water will often prevent episodes.
• Allow sufficient daily exercise.
• Prevent obesity.
• Be certain that all postoperative patients are eating and passing feces prior to release.

• Regularly brush rabbits to remove shed hair and prevent ingestion.

### POSSIBLE COMPLICATIONS
• Persistent ileus and death
• Postoperative gastrointestinal stasis and subsequent overgrowth of bacterial pathogens
• Stricture formation at the site of removal; intraabdominal adhesions postoperatively
• Death due to gastric rupture

### EXPECTED COURSE AND PROGNOSIS
• Early medical management of animals with gastrointestinal hypomotility usually carries a good to excellent prognosis.
• The prognosis following surgical removal of foreign material or acute small intestinal obstructions is guarded to poor. Patients recovering well after 7 days appear to have a good prognosis for complete recovery.

 MISCELLANEOUS

### ASSOCIATED CONDITIONS
• Dental disease
• Hypercalciuria
• Hepatic lipidosis

### AGE-RELATED FACTORS
Middle-aged to older rabbits are more likely to develop gastrointestinal hypomotility or neoplasia.

### ZOONOTIC POTENTIAL
N/A

### PREGNANCY
N/A

### SYNONYMS
• Hairballs
• Wool block

### SEE ALSO
• Clostridial enterotoxicosis/enterotoxicosis
• Diarrhea, acute
• Diarrhea, chronic
• Gastrointestinal hypomotility and gastrointestinal stasis

### ABBREVIATIONS
• ALT = alanine aminotransferase
• LRS = lactated Ringer's solution
• NPO = nothing by mouth
• NSAIDs = nonsteroidal antiinflammatory drugs
• PCV = packed cell volume
• TS = total solids

*Suggested Reading*
Brown SA, Rosenthal KL. The anorexic rabbit. Proc North Am Vet Conf 1997:788.
Cheeke PR. Rabbit Feeding and Nutrition. Orlando, FL: Academic Press, 1987.
Donoghue S. Nutrition and pet rabbits. In: Rosenthal KL, ed. Practical Exotic Animal Medicine: The Compendium Collection. Trenton, NJ: Veterinary Learning Systems, 1997:107.
Jenkins JR. Feeding recommendations for the house rabbit. Vet Clin North Am Exotic Anim Pract 1999;2(1):143–151.
Jenkins JR. Gastrointestinal diseases. In: Quesenberry KE, Carpenter JW, eds. Ferrets, Rabbits and Rodents: Clinical Medicine and Surgery. 2nd Ed. Philadelphia: WB Saunders, 2004:161–171.
Paul-Murphy JA, Ramer JC. Urgent care of the pet rabbits. Vet Clin North Am Exotic Anim Pract 1998;1(1):127–152.
Rees Davies R, Rees Davies JAE. Rabbit gastrointestinal physiology. Vet Clin North Am Exotic Anim Pract 2003;6(1):139–153.

# ULCERATIVE PODODERMATITIS (SORE HOCKS)

## BASICS

### DEFINITION
• Avascular necrosis, usually followed by abscessation, cellulitis, osteomyelitis, and synovitis occurring on the plantar or palmar aspect of the feet. Ulcerative pododermatitis occurs more commonly on the rear feet, hence the lay term "sore hocks"; however, the front feet or any portion of the plantar surface can be affected.
• Deep pyoderma/cellulitis secondary to prolonged contact with abrasive, wet, or urine/feces-soaked surfaces, hard or rough surfaces, or excessive weight bearing
• Ulcerative pododermatitis is a painful and often irreversible condition.

### PATHOPHYSIOLOGY
• During locomotion, rabbits normally bear weight on the hind digits (digitigrade stance). At rest, weight is borne in the area between the hind claws and hock (plantigrade stance). Rabbits do not have foot pads, but instead rely on a covering of thick fur on the plantar aspect of the feet, combined with a compliant surface, to protect the feet. Any condition that disrupts normal digitigrade locomotion or cushioning of the plantar aspect of the feet may lead to the formation of pressure sores on the feet. Increased pressure often occurs due to obesity or decreased weight bearing on other feet.
• Avascular necrosis occurs as a consequence of constant pressure applied to skin and soft tissues pressed between the bones of the feet and a hard surface. Necrosis of these tissues is followed by sloughing, ulceration, and secondary bacterial infection.
• Dermatitis on the plantar aspect of the foot is common in rabbits housed on abrasive surfaces (wire, carpeting, or Astroturf) or those that sit in soiled cat litter or corn cob litter or on soiled bedding. Prolonged contact with wire, abrasive, or moist surfaces leads first to hair loss, followed by superficial dermatitis, deep pyoderma, cellulitis, and abscess formation. Untreated, it may progress to osteomyelitis and synovitis.
• Pain associated with necrosis and infection often causes affected rabbits to remain sedentary; continued weight bearing on affected feet in sedentary rabbits extends areas of pressure necrosis, exacerbating the condition. Eventually, some affected rabbits develop osteomyelitis and synovitis with permanent damage to tendons, so that maintenance of a normal stance is no longer possible. In these rabbits, damage is often irreversible.
• Conditions leading to ulcerative pododermatitis may be environmental (e.g., wire cages; hard surfaces; soiled, damp bedding), or may be an underlying condition (e.g., obesity, urine scald, spondylosis).

### SYSTEMS AFFECTED
• Skin/exocrine—percutaneous
• Musculoskeletal—osteomyelitis, tendonitis

### INCIDENCE/PREVALENCE
Extremely common in commercial rabbits or pet/show rabbits housed in wire cages or hutches. Frequently seen in house rabbits housed on hard floors or carpeting

### SIGNALMENT
• No age or sex predilection
• Rex, angoras, and large breeds may be more susceptible.

### SIGNS

#### Historical Findings
• Husbandry history—very important in determining underlying cause. Seen in rabbits confined to small, wire cages or hutches; rabbits housed on noncompliant surfaces such as bare floors or carpeting; rabbits kept on soiled, feces- and urine-soaked bedding
• History of sitting in the litter box—sitting on soiled litter, especially corn cob litter and scoopable litters
• A history of shaving the thick, protective hair on the plantar aspect of the hocks
• History of obesity, musculoskeletal disorder causing sedentary life, decreased weight bearing on the contralateral limb, or urine scalding in the perineal and hind limb region
• History of alopecia on the plantar surface of the hock early in the course of disease; progresses to erythema, ulceration, scab formation, abscess
• Anorexia, depression, lameness, reluctance to move—from pain

#### Physical Examination Findings
• Early, asymptomatic disease (Grade I)—hair loss on the plantar or palmar aspect of the feet or hocks
• Mild disease (Grade II)—erythema, swelling with overlying skin intact
• Moderate disease (Grade III)—ulceration, scab formation
• Severe disease (Grade IV)—abscess, inflammation of tendons or deeper tissues
• Severe, often irreversible disease (Grade V)—osteomyelitis; synovitis and tendonitis leading to abnormal stance and gait

#### Other Findings
• Anorexia, depression, lameness, reluctance to move—from pain
• Obesity
• Examine other limbs for musculoskeletal disorders causing a decrease in weight bearing.

### CAUSES
• Pressure sores; avascular necrosis caused by entrapment of soft tissues of the limb between bone and hard surfaces

• Excoriation, friction, or constant moisture on the skin and soft tissues of the plantar aspect of the hock is caused by lack of protective fur covering and/or feces, urine, or water coating the feet.
• Pyogenic bacteria—secondary infection with *Staphylococcus aureus* most common; *Pseudomonas*; *Escherichia coli*; b-hemolytic *Streptococcus* spp.; *Proteus* spp.; *Bacteroides* spp.; *Pasteurella multocida*

### RISK FACTORS
• Environmental—sitting on soiled litter (cat litter, corn cob litter); wire-floored cages, hard floor surfaces, abrasive carpeting, soiled bedding. A lack of footpads requires a soft, compliant surface (grass, dirt in nature; hay or other dry, soft bedding in captivity) for protection of the feet.
• Lack of exercise—small cages or housing; abnormal amount of time spent with weight borne on the hocks; this combined with an abrasive/hard surface or soiled litter/bedding will predispose to disease.
• Obesity—increased amount of weight supported by hocks; long periods of recumbency
• Musculoskeletal disease or other painful conditions (dental disease, urolithiasis)—reluctance to move increases time spent on hocks; may prevent rabbit from adopting a normal stance while micturating, resulting in urine scalding; may prevent eating of cecotrophs and accumulation of cecotrophs on perineal region and feet; may prevent normal locomotion or weight bearing at rest
• Urinary tract disease or gastrointestinal disease—may cause polyuria or diarrhea leading to urine scald or pasting of feces on feet and perineal region
• Clipping or shaving the protective layer of fur on the plantar or palmar aspect of the hock or feet
• Nervous, stressed rabbits—thumping and stamping the rear limbs
• Trauma or puncture wounds to the plantar or palmar aspect of the hock or feet

## DIAGNOSIS

### DIFFERENTIAL DIAGNOSIS
• Abscess secondary to bacteremia or trauma
• Neoplasia
• Granuloma
• Fracture

### CBC/BIOCHEMISTRY/URINALYSIS
• CBC—normal or relative neutrophilia and lymphopenia; TWBC elevations not usually seen in rabbits with abscesses
• Urinalysis and serum chemistry profile—depend on underlying cause and system affected

# ULCERATIVE PODODERMATITIS (SORE HOCKS)

### OTHER LABORATORY TESTS
N/A

### IMAGING
• Radiography—to determine the extent of bone involvement; essential in guidance of treatment plan and expected prognosis; osteomyelitis carries poorer prognosis, prolonged treatment
• Skull radiographs—to rule out dental disease as a cause of pain and reluctance to groom or ambulate
• Whole body radiographs—to rule out other causes of pain and reluctance to groom or ambulate (arthritis, urolithiasis, problems with contralateral limb).
• Ultrasonography—to determine underlying causes, organ system affected, extent of disease

### DIAGNOSTIC PROCEDURES
• Aspiration—may reveal a thick, creamy to caseous, white exudate in rabbits with secondary bacterial infection; high nucleated cell count; primarily degenerative neutrophils with lesser numbers of macrophages and lymphocytes
• Biopsy if mass lesion is present—to rule out neoplasia, granuloma, and other causes of masses; sample should contain both normal and abnormal tissue in the same specimen; submit for histopathologic examination and culture.
• Culture—sterile, deep sample from affected tissue and/or exudate—aerobic and anaerobic bacteria; bacterial susceptibility testing to direct antibiotic therapy

### PATHOLOGIC FINDINGS
• Exudate—large numbers of neutrophils in various stages of degeneration, other inflammatory cells, necrotic tissue
• Surrounding tissue—avascular or suppurative necrosis, ulceration, large number of neutrophils, variable number of lymphocytes, plasma cells, macrophages, fibrous connective tissue
• Osteomyelitis—bone resorption, severe septic arthritis

# TREATMENT

### APPROPRIATE HEALTH CARE
• It is essential to remove/correct the underling cause for long-term success.
• Outpatient—early disease (erythema, alopecia)
• Inpatient—surgical procedures; daily debridement and bandaging

### NURSING CARE
• Depends on severity of disease
• Caging on soft, dry bedding alone may be effective in early disease (erythema, alopecia prior to ulceration or abscess). Clean hay, pine shavings, or shredded paper over a

padded surface that can be completely cleaned and dried works well.
• More severe disease—requires frequent debridement and flushing of exudate and necrotic tissue (daily in severe cases), frequent bandage changes, long-term antibiotics, and pain control
• Bandaging—depends on severity of disease. Usually only necessary in rabbits with open wounds or following debridement. Severely affected rabbits may require daily debridement or flushing. This is a painful procedure requiring general anesthesia (isoflurane). Following debridement, application of wet-to-dry bandages may be required initially until a granulation bed is formed; postdebridement application of silver sulfadiazine cream followed by bandaging may also be effective. Bandage change interval increases with improvement; wet bandages should be changed immediately.

### ACTIVITY
• Restrict until adequate healing of tissues has taken place.
• Long term—encourage activity; prolonged inactivity may cause or exacerbate pododermatitis.

### DIET
• It is absolutely imperative that the rabbit continue to eat during and following treatment. Anorexia will often cause gastrointestinal hypomotility, derangement of the gastrointestinal microflora, and overgrowth of intestinal bacterial pathogens.
• Offer a large selection of fresh, moistened greens such as cilantro, romaine lettuce, parsley, carrot tops, dandelion greens, spinach, collard greens, etc., and good-quality grass hay. Many rabbits will begin to eat these foods, even if they were previously anorectic.
• If the patient refuses these foods, syringe feed a gruel such as Critical Care for Herbivores (Oxbow Pet Products, Murdock, NE) 10–15 mL/kg PO q6–8h. Alternatively, pellets can be ground and mixed with fresh greens, vegetable baby foods, water, or juice to form a gruel.
• High-carbohydrate, high-fat nutritional supplements are contraindicated.
• Encourage oral fluid intake by offering fresh water, wetting leafy vegetables, or flavoring water with vegetable juices.
• Dietary modification to correct underlying obesity, when present is helpful.

### CLIENT EDUCATION
• Discuss need to correct or prevent risk factors. Correction of underlying disease and husbandry problems is imperative for a successful outcome. Discuss appropriate bedding material; do not house rabbits on wire flooring.

• Severe disease, involving bone and tendon, carries a guarded to poor prognosis for complete resolution. Most will require surgical debridement, sometimes multiple surgeries and multiple follow-up visits. Recurrences are common, especially if the underlying cause cannot be corrected. Clients must be aware of the monetary and time investment.

### SURGICAL CONSIDERATIONS
• Debride all visibly necrotic tissue.
• Simple lancing and draining is not adequate to treat abscesses in rabbits. Thick exudates do not drain well, and the abscess will recur. Instead of draining, curette all visible exudates and flush copiously. Repeated, sometimes daily, debridement and flushing are often required.
• Treat as open wound—flush and debride wound daily initially, followed by twice weekly to weekly debridement as healing occurs. Irrigate wound with dilute antiseptic solution (chlorhexidine or iodine) daily until healthy granulation bed forms, followed by silver sulfadiazine cream until reepithelialization occurs. Follow debridement with application of soft, padded bandages. Bandages must be changed immediately if they become wet.
• Remove any foreign objects(s) or nidus of infection.
• Feet that are extensively diseased or abscessed often respond well to filling the defect with antibiotic-impregnated polymethyl methacrylate (AIPMMA) beads.
• AIPMMA beads release a high concentration of antibiotic into local tissues for several months. Selection of antibiotic is limited to those known to elute appropriately from bead to tissues and should be based on culture and susceptibility testing. AIPMMA beads are not commercially available, but can be made using PMMA by Surgical Simplex Bone Cement (Howmedica, Rutherford, NJ) or Bone Cement (Zimmer, Charlotte, NC). Antibiotics successfully used include cephalothin, cefazolin, or ceftiofur (2 g/20 g PMMA); gentamicin or tobramycin (1 g/2 g PMMA); or amikacin (1.25 g/2 g PMMA). Antibiotic is added to the copolymer powder before adding the liquid and formed into small, spherical beads. Beads must be inserted aseptically, and unused beads should be gas sterilized prior to future use. Beads should be left in the incision site for at least 2 months, but can be left in indefinitely.
• Given the expense and pain involved in these procedures, the author recommends referral to a specialist if surgical expertise or AIPMMA beads are not available.
• Place on long-term antibiotic therapy; appropriate pain management
• Severe osteomyelitis may require amputation; midfemoral amputation of hind limb

better tolerated; may be precluded by the presence of bilateral disease
• Correct underlying cause—provide soft bedding, improve husbandry, promote weight loss.

## MEDICATIONS

### DRUG(S) OF CHOICE

Antimicrobial drugs are effective against the infectious agent; gain access to site of infection. Choice of antibiotic is ideally based on results of culture and susceptibility testing. Depending on the severity of infection, long-term antibiotic therapy is required (4–6 weeks minimum to several months or years). Use broad-spectrum antibiotics such as enrofloxacin (5–20 mg/kg PO, SC, IM q12–24h) or trimethoprim sulfa (30 mg/kg PO q12h); if anaerobic infections are suspected use chloramphenicol (50 mg/kg PO q8h); metronidazole (20 mg/kg PO q12–24h) or azithromycin (30 mg/kg PO q24h, can be used alone or combined with metronidazole [20 mg/kg PO q12h]). Alternatively, use penicillin g (40,000–60,000 IU/kg SC q2–7d). Combine with topical treatment listed above.

#### Acute Pain Management
• Butorphanol (0.1–1.0 mg/kg SC, IM, IV q4–6h)—may cause profound sedation; short-acting
• Buprenorphine (0.01–0.05 mg/kg SC, IM, IV q8–12h); less sedating, longer-acting than butorphanol
• Morphine (2–5 mg/kg SC, IM q2–4h) or oxymorphone (0.05–0.2 mg/kg SC, IM q8–12h); use with caution; more than one to two doses may cause gastrointestinal stasis.
• Meloxicam (0.2 mg/kg SC, IM q24h)
• Carprofen (1–4 mg/kg SC q12h)

#### Long-Term Pain Management
• NSAIDs—have been used for short- or long-term therapy to reduce pain and inflammation in rabbits with spinal cord disease: meloxicam (0.2–0.5 mg/kg PO q24h) or carprofen (2.2 mg/kg PO q12–24h)
• For sedation—light sedation with midazolam (1–2 mg/kg IM) or diazepam (1–3 mg/kg IM); for deeper sedation and longer procedures, the author prefers ketamine (15–20 mg/kg IM) plus midazolam (0.5 mg/kg IM); many other sedation protocols exist.

### CONTRAINDICATIONS
• Oral administration of antibiotics that select against Gram-positive bacteria (penicillins, macrolides, lincosamides, and cephalosporins) can cause fatal enteric dysbiosis and enterotoxemia.
• The use of corticosteroids (systemic or topical preparations) can severely exacerbate infection.

### PRECAUTIONS
If amputation of a limb is necessary, the contralateral limb will be at increased risk of developing pododermatitis due to increase in weight bearing.

### POSSIBLE INTERACTIONS
N/A

### ALTERNATIVE DRUGS
50% dextrose or honey have been used successfully as topical abscess treatment following surgical debridement. These have bactericidal properties and promote granulation bed formation. The abscess cavity is filled with honey or dextrose-soaked gauze daily. Old gauze is removed from the cavity prior to instillation of fresh gauze. Treatment is continued for weeks. Effectiveness varies, depending on the severity of disease and owner compliance.

## FOLLOW-UP

### PATIENT MONITORING
Monitor for progressive decrease in exudate, resolution of inflammation, and improvement of clinical signs.

### PREVENTION/AVOIDANCE
• Provide clean, appropriate surface substrates; provide separate litter box and hide box or bed to prevent prolonged sitting on soiled litter; clean soiled substrates daily; avoid wet bedding (rain, spilled water bowls or bottles).
• Prevent obesity.
• Encourage exercise; provide large spaces to encourage movement.

### POSSIBLE COMPLICATIONS
• Severe osteomyelitis; irreversible tendon damage
• Sepsis
• Development of pododermatitis on other feet due to increase in weight bearing
• Urine scald from immobility; myiasis

### EXPECTED COURSE AND PROGNOSIS
Depend on the amount of tissue destruction
• Alopecia of weight bearing foot surfaces (Grade I)—hair often will not regrow; these animals are at risk lifelong; closely control environmental factors and monitor feet.
• Superficial disease (Grade II–III erythema, alopecia, swelling without involvement of deeper tissues)—good to fair prognosis; recurrence if husbandry problems are not addressed
• Osteomyelitis, tendon damage, extensive abscesses (Grade IV–V)—prognosis for return to normal anatomy is grave; prognosis for return to functional weight bearing depends on the severity of bone involvement and extent of abscesses. Multiple surgical debridement, AIPMMA beads, and follow-

up treatments are usually required; recurrence rates are high. Amputation or euthanasia may be warranted in animals with intractable pain.

## MISCELLANEOUS

### ASSOCIATED CONDITIONS
• Immunosuppression
• Gastrointestinal hypomotility

### AGE-RELATED FACTORS
N/A

### ZOONOTIC POTENTIAL
N/A

### PREGNANCY
N/A

### SEE ALSO
• Abscessation
• Obesity

### ABBREVIATIONS
• CBC = complete blood count
• NSAIDs = nonsteroidal antiinflammatory drugs
• TWBC = total white blood cell

*Suggested Reading*
Bennet RA. Treatment of abscesses in the head of rabbits. Proc North Am Vet Conf 1999;821–823.
Deeb BJ, Carpenter JW. Neurologic and musculoskeletal diseases. In: Quesenberry KE, Carpenter JW, eds. Ferrets, Rabbits and Rodents: Clinical Medicine and Surgery. 2nd Ed. Philadelphia: WB Saunders, 2004:203–210.
Ethell MT, Bennett RA, Brown MP, et al. In vitro elution of gentamicin, amikacin, and ceftiofur from polymethylmethacrylate and hydroxyapatite cement. Vet Surg 2000;29:375–382.
Harcourt-Brown F. Neurological and locomotor diseases. In: Harcourt-Brown F, ed. Textbook of Rabbit Medicine. Oxford: Butterworth-Heinemann, 2002:307–323.
Hess L. Dermatologic diseases. In: Quesenberry KE, Carpenter JW, eds. Ferrets, Rabbits and Rodents: Clinical Medicine and Surgery. 2nd Ed. Philadelphia: WB Saunders, 2004:194–202.
Kapatkin A. Orthopedics in small mammals. In: Quesenberry KE, Carpenter JW, eds. Ferrets, Rabbits and Rodents: Clinical Medicine and Surgery. 2nd Ed. Philadelphia: WB Saunders, 2004:383–391.
Lukehart SA, Fohn MJ, Baker-Zander SA. Efficacy of azithromycin for therapy of active syphilis in the rabbit model. J Antimicrob Chemother 1990;25 Suppl A:91–99.

# URINARY TRACT OBSTRUCTION

## BASICS

### DEFINITION
Restricted flow of urine from the kidneys through the urinary tract to the external urethral orifice

### PATHOPHYSIOLOGY
• Excess resistance to urine flow through the urinary tract develops because of lesions affecting the excretory pathway, which cause increased pressure in the urinary space proximal to the obstruction and may cause abnormal distension of this space with urine. Ensuing pathophysiologic consequences depend on the site, degree, and duration of obstruction. Complete obstruction produces a pathophysiologic state equivalent to oliguric acute renal failure.
• The most common cause of urinary tract obstruction in rabbits is hypercalciuria and the subsequent formation of uroliths or calcium "sand" or "sludge" blocking the urethra. In rabbits, intestinal calcium absorption is not dependent on vitamin D, and nearly all calcium in the diet is absorbed. Calcium excretion occurs primarily through the kidneys (vs. the gallbladder in other mammals); the fractional urinary excretion is 45–60% in rabbits compared to less than 2% in other mammals.
• Rabbits normally eat a diet high in calcium; however, not all rabbits develop hypercalciuria.
• The factors leading to hypercalciuria and urolith formation in rabbits are unclear; however, the disease is seen more commonly in obese, sedentary rabbits fed a diet composed primarily of alfalfa-based commercial pellets. Most commercial diets contain excessive amounts of calcium. However, it is unlikely that high dietary calcium content alone is the cause of hypercalciuria, but may exacerbate urinary sludge formation when combined with other factors leading to urine retention.
• Inadequate water intake leading to a more concentrated urine and factors that impair complete evacuation of the bladder, such as lack of exercise, obesity, cystitis, neoplasia or neuromuscular disease, may also contribute. Without frequent urination and dilute urine, calcium crystals may precipitate out of solution within the bladder. Precipitated crystals form a thick sand or sludge within the bladder that does not mix normally with urine and is not eliminated during voiding.
• Uroliths may also form in the renal pelvis or ureters.

### SYSTEMS AFFECTED
• Renal/urologic
• Gastrointestinal, cardiovascular, nervous, and respiratory systems as uremia develops

### SIGNALMENT
Seen most commonly in middle-aged rabbits 3–5 years old

### SIGNS
• Some animals remain asymptomatic, despite large amounts of calcium sludge accumulation in the bladder.
• Depend on location, size, and amount of material in the bladder

#### Historical Findings
• Pollakiuria (common) or stranguria
• Owners may report thick, pasty beige- to brown-colored urine; sometimes this urine is so thick that it is mistaken for diarrhea.
• Abnormal-appearing urine is not always reported. Some rabbits void clear urine while sludge remains in the bladder; sometimes cloudy urine is reported.
• Hunched posture, ataxia, or difficulty ambulating in rabbits with neurologic or orthopedic disorders leading to urine retention
• Urine scald, moist pyoderma
• Reduced velocity or caliber of the urine stream or no urine flow during voiding
• Gross hematuria
• Signs of uremia that develop when urinary tract obstruction is complete (or nearly complete)—anorexia, weight loss, lethargy, tooth grinding, tenesmus, and a hunched posture

#### Physical Examination Findings
• Excessive (i.e., overly large or turgid) or inappropriate (i.e., remaining after voiding efforts), palpable distension of the urinary bladder
• Detect urocystoliths by abdominal palpation; failure to palpate uroliths does not exclude them from consideration. Usually one single, large calculus is palpated. In rabbits with crystalluria, the bladder palpates as a soft, doughy mass.
• Manual expression of the bladder may reveal thick, beige- to brown-colored urine. Manual expression of the bladder may expel thick, brown urine even in rabbits that have normal-appearing voided urine.
• A large kidney may be palpated in rabbits with ureteroliths and subsequent hydronephrosis (rare).
• Signs of severe uremia—dehydration, weakness, hypothermia, bradycardia, high rate of shallow respirations, stupor or coma, seizures sometimes occurring terminally, tachycardia resulting from ventricular dysrhythmias induced by severe hyperkalemia

### CAUSES

#### Intraluminal Causes
Solid or semisolid structures including calcium oxalate and calcium carbonate uroliths or precipitated "sand," blood clots, and sloughed tissue fragments

#### Intramural Causes
• Neoplasia of the bladder neck or urethra—rare
• Fibrosis at a site of prior injury or inflammation can cause stricture or stenosis, which may impede urine flow or may be a site where intraluminal debris becomes lodged.
• Ruptures, lacerations, and punctures—usually caused by traumatic incidents

### RISK FACTORS CONTRIBUTING TO HYPERCALCIURIA, UROLITHS, CALCIUM "SAND" IN THE BLADDER
• Inadequate water intake—dirty water bowls, unpalatable water, changing water sources, inadequate water provision
• Urine retention—underlying bladder pathology, neuromuscular disease, painful conditions causing a reluctance to ambulate (musculoskeletal disease, dental disease, abscess)
• Inadequate cleaning of litter box or cage may cause some rabbits to avoid urinating for abnormally long periods
• Obesity
• Lack of exercise
• Feeding of exclusively alfalfa-based commercial pelleted diets
• Renal disease
• Calcium or vitamin/mineral supplements added to diet

## DIAGNOSIS

### DIFFERENTIAL DIAGNOSIS
• Repeated unproductive squatting in the litter box by a rabbit that has a urethral obstruction can be misinterpreted as constipation.
• Animals whose efforts to urinate are not observed by their owners can be examined because of signs referable to uremia without a history of possible obstruction.
• Evaluation of any patient with azotemia should include consideration of possible postrenal causes (e.g., urinary obstruction).
• Once existence of urinary obstruction is recognized, diagnostic efforts focus on detecting the presence and evaluating the magnitude of abnormalities secondary to obstruction and identifying the location, cause, and completeness of the impediment(s) to urine flow.

### CBC/BIOCHEMISTRY/URINALYSIS
• Results of a hemogram are usually normal.
• Most affected rabbits are hypercalcemic (normal range 12–16 mg/dL); however, the significance of this is unclear since many normal rabbits have high serum calcium concentration and never develop hypercalciuria.

• With urinary tract infection, leukocytosis may be seen, but this finding is rare.
• Complete urinary outflow obstruction can cause postrenal azotemia (e.g., high BUN, creatinine, potassium, or phosphorus).
• Urinary sediment evaluation reveals calcium oxalate or calcium carbonate crystals; however, this is a normal finding in rabbits, and the presence of large amounts of crystals in the urine does not necessarily indicate disease. Disease occurs only when the concentration of crystals is excessive, forming thick, white to brown, sandlike urine and subsequent inflammatory cystitis or partial to complete blockage of the urethra.
• Pyuria (normal value 0–1 WBC/hpf), hematuria (normal value 0–1 RBC/hpf), and proteinuria (normal value 0–33 mg/dL) indicate urinary tract inflammation, but these are nonspecific findings that may result from infectious and noninfectious causes of lower urinary tract disease.

## OTHER LABORATORY TESTS
Uroliths retrieved should be sent for crystallographic analysis to determine their composition.

## IMAGING
### Abdominal Radiography
• Calcium oxalate uroliths and "sand" are radiopaque and usually detected by survey radiography. Uroliths must be differentiated from calcium "sand" or "sludge" in the bladder, which resembles a bladder full of contrast material. Ultrasonic examination of the bladder and palpation can be helpful to distinguish solitary calculi from amorphous "sand."
• Occasionally, relatively large uroliths can be found in the urethra and may cause only partial obstruction.

### Abdominal Ultrasonography
Ultrasonography is highly sensitive for detecting lesions of the bladder and proximal urethra and upper urinary tract (i.e., ureter or renal pelvis) obstruction.

## DIAGNOSTIC PROCEDURES
• Urinary catheterization has diagnostic and therapeutic value. As the catheter is inserted, the location and nature of obstructing material may be determined. Some or all of the obstructing material (e.g., small uroliths and urethral sludge) may be induced to pass out of the urethra distally for identification and analysis. Retrograde irrigation of the urethral lumen may propel intraluminal debris toward the bladder. Although intramural lesions sometimes are detected during catheterization, catheter insertion can be normal. Animals that cannot urinate despite generating adequate intravesicular pressure (i.e., excessive outlet resistance) and have urethras that can be readily catheterized and irrigated either have intramural lesions or functional urinary retention.

• Abdominocentesis is required if rupture of the bladder or ureter is suspected.

# TREATMENT

## APPROPRIATE HEALTH CARE
• Complete obstruction is a medical emergency that can be life threatening; treatment should usually be started immediately.
• Partial obstruction—not necessarily an emergency, but these patients may be at risk for developing complete obstruction; may cause irreversible urinary tract damage if not treated promptly
• Treat as an inpatient until the patient's ability to urinate has been restored.
• Surgery is sometimes required.
• Long-term management and prognosis depend on the cause of the obstruction and resulting damage to the bladder wall or renal parenchyma.
• Treatment has three major components: combating the metabolic derangements associated with postrenal uremia; restoring and maintaining a patent pathway for urine outflow; and implementing specific treatment for the underlying cause of urine retention.
• Ureteroliths can be surprisingly large and may nevertheless cause only partial obstruction. Retrograde urohydropropulsion can sometimes be used to push small stones back into the bladder, then removed via cystotomy.

## NURSING CARE
Give fluid therapy to patients with dehydration or azotemia. Give fluids intravenously if systemic derangements are moderately severe or worse. Fluid therapy for rabbits with urinary obstruction should be based on treatment modalities used in cats with obstructive urinary tract disease.

## ACTIVITY
• Reduce during the period of tissue repair after surgery.
• Long term—increase activity level by providing large exercise areas to encourage voiding and prevent recurrence.

## DIET
• It is absolutely imperative that the rabbit continue to eat during and following treatment. Many rabbits with urinary tract obstruction have a decreased appetite. Anorexia may cause or exacerbate gastrointestinal hypomotility and cause derangement of the gastrointestinal microflora and overgrowth of intestinal bacterial pathogens.
• Offer a large selection of fresh, moistened greens such as cilantro, romaine lettuce, parsley, carrot tops, dandelion greens, spinach, or collard greens and good-quality grass hay. Many rabbits will begin to eat these foods, even if they were previously anorectic.

• If the patient refuses these foods, syringe feed a gruel such as Critical Care for Herbivores (Oxbow Pet Products, Murdock, NE) 10–15 mL/kg PO q6–8h. Larger volumes and more frequent feedings are often accepted; feed as much as the rabbit will readily accept. Alternatively, pellets can be ground and mixed with fresh greens, vegetable baby foods, water, or juice to form a gruel. The addition of canned pumpkin to this gruel is a palatable source of fiber and calories. If sufficient volumes of food are not accepted in this manner, nasogastric intubation is indicated.
• High-carbohydrate, high-fat nutritional supplements are contraindicated.
• Increasing water consumption is essential to prevention and treatment of hypercalciuria. Provide multiple sources of fresh water. Automatic, continuously pouring water fountains available for cats entice some rabbit to drink. Flavoring the water with fruit or vegetable juices (with no added sugars) may be helpful. Provide a variety of clean, fresh, leafy vegetables sprayed or soaked with water.
• No reports of dissolution of calcium oxalate uroliths with special diets
• Following treatment, reduction in the amount of calcium in the diet may help to prevent or delay recurrence. Eliminate feeding of alfalfa pellets and switch to a high-fiber timothy-based pellet (Oxbow Pet Products, Murdock, NE). The form of calcium found in alfalfa-based commercial pellets and alfalfa hay is calcium carbonate, which is 50% more bioavailable than the calcium oxalate found in most green, leafy vegetables. Feed timothy and grass hay instead of alfalfa hay, and offer large volumes of fresh, green, leafy vegetables.

## CLIENT EDUCATION
Urolith removal or removal of calcium "sand" does not alter the factors responsible for their formation; eliminating risk factors such as obesity, sedentary life, and poor diet combined with increasing water consumption is necessary to minimize or delay recurrence. Even with these changes, however, recurrence is likely.

## SURGICAL CONSIDERATIONS
• Uroliths within the bladder, ureters, or renal pelvis must be removed surgically. The procedures are similar to those performed on dogs or cats.
• Large urethral calculi may require surgical removal.
• Calcium "sludge" in the bladder that does not respond to medical therapy may require cystotomy for removal.

# URINARY TRACT OBSTRUCTION

## MEDICATIONS

### DRUG(S) OF CHOICE
• Medical dissolution is ineffective.
• Dietary therapy aimed at prevention of recurrent disease (See Diet above) is imperative following relief of obstruction.
• Pain management is essential during and following surgery or if pain is causing reduced frequency of voiding. Perioperative choices include butorphanol (0.1–1.0 mg/kg SC, IM, IV q4–6h) or buprenorphine (0.01–0.05 mg/kg SC, IM, IV q6–12h). Meloxicam (0.2–0.5 mg/k PO q24h) and carprofen (1–2.2 mg/kg PO q12h) have been used for long-term pain management.
• Procedures for relief of obstruction often require, or are facilitated by, giving sedatives or anesthetics. When substantial systemic derangements exist, start fluid administration and other supportive measures first. Calculate the dosage of sedative or anesthetic drug using the low end of the recommended range or give only to effect. Isoflurane is the anesthetic of choice.

### CONTRAINDICATIONS
Avoid intramuscular ketamine in patients with complete obstruction, because it is excreted through the kidneys. If the obstruction cannot be eliminated, prolonged sedation may result.

### PRECAUTIONS
• Avoid drugs that reduce blood pressure or induce cardiac dysrhythmia until dehydration is resolved.
• Modify dosages of all drugs that require renal metabolism or elimination.
• Avoid nephrotoxic agents (NSAIDs, aminoglycosides).

### POSSIBLE INTERACTIONS
None

### ALTERNATIVE DRUGS
N/A

## FOLLOW-UP

### PATIENT MONITORING
• Gastrointestinal hypomotility and stasis are common postoperatively. Make sure that the rabbit is eating, well hydrated, and passing normal stool prior to release.
• Assess urine production and hydration status frequently, and adjust fluid administration rate accordingly.
• Verify ability to urinate adequately or use urinary catheterization to combat urine retention.

### PREVENTION/AVOIDANCE
• Increase water consumption for the remainder of the rabbit's life.
• Place patients on a lowered calcium diet (described above).
• Increase exercise.

### POSSIBLE COMPLICATIONS
• Bladder rupture, uroabdomen
• Trauma to the excretory pathway while trying to relieve obstruction
• Ureteral or urethral stricture formation
• Bradycardia secondary to hyperkalemia
• Renal failure
• Recurrence of obstruction

### EXPECTED COURSE AND PROGNOSIS
• Highly variable; depends on urolith location and size and the presence of secondary complications (e.g., obstruction, infection, renal failure)
• The prognosis following surgical removal of uroliths is usually fair to good. Although husbandry changes and dietary management may decrease the likelihood of recurrence, many rabbits will develop clinical disease again within 1–2 years.

## MISCELLANEOUS

### ASSOCIATED CONDITIONS
• Gastrointestinal hypomotility
• Dental disease
• Lower urinary tract infections

### AGE-RELATED FACTORS
• Neoplasia tends to occur in middle-aged to older rabbits.
• Hypercalciuria tends to occur in middle-aged to older rabbits.

### ZOONOTIC POTENTIAL
N/A

### PREGNANCY
N/A

### SYNONYMS
Urethral obstruction

### SEE ALSO
• Hypercalciuria and urolithiasis
• Lower urinary tract infection

### ABBREVIATIONS
• BUN = blood urea nitrogen
• NSAIDs = nonsteroidal antiinflammatory drugs
• RBC = red blood cell
• WBC = white blood cell

### Suggested Reading
Brown SA. Rabbit urinary tract disease. Proc North Am Vet Conf 1997;785–787.
Cheeke PR, Amberg JW. Comparative calcium excretion by rats and rabbits. J Anim Sci 1973;37:450–454.
Donoghue S. Nutrition and pet rabbits. In: Rosenthal KL, ed. Practical Exotic Animal Medicine: The Compendium Collection. Trenton, NJ: Veterinary Learning Systems, 1997:107.
Garibaldi BA, Pecquet-Goad ME. Hypercalcemia with secondary nephrolithiasis in a rabbit. Lab Anim Sci 1988;38:331–333.
Harcourt-Brown F. Urogenital disease. In: Harcourt-Brown F, ed. Textbook of Rabbit Medicine. Oxford: Butterworth-Heinemann, 2002:335–351.
Harkness JE, Wagner JE. The Biology and Medicine of Rabbits and Rodents. 3rd Ed. Baltimore: Williams & Wilkins, 1989.
Kampheus J. Calcium metabolism of rabbits as an etiological factor for urolithiasis. J Nutr 1991;121:595–596.
Pare JA, Paul-Murphy J. Disorders of the reproductive and urinary systems. In: Quesenberry KE, Carpenter JW, eds. Ferrets, Rabbits and Rodents: Clinical Medicine and Surgery. 2nd Ed. Philadelphia: WB Saunders, 2004:183–193.
Paul-Murphy J, Ramer JC. Urgent care of the pet rabbits. Vet Clin North Am Exotic Anim Pract 1998;1(1):127–152.
Redrobe S. Calcium metabolism in rabbits. Semin Avian Exotic Pet Med 2002;11(2):94–101.

### Portions Adapted From
Lees GE. Urinary Tract Obstruction. In: Tilley LP, Smith FWK, Jr., eds. The 5-Minute Veterinary Consult: Canine and Feline, 3rd Ed. Baltimore: Lippincott Williams & Wilkins, 2004.

## BASICS

### OVERVIEW
• Most common neoplasm in rabbits; incidence of up to 60% in females >3 years old; higher incidence in some breeds.
• Arises from the endometrial glandular epithelium
• May be preceded by endometriosis, endometritis, endometrial hyperplasia, or endometrial venous aneurysms
• Tumors or associated venous aneurysms frequently bleed. Hemorrhage may become life threatening.
• No difference in incidence in breeding vs. nonbreeding does
• Age is the most significant risk factor.
• Relatively slow-growing, but will eventually metastasize locally by extension into the myometrium and peritoneum, or will metastasize hematogenously
• Most common site of distal metastasis is the lung; brain, ocular, cutaneous, bone, and hepatic metastasis may also occur.
• Average interval between onset of clinical signs and death from metastasis is 12–24 months.
• Tumors are usually multicentric; present in both uterine horns
• Tumors may occur simultaneously with endometrial venous aneurysms, pyometra, or pregnancy.
• Mammary neoplasia or cystic mastitis often found in does with uterine neoplasia

### SIGNALMENT
• Intact females
• Highest incidence in does >3–4 years old
• All breeds are at risk; highest incidence reported in tan, French silver, Havana, and Dutch breed (up to 80%)

### SIGNS

#### Historical Findings
• Hematuria—most common presenting complaint. Not true hematuria, since blood originates from the uterus, but is released during micturition. Hematuria is often reported as intermittent or cyclic; usually occurs at the end of micturition; blood clots sometimes seen
• Serosanguineous to purulent, blood-tinged vaginal discharge
• Mastitis (mammary gland cysts)—usually cystic, involving one or more mammary glands; cysts contain clear to cloudy fluid; may be seen in up to 30% of rabbits with uterine adenocarcinoma
• Mammary gland neoplasia
• Increased aggressiveness
• Breeding does—small litter size; increased number of stillborn or resorbed fetuses; infertility; dystocia; abandonment of litters

• Late disease, with metastasis—lethargy, anorexia, pale mucous membranes, dyspnea (pulmonary metastasis)

#### Physical Examination Findings
• Firm, often multiple midcaudal abdominal masses; usually palpable dorsal to the bladder between the bladder and the colon
• Abdominal masses may not be palpable until up to 6 months following the onset of reproductive dysfunction.
• Mammary masses
• Blood-stained perineum

### CAUSES AND RISK FACTORS
Intact sexual status

## DIAGNOSIS

### DIFFERENTIAL DIAGNOSIS
• Endometrial venous aneurysms (especially if blood passed with micturition)
• Pregnancy
• Endometrial hyperplasia, hydrometra, or mucometra
• Pyometra
• Other uterine tumors
• Other midcaudal abdominal masses

### CBC/BIOCHEMISTRY/URINALYSIS
• Anemia with significant uterine hemorrhage
• May see increased liver enzymes with metastasis

### OTHER LABORATORY TESTS
N/A

### IMAGING
• Abdominal radiographs—may detect a caudal abdominal mass, usually dorsal to the bladder
• Thoracic radiographs—always recommended; assess for metastasis.
• Ultrasonography—very useful to delineate uterine mass and to differentiate between uterine bleeding and hematuria if blood is expelled during micturition

### DIAGNOSTIC PROCEDURES
• Ultrasound-guided cystocentesis—to differentiate hematuria from uterine blood expelled with urination
• Cytologic evaluation—of associated mammary masses
• Histopathologic examination—necessary for definitive diagnosis

### PATHOLOGIC FINDINGS
• Gross—usually multicentric; may involve one or both horns; may appear as cauliflower-like or papillary- or polyplike projections into the uterine lumen. Often have necrotic or hemorrhagic center, or may secrete mucus. Tumors may occur simultaneously with endometriosis, endometrial venous aneurysms, pyometra, or pregnancy. May

find metastases in local lymph nodes, peritoneum, liver, lung, bone, eyes, or skin
• Histologic—usually well-differentiated adenocarcinoma

## TREATMENT
• Ovariohysterectomy—treatment of choice; usually curative if metastasis has not occurred
• Examine and biopsy the liver to check for metastases.
• Occasionally, local metastasis is not yet grossly visible at time of surgery; give owner a guarded prognosis and recheck at 3- to 6-month intervals.
• Assist-feed any rabbit that is anorectic or inappetent to avoid secondary gastrointestinal disorders.
• Blood transfusion may be indicated in rabbits with significant uterine hemorrhage.
• Excise neoplastic or abscessed mammary glands; cystic mastitis will resolve with ovariohysterectomy alone and does not require excision.

## MEDICATIONS

### DRUG(S) OF CHOICE
• Chemotherapy—success in metastatic disease has not been reported in rabbits. Doxorubicin, cisplatin, and carboplatin are used in cats/dogs. Consult with oncologist.
• Postoperative pain management—choices include butorphanol (0.1–1.0 mg/kg SC, IM, IV q4–6h) or buprenorphine (0.01–0.05 mg/kg SC, IM, IV q6–12h). Meloxicam (0.2–0.5 mg/k PO q24h) and carprofen (1–2.2 mg/kg PO q12h) have been used for long-term pain management.

### CONTRAINDICATIONS/POSSIBLE INTERACTIONS
Chemotherapy may be toxic; seek advice if unfamiliar with these agents.

## FOLLOW-UP

### PATIENT MONITORING
Consider thoracic and abdominal radiographs every 3 months for the first 1–2 years postovariohysterectomy. Not all metastases are grossly visible at the time of surgery.

### PREVENTION/AVOIDANCE
Ovariohysterectomy is recommended for all nonbreeding rabbits; usually performed between 6 months and 2 years of age. For breeding rabbits—recommend stop breeding and spay before 4 years of age, as this is when most tumors occur.

## UTERINE ADENOCARCINOMA

### EXPECTED COURSE AND PROGNOSIS
• Excellent (cure) if ovariohysterectomy prior to metastasis or mammary neoplasia; poor to grave if metastasis has occurred (5 month to 2 years to metastasize); after chemotherapy, unknown
• Without ovariohysterectomy—metastasis, death in 12–24 months
• Associated cystic mastitis will resolve with ovariohysterectomy alone, unless secondary infection has developed.

 **MISCELLANEOUS**

### ASSOCIATED CONDITIONS
• Mammary neoplasia
• Mastitis
• Pyometra or other nonneoplastic endometrial disorders
• Ovarian neoplasia

### AGE-RELATED FACTORS
Rare in rabbits under 2 years of age; risk increases with age; seen in up to 60% of does over 3 years old.

### ZOONOTIC POTENTIAL
N/A

### PREGNANCY
Uterine neoplasia may be concurrent with pregnancy.

### SEE ALSO
• Mastitis, septic and cystic
• Pyometra and nonneoplastic endometrial disorders

### Suggested Reading
Baba N, von Haam E. Animal model for human disease: spontaneous adenocarcinoma in aged rabbits. Am J Pathol 1972;68:653–656.
Jenkins JR. Surgical sterilization in small mammals: spay and castration. Vet Clin North Am Exotic Anim Pract 2000;3(3):617–627.
Lewis B. Uterine adenocarcinoma in a rabbit. Exotic DVM 2003;5(1):11.
Pare JA, Paul-Murphy J. Disorders of the reproductive and urinary systems. In: Quesenberry KE, Carpenter JW, eds. Ferrets, Rabbits and Rodents: Clinical Medicine and Surgery. 2nd Ed. Philadelphia: WB Saunders, 2004:183–193.
Saito K, Nakanishi M, Hasegawa A. Uterine disorders diagnosed by ventrotomy in 47 rabbits. J Vet Med Sci 2002;64(6):495–497.

# BASICS

### DEFINITION
Any substance emanating from the vulvar labia; in rabbits fresh blood or serosanguineous discharge is most common.

### PATHOPHYSIOLOGY
• It may originate from several distinct sources, depending in part on the age and reproductive status of the patient; from uterus (most common), urinary tract, vagina, vestibule or perivulvar skin; except for a small amount of lochia postpartum, vaginal discharge is always abnormal.
• No discharge is seen during estrus in normal does (female rabbit is called a doe). When receptive, the vulva may be slightly swollen, moist, and deep red to purple in color.
• Normal cycling rabbit—induced ovulators with silent estrus; estrous cycles last 7–14 days.
• Serosanguineous discharge or fresh blood is usually mistaken for hematuria, since blood is often expelled from the uterus during micturition.

### SYSTEMS AFFECTED
• Reproductive
• Renal/urologic
• Skin/exocrine

### SIGNALMENT
• Intact females
• Highest incidence of uterine disorders is seen in does >3–4 years old.
• All breeds are at risk.
• Postpartum does—normal bloody or greenish discharges common

### SIGNS

#### Historical Findings
• Hematuria—most common presenting complaint. Not true hematuria, since blood originates from the uterus, but is expelled during micturition. Hematuria is often reported as intermittent or cyclic; it usually occurs at the end of micturition
• Discharge from the vulva adhering to perineal fur
• Spotting—usually bloody
• May have had signs of pseudopregnancy—pulling hair, nest building
• Increased aggressiveness
• Recent parturition—with postpartum discharge
• Breeding does—may have history of small litter size; increased number of stillborn or resorbed fetuses; infertility; dystocia; abandonment of litters

#### Physical Examination Findings
• Blood or serosanguineous discharge—most commonly expelled during urination,

but can appear independent of micturition; may see discharge adhered to fur
• Purulent discharge is extremely uncommon.
• Uterus—may be palpably large; careful palpation may allow determination of size; overly aggressive palpation may induce rupture in rabbits with pyometra.
• Enlarged mammary gland—one or multiple, may be firm and multilobulated (mammary tumors) or fluid filled (cystic)
• Pale mucous membranes and tachycardia in rabbits that have had significant uterine hemorrhage
• Depression, lethargy, and anorexia in rabbits with pyometra or uterine hemorrhage

### CAUSES

#### Serosanguineous or Frank Blood
• Uterine adenocarcinoma—most common cause; other uterine neoplasia possible
• Endometrial disorders—extremely common; endometrial hyperplasia (most common), endometrial venous aneurysms, endometriosis, and endometritis
• Foreign body—rare
• Vaginal neoplasia or vaginal hematoma—rare
• Vaginal trauma
• Urinary tract infection (unusual)

#### Greenish Discharge/Lochia
• Immediately postpartum
• Dystocia

#### Purulent Exudate
• Usually not seen with pyometra or vaginitis since exudate is thick and does not drain well
• Acquired perivulvar dermatitis can also be mistaken for vaginal discharge.
• Vaginitis—rare in rabbits
• Fetal death

### RISK FACTORS
• Intact sexual status
• Risk for uterine disorders, including neoplasia, increases with age—seen more often in rabbits over 3 years of age
• Risk may increase with sterile mating or when does mount each other.

# DIAGNOSIS

### DIFFERENTIAL DIAGNOSES
• Perivulvar dermatitis—moist dermatitis (urine scald); feces pasted around perineum. *Treponema cuniculi* (rabbit syphilis) or myxomatosis—similar lesions in periocular or perioral regions
• Serosanguineous or bloody discharge—may be difficult clinically to differentiate nonneoplastic endometrial disorders from uterine adenocarcinoma prior to ovariohysterectomy. Frequently there are more than

one disorder in the same rabbit, especially in rabbits with uterine adenocarcinoma. For instance, many rabbits with uterine neoplasia also have areas of cystic endometrial hyperplasia.
• Hematuria—use ultrasound-guided cystocentesis to collect urine; differentiates true hematuria from blood expelled from the uterus

### CBC/BIOCHEMISTRY/URINALYSIS
• Often unremarkable in rabbits with uterine adenocarcinoma or other uterine disorders
• Neutrophilia—sometimes seen in rabbits with pyometra
• Regenerative anemia possible in rabbits with uterine hemorrhage
• Azotemia, increases in ALT, electrolyte disturbances—all can be abnormal in rabbits with pyometra, septicemia, or severe dehydration, depending on clinical course
• Urinalysis—sample collected by ultrasound-guided cystocentesis to differentiate hematuria from uterine bleeding

### OTHER LABORATORY TESTS
Histopathologic examination of uterus following ovariohysterectomy—necessary for definitive diagnosis

### IMAGING
• Abdominal radiography—may detect a large uterus in patients with uterine adenocarcinoma, endometrial disorder, or pyometra and later stages of fetal death
• Thoracic radiographs—always recommended; assess for metastasis

#### Ultrasonography
• Assess size of uterus and nature of uterine contents.
• Rule out pregnancy.

### DIAGNOSTIC PROCEDURES
• Vaginal bacterial culture—via guarded culturette (AccuCulShure); perform before doing any other vaginal procedure; may not be helpful in confirming diagnosis (bacteria cultured are usually normal vaginal flora)
• Vaginal cytologic examination—may be helpful in determining if the discharge is purulent or bloody; cytology does not establish stage of estrus.
• Cystocentesis and bacterial culture—help rule out urinary tract disorders
• Biopsy of vaginal mass—rules out neoplasia, if suspected.
• Fine needle aspirate or biopsy of mammary masses, if present

# TREATMENT
• Ovariohysterectomy—treatment of choice for uterine adenocarcinoma; usually curative if metastasis has not occurred

## VAGINAL DISCHARGE

• Ovariohysterectomy—treatment of choice for most uterine disorders. Most uterine disorders carry risk of hemorrhage into the uterus; can become life threatening; can progress; all are at risk for developing uterine adenocarcinoma; reproductive performance is reduced in does with endometrial disorders.

• In does with neoplasia, local metastases are sometimes not grossly visible at time of surgery; give owner a guarded prognosis and recheck at 3- to 6-month intervals.

• Assist-feed any rabbit that is anorectic or inappetent to avoid secondary gastrointestinal disorders.

• Blood transfusion may be indicated in rabbits with significant uterine hemorrhage.

• Excise neoplastic or abscessed mammary glands; cystic mastitis will resolve with ovariohysterectomy alone and does not require excision.

## MEDICATIONS

### DRUG(S) OF CHOICE
• Bacterial vaginitis, pyometra, or endometritis—antibiotics; empirical pending results of bacterial culture and sensitivity test. Use broad-spectrum antibiotics such as enrofloxacin (5–20 mg/kg PO, SC, IM q12–24h), trimethoprim sulfa (30 mg/kg PO q12h), or chloramphenicol (50 mg/kg PO q8h).

• Acute pain management—buprenorphine (0.01–0.05 mg/kg SC, IM, IV q8–12h); use preoperatively.

• Postoperative or long-term pain management—meloxicam (0.2–0.5 mg/kg PO q24h) or carprofen (2.2 mg/kg PO q12–24h)

• Sedation or premedication—ketamine (15–20 mg/kg IM) plus midazolam (0.5–1.0 mg/kg IM); many other protocols exist.

### CONTRAINDICATIONS
• Oral administration of most antibiotics effective against anaerobes will cause a fatal gastrointestinal dysbiosis in rabbits. Do not administer penicillins, macrolides, lincosamides, and cephalosporins by oral administration.

• Corticosteroids—associated with gastrointestinal ulceration and hemorrhage, delayed wound healing, and heightened susceptibility to infection; rabbits are very sensitive to the immunosuppressive effects of both topical and systemic corticosteroids; use may exacerbate subclinical bacterial infection.

### PRECAUTIONS
• Chloramphenicol—avoid human contact with chloramphenicol due to potential blood dyscrasia. Advise owners of potential risks.

• Meloxicam—use with caution in rabbits with compromised renal function.

### POSSIBLE INTERACTIONS
N/A

### ALTERNATIVE DRUGS
Prostaglandins—PGF2α has not been used successfully in rabbits for treatment of pyometra.

## FOLLOW-UP

### PATIENT MONITORING
• Monitor carefully for signs of pain (reluctance to move, teeth grinding) postoperatively.

• Make certain the doe continues to eat postoperatively.

• If owners elect not to perform surgery to treat endometrial disorders—monitor carefully for signs of uterine hemorrhage (blood passed during micturition) or sepsis in rabbits with endometritis or mastitis.

### PREVENTION/AVOIDANCE
• Ovariohysterectomy, for all nonbreeding rabbits; usually performed between 6 months and 2 years of age

• For breeding rabbits—recommend breeding be stopped and spay after 4 years of age, as this is when most endometrial disorders (including adenocarcinoma) occur.

### POSSIBLE COMPLICATIONS
• Peritonitis, sepsis in does with endometritis or pyometra

• Postoperative intraabdominal adhesions—may contribute to chronic pain, gastrointestinal motility disorders

• Uterine adenocarcinoma, metastasis, and mammary neoplasia in does over 3 years of age

• Hemorrhage, possible death in rabbits with bleeding uterine disorders

### EXPECTED COURSE AND PROGNOSIS
• Good prognosis with timely ovariohysterectomy for most uterine disorders, including adenocarcinoma that has not metastasized

• Guarded prognosis in does presented with vigorous vaginal hemorrhage; emergency stabilization and hysterectomy is indicated to control hemorrhage.

• Guarded to poor in does with pyometra that is not treated early; sepsis or peritonitis may follow.

• Excellent (cure) of uterine adenocarcinoma with ovariohysterectomy prior to metastasis or mammary neoplasia; poor to grave if metastasis has occurred (5 month to 2 years to metastasize); after chemotherapy, unknown; without ovariohysterectomy—metastasis, death in 12–24 months.

• Associated cystic mastitis will resolve with ovariohysterectomy alone, unless secondary infection has developed.

## MISCELLANEOUS

### ASSOCIATED CONDITIONS
• Mammary neoplasia
• Mastitis
• Ovarian neoplasia
• Ovarian abscess

### AGE-RELATED FACTORS
Uterine neoplasia—rare in rabbits under 2 years of age; risk increases with age; seen in up to 60% of does over 3 years old

### ZOONOTIC POTENTIAL
N/A

### PREGNANCY
Many antibiotics and corticosteroids are contraindicated during pregnancy.

### SEE ALSO
• Mastitis, cystic and septic
• Pyometra and nonneoplastic endometrial disorders
• Uterine adenocarcinoma

### ABBREVIATIONS
• ALT = alanine aminotransferase
• PGF2α = prostaglandin F2-alpha

### Suggested Reading
Baba N, von Haam E. Animal model for human disease: spontaneous adenocarcinoma in aged rabbits. Am J Pathol 1972;68:653–656.

Jenkins JR. Surgical sterilization in small mammals: spay and castration. Vet Clin North Am Exotic Anim Pract 2000;3(3):617–627.

Lewis B. Uterine adenocarcinoma in a rabbit. Exotic DVM 2003;5(1):11.

Pare JA, Paul-Murphy J. Disorders of the reproductive and urinary systems. In: Quesenberry KE, Carpenter JW, eds. Ferrets, Rabbits and Rodents: Clinical Medicine and Surgery. 2nd Ed. Philadelphia: WB Saunders, 2004:183–193.

Saito K, Nakanishi M, Hasegawa A. Uterine disorders diagnosed by ventrotomy in 47 rabbits. J Vet Med Sci 2002;64(6):495–497.

### Portions Adapted From
Eilts BE. Vaginal Discharge. In: Tilley LP, Smith FWK, Jr., eds. The 5-Minute Veterinary Consult: Canine and Feline, 2nd Ed. Baltimore: Lippincott Williams & Wilkins, 2004.

# VERTEBRAL FRACTURE OR LUXATION

## BASICS

### OVERVIEW
• Extremely common cause of posterior paresis and paralysis in pet rabbits
• Rabbits have strong muscles in the hindquarters, used for hopping. With improper handling, or when caged rabbits are suddenly startled and jump, the hindquarters may twist at the lumbosacral junction, resulting in vertebral fracture or luxation, most commonly at L7.
• Fractures occur more often than dislocations.
• Many affected rabbits are unable to voluntarily express their bladder and may lose anal sphincter tone. Complications secondary to urine retention or urinary/fecal incontinence (uremia, hypercalciuria, moist dermatitis, fly strike) and decubital ulcer formation are common, and often lead to the decision to euthanize.

### SIGNALMENT
No specific age, breed, or gender predisposition

### SIGNS

#### General Comments
Acute onset of posterior paresis—most common finding

#### Historical Findings
• Owner may describe an abnormal gait; the rabbit may be unable to hop, may drag the affected limbs, or may be unable to get up.
• Sudden onset of paresis/paralysis
• History of improper restraint—inexperienced handlers or owners; restraint for mask induction of anesthesia; very nervous animals escaping from inappropriate restraint
• Trauma may not have been witnessed. Many rabbits fracture or luxate vertebrae by suddenly jumping while in their cages. History may include startling event such as a loud thunderstorm or fireworks or unfamiliar people or pets in the house.

#### Physical Examination Findings
• Patient usually alert
• Pain or hyperesthesia can usually be elicited at site of spinal cord damage.
• If in pain, patient may resent handling and manipulation during the examination.
• Superficial and deep pain perception may be decreased or absent in the rear limbs.
• Decreased or absent anal tone
• Decreased or absent proprioception in the rear limbs
• Decreased or absent voluntary movement in the rear limbs and/or tail
• Forelimb function is normal; occasionally Schiff-Sherrington phenomena may cause increased muscle tone in the forelimbs.
• Bladder may also be paralyzed in rabbits with severe spinal cord damage, negating voluntary urination.
• Urine scald in the perineal region; dermatitis or alopecia due to inappropriate grooming or urinary incontinence—sequela to vertebral trauma, days to months following event

### CAUSES AND RISK FACTORS

#### Inappropriate Restraint
• Rabbits often try to jump or twist free of restraint. Injury to L7 is most common result.
• When restraining rabbits, always restrain both front and rear quarters simultaneously. Rabbits can be restrained by using one hand to hold the scruff or hold between the front limbs and one hand to hold the hindquarters, or by tucking the head under one arm while holding the hindquarters with the other hand and holding the rabbit against your body.
• On an examination table, always apply pressure to the front and hindquarters simultaneously; use a towel to firmly wrap the body.
• Covering the eyes will calm some rabbits.
• Cradle the rabbit on its back to examine ventral areas; hold nervous rabbits close to the floor as they may jump during examination.
• Use a well-trained assistant for restraint.
• Most rabbits particularly object to examination of the mouth and ears. Be especially cautious with restraint during these procedures.
• When in doubt, administer sedation or anesthesia to perform noxious procedures.

#### Trauma During Anesthetic Induction
• Many rabbits object to the odor of gas anesthetics. They often appear calm, then suddenly and forcibly jump or kick.
• To prevent injury, be certain that the rabbit is securely restrained, administer preanesthetic sedation prior to mask induction, or use a chamber for induction.
• Even with preanesthetic sedation, be prepared for sudden, unexpected jumping or kicking.

#### Trauma in Cage
• Caged rabbits can injure themselves when startled.
• Usually follows an event such a noisy thunderstorms, fireworks, or the appearance of unfamiliar people or pets
• Return a hospitalized rabbit to the cage rear-end first to prevent jumping.

## DIAGNOSIS

### DIFFERENTIAL DIAGNOSIS

#### Weak Pelvic Limbs
• Pain or hyperesthesia elicited at site of spinal cord damage usually seen with trauma, IVD disease, discospondylitis, and, rarely, bone tumors
• Lack of pain along spinal column—consider *Encephalitozoon cuniculi*, CNS lesions, systemic or metabolic disease; vascular disease (rare), degenerative myelopathy, neoplasia
• Acute onset—most common with spinal cord trauma, but has been anecdotally reported with *E. cuniculi*
• Gradual onset or intermittent weakness—usually systemic or metabolic disease; occasionally seen with IVD extrusion, if extrusion is gradual
• Other clinical signs—lethargy, weight loss, signs referable to a specific system seen in rabbits with metabolic disease causing weakness
• Severe obesity—can cause rear limb weakness
• Spinal reflexes—localized weakness to the thoracolumbar or lower lumbar cord segments.
• Musculoskeletal disorders—typically produce lameness and a reluctance to move; rule out bilateral hind limb fracture or coxofemoral luxation.

### CBC/BIOCHEMISTRY/URINALYSIS
Usually normal

### OTHER LABORATORY TESTS
N/A

### IMAGING
• Spinal radiographs—lesion localized to the spinal cord; usually reveals fracture or luxation; occasionally spinal column luxates, damaging the cord, then returns to normal-appearing radiographic position; prognosis in these cases can vary widely. Severely displaced, overriding segments or compression fractures generally result in more severe spinal cord injury and poorer prognosis. Use spinal radiographs to rule out other causes, such as intravertebral disc disease, discospondylitis, bony tumor, and congenital vertebral malformation.
• Skull films or thoracic radiographs—to rule out other causes of weakness if vertebral abnormalities are not seen
• Myelography—if survey radiography is not diagnostic

## VERTEBRAL FRACTURE OR LUXATION

• CT or MRI—CT is of limited value for evaluation of spine in rabbits; MRI is more accurate, but may not be widely available.

### DIAGNOSTIC PROCEDURES
N/A

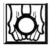

## TREATMENT

• Inpatient—with severe weakness/paralysis or until bladder function can be ascertained
• Bedding—move paralyzed, paretic, or painful rabbits away from soiled bedding; check and clean frequently to prevent urine scalding and moist pyoderma; use padded bedding to help prevent decubital ulcer formation.
• Keep fur clean and dry.
• Turning—turn recumbent patients from side to side four to eight times daily; prevent hypostatic lung congestion and decubital ulcer formation.
• Manual expression of the bladder if unable to urinate
• Carts available for small breed dogs can sometimes be fitted for larger rabbits and may be tolerated for limited periods.

### ACTIVITY
Restricted to cage rest only in rabbits with spinal trauma

### DIET
• It is absolutely imperative that the rabbit continue to eat during and following treatment. Rabbits in pain may become anorectic. Anorexia will often cause gastrointestinal hypomotility, derangement of the gastrointestinal microflora, and overgrowth of intestinal bacterial pathogens. Hand-feed or bring food to nonambulatory rabbits.
• Offer a large selection of fresh, moistened greens such as cilantro, romaine lettuce, parsley, carrot tops, dandelion greens, spinach, collard greens, etc., and good-quality grass hay. Place the food in front of recumbent rabbits or feed by hand.
• If the patient refuses these foods, syringe feed a gruel such as Critical Care for Herbivores (Oxbow Pet Products, Murdock, NE) 10–15 mL/kg PO q6–8h. Alternatively, pellets can be ground and mixed with fresh greens, vegetable baby foods, water, or juice to form a gruel.
• High-carbohydrate, high-fat nutritional supplements are contraindicated.
• Encourage oral fluid intake by offering fresh water, wetting leafy vegetables, or flavoring water with vegetable juices. Place water bottles or dishes within reach of recumbent rabbits.

## MEDICATIONS

### DRUG(S) OF CHOICE

#### For Spinal Trauma
• No drugs are recommended until the source or cause of the problem is identified.
• Corticosteroids have been used in rabbits with acute spinal cord trauma with some success. Although clinical improvement has been anecdotally reported, rabbits are very sensitive to the immunosuppressive and gastrointestinal side effects of corticosteroids; immunosuppression may exacerbate subclinical bacterial infections or *E. cuniculi*.
• The use of corticosteroids in rabbits with acute spinal trauma is controversial. Methylprednisolone sodium succinate administered in IV doses may be of benefit with acute fracture or luxation. Reported canine dose—30 mg/kg IV followed by 15 mg/kg 2 and 6 hours later; doses for rabbits not reported.
• Administer with gastrointestinal protectant to reduce risk of ulceration: cimetidine (5–10 mg/kg PO, SC, IM, IV q8–12h) or ranitidine (2 mg/kg IV q24h or 2–5 mg/kg PO q12h)

#### Acute Pain Management
• Butorphanol (0.1–1.0 mg/kg SC, IM, IV q4–6h)—may cause profound sedation; short-acting
• Buprenorphine (0.01–0.05 mg/kg SC, IM, IV q8–12h)—less sedating, longer-acting than butorphanol
• Morphine (2–5 mg/kg SC, IM q2–4h) or oxymorphone (0.05–0.2 mg/kg SC, IM q8–12h)—use with caution; more than one to two doses may cause gastrointestinal stasis.
• Meloxicam (0.2 mg/kg SC, IM q24h)
• Carprofen (1–4 mg/kg SC q12h)

#### Long-Term Pain Management
NSAIDs—have been used for short- or long-term therapy to reduce pain and inflammation in rabbits with spinal cord disease: meloxicam (0.2–0.5 mg/kg PO q24h) or carprofen (2.2 mg/kg PO q12–24h).

#### Sedation
Midazolam (1–2 mg/kg IM) or diazepam (1–3 mg/kg IM, IV)

#### Preanesthetics
• Butorphanol (0.2–0.4 mg/kg SC, IM) or buprenorphine (0.01–0.05 mg/kg IM), plus ketamine (20–30 mg/kg IM), followed by diazepam or midazolam (0.5 mg/kg IV after 10 minutes)
• Alternatively, ketamine (10–20 mg/kg IM) plus midazolam (0.25 mg/kg IM), or ketamine (10–15 mg/kg IM) plus diazepam (0.3–0.5 mg/kg IV, IM) if no preoperative analgesic is required

• Many other preanesthetic protocols exist; choice depends on patient status; use lower doses in debilitated, obese, or geriatric patients.

#### Antibiotics
For treatment of secondary bacterial dermatitis or cystitis. Use broad-spectrum antibiotics such as enrofloxacin (5–15 mg/kg PO, IM, SC q12h) or trimethoprim sulfa (30 mg/kg PO q12h); if anaerobic infections are suspected use chloramphenicol (50 mg/kg PO q8h) or metronidazole (20 mg/kg PO q12–24h)

### CONTRAINDICATIONS
• Oral administration of antibiotics that select against Gram-positive bacteria (penicillins, macrolides, lincosamides, and cephalosporins) can cause fatal enteric dysbiosis and enterotoxemia.
• Corticosteroids—do not use with NSAIDs because of combined negative effects on the gastrointestinal tract.

### PRECAUTIONS
Corticosteroids—use with caution, only in acute spinal trauma; associated with gastrointestinal ulceration and hemorrhage, delayed wound healing, and heightened susceptibility to infection; rabbits are very sensitive to the immunosuppressive effects of both topical and systemic corticosteroids; use may exacerbate subclinical bacterial infection.

### ALTERNATIVE DRUGS
• For acute spinal trauma—prednisolone (0.25 mg/kg PO q12h × 5 days); dexamethasone (0.5–2 mg/kg IV, IM); use with caution, if at all.
• Acupuncture may be effective for rabbits with chronic pain.

## FOLLOW-UP

### PATIENT MONITORING
• Neurologic examinations—daily to monitor status
• Bladder—evacuate (via manual expression or catheterization) three to four times a day to prevent overdistension and subsequent bladder atony; patient can be managed at home if bladder function returns, or owners can be taught to express the bladder. Monitor for bladder enlargement, bladder atony, or uremia secondary to urine retention.

### POSSIBLE COMPLICATIONS
• Urinary tract infection, bladder atony, urine scalding and pyoderma, constipation, decubital ulcer formation
• Exacerbation of bacterial infections (possibly life threatening), hepatic abscess, and gastric ulceration with corticosteroid usage
• Permanent paralysis warranting euthanasia

# VERTEBRAL FRACTURE OR LUXATION

## EXPECTED COURSE AND PROGNOSIS
- Depends on the severity of spinal cord injury
- Rabbits with rear limb paresis or paralysis due to mild to moderate spinal cord trauma may regain partial or full function with exercise restriction, supportive care, and long-term administration of NSAIDs.
- Most paralyzed rabbits with severe spinal trauma do not regain mobility; euthanasia may be warranted; rate of complicating conditions (bladder, cutaneous) is very high; quality of life is often poor.
- Wheeled carts manufactured for small dogs have been used successfully in a limited number of rabbits.

 **MISCELLANEOUS**

## ASSOCIATED CONDITIONS
Gastrointestinal hypomotility

## ABBREVIATIONS
- CNS = central nervous system
- CT = computed tomography
- IVD = intervertebral disc disease
- MRI = magnetic resonance imaging
- NSAIDs = nonsteroidal antiinflammatory drugs

*Suggested Reading*

Deeb BJ, Carpenter JW. Neurologic and musculoskeletal diseases. In: Quesenberry KE, Carpenter JW, eds. Ferrets, Rabbits and Rodents: Clinical Medicine and Surgery. 2nd Ed. Philadelphia: WB Saunders, 2004:194–210.

Greenaway JB, Partlow GD, Gonsholt NL, et al. Anatomy of the lumbosacral spinal cord in rabbits. J Am Anim Hosp Assoc 2001;37(1):27–34.

Harcourt-Brown F. Neurological and loco-motor diseases. In: Harcourt-Brown F, ed. Textbook of Rabbit Medicine. Oxford: Butterworth-Heinemann, 2002:307–323.

Paul-Murphy J, Ramer JC. Urgent care of the pet rabbits. Vet Clin North Am Exotic Anim Pract 2998;1(1):127–152.

# WEIGHT LOSS AND CACHEXIA

## BASICS

### DEFINITION
• Weight loss is considered clinically important when it exceeds 10% of the normal body weight and is not associated with fluid loss.
• Cachexia is defined as the state of extremely poor health and is associated with anorexia, weight loss, weakness, and mental depression.

### PATHOPHYSIOLOGY
• Weight loss can result from many different pathophysiologic mechanisms that share a common feature—insufficient caloric intake or availability to meet metabolic needs.
• Insufficient caloric intake or availability can be caused by (1) a high energy demand (e.g., that characteristic of a hypermetabolic state); (2) inadequate energy intake, including insufficient quantity or quality of food, or inadequate nutrient assimilation (e.g., with anorexia, dysphagia or malabsorptive disorders); (3) excessive loss of nutrients or fluid, which can occur in patients with gastrointestinal losses, glucosuria, or proteinuria.
• Caloric requirements reported for rabbits: 150–175 kcal/kg for growing, pregnant, lactating or small breed rabbits; 40–50 kcal/kg for large breed adult maintenance.

### SYSTEMS AFFECTED
Any can be affected by weight loss, especially if severe or the result of systemic disease.

### SIGNALMENT
No age or sex predilection

### SIGNS

#### Historical Findings
• Clinical signs of particular diagnostic value in patients with weight loss are whether the appetite is normal, increased, decreased, or absent.
• Historical information is very important, especially regarding type of diet, environment (chewing habits and access to potential gastrointestinal foreign bodies), signs of dental disease, chronic respiratory disease, abscesses, signs of gastrointestinal disease (including lack of fecal production or scant feces), diarrhea, or signs of any specific disease.
• Signs of pain, such as teeth grinding, a hunched posture, and reluctance to move, are extremely common in rabbits with oral disease or gastrointestinal hypomotility.
• Pseudoanorectic patients commonly display excessive drooling, difficulty in prehension and mastication of food, halitosis, dysphagia, bruxism, and odynophagia (painful eating).

#### Physical Examination Findings
• Most underlying causes of pseudoanorexia can be identified by a thorough examination of the face, mandible, teeth, neck, oropharynx, and esophagus for dental disease, ulceration, traumatic lesions, masses, foreign bodies, and neuromuscular dysfunction.
• A thorough examination of the oral cavity, including the incisors, molars, and mucosa, is necessary to rule out dental disease. Use of an otoscope or speculum is required to adequately perform an examination of the molars. Sedation or anesthesia may be necessary.
• Examine the face for evidence of chronic upper respiratory disease, such as secretions or dried discharges around the nose and front limbs, ocular discharge, exophthalmos, facial swelling, or pain.
• Abdominal palpation is a valuable tool in the diagnosis of gastrointestinal stasis. Ingesta, including hair, are nearly always palpable in the stomach of a normal rabbit. The normal stomach should be easily deformable, feel soft and pliable, and not remain pitted on compression. A firm, noncompliant stomach or stomach contents that remain pitted on compression is an abnormal finding.
• Gas distension of the intestines or cecum is common in rabbits with gastrointestinal tract disease.
• Abdominal palpation may also reveal the presence of organomegaly, masses, or gastrointestinal foreign bodies.
• Auscultation of the thorax may reveal cardiac murmurs, arrhythmias, or abnormal breath sounds.
• Auscultation of the abdomen reveals decreased borborygmus in most rabbits with gastrointestinal hypomotility.

### CAUSES AND RISK FACTORS

#### Excessive Use of Calories
• Increased catabolism—fever, inflammation, cancer; very common, especially chronic upper respiratory disease, abscesses (subcutaneous, joint, facial, intrathoracic, intraabdominal)
• Increased physical activity
• Pregnancy or lactation

#### Pseudoanorexia
• Inability to prehend or chew food—dental disease is extremely common.
• Dysphagia

#### Maldigestive/Malabsorptive Disorders
• Gastrointestinal hypomotility/gastrointestinal stasis—very common
• Intestinal dysbiosis/chronic intermittent diarrhea—very common
• Coccidiosis—young or debilitated animals

#### Metabolic Disorders
• Organ failure—cardiac failure, hepatic failure, and renal failure; common
• Cancer cachexia—lymphoma, uterine adenocarcinoma; common

#### Dietary Causes
• Insufficient long-stemmed hay and excessive simple carbohydrate—very common, lead to secondary gastrointestinal disorders and dental disease
• Insufficient quantity
• Poor quality

#### Neuromuscular Disease and Pain
• Degenerative joint disease
• Spinal luxation, fracture, or intervertebral disc disease—common
• Joint or facial abscesses—very common
• Ulcerative pododermatitis (sore hocks)—very common
• Otitis interna/media; vestibular disorders—very common
• Dental disease—extremely common
• Urolithiasis/hypercalciuria—very common
• CNS disease—brain abscess (and, possibly, *Encephalitozoon cuniculi*); can be associated with anorexia or pseudoanorexia

#### Excessive Nutrient Loss
• Protein-losing enteropathy (secondary to infectious or infiltrative diseases)
• Protein-losing nephropathy—rare

## DIAGNOSIS
• If previous weights are not available, subjectively assess the patient for cachexia, emaciation, dehydration, or other clues that would confirm the owner's complaint of weight loss.
• After weight loss is confirmed, seek the underlying cause.

### DIFFERENTIAL DIAGNOSIS
• First categorize the weight loss as occurring with a normal, increased, or decreased appetite.
• The list of likely differential diagnoses for a patient with weight loss despite a normal or increased appetite is much different and much shorter than that for patients with decreased appetite or anorexia.
• Determine what the patient's appetite was at the onset of weight loss; any condition can lead to anorexia if it persists long enough for the patient to become debilitated.
• Seek causes of pseudoanorexia—dental disease is one of the most common causes of weight loss in rabbits.
• Some loss of muscle mass may be a normal aging change.

## CBC/BIOCHEMISTRY/URINALYSIS
• Help identify infectious, inflammatory, and metabolic diseases, including organ failure.
• Especially helpful when the history and physical examination do not provide much useful information

## OTHER LABORATORY TESTS
• Determined by the clinician's list of most likely differential diagnoses on the basis of the specific findings of the history and physical examination
• Fecal direct examination, fecal flotation to rule out coccidians

## IMAGING
• If underlying disease is suspected but no abnormalities are revealed by the physical examination or minimum database, perform abdominal radiography and abdominal ultrasonography to identify hidden conditions such as gastrointestinal tract disease, hepatic disease, uterine adenocarcinomas, or internal abscesses. Consider thoracic radiography to rule out cardiac or pulmonary disease.
• Obtain skull radiographs to rule out dental disease.
• The need for further diagnostic imaging varies with the underlying condition suspected (see other topics on specific diseases).

## DIAGNOSTIC PROCEDURES
• Vary depending on initial diagnostic findings and the suspected underlying cause of weight loss
• A thorough examination of the oral cavity is indicated in every rabbit with epiphora. A thorough examination includes the incisors, molars, and buccal and lingual mucosa to rule out dental disease. Use of an otoscope or speculum may be useful in identifying severe abnormalities; however, many problems will be missed by using this method alone. Complete examination requires heavy sedation or general anesthesia and specialized equipment.

## TREATMENT
• The most important treatment principle is to treat the underlying cause of the weight loss.
• Symptomatic therapy includes attention to fluid and electrolyte derangements, reduction in environmental stressors, and modification of the diet to improve palatability.

## DIET
• It is absolutely imperative that the rabbit begin eating as soon as possible, regardless of the underlying cause. Continued anorexia will exacerbate gastrointestinal hypomotility and cause further derangement of the gastrointestinal microflora and overgrowth of intestinal bacterial pathogens.
• Offer a large selection of fresh, moistened greens such as cilantro, romaine lettuce, parsley, carrot tops, dandelion greens, spinach, collard greens, etc., and good-quality grass hay. Many rabbits will begin to eat these foods, even if they were previously anorectic. Also offer the rabbit's usual pelleted diet, as the initial goal is to get the rabbit to eat.
• If the patient refuses these foods, syringe feed a gruel such as Critical Care for Herbivores (Oxbow Pet Products, Murdock, NE) 10–15 mL/kg PO q6–8h. Larger volumes and more frequent feedings are often accepted; feed as much as the rabbit will readily accept. Alternatively, pellets can be ground and mixed with fresh greens, vegetable baby foods, water, or juice to form a gruel. The addition of canned pumpkin to this gruel is a palatable source of fiber and calories. If sufficient volumes of food are not accepted in this manner, nasogastric intubation is indicated.
• High-carbohydrate, high-fat nutritional supplements are contraindicated.

## MEDICATIONS
### DRUG(S) OF CHOICE
• Depend on the underlying cause of the weight loss; see specific topic for each condition, including anorexia.
• See other sections regarding specific disorders or problems.

### CONTRAINDICATIONS
N/A

### PRECAUTIONS
N/A

### POSSIBLE INTERACTIONS
N/A

### ALTERNATIVE DRUGS
N/A

## FOLLOW-UP
### PATIENT MONITORING
The necessity for frequent patient monitoring and the methods required depend on the underlying cause of the weight loss; however, the patient should be weighed regularly and often.

### POSSIBLE COMPLICATIONS
See Causes and Risk Factors.

## MISCELLANEOUS
### ASSOCIATED CONDITIONS
See Causes and Risk Factors.

### AGE-RELATED FACTORS
N/A

### ZOONOTIC POTENTIAL
N/A

### PREGNANCY
Pregnancy and lactation can be associated with weight loss due to increased calorie expenditure.

### SYNONYMS
N/A

### SEE ALSO
• Abscessation
• Anorexia
• Gastrointestinal hypomotility
• Tooth root abscess

*Suggested Reading*
Brown SA, Rosenthal KL. The anorexic rabbit. Proc North Am Vet Conf 1997:788.
Donoghue S. Nutrition and pet rabbits. In: Rosenthal KL, ed. Practical Exotic Animal Medicine: The Compendium Collection. Trenton, NJ: Veterinary Learning Systems, 1997:107.
Jenkins JR. Gastrointestinal diseases. In: Hillyer EV, Quesenberry KE, eds. Ferrets, Rabbits and Rodents: Clinical Medicine and Surgery. Philadelphia: WB Saunders, 1997:160.
Jenkins JR. Soft tissue surgery and dental procedures. In: Hillyer EV, Quesenberry KE, eds. Ferrets, Rabbits and Rodents: Clinical Medicine and Surgery. Philadelphia: WB Saunders, 1997:227.

*Portions Adapted From*
Cranell J. Weight Loss and Cachexia. In: Tilley LP, Smith FWK, Jr., eds. The 5-Minute Veterinary Consult: Canine and Feline, 3rd Ed. Baltimore: Lippincott Williams & Wilkins, 2004.

Appendix I    Common Dosages for Ferrets                                                      388
Appendix II   Normal Values for Ferrets                                                       392
Appendix III  Common Dosages for Rabbits                                                      394
Appendix IV   Normal Values for Rabbits                                                       397
Appendix V    Toxic Plants and Their Clinical Signs—Antidotes and Treatment                   399

# APPENDIX I

## COMMON DOSAGES FOR FERRETS

| Drug | Dosage | Indication |
|------|--------|------------|
| Acepromazine | 0.01–0.25 mg/kg; SC, IM | Light sedation |
| Acetylsalicylic acid | 10–20 mg/kg bid to q48h; PO | Analgesia, antiinflammatory, anticoagulant |
| Amikacin | 8–16 mg/kg total per day, divided q8–24h; SC, IM, IV | General antibiotic therapy. See precautions for aminoglycosides |
| | 10–15 mg/kg bid; SC, IM | |
| Aminophylline | 4–6.5 mg/kg bid; PO, IM | Bronchodilation |
| Amitraz | Apply to affected skin 3–6 times at 14-day intervals | Ectoparasite control, especially mites |
| Amoxicillin | 10–20 mg/kg bid; PO, SC | General antibiotic therapy |
| | 10 mg/kg q12h + metronidazole (20 mg/kg q12h) + bismuth subsalicylate (17.5 mg/kg q12h, Pepto-Bismol original formula); PO | Treatment of *Helicobacter pylori* gastritis, can be combined with $H_2$-receptor blockers; treat for at least 2 weeks |
| Amoxicillin + clavulanic acid | 12.5 mg/kg bid; PO | General antibiotic therapy (dose of combined drugs) |
| Amphotericin B | 0.4–0.8 mg/kg once weekly to a total cumulative dose of 7–25 mg; IV | Systemic antifungal therapy |
| | 0.25 mg/kg on alternate days until total cumulative dose of 7–25 mg given; IV | |
| | **OR** Follow published canine/feline protocols | |
| Ampicillin | 5–30 mg/kg bid; PO, SC, IM, IV | General antibiotic therapy |
| Anastrozole | 0.1 mg/kg PO once daily until signs resolve, then sid on a week on/week off basis | Adrenal disease in females; estrogen inhibitor |
| Apomorphine | 5 mg/kg single dose; SC | To stimulate emesis |
| Aspirin | See acetylsalicylic acid | |
| Atenolol | 3.125–6.25 mg/kg once daily; PO | β-Adrenergic receptor blocker used in treatment of cardiomyopathy |
| Atipamezole | 0.4–1 mg/kg; IM | Reversal agent for medetomidine |
| | 5 times dose of medetomidine on a milligram-to-milligram basis | Reversal agent for medetomidine |
| | 2–10 mg/kg as needed; SC, IM | Treatment for organophosphate toxicity |
| Azathioprine | 0.9 mg/kg q24, 48, or 72h (for severe, moderate, or mild gastroenteritis, respectively); PO | For the treatment of inflammatory bowel disease |
| Barium sulfate | 10–15 mL/kg; PO | Gastrointestinal contrast radiography (dilute as per product directions for varying opacity) |
| Bismuth subsalicylate | 0.25–1 mL/kg of regular strength formula tid to qid; PO | Gastric protectant |
| | 17.5 mg/kg bid (Pepto-Bismol original formula) + amoxicillin (10 mg/kg bid) + metronidazole (20 mg/kg bid); PO | Treatment of *H. pylori* gastritis, can be combined with $H_2$-receptor blockers; treat for at least 2 weeks |
| | 24 mg/kg ranitine bismuth citrate + 12.5 mg/kg clarithromycin tid, for 14 days; PO | Treatment of *H. pylori* gastritis |
| Buprenorphine | 0.01–0.05 mg/kg q12h as needed; SC, IM, IV | Analgesic |
| Butorphanol | 0.05–0.5 mg/kg q8–12h as needed; SC, IM, IV | Analgesic |
| Carbaryl (0.5% w/v shampoo, 5.0% w/w powder) | Treat once weekly for 3–6 weeks | Ectoparasite control |
| Captopril | 1/8 of a 12.5-mg tablet q48h to start; PO | Vasodilator as part of therapy for congestive heart failure |
| Cefadroxil | 15–20 mg/kg bid; PO | General antibiotic therapy |
| Cephalexin | 15–25 mg/kg bid to tid; PO | General antibiotic therapy |
| Chloramphenicol | 25–50 mg/kg bid; PO (palmitate), SC, IM (succinate) | General antibiotic therapy; treatment of choice for proliferative bowel disease with minimum treatment period of 14 days |
| | 50 mg/kg tid for 2 weeks; PO (palmitate) | Proliferative bowel disease |
| Chlorpheniramine | 1–2 mg/kg bid to tid; PO | Antihistamine |
| Chorionic gonadotropin | 100 IU once after second week of estrus, repeat in 2 weeks if needed; IM | To terminate estrus |
| Cimetidine | 5–10 mg/kg tid; PO, SC, IM, slow IV | $H_2$-receptor blocking agent for gastric ulcer therapy |
| Ciprofloxacin | 5–15 mg/kg bid; PO | General antibiotic therapy |
| Cisapride | 0.5 mg/kg bid to tid; PO | Gastrointestinal motility stimulant |
| Clarithromycin | 12.5 mg/kg tid + 24 mg/kg ranitine bismuth citrate for 14 days; PO | Treatment of *H. pylori* gastric infection |
| Clavulanic acid and amoxicillin | See amoxicillin + clavulanic acid | |

## COMMON DOSAGES FOR FERRETS (CONTINUED)

| Drug | Dosage | Indication |
|------|--------|------------|
| Clindamycin | 5.5–10 mg/kg bid; PO | General antibiotic therapy |
| Cloxacillin | 10 mg/kg qid; PO, IM, IV | General antibiotic therapy |
| Desoxycorticosterone pivalate (DOCP) | 2 mg/kg IM q21d | Mineralocorticoid for treatment of Addison's disease after bilateral adrenal surgery |
| Dexamethasone | 0.5–2.0 mg/kg once; IM, IV | Therapy for shock, antiinflammatory, after bilateral adrenalectomy |
| Dexamethasone sodium phosphate | 4–8 mg/kg once; IM, IV | As above, also prior to blood transfusion |
| Dextrose | 0.5–2 mL of 50% in slow IV bolus to effect | Hypoglycemia caused by insulinoma |
| | Continuous IV infusion of 5% dextrose in crystalloid fluids | |
| Diazepam | 0.2–1 mg/kg as needed; IV | For sedation |
| | 0.25–1 mg/kg as needed; IV | For seizure control |
| Diazoxide | 5–20 mg/kg daily dose initially, divided bid to tid as necessary, increasing up to 60 mg/kg daily total dose; PO | For treatment of insulinoma, in combination with prednisone |
| Digoxin elixir | 0.005–0.01 mg/kg once daily to bid; PO. Adjust dose as necessary | Management of congestive heart failure and cardiomyopathy |
| Diltiazem | 1.5–7.5 mg/kg once daily to qid; PO. Adjust dose as necessary | Management of congestive heart failure and cardiomyopathy |
| Diphenhydramine | 0.5–2 mg/kg bid to tid; PO q12h; IM | Antihistamine |
| Doxapram | 5–11 mg/kg; IV | Respiratory stimulant |
| Enalapril | 0.25–0.5 mg/kg q48h initially, increase to q24h clinically appropriate; PO | Management of congestive heart failure and cardiomyopathy |
| Enilconazole | Apply topically as required | |
| Enrofloxacin | 10–20 mg/kg sid; PO, SC, IM | General antibiotic therapy |
| Epoetin alpha | 50–150 IU/kg 3 times per week until packed cell volume is stable, then 1–2 times per week | Stimulates erythropoiesis |
| Erythromycin | 10 mg/kg qid; PO | General antibiotic therapy |
| Famotidine | 0.25–0.5 mg/kg once daily; PO, SC, IV | $H_2$-receptor blocking agent for gastric ulcer therapy |
| Fenbendazole | 20 mg/kg once daily for 5 days; PO | Endoparasites |
| Fludrocortisone | 0.05–0.1 mg/kg once daily or divided twice daily; PO. Adjust according to patient's response | Mineralocorticoid; support for Addison's disease after bilateral adrenalectomy |
| Flunixin meglumine | 0.3–2 mg/kg once daily to bid; PO, SC, deep IM, IV; maximum of 3 days treatment | Nonsteroidal antiinflammatory |
| Flutamide | 10 mg/kg PO once to twice daily | Inhibits androgens; treatment of prostatomegaly in adrenal disease |
| Furosemide | 1–4 mg/kg bid to tid; PO, SC, IM, IV | Diuretic, initial management of congestive heart failure |
| | 1–2 mg/kg bid to tid; PO | Long-term maintenance therapy of congestive heart failure |
| Glycopyrrolate | 0.01–0.02 mg/kg; SC, IM, IV | Anticholinergic preanesthetic |
| GnRH | 20 μg once after second week of estrus, repeat in 2 weeks if needed; SC, IM | To terminate estrus |
| Griseofulvin | 25 mg/kg once daily for 3–6 weeks; PO | Systemic antifungal therapy |
| HCG | See chorionic gonadotropin | To induce ovulation and terminate estrus |
| Hydrocortisone sodium succinate | 25–40 mg/kg single dose; IV | Treatment of shock, adrenal insufficiency |
| Hydroxyzine hydrochloride | 2 mg/kg tid; PO | Antihistamine |
| Imidacloprid | Treat as for small cat | Flea control |
| Insulin, NPH | 0.1–5 U/kg bid; SC, IM; start with low dose and increase according to patient's response | For treatment of diabetes mellitus; monitor blood/urine glucose |
| Iron dextran | 10 mg/kg once; IM | For iron deficiency anemia |
| Isoflurane | 3–5% for induction, 0.5–2.5% or as required for maintenance | Inhalant anesthetic of choice |
| Ivermectin | 200–400 μg/kg twice at 14-day intervals; PO, SC | General parasite control; sarcoptic mange |
| | Dilute 1:10 in propylene glycol; 400 μg/kg; instill half of dose into each ear; massage in well | Control of ear mites |
| | 0.05 mg/kg once monthly; PO, SC | Heartworm microfilaricide |
| | 0.055 mg/kg once monthly; PO | Heartworm prevention |
| | 1/4 of a 68-μg canine Heartgard tablet | Heartworm prevention |
| Kaolin-pectin products | 1–2 mL/kg of regular strength product; q2–6h as needed; PO | Gastrointestinal protectant |

## COMMON DOSAGES FOR FERRETS (CONTINUED)

| Drug | Dosage | Indication |
|------|--------|------------|
| Ketamine + acepromazine | 10–35 mg/kg + 0.05–0.35 mg/kg; IM, SC | Anesthesia |
| Ketamine + diazepam | 10–20 mg/kg + 1–2 mg/kg; IM | Anesthesia |
| | 5–10 mg/kg + 0.5–1 mg/kg; IV | Anesthesia |
| Ketamine + medetomidine | 5–8 mg/kg + 60–80 μg/kg; IM | Anesthesia |
| Ketamine + medetomidine + butorphanol | 5 mg/kg +80 μg/kg + 0.1 mg/kg; IM | Anesthesia (use separate syringe for butorphanol) |
| Ketamine + midazolam | 5–10 mg/kg + 0.25–0.5 mg/kg; IV | Anesthetic induction |
| Ketoconazole | 10–30 mg/kg once daily to bid; PO | Systemic antifungal therapy |
| Lactulose (syrup—15 mg/10 mL) | 0.1–0.75 mL/kg bid; PO | In hepatic disease to decrease blood ammonia levels; laxative |
| Leuprolide acetate (Lupron) 30-day depot | 100–250 μg/ferret once monthly; IM; may decrease to q6–8w | Ferret adrenal disease (1-month depot formulation) |
| Lime sulfur | Dilute 1:40 in water, wash once weekly for 6 weeks | Ectoparasite control (especially mites) |
| Medetomidine | See ketamine + medetomidine | |
| | 0.08–0.2 mg/kg; SC, IM | Dose dependent sedation and immobilization |
| Melarsomine dihydrochloride | 2.5 mg/kg IM once; repeat 1 month later with 2 injections 24 hours apart | Heartworm adulticide treatment; deep IM injection |
| Melatonin | 0.5–1.0 mg/ferret q24h; inject 7–9 hours after sunrise | Symptomatic treatment of ferret adrenal disease |
| Meloxicam | 0.2 mg/kg initial dose, then 0.1 mg/kg once daily for 2–3 days. Reduce to 0.025 mg/kg q24–48h for long-term use; PO, SC, IM, IV | Analgesic and antiinflammatory |
| Metoclopramide | 0.2–1 mg/kg bid to qid; PO, SC | Gastric motility disorders, vomiting and nausea associated with gastritis |
| Metronidazole | 15–20 mg/kg bid; PO | Antibacterial agent with good anaerobic spectrum |
| | 20 mg/kg bid; PO for 10 days | Giardiasis |
| | 20 mg/kg bid + amoxicillin (10 mg/kg bid) + bismuth subsalicylate (17.5 mg/kg bid, Pepto-Bismol original formula); PO for at least 2 weeks | Treatment of *H. pylori* gastritis, can be combined with $H_2$-receptor blockers |
| Midazolam | 0.3–1.0 mg/kg; SC, IM | Sedation |
| Morphine | 0.1–2 mg/kg q4–6h as needed; SC, IM | Analgesia |
| Naloxone | 0.01–0.03 mg/kg or to effect; SC, IM, IV | Opioid reversal by titration |
| Neomycin | 10–20 mg/kg bid to qid; PO | Local antibiotic therapy in the gastrointestinal tract |
| Nitroglycerine | 1/8-in. length of 2% ointment applied topically; once daily to bid | Management of congestive heart failure |
| Omeprazole | 0.7 mg/kg sid; PO | Proton pump inhibitor; for gastric ulcer therapy |
| Oxymorphone | 0.05–0.2 mg/kg q2–6h as needed; SC, IM, IV | Analgesia |
| Oxytetracycline | 20 mg/kg tid; PO | General antibiotic therapy |
| Oxytocin | 0.2–3 IU/kg once; SC, IM | To stimulate uterine motility or milk letdown |
| Phenobarbital elixir | 1–2 mg/kg bid to tid for seizure control, titrate dose for maintenance; PO | Control and prevention of seizures |
| Prednisone, prednisolone | 0.5–1.0 mg/kg bid, reduce dose and frequency for long-term therapy; PO, IM | Antiinflammatory |
| | 0.5–2.5 mg/kg bid; PO, IM; start at low dose, increase as necessary | Treatment of hypoglycemia due to insulinoma; reduce dosage if combined with diazoxide therapy |
| | 1.25–2.5 mg/kg once daily; taper dose to 0.5–1.25 every other day or lowest dose possible | Inflammatory bowel disease |
| | 1 mg/kg once daily or divided bid, for 3 months; PO; taper dose to wean animal at completion of therapy | In conjunction with adulticide treatment for heartworm disease |
| | 1–2 mg/kg once daily; PO | Chemotherapy for lymphoma; palliative alone or used with other protocols |
| Prednisolone sodium succinate | 22 mg/kg; slow IV | Therapy for shock |
| Propranolol | 0.2–1 mg/kg bid to tid; PO, SC | Medical management of cardiomyopathy |
| Prostaglandin F2-α | 0.5–1.0 mg/ferret as needed; IM | Treatment of dystocia or metritis |
| Pyrantel pamoate | 4.4 mg/kg once, repeat in 2 weeks; PO | Treatment of gastrointestinal nematodes |
| Pyrethrin products | Use topically as directed; treat once weekly as needed | Treatment of ectoparasites, especially fleas |
| Ranitidine bismuth citrate | 24 mg/kg tid; PO | Combine with clarithromycin for treatment of *Helicobacter pylori* gastritis |
| Ranitidine HCl | 3.5 mg/kg bid; PO | $H_2$-receptor blocking agent for gastric ulcer therapy |

## Common Dosages for Ferrets (continued)

| Drug | Dosage | Indication |
|------|--------|------------|
| Selamectin | Treat topically with 6–10 mg/kg as directed, once monthly | Treatment of ectoparasites and endoparasites, heartworm prevention |
| Stanozolol | 0.5 mg/kg bid; PO, SC, IM | Anabolic steroid |
| Sucralfate | 25 mg/kg bid to qid; PO | Treatment of gastric ulceration and gastritis |
| Sulfadimethoxine | 50 mg/kg once, then 25 mg/kg daily for 9 days; PO | Treatment of gastrointestinal coccidiosis |
| Tetracycline | 25 mg/kg bid to tid; PO | General antibiotic therapy |
| Theophylline (elixir) | 4.25 mg/kg bid to tid; PO | Bronchodilation |
| Trimethoprim sulfonamide combinations | 15–30 mg/kg bid; PO, SC | General antibiotic therapy |
| | 30 mg/kg once daily for 2 weeks; PO | Treatment of gastrointestinal coccidiosis |
| Ursodiol | 15–20 mg/kg once daily to bid; PO | Treatment of cholangiolar and gallbladder disorders |
| Vitamin B complex | Dose to thiamine content at 1–2 mg/kg as needed; IM | Vitamin B supplementation |
| Vitamin C | 50–100 mg/kg bid; PO | Supportive therapy, as an antioxidant |

Adapted from Allen DG, Dowling PM, Smith DA, et al. Handbook of Veterinary Drugs. 3rd Ed. Baltimore: Lippincott Williams & Wilkins, 2005.

# APPENDIX II

## NORMAL VALUES FOR FERRETS

Table 1.

| Reference Ranges for Serum Biochemistry Values: Ferrets | | |
|---|---|---|
| Parameter | Albino Ferrets | Fitch Ferets |
| Sodium (mmol/L) | 137–162 | 146–160 |
| Potassium (mmol/L) | 4.5–7.7 | 4.3–5.3 |
| Chloride (mmol/L) | 106–125 | 102–121 |
| Calcium (mg/dL) | 8.0–11.8 | 8.6–10.5 |
| Phosphorus (mg/dL) | 4.0–9.1 | 5.6–8.7 |
| Glucose (mg/dL) | 94–207 | 62.5–134 |
| BUN (mg/dL) | 10–45 | 12–43 |
| Creatinine (mg/dL) | 0.4–0.9 | 0.2–0.6 |
| Total protein (g/dL) | 5.1–7.4 | 5.3–7.2 |
| Albumin (g/dL) | 2.6–3.8 | 3.3–4.1 |
| Globulin (g/dL) | — | 2.0–2.0 |
| Total bilirubin (mg/dL) | <1.0 | <1.0 |
| Cholesterol | 64–296 | 119–201 |
| Alkaline phosphatase (SAP) (IU/L) | 9–84 | 30–120 |
| Alanine aminotransferase (ALT) (IU/L) | — | 82–289 |
| Aspartate aminotransferase (AST) (IU/L) | 28–120 | 74–248 |

Adapted from Fox, JG. Normal clinical and biologic parameters. In: Fox JG, ed. Biology and Disease of the Ferret. 2nd Ed. Baltimore: Williams & Wilkins, 1998.

Table 2.

| Hematologic Values: Ferrets | | |
|---|---|---|
| Parameter | Male Albino | Male Fitch |
| PCV% | 44–61 | 48–59 |
| Hemoglobin (g/dL) | 16.3–18.2 | 15.4–18.5 |
| RBC ($\times 10^6$/mm$^3$) | 7.3–12.18 | 10.1–13.2 |
| MCV | — | 42.6–51 |
| MCH | — | 13.7–16 |
| MCHC | — | 30.3–34.9 |
| Reticulocytes % | 1–12 | — |
| Platelets (10$^3$/mm$^3$) | 297–730 | — |
| WBC ($\times 10^3$/mm$^3$) | 4.4–19.1 | 1.7–11.9 |
| Differential (%) | | |
| Bands | — | 0–1 |
| Neutrophils | 11–82 | 24–72 |
| Lymphocytes | 12–54 | 26–73 |
| Monocytes | 0–9 | 1–4 |
| Eosinophils | 0–7 | 0–3 |
| Basophils | 0–2 | 0–2.7 |

Adapted from Fox, JG. Normal clinical and biologic parameters. In: Fox JG, ed. Biology and Disease of the Ferret. 2nd Ed. Baltimore: Williams & Wilkins, 1998.

Table 3.

| Selective Normative Data | |
| --- | --- |
| Adult weight | |
|   Male | 1–2 kg |
|   Female | 600–950 g |
| Life span (average) | 5–11 years |
| Body temperature | 37.8–40°C (100–104°F) |
| Dental formula | 2 (I 3/3, C 1/1, P 4/3, M 1/2) |
| Vertebral formula | $C_7T_{15}L_5S_3Cd_{14}$ |
| Age of sexual maturity | 6–12 months |
| Length of breeding life | 2–5 years |
| Gestation | 42 +/– 2 days |
| Litter size | average 8 (range 1–18) |
| Birth weight | 6–12 g |
| Eyes open | 34 days |
| Onset of hearing | 32 days |
| Weaning | 6–8 weeks |
| Food consumption | 140–190 g/24 h |
| Water intake | 75–100 mL/24 h |
| Arterial blood pressure: | |
|   Mean systolic | Female 133; male 161 mm Hg (conscious) |
|   Mean diastolic | 110–125 mm Hg (anesthetized) |
| Heart rate | 200–400 bpm |
| Cardiac output | 139 mL/min |
| Blood volume | Male 60 mL, female 40 mL (approximate) |
| Respiration | 33–36 breaths/min |

Adapted from Fox, JG. Normal clinical and biologic parameters. In: Fox JG, ed. Biology and Disease of the Ferret. 2nd Ed. Baltimore: Williams & Wilkins, 1998.

# APPENDIX III

## COMMON DOSAGES FOR RABBITS

| Drug | Dosage | Indication |
|------|--------|------------|
| Acepromazine | 0.25–1 mg/kg; SC, IM | Light sedation |
| Activated charcoal | 1–3 g/kg every 4–6 hours as needed; PO | To decrease toxin absorption |
| | Dilute 1 g charcoal/5–10 mL water | |
| Albendazole | 20–30 mg/kg once daily; PO for 30 days, then reduce to 15 mg/kg once daily PO for 30 days | To treat *Encephalitozoon cuniculi* |
| Amikacin | 2 mg/kg tid; SC, IM, IV | General antibiotic therapy |
| Amoxicillin | DO NOT USE | DO NOT USE |
| Ampicillin | DO NOT USE | DO NOT USE |
| Amprolium 9.6% solution | 0.5 mL/500 mL of drinking water for 10 days | Coccidiostat |
| Atropine | 0.1–0.5 mg/kg; IM, SC | Bradycardia |
| | 2–10 mg/kg q20min as necessary for organophosphate toxicity; IM, SC | Organophosphate toxicity |
| | 1% atropine ophthalmic drops to dilate eyes in albino animals | Mydriasis |
| Atropine + phenylephrine | 1 drop of 1% atropine + 1 drop of 10% phenylephrine ophthalmic drops 3 to 4 times over 15 minutes to dilate eyes in animals with ocular pigmentation | Mydriasis |
| Azithromycin | 30 mg/kg PO once daily; can combine with metronidazole 20 mg/kg sid to bid; PO | Treatment of anaerobic infections |
| Barium sulfate | 10–15 mL/kg; PO | Gastrointestinal contrast radiography (dilute as per product directions for varying opacity) |
| Buprenorphine | 0.01–0.05 mg/kg bid to tid; SC, IM, IV | Analgesia |
| Butorphanol | 0.1–1.0 mg/kg q4–6h; SC, IM, IV | Analgesia, can cause sedation |
| Calcium EDTA | 25 mg/kg bid to qid for 5 days; SC; dilute to 10 mg/mL with saline. Repeat if necessary | Chelation, lead toxicosis |
| Carbaryl 5% powder | Dust lightly once weekly | Ectoparasites |
| Carprofen | 2.2 mg/kg sid to bid; PO | Analgesia |
| | 1–4 mg/kg bid; SC | |
| Cefazolin | 2 g/20 g PMMA | Local treatment in abscess cavities |
| Ceftiofur | 2 g lyophilized drug/20 g PMMA | Local treatment in abscess cavities |
| Cephalexin | 15 mg/kg bid; IM; DO NOT administer orally | Antibiotic—parenteral use only |
| Chloramphenicol palmitate | 50 mg/kg bid; PO | General antibiotic therapy |
| Chloramphenicol succinate | 30–50 mg/kg bid to tid; IM, SC | General antibiotic therapy |
| Cholestyramine | 2 g in 20 mL water once daily by gavage (2.5–3.8 kg animal) | Absorption of clostridial enterotoxins |
| Cimetidine | 5–10 mg/kg bid to tid; PO, SC, IM, IV | Gastric protectant |
| Ciprofloxacin | 10–20 mg/kg bid; PO | General antibiotic therapy |
| | 15–20 mg/kg once daily to tid; PO | |
| Cisapride | 0.5 mg/kg once daily to tid; PO, SC | Gastrointestinal promotility agent |
| Clindamycin | DO NOT USE | DO NOT USE |
| Clotrimazole | Topical application to clipped skin as needed | Topical antifungal |
| Cyproheptadine | 1 mg/rabbit once daily to bid; PO | Appetite stimulant |
| Dexamethasone | 0.5–2.0 mg/kg bid; PO, SC, IM. Wean off dosage at end of treatment. Seldom indicated in rabbits | Antiinflammatory. Rarely indicated in rabbits. Use with caution |
| Diazepam | 1–2 mg/kg; IM, IV | Seizures |
| | 0.5–1.0 mg/kg; IV for seizures; may repeat PRN up to 5 mg/kg total dose; may be administered rectally if IV access cannot be achieved | |
| Digoxin | 0.005–0.01 mg/kg PO once daily to every other day | Management of congestive heart failure and cardiomyopathy |
| Diphenhydramine | 2 mg/kg bid to tid; PO, SC | Antihistamine |
| Doxapram | 2–5 mg/kg as needed; SC, IV | Respiratory stimulant |
| Enalapril | 0.25–0.5 mg/kg once daily to every other day; PO | Management of congestive heart failure and cardiomyopathy |
| Enilconazole | Apply topically as required | Antifungal |
| Enrofloxacin | 5–20 mg/kg sid to bid; PO, SC, IM | General antibiotic treatment |
| Enrofloxacin (Baytril Otic) | Apply topically as directed, adjust dose to body size of patient | Topical otic antibiotic |
| Erythromycin | DO NOT USE | DO NOT USE |
| Epoetin alpha | 50–150 IU/kg every 2–3 days; SC | Stimulates erythropoiesis |
| Epinephrine | 0.2 mg/kg IV; cardiac arrest | Cardiac arrest |

# Common Dosages for Rabbits (continued)

| Drug | Dosage | Indication |
|------|--------|------------|
| Fenbendazole | 20 mg/kg once daily for 5–28 days; PO. | For treatment of *E. cuniculi* |
| Fipronil | DO NOT USE | DO NOT USE |
| Flunixin | 0.3–2.0 mg/kg once daily to bid for no more than 3 days; PO, deep IM | Analgesia; use for no more than 3 days |
| Furosemide | 1–4 mg/kg bid to tid; IM, IV | Diuretic |
| | 1–2 mg/kg bid to tid; PO long-term use | |
| Gentamicin | 1 g/20 g PMMA | Local treatment in abscess cavity |
| Glycopyrrolate | 0.01–0.1 mg/kg; SC | Anticholinergic preanesthetic |
| Griseofulvin | 25 mg/kg once daily or divided bid for 28–40 days; PO | Systemic antifungal therapy |
| Hetastarch | 20 mL/kg IV | Volume expansion |
| Hydroxyzine | 2 mg/kg bid to tid; PO | Antihistamine |
| Imidacloprid | Treat as per cats | Topical flea treatment |
| Iron dextran | 4–6 mg/kg once; IM | Iron deficient anemia |
| Isoflurane | Anesthetic of choice | Anesthesia |
| Itraconazole | 5 mg/kg daily for 3–4 weeks | Systemic antifungal therapy |
| Ivermectin | 200–400 µg/kg once, repeat in 10–14 days for a total of 2–3 treatments as needed; SC | Ectoparasites |
| Ketamine | 20–50 mg/kg; IM | Anesthesia |
| Ketamine + acepromazine | 25–40 mg/kg + 0.25–1.0 mg/kg; IM | Anesthesia |
| Ketamine + diazepam | 15–20 mg/kg + 1–3 mg/kg; IM | Sedation |
| Ketamine + midazolam | 15–20 mg/kg + 0.5–1.0 mg/kg; IM | Sedation |
| Ketoconazole | 10–15 mg/kg once daily for 3–4 weeks | Systemic antifungal therapy |
| Ketoprofen | 1 mg/kg sid to bid; IM | Analgesia |
| Lidocaine | 1–2 mg/kg IV or 2–4 mg/kg IT | Antiarrhythmia |
| Lime sulfur 2.5% solution | Apply once weekly for 4–6 weeks | Ectoparasites |
| Lufenuron | Treat as per cat; 30 mg/kg PO every 30 days | Flea treatment |
| Meclizine | 2–12 mg/kg sid; PO | Vestibular disorders |
| Meloxicam | 0.2 mg/kg once daily; SC, IM | Analgesia |
| | 0.2–0.5 mg/kg once daily; PO | |
| Metoclopramide | 0.2–0.5 mg/kg tid to qid; PO, SC | Gastrointestinal promotility agent |
| Metronidazole | 20 mg/kg bid; PO | For anaerobic infections; treat for 2 weeks for *Clostridium* spp. |
| Miconazole (cream or 2% shampoo) | Apply topically as required | Topical antifungal |
| Midazolam | 0.5–2 mg/kg; IM | Sedation |
| Morphine | 2–5 mg/kg q2–4h; IM, SC | Analgesia |
| Naloxone (titrate to effect) | 0.01–0.1 mg/kg; IM, IV | Opioid reversal by titration |
| Oxibendazole | 20 mg/kg once daily for 7–14 days; PO; then reduce to 15 mg/kg once daily for 30–60 days | For treatment of *E. cuniculi* |
| Oxymorphone | 0.05–0.2 mg/kg bid to tid; SC, IM | Analgesia |
| Oxytocin | 0.1–3 U/kg; SC, IM | To stimulate uterine motility or milk letdown |
| Penicillin g, procaine | 40,000–60,000 U/kg once daily every 2–7 days; SC, IM | General antibiotic treatment. Do not administer orally |
| Penicillin g, benzathine | 42,000–84,000 U/kg once per week for 3 treatments; SC, IM | For treatment of *Treponema cuniculi*. Do not administer orally |
| Piperazine adipate | 500 mg/kg once daily for 2 days; PO | Antiparasitic |
| Polysulfate glycosaminoglycans | 2.2 mg/kg q3d for 21–28 days, then q14d; SC, IM | Nutraceutical treatment for joint inflammation |
| Praziquantel | 5–10 mg/kg once, repeat in 10 days; PO, SC, IM | Antiparasitic |
| Prednisone | 0.5–2 mg/kg; PO | Few indications in rabbits; use with extreme caution |
| Propofol | 2–6 mg/kg; IV slowly | Anesthesia |
| Pyrethrin products (0.05% shampoo) or use as directed for cats | Once weekly for 4 weeks | Treatment of ectoparasites, especially fleas |
| Ranitidine HCl | 2 mg/kg once daily IV or 2–5 mg/kg twice daily PO | $H_2$-receptor blocking agent for gastric ulcer therapy |
| Selamectin | Treat as per cat; 6–10 mg/kg applied topically every 30 days | Treatment of ectoparasites and endoparasites |
| Sevoflurane | Inhalant anesthetic used to effect | Anesthesia |
| Simethicone | 65–130 mg/animal q1h as needed; PO | Alleviation of gastrointestinal gas |
| Stanozolol | 1–2 mg/rabbit; PO, once | Anabolic steroid |
| Sodium bicarbonate | 2 mEq/kg IV, IP | Treatment of acidosis |

## COMMON DOSAGES FOR RABBITS (CONTINUED)

| Drug | Dosage | Indication |
| --- | --- | --- |
| Sucralfate | 25 mg/kg bid to tid; PO | Treatment of gastric ulceration and gastritis |
| Sulfadimethoxine | 25–50 mg/kg once daily, or 50 mg/kg loading dose followed by 25 mg/kg for 9 days; PO | Treatment of gastrointestinal coccidiosis |
| Tiletamine-zolazepam | DO NOT USE | DO NOT USE |
| Trimethoprim sulfadiazine | 30 mg/kg bid; SC, PO | General antibiotic therapy |
| Tropicamide 1% eye drops | Topically to dilate eyes in albino animals | Mydriasis |
| Verapamil | 200 $\mu$g/kg at surgery and tid for 9 doses total; IV, IP | May decrease postsurgical peritoneal adhesion formation |
| Vitamin B complex | Dose to thiamine content at 1–2 mg/kg as needed; IM | Thiamine deficiency |
| Vitamin K$_1$ | 2.5 mg/kg once daily; PO for 10–30 days | Treatment of anticoagulant rodenticide toxicosis |
| | 2–10 mg/kg as needed; IM | Use with caution; anaphylaxis reported |

Adapted from Allen DG, Dowling PM, Smith DA, et al. Handbook of Veterinary Drugs. 3rd Ed. Baltimore: Lippincott Williams & Wilkins, 2005.

# Appendix IV

## Normal Values for Rabbits

Table 1.

| Reference Ranges for Serum Biochemistry Values: Rabbits | |
|---|---|
| Serum protein | 2.8–10.0 g/dL^ |
| Albumin | 2.7–4.6 g/dL^ |
| Globulin | 1.5–2.8 g/dL^ |
| Fibrinogen | 0.2–0.4 g/dL^ |
| Serum glucose | 75–150 mg/dL^ |
| Blood urea nitrogen | 15.0–23.5 mg/dL^ |
| Creatinine | 0.5–2.5 mg/dL* |
| Total bilirubin | 0.25–0.74 mg/dL^ |
| Serum lipids | 280–350 mg/dL^ |
| Phospholipids | 75–113 mg/dL^ |
| Triglycerides | 124–156 mg/dL^ |
| Cholesterol | 18–35 mg/dL^ |
| Calcium | 5.6–12.5 mg/dL* |
| Phosphorus | 4.0–6.9 mg/dL* |
| Alanine aminotransferase (ALT) | 48–80 U/L* |
| Aspartate aminotransferase (AST) | 14–113 U/L* |
| Alkaline phosphatase (AP) | 4–16 U/L* |

^Harkness JE, Wagner JE. The Biology and Medicine of Rabbits and Rodents. 4th Ed. Baltimore: Williams & Wilkins, 1995.
*Okerman L. Diseases of Domestic Rabbits. 2nd Ed. Oxford: Blackwell Scientific Publications, 1994.

Table 2.

| Hematologic Values: Rabbit | |
|---|---|
| Erythrocytes | $4–7.2 \times 10^6$/mm$^3$ |
| Hematocrit | 36–48% |
| Hemoglobin | 10.0–15.5 mg/dL |
| Leukocytes | $7.5–13.5 \times 10^3$/mm$^3$ |
| Neutrophils | 20–35% |
| Lymphocytes | 55–80% |
| Monocytes | 1–4% |
| Basophils | 2–10% |
| Platelets | $200–1000 \times 10^3$/mm$^3$ |

Adapted from Harkness JE, Wagner JE. The Biology and Medicine of Rabbits and Rodents. 4th Ed. Baltimore: Williams & Wilkins, 1995.

Table 3.

| Physiologic Values: Rabbits | |
|---|---|
| Body weight | 2–6 kg |
| Respiratory rate | 30–60 breaths/min |
| Tidal volume | 4–6 mL/kg |
| Oxygen use | 0.4—0.85 mL/g/hr |
| Heart rate | 103–325 beats/min |
| Blood volume | 57–78 mL/kg |
| Blood pressure | 90–130/60–90 mm Hg |
| Rectal temperature | 38.5–40.0°C (101–104° F) |
| Life span | 5–6 years or more |
| Water consumption | 5–10 mL/100 g/day |
| Gastrointestinal transit time | 4–5 hours |
| Breeding onset: Male | 6–10 months |
| Breeding onset: Female | 4–9 months |
| Cycle length | Induced ovulator |
| Gestation period | 29–35 days |
| Postpartum estrus | None |
| Litter size | 4–10 |
| Weaning age | 4–6 weeks |
| Breeding duration | 1–3 years |
| Milk composition | 12.2% fat, 10.4% protein, 1.8% lactose |

Adapted from Harkness JE, Wagner JE. The Biology and Medicine of Rabbits and Rodents. 4th Ed. Baltimore: Williams & Wilkins, 1995.

# APPENDIX V

## TOXIC PLANTS AND THEIR CLINICAL SIGNS—ANTIDOTES AND TREATMENT

| Mon Tilley ed. 3–5 Min Consultr | | |
|---|---|---|
| Plant and characteristics | Clinical signs | Antidotes and treatment |
| Angol's trumpet (*Datura* spp.)<br>Garden annual with white trumpet-shaped flowers<br>Whole plant toxic; toxicity highest in seeds | Thirst, GI atony, disturbed vision, delirium, hallucinations | Parasympathomimetic drugs |
| Autumn crocus (*Colchicum autumnale*)<br>Houseplant<br>Whole plant toxic; toxicity highest in bulbs | Burning sensation in throat and mouth, thirst, nausea, diarrhea | Fluids; analgesics and atropine to alleviate colic and diarrhea |
| Azalea (*Rhododendron* spp.)<br>Garden, landscape plant<br>Leaves and flowers are toxic<br>Honey made from flower nectar is toxic | Burning sensation in mouth, salivation, emesis, diarrhea, muscular weakness, dimness of vision, bradycardia, arrythmia, hypotension EMERGENCY CONDITION | Do not use emetics. Use activated charcoal. Fluid replacement and respiratory support are required. Treat heart block with isoproterenol. |
| Belladonna lily (*Amaryllis* spp.)<br>Garden, potted plant<br>Bulbs are most toxic | Nausea, diarrhea, hypotension, depression, liver damage | Gastric lavage, charcoal, fluids, and supportive treatment |
| Bittersweet (*Celastrus* spp.)<br>Weed, vine with red berries<br>Immature fruits are toxic | Gastric irritation, fever, diarrhea | Fluids |
| Bleeding heart (*Dicentra* spp.)<br>Garden, woods, pottted plant<br>Roots more toxic than leaves | Vomiting, diarrhea, convulsions or paralysis | Fluids and seizure control |
| Castor bean (*Ricinus communis*)<br>Garden annual, grows to 2 m<br>Seeds are 1 cm, dark and light motted, and highly toxic | Latent period; colic, emesis, diarrhea, thirst | Emesis, charcoal, fluids, and electrolytes |
| Chinaberry tree (*Melia azedarach*)<br>Ornamental tree in temperate to subtropical areas<br>Fruit and bark are most toxic | Faintness, ataxia, mental confusion, intense gastritis, emesis, diarrhea | Fluid and electrolyte replacement |
| Christmas rose (*Helleborus niger*)<br>Houseplant<br>Entire plant is toxic | Pain in mouth and abdomen, nausea, emesis, colic, diarrhea, arrhythmia, hypotension | Gastric lavage or emesis: activated charcoal or saline cathartics to decontaminate the GI tract |
| Daphne (*Daphne mezereum*)<br>Landscape shrub<br>Entire plant is toxic | Vesication and edema of the lips and oral cavity, salivation, thirst, abdominal pain, emesis, hemorrhagic diarrhea | Fluid and electrolyte replacement |
| Delphinium or larkspur (*Delphinium* spp.)<br>Outdoor garden, mountains; tall with blue flowers<br>Seeds more toxic than leaves | Trembling, ataxia, weakness, salivation | GI detoxification; physostigmine to treat muscarinic signs |
| English holly (*Ilex* spp.)<br>Landscape plant<br>Fruit is toxic | Nausea, vomiting, diarrhea | Fluid and electrolyte replacement |
| English ivy (*Hedera helix*)<br>Houseplant<br>Fruit and leaves are toxic | Salivation, thirst, emesis, gastroenteritis, diarrhea, dermatitis | Corticosteroids to treat dermal response; treat other signs symptomatically |

## TOXIC PLANTS AND THEIR CLINICAL SIGNS—ANTIDOTES AND TREATMENT (CONTINUED)

| Plant and characteristics | Clinical signs | Antidotes and treatment |
|---|---|---|
| Foxglove (*Digitalis purpurea*) Outdoor gardens Entire plant is toxic (especially leaves) | Nausea, emesis, abdominal pain, diarrhea, bradycardia, arrhythmia with prolonged P-R interval and hypokalemia | GI decontamination with activated charcoal or saline cathartics. Treat hypokalemia and give lidocaine for ventricular arrhythmia. |
| Golden chain (*Laburnum anagyroides*) Landscape tree with long chains of yellow flowers Entire plant is toxic | Emesis, depression, weakness, incoordination, mydriasis, tachycardia | GI decontamination with lavage or emesis followed by activated charcoal |
| Horse chestnut or buckeye (*Aesculus* spp.) Landscape or forest tree; palmate leaves Nuts and twigs most toxic | Gastroenteritis, diarrhea, dehydration, electrolyte imbalance | Fluid and electrolyte replacement, demulcents, and therapy for gastroenteritis |
| Iris or flag (*Iris* spp.) Perennial garden flower Rootstock most toxic | Colic, nausea, vomiting, diarrhea | Fluid and electrolyte replacement |
| Irish potato (*Solanum tuberosum*) Vegetable garden Vines, green skin, and sprouts are toxic | Colic, diarrhea, salivation, ataxia, weakness, bradycardia, hypotension. Signs may vary from atropine-like to cholinesterase inhibition. Use antidotes accordingly and with caution. | GI decontamination. If atropine-like signs predominate, use physostigmine. If salivation and diarrhea are present, use atropine cautiously. |
| Jack-in-the-pulpit (*Arisaema triphyllum*) Woods and gardens or temperate zones Entire plant is toxic | Glossitis, pharyngitis, oral inflammation, edema, salivation | Irrigate mouth with water. Cool liquids or demulcents held in mouth may relieve signs. |
| Lantana (*Lantana camara*) Garden and wild in mild temperate to tropical areas; bright orange and yellow flowers Foliage and immature berries are toxic | Weakness, lethargy, vomiting, diarrhea, mydriasis, bradypnea. Advanced signs are cholestasis, bilirubinemia, and photosensitization. | GI decontamination, fluids, and respiratory support. Protect from sunlight and treat for hepatic insufficiency. |
| Lily, including Easter lily, tiger lily (*Lilium* spp.). daylily (*Hemerocallis* spp.) | Depression, oliguria, renal failure in cats as a result of toxic tubular necrosis | Prompt GI decontamination and supportive therapy for renal failure. Toxin presently is unknown. |
| Lily-of-the-valley (*Convallaria majalis*) Garden ornamental Seeds and flowers more toxic than leaves | Colic, vomiting, diarrhea, bradycardia, arrhythmia | Decontaminate GI tract with lavage and charcoal. Avoid emetics. Lidocaine to treat ventricular arrhythmias; treat as for other digitalis glycoside overdose, including correction of hyperkalemia. |
| Lupine (*Lupinus* spp.) Garden ornamental Seeds more toxic than leaves | Salivation, ataxia, seizures, dyspnea | GI decontamination, control of seizures |
| Mistletoe (*Phoradendron* spp.) Parasitic shrub on other trees Access to pets in homes at holiday time Leaves, stems, and berries are moderately toxic | Emesis, colic, diarrhea, mydriasis, hypovolemia | Fluid and electrolyte replacement; demulcents for gastroenteritis |
| Monkshood (*Aconitum* spp.) Perennial garden ornamental Entire plant is toxic | Glossitis, pharyngitis, salivation, nausea, emesis, impaired vision, bradycardia | GI decontamination, fluid and electrolyte replacement. Manage similar to digitalis glycoside overdose, with caution about potassium administration. |

## TOXIC PLANTS AND THEIR CLINICAL SIGNS—ANTIDOTES AND TREATMENT (CONTINUED)

| Plant and characteristics | Clinical signs | Antidotes and treatment |
| --- | --- | --- |
| Moonseed (*Menispermum canadense*) Woody vine of forests Fruit is most toxic | Convulsions | Maintain airway and support respiration as needed. Control seizures with least medication possible (e.g., diazepam) |
| Morning glory (*Ipomoea purpurea* and *Ipomoea tricolor*) Garden annual, potted plant Seeds most toxic Occasionally used as hallucinogen | Nausea, mydriasis, hallucinations, decreased reflexes, diarrhea, hypotension | Activated charcoal; dark, quiet surroundings; tranquilization with diazepam |
| Mountain laurel (*Kalmia* spp.) Native of eastern and southeastern woods, mountains Leaves and flowers are toxic Honey from nectar also toxic | Oral irritation, salivation, emesis, diarrhea, weakness, impaired vision, bradycardia, hypotension, AV block | Emetics are contraindicated. Use activated charcoal, fluid replacement, and respiratory support as needed. Isoproterenol to treat AV block as needed. |
| Narcissus, daffodil, jonquil (*Narcissus* spp.) Garden ornamental bulb Bulb is most toxic | Nausea, emesis, hypotension, diarrhea | Gastric lavage, charcoal, fluid replacement, supportive treatment for gastroenteritis |
| Nettle (*Urtica dioica*) Garden weed Hairs on leaves contain toxin that enters skin on contact | Oral irritation and pain, salivation, swelling and edema of nose and periocular areas or other areas of skin contact | Antihistamines and atropine may control appropriate signs. Local or systemic anti-inflammatory supportive therapy to treat affected contacts areas. |
| Oleander (*Nerium oleander*) Landscape shrub 1–3 m tall Whole plant is extremely toxic | Nausea, early signs of vomiting, colic, diarrhea; bradycardia and arrythmia with hyperkalemia develop soon after; EMERGENCY CONDITION | Gastric lavage or induced emesis; activated charcoal or saline cathartics. Treat as for digitalis glycoside overdose, including correction of hyperkalemia. Lidocaine or other appropiriate drugs for arrhythmia. |
| Philodendron (*Monstera* and *Philodendron* spp). Houseplant Leaves are slightly to moderately toxic | Painful irritation, edema of lips, mouth, tongue, and throat; reported nephrotoxic to cats | Cool liquids or demulcents held in mouth may aid relief. |
| Poinsettia (*Euphorbia pulcherrima*) Garden or potted plant, especially at Christmas holidays Sap of stem and leaves is mildly to moderately irritant or toxic | Irritation of mouth; may cause vomiting, diarrhea, and dermatitis | Demulcents and fluids to prevent dehydration |
| Rhubarb (*Rheum rhaponticum*) Garden plant Raw or canned Leaves are high in oxalates | Vomiting, diarrhea, and occasionally icterus. Renal failure develops from oxalate nephrosis. | Early GI decontamination is important. Demulcents and fluid replacement. Treat possible oxalate nephrosis. |
| Rosary pea or precatory bean (*Abrus precatorius*) Native of Caribbean Islands Seeds (when broken or chewed) are highly toxic Illegal to import into United States | Nausea, vomiting, diarrhea, weakness, tachycardia, possible renal failure, coma, death | Emesis or lavage followed with charcoal, demulcents, fluids, and electrolytes. Vitamin C may improve survival. |

## TOXIC PLANTS AND THEIR CLINICAL SIGNS—ANTIDOTES AND TREATMENT (CONTINUED)

| Plant and characteristics | Clinical signs | Antidotes and treatment |
| --- | --- | --- |
| Thorn apple or jimsonweed (*Datura stramonium*) Annual weed, some species are ornamental (*Datura metal*) Entire plant is toxic, but seeds are most toxic and available Relatively common drug abuse plant used as hallucinogen | Thirst, disturbances of vision, delirium, mydriasis, GI atony. Signs similar to atropine overdose. | Parasympathomimetic drug (e.g., physostigmine) |
| Tobacco (*Nicotiana tabacum*) Garden plant, weed, cigarettes Whole plant is toxic | Rapid onset of salivation, nausea, emesis, tremora. Incoordination, and ataxia, followed by collapse and respiratory failure: EMERGENCY CONDITION | Assist ventilation and vascular support first to save the animal. After respiratory support, decontaminate the GI tract with lavage and activated charcoal. |
| Wisteria (*Wisteria* spp.) Woody vine or shrub with blue to white legume flowers Entire plant is toxic | Nausea, abdominal pain, prolonged vomiting | Antiemetics and fluid replacement therapy |
| Yellow jessamino (*Gelsemium sempervirens*) Mild temperate to subtropical climates Yellow trumpet-shaped flowers grow on evergreen vines | Abdominal pain, bradypnea, paresis, seizures, hypothermia | Symptomatic and supportive therapy of respiration and cardiovascular function. GI decontamination and fluid replacement therapy. |
| Yew (*Taxus cuspidata* and *Taxus baccata*) Evergreen landscape shrub with two-ranked flat needle Whole plant (except ripe fruit) is toxic | Acute onset or sudden death. Affected animals show trembling, muscle weakness, dyspnea, collapse, arrhythmia, and heart block. | Symptomatic and supportive therapy of respiration and cardiovascular function. GI decontamination and fluid replacement therapy. |

Contributed by Gary Osweiler, College of Veterinary Medicine, Iowa State University, Ames, IA.
Reprinted with permission from Tilley LP, Smith FWK Jr. The 5-Minute Veterinary Consult: Cannine and Feline, 3rd ed. Baltimore: Lippincott Williams & Wilkins, 2004.

# INDEX

Text in **boldface** denote chapter discussions. Page numbers followed by a t denote tables.

## A

Abdominal effusion. See Ascites
Abdominocentesis
  in ascites, 9
  in clostridial enterotoxicosis, 21
  in congestive heart failure, 25, 213
  in hepatomegaly, 72
  in lymphosarcoma, 95
  in proliferative bowel disease, 132
  in urinary tract obstruction, 375
**Abscessation**
  in exophthalmos and orbital diseases, 250–252
  in malocculsion, 201–204
  in pasteurellosis, 317–319
  in rabbits, 178–181
  tooth root abscesses (apical abscesses), 360–363
ACE inhibitors
  for congestive heart failure, 25, 213–214
  for dilated cardiomyopathy, 18
  for renal failure, 151
Acepromazine
  dosage in ferrets, 388t
  dosage in rabbits, 394t
Acetylsalicylic acid
  dosage in ferrets, 388t
Activated charcoal
  for anticoagulant rodenticide poisoning, 190–191
  dosage in rabbits, 394t
  for poisoning in rabbits, 324
Acupunture
  for lameness, 287
  for osteoarthritis, 193
  for spondylosis deformans, 355
  for vertebral fracture or luxation, 382
Adenoma/adenocarcinoma, 106, 107
**Adrenal disease**
  alopecia, 2, 5
  in ferrets, 2–4, 5
  prostatitis and prostatic abscesses and, 134
  prostatomegaly and, 136
  pruritus and, 138, 139
  in urogenital cysts, 164–166
Adrenalectomy, 3, 75, 134, 135, 162, 165
AIPMMA (antibiotic-impregnated polymethyl methacrylate) beads
  for abscessation, 180, 203, 363
  after enucleation, 251–252
  for otitis, 309, 312–313
  for pasteurellosis, 319
  for septic arthritis, 195
  for ulcerative pododermatitis, 372
Albendazole
  dosage in rabbits, 394t
  for encephalitozoonosis, 188, 199–200, 239, 242, 271, 351
Albumin levels, in ascites, 9
**Aleutian Disease Virus (ADV)**, 115–116

Alopecia
  in bacterial folliculitis, 5, 6, 183
  in cheyletiellosis, 205
  in conjunctivitis, 215
  in dermatophytosis, 5, 6, 30, 182, 183, 223
  ear mites and, 5, 47, 182, 236
  in epiphora, 245
  in ferrets, 5–6
  fleas and, 5–6, 182, 183, 257
  in gastroduodenal ulcers, 58
  in *Helicobacter mustelae* infection, 68
  in hyperadrenocorticism, 2, 5
  in hyperestrogenism, 5, 74
  in insulinoma, 85
  in mast cell tumor, 97
  melena and, 100
  in neoplasia, 5, 6, 182, 183
  in otitis, 111, 308
  in pruritus, 138, 328
  in pyometra, 142
  in rabbits, 182–183
  sarcoptic mange, 5, 6, 157, 182, 183
  seasonal flank, 5
  in treponematosis (rabbit syphillis), 182, 183
  in ulcerative pododermatitis, 371
  with vaginal discharge, 170
Amantadine, for influenza, 84
Amikacin
  in AIPMMA (antibiotic-impregnated polymethyl methacrylate) beads, 195, 252, 309, 313, 319, 362, 372
  dosage
    in ferrets, 388t
    in rabbits, 394t
Aminophylline
  dosage in ferrets, 388t
Amitraz
  for demodicosis, 6, 139
  dosage in ferrets, 388t
  for sarcoptic mange, 157
Amoxicillin
  for clostridial enterotoxicosis, 22
  for cystitis, 46
  for diarrhea, 36
  dosage
    in ferrets, 388t
    in rabbits, 394t
  for dyschezia and hematochezia, 38
  for epizootic catarrhal enteritis, 51
  for gastritis, 56
  for gastrodoudenal ulcers, 59
  for gastrointestinal and esophageal foreign bodies, 62
  for *Helicobacter mustelae,* 36, 56, 59, 62, 69, 92, 100, 173
  for lymphoplasmacytic enteritis and gastroenteritis, 93
  for megaesophagus, 99
  for melena, 100–101
  for pneumonia, aspiration, 121
  for pneumonia, bacterial, 123

  for regurgitation, 149
  for vomiting, 173
Amoxicillin/clavulanate
  for bacterial folliculitis, 6
  dosage in ferrets, 388t
  for gingivitis and periodontal disease, 65
  for lower urinary tract disease, 88
Amphotericin B
  dosage in ferrets, 388t
  for nasal discharge, 105
  for pneumonia, mycotic, 125–126
Ampicillin
  in AIPMMA (antibiotic-impregnated polymethyl methacrylate) beads, 180
  for campylobacteriosis, 13
  dosage
    in ferrets, 388t
    in rabbits, 394t
  for tooth root abscesses, 362
Amprolium
  for coccidiosis, 211, 227
  dosage in rabbits, 394t
Anabolic steroids, for hyperestrogenism, 75
Anal prolapse, in ferrets, 147
Anal sacculectomy, 147
Analgesics. *See specific drugs*
Anastrozole
  dosage in ferrets, 388t
  for hyperadrenocorticism, 4
Androstenedione
  elevation in hyperadrenocorticism, 2, 136
  elevation in prostatic disease, 134
Anemia
  in Aleutian disease virus, 115
  in anticoagulant rodenticide poisoning, 190
  ataxia from, 11, 196
  in dyspnea and tachypnea, 42
  in endometrial disorders, 336
  from fleas and flea infestation, 53, 257
  in gastritis, 55
  in gastroduodenal ulcers, 58
  in heat stroke and heat stress, 273
  in *Helicobacter mustelae* infection, 68
  in hematuria, 275
  in hepatomegaly, 71
  in hyperestrogenism, 74
  in lead toxicity, 288
  in lymphoplasmacytic enteritis and gastroenteritis, 92
  in lymphosarcoma, 94
  in melena, 100, 295
  in neoplasia, digestive system, 106
  in paresis, 113, 114
  in pneumonia, aspiration, 121
  in pregnancy toxemia, 131
  in prostatitis, 134
  in pyometra, 142, 336
  in renal failure, 150, 344, 345
  in renomegaly, 153
  in salmonellosis, 155
  in splenomegaly, 159

Anemia *(continued)*
    in urinary tract obstruction, 161
    in uterine adenocarcinoma, 377
    in vaginal discharge, 170, 379
    in vomiting, 172
**Anorexia**
    in abscessation, 178
    in Aleutian disease virus, 115
    in clostridial enterotoxicosis, 207
    in congestive heart failure, 212
    in conjunctivitis, 216
    in constipation, 219
    in diarrhea, 228, 229
    in dyspnea and tachypnea, 231
    in dysuria and pollakiuria, 234
    in encephalitozoonosis, 238
    in eosinophilic gastroenteritis, 48
    in epistaxis, 248
    in epizootic catarrhal enteritis, 50–51
    in ferrets, 7–8
    in gastric dilation, 259
    in gastritis, 55–56
    in gastroduodenal ulcers, 58
    in gastrointestinal and esophageal foreign
        bodies, 61, 262
    in gastrointestinal hypomotility and
        gastrointestinal stasis, 266, 267
    in head tilt, 270, 271
    in heartworm disease, 66
    in *Helicobacter mustelae* infection, 68
    in hypercalciuria, 277
    in hyperestrogenism, 74
    in inflammatory bowel disease, 81
    in influenza, 83
    in lead toxicity, 288
    in lymphoplasmacytic enteritis and
        gastroenteritis, 92
    in lymphosarcoma, 94
    in malocclusion, 201–202, 280–281
    in mast cell tumor, 97
    in mastitis, 293
    in megaesophagus, 98
    melena and, 100, 295
    in myxomatosis, 297
    in nephrolithiasis and ureterolithiasis, 303
    in otitis, 311
    in pasteurellosis, 317
    in pleural effusion, 119
    in pneumonia
        bacterial, 123
        in rabbits, 321
    in pregnancy toxemia, 131
    in proliferative bowel disease, 132
    in prostatomegaly, 136
    in ptyalism, 140, 330
    in pyometra and endometrial disorders,
        336
    in rabbits, 184–186
    in renal failure, 150, 151, 344
    in rhinitis and sinusitis, 347
    in septic arthritis, 194
    in stertor and stridor, 356
    in tooth root abscessation, 360, 361
    trichobezoars and, 367, 369
    in ulcerative pododermatitis, 371
    in urinary tract obstruction, 161, 374
    in urogenital cysts, 164
    in urolithiasis, 167
    vaginal discharge and, 379
    in weight loss, 174
**Anterior uveitis**
    epiphora in, 245
    in rabbits, 187–189
    red eye, 341

Antibiotic therapy
    for abscessation, 180, 203, 282, 331, 362
    AIPMMA (antibiotic-impregnated polymethyl
        methacrylate) beads, 180, 195, 203,
        251–252, 309, 312–313, 319, 362, 372
    for anterior uveitis, 188
    for ascites, 10
    for bacterial folliculitis, 6, 183
    for bacterial meningoencephalitis and abscess,
        351
    for campylobacteriosis, 13
    for clostridial enterotoxicosis, 22, 208
    clostridial enterotoxicosis from, 207
    for coccidiosis-associated infection, 211
    for conjunctivitis, 217
    for constipation, 221
    for cough, 27
    for cystitis, 46
    for dermatitis, 354
    for diarrhea, 36, 227, 229
    for dyschezia and hematochezia, 38
    for dysuria and pollakiuria, 235
    for endometrial disorders, 337
    for enteric dysbiosis, 325
    for epiphora, 246
    for epistaxis, 249
    for epizootic catarrhal enteritis, 51
    for exophthalmos and orbital diseases, 252
    for facial and dental abscesses, 203
    for gastric dilation, 260
    for gastrodoudenal ulcers, 59
    for gastrointestinal and esophageal foreign
        bodies, 62, 264
    for gastrointestinal hypomotility and
        gastrointestinal stasis, 268
    for gingivitis and periodontal disease, 65
    for head tilt, 271
    for *Helicobacter mustelae,* 36, 56, 69
    for influenza-associated bacterial infections, 83
    for lameness, 287
    for lower urinary tract disease, 88–89, 291
    for lymphoplasmacytic enteritis and
        gastroenteritis, 92
    for mastitis, 294
    for megaesophagus, 99
    for melena, 100–101, 296
    for meningoencephalitis, 242
    for moist pyoderma, 331
    for nasal discharge, 105, 299
    for otitis, 111, 310, 313
    for pasteurellosis, 319
    for pneumonia
        aspiration, 121
        bacterial, 123
        in rabbits, 322
    for pododermatitis and nail bed disorders, 127
    for proliferative bowel disease, 132
    for prostatitis and prostatic abscesses,
        134, 162
    for prostatomegaly, 137
    for pyoderma, 334
    for pyometra, 143, 337
    for red eye, 343
    for regurgitation, 149
    for rhinitis and sinusitis, 348, 349
    for salmonellosis, 155
    for septic arthritis, 180
    for stertor and stridor, 357
    for tooth root abscesses, 362
    for *Treponema cuniculi,* 366
    for treponematosis, 183
    for trichobezoars, 369
    for ulcerative pododermatitis, 373
    for urogenital cysts, 166

    for vaginal discharge, 171, 380
    for vomiting, 173
Anticholinergics, for diarrhea, 36
**Anticoagulant rodenticide poisoning**
    epistaxis and, 248–249
    in rabbits, 190–191, 325
Antiemetics
    for gastritis, 56
    for uremic crisis, 151
    for vomiting, 173
Antihistamines
    for fleas, 53
    for influenza-associated nasal discharge, 83
    for nasal discharge, 105, 299
    for pododermatitis and nail bed disorders, 128
    for pruritus, 139, 328
    for rhinitis and sinusitis, 349
    for sarcoptic mange, 157
Anuria, 150–151, 344–346
Aplastic anemia, in hyperestrogenism, 74
Apomorphine
    dosage in ferrets, 388t
APTT, in rabbits, 248
Arrhythmias
    in congestive heart failure, 24, 25, 212
    in dilated cardiomyopathy, 18
    in heartworm disease, 66
    in heat stroke and heat stress, 273, 274
    in hypertrophic cardiomyopathy, 19
**Arthritis**
    osteoarthritis in rabbits, 192–193
    septic in rabbits, 194–195
Arthrocentesis, 192
Arthrodesis, 192
Arthroplasty, 192
Arthrotomy, 192, 194
Artificial tears, 217
**Ascites**
    in coccidiosis, 210
    in congestive heart failure, 24, 212, 213
    in ferrets, 9–10
    in heartworm disease, 66
Asparaginase, for lymphosarcoma, 95
Aspirates
    in abscessation, 179
    in exophthalmos and orbital diseases, 251
    in lymphadenomegaly, 90–91
    in malocclusion, 202, 281
    in mastitis, 293
    in neoplasia
        digestive system, 106
        musculoskeletal and nervous system, 108
    in pneumonia
        bacterial, 123
        mycotic, 125
    in ptyalism, 331
    in renal failure, 345
    in thymoma/thymic lymphoma, 359
    in tooth root abscessation, 361
    in ulcerative pododermatitis, 372
    in vaginal discharge, 379
Aspirin
    dosage in ferrets, 388t
**Ataxia**
    in encephalitozoonosis, 238
    in ferrets, 11–12
    in heat stroke and heat stress, 273
    in hypercalciuria, 277
    in hyperestrogenism, 74
    in hypoglycemia, 79
    in insulinoma, 85
    in lead toxicity, 288
    in neck and back pain, 301
    in otitis, 308

in proliferative bowel disease, 132
in rabbits, 196–198
in renal failure, 150, 344
in spondylosis deformans, 354
in toxoplasmosis, 364
in urinary tract obstruction, 374
Atenolol
for congestive heart failure, 25, 26, 214
for dilated cardiomyopathy, 18
dosage in ferrets, 388t
for hypertrophic cardiomyopathy, 19
Atipamezole
dosage in ferrets, 388t
Atrial fibrillation
in congestive heart failure, 25, 26
in dilated cardiomyopathy, 18
Atropine
for anterior uveitis, 188
for ciliary spasm, 252, 343
dosage in rabbits, 394t
Auscultation
in anticoagulant rodenticide poisoning, 190
in congestive heart failure, 24, 212
in constipation, 219
in dilated cardiomyopathy, 17
gastrointestinal foreign bodies and, 262
in gastrointestinal hypomotility and
gastrointestinal stasis, 266
in heartworm disease, 66
in hypertrphic cardiomyopathy, 19
in pneumonia
bacterial, 123
mycotic, 125
in rabbits, 321
in stertor and stridor, 356
Azathioprine
dosage in ferrets, 388t
for eosinophilic gastroenteritis, 49
for inflammatory bowel disease, 81
for lymphoplasmacytic enteritis and
gastroenteritis, 93
Azithromycin
for abscessation, 180, 331
for anterior uveitis, 188
for bacterial meningoencephalitis and abscess,
351
dosage in rabbits, 394t
for epistaxis, 249
for exophthalmos and orbital diseases, 252
for facial and dental abscesses,
203, 282
for head tilt, 271
for nasal discharge, 299
for otitis, 310, 313
for pasteurellosis, 319
for pneumonia in rabbits, 322
for rhinitis and sinusitis, 348
for septic arthritis, 195
for stertor and stridor, 357
for tooth root abscesses, 362
for ulcerative pododermatitis, 373
Azotemia
in diarrhea, 226
in dysuria and pollakiuria, 234
in hematuria, 275
in lower urinary tract infection, 290
in mastitis, 293
in nephrolithiasis and ureterolithiasis, 303
in polyuria and polydipsia (PU/PD), 129
in pregnancy toxemia, 131
in pyometra and endometrial disorders, 336
in renal failure, 150, 344
in renomegaly, 153
in urinary tract obstruction, 161, 375

in urolithiasis, 167
in vaginal discharge, 379

B

Bacitracin, for ocular ulceration, 252
**Back pain**, in rabbits, 301–302
Bacteremia/septicemia, in salmonellosis, 155
Bacterial folliculitis, 5, 6, 183, 329
Barbering, 219, 266
Barium sulfate
dosage in ferrets, 388t
dosage in rabbits, 394t
Basal cell tumor, 107
Bathing rabbits, 324, 334
*Baylisascaris procyonis,* 244
Benazepril, for renal failure, 151
Benzimidazole antihelmintics, for encephalitozoonosis, 239, 242, 271, 351
Beta blockers
for congestive heart failure, 25, 26, 213–214
for dilated cardiomyopathy, 18
for hypertrophic cardiomyopathy, 19
Bethanechol chloride, 279
Bicalutamide, for hyperadrenocorticism, 4
Biliary obstruction, hepatomegaly from, 71
Biochemistry
in abscessation, 179
in Aleutian disease virus, 115
in ascites, 9
in campylobacter, 13
in congestive heart failure, 24, 212
in constipation, 220
in cough, 27–28
in diabetes mellitus, 32
in diarrhea, 35, 226, 228
in dysphagia, 40
in dyspnea and tachypnea, 42, 231
in dystocia, 44
in dysuria and pollakiuria, 45, 234
in encephalitozoonosis, 238
in eosinophilic gastroenteritis, 48
in epizootic catarrhal enteritis, 50
in gastric dilation, 259
in gastritis, 55
in gastroduodenal ulcers, 58
in gastrointestinal hypomotility and
gastrointestinal stasis, 267
in heat stroke and heat stress, 273
in hepatomegaly, 71
in hypoglycemia, 79
in mastitis, 293
in melena, 100, 295
in multiple myeloma, 102
in neoplasia, digestive system, 106
in nephrolithiasis and ureterolithiasis, 304
in patechia/eccymosis/bruising, 117
in polyuria and polydipsia (PU/PD),
129, 326
in pregnancy toxemia, 131
in ptyalism, 140
reference ranges
in ferrets, 392t
in rabbits, 397t
in renal failure, 150, 344
in renomegaly, 153
trichobezoars and, 368
in urinary tract obstruction, 161, 375
in urolithiasis, 167
in vaginal discharge, 170, 379
in vomiting, 172
Biopsy
in abscessation, 179
in conjunctivitis, 216

in cryptosporidiosis, 29
in dermatophytosis, 223
in diarrhea, 36
in dyspnea and tachypnea, 232
in eosinophilic gastroenteritis, 48
in epistaxis, 248
in epizootic catarrhal enteritis, 50
in exophthalmos and orbital diseases, 251
gastric, 58, 59, 68
in *Helicobacter mustelae* infection, 68
in hepatomegaly, 71
in lameness, 286
in lymphadenomegaly, 90–91
in lymphosarcoma, 95
in mastitis, 293
nasal cavity, 105
in nasal discharge, 299
in neck and back pain, 301
in neoplasia, digestive system, 106
in osteoarthritis, 192
in otitis, 312
in pleural effusion, 120
in pneumonia, mycotic, 125
in pododermatitis and nail bed disorders,
127
in proliferative bowel disease, 132
in pruritus, 138, 328
in pyoderma, 334
in red eye, 342
in renal failure, 150, 345
in renomegaly, 153
in rhinitis and sinusitis, 348
in stertor and stridor, 357
in treponematosis, 366
in ulcerative pododermatitis, 372
in vaginal discharge, 379
in weight loss, 174
Bismuth subsalicylate
for diarrhea, 36
dosage in ferrets, 388t
for gastritis, 56
for gastrodoudenal ulcers, 59
for gastrointestinal and esophageal foreign
bodies, 62
for *Helicobacter mustelae,* 36, 56, 59, 62, 69,
92, 101, 173
for lymphoplasmacytic enteritis and
gastroenteritis, 93
for melena, 101
Blastomycosis, 125–126
Bleeding time
in anticoagulant rodenticide poisoning, 190
in patechia/eccymosis/bruising, 117
Blepharitis, 245, 341
Blepharospasm, 341
Bloat. *See* Gastric dilation
Bloat syndrome, in clostridial enterotoxicosis,
21–22
Bone marrow aspirate
in hyperestrogenism, 74
in lymphosarcoma, 95
in patechia/eccymosis/bruising, 117
in splenomegaly, 159, 160
Bone marrow suppression, in hyperestrogenism,
74, 75
Borborygmus, 219, 262, 266, 384
Bronchodilators
for cough, 27–28
for pneumonia, aspiration, 121
Bronchoscopy, in aspiration pneumonia, 121
Bruising, 117–118
Bruxism
in constipation, 219
in dysuria and pollakiuria, 234

Bruxism *(continued)*
 in exophthalmos and orbital diseases, 250
 in gastroduodenal ulcers, 58
 in gastrointestinal and esophageal foreign
 bodies, 61, 262
 in gastrointestinal hypomotility and
 gastrointestinal stasis, 266
 in *Helicobacter mustelae* infection, 68
 in hypercalciuria, 277
 in malocclusion, 201, 280
 in megaesophagus, 98
 melena and, 100, 295
 in nephrolithiasis and ureterolithiasis, 303
 in otitis, 311
 in ptyalism, 140, 330
 in stertor and stridor, 356
 in tooth root abscessation, 360
 trichobezoars and, 367
 in urinary tract obstruction, 374
Bulla osteotomy, 255, 271, 312
BUN
 in ascites, 9
 in polyuria and polydipsia (PU/PD),
 129, 326
 in pregnancy toxemia, 131
 in renal failure, 150, 344
 with vaginal discharge, 170
Buprenorphine
 dosage
 in ferrets, 388t
 in rabbits, 394t
 for pain
 in abscessation, 180, 203, 282
 in anorexia, 185
 in clostridial enterotoxicosis, 208
 in constipation, 221
 in diarrhea, 227, 229
 in exophthalmos and orbital diseases, 252
 in gastric dilation, 260
 in gastric distention, 22
 with gastrointestinal foreign bodies, 264
 in gastrointestinal hypomotility, 268
 in hypercalciuria management, 279
 in lameness, 287
 in nephrolithiasis and ureterolithiasis, 305
 in poisonings, 325
 postoperative, 377
 in pyometra and endometrial disorders,
 337
 in septic arthritis, 195
 in tooth root abscesses, 362
 in trichobezoars, 369
 in ulcerative pododermatitis, 373
 in urinary tract obstruction, 376
 with vaginal discharge, 380
 in vertebral fracture or luxation, 382
Butorphanol
 dosage
 in ferrets, 388t
 in rabbits, 394t
 for pain
 in abscessation, 180, 203
 in exophthalmos and orbital diseases, 252
 in gastric distention, 22
 in hypercalciuria management, 279
 in lameness, 287
 in nephrolithiasis and ureterolithiasis, 305
 postoperative, 377
 in pyometra and endometrial disorders,
 337
 in tooth root abscesses, 362
 in ulcerative pododermatitis, 373
 in urinary tract obstruction, 376
 in vertebral fracture or luxation, 382

C

Cachexia
 in encephalitozoonosis, 238
 in ferrets, 174–175
 in rabbits, 384–386
 in renal failure, 150, 344
CaEDTA, 288–289, 325, 394t
Calcium channel blockers, for congestive heart
 failure, 25, 213
Calcium oxalate urolithiasis. *See* Hypercalciuria;
 Nephrolithiasis and ureterolithiasis; Urolithiasis
**Campylobacteriosis**, in ferrets, 13–14
**Canine distemper virus**
 in ferrets, 15–16
 pododermatitis from, 127
Captopril
 dosage in ferrets, 388t
Carbamide peroxide, 112
Carbaryl
 for cheyletiellosis, 205
 dosage
 in ferrets, 388t
 in rabbits, 394t
 for fleas, 6, 53, 139, 257
**Cardiomyopathy**
 dilated in ferrets, 17–18
 hypertrophic in ferrets, 19–20
Carprofen
 for anorexia, 8
 dosage in rabbits, 394t
 for pain
 in abscessation, 180, 203, 282
 in anterior uveitis, 185
 in conjunctivitis, 217
 in dental disease, 331, 343
 in diarrhea, 227, 229
 in dysuria and pollakiuria, 235
 in epiphora, 247
 in exophthalmos and orbital diseases, 252
 in gastric dilation, 260
 in hematuria, 276
 in hypercalciuria management, 279
 in lameness, 287
 in mastitis, 294
 in neck and back, 302
 in nephrolithiasis and ureterolithiasis, 305
 in osteoarthritis, 192
 in otitis, 310, 313
 in paresis and paralysis, 315
 in pasteurellosis, 319
 postoperative, 377
 in pyoderma, 334
 in pyometra and endometrial disorders,
 337
 in septic arthritis, 195
 in spondylosis deformans, 354
 in tooth root abscesses, 362
 in ulcerative pododermatitis, 373
 in urinary tract obstruction, 376
 with vaginal discharge, 380
 in vertebral fracture or luxation, 382
Carvedilol
 for congestive heart failure, 26, 214
 for dilated cardiomyopathy, 18
**Cataracts**
 in encephalitozoonosis, 238
 in rabbits, 199–200
CBC
 in abscessation, 179
 in Aleutian disease virus, 115
 in alopecia, 5
 in anticoagulant rodenticide poisoning, 190
 in ascites, 9

 in canine distemper virus infection, 15
 in clostridial enterotoxicosis, 21, 207
 in coccidiosis, 23
 in congestive heart failure, 24
 in cough, 27–28
 in diabetes mellitus, 32
 in diarrhea, 35, 226, 228
 in dysphagia, 40
 in dyspnea and tachypnea, 42, 231
 in dysuria and pollakiuria, 45
 in encephalitozoonosis, 238
 in endometrial disorders, 336
 in eosinophilic gastroenteritis, 48
 in epizootic catarrhal enteritis, 50
 in gastric dilation, 259
 in gastritis, 55
 in gastroduodenal ulcers, 58
 in gastrointestinal hypomotility and gastrointestinal stasis, 267
 in heartworm disease, 66
 in heat stroke and heat stress, 273
 in *Helicobacter mustelae* infection, 68
 hematologic values
 in ferrets, 392t
 in rabbits, 397t
 in hematuria, 275
 in hepatomegaly, 71
 in hyperadrenocorticism, 2
 in hyperestrogenism, 74
 in hypoglycemia, 79
 in inflammatory bowel disease, 81
 in insulinoma, 85
 in lead toxicity, 288
 in lymphadenomegaly, 90
 in lymphoplasmacytic enteritis and
 gastroenteritis, 92
 in lymphosarcoma, 94
 in mastitis, 293
 in megaesophagus, 98
 in melena, 100, 295
 in multiple myeloma, 102
 in nasal discharge, 104
 in nephrolithiasis and ureterolithiasis, 304
 in patechia/eccymosis/bruising, 117
 in pneumonia
 aspiration, 121
 bacterial, 123
 mycotic, 125
 in polyuria and polydipsia (PU/PD),
 129, 326
 in pregnancy toxemia, 131
 in proliferative bowel disease, 132
 in prostatitis, 134
 in prostatomegaly, 136
 in ptyalism, 140
 in pyometra, 142, 336
 in regurgitation, 148
 in renal failure, 150, 344
 in renomegaly, 153
 in rhinitis and sinusitis, 347
 in salmonellosis, 155
 in septic arthritis, 194
 in splenomegaly, 159
 in tooth root abscessation, 361
 trichobezoars and, 368
 in urinary tract obstruction, 161
 in urolithiasis, 167
 in uterine adenocarcinoma, 377
 in vaginal discharge, 170, 379
 in vomiting, 172
 in weight loss, 174
Cecotrophs, 225, 228
Cefadroxil
 dosage in ferrets, 388t

Cefazolin
  in AIPMMA (antibiotic-impregnated
    polymethyl methacrylate) beads, 180, 195,
    252, 309, 312, 319, 362, 372
  dosage in rabbits, 394t
  for tooth root abscesses, 362
Ceftiofur
  in AIPMMA (antibiotic-impregnated
    polymethyl methacrylate) beads, 195, 252,
    309, 312, 319, 362, 372
  dosage in rabbits, 394t
Cell culture, for influenza, 83
Cephalexin
  for bacterial folliculitis, 6
  dosage
    in ferrets, 388t
    in rabbits, 394t
  for lower urinary tract disease, 88
  for nasal discharge, 105
  for otitis, 111
Cephalosporin
  for cough, 27
  for influenza-associated bacterial infections, 83
  for nasal discharge, 105
  for vaginal discharge, 171
Cephalothin, in AIPMMA (antibiotic-
  impregnated polymethyl methacrylate) beads,
  195, 252, 309, 312, 319, 362, 372
Cerebellar disease, ataxia from, 11, 196
Cerebral edema, 274
Cerumenolytics, 112
Cesarean section, 44, 131
**Cheek teeth (molar and premolar) malocclusion
  and elongation,** 201–204
Chemosis, 341
Chemotherapy
  for lymphosarcoma, 95
  for mast cell tumor, 97
  for multiple myeloma, 102
  for neoplasia, integumentary, 107
  for uterine adenocarcinoma, 377
Chest tap. *See* Thoracocentesis
**Cheyletiellosis (fur mites),** 182, 205–206
Chloramphenicol
  for abscessation, 180, 331
  for anterior uveitis, 188
  for bacterial meningoencephalitis and abscess,
    351
  for campylobacteriosis, 13
  for conjunctivitis, 217
  for diarrhea, 36
  dosage
    in ferrets, 388t
    in rabbits, 394t
  for epiphora, 246
  for epistaxis, 249
  for exophthalmos and orbital diseases, 252
  for facial and dental abscesses,
    203, 282
  for head tilt, 271
  for mastitis, 294
  for meningoencephalitis, 242
  for nasal discharge, 299
  for ocular ulceration, 252
  for otitis, 310, 313
  for pasteurellosis, 319
  for pneumonia in rabbits, 322
  for proliferative bowel disease, 36, 38, 100,
    132
  for pyometra and endometrial disorders, 337
  for red eye, 343
  for rhinitis and sinusitis, 348
  for salmonellosis, 155
  for septic arthritis, 195

  for tooth root abscesses, 362
  for ulcerative pododermatitis, 373
  for urogenital cysts, 166
  for vaginal discharge, 380
Chlorhexidine, for gingivitis and periodontal
  disease, 65
Chlorpheniramine
  dosage in ferrets, 388t
  for fleas, 53
  for influenza-associated nasal discharge, 83
  for nasal discharge, 105
  for pododermatitis and nail bed disorders, 128
  for pruritus, 139
  for sarcoptic mange, 157
Chlorpromazine
  for gastritis, 56
  for vomiting, 173
Cholestyramine
  for clostridial enterotoxicosis, 208, 227
  dosage in rabbits, 394t
  for enteric dysbiosis, 325
Chondroitin sulfate
  for neck and back pain, 302
  for osteoarthritis, 193
  for spondylosis deformans, 355
Chondroma/chondrosarcoma, 108
Chordoma, 108
Chorionic gonadotropin
  dosage in ferrets, 388t
Chylothorax, in pleural effusion, 119, 120
Cimetidine
  dosage
    in ferrets, 388t
    in rabbits, 394t
  for esophagitis, 99, 148
  for gastric ulceration, 59, 131, 185, 260, 264,
    268, 315, 325, 369, 382
  for gastritis, 8, 36, 51, 56, 59, 62, 69, 173
  for melena, 296
  for renal failure, 151, 345
  for uremic crisis, 151
Ciprofloxacin
  for anterior uveitis, 188
  for conjunctivitis, 217
  dosage
    in ferrets, 388t
    in rabbits, 394t
  for epiphora, 246
  for nasal discharge, 299
  for red eye, 343
  for rhinitis and sinusitis, 349
Cirrhosis, hypoglycemia in, 79
Cisapride
  for anorexia, 8, 185
  for constipation, 221
  dosage
    in ferrets, 388t
    in rabbits, 394t
  for gastritis, 56
  for gastrointestinal hypomotility, 264, 268,
    289, 325, 369
  for megaesophagus, 99
  for regurgitation, 149
Clarithromycin
  dosage in ferrets, 388t
  for gastroduodenal ulcers, 59
  for gastrointestinal and esophageal foreign
    bodies, 62
  for *Helicobacter mustelae,* 36, 59, 62, 69, 92,
    101
  for lymphoplasmacytic enteritis and
    gastroenteritis, 93
Clavulanic acid and amoxicillin. *See*
  Amoxicillin/clavulanate

Clindamycin
  for clostridial enterotoxicosis, 22
  dosage
    in ferrets, 389t
    in rabbits, 394t
  for gingivitis and periodontal disease, 65
CLO test, in *Helicobacter mustelae* infection, 69
**Clostridial enterotoxicosis**
  in ferrets, 21–22
  in rabbits, 207–209
Clotrimazole
  for dermatophytosis, 183, 223, 329
  dosage in rabbits, 394t
Cloxacillin
  dosage in ferrets, 389t
Coagulation study
  in anticoagulant rodenticide poisoning,
    190
  in epistaxis, 248
  in hepatomegaly, 72
  in melena, 100
  in patechia/eccymosis/bruising, 117
Coccidiodomycosis, 125
**Coccidiosis**
  in ferrets, 23
  in rabbits, 210–211
  rectal and anal prolapse in, 147
Collapse
  in Aleutian disease virus, 115
  gastrointestinal foreign bodies and, 262
  in insulinoma, 85
Colopexy, 147
Computed tomography. *See* CT (computed
  tomography)
**Congestive heart failure**
  in ferrets, 24–26
  in heartworm disease, 66
  in rabbits, 212–214
**Conjunctivitis**
  epiphora in, 245
  in influenza, 83
  in rabbits, 215–218
  red eye, 341
**Constipation,** in rabbits, 219–222
Contact dermatitis, 138, 182, 328
Corneal ulcers, 341, 342
Coronavirus, 50
Corticosteroids
  for anterior uveitis, 188
  for diarrhea, 36
  for eosinophilic gastroenteritis, 49
  for fleas, 53
  for gastric bloat, 22
  for lymphosarcoma, 95
  for megaesophagus, 99
  for melena, 101
  for otitis, 111
  for paresis and paralysis, 114, 315
  for pneumonia, aspiration, 121
  for pododermatitis and nail bed disorders,
    128
  for pruritus, 139
  for regurgitation, 149
  for vertebral fracture or luxation, 382
Cough
  in Aleutian disease virus, 115
  in canine distemper virus, 15
  in congestive heart failure, 24
  in ferrets, 27–28
  in heartworm disease, 66
  in influenza, 83
  in lymphosarcoma, 94
  in megaesophagus, 98
  in pleural effusion, 119

**Cough** (continued)
　in pneumonia
　　aspiration, 121
　　bacterial, 123
　　mycotic, 125
　in regurgitation, 148
Cough suppressants, 27–28
Counterimmunoelectrophoresis (CEP), in
　Aleutian disease virus, 115
Coupage
　in pneumonia, aspiration, 121
　in pneumonia, bacterial, 123
Cranial nerve deficits, 330
Creatine kinase, 40, 301
Creatinine
　in ascites, 9
　in polyuria and polydipsia (PU/PD), 129
　in renal failure, 150, 344
　with vaginal discharge, 170
Cryptococcosis, 125
Cryptosporidiosis, 29
Crystalluria, in dysuria and pollakiuria, 45
CSF analysis
　in ataxia, 12, 197
　in encephalitis and meningoencephalitis, 242
　in facial nerve paresis/paralysis, 255
　in head tilt, 271
　in neck and back pain, 301
　in paresis and paralysis, 114, 315
　in pneumonia, mycotic, 125
　in seizures, 350
CT (computed tomography)
　in abscessation, 179
　in anterior uveitis, 188
　in ataxia, 11–12, 197
　in conjunctivitis, 216
　in cough, 27
　in dysphagia, 40
　in dyspnea and tachypnea, 232
　in encephalitis and meningoencephalitis, 241,
　　244
　in epiphora, 246
　in epistaxis, 248
　in exophthalmos and orbital diseases, 251
　in facial nerve paresis/paralysis, 255
　in head tilt, 271
　in lameness, 286
　in malocclusion, 202, 281
　in nasal discharge, 104, 299
　in neck and back pain, 301
　in otitis, 308, 312
　in paresis and paralysis, 114, 315
　in pasteurellosis, 318
　in ptyalism, 331
　in red eye, 342
　in rhinitis and sinusitis, 348
　in seizures, 350
　in spondylosis deformans, 354
　in stertor and stridor, 357
　in tooth root abscessation, 361
　in toxoplasmosis, 364
　in vertebral fracture or luxation, 382
Culture
　in abscessation, 179
　in conjunctivitis, 216
　in dermatophytosis, 30, 223
　in dyspnea and tachypnea, 232
　in dysuria and pollakiuria, 234
　in encephalitis and meningoencephalitis,
　　241–242
　in endometrial disorders, 336
　in epiphora, 246
　in exophthalmos and orbital diseases, 251
　in facial nerve paresis/paralysis, 255

　in head tilt, 271
　in *Helicobacter mustelae* infection, 68
　in hematuria, 275
　in hepatomegaly, 71
　in hypercalciuria, 278
　in lower urinary tract disease, 88, 290
　in malocclusion, 202, 281
　in mastitis, 293
　in nasal discharge, 104–105, 299
　in osteoarthritis, 192
　in otitis, 111, 309, 312
　in pasteurellosis, 318
　in pneumonia
　　aspiration, 121
　　bacteria, 123
　　mycotic, 125
　　in rabbit, 321
　in polyuria and polydipsia (PU/PD), 326
　in prostatitis and prostatic abscesses, 134
　in pyoderma, 334
　in pyometra, 142, 336
　in red eye, 342
　in rhinitis and sinusitis, 348
　in septic arthritis, 194
　in stertor and stridor, 357
　in tooth root abscessation, 361
　in ulcerative pododermatitis, 372
　in urogenital cysts, 164
　in urolithiasis, 168
　in vaginal discharge, 379
Cutaneous hyperpigmentation, in hyperestro-
　genism, 74
Cyanosis
　in pleural effusion, 119
　in pneumonia, aspiration, 121
Cyclophosphamide
　for Aleutian disease virus infection, 116
　for lymphosarcoma, 95
　for multiple myeloma, 102
Cycloplegic drugs, 188
Cyclosporine A, for conjunctivitis, 217
Cyproheptadine
　dosage in rabbits, 394t
Cystic mastitis, 293–294
Cystitis. *See* Lower urinary tract infection
Cystocentesis, 88, 162, 168
Cystotomy, 162, 168
Cytology
　in conjunctivitis, 216
　in dyspnea and tachypnea, 42, 232
　in dysuria and pollakiuria, 45
　in endometrial disorders, 336
　in epiphora, 246
　in epistaxis, 248
　in exophthalmos and orbital diseases, 251
　in hepatomegaly, 71
　of joint fluid in lameness, 286
　in lymphadenomegaly, 90–91
　in nasal discharge, 104, 299
　in neoplasia, digestive system, 106
　in neoplasia, musculoskeletal and nervous
　　system, 108
　in otitis, 313
　in pasteurellosis, 318
　in pneumonia
　　bacterial, 123
　　mycotic, 125
　　in rabbits, 321
　in polyuria and polydipsia (PU/PD), 129
　in proliferative bowel disease, 132
　in prostatomegaly, 136
　in ptyalism, 141, 331
　in pyometra, 142, 336
　in red eye, 342

　in renomegaly, 153
　in rhinitis and sinusitis, 348
　in stertor and stridor, 357
　in uterine adenocarcinoma, 377
　in vaginal discharge, 170, 379

**D**

Dacryocystitis
　epiphora in, 245–247
　red eye in, 341, 343
Dacryocystorhinography, 216, 246, 342
Decongestants, for nasal discharge, 105
Dehydration, in epizootic catarrhal enteritis, 50
Demodicosis, 6, 139
Dental disease
　abscessation, 178–179
　anorexia in, 8, 184, 185
　cheek teeth (molar and premolar) malocclu-
　　sion and elongation, 201–204
　conjunctivitis and, 215–217
　constipation in, 220
　epiphora in, 245–247
　epistaxis in, 248
　in exophthalmos and orbital diseases,
　　250–252
　gingivitis and periodontal disease, 65
　incisor extraction, 282
　incisor malocclusion and overgrowth, 280–283
　molar extraction, 203
　nasal discharge in, 104, 105, 298, 299
　in ptyalism, 140, 330–331
　pyoderma in, 333
　red eye and, 341, 342, 343
　rhinitis and sinusitis and, 347
　stertor and stridor and, 356
　tooth root abscesses (apical abscesses) in
　　rabbits, 360–363
　trimming teeth, 203, 281–282, 331
Depression
　in abscessation, 178
　in anticoagulant rodenticide poisoning, 190
　in clostridial enterotoxicosis, 207
　in coccidiosis, 210
　in diarrhea, 225, 228
　in encephalitis and meningoencephalitis, 241
　in encephalitozoonosis, 238
　in endometrial disorders, 336
　in gastric dilation, 259
　in hyperestrogenism, 74
　in hypoglycemia, 79
　in insulinoma, 85
　in lead toxicity, 288
　in mastitis, 293
　in pasteurellosis, 317
　in pneumonia, mycotic, 125
　in pregnancy toxemia, 131
　in prostatomegaly, 136
　in pyometra, 142, 336
　in renal failure, 344
　in ulcerative pododermatitis, 371
　in urogenital cysts, 164
　in urolithiasis, 167
　vaginal discharge and, 379
Dermatitis
　contact, 138, 182, 328
　pododermatitis and nail bed disorders in
　　ferrets, 127–128
　ulcerative pododermatitis (sore hocks) in
　　rabbits, 314, 370–373
**Dermatophytosis**
　alopecia, 5, 6, 182
　in ferrets, 5, 6, 30–31
　pruritus, 138, 139, 328, 329
　in rabbits, 223–224

Desoxycorticosterone pivalate (DOCP)
    dosage in ferrets, 389t
    for hyperadrenocorticism, 4
*Desulfovibrio* sp., 23, 38
Dewlap pyoderma, 330, 333
Dexamethasone
    after adrenalectomy, 165
    dosage
        in ferrets, 389t
        in rabbits, 394t
    for paresis and paralysis, 315
    for vaccine reaction, 101
    for vertebral fracture or luxation, 382
Dexamethasone sodium phosphate
    dosage in ferrets, 389t
    for gastric bloat, 22
Dextrose
    dosage in ferrets, 389t
    for hypoglycemia, 79–80, 85–86, 351
    for tooth abscessation, 362
    for topical abscessation, 180–181, 373
**Diabetes mellitus**, in ferrets, 32–34
Diaphragmatic hernia, 119, 120
**Diarrhea**
    acute in rabbits, 225–227
    in campylobacteriosis, 13
    in canine distemper virus, 15
    chronic in rabbits, 228–230
    in clostridial enterotoxicosis, 21–22, 207
    in coccidiosis, 23, 210
    in cryptosporidiosis, 29
    in eosinophilic gastroenteritis, 48–49
    in epizootic catarrhal enteritis, 50–51
    in ferrets, 35–37
    in gastritis, 55
    in gastroduodenal ulcers, 58
    in gastrointestinal and esophageal foreign
        bodies, 61, 262
    in gastrointestinal hypomotility and gastroin-
        testinal stasis, 266
    in giardiasis, 64
    in *Helicobacter mustelae* infection, 68
    in inflammatory bowel disease, 81
    in lymphoplasmacytic enteritis and gastroen-
        teritis, 92
    in lymphosarcoma, 94
    melena and, 100, 295
    in proliferative bowel disease, 132
    in ptyalism, 140
    rectal and anal prolapse and, 147
    in renal failure, 150, 344
    in salmonellosis, 155
    trichobezoars and, 367
Diazepam
    dosage
        in ferrets, 389t
        in rabbits, 394t
    for sedation
        in ferrets, 66, 168
        in rabbits, 180, 217, 247, 260, 264, 310,
            319, 322, 334, 343, 369, 373, 382
    for seizures
        cluster seizures and status epilepticus, 351
        in encephalitis and meningoencephalitis,
            242
        in encephalitozoonosis, 239
        in head tilt, 271
        in heat stroke and heat stress, 273
        in lead toxicity, 288
        in otitis, 313
        in poisonings, 325
    for vestibular signs
        in encephalitis and meningoencephalitis,
            242

    in encephalitozoonosis, 239
    in head tilt, 271
    in otitis, 313
Diazoxide
    dosage in ferrets, 389t
    for insulinoma, 86
Diclofenac
    for anterior uveitis, 188
    for cataracts, 199
    for conjunctivitis, 217
    for epiphora, 246
    for red eye, 343
Diet
    in abscessation, 179
    in Aleutian disease virus infection, 116
    in anorexia, 185
    in ataxia, 197
    in clostridial enterotoxicosis, 208
    in coccidiosis, 210
    in congestive heart failure, 213
    in conjunctivitis, 216
    in constipation, 220–221
    in diabetes mellitus, 32
    in diarrhea, 36, 226, 229
    diarrhea caused by, 36
    in dyspnea and tachypnea, 232
    in encephalitis and meningoencephalitis, 242
    in encephalitozoonosis, 238
    in endometrial disorders, 336–337
    in eosinophilic gastroenteritis, 48
    in epizootic catarrhal enteritis, 51
    in exophthalmos and orbital diseases, 251
    in facial nerve paresis/paralysis, 255
    in gastric dilation, 260
    in gastritis, 55
    in gastrodoudenal ulcers, 59
    in gastrointestinal and esophageal foreign
        bodies, 62, 264
    in gastrointestinal hypomotility and gastroin-
        testinal stasis, 267
    in head tilt, 271
    in *Helicobacter mustelae* infection, 69
    in hepatomegaly, 72
    in hypercalciuria, 278–279
    in hyperestrogenism, 75
    in inflammatory bowel disease, 81
    in influenza, 83
    in insulinoma, 86
    in lameness, 286–287, 287
    in lead toxicity, 288
    in lower urinary tract infection, 291
    in lymphoplasmacytic enteritis and
        gastroenteritis, 92
    in malocclusion, 202, 281
    in melena, 295–296
    in nasal discharge, 105, 299
    in neck and back pain, 301–302
    in nephrolithiasis and ureterolithiasis, 304
    in obesity, 109–110, 306
    in osteoarthritis, 192
    in otitis, 312
    in paresis and paralysis, 315
    in pasteurellosis, 317
    in pneumonia in rabbits, 322
    in polyuria and polydipsia (PU/PD), 326–327
    in pregnancy toxemia, 131
    in proliferative bowel disease, 132
    in ptyalism, 331
    in pyometra, 143, 336–337
    in regurgitation, 148
    in renal failure, 151, 345
    in rhinitis and sinusitis, 348
    in septic arthritis, 194
    in tooth root abscessation, 361

    in toxoplasmosis, 364
    in trichobezoars, 368
    in ulcerative pododermatitis, 372
    in urinary tract obstruction, 375, 376
    in urolithiasis, 168
    in vertebral fracture or luxation, 382
    in vomiting, 173
    in weight loss, 175, 385
Diethylstilbesterol, for urinary incontinence, 285
Digitalis, for dilated cardiomyopathy, 18
Digoxin
    for congestive heart failure, 25, 213
    for dilated cardiomyopathy, 18
    dosage
        in ferrets, 389t
        in rabbits, 394t
**Dilated cardiomyopathy**, in ferrets, 17–18
Diltiazem
    for congestive heart failure, 25
    dosage in ferrets, 389t
    for hypertrophic cardiomyopathy, 19
Dioctyl sodium sulfosuccinate, 112
Diphenhydramine
    dosage
        in ferrets, 389t
        in rabbits, 394t
    for fleas, 53
    for influenza-associated nasal discharge, 83
    for nasal discharge, 105
    for pododermatitis and nail bed disorders, 128
    for pruritus, 139, 328
    for rhinitis, 299, 349
    for sarcoptic mange, 157
    for sinusitis, 349
    for vaccine reaction, 101
*Dirofilaria immitis,* 66
Distichiasis, 245
Diuretics
    for congestive heart failure, 25, 26, 213–214
    for diuresis induction in renal failure, 345
    for heartworm disease, 67
    for pleural effusion, 120
    for poisoning in rabbits, 325
DNA probe test, for Aleutian disease virus, 116
DOCP
    dosage in ferrets, 389t
    for hyperadrenocorticism, 4
Dopamine, in renal failure, 151
Doxapram
    dosage in ferrets, 389t
    dosage in rabbits, 394t
Doxorubicin, for lymphosarcoma, 95
Doxycycline, for toxoplasmosis, 364
Drooling. *See also* Ptyalism
    in tooth root abscessation, 360
Drug dosages
    for ferrets, 388t–391t
    for rabbits, 394t–396t
**Dyschezia and hematochezia**, in ferrets, 38–39
**Dysphagia**
    in ferrets, 40–41
    in megaesophagus, 98
    in ptyalism, 140
    in regurgitation, 148
**Dyspnea**
    in abscessation, 178
    in Aleutian disease virus, 115
    in anticoagulant rodenticide poisoning, 190
    in congestive heart failure, 24, 212
    in ferrets, 42–43
    in heartworm disease, 66
    in influenza, 83
    in myxomatosis, 297
    nasal discharge and, 298

**Dyspnea** *(continued)*
in pasteurellosis, 317
in pleural effusion, 119
in pneumonia
aspiration, 121
bacterial, 123
mycotic, 125
in rabbits, 321
in rabbits, 231–233
in regurgitation, 148
in thymoma/thymic lymphoma, 359
**Dystocia and fetal death,** in ferrets, 44
**Dysuria**
in ferrets, 45–46
in hypercalciuria, 277
in lower urinary tract disease, 88
in nephrolithiasis and ureterolithiasis, 303
in prostatitis, 134
in prostatomegaly, 136
in rabbits, 234–235
in urogenital cysts, 164
in urolithiasis, 167

E

Ear canal ablation, 271, 312
**Ear mites**
alopecia, 5, 182
in ferrets, 5, 47, 111
pruritus, 138, 139
in rabbits, 236–237
Ecchymosis, 117–118
Echocardiography
in ataxia, 12
in congestive heart failure, 25, 213
in dilated cardiomyopathy, 17
in heartworm disease, 66
in hypertrophic cardiomyopathy, 19
in paresis and paralysis, 114
in pericardial abscessation, 179
in pleural effusion, 119
Ectopic ureters, 284–285
Edema, stertor and stridor and, 356
EDTA, 288–289, 325, 394t
*Eimeria*
in ferrets, 23
in rabbits, 210
Electrocardiography
in congestive heart failure, 25, 213
in dilated cardiomyopathy, 17
in hypertrophic cardiomyopathy, 19
Electromyography (EMG)
in dysphagia, 40
in lameness, 286
in neck and back pain, 301
Electron microscopy, in epizootic catarrhal
enteritis, 51
Electrophoresis
in Aleutian disease virus, 115
counterimmunoelectrophoresis (CEP) in
Aleutian disease virus, 115
in multiple myeloma, 102
in paresis and paralysis, 114
in renal failure, 150
ELISA test
for Aleutian disease virus, 115
for *Pasteurella,* 179, 231, 241, 244, 251, 255,
271, 293, 308, 312, 318, 347, 350, 356–357
Enalapril
for congestive heart failure, 25, 213
for dilated cardiomyopathy, 18
dosage
in ferrets, 389t
in rabbits, 394t

for heartworm disease, 67
for hypertrophic cardiomyopathy, 20
for renal failure, 151
**Encephalitis and meningoencephalitis,** in rabbits,
241–243
**Encephalitis secondary to parasitic migration,** in
rabbits, 244
**Encephalitozoonosis**
anterior uveitis in, 187–189
in rabbits, 238–240
Endometrial disorders, in rabbits, 336–338
Endoscopy
in gastrodoudenal ulcers, 59
gastrointestinal foreign bodies and, 55, 62,
263, 264
in megaesophagus, 98
in melena, 295
in vomiting, 173
Endotracheal tube placement in rabbits, 324
Enilconazole
dosage in ferrets, 389t
dosage in rabbits, 394t
Enophthamos, 250–251
Enrofloxacin
for abscessation, 180
for anterior uveitis, 188
for bacterial folliculitis, 183, 329
for bacterial meningoencephalitis and abscess,
351
for coccidiosis-associated infection, 211
for constipation, 221
for cough, 27
for cystitis, 46
for dermatitis, 354
for diarrhea, 36, 227, 229
dosage
in ferrets, 389t
in rabbits, 394t
for dyschezia and hematochezia, 38
for dysuria and pollakiuria, 235
for endometrial disorders, 337
for epistaxis, 249
for epizootic catarrhal enteritis, 51
for exophthalmos and orbital diseases, 252
for facial and dental abscesses, 203, 282
for gastric dilation, 260
for gastrointestinal foreign bodies, 264
for gastrointestinal hypomotility and
gastrointestinal stasis, 268
for head tilt, 271
for influenza-associated bacterial infections, 83
for lameness, 287
for lower urinary tract infection, 88, 291
for mastitis, 294
for megaesophagus, 99
for melena, 100, 296
for meningoencephalitis, 242
for moist pyoderma, 331
for nasal discharge, 105, 299
for otitis, 111, 310, 313
for pasteurellosis, 319
for pneumonia
aspiration, 121
bacterial, 123
in rabbits, 322
for pododermatitis and nail bed disorders,
127
for prostatitis and prostatic abscesses, 134,
162
for pyoderma, 334
for pyometra, 143, 337
for regurgitation, 149
for rhinitis and sinusitis, 348
for salmonellosis, 155

for septic arthritis, 195
for stertor and stridor, 357
for tooth root abscesses, 362
for trichobezoars, 369
for ulcerative pododermatitis, 373
for urogenital cysts, 166
for vaginal discharge, 171, 380
for vomiting, 173
Enterotoxicosis, clostridial
in ferrets, 21–22
in rabbits, 207–209
Entropion, 245–246, 250
Enucleation, 188, 251–252
Enzymatic digestion of trichobezoars, 221, 265,
268, 369
Eosinophilia
in eosinophilic gastroenteritis, 48
in lymphadenomegaly, 90
in melena, 100
in splenomegaly, 159
in vomiting, 172
**Eosinophilic gastroenteritis,** 48–49, 55
Epaxial muscles, pain from, 301
Epilepsy, 350–351. *See also* Seizures
Epinephrine
dosage in rabbits, 395t
**Epiphora**
in malocclusion, 201, 202
in pasteurellosis, 317
pyoderma and, 333
in rabbits, 245–247
in rhinitis and sinusitis, 347
in stertor and stridor, 356
**Epistaxis**
in rabbits, 248–249
in rhinitis and sinusitis, 347
in stertor and stridor, 356
**Epizootic catarrhal enteritis,** in ferrets, 50–52
Epoetin alfa
dosage in ferrets, 389t
dosage in rabbits, 395t
Erythromycin
for campylobacteriosis, 13
dosage
in ferrets, 389t
in rabbits, 394t
Erythropoietin, for anemia in renal failure, 151,
345
Esophageal foreign body, 61–63
Esophagitis, 55, 99, 148
Esophagoscopy, 141, 149
Esophagram, 98
Estrogen-responsive urinary incontinence,
284–285
Estrogens
elevation in hyperadrenocorticism, 2, 136
elevation in prostatic disease, 134
hyperestrogenism, 5, 74–76
Estrus, prolonged, 74–75
Exenteration, 251, 252
**Exophthalmos**
in malocclusion, 201, 202, 280
ptyalism and, 330
in rabbits, 250–253
in thymoma/thymic lymphoma, 359
in tooth root abscessation, 360, 361
Exudate
in abscessation, 179
in ascites, 9
in otitis, 308, 309
in pleural effusion, 119–120
in ulcerative pododermatitis, 372
vaginal discharge, 379
Eyelid abnormalities, 246, 297

# F

**Facial nerve paresis/paralysis**
epiphora and, 246
in otitis, 311
in rabbits, 254–256
Facial pyoderma, 333
Famotidine
dosage in ferrets, 389t
for esophagitis, 99, 148
for gastric ulceration, 59, 131
for gastritis, 8, 36, 51, 56, 59, 62, 69, 173
for renal failure, 151
Fecal antigen detection, for cryptosporidiosis, 29
Fecal culture
in campylobacteriosis, 13
in clostridial enterotoxicosis, 21, 207
in diarrhea, 36, 226, 229
in dyschezia and hematochezia, 38
in epizootic catarrhal enteritis, 51
in inflammatory bowel disease, 81
in lymphoplasmacytic enteritis and
gastroenteritis, 92
in melena, 100, 295
in proliferative bowel disease, 132
in salmonellosis, 155
in vomiting, 172
Fecal cytology
in campylobacteriosis, 13
in clostridial enterotoxicosis, 21, 207
in diarrhea, 36, 226, 229
in dyschezia and hematochezia, 38
in epizootic catarrhal enteritis, 51
in inflammatory bowel disease, 81
in lymphoplasmacytic enteritis and gastroenteritis, 92
in melena, 100, 295
in proliferative bowel disease, 132
in vomiting, 172
in weight loss, 174
Fecal examination
for campylobacteriosis, 13
for coccidiosis, 23, 210
for cryptosporidiosis, 29
in diarrhea, 35, 226, 229
in gastroduodenal ulcers, 58
for giardiasis, 64
in inflammatory bowel disease, 81
in lymphoplasmacytic enteritis and gastroenteritis, 92
for pinworms, 320
in weight loss, 174
Fecal Gram's stain
diarrhea and, 226, 229
melena and, 295
Fecal occult blood testing
in diarrhea, 226, 229
in melena, 295
Fenbendazole
dosage
in ferrets, 389t
in rabbits, 395t
for encephalitozoonosis, 188, 199, 239, 242,
271, 351
for pinworms, 320, 329
Fetal death, 44
Fever
in diarrhea, 225
in dyspnea and tachypnea, 231
in influenza, 83
in mastitis, 293
in myxomatosis, 297
in pneumonia
aspiration, 121

bacterial, 123
mycotic, 125
in rabbits, 321
in pyometra, 142
in regurgitation, 148
in renal failure, 150, 344
Fibroma/fibrosarcoma, 107, 108
Fine needle aspirate
in exophthalmos and orbital diseases, 251
in hepatomegaly, 71
in lymphosarcoma, 95
in malocclusion, 202, 281
in mastitis, 293
in pneumonia
mycotic, 125
in rabbits, 322
in pododermatitis and nail bed disorders, 127
in pruritus, 328
in ptyalism, 331
in renal failure, 150, 345
in renomegaly, 153
in splenomegaly, 159
in thymoma/thymic lymphoma, 359
in tooth root abscessation, 361
in vaginal discharge, 379
Fipronil
dosage in rabbits, 395t
for fleas, 5, 53, 139, 257
**Fleas and flea infestation**
alopecia, 5–6, 182, 183
in ferrets, 5–6, 53–54
pruritus, 53, 138, 139, 257
in rabbits, 257–258
Florinef (fludrocortisone acetate)
after adrenalectomy, 165–166
for hyperadrenocorticism, 4
Fluconazole, for mycotic pneumonia, 125–126
Fludrocortisone
dosage in ferrets, 389t
Fluid therapy
in anorexia, 185
in clostridial enterotoxicosis, 208
in coccidiosis, 210
in constipation, 220
in diarrhea, 36, 226
in dystocia, 44
in epizootic catarrhal enteritis, 51
in gastric dilation, 259
in gastritis, 55
in gastrodoudenal ulcers, 59
in gastrointestinal and esophageal foreign
bodies, 62, 263
in gastrointestinal hypomotility and gastrointestinal stasis, 267
in heat stroke and heat stress, 273–274
in *Helicobacter mustelae* infection, 69
in hepatomegaly, 72
in influenza, 83
in insulinoma, 86
in lymphosarcoma, 95
in poisoning in rabbits, 325
in polyuria and polydipsia (PU/PD), 130
in pregnancy toxemia, 131
in prostatomegaly, 136–137
in pyometra, 143, 171
in regurgitation, 148
in renal failure, 150–151, 345
for trichobezoars, 368
in urinary tract obstruction, 161
in urogenital cysts, 165
in urolithiasis, 168
Flunixin meglumine
dosage
in ferrets, 389t

in rabbits, 395t
for gastrointestinal foreign bodies, 264
for pyometra, 143
Fluorescein stain, 188, 202, 216, 246, 342
Fluoroscopy
in dysphagia, 40
in megaesophagus, 98
in regurgitation, 148
Flurbiprofen
for anterior uveitis, 188
for cataracts, 199
for conjunctivitis, 217
for epiphora, 246
for red eye, 343
Flutamide
dosage in ferrets, 389t
for hyperadrenocorticism, 3
for prostatic disease, 134–135, 137, 163,
166
Food allergy, in eosinophilic gastroenteritis,
48
Footpad hyperkeratosis, 15
Foreign body
dysphagia from, 40
esophageal, 61–63
gastric, 55, 58, 61–63
nasal discharge and, 104
stertor and stridor and, 356
Fungal culture, in dermatophytosis, 30, 223
Fungal infections
dermatophytosis, 5, 6, 30–31, 223–224
nasal discharge in, 104, 105
pneumonia, mycotic, 125–126
in pododermatitis and nail bed disorders, 127
Fur mites. *See* Cheyletiellosis
Furosemide
for ascites, 10
for congestive heart failure, 25, 213–214
for dilated cardiomyopathy, 18
for diuresis induction in renal failure, 345
dosage
in ferrets, 389t
in rabbits, 395t
for heartworm disease, 67
for hypertrophic cardiomyopathy, 20
for poisoning in rabbits, 325
for renal failure, 151

# G

Gagging, 98, 104–105
Gastric decompression, 22, 259, 263–264,
368–369
**Gastric dilation**, in rabbits, 259–261
Gastric foreign body, 55, 58
Gastric lavage, for poisoning in rabbits, 325
**Gastritis**, in ferrets, 55–57
**Gastroduodenal ulcers**
in ferrets, 58–60
melena and, 295
Gastrointestinal antisecretory agents, for gastritis,
56
in anorexia, 8
in diarrhea, 36
in epizootic catarrhal enteritis, 51
in gastrodoudenal ulceration, 59
in gastrointestinal foreign body, 62
in *Helicobacter mustelae* infection, 69
in melena, 101
in vomiting, 173
**Gastrointestinal foreign bodies**
in ferrets, 61–63
in rabbits, 262–265
trichobezoars, 367–370

**Gastrointestinal hypomotility**
constipation and, 219–221
gastrointestinal foreign bodies and, 262–265
in lead toxicity, 288, 289
in poisonings, 325
in rabbits, 266–269
in renal failure, 344
in tooth root abscessation, 361
trichobezoars and, 367, 368, 369
**Gastrointestinal stasis**, in rabbits, 266–269
Gastrointestinal tumors, 106
Gastroscopy, 141, 172–173
Gastrotomy, for gastric foreign body removal, 56
Gentamicin
in AIPMMA (antibiotic-impregnated poly-methyl methacrylate) beads, 195, 252, 309, 313, 319, 362, 372
for anterior uveitis, 188
for conjunctivitis, 217
dosage in rabbits, 395t
for epiphora, 246
for red eye, 343
**Giardiasis**, in ferrets, 64
**Gingivitis**
in ferrets, 65
ptyalism, 330
Glaucoma, 245, 341
Glucagon, plasma concentration, 32
Glucagonoma, 32
Glucocorticoids
after adrenalectomy, 165–166
for gastritis, 56
for insulinoma, 86
for neck and back pain, 302
Glucose
curve, 33
serum concentration in insulinoma, 85, 86
Glucosuria
in diabetes mellitus, 32, 33
in polyuria and polydipsia (PU/PD), 129
Glycopyrrolate
dosage
in ferrets, 389t
in rabbits, 395t
in poisoning, 325
Glycosaminoglycans
dosage in rabbits, 395t
for lameness, 287
for neck and back pain, 302
for spondylosis deformans, 355
GnRH
dosage in ferrets, 389t
for hyperestrogenism, 75
Green slime disease. *See* Epizootic catarrhal enteritis
Griseofulvin
for dermatophytosis, 31, 183, 223–224, 329
dosage
in ferrets, 389t
in rabbits, 395t

H

Hair balls. *See* Trichobezoars
Halitosis
in megaesophagus, 98
in periodontal disease, 65
in ptyalism, 140, 330
in renal failure, 150
in tooth root abscessation, 360
Hard pad disease. *See* Canine distemper virus
HCG
dosage in ferrets, 389t
for hyperestrogenism, 75, 171
for pyometra, 143

Head shaking, in otitis, 111, 308
**Head tilt**
in ataxia, 11, 196
in encephalitis and meningoencephalitis, 241–243
in encephalitozoonosis, 238
nasal discharge and, 298
in otitis, 308, 311
in pasteurellosis, 317
in rabbits, 270–272
in rhinitis and sinusitis, 347
seizures and, 350
Heart disease
congestive heart failure
in ferrets, 24–26
in rabbits, 212–214
dilated cardiomyopathy in ferrets, 17–18
dyspnea and tachypnea in, 42
heartworm disease, 66–67
hypertriophic cardiomyopathy in ferrets, 19–20
**Heartworm disease**, in ferrets, 66–67
**Heat stroke and heat stress**, in rabbits, 273–274
*Helicobacter mustelae*
diarrhea, 35–37
in ferrets, 68–70
gastritis, 55–56
gastroduodenal ulcers, 58–59
ptyalism and, 141
Hemangioma/hemangiosarcoma, 71, 107, 127
Hematemesis, with gastrointestinal and esophageal foreign bodies, 61
**Hematochezia**
in anticoagulant rodenticide poisoning, 190
epistaxis and, 248
in ferrets, 38–39
in heat stroke and heat stress, 273
Hematologic values
in ferrets, 392t
in rabbits, 397t
Hematoma, with anticoagulant rodenticide poisoning, 190
**Hematuria**
in anticoagulant rodenticide poisoning, 190
in dysuria and pollakiuria, 45, 234
epistaxis and, 248
in hypercalciuria, 277
in hyperestrogenism, 74
in lower urinary tract disease, 88, 290
in nephrolithiasis and ureterolithiasis, 303
in polyuria and polydipsia (PU/PD), 326
in pyometra and endometrial disorders, 336
in rabbits, 275–276
in urinary tract obstruction, 161, 374
in urolithiasis, 167
in uterine adenocarcinoma, 377
vaginal discharge and, 379
Hemorrhage
in anticoagulant rodenticide poisoning, 190
in ascites, 9
epistaxis, 248–249
in pleural effusion, 119–120
Hemostasis disorders, patechia/eccymosis/bruising in, 117–118
Hemothorax, in pleural effusion, 119
Hepatic lipidosis
hepatomegaly from, 71
in pregnancy toxemia, 131
Hepatitis
hepatomegaly in, 71
hypoglycemia in, 79
Hepatobiliary tumors, 106
**Hepatomegaly**
in coccidiosis, 210
in congestive heart failure, 24, 212–213

in diabetes mellitus, 32
in dilated cardiomyopathy, 17
in eosinophilic gastroenteritis, 48
in ferrets, 71–72
in heartworm disease, 66
Hetastarch
for ascites, 10
for diarrheal hypoproteinemia, 36, 51
dosage in rabbits, 395t
Histiocytoma, 107
Histopathology
in Aleutian disease virus, 116
in anterior uveitis, 188
in canine distemper virus infection, 15
in clostridial enterotoxicosis, 207
in diabetes mellitus, 32
in encephalitozoonosis, 238
in eosinophilic gastroenteritis, 48
in epistaxis, 248
in epizootic catarrhal enteritis, 51
in gastritis, 55
in gastrodoudenal ulcers, 59
in *Helicobacter mustelae* infection, 69
in hyperestrogenism, 74
in influenza, 83
in insulinoma, 85
in lymphoplasmacytic enteritis and gastroenteritis, 92
in mast cell tumor, 97
in multiple myeloma, 102
in myxomatosis, 297
in neoplasia
digestive system, 106
integumentary, 107
musculoskeletal and nervous system, 108
in papilloma virus infection, 353
in proliferative bowel disease, 132
in pyometra and endometrial disorders, 336
in rabies, 145, 339
in renal failure, 150, 345
in treponematosis, 366
in urogenital cysts, 164
in uterine adenocarcinoma, 377
in vaginal discharge, 379
Histoplasmosis, 125
Honey. *See* Dextrose
Human chorionic gonadotropin (hCG) challenge test, 2, 74, 170
Hydralazine
for congestive heart failure, 25, 214
for dilated cardiomyopathy, 18
Hydrocortisone sodium succinate
dosage in ferrets, 389t
**Hydronephrosis**, in ferrets, 73, 153
17-hydroxyprogesterone
elevation in hyperadrenocorticism, 2, 136
elevation in prostatic disease, 134
Hydroxyzine
dosage
in ferrets, 389t
in rabbits, 395t
for fleas, 53
for pododermatitis and nail bed disorders, 128
for pruritus, 139, 328
for rhinitis, 299, 349
for sarcoptic mange, 157
for sinusitis, 349
Hyperadrenocorticism, in ferrets, 2–4
Hypercalcemia
in hematuria, 275
in nephrolithiasis and ureterolithiasis, 304
in polyuria and polydipsia (PU/PD), 129, 326
in urinary tract obstruction, 374

**Hypercalciuria**
in dysuria and pollakiuria, 234–235
in hematuria, 275–276
in lower urinary tract infection, 290
in nephrolithiasis and ureterolithiasis, 303–304
in rabbits, 277–279
in spondylosis deformans, 354
in urinary incontinence, 284–285
in urinary tract obstruction, 374
Hyperesthesia, in paresis and paralysis, 113
**Hyperestrogenism**
alopecia, 5
in ferrets, 5, 74–76
patechia/eccymosis/bruising in, 117
pyometra in, 142–143
with vaginal discharge, 170
Hyperglobulinemia
in Aleutian disease virus, 115
in lymphadenomegaly, 90
in pyometra, 142
in splenomegaly, 159
Hyperglycemia
in diabetes mellitus, 32, 33
in polyuria and polydipsia (PU/PD), 129
stress, 32
Hyperkalemia
in polyuria and polydipsia (PU/PD), 129
in renal failure, 344
Hyperkeratosis
in dermatophytosis, 30
footpad in canine distemper virus infection, 15
Hypermetria, 196
Hyperphosphatemia, in renal failure, 344
Hyperproteinemia, in pyometra, 142
Hypersalivation. *See* Ptyalism
Hypersensitivity/contact irritant
in pododermatitis and nail bed disorders, 127, 128
**Hypersplenism,** 77–78, 159
Hyperthermia, 273
**Hypertrophic cardiomyopathy, in ferrets,** 19–20
Hypoadrenocorticism, iatrogenic, 79
Hypoalbuminemia
in hepatomegaly, 71
in inflammatory bowel disease, 81
in melena, 100
in pleural effusion, 119
in polyuria and polydipsia (PU/PD), 129, 326
in salmonellosis, 155
in vomiting, 172
Hypocalcemia, seizures and, 350
**Hypoglycemia**
ataxia from, 11
in dysuria and pollakiuria, 45
in ferrets, 2, 79–80
in hyperadrenocorticism, 2
in paresis, 113–114
in pregnancy toxemia, 131
seizures and, 350
Hypokalemia
in epizootic catarrhal enteritis, 51
in renal failure, 151
Hyponatremia, in polyuria and polydipsia (PU/PD), 326
Hypoproteinemia
in ascites, 9–10
in diarrhea, 36
in epizootic catarrhal enteritis, 50, 511
in gastroduodenal ulcers, 58
in hepatomegaly, 71
in inflammatory bowel disease, 81
in lymphoplasmacytic enteritis and gastroenteritis, 92
in proliferative bowel disease, 132

Hypopyon, in encephalitozoonosis, 238
Hypothermia
in clostridial enterotoxicosis, 207
in diarrhea, 225
in renal failure, 344

I

Icterus, 71
Ileus, in renal failure, 344
Imaging. *See* CT; MRI; Radiography; Ultrasonography
Imidacloprid
dosage
in ferrets, 389t
in rabbits, 395t
for fleas, 5–6, 53, 139, 183, 257, 328
Immunofluorescent antibody (IFA) test
in Aleutian disease virus, 115
canine distemper virus, 15, 127
Immunohistochemical staining, in diabetes mellitus, 32
Inappetence. *See* Anorexia
**Incisor malocclusion and overgrowth,** in rabbits, 280–283
**Incontinence,** urinary in rabbits, 284–285
**Inflammatory bowel disease,** in ferrets, 81–82
**Influenza virus,** in ferrets, 83–84
Insulin
for diabetes mellitus, 32
dosage in ferrets, 389t
plasma concentration, 32
serum concentration in insulinoma, 85
Insulin deficiency, in diabetes mellitus, 32
**Insulinoma,** 32, 79, 85–87
Intention tremors, 11, 196
Intestinal protectants, for melena, 101
Intoxication. *See* Poisoning
Intubation of rabbits, 324, 357
Iridocyclitis. *See* Anterior uveitis
Iron dextran
dosage
in ferrets, 389t
in rabbits, 395t
in hyperestrogenism, 75
Isoflurane
for anesthesia
in ferrets, 17, 25, 66, 120, 131
in rabbits, 203, 217, 247, 252, 282
dosage
in ferrets, 389t
in rabbits, 395t
*Isospora,* 23
Isotretinoin, for cutaneous lymphosarcoma, 95
Itraconazole
for dermatophytosis, 183, 223, 329
dosage in rabbits, 395t
for pneumonia, mycotic, 125
Ivermectin
for cheyletiellosis, 182, 205, 328
dosage
in ferrets, 389t
in rabbits, 395t
for ear mites, 5, 47, 111, 139, 182, 236, 310, 328
for eosinophilic gastroenteritis, 49
for heartworm disease, 66, 67
for otitis, 111
for sarcoptic mange, 6, 127, 139, 157, 183, 329

J

Joint swelling
in anticoagulant rodenticide poisoning, 190

in osteoarthritis, 192
in septic arthritis, 194

K

Kaolin-pectin products
dosage in ferrets, 389t
Keratitis
epiphora in, 245
in exophthalmos and orbital diseases, 252
red eye, 341
Keratoconjunctivitis sicca (KCS), 215, 216, 217
Ketamine
dosage in rabbits, 395t
for sedation in ferrets, 17, 25, 66, 120
for sedation in rabbits, 180, 203, 247, 252, 282, 310, 319, 322, 331, 334, 337, 343, 362, 380
Ketamine and acepromazine
dosage in ferrets, 390t
dosage in rabbits, 395t
Ketamine and diazepam
dosage in ferrets, 390t
dosage in rabbits, 395t
Ketamine and medetomidine
dosage in ferrets, 390t
Ketamine and medetomidine and midazolam
dosage in ferrets, 390t
Ketamine and midazolam
dosage in rabbits, 395t
Ketoconazole
for dermatophytosis, 31, 183, 224
dosage
in ferrets, 390t
in rabbits, 395t
for nasal discharge, 105
Ketonuria, in diabetes mellitus, 32
Ketoprofen
dosage in rabbits, 395t
Kidney disease
hydronephrosis, 73
renal failure, 150–152
renomegaly, 73, 150, 153–154

L

Lactoperoxidase, for gingivitis and periodontal disease, 65
Lactulose syrup
dosage in ferrets, 390t
Lagophthalmos, 252
**Lameness**
in abscessation, 178
in osteoarthritis, 192
in pasteurellosis, 317
in pododermatitis and nail bed disorders, 127
in rabbits, 286–287
in septic arthritis, 194
in ulcerative pododermatitis, 371
Laparotomy
in clostridial enterotoxicosis, 21
in diarrhea, 36
in epizootic catarrhal enteritis, 50
in gastritis, 55
in gastrodoudenal ulcers, 58
in *Helicobacter mustelae* infection, 68
in lymphoplasmacytic enteritis and gastroenteritis, 92
in melena, 100, 295
in neoplasia, digestive system, 106
in neoplasia, musculoskeletal and nervous system, 108
in proliferative bowel disease, 132

Laparotomy *(continued)*
　　in rectal and anal prolapse, 147
　　in vomiting, 173
　　in weight loss, 174
Laryngopharyngoscopy, 232
Laryngoscopy, in stertor and stridor, 357
Lateral ear canal resection, 309
Latex agglutination test, in mycotic pneumonia, 125
Lavage
　　in aspiration pneumonia, 121
　　in bacterial pneumonia, 123
**Lead toxicity**, 58, 288–289, 325
Lens removal, 188
*Leporacarus gibbus,* 205
Lethargy
　　in Aleutian disease virus, 115
　　in anticoagulant rodenticide poisoning, 190
　　in coccidiosis, 210
　　in congestive heart failure, 212
　　in diarrhea, 225, 228
　　in dyspnea and tachypnea, 231
　　in dysuria and pollakiuria, 234
　　in encephalitozoonosis, 238
　　in endometrial disorders, 336
　　in gastritis, 55
　　in gastrointestinal and esophageal foreign
　　　bodies, 61
　　in heartworm disease, 66
　　in hypercalciuria, 277
　　in hyperestrogenism, 74
　　in hypoglycemia, 79
　　in influenza, 83
　　in lead toxicity, 288
　　in lymphosarcoma, 94
　　in mastitis, 293
　　in myxomatosis, 297
　　in nephrolithiasis and ureterolithiasis, 303
　　in obesity, 109, 306
　　in pleural effusion, 119
　　in pneumonia
　　　aspiration, 121
　　　bacterial, 123
　　　in rabbits, 321
　　in pregnancy toxemia, 131
　　in pyometra, 142, 336
　　in rabies, 145
　　in renal failure, 150, 344
　　in salmonellosis, 155
　　in septic arthritis, 194
　　in urinary tract obstruction, 161, 374
　　in urogenital cysts, 164
　　in urolithiasis, 167
　　vaginal discharge and, 379
Leukocytosis
　　in ascites, 9
　　in dyspnea and tachypnea, 42
　　in epizootic catarrhal enteritis, 50
　　in gastritis, 55
　　in gastroduodenal ulcers, 58
　　in *Helicobacter mustelae* infection, 68
　　in hepatomegaly, 71
　　in hyperadrenocorticism, 2
　　in megaesophagus, 98
　　in pneumonia, bacterial, 123
　　in proliferative bowel disease, 132
　　in prostatitis, 134
　　in prostatomegaly, 136
　　in ptyalism, 140
　　in pyoderma, 5
　　in renomegaly, 153
　　in splenomegaly, 159
　　in urinary tract obstruction, 161
　　with vaginal discharge, 170

Leukopenia, in splenomegaly, 159
Leuprolide acetate
　　for adrenal disease, 3, 6, 139
　　dosage in ferrets, 390t
　　for prostatic hyperplasia, 134, 137, 162, 165
Lidocaine
　　dosage in rabbits, 395t
　　for urinary catheterization, 168
　　for ventricular arrhythmia, 274
Lime sulfur dip
　　for cheyletiellosis, 205
　　for dermatophytosis, 6, 30, 127, 139, 183, 223, 329
　　dosage
　　　in ferrets, 390t
　　　in rabbits, 395t
　　for sarcoptic mange, 157
Liver disease. *See also* Hepatomegaly
　　hepatic lipidosis, 71, 131
　　hepatitis, 71, 79
　　hepatobiliary tumors, 106
　　in polyuria and polydipsia (PU/PD), 326
　　seizures and, 350
Liver enzymes
　　in abscessation, 179
　　in Aleutian disease virus, 115
　　in ascites, 9
　　in coccidiosis, 23
　　in cough, 27–28
　　in diarrhea, 226
　　in epizootic catarrhal enteritis, 50
　　in gastroduodenal ulcers, 58
　　gastrointestinal foreign bodies and, 263
　　in gastrointestinal hypomotility and gastroin-
　　　testinal stasis, 267
　　in hepatomegaly, 71
　　in lymphosarcoma, 94
　　in megaesophagus, 98
　　in neoplasia, digestive system, 106
　　in tooth root abscessation, 361
　　trichobezoars and, 368
　　in uterine adenocarcinoma, 377
Loperamide, for diarrhea, 36, 51
Lower motor neurons, 113
**Lower urinary tract infection**
　　in ferrets, 88–89
　　in rabbits, 290–292
Lubricants, intestinal, 221, 265, 268, 370
Lufenuron
　　dosage in rabbits, 395t
　　for fleas, 53, 257
Lupron
　　for hyperadrenocorticism, 3, 6, 139
　　for prostatic hyperplasia, 134, 137, 162, 165
Lymphadenitis, 90
**Lymphadenopathy (lymphadenomegaly)**
　　in ferrets, 90–91
　　in salmonellosis, 155
　　in sarcoptic mange, 157
Lymphocytosis
　　in lymphadenomegaly, 90
　　in lymphosarcoma, 94
　　in splenomegaly, 159
Lymphoid hyperplasia, 90
Lymphoma
　　cutaneous, 107
　　foot, 127
　　hepatomegaly in, 71
　　lymphadenomegaly in, 90–91
　　thymic, 359
Lymphopenia
　　in canine distemper virus infection, 15
　　in mastitis, 293

　　in tooth root abscessation, 361
**Lymphoplasmacytic enteritis and gastroenteritis,**
　　in ferrets, 92–93
**Lymphosarcoma,** in ferrets, 94–96

M

Magnetic resonance imaging. *See* MRI (magnetic
　　resonance imaging)
*Malassezia* sp., 111
Maldigestive/malabsorptive disorders, 384
Malocclusion in rabbits
　　cheek teeth, 201–204
　　incisor, 280–281
Mannitol
　　for cerebral edema, 274
　　for diuresis induction in renal failure, 345
**Mast cell tumor**
　　alopecia from, 5
　　in ferrets, 97, 107
　　foot, 127
　　pruritus from, 138
Mastectomy, 294
**Mastitis**
　　cystic and septic in rabbits, 293–294
　　uterine adenocarcinoma and, 377, 378
Meclizine
　　dosage in rabbits, 395t
　　for head tilt, 271
　　for otitis, 313
　　for vestibular signs in encephalitozoonosis, 239
Medetomidine
　　dosage in ferrets, 390t
Mediastinal mass, dyspnea and tachypnea and, 42
**Megaesophagus**, 40, 98–99, 148
Melarsomine dihydrochloride (Immiticid)
　　dosage in ferrets, 390t
　　for heartworm disease, 67
Melatonin
　　dosage in ferrets, 390t
　　for hyperadrenocorticism, 3
**Melena**
　　in Aleutian disease virus, 115
　　in canine distemper virus, 15
　　in epistaxis, 248
　　in ferrets, 100–101
　　in gastritis, 55
　　in gastroduodenal ulcers, 58
　　in gastrointestinal and esophageal foreign
　　　bodies, 61
　　in heartworm disease, 66
　　in heat stroke and heat stress, 273
　　in *Helicobacter mustelae* infection, 68
　　in hyperestrogenism, 74
　　in inflammatory bowel disease, 81
　　in lymphoplasmacytic enteritis and
　　　gastroenteritis, 92
　　in lymphosarcoma, 94
　　in pregnancy toxemia, 131
　　in ptyalism, 140
　　in rabbits, 295–296
Meloxicam
　　dosage
　　　in ferrets, 390t
　　　in rabbits, 395t
　　for pain
　　　in abscessation, 180, 203, 282
　　　in anorexia, 185
　　　in anterior uveitis, 185
　　　in clostridial enterotoxicosis, 208
　　　in conjunctivitis, 217
　　　in dental disease, 331, 343
　　　in diarrhea, 227, 229

in dysuria and pollakiuria, 235
in epiphora, 247
in exophthalmos and orbital diseases, 252
in gastric dilation, 260
with gastrointestinal foreign bodies, 264
in gastrointestinal hypomotility, 268
in hematuria, 276
in hypercalciuria management, 279
in lameness, 287
in mastitis, 294
in neck and back, 302
in nephrolithiasis and ureterolithiasis, 305
in osteoarthritis, 192
in otitis, 310, 313
in paresis and paralysis, 315
in pasteurellosis, 319
postoperative, 377
in pyoderma, 334
in pyometra and endometrial disorders, 337
in septic arthritis, 195
in spondylosis deformans, 354
in tooth root abscesses, 362
in trichobezoars, 369
in ulcerative pododermatitis, 373
in urinary tract obstruction, 376
with vaginal discharge, 380
in vertebral fracture or luxation, 382
Melphalan, for multiple myeloma, 102
Meningoencephalitis in rabbits, 241–243
Metastatic calcification, 345
Methylprednisolone sodium succinate
for paresis and paralysis, 114, 315
for vertebral fracture or luxation, 382
Metoclopramide
for anorexia, 8, 185
for constipation, 221
dosage
in ferrets, 390t
in rabbits, 395t
for gastritis, 56
for gastrointestinal hypomotility, 264, 268,
325, 369
for megaesophagus, 99
for regurgitation, 149
for uremic crisis, 151
for vomiting, 173
Metoprolol
for congestive heart failure, 26, 214
for dilated cardiomyopathy, 18
Metritis, 171
Metronidazole
for abscessation, 180, 331
in AIPMMA (antibiotic-impregnated
polymethyl methacrylate) beads, 180
for anterior uveitis, 188
for bacterial meningoencephalitis and abscess,
351
for campylobacteriosis, 13
for clostridial enterotoxicosis, 22, 208
for coccidiosis-associated infection, 211
for constipation, 221
for diarrhea, 36, 227, 229
dosage
in ferrets, 390t
in rabbits, 395t
for enteric dysbiosis, 325
for eosinophilic gastroenteritis, 49
for epistaxis, 249
for exophthalmos and orbital diseases, 252
for facial and dental abscesses, 203, 282
for gastritis, 56
for gastrodoudenal ulcers, 59
for gastrointestinal and esophageal foreign
bodies, 62, 264

for gastrointestinal hypomotility and gastrointestinal stasis, 268
for giardiasis, 36, 64, 100
for head tilt, 271
for *Helicobacter mustelae,* 36, 56, 59, 62, 69,
92, 100–101, 173
for inflammatory bowel disease, 81
for lameness, 287
for lymphoplasmacytic enteritis and
gastroenteritis, 92, 93
for melena, 296
for nasal discharge, 299
for otitis, 310, 313
for pneumonia in rabbits, 322
for proliferative bowel disease, 132
for rhinitis and sinusitis, 348
for septic arthritis, 195
for stertor and stridor, 357
for tooth root abscesses, 362
for trichobezoars, 369
for ulcerative pododermatitis, 373
Miconazole
for dermatophytosis, 6, 139
dosage in rabbits, 395t
for otitis, 310, 313
Microalbuminuria, in renal failure, 150
*Microsporum canis,* 30, 223
*Microsporum gypseum,* 223
Midazolam
dosage
in ferrets, 390t
in rabbits, 395t
for sedation
in ferrets, 17, 25, 66, 120
in rabbits, 180, 203, 217, 246–247, 252,
260, 264, 282, 310, 319, 322, 331, 334,
337, 343, 362, 369, 373, 380, 382
for seizures
in encephalitozoonosis, 239
in head tilt, 271
in otitis, 313
for vestibular signs
in encephalitis and meningoencephalitis,
242
in encephalitozoonosis, 239
in head tilt, 271
in otitis, 313
Milbemycin, for sarcoptic mange, 157
Mink parvovirus. *See* Aleutian Disease Virus (ADV)
Mitodane, for hyperadrenocorticism, 4
Modified Knott's test, 66
Modified transudate
in ascites, 9
in congestive heart failure, 25
in dilated cardiomyopathy, 17
in pleural effusion, 119
Molar extraction, 203
Morphine
dosage
in ferrets, 390t
in rabbits, 395t
for pain
in abscessation, 180, 203
in exophthalmos and orbital diseases, 252
in gastric dilation, 260
in lameness, 287
in pyometra and endometrial disorders,
337
in tooth root abscesses, 362
in ulcerative pododermatitis, 373
in vertebral fracture or luxation, 382
MRI (magnetic resonance imaging)
in abscessation, 179
in ataxia, 11–12, 197

in dysphagia, 40
in dyspnea and tachypnea, 232
in encephalitis and meningoencephalitis, 241,
244
in epistaxis, 248
in head tilt, 271
in lameness, 286
in nasal discharge, 299
in neck and back pain, 301
in otitis, 308
in paresis and paralysis, 114, 315
in pasteurellosis, 318
in rhinitis and sinusitis, 348
in seizures, 350
in spondylosis deformans, 354
in stertor and stridor, 357
in toxoplasmosis, 364
in vertebral fracture or luxation, 382
Mucoid enteritis. *See* Clostridial enterotoxicosis
**Multiple myeloma**, in ferrets, 102–103
Muscle fasiculations, insulinoma and, 85
Musculoskeletal neoplasia, 108
Myasis, 244
Mydriatic drugs, 188
Myelography
in ataxia, 12
in neck and back pain, 301
in neoplasia, musculoskeletal and nervous
system, 108
in paresis and paralysis, 114, 314
in spondylosis deformans, 354
in vertebral fracture or luxation, 381
Myxoma/myxosarcoma, 107
**Myxomatosis,** 297

N

**Nail bed disorders,** 127–128
Naloxone
dosage in ferrets, 390t
dosage in rabbits, 395t
**Nasal discharge**
in ataxia, 196
in canine distemper virus infection, 15–16
in dyspnea and tachypnea, 231
in epiphora, 245
in epistaxis, 248
in exophthalmos and orbital diseases, 250
in ferrets, 104–105
in head tilt, 270
in influenza, 83
in malocclusion, 201–202, 280
in megaesophagus, 98
in pasteurellosis, 317
in pneumonia
aspiration, 121
bacterial, 123
mycotic, 125
in rabbits, 321
ptyalism and, 330
in rabbits, 298–300
in rhinitis and sinusitis, 347–349
in stertor and stridor, 356
in tooth root abscessation, 360, 361
Nasolacrimal duct flush, 188, 216, 246, 318, 342,
348
Nausea
in hypoglycemia, 79
in insulinoma, 85
in vomiting, 172
Nebulization therapy
for pneumonia, aspiration, 121
for pneumonia, bacterial, 123
for rhinitis and sinusitis, 349

**Neck and back pain,** in rabbits, 301–302
Neomycin
    for campylobacteriosis, 13
    dosage in ferrets, 390t
    for ocular ulceration, 252
**Neoplasia**
    adrenal, 2–4
    alopecia in, 5, 6, 182, 183
    anorexia in, 184, 185
    ascites in, 9
    ataxia in, 11–12, 196–197
    diarrhea in, 228
    of digestive system, in ferrets, 106
    dyschezia and hematochezia in, 38
    dysuria and pollakiuria in, 45, 234
    ear canal, 111
    epiphora in, 245
    in exophthalmos and orbital diseases,
        250–252
    in ferrets
        digestive system, 106
        integumentary, 107
        musculoskeletal and nervous system, 108
    gastric, 58
    head tilt in, 270
    hematuria in, 275–276
    hepatomegaly in, 71
    hypoglycemia in, 79
    insulinoma, 85–87
    integumentary, in ferrets, 107
    lymphadenopathy in, 90
    lymphosarcoma, 94–96
    mammary, 294
    mast cell tumor, 97
    multiple myeloma, 102–103
    musculoskeletal and nervous system, in ferrets,
        108
    nasal discharge in, 104, 298, 299
    in paresis and paralysis, 113
    pleural effusion in, 119
    in pododermatitis and nail bed disorders, 127
    pruritus from, 138
    ptyalism in, 330
    in renomegaly, 153
    rhinitis and sinusitis in, 347, 348
    in splenomegaly, 159
    thymoma/thymic lymphoma, 359
    urinary tract obstruction in, 161, 374
    uterine adenocarcinoma in rabbits, 377–378
    vaginal, 379–380
    vomiting in, 172
    weight loss in, 174
Nephrectomy, 73
**Nephrolithiasis and ureterolithiasis,** 167, 168,
    303–305
Nervous system tumors, 108
Neurological diseases
    ataxia from, 11, 196
    canine distemper virus, 15–16
    dysuria and pollakiuria in, 45
    encephalitis and meningoencephalitis, in
        rabbits, 241–243
    encephalitis secondary to parasitic migration,
        in rabbits, 244
    encephalitozoonosis, 238–240
    facial nerve paresis/paralysis, 254–256
    head tilt in rabbits, 270–272
    neck and back pain in, 301
    paresis and paralysis, 113–114, 314–316
    pasteurellosis, 317
    ptyalism in, 140, 330
    rabies, 145–146, 339–340
    toxoplasmosis, 364–365
    in urinary incontinence, 284–285

Neuromuscular disorders
    constipation in, 220
    in dysphagia, 40
    dyspnea and tachypnea in, 42
    in megaesophagus, 98
Neutrophilia
    in endometrial disorders, 336
    in lymphadenomegaly, 90
    in polyuria and polydipsia (PU/PD), 129, 326
    in pyometra, 142, 336
    in vaginal discharge, 379
Nitroglycerin
    for congestive heart failure, 25, 213
    for dilated cardiomyopathy, 18
    dosage in ferrets, 390t
    for hypertrophic cardiomyopathy, 20
*Notoedres cati,* 182
NPH insulin, 33
NSAIDs
    for anterior uveitis, 188
    for cataracts, 199
    for conjunctivitis, 217
    for osteoarthritis, 192
    for pain
        in abscessation, 180, 203, 282
        in dental disease, 331
        in dysuria and pollakiuria, 235
        in epiphora, 246, 247
        in exophthalmos and orbital diseases, 252
        in hematuria, 275–276
        in lameness, 287
        in mastitis, 294
        in neck and back, 302
        in paresis and paralysis, 315
        in pyometra and endometrial disorders, 337
        in spondylosis deformans, 354
        in tooth root abscesses, 362
        in ulcerative pododermatitis, 373
        in vertebral fracture or luxation, 382
    for red eye, 343
    ulcers from, 58, 59, 325
Nystagmus
    in ataxia, 11, 196
    in encephalitis and meningoencephalitis, 241
    in encephalitozoonosis, 238
    in otitis, 308, 311
    in pasteurellosis, 317

## O

**Obesity**
    in cheyletiellosis, 205
    in constipation, 219
    in ferrets, 109–110
    in gastrointestinal hypomotility and gastroin-
        testinal stasis, 266
    in heat stroke and heat stress, 273
    in lower urinary tract infection, 290
    in neck and back pain, 301
    in nephrolithiasis and ureterolithiasis, 303
    in osteoarthritis, 192
    in paresis, 113, 314
    in pyoderma, 333
    in rabbits, 306–307
    in spondylosis deformans, 354
    trichobezoars and, 367
    in ulcerative pododermatitis, 371
Obstipation, 219
Ocular discharge
    in ataxia, 196
    in canine distemper virus, 15
    in conjunctivitis, 215
    in dyspnea and tachypnea, 231
    in epistaxis, 248

    in head tilt, 270
    in influenza, 83
    in malocclusion, 202, 280
    nasal discharge and, 104, 298
    in pasteurellosis, 317
    in pneumonia
        mycotic, 125
        in rabbits, 321
    in red eye, 341
    in rhinitis and sinusitis, 347
    in stertor and stridor, 356
    in tooth root abscessation, 361
Oliguria, 150–151, 344–346
Omeprazole
    dosage in ferrets, 390t
    for esophagitis, 99, 148
    for gastric ulceration, 59, 131
    for gastritis, 8, 36, 51, 56, 59, 62, 69, 173
    for melena, 101
    for uremic crisis, 151
Oral examination in rabbits, 201, 215, 245, 250,
    330, 341, 385
Orbital diseases, in rabbits, 250–253
Organophosphates
    for fleas, 53, 257
    poisoning from, 325
Orogastric intubation, for gastric decompression,
    22
Orthopnea, 42, 231
Osteoarthritis, in rabbits, 192–193
Osteoma, 108
Osteomyelitis
    in tooth abscessation, 360, 363
    in ulcerative pododermatitis, 372, 373
**Otitis externa and media**
    in ferrets, 111–112
    in rabbits, 308–310
**Otitis media and interna**
    in rabbits, 311–313
*Otodectes cynotis,* 47, 111, 138, 139
Ovarian remnant, 74, 75, 143
Ovariohysterectomy, 75, 337, 377–380
Oxibendazole
    dosage in rabbits, 395t
    for encephalitis secondary to parasitic
        migration, 244
    for encephalitozoonosis, 239, 242, 271, 351
Oxygen therapy
    for congestive heart failure, 213
    for dyspnea and tachypnea, 43, 232
    for heartworm disease, 67
    for pneumonia, aspiration, 121
    for pneumonia, bacterial, 123
    for stertor and stridor, 357
Oxyglobin
    for gastrodoudenal hemorrhage, 59
    for hyperestrogenism, 75
Oxymorphone
    dosage
        in ferrets, 390t
        in rabbits, 395t
    for pain
        in abscessation, 180
        in exophthalmos and orbital diseases, 252
        in gastric dilation, 260
Oxytetracycline
    dosage in ferrets, 390t
Oxytocin
    dosage
        in ferrets, 390t
        in rabbits, 395t
    for parturition induction, 44
    for pyometra, 171
Oxyurids, 320

**P**

Pain
in abscessation, 178
anorexia in, 184
in clostridial enterotoxicosis, 22, 207, 208
in conjunctivitis, 215–216
in constipation, 219
in diarrhea, 225, 228
in dysphagia, 40
in dysuria and pollakiuria, 235
in endometrial disorders, 337
in epiphora, 245
in exophthalmos and orbital diseases, 250–252
in gastric dilation, 259
in gastritis, 55
in gastroduodenal ulcers, 58
gastrointestinal foreign bodies and, 262
in gastrointestinal hypomotility and
gastrointestinal stasis, 266
in *Helicobacter mustelae* infection, 68
in hematuria, 275–276
in malocclusion, 201, 203, 280, 282
in mastitis, 294
in multiple myeloma, 102
neck and back, 301–302
in nephrolithiasis and ureterolithiasis, 303, 305
in otitis, 111, 308, 310, 311, 313
in paresis and paralysis, 113
in pasteurellosis, 317
in pododermatitis and nail bed disorders, 127
in ptyalism, 140, 330, 331
in pyoderma, 334
in pyometra, 142, 337
in red eye, 341, 343
in salmonellosis, 155
in spondylosis deformans, 354
in tooth root abscessation, 360, 362
trichobezoars and, 367
in ulcerative pododermatitis, 371, 373
in vertebral fracture or luxation, 381
Pain relief. *See specific conditions; specific medications*
2-PAM, 325
Pancreatectomy, 32, 33
Pancreatic tumors, 106
Pancytopenia, in pyometra, 142–143
Papilloma virus, 353
Paracentesis, aqueous humor, 188
Paralysis. *See* Paresis/paralysis
Paramyovirus. *See* Canine distemper virus
Paraplegia, 314
**Parasitic migration, encephalitis secondary to,**
244
**Paraurethral cysts,** 164–166. *See also* Urogenital
cysts
**Paresis/paralysis**
in Aleutian disease virus, 115
in ataxia, 11
in dilated cardiomyopathy, 17
in encephalitis and meningoencephalitis, 241
in encephalitozoonosis, 238
in ferrets, 113–114
in hyperestrogenism, 74
in hypoglycemia, 79
in insulinoma, 85
in multiple myeloma, 102
in rabbits, 314–316
in rabies, 145
in toxoplasmosis, 364
in urinary incontinence, 284
in vertebral fracture or luxation, 381
Parturition
for dystocia and fetal death in ferrets, 44
induction, 44

**Parvovirus infection,** in ferrets, 115–116
**Pasteurellosis,** in rabbits, 178, 179, 317–319
PCR, for *Pasteurella,* 318
Penicillin
for abscessation, 180, 331
in AIPMMA (antibiotic-impregnated polymethyl methacrylate) beads, 180
for bacterial meningoencephalitis and abscess,
351
for campylobacteriosis, 13
dosage in rabbits, 395t
for epistaxis, 249
for exophthalmos and orbital diseases, 252
for facial and dental abscesses, 203, 282
for head tilt, 271
for lameness, 287
for mastitis, 294
for meningoencephalitis, 242
for nasal discharge, 299
for otitis, 310, 313
for pasteurellosis, 319
for pneumonia in rabbits, 322
for rhinitis and sinusitis, 348
for septic arthritis, 195
for stertor and stridor, 357
for tooth root abscesses, 362
for *Treponema cuniculi,* 366
for treponematosis, 183
for ulcerative pododermatitis, 373
Perineal dermatitis, 333, 334
Periodontal disease, 65, 140. *See also* Dental
disease
Periprostatic cysts, in lower urinary tract disease,
88
Periurethral cysts, in hyperestrogenism, 75
Perivulvar dermatitis, 170
Permethrin, for fleas, 53
**Petechia/eccymosis/bruising**
in ferrets, 117–118
in heat stroke and heat stress, 273
hematuria and, 275
PGα. *See* Prostaglandin α (Lutalyse)
Phacoclastic uveitis, 238, 239
Phacoemulsification, 188, 199, 239
Pharyngoscopy
in dysphagia, 40
in stertor and stridor, 357
Phenobarbital
dosage in ferrets, 390t
for seizures, 351
Phenylephrine
for anterior uveitis, 188
dosage in rabbits, 394t
Physiologic values
in ferrits, 393t
in rabbits, 398t
**Pinworms (oxyurids),** in rabbits, 320
Piperazine
dosage in rabbits, 395t
for pinworms, 320
Plants, toxic, 399t–402t
Plasma electrophoresis, in renal failure, 150
**Pleural effusion**
in congestive heart failure, 24, 25, 212, 213
in ferrets, 119–120
in heartworm disease, 66
Pleural effusion analysis
in congestive heart failure, 213
in dilated cardiomyopathy, 17
**Pneumonia**
aspiration
in ferrets, 121–122
in megaesophagus, 98–99
in rabbits, 321

bacterial
in ferrets, 123–124
in rabbits, 123–124
in canine distemper virus infection, 15
in ferrets, 121–126
mycotic
in ferrets, 125–126
in rabbits, 321
in rabbits, 321–323
**Pododermatitis**
in ferrets, 127–128
ulcerative pododermatitis (sore hocks) in
rabbits, 314, 370–373
**Poisoning (intoxication)**
in rabbits, 324–325
seizures and, 350
toxic plants, 399t–402t
**Pollakiuria**
in ferrets, 45–46
in hematuria, 275
in hypercalciuria, 277
in lower urinary tract disease, 88, 290
in nephrolithiasis and ureterolithiasis, 303
in prostatitis, 134
in prostatomegaly, 136
in rabbits, 234–235
in urinary tract obstruction, 161, 374
in urogenital cysts, 164
in urolithiasis, 167
Polymyxin, for ocular ulceration, 252
Polyphagia, in diabetes mellitus, 32
Polysulfate glycosaminoglycans
dosage in rabbits, 395t
for neck and back pain, 302
for osteoarthritis, 193
for spondylosis deformans, 355
**Polyuria and polydipsia (PU/PD)**
in diabetes mellitus, 32
in ferrets, 129–130
in insulinoma, 85
in mastitis, 293
in pyometra and endometrial disorders, 336
in rabbits, 326–327
in renal failure, 150, 344
in urinary incontinence, 284
Posterior paresis. *See* Paresis/paralysis
Potassium supplementation, 26, 151, 214
Praziquantel
dosage in rabbits, 395t
Preanesthetics, 382
Prednisolone
for anterior uveitis, 188
dosage in ferrets, 390t
for inflammatory enterocolitis, 173
for paresis and paralysis, 315
for vertebral fracture or luxation, 382
Prednisolone acetate
for cataracts, 199
for encephalitozoonosis, 239
Prednisolone sodium succinate
dosage in ferrets, 390t
for gastric bloat, 22
for vaccine reaction, 101
Prednisone
after adrenalectomy, 165
for Aleutian disease virus infection, 116
for diarrhea, 36
dosage
in ferrets, 390t
in rabbits, 395t
for eosinophilic gastroenteritis, 49
for epizootic catarrhal enteritis, 51
for fleas, 53
for gastritis, 56

Prednisone *(continued)*
    for heartworm disease, 66, 67
    for hyperadrenocorticism, 3–4
    for inflammatory bowel disease, 81
    for insulinoma, 86
    for lymphoplasmacytic enteritis and
        gastroenteritis, 92
    for lymphosarcoma, 95
    for melena, 101
    for multiple myeloma, 102
    for otitis, 111
    for pododermatitis and nail bed disorders, 128
    for pruritus, 139
    for sarcoptic mange, 157
    for thymoma/thymic lymphoma, 359
**Pregnancy toxemia**, in ferrets, 131
Prokinetics, for gastritis, 56
**Proliferative bowel disease**
    in ferrets, 132–133
    rectal and anal prolapse and, 147
Promotility agents, for anorexia, 185
Propofol
    dosage in rabbits, 395t
Propranolol
    for congestive heart failure, 25
    for dilated cardiomyopathy, 18
    dosage in ferrets, 390t
    for hypertrophic cardiomyopathy, 19
Prostaglandin α (Lutalyse)
    dosage in ferrets, 390t
    for parturition induction, 44
    for pyometra, 143, 171, 380
Prostatic disease, dysuria and pollakiuria in, 45
**Prostatitis and prostatic abscesses**, in ferrets,
    134–135
**Prostatomegaly**
    in ferrets, 136–137
    in hyperadrenocorticism, 2
    in urinary tract obstruction, 161
Protein-losing enteropathy, hepatomegaly in, 71
Proteinuria
    in dysuria and pollakiuria, 45, 234
    in polyuria and polydipsia (PU/PD), 326
    in renal failure, 344
    in urolithiasis, 167
**Pruritus**
    in cheyletiellosis, 205
    in dermatophytosis, 223
    from ear mites, 47, 236
    in ferrets, 2, 138–139
    from fleas and flea infestation, 53, 138, 139,
        257
    in hyperadrenocorticism, 2
    in lymphosarcoma, 94
    in mast cell tumor, 97
    in otitis, 111
    in pinworm parasitism, 320
    in rabbits, 328–329
    in sarcoptic mange, 157
    with vaginal discharge, 170
Pseudoanorexia
    in ferrets, 7
    in rabbits, 184–186, 384
Pseudopregnancy
    in ferrets, 44
    in rabbits, 336
Pseudoptyalism, 140
*Psoroptes cuniculi*, 223, 236
PT (prothrombin time)
    in anticoagulant rodenticide poisoning, 190
    in epistaxis, 248
Ptosis, 250
PTT (partial thromboplastin time), in anticoagu-
    lant rodenticide poisoning, 190

**Ptyalism**
    in dyspnea and tachypnea, 231
    in epistaxis, 248
    in exophthalmos and orbital diseases, 250
    in ferrets, 140–141
    in gastritis, 55
    in gastroduodenal ulcers, 58
    in gastrointestinal and esophageal foreign
        bodies, 61, 262
    in *Helicobacter mustelae* infection, 68
    in hypoglycemia, 79
    in inflammatory bowel disease, 81
    in insulinoma, 85
    in lymphoplasmacytic enteritis and
        gastroenteritis, 92
    in malocclusion, 202, 280
    in megaesophagus, 98
    nasal discharge and, 298
    in pasteurellosis, 317
    in pneumonia in rabbits, 321
    in rabbits, 330–332
    in regurgitation, 148
    in rhinitis and sinusitis, 347
    in stertor and stridor, 356
    in tooth root abscessation, 360
Pulmonary hypertension, in heartworm disease, 66
Pulse deficits, in dilated cardiomyopathy, 17
Pyelonephritis, 73
**Pyoderma**
    dewlap, 330, 333
    in rabbits, 333–335
    in sarcoptic mange, 157
**Pyometra**
    in ferrets, 142–144
    in hyperestrogenism, 75
    in rabbits, 336–338
    with vaginal discharge, 170–171
Pyrantel pamoate
    dosage in ferrets, 390t
Pyrethrin
    dosage
        in ferrets, 390t
        in rabbits, 395t
    for fleas, 6, 53, 139, 257, 258
Pyrexia, in pyometra, 142
Pyrimethamine, for toxoplasmosis, 242, 364
Pyuria
    in dysuria and pollakiuria, 45, 234
    in hematuria, 275
    in hypercalciuria, 278
    in lower urinary tract disease, 88, 290
    in nephrolithiasis and ureterolithiasis, 304
    in polyuria and polydipsia (PU/PD), 326
    in urinary incontinence, 284
    in urinary tract obstruction, 375
    in urolithiasis, 167

Q

Quadriplegia, 314. *See also* Paresis/paralysis

R

Rabbit syphillis, 182, 183, 366
**Rabies**
    dysphagia in, 40, 41
    in ferrets, 145–146
    in rabbits, 339–340
Radiography
    in abscessation, 179
    in Aleutian disease virus, 116
    in alopecia, 182
    in anorexia, 7, 185
    in anterior uveitis, 188

    in anticoagulant rodenticide poisoning, 190
    in ascites, 9
    in ataxia, 11–12, 197
    in clostridial enterotoxicosis, 21, 207
    in coccidiosis, 210
    in congestive heart failure, 24, 212–213
    in conjunctivitis, 216
    in constipation, 220
    in cough, 27
    in diarrhea, 36, 226, 229
    in dilated cardiomyopathy, 17
    in dyschezia and hematochezia, 38
    in dysphagia, 40
    in dyspnea and tachypnea, 42, 43, 232
    in dystocia, 44
    in dysuria and pollakiuria, 46, 235
    in encephalitis and meningoencephalitis, 241,
        244
    in encephalitozoonosis, 238
    in endometrial disorders, 336
    in eosinophilic gastroenteritis, 48
    in epiphora, 246
    in epistaxis, 248
    in exophthalmos and orbital diseases, 251
    in facial nerve paresis/paralysis, 255
    in gastric dilation, 259
    in gastritis, 55
    in gastroduodenal ulcers, 58
    in gastrointestinal and esophageal foreign
        bodies, 61–62, 263
    in gastrointestinal hypomotility and
        gastrointestinal stasis, 267
    in head tilt, 271
    in heartworm disease, 66
    in heat stroke and heat stress, 273
    in *Helicobacter mustelae* infection, 68
    in hepatomegaly, 71
    in hydronephrosis, 73
    in hyperadrenocorticism, 2
    in hypercalciuria, 278
    in hyperestrogenism, 74
    in hypertrophic cardiomyopathy, 19
    in hypoglycemia, 79
    in inflammatory bowel disease, 81
    in influenza, 83
    in insulinoma, 85
    in lameness, 286
    in lead toxicity, 288
    in lower urinary tract disease, 88, 290
    in lymphadenomegaly, 90
    in lymphosarcoma, 95
    in malocclusion, 202, 281
    in mast cell tumor, 97
    in mastitis, 293
    in megaesophagus, 98
    in melena, 100, 295
    in multiple myeloma, 102
    in nasal discharge, 104, 298–299
    in neck and back pain, 301
    in neoplasia
        digestive system, 106
        integumentary, 107
        musculoskeletal and nervous system,
        108
    in nephrolithiasis and ureterolithiasis, 304
    in osteoarthritis, 192
    in otitis, 111, 308, 312
    in paresis and paralysis, 114, 314
    in pasteurellosis, 318
    in periodontal disease, 65
    in pleural effusion, 119
    in pneumonia
        aspiration, 121
        bacterial, 123

mycotic, 125
  in rabbits, 321
in polyuria and polydipsia (PU/PD), 129, 326
in pregnancy toxemia, 131
in proliferative bowel disease, 132
in prostatitis and prostatic abscesses, 134
in prostatomegaly, 136
in pruritus, 328
in ptyalism, 141, 331
in pyoderma, 334
in pyometra, 142, 336
in rectal and anal prolapse, 147
in red eye, 342
in regurgitation, 148
in renal failure, 150, 344–345
in renomegaly, 153
in rhinitis and sinusitis, 347–348
in seizures, 350
in septic arthritis, 194
in splenomegaly, 159
in spondylosis deformans, 354
in stertor and stridor, 357
in thymoma/thymic lymphoma, 359
in tooth root abscession, 361
in toxoplasmosis, 364
trichobezoars and, 368
in ulcerative pododermatitis, 372
in urinary incontinence, 285
in urinary tract obstruction, 161, 375
in urogenital cysts, 164
in urolithiasis, 168
in uterine adenocarcinoma, 377
in vaginal discharge, 170, 379
in vertebral fracture or luxation, 381
in vomiting, 172
in weight loss, 174, 385
Radiotherapy, for integumentary neoplasia, 107
Ranitidine bismuth citrate
  for diarrhea, 36
  dosage in ferrets, 390t
  for gastrodoudenal ulcers, 59
  for gastrointestinal and esophageal foreign
    bodies, 62
  for *Helicobacter mustelae*, 36, 59, 69, 92, 101
  for lymphoplasmacytic enteritis and
    gastroenteritis, 93
Ranitidine HCl
  dosage
    in ferrets, 390t
    in rabbits, 395t
  for gastric ulceration, 59, 131, 185, 260, 264,
    268, 315, 369, 382
  for gastritis, 59, 62
  for *Helicobacter mustelae*, 69
  for melena, 296
  for renal failure, 345
Rear limb weakness. *See* Paresis/paralysis;
  Weakness
**Rectal prolapse**
  in coccidiosis, 23, 147
  in ferrets, 147
  in pinworm parasitism, 320
  in proliferative bowel disease, 132
**Red eye**, in rabbits, 341–343
**Regurgitation**
  in ferrets, 148–149
  with gastrointestinal and esophageal foreign
    bodies, 61
  in megaesophagus, 98
  melena and, 100
  in ptyalism, 140
Renal cysts, 153
**Renal failure**
  in ferrets, 150–152

in rabbits, 344–346
Renoliths. *See* Nephrolithiasis and ureterolithiasis
**Renomegaly**
  in ferrets, 153–154
  in hydronephrosis, 73, 153
  in nephrolithiasis and ureterolithiasis, 303, 305
  in renal failure, 150
Respiratory disease. *See also specific diseases and
  symptoms*
    cough, 27–28
    dyspnea and tachypnea
      in ferrets, 42–43
      in rabbits, 231–233
    influenza, 83–84
    pneumonia
      aspiration, 121–122
      bacterial, 123–124
      mycotic, 125–126
      in rabbits, 321–323
    rhinitis, 347–349
    sneezing
      in ferrets, 104–105
      in rabbits, 298–300
    stertor and stridor in, 356–358
Retinoids, for cutaneous lymphosarcoma, 95
**Rhinitis**
  epiphora in, 245
  in pasteurellosis, 317
  in rabbits, 347–349
  stertor and stridor and, 356
Rhinoscopy, 104, 216, 232, 246, 299, 348
Ringworm. *See* Dermatophytosis
Rodenticide poisoning, in rabbits, 190–191

### S

Salivary gland disease, ptyalism in, 140
**Salmonellosis**, in ferrets, 155–156
Salt restriction, for ascites, 10
**Sarcoptic mange**
  alopecia, 5, 6, 182, 183
  in ferrets, 5, 6, 157–158
  in pododermatitis, 127
  pruritus, 138, 139
Schiff-Sherrington phenomena, 381
Schirmer tear test, 216, 255, 342
Secondary hyperparathyroidism, 201
**Seizures**
  in encephalitis and meningoencephalitis,
    241–242
  in encephalitozoonosis, 238, 239
  in heat stroke and heat stress, 273, 274
  in hypoglycemia, 79
  in insulinoma, 85
  in lead toxicity, 288
  in myxomatosis, 297
  in rabbits, 350–352
  in rabies, 145
  in renal failure, 150, 344
  in toxoplasmosis, 364
Selamectin
  for cheyletiellosis, 182, 328
  dosage
    in ferrets, 391t
    in rabbits, 395t
  for ear mites, 5, 111, 139, 182, 236, 310, 328
  for fleas, 6, 53, 139, 183, 257, 329
  for otitis, 111
  for sarcoptic mange, 6, 157
Sepsis, hypoglycemia in, 79
Septic arthritis, in rabbits, 194–195
Septic mastitis, 293–294
Serology
  for Aleutian disease virus, 115

for *Encephalitozoon cuniculi*, 187, 194,
    196–197, 199, 238, 241, 244, 254, 271,
    284, 311–312, 342, 350, 364
  in heartworm disease, 66
  for *Helicobacter mustelae*, 68
  in myxomatosis, 297
  for *Pasteurella*, 179, 187–188, 194, 197, 231,
    241, 244, 251, 255, 271, 293, 298, 308,
    312, 318, 321, 347, 350, 356–357, 364
  in pneumonia, mycotic, 125
  for *Treponema cuniculi*, 366
Serum protein electrophoresis
  in Aleutian disease virus, 115
  in multiple myeloma, 102
  in paresis and paralysis, 114
Sevoflurane
  dosage in rabbits, 395t
Sexual aggression, in hyperadrenocorticism, 2
Sialorrhea. *See* Ptyalism
Simethicone
  for constipation, 221
  dosage in rabbits, 395t
  for gastrointestinal foreign bodies, 264
  for gastrointestinal hypomotility, 268
  for trichobezoars, 369
**Sinusitis**
  epiphora in, 245
  in pasteurellosis, 317
  in rabbits, 347–349
  stertor and stridor and, 356
Skin scrapping
  in cheyletiellosis, 205
  in ear mites, 47, 236
  in pododermatitis and nail bed disorders, 127
  in pruritus, 138, 328
  in pyoderma, 334
  in sarcoptic mange, 157
Slobbers, in rabbits, 330–332
**Sneezing**
  in dyspnea and tachypnea, 231
  epistaxis and, 248
  in ferrets, 104–105
  in influenza, 83
  in pasteurellosis, 317
  in rabbits, 298–300
  in rhinitis and sinusitis, 347
  in stertor and stridor, 356
Snuffles. *See* Nasal discharge, in rabbits
Sodium bicarbonate
  dosage in rabbits, 395t
  for metabolic acidosis, 274
Sodium concentration, in polyuria and polydipsia
  (PU/PD), 129
Sore hocks (ulcerative pododermatitis), 314,
  370–373
Spinal cord disease
  in ataxia, 11–12, 196–197
  in paresis and paralysis, 113–114
Spironolactone, for congestive heart failure, 25, 214
Splenectomy, 160
Splenitis, 159
**Splenomegaly**
  in Aleutian disease virus, 115
  in congestive heart failure, 24, 212
  in diabetes mellitus, 32
  in dilated cardiomyopathy, 17
  in eosinophilic gastroenteritis, 48
  in epizootic catarrhal enteritis, 50
  in ferrets, 159–160
  in gastroduodenal ulcers, 58
  in heartworm disease, 66
  in *Helicobacter mustelae* infection, 68
  in hyperadrenocorticism, 2
  in hyperestrogenism, 74

**Splenomegaly** *(continued)*
   in insulinoma, 85
   in lymphoplasmacytic enteritis and
      gastroenteritis, 92
   in lymphosarcoma, 94
   in mast cell tumor, 97
   in patechia/eccymosis/bruising, 117
**Spondylosis deformans,** in rabbits, 354–355
Squamous cell carcinoma, 107, 127
Stannous fluoride gel, for gingivitis and periodontal disease, 65
Stanozolol
   dosage
      in ferrets, 391t
      in rabbits, 395t
   for hyperestrogenism, 75
Status epilepticus, 351
**Stertor and stridor,** in rabbits, 356–358
*Stinerma carpocapsae,* 257
Stomach tube placement in rabbits, 325
Stomatitis, in ptyalism, 140, 330
Strabismus, 250–251, 311
Stranguria
   in hyperadrenocorticism, 2
   in prostatitis, 134
   in prostatomegaly, 136
   in urinary tract obstruction, 374
   in urogenital cysts, 164
   in urolithiasis, 167
Stridor, in rabbits, 356–358
Stump pyometra. *See* Pyometra
Sucralfate
   dosage
      in ferrets, 391t
      in rabbits, 396t
   for esophagitis, 99, 148
   for gastric ulceration, 59, 131, 173, 325
   for gastritis, 56, 59, 69
   for melena, 296
   for uremic crisis, 151
Sulfadiazine, for toxoplasmosis, 242, 364
Sulfadimethoxine
   for coccidiosis, 23, 38, 211, 227
   dosage
      in ferrets, 391t
      in rabbits, 396t
Surgery. *See also* Laparotomy
   for abscessation, 179–180, 318–319
   adrenalectomy, 3, 75, 134, 135, 162, 165
   for anterior uveitis, 188
   arthrodesis, 192
   arthroplasty, 192
   arthrotomy, 192, 194
   bulla osteotomy, 255, 271, 312
   for cataracts, 199
   cesarean section, 44
   for conjunctivitis, 216–217
   for constipation, 221
   cystotomy, 162, 168
   for dysphagia, 40
   for dyspnea and tachypnea, 43
   for dystocia and fetal death, 44
   ear canal ablation, 271, 312
   for endometrial disorders, 337
   enucleation, 188, 251–252
   exenteration, 251, 252
   for exophthalmos and orbital diseases, 251–252
   for facial nerve paresis/paralysis, 255
   for fold pyoderma, 34
   for gastric dilation, 260
   for gastrodoudenal ulcers, 59
   for gastrointestinal and esophageal foreign bodies, 62, 264

for gastrointestinal hypomotility and gastrointestinal stasis, 268
gastrotomy for foreign body removal, 56
head tilt and, 271
for hydronephrosis, 73
for hyperestrogenism, 75
for insulinoma, 86
for lameness, 287
lateral ear canal resection, 309
lens removal, 188
for malocclusion, 203, 281–282
for mast cell tumor, 97
mastectomy, 294
molar extraction, 203
for multiple myeloma, 102
for nasal discharge, 105
for neoplasia
   digestive system, 106
   integumentary, 107
   musculoskeletal and nervous system, 108
nephrectomy, 73
for nephrolithiasis and ureterolithiasis, 304–305
for osteoarthritis, 192
for otitis, 309, 312–313
ovariohysterectomy, 75, 337, 377–380
pancreatectomy, 32, 33
in papilloma virus infection, 353
for pasteurellosis, 318–319
for pleural effusion, 120
for pododermatitis and nail bed disorders, 127, 128
for prostatitis and prostatic abscesses, 134
for pyometra, 143, 337
for rectal and anal prolapse, 147
in septic arthritis, 194–195
splenectomy, 160
for tooth root abscessation, 361–362
for trichobezoars, 369
urethrostomy, 162, 168
for urinary tract obstruction, 162, 375
for urogenital cysts, 165
for urolithiasis, 168
for uterine adenocarcinoma, 377
Swallowing difficulties, 40–41
Syncope, in congestive heart failure, 212
Synovial fluid analysis
   in osteoarthritis, 192
   in septic arthritis, 194

### T

**Tachypnea**
   in clostridial enterotoxicosis, 207
   in congestive heart failure, 212
   in ferrets, 42–43
   in gastric dilation, 259
   gastrointestinal foreign bodies and, 262
   in heartworm disease, 66
   in heat stroke and heat stress, 273
   in pasteurellosis, 317
   in pleural effusion, 119
   in pneumonia, aspiration, 121
   in rabbits, 231–233
   in renal failure, 344
   in thymoma/thymic lymphoma, 359
   trichobezoars and, 367
Tenesmus
   in campylobacteriosis, 13
   in coccidiosis, 23, 210
   in dysuria and pollakiuria, 234
   in hypercalciuria, 277
   in nephrolithiasis and ureterolithiasis, 303
   in prostatitis, 134

in prostatomegaly, 136
in rectal and anal prolapse, 147
in salmonellosis, 155
in urinary tract obstruction, 374
in urogenital cysts, 164
Terbutaline, for bronchoconstriction, 357
Tetracycline
   dosage in ferrets, 391t
Theophylline
   for cough, 27
   dosage in ferrets, 391t
   for heartworm disease, 67
   for pneumonia, aspiration, 121
Thiabendazole
   for ear mites, 5, 47, 111, 139
   for otitis, 111
   for pinworms, 320, 329
Thiacetarsemide (Caparsolate), for heartworm disease, 67
Third eyelid protrusion, 250
Thoracocentesis
   in anticoagulant rodenticide poisoning, 190
   for congestive heart failure, 25, 213
   in cough, 27
   for dilated cardiomyopathy, 17
   in dyspnea and tachypnea, 42, 43, 232
   for heartworm disease, 66
   for hypertrophic cardiomyopathy, 19
   in lymphosarcoma, 95
   in pleural effusion, 119–120
Thrombocytopenia
   in heat stroke and heat stress, 273
   in hematuria, 275
   patechia/eccymosis/bruising and, 117–118
   in pyometra, 142
   in splenomegaly, 159
**Thymoma/thymic lymphoma,** in rabbits, 359
Tiletamine-zolazepam
   dosage in rabbits, 396t
Tobramycin, in AIPMMA (antibiotic-impregnated polymethyl methacrylate) beads, 195, 252, 309, 313, 319, 362, 372
Tonometry, 188, 342
Tooth extraction, 203, 282, 331, 361–362
Tooth grinding. *See* Bruxism
**Tooth root abscesses (apical abscesses),** in rabbits, 360–363
Torticollis
   in encephalitozoonosis, 238, 239
   in otitis, 311
   in pasteurellosis, 317
   in toxoplasmosis, 364
Total ear canal ablation, 271, 312
Toxicity
   lead, 58, 288–289, 325
   poisoning (intoxication), in rabbits, 324–325
   ptyalism and, 140
   toxin plants, 399t–402t
**Toxoplasmosis,** in rabbits, 364–365
Tracheal wash
   in dyspnea and tachypnea, 42
   in pneumonia, aspiration, 121
   in pneumonia, bacterial, 123
Tracheostomy, 357
Transfusions
   for anticoagulant rodenticide poisoning, 190, 325
   for gastrodoudenal ulcers, 59
   for hyperestrogenism, 75
   for patechia/eccymosis/bruising, 117
   for pyometra, 143
   for uterine hemorrhage, 380
Transudate
   in ascites, 9

in pleural effusion, 119
**Treponematosis (rabbit syphillis)**
    alopecia, 182, 183
    in rabbits, 366
**Trichobezoars**
    in constipation, 221
    in ferrets, 61
    as gastrointestinal foreign bodies, 262, 264
    in gastrointestinal hypomotility and gastrointestinal stasis, 266, 268
    in rabbits, 367–370
*Trichophyton mentagrophytes*, 30, 223
Trimethoprim/sulfa
    for abscessation, 180
    for anterior uveitis, 188
    for bacterial folliculitis, 6, 183, 329
    for bacterial meningoencephalitis and abscess, 351
    for coccidiosis, 211, 227
    for constipation, 221
    for cough, 27
    for cystitis, 46
    for dermatitis, 354
    for diarrhea, 36, 227, 229
    dosage
        in ferrets, 391t
        in rabbits, 396t
    for dyschezia and hematochezia, 38
    for dysuria and pollakiuria, 235
    for endometrial disorders, 337
    for epistaxis, 249
    for epizootic catarrhal enteritis, 51
    for exophthalmos and orbital diseases, 252
    for facial and dental abscesses, 203, 282
    for gastric dilation, 260
    for gastrointestinal foreign bodies, 264
    for gastrointestinal hypomotility and gastrointestinal stasis, 268
    for head tilt, 271
    for influenza-associated bacterial infections, 83
    for lameness, 287
    for lower urinary tract disease, 88, 291
    for mastitis, 294
    for melena, 100, 296
    for meningoencephalitis, 242
    for moist pyoderma, 331
    for nasal discharge, 105, 299
    for otitis, 111, 310, 313
    for pasteurellosis, 319
    for pneumonia in rabbits, 322
    for pododermatitis and nail bed disorders, 127
    for prostatitis and prostatic abscesses, 134, 162
    for pyoderma, 334
    for pyometra, 143, 337
    for rhinitis and sinusitis, 348
    for salmonellosis, 155
    for septic arthritis, 195
    for stertor and stridor, 357
    for tooth root abscesses, 362
    for toxoplasmosis, 242, 351, 364
    for trichobezoars, 369
    for ulcerative pododermatitis, 373
    for urogenital cysts, 166
    for vaginal discharge, 171, 380
    for vomiting, 173
Trimming teeth, 203, 281–282
Tropicamide 1% eye drops
    dosage in rabbits, 396t

**U**

**Ulcerative pododermatitis (sore hocks)**, 314, 370–373
Ultralente insulin, 33

Ultrasonography
    in abscessation, 179
    in anorexia, 185
    in anterior uveitis, 188
    in ascites, 9
    in ataxia, 12, 197
    in conjunctivitis, 216
    in constipation, 220
    in cough, 27
    in diarrhea, 36, 226, 229
    in dyschezia and hematochezia, 38
    in dysphagia, 40
    in dyspnea and tachypnea, 42, 43, 232
    in dystocia, 44
    in dysuria and pollakiuria, 46, 235
    in endometrial disorders, 336
    in eosinophilic gastroenteritis, 48
    in exophthalmos and orbital diseases, 251
    in gastric dilation, 259
    in gastritis, 55
    in gastroduodenal ulcers, 58
    in gastrointestinal and esophageal foreign bodies, 62, 263
    guided biopsy, 79
    in hepatomegaly, 71
    in hydronephrosis, 73
    in hyperadrenocorticism, 2, 5
    in hyperestrogenism, 74
    in inflammatory bowel disease, 81
    in lower urinary tract disease, 88
    in lymphadenomegaly, 90
    in lymphosarcoma, 95
    in mastitis, 293
    in melena, 100, 295
    in multiple myeloma, 102
    in neck and back pain, 301
    in neoplasia, digestive system, 106
    in neoplasia, musculoskeletal and nervous system, 108
    in nephrolithiasis and ureterolithiasis, 304
    in paresis and paralysis, 114, 315
    in pasteurellosis, 318
    in pleural effusion, 119
    in pneumonia, mycotic, 125
    in polyuria and polydipsia (PU/PD), 129, 326
    in pregnancy toxemia, 131
    in prostatitis and prostatic abscesses, 134
    in prostatomegaly, 136
    in ptyalism, 331
    in pyoderma, 334
    in pyometra, 142, 336
    in rectal and anal prolapse, 147
    in red eye, 342
    in renal failure, 150, 345
    in renomegaly, 153
    in splenomegaly, 159
    trichobezoars and, 368
    in ulcerative pododermatitis, 372
    in urinary incontinence, 285
    in urinary tract obstruction, 161, 162, 375
    in urogenital cysts, 164, 166
    in urolithiasis, 168
    in uterine adenocarcinoma, 377
    in vaginal discharge, 170, 379
    in vomiting, 172
    in weight loss, 174
Upper motor neurons, 113
Urease test, in *Helicobacter mustelae* infection, 69
Uremia
    in urinary tract obstruction, 161, 374
    in urolithiasis, 167
**Ureterolithiasis**, in rabbits, 303–305
Urethral plugs, dysuria and pollakiuria from, 45

Urethrostomy, 162, 168
Urinalysis
    in diabetes mellitus, 32
    in dysuria and pollakiuria, 45
    in hydronephrosis, 73
    in hypercalciuria, 277–278
    in lower urinary tract infection, 290
    in mastitis, 293
    in multiple myeloma, 102
    in nephrolithiasis and ureterolithiasis, 304
    in polyuria and polydipsia (PU/PD), 326
    in pregnancy toxemia, 131
    in prostatitis, 134
    in prostatomegaly, 136
    in pyometra and endometrial disorders, 336
    in renal failure, 344
    in urinary incontinence, 284
    in urinary tract obstruction, 161
    in urolithiasis, 167
    in vaginal discharge, 379
Urinary catheterization, in urinary tract obstruction, 161–162, 168
**Urinary incontinence**, in rabbits, 284–285, 314
Urinary protein:creatinine ratio, in renal failure, 150
**Urinary tract infection**
    dysuria and pollakiuria in, 45–46
    in ferrets, 88–89
    in rabbits, 290–292
**Urinary tract obstruction**
    in ferrets, 161–163
    in rabbits, 374–376
Urine culture
    in dysuria and pollakiuria, 45, 234
    in hypercalciuria, 278
    in lower urinary tract infection, 88, 290
    in polyuria and polydipsia (PU/PD), 129, 326
Urine protein electrophoresis, in multiple myeloma, 102
Urine sedimentation
    in encephalitozoonosis, 238
    in nephrolithiasis and ureterolithiasis, 304
    in renal failure, 344
**Urogenital cysts**
    dysuria and pollakiuria from, 45
    in ferrets, 164–166
    in hyperadrenocorticism, 2
    in lower urinary tract disease, 88
    in urinary tract obstruction, 161
**Urolithiasis**
    dysuria and pollakiuria in, 45, 234
    in ferrets, 167–169
    in lower urinary tract infection, 290–291
    in rabbits, 277–279
Ursodiol
    dosage in ferrets, 391t
**Uterine adenocarcinoma**, in rabbits, 377–378
Uveitis
    anterior, 187–189
        epiphora in, 245
        red eye, 341
    in encephalitozoonosis, 238, 239

**V**

Vaccination
    canine distemper virus, 16
    myxomatosis, 297
    rabies, 146, 340
Vaginal cytology, 74, 170
**Vaginal discharge**
    in endometrial disorders, 336
    in ferrets, 170–171

**Vaginal discharge** *(continued)*
in pyometra, 142, 336
in rabbits, 379–380
Venodilators, for congestive heart failure, 25, 213–214
Verapamil
dosage in rabbits, 396t
**Vertebral fracture or luxation**, in rabbits, 381–383
**Vestibular disease**
ataxia from, 11, 196
encephalitis and meningoencephalitis, 241–243
encephalitozoonosis, 238, 239
head tilt, 270–272
nasal discharge and, 298
otitis and, 111, 308, 311
in rabbits, 270–272
seizures and, 350
Vincristine, for lymphosarcoma, 95
Vitamin B complex
dosage in ferrets, 391t
dosage in rabbits, 396t
Vitamin C
dosage in ferrets, 391t
Vitamin K₁
for anticoagulant rodenticide poisoning, 190–191, 248–249, 325
dosage in rabbits, 396t
**Vomiting**
in canine distemper virus, 15
in eosinophilic gastroenteritis, 48
in epizootic catarrhal enteritis, 50
in ferrets, 172–173
in gastritis, 55–56
in gastroduodenal ulcers, 58
in gastrointestinal and esophageal foreign bodies, 61
in *Helicobacter mustelae* infection, 68, 69
in inflammatory bowel disease, 81
in insulinoma, 85
in lymphoplasmacytic enteritis and gastroenteritis, 92
in lymphosarcoma, 94
in mast cell tumor, 97
melena and, 100
in ptyalism, 140
in pyometra, 142
in renal failure, 150, 151

in salmonellosis, 155
urinary tract obstruction, 161
Vulva, swollen
in hyperadrenocorticism, 2
in hyperestrogenism, 74
in pyometra, 142
with vaginal discharge, 170

$\boxed{\text{W}}$

Weakness
in coccidiosis, 210
in congestive heart failure, 212
in diarrhea, 228
in gastric dilation, 259
in gastroduodenal ulcers, 58
in gastrointestinal and esophageal foreign bodies, 61, 262
in heartworm disease, 66
in heat stroke and heat stress, 273
in *Helicobacter mustelae* infection, 68
in hyperestrogenism, 74
in hypoglycemia, 79
in insulinoma, 85
in lead toxicity, 288
in multiple myeloma, 102
in neck and back pain, 301
in obesity, 109, 306
paresis, 113–114, 314
in pleural effusion, 119
in pneumonia, aspiration, 121
in pneumonia, bacterial, 123
in pregnancy toxemia, 131
in proliferative bowel disease, 132
in regurgitation, 148
in salmonellosis, 155
in spondylosis deformans, 354
in toxoplasmosis, 364
trichobezoars and, 367
in vertebral fracture or luxation, 381
**Weight loss and cachexia**
in Aleutian disease virus, 115
in coccidiosis, 210
in congestive heart failure, 212
in constipation, 219
in diabetes mellitus, 32
in diarrhea, 228
in dyspnea and tachypnea, 231

in dysuria and pollakiuria, 234
in eosinophilic gastroenteritis, 48
in ferrets, 174–175
in gastritis, 55–56
in gastroduodenal ulcers, 58
in gastrointestinal and esophageal foreign bodies, 61
in gastrointestinal hypomotility and gastrointestinal stasis, 266
in giardiasis, 64
in *Helicobacter mustelae* infection, 68
in hypercalciuria, 277
in inflammatory bowel disease, 81
in lead toxicity, 288
in lymphoplasmacytic enteritis and gastroenteritis, 92
in lymphosarcoma, 94
in malocclusion, 201–202, 280–281
in megaesophagus, 98
melena and, 100, 295
in nephrolithiasis and ureterolithiasis, 303
in pinworm parasitism, 320
in pneumonia
bacterial, 123
mycotic, 125
in rabbits, 321
in proliferative bowel disease, 132
in prostatomegaly, 136
in ptyalism, 140, 330
in rabbits, 384–386
in regurgitation, 148
in renal failure, 150, 344
in salmonellosis, 155
in tooth root abscessation, 360, 361
trichobezoars and, 367
in urinary tract obstruction, 374
in urogenital cysts, 164
in vomiting, 172
Wood's lamp examination, 30, 127, 138, 223, 328
Wool block. *See* Gastrointestinal foreign bodies; Trichobezoars
Wry neck. *See* Head tilt

$\boxed{\text{Z}}$

Zinc oxide, 331, 334, 354